STOLLER'S
Orthopaedics and Sports Medicine

David W. Stoller, MD • Cloyce Martin, MD • John V. Crues III, MD
• Leo Kaplan, MD • Jerrold H. Mink, MD

Meniscal Tears: Pathologic Correlation with MR Imaging[1]

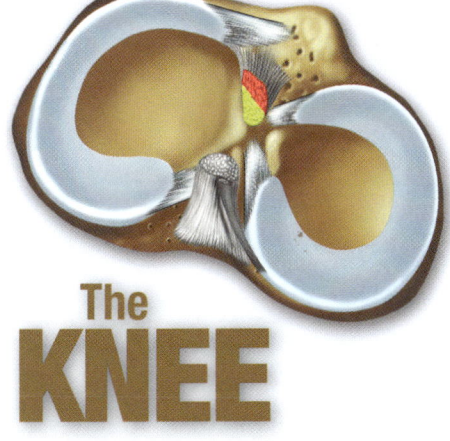

The KNEE

Menisci from 12 autopsies and above-knee amputations were imaged with magnetic resonance (MR) at 1.5 T and then sectioned for gross and histologic examination. A histologic staging system was developed and showed a one-to-one correlation with corresponding grades of MR signal intensities. Histologic stages 1 and 2 represented a continuum of degeneration culminating in stage 3 fibrocartilaginous tears, seen most frequently in posterior-horn segments of the medial meniscus. Correlation of histologic stages with MR signal intensity allows for an improved diagnostic reading of MR images.

Index terms: Knee, MR studies, 452.1214
• Knee, injuries, 452.4852

Radiology 1987;
163:731-735

MAGNETIC resonance (MR) imaging has emerged as an important modality in the noninvasive evaluation of osseous and soft-tissue structures in and around the knee (1-3). Initial reports of increased signal intensities within normally low-signal-intensity menisci have been used to show the sensitivity of MR imaging in the detection of meniscal tears (3-5). To increase diagnostic specificity, preliminary reports suggested a subjective grading system for meniscal signal intensity with arthroscopic validation (5); a more objective grading of the meniscal signal by Lotysch et al. (4) was also developed and compared with results from arthroscopy. True sensitivity and specificity are difficult to assess, however, as both grading systems were compared with an arthroscopic standard reported to be 69%-90% (6, 7) sensitive and unable to evaluate the significance of signal intensities in menisci without surface tears (6-9). The present study was undertaken to improve diagnostic interpretation by classifying the gross and histologic changes within menisci, and to correlate this with the grading of the MR signal independent of the limitations of arthroscopy. The use of a histologic model affords the advantage of understanding the representation of MR signal at a cellular and tissue level before a tear can be arthroscopically detected.

MATERIALS AND METHODS

MR imaging of 12 menisci (six medial and six lateral) was performed within 12 hours of obtaining each knee specimen from eight human autopsies and four above-knee amputations. Subjects ranged in age from 50 to 89 years with equal representation of men and women. Coronal and sagittal images were obtained with a 5.5-inch flat surface coil placed posterior to the knee and a 1.5-T MR imager (General Electric, Milwaukee). A spin echo of 800/25 (repetition time [TR] msec/echo time [TE] msec) was used with a 256 X 128 matrix displayed

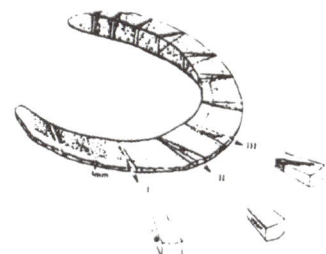

Figure 1. Illustration of surgically removed meniscus with 3-mm radial sections shows representative stages of tear.

on a 16-cm field of view format. Contiguous 5-mm interleaved sections were imaged with the knee in 10°-15° of external rotation. In subsequent clinical studies, we have used a circumferential extremity coil with a 256 X 256-pixel display (10).

Following MR imaging of the knee, menisci were surgically removed in total after a U-shaped incision was made to expose and open the joint capsule. Surgical 3-mm radial sections were then made perpendicular to the horizontal (axial) anatomic plane of the meniscus (Fig. 1). Each of approximately 20 radially performed sections in each meniscus was stained with hematoxylin and eosin for microscopic examination. For pathologic correlation, the radial sections from each of the 12 menisci in the study were grouped into three segments, consisting of an anterior horn, body, and posterior horn, for a total of 36 meniscal segments. In the case of a bucket-handle tear, MR imaging could not resolve the normally visualized body segment of the meniscus, since the attenuated width of the tear approximated the 5-mm resolution thickness of the sagittal-plane images.

An MR grading system was used that is based on the distribution of meniscal signal in relation to an articular surface. The sagittal imaging plane best defined meniscal abnormalities, which could be corroborated in coronal imaging. MR grade 1 (Fig. 2a) represented one or

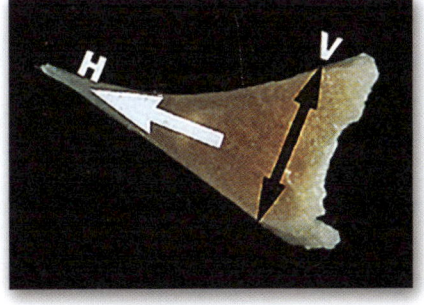

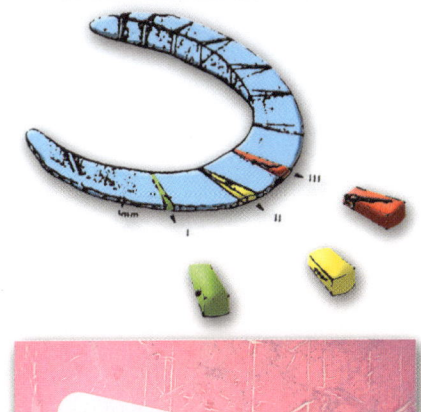

---

[1] From the Department of Radiology, University of California, School of Medicine, San Francisco, CA 94143 (D.W.S.), and the Departments of Pathology (C.M., L.K.) and Radiology (J.V.C., J.H.M.), Cedars-Sinai Medical Center, Los Angeles. Received October 9, 1986; revision requested November 11; revision received February 3, 1987; accepted February 9. Address reprint requests to D.W.S.
© RSNA, 1987
See also the article by Manco et al. (pp. 727-730) in this issue.

STOLLER'S
Orthopaedics and Sports Medicine

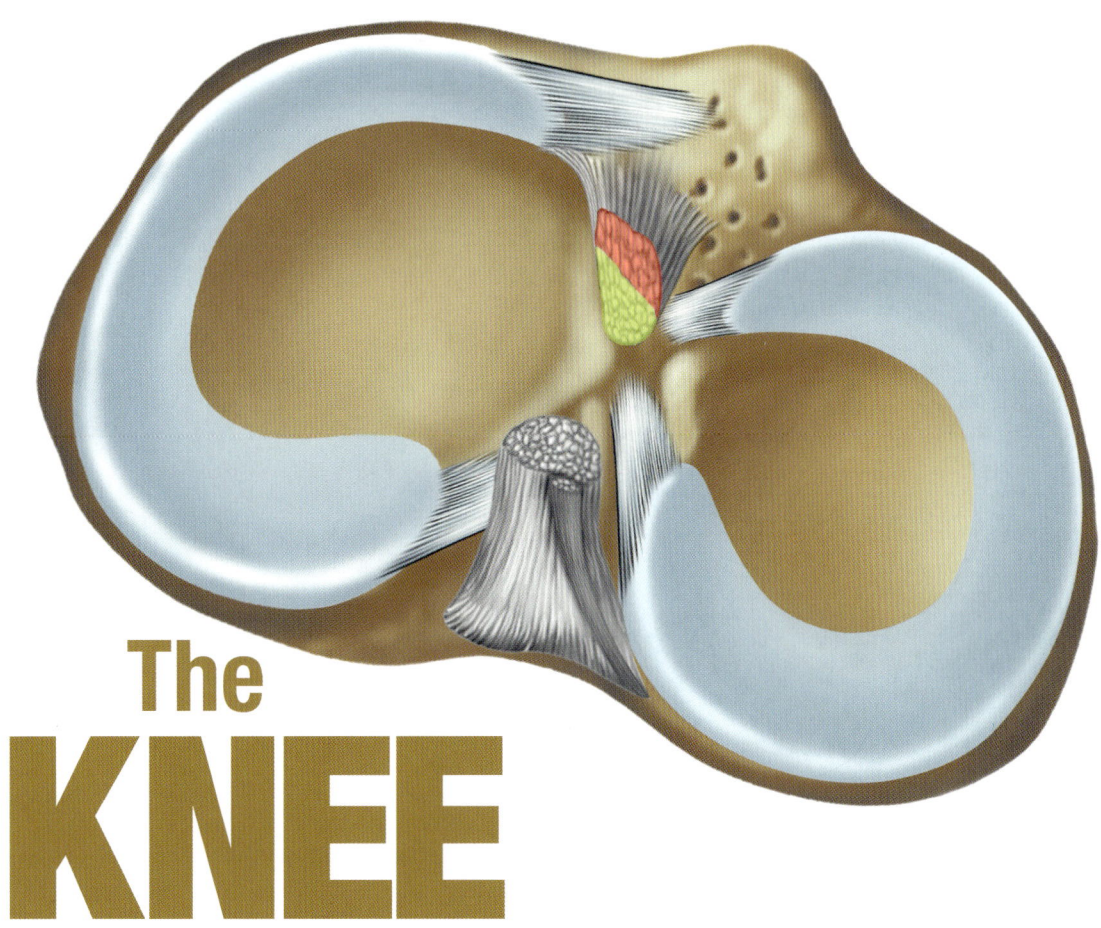

The KNEE

David W. Stoller, MD, FACR

National Director,
  Orthopaedic and Musculoskeletal Imaging, RadNet
Medical Director,
  *Orthopaedic and Musculoskeletal Imaging, Beverly Radiology,
  Northern California, San Francisco, California*
Affiliate Member,
  American Shoulder and Elbow Surgeons

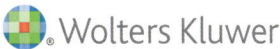. Wolters Kluwer

Philadelphia • Baltimore • New York • London
Buenos Aires • Hong Kong • Sydney • Tokyo

Acquisitions Editor: Ryan Shaw
Product Development Editor: Kate Heaney
Production Project Manager: Alicia Jackson
Designer: Larry Pezzato
Senior Manufacturing Coordinator: Beth Welsh
Marketing Manager: Dan Dressler
Prepress Vendor: Absolute Service, Inc.

Copyright © 2017 Wolters Kluwer

All rights reserved. This book is protected by copyright. No part of this book may be reproduced or transmitted in any form or by any means, including as photocopies or scanned-in or other electronic copies, or utilized by any information storage and retrieval system without written permission from the copyright owner, except for brief quotations embodied in critical articles and reviews. Materials appearing in this book prepared by individuals as part of their official duties as U.S. government employees are not covered by the above-mentioned copyright. To request permission, please contact Wolters Kluwer Health at Two Commerce Square, 2001 Market Street, Philadelphia, PA 19103, via email at permissions@lww.com, or via our website at lww.com (products and services).

9 8 7 6 5 4 3 2 1

Printed in the United States of America

Library of Congress Cataloging-in-Publication Data

Stoller, David W., author.
  Stoller's orthopaedics and sports medicine. The knee / David W. Stoller.
      p. ; cm.
  Orthopaedics and sports medicine. The knee
  Knee
    ISBN 978-1-4963-1828-2 (hardback)
  I. Title. II. Title: Orthopaedics and sports medicine. The knee. III. Title: Knee.
  [DNLM: 1. Knee Injuries—Atlases. 2. Knee—pathology—Atlases. 3. Knee Joint—pathology—Atlases. 4. Magnetic Resonance Imaging—Atlases. WE 17]
  RD561
  617.5'82—dc23
                        2015024070

This work is provided "as is," and the publisher disclaims any and all warranties, express or implied, including any warranties as to accuracy, comprehensiveness, or currency of the content of this work.

This work is no substitute for individual patient assessment based upon healthcare professionals' examination of each patient and consideration of, among other things, age, weight, gender, current or prior medical conditions, medication history, laboratory data and other factors unique to the patient. The publisher does not provide medical advice or guidance and this work is merely a reference tool. Healthcare professionals, and not the publisher, are solely responsible for the use of this work including all medical judgments and for any resulting diagnosis and treatments.

Given continuous, rapid advances in medical science and health information, independent professional verification of medical diagnoses, indications, appropriate pharmaceutical selections and dosages, and treatment options should be made and healthcare professionals should consult a variety of sources. When prescribing medication, healthcare professionals are advised to consult the product information sheet (the manufacturer's package insert) accompanying each drug to verify, among other things, conditions of use, warnings and side effects and identify any changes in dosage schedule or contraindications, particularly if the medication to be administered is new, infrequently used or has a narrow therapeutic range. To the maximum extent permitted under applicable law, no responsibility is assumed by the publisher for any injury and/or damage to persons or property, as a matter of products liability, negligence law or otherwise, or from any reference to or use by any person of this work.

LWW.com

DEDICATION

To my family and friends for their support and understanding. To my parents for their inspiration, love, and encouragement.

I have always been cognizant and thankful for the opportunity to contribute to the specialties of orthopaedics and radiology. The respect shown by my colleagues and students has and continues to be a humbling and motivating force in my life.

The veracity of truth is a trenchant ally against the consensus who follow convention as if dogma.

The model checklist:
- Honesty, humility in thought and action
- Excel for others through example.
- Never compromise on the truth for without honesty we cannot build knowledge.
- Change of heart and mind through teaching others is the most powerful and natural healing force of the human spirit.

To Howard Berger, MD, President of RadNet, for supporting the development of a world class orthopaedic imaging program.

CONTRIBUTORS

David W. Stoller, MD, FACR
National Director Orthopaedic and Musculoskeletal Imaging, RadNet Medical
Director Orthopaedic and Musculoskeletal Imaging, Beverly Radiology—
Northern California San Francisco, California
Affiliate Member, American Shoulder and Elbow Surgeons

CASE CONTRIBUTORS

Lesley J. Anderson, MD
Assistant Clinical Professor of Orthopaedic Surgery
University of California, San Francisco
Orthopaedic Surgeon
California Pacific Medical Center
San Francisco, California

Piers Barry, MD
Orthopaedic Surgeon
Post Street Orthopaedics and Sports Medicine
San Francisco, California

W. Dilworth Cannon, MD
Professor of Clinical Orthopaedic Surgery
UCSF Sports Medicine Center
University of California
San Francisco, California

James L. Chen, MD
Orthopaedic Surgeon
SportsMed Orthopaedic Group
Faculty, San Francisco Orthopaedic Residency
Clinical Preceptor, University of California San Francisco
San Francisco, California

Garry E. Gold, MD
Professor of Radiology and (by courtesy) Bioengineering and Orthopaedic Surgery
Associate Chair for Research, Radiology
Stanford University
Palo Alto, California

Hollis G. Potter, MD
Chairman, Department of Radiology & Imaging
Hospital for Special Surgery
Professor of Radiology
Weill Medical College of Cornell University

Edward Shin, MD
Orthopaedic Surgeon
Orthopaedic SportsMed Group
San Francisco, California

Kevin R. Stone, MD
Orthopaedic Surgeon
The Stone Clinic
San Francisco, California

Eugene M. Wolf, MD
Department of Orthopaedic Surgery
St. Mary's Medical Center
San Francisco, California

SCIENTIFIC/RESEARCH CONTRIBUTORS

Weitian Chen
Assistant Professor
Department of Imaging & Interventional Radiology
Faculty of Medicine
The Chinese University of Hong Kong

Adriana Kanwischer, BS
Global Product Marketing Leader
MR Premium Segment
GE Healthcare

Jose G. Tamez-Peña, PhD
Chief Technology Officer
Qmetrics Technologies

Melissa E. Sims, MD, MPH
Musculoskeletal Radiologist
San Mateo, California

PREFACE

Stoller's Orthopaedics and Sports Medicine: The Knee represents an ambitious and comprehensive undertaking for both myself and Wolters Kluwer. In order to organize this wealth of information and images in an accessible manner, a unique new format has been developed. A bulleted text that is concise provides for direct and rapid comprehension of a wealth of orthopaedic advancements. Our knowledge of knee anatomy and pathology is a rapidly changing and fluid body of knowledge. **For example, Dr. Freddie Fu's most recent work (2016) on the anterolateral complex has shown that the anterolateral ligament is a disputed structure and is in fact part of the ITB deep capsulo-osseous layer.**

Special features include:
- Comprehensive collections of color illustrations and arthroscopic cases of orthopaedic pathoanatomy
- Key concepts section introductions to emphasize and reinforce critical information
- Detailed figure legends rich in content provide descriptive information and introduce novel concepts.
- 3T and high resolution MR images to demonstrate critical structures in functional knee anatomy and pathology.
- Evolved checklist approach as the keystone for accurate and reproducible image interpretation
- Updated concepts in the knee including:
  - Prospective diagnosis of meniscal tear patterns
  - Meniscal allograft transplantation
  - ACL graft isometry and anatomic double-bundle ACL reconstruction
  - Posterolateral corner and posteromedial corner
  - Multiple–ligament injuries
  - Restorative techniques for articular cartilage

David W. Stoller, MD, FACR
National Director
   Orthopaedic and Musculoskeletal Imaging, RadNet
Medical Director
   Orthopaedic and Musculoskeletal Imaging, Beverly Radiology, Northern California
   San Francisco, California
Affiliate Member
   American Shoulder and Elbow Surgeons

ACKNOWLEDGMENTS

Undertaking the writing of this text has provided a unique opportunity to contribute to the emerging field of orthopaedic magnetic resonance imaging (MRI). Orthopaedic MRI has earned respect as a distinct subspecialty and is now a primary modality in the diagnosis of internal derangement of the joints. I would like to acknowledge the contributions of the following individuals:

> J.A. Gosling, MD, MB, ChB; P.F. Harris, MD, MB, ChB, MSc; J.R. Humpherson, MB, ChB; J. Whitmore, MD, MB, BS, LRCP, MRCS; and P.L.T. Willan, MB, ChB, FRCS, for providing quality gross anatomic color plates from their text, *Human Anatomy*, Second Edition, Gower Medical Publishing.

The expert staff at Wolters Kluwer, for their efforts and appreciation of the necessary quality required to bring this text to fruition, including Lisa McAllister, VP & Publisher, Medicine & Advanced Practice; Ryan Shaw, Acquisitions Editor; Kate Heaney, Product Development Editor; Larry Pezatto, Creative Services Director; and Crystal Perkins, West Coast production liaison for Wolters Kluwer.

Special acknowledgment for Doug Smock for a lifetime of excellence as a creative force in design and creative services for my books with LWW and Wolters Kluwer over the past two decades.

Qmetrics Technologies

Melissa E. Sims, MD, MPH for reference compilation.

Brent Berthy, General Manager, Invivo for his innovative MR coil development and support of MR education.

Robert Hoffman and Intelerad for their support in the storage of MR cases.

Ralph Stubenrauch, Clinical Applications Manager, RadNet for computer and PACs processing of 3T images.

W. Dilworth Cannon, MD; Scott Dye, MD; Greg Ondera, MD; and Plexus Communications for knee dissection and arthroscopy.

I would like to recognize the work of Michel Bonnin, MD and Freddie Fu, MD

> *The Knee Joint: Surgical Techniques and Strategies,*
> Michel Bonnin, MD
>
> *Master Techniques in Orthopaedic Surgery: Sports Medicine,*
> Freddie H. Fu, MD, DSci(Hon), DPs(Hon)

CONTENTS

- **Practical Guide to Knee MR Imaging** 1
- **Knee Anatomy** 29
- **Stoller's Knee Checklist and Protocols** 95
- **The Meniscus** 151
- **Cruciate Ligaments** 395
- **Collateral Ligaments** 579
- **Patellofemoral Joint and the Extensor Mechanism** 695
- **General Pathologic Conditions Affecting the Knee** 843

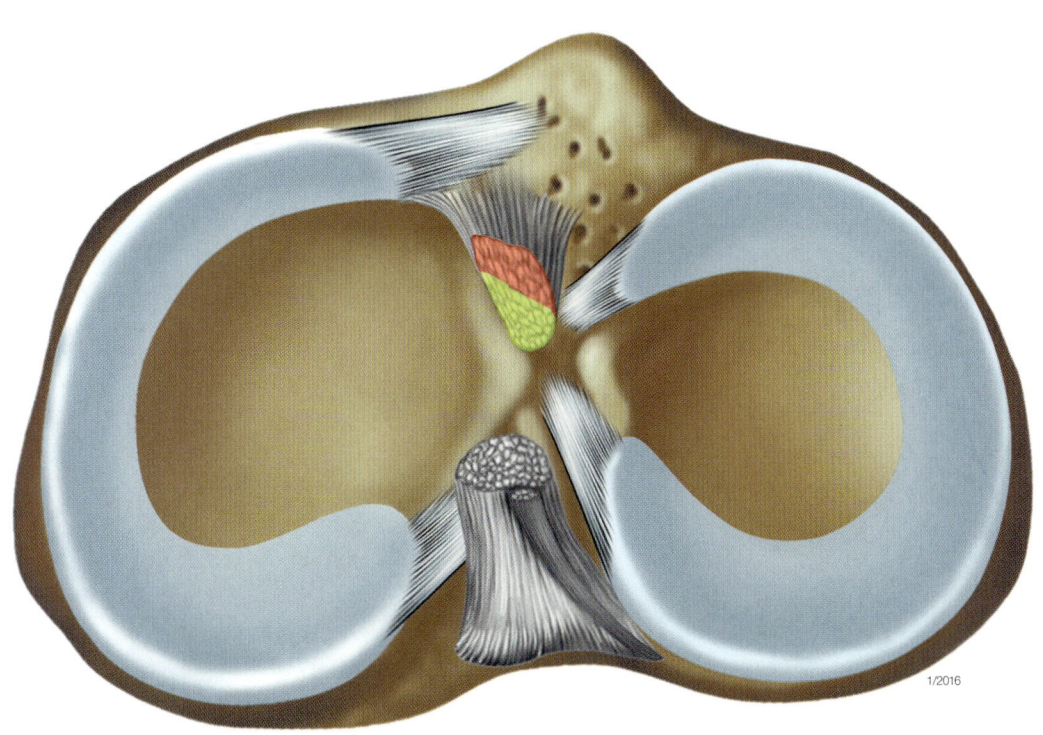

1
Practical Guide to Knee MR Imaging

Key Factors to Clinical Diagnostics (page 3)

Positioning (page 4)

Basic Pulse Sequences (pages 5-6)

Scan Parameters (pages 7-9)

Advanced Applications (pages 10-18)

3-T Imaging Considerations (pages 18-20)

Parallel Imaging (pages 20-21)

Fat Suppression (pages 21-23)

Uniformity Corrections: Image Enhancement Filters (pages 23-24)

Segmentation (pages 25-26)

Sequence and Parameter Acronyms (page 27)

Practical Guide to Knee MR Imaging

Key Factors to Clinical Diagnostics

Motion Insensitivity
- Sequences and parameters that eliminate or reduce patient motion and flow-related artifacts

Uniform Fat Suppression
- Techniques insensitive to B_0 and B_1 inhomogeneity, preferably flexible on the amount of saturation

Contrast
- Consisting of T1, proton density (PD), and T2* weighting

High Resolution
- Required for visualizing submillimeter structures

Isotropic Resolution
- 3D imaging techniques for postacquisition reformatting

Off-Isocenter Image Quality
- Consistent image quality even when the knee is positioned away from isocenter

Reduced Distortion Around Metal
- Availability of advanced techniques for imaging around total knee arthroplasties as well as fixation screws

Efficient Surface Coils
- Coils that support parallel imaging, possess sufficient signal-to-noise ratio (SNR) with tissue depth, provide stability and comfort to the patient, and are easy to set up

Positioning

Radiofrequency (RF) Coils

- There are several commercial knee coil options to choose from, though compatibility will depend on the specific MR system vendor, model, and field strength. The most common are transmit/receive (TR) coils, which typically consist of a local transmit birdcage coil coupled with an array of receive elements. The benefits of a TR knee coil include reduced specific absorption rate (SAR) deposition to the patient, reduced signal wrapping from adjacent anatomy, and some performance improvement on the specific sequences.

- Whether TR or receive-only, the number of receive channels varies between eight and 18, with a trend to higher channel counts. Higher receive channel counts will provide higher SNR closer to the surface and enable higher acceleration factors with parallel imaging. However, the drawback with higher channels is the need for intensity correction due to intense signal closer to the surface coils.

- Most TR knee coils have rigid enclosures, with a split-top design, making patient positioning relatively straightforward. Some receive-only coils may require additional fixation structures to support the patient's knee and the coil. As such, positioning of the patient's knee typically consists of centering the knee within the superior/inferior extent of the coil. Most often, this is best accomplished by centering the tibial plateau with the patient lying supine. Some flexible coils will be able to accommodate larger patients who might not fit within rigid coils.

Immobilization

- Patients will almost always be positioned supine, with the knee to be imaged located as close to right/left isocenter as possible, though this will be limited by the size of the nonimaged knee. Wedge pads will often be placed within the coil to keep the knee immobilized, with a slight bend for comfort, though some radiologists may prefer a straighter knee. Depending on the MR system, either a feet first or head first orientation can be used, though most patients will prefer feet first.

Basic Pulse Sequences

FSE

- The most commonly used sequence for musculoskeletal imaging is fast spin-echo or turbo spin-echo. Most vendors have versions for 2D and 3D acquisitions, but multiplanar 2D is primarily used, though there is an increasing trend toward 3D. FSE provides spin-echo type contrast with faster scan times by acquiring multiple echoes in each shot. PD, T1, or T2 image contrast can be obtained, determined by the TR, echo time (TE), and echo train length (ETL) parameters. FSE protocols typically focus on controlling echo spacing (time between echoes) to avoid blurring and flow artifacts. The minimum TE is an indicator of echo spacing, and shorter values are desired to provide good image quality.

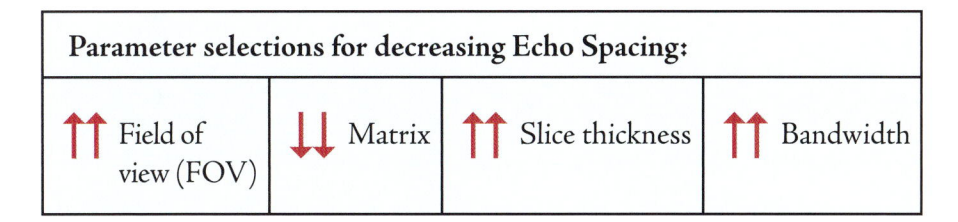

Parameter selections for decreasing Echo Spacing:			
↑↑ Field of view (FOV)	↓↓ Matrix	↑↑ Slice thickness	↑↑ Bandwidth

FRFSE

- The fast recovery fast spin-echo (FRFSE) sequence produces images with more T2 contribution with the same TR as FSE. It is a modified FSE sequence using additional RF pulses after the acquisition window to hasten recovery of longitudinal magnetization from signal with long T2.

- FRFSE is commonly used to reduce scan time by using a shorter TR, while maintaining T2 contrast.

Recommended TR, TE, and ETL values for FSE and FRFSE:			
Pulse Sequence	TR	TE	ETL
FRFSE PD	2000–3000ms	30–60ms	6–10
FRFSE T2	2000–3000ms	85ms	12–14
FSE T1	500–900ms	Min.	2–4

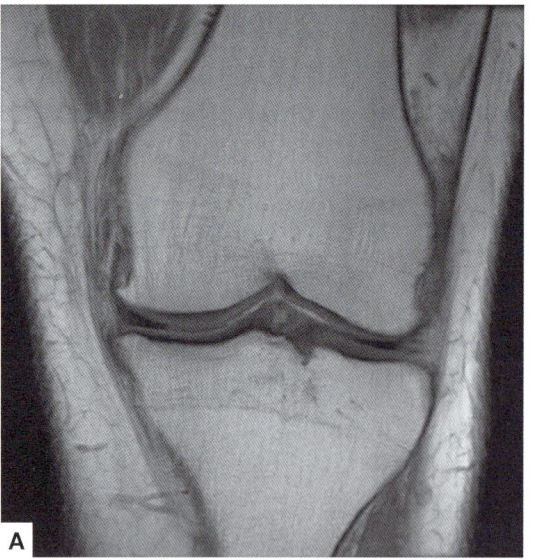 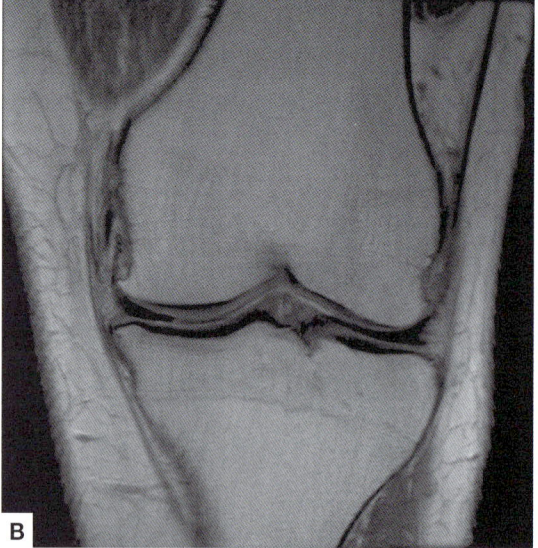

FIGURE 1.1 (**A**, **B**) Image on the left with an echo spacing of 8ms compared to an echo spacing of 16ms resulting in image blurring.

GRE

■ Gradient echo (GRE) sequences are used to provide T1 and T2* contrast, which can complement spin-echo based acquisitions. Most practical uses in the knee are with 3D sequences, such as spoiled gradient echo (SPGR) for assessing physes. Generally, the key parameter for managing contrast with GRE sequences is flip angle:

Sequence	Contrast	Flip Angle
2D GRE/SPGR	T1 T2*	40–60 20–30
3D GRE/SPGR	T1 T2*	25–45 5–8

An increase in flip angle:	
⇈ T1 contrast	⇈ SNR

Inversion Recovery

■ Inversion recovery sequences are frequently used for uniform suppression of fat signal by acquiring data at the null point of the T1 recovery, with the key parameter being the TI (inversion time).

Scan Parameters

Spatial Resolution

- Determined by voxel size, which depends on the FOV, acquisition matrix, and slice thickness

Calculating Voxel Size

$$\frac{\text{Phase FOV}}{\text{\# Phase matrix}} = \text{Phase dimension}$$

$$\frac{\text{Frequency FOV}}{\text{\# Frequency matrix}} = \text{Frequency dimension}$$

Phase dimension × Frequency dimension × Slice thickness = Voxel volume

- High resolution may add valuable information for musculoskeletal imaging.

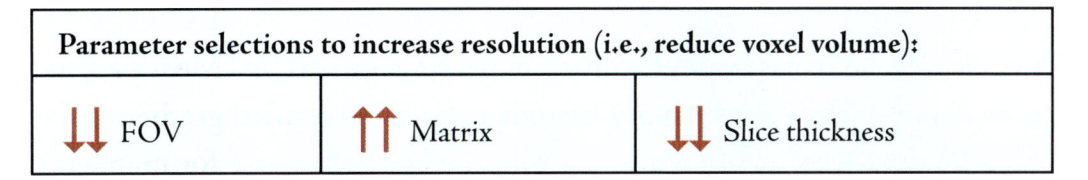

Parameter selections to increase resolution (i.e., reduce voxel volume):		
⇓ FOV	⇑⇑ Matrix	⇓⇓ Slice thickness

Acquisition Time

- Typically, the SNR is proportional to the acquisition time. However, longer scans are more prone to motion artifacts. The primary parameters that impact acquisition times are TR, phase matrix, and the number of excitations (NEX) or averages. For 3D sequences, phase matrix includes both the in-plane and slice direction, which is typically the number of slices.

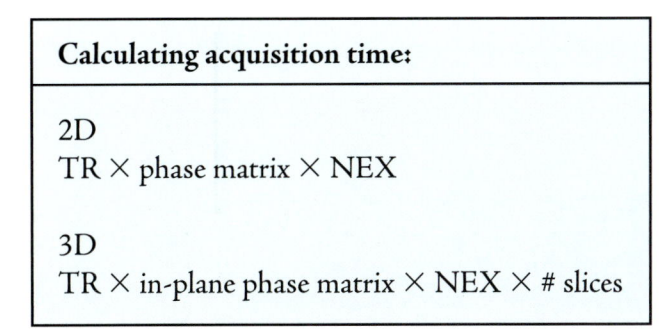

Calculating acquisition time:

2D
TR × phase matrix × NEX

3D
TR × in-plane phase matrix × NEX × # slices

SNR

- Noise is the nondiagnostic signal that is generated from the patient, the environment, and the system electronics. The goal of sequence parameter optimization is to increase signal, which is proportional to field strength, voxel volume, and the time spent acquiring the signal.

- Parameter selection to increase SNR:

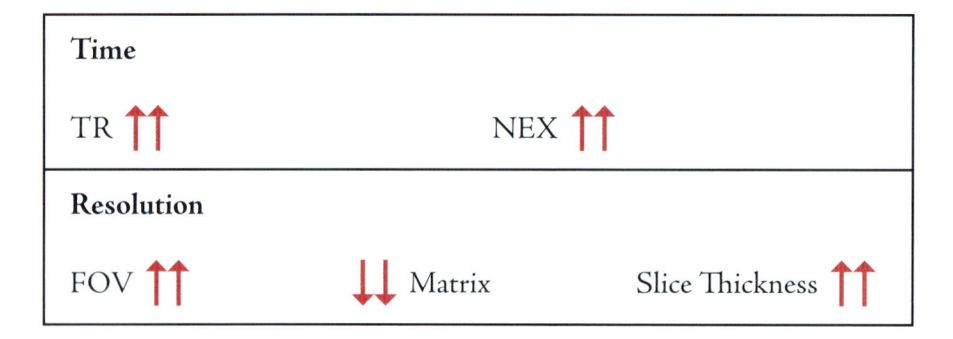

Time		
TR ⇈		NEX ⇈
Resolution		
FOV ⇈	⇊ Matrix	Slice Thickness ⇈

Trade-Offs

- In the clinical environment, the imaging protocol parameters will be determined according to many different goals. Understanding the parameter trade-offs is the only way to achieve good image quality, whether there is patient motion or anxiety, positioning limitations, anatomic variations, time restrictions, or any other challenges.

- The table below is designed to provide guidance to adjust protocols without compromising the exam objectives.

Parameters	Resolution	Time	SNR
⇈ TR	–	⇈	⇈
⇈ TE	–	–	⇊
⇈ NEX	–	⇈	⇈
⇈ Slice Thickness	⇊	–	⇈
⇈ FOV	⇊	–	⇈
⇈ Bandwidth	–	–	⇊
⇈ Frequency	⇈	–	⇊
⇈ Phase	⇈	⇈	⇊

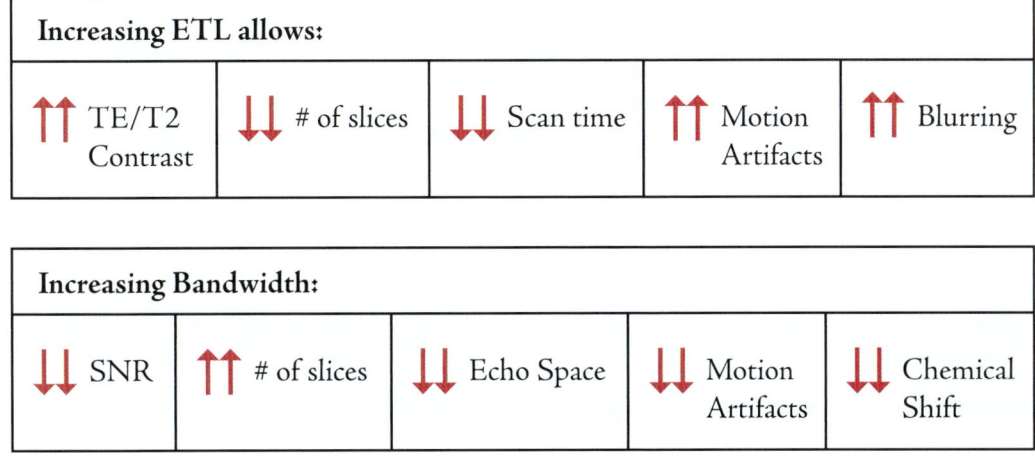

- ETL and bandwidth are parameters that affect protocols in a wider manner and deserve special mention.

Increasing ETL allows:				
↑↑ TE/T2 Contrast	↓↓ # of slices	↓↓ Scan time	↑↑ Motion Artifacts	↑↑ Blurring

Increasing Bandwidth:				
↓↓ SNR	↑↑ # of slices	↓↓ Echo Space	↓↓ Motion Artifacts	↓↓ Chemical Shift

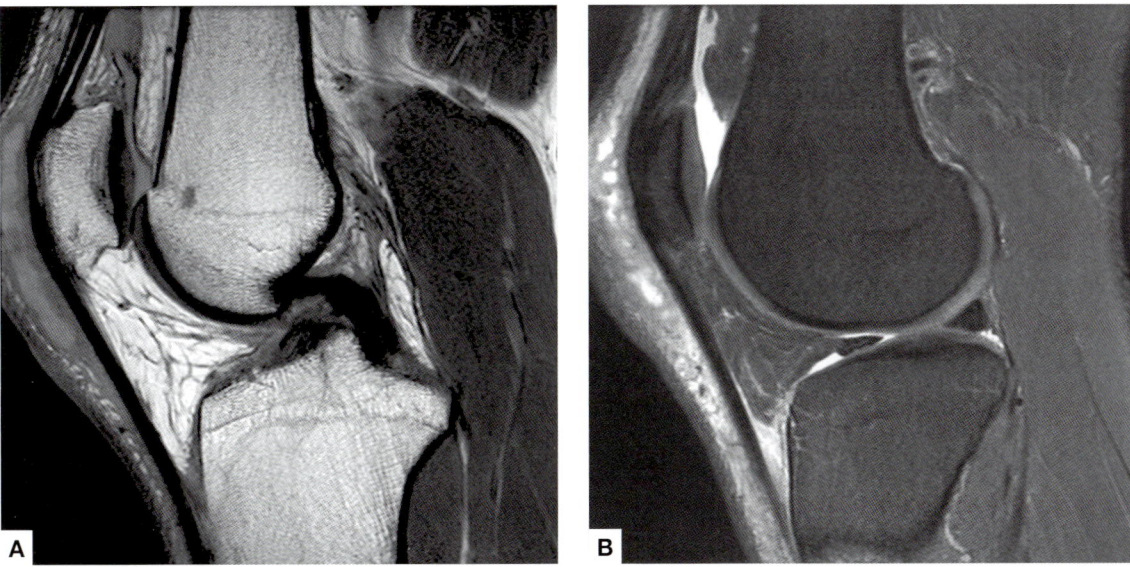

FIGURE 1.2 (**A**) Sagittal FR FSE PD and (**B**) sagittal FR FSE PD fat saturation images.

Advanced Applications

CartiGram—T2 Mapping (GE Healthcare)

- CartiGram (T2 mapping) is a technique that is used to noninvasively detect changes in the collagen component of the extracellular matrix of cartilage. This application acquires multiple scans at each slice location; each set of scans has a unique TE, resulting in a set of gray scale images that represent different T2 weighting. The acquired data can be processed to produce T2 color maps, which demonstrate more subtle changes in cartilage ultrastructure that are not visible on gray scale MR images.

- The collagen in the radial zone of articular cartilage, close to the subchondral bone, is highly ordered, with only small quantities of mobile water. By contrast, the collagen in the transitional zone is more randomly oriented, with increased mobile water and more prolonged T2 values. Increased T2 relaxation times within cartilage have been associated with matrix damage, particularly loss of the orientation of the collagen matrix.

- CartiGram can be used as a "quantitative" prescription. It is essential that the parameters are not significantly modified. The acquisition scan plane is decided according to the clinical need. Axial slices are prescribed on the patellofemoral joint, whereas sagittal or coronal slices are prescribed on the femoral condyle and tibial plateau.

- Choose the appropriate number of slices to cover the area of interest. The number of TE's per scan is the selection that determines the number of images acquired at each location. For example, if 10 slices are prescribed and eight TE's per scan are prescribed, then there are 10 data sets with eight images per location. Each image within a data set or location has eight unique images with variable T2 weighting. The acquired data set is processed (FuncTool) to generate automatic calculations of the functional maps.

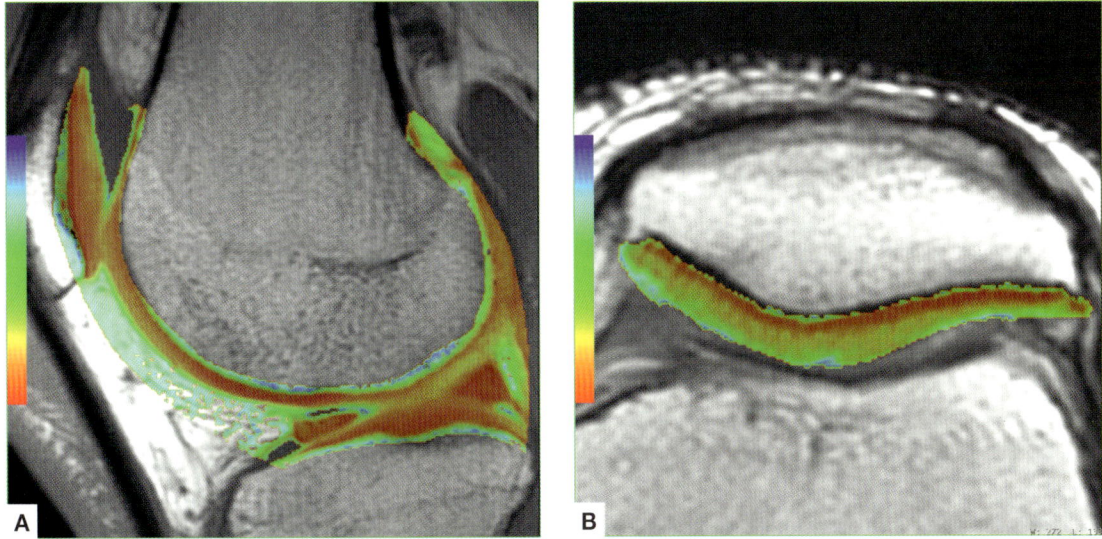

FIGURE 1.3   CartiGram T2 mapping sagittal (**A**) and axial (**B**) images.

3.0T

Pulse Sequence Definition (PSD)	TR (ms)	TE (ms)	Bandwidth (BW) (kHz)	NEX	FOV (cm)	Matrix	Thick (mm)	Imaging Options
T2MAP	1000	20.1	62.5	1	16	320 × 224	3.0	Fast, ASSET

CUBE (GE Healthcare)

- CUBE is a 3D FSE pulse sequence that applies modified refocusing pulses for better SNR and SAR efficiency. It can be used to generate PD and T2 contrasts. It is always combined with acceleration techniques to avoid long scan times. CUBE allows isotropic volume acquisitions that can be reformatted in any plane with the same resolution as the original plane.

- CUBE image quality is very dependent on protocol parameters. Settings enhanced for the musculoskeletal system (MSK) provide for shorter gradients, reducing echo spacing and consequently decreased blurring. CUBE also allows a choice for the refocusing flip angle. Recommendations are 90 for 1.5T and 70 for 3.0T, increasing SNR when relatively shorter ETL (~32 to 36) is used. Whole-volume excitation improves signal intensity uniformity across all slices.

- CUBE protocols allow no phase wrap (NPW) and multi-NEX. Fat saturation uses an adiabatic spectral inversion recovery technique (ASPIR), and the fat saturation efficiency can be modified by percentage, providing lighter to stronger fat suppression according to the user preference. Selecting fat saturation will minimize possible wrap artifacts in the slice direction that are visible in reformatted images.

- Banding or shading may be observed on off-center imaging so the anatomy must always be positioned as close as possible to the isocenter. Longer scan times when using NPW and multi-NEX are expected.

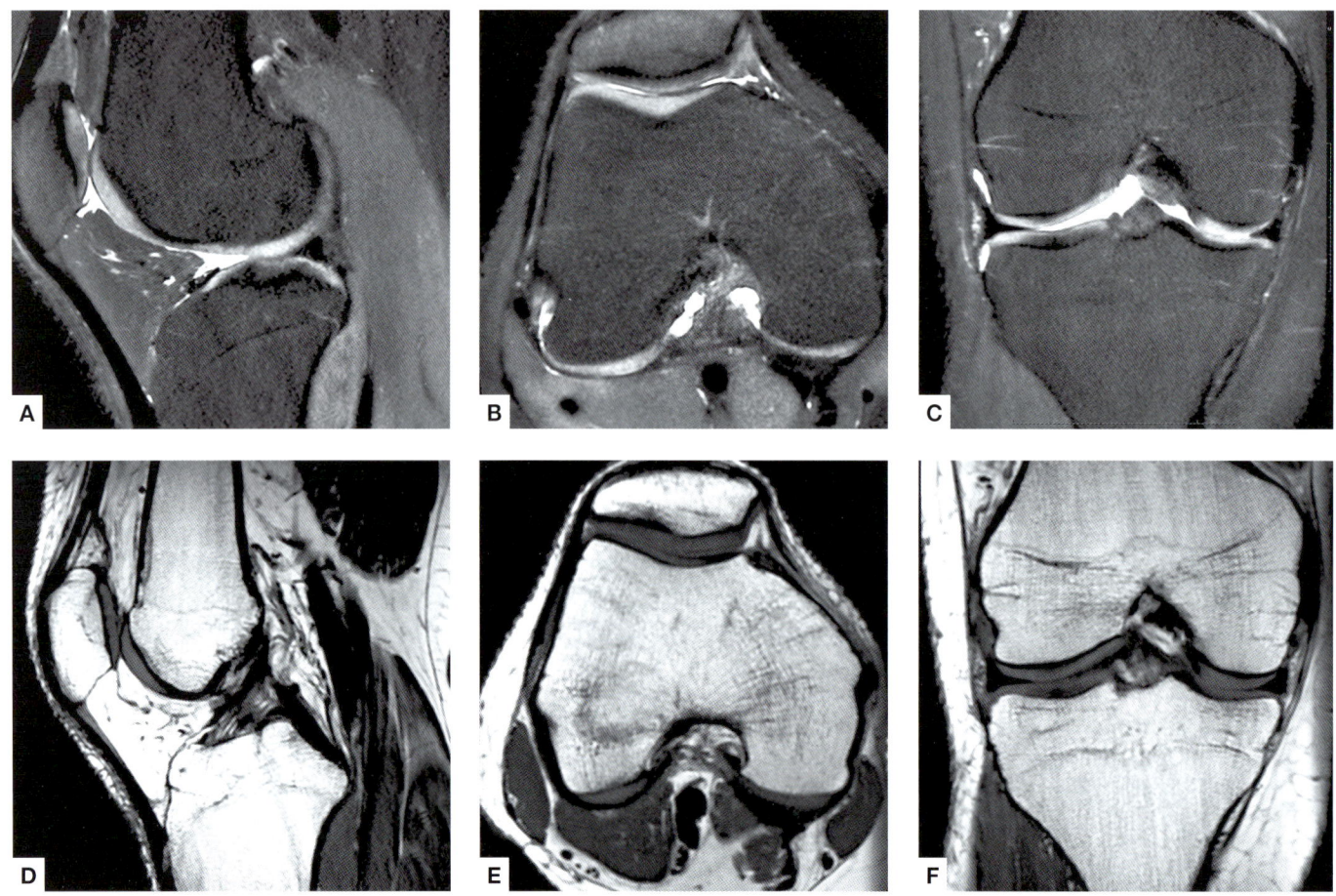

FIGURE 1.4 3D CUBE images: (**A**) 3D CUBE PD fat saturation (Fat Sat) sagittal, (**B**) 3D CUBE PD Fat Sat axial, (**C**) 3D CUBE PD Fat Sat coronal, (**D**) 3D CUBE T1 sagittal, (**E**) 3D CUBE T1 axial, and (**F**) 3D CUBE T1 coronal images.

3.0T

PSD	TR (ms)	TE (ms)	BW (kHz)	ETL	NEX	FOV (cm)	Matrix	Thick (mm)	Imaging Options
CUBE	1600	40	50	32	1	16	384 × 384	1.2	Fat Sat, EDR, ARC

IDEAL (GE Healthcare)

- IDEAL is a three-point Dixon technique that acquires three images at slightly different echo times to generate phase shifts between water and fat. The water/fat separation method is very efficient at providing homogeneous image quality.

- One acquisition provides four contrasts: water, fat, in-phase, and out-of-phase images. Available for 2D FSE, 2D FRFSE, 3D Fast GRE, and 3D Fast SPGR sequences, it can be combined with acceleration (ARC) for faster acquisition times. IDEAL is part of the imaging options list, and when selected, it will open a new tab on the protocol for a choice of which of the four contrasts should be reconstructed.

- The typical IDEAL bandwidth is the pre-IDEAL sequence value multiplied by two. The FOV must include all the anatomy of interest since phase wrap artifacts may cause fat and water signal to be swapped.

- To prevent blurring and maintain resolution, place the center of the effective TE between the minimum (Min) and maximum (Max) TE values by adjusting ETL to reduce the Max TE. The minimum and maximum TE values are annotated at the bottom of the protocol page. IDEAL reduces image artifacts caused by chemical shift and magnetic susceptibility.

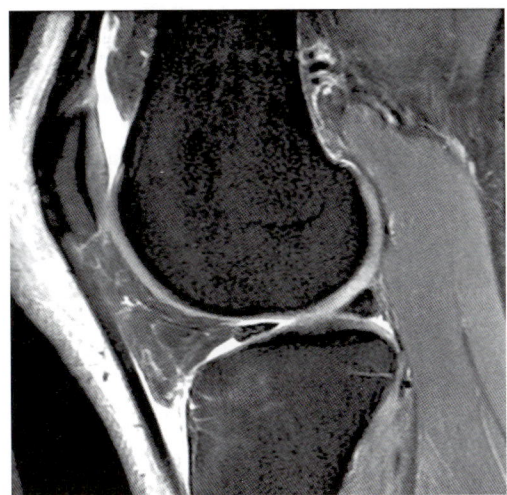

FIGURE 1.5   IDEAL sagittal water image.

3.0T

PSD	TR (ms)	TE (ms)	BW (kHz)	ETL	NEX	FOV (cm)	Matrix	Thick (mm)	Imaging Options
IDEAL	3250	35	62.5	9	1	14	320 × 224	3.0	FC, IDEAL, EDR, TRF

3D MERGE (GE Healthcare)

■ 3D MERGE is a 3D Fast GRE pulse sequence that acquires multiple echoes at several different TEs and then average those echoes to form a single T2*-weighted image. This technique can be used when susceptibility weighting is desired. It maintains visualization of ligaments while adding soft tissue contrast. Water excitation is available for robust fat suppression.

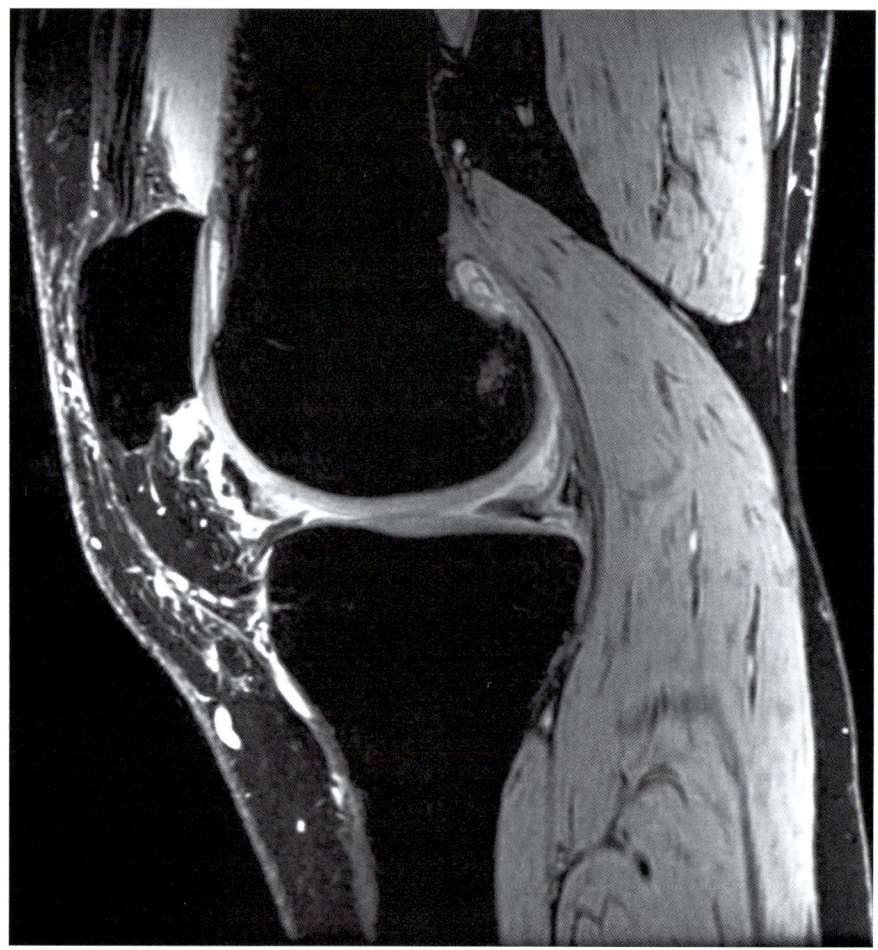

FIGURE 1.6   3D MERGE water excitation.

3.0T

PSD	TR (ms)	TE (ms)	BW (kHz)	Flip Angle	NEX	FOV (cm)	Matrix	Thick (mm)	Imaging Options
MERGE	30	Min Full	41.67	9	1	18	288 × 288	1.2	FC, EDR, ZIP2, ASSET, ZIP2, SSRF

PROPELLER (GE Healthcare)

- PROPELLER is a pulse sequence designed for motion correction. The technique is based on periodically rotated overlapping parallel lines with enhanced reconstruction. It uses radial k-space filling with an arrangement of blades resulting in oversampling the center of k-space and providing images with high signal. The radial trajectory removes structured motion artifacts.

- Acceleration is used to increase blade width and reduce scan times. It can be used for any scan plane and is an excellent choice of sequence when imaging through motion is needed due to breathing, flow, or uncooperative patients. It is compatible with fat saturation and can produce PD and T2 contrast for MSK imaging.

- PROPELLER image quality is very dependent of scan parameters. Blade width (ETL × phase acceleration), oversampling factor, and refocusing flip angle are concepts that deserve special attention for obtaining good image quality. The oversampling factor (OSF) works as the analogue to NPW for PROPELLER.

- Blade width must be adjusted properly to prevent streaking artifacts. Increase ETL, use acceleration, and decrease OSF to keep the minimum blade width equal to at least 12 for musculoskeletal imaging.

- Contrast can be adjusted by modifying the refocusing flip angle value. Decreasing the refocusing flip angle will provide brighter cartilage signal. It will also allow higher TE and ETL values while still avoiding artifacts. Proper prescan values must be obtained before scanning PROPELLER. Prescribe a shim volume on the area of interest for the series that will be scanned previously to PROPELLER.

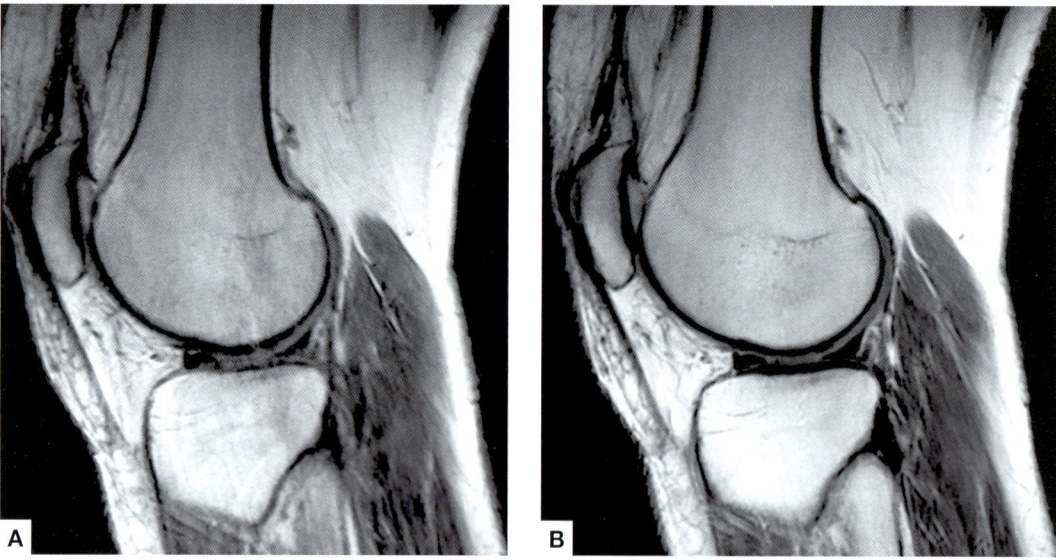

FIGURE 1.7 Same study comparison of FSE image with motion (**A**) and PROPELLER with motion correction (**B**).

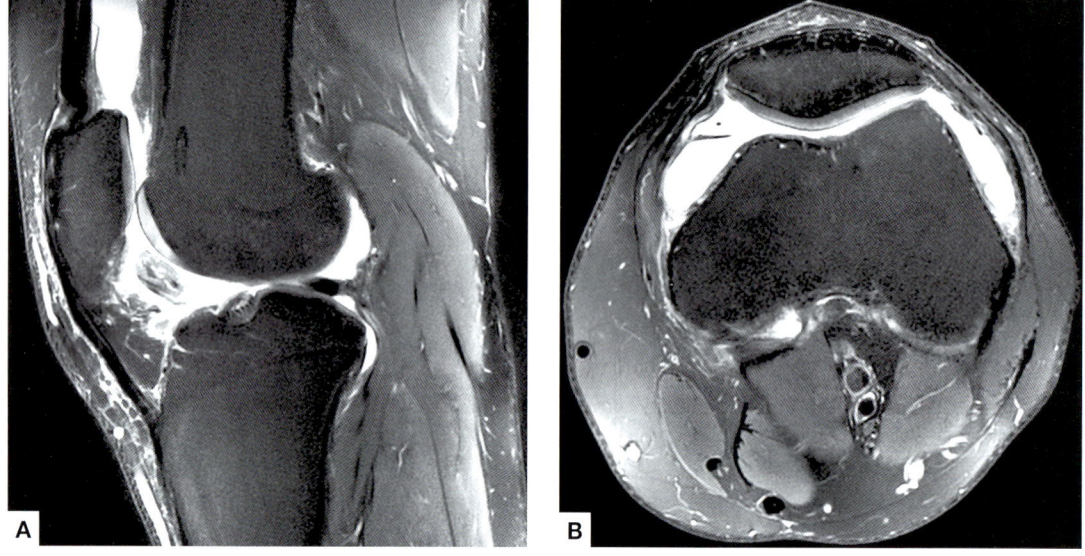

FIGURE 1.8 PROPELLER images: PROPELLER sagittal Fat Sat (**A**) and PROPELLER axial Fat Sat (**B**) images.

3.0T

PSD	TR (ms)	TE (ms)	BW (kHz)	ETL	NEX	FOV (cm)	Matrix	Thick (mm)	Imaging Options
PROPELLER	6800	105	83.3	22	3	17	416 × 416	3.0 × 0.3	Fat Sat, NP2.0, ARC, TRF

MAVRIC SL (GE Healthcare)

- MAVRIC SL is a pulse sequence designed to reduce susceptibility artifacts. It is used for imaging soft tissue and bone near MR conditional metal implants. MAVRIC SL is a multispectral 3D imaging technique that acquires multiple 3D FSE images at discrete transmit and receive frequency offsets. All data acquired are then added together to form a final composite image.

- The recommended protocol for MR conditional implant imaging includes MAVRIC SL PD, MAVRIC SL Fluid, and MARS (high-bandwidth FSE) protocols.

- The MAVRIC SL PD sequence is used for evaluating the tissue in the immediate vicinity of the implant, and the MAVRIC SL Fluid (inversion recovery [IR]-based fat suppression) sequence is used as a low-resolution fluid detection mechanism replacing the conventional 2D FSE STIR sequence. MAVRIC SL T1 contrast images can be achieved by decreasing TR and ETL with the advantage that shorter ETL values decrease blurring. A high-resolution MARS sequence is used for evaluating the soft tissue located away from the implant. The MARS technique is a 2D FSE protocol with a high bandwidth value.

- Prescribing a wide enough FOV to cover the sensitivity region is recommended to avoid image wrap. Or, leave enough space away from the implant for fold-over to occur without impinging on the metal-distorted region. Aggressive parallel imaging (ARC) is used to maintain low scan times and is not limited by coil configurations like other applications. Residual metal artifacts may occur. They are different from conventional susceptibility distortions and could occasionally appear as "ringing" near the corners of the implants.

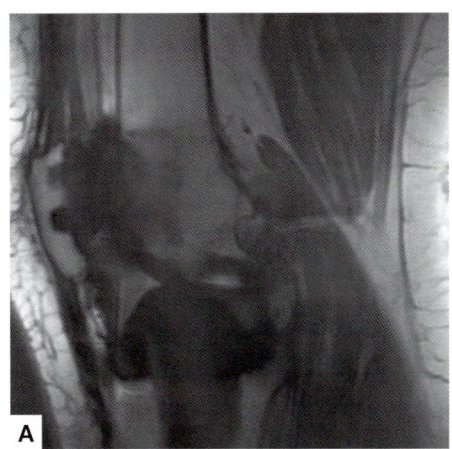 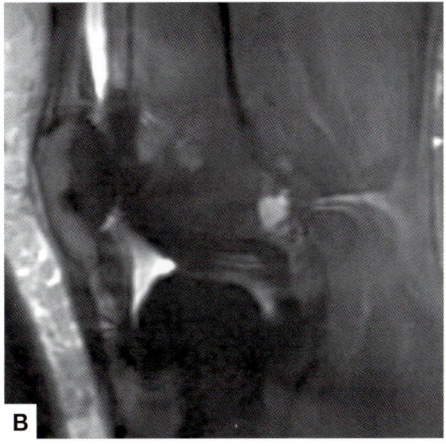 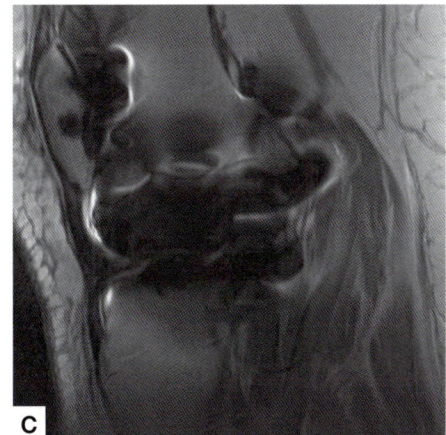

FIGURE 1.9   (A) MAVRIC SL PD, (B) MAVRIC SL Fluid, and (C) MARS images.

3.0T

PSD	TR (ms)	TE/TI (ms)	BW (kHz)	ETL	NEX	FOV (cm)	Matrix	Thick (mm)	Imaging Options
MAVRIC SL PD	3000	7.5	125	20	0.5	20	320 × 256	4.0	ARC, EDR
MAVRIC SL Fluid	5000	7/175	125	20	0.5	20	256 × 192	4.0	ARC, EDR
MARS	7000	25	100	20	2	20	512 × 320	3.5	NPW, EDR, TRF

3-T Imaging Considerations

Advantages

- High-field MR imaging at 3.0T allows for up to 100% SNR increase when compared to 1.5T systems. The extra SNR can be used to decrease scan times and increase resolution: increasing matrix, decreasing FOV, or decreasing slice thickness. Decreasing NEX will reduce scan acquisition time.

- T1 relaxation times are longer at 3.0T. Increasing the TR for acquiring the desired contrast must be considered.

Challenges

- Chemical Shift:
    - Chemical shift is a misregistration artifact in the frequency encoding direction caused by the frequency difference between fat and water signals.
    - Precessional frequencies are proportional to the magnetic field, and since they double from 1.5T to 3.0T (220Hz /440Hz), chemical shift artifacts are twice as bad at 3.0T.
    - Increasing the bandwidth reduces the number of pixels of the shift between fat and water, minimizing the appearance of the chemical shift artifact; therefore, 3.0T protocols have higher bandwidth when compared to 1.5T protocols.

- **Magnetic Susceptibility:**
  - The ability of the magnetic field to penetrate different substances is called susceptibility, and it induces magnetic field perturbations resulting in distortion artifacts. The appearance of the artifacts is the result of the sum of surrounding tissues with different magnetic susceptibilities. Susceptibility artifacts cause signal loss and distortions and will be observed in interfaces like bone/tissue, air/tissue, and presence of metal. Since susceptibility is proportional to the magnetic field, the artifacts will be twice as severe at 3.0T as at 1.5T.
  - Increasing bandwidth can help minimize susceptibility artifacts. Inversion recovery techniques are recommended because GRE sequences and fat suppression methods are more sensitive to susceptibility artifacts.

- **Specific Absorption Rate:**
  - Specific absorption rate (SAR) is a measurement of the RF energy deposition.
  - SAR is dependent on the square of the B_0 field strength; therefore, it is four times higher at 3.0T than at 1.5T.
  - SAR values may restrict minimum TR values and the number of slices per TR for FSE sequences. Increasing TR, decreasing refocusing flip angles, and using GRE sequences are efficient ways of decreasing SAR values.

- **Dielectric Effect:**
  - Dielectric artifacts are represented by areas of inhomogeneity, shading, or lower SNR. They are caused by the interaction by the RF field and increased conductivity of the body tissue. Because the RF wavelength on the 3.0T magnetic field strength is comparable to the patient diameter, the dielectric effect is more evident on 3.0T systems.
  - The artifacts are seen mostly on abdominal imaging and are related to patient size, being more evident on smaller and thinner individuals.
  - Presence of fluid can also exacerbate the shading, for example, on patients with ascites.

- Multichannel coils may also intensify dielectric effect due to the higher signal intensity, making nonuniformity areas more apparent.

- Dielectric pads may be used between the coil and the patient to minimize shading, but with limited success. They are made of a dilute manganese chloride solution.

- Uniformity correction methods can be applied, reducing dielectric effect. Commonly used mitigation at 3.0T for reducing dielectric shading is "dual drive" or "RF shimming," which modifies the transmit RF field polarization.

Parallel Imaging

- Parallel imaging is a method that allows rapid MR data acquisition by using the spatial information in multichannel coils combined with mathematical techniques such as ASSET and ARC. Acquisition times are shorter since only partial data are acquired. The rest of the information is completed using spatial information obtained by coil sensitivity.

- Parallel imaging comes at the expense of SNR loss, but it includes other benefits such as the reduction of image blurring, motion artifacts, and geometric distortion.

- Parallel imaging performance is improved by optimized coil designs with more receiver channels and is also dependent of the distance that separates elements in the phase encoding direction.

ASSET

- Array Spatial Sensitivity Encoding Technique (ASSET) is an externally calibrated parallel imaging method whose generic name is SENSE. The calibration acquisition provides the coil sensitivity maps and is acquired separately from the ASSET acquisition. Incomplete calibration coverage, calibration wrap, area of interest mismatch, and poor coil positioning are the most common causes of artifacts.

ARC

- Autocalibrating Reconstruction for Cartesian imaging (ARC) is an auto-calibrated parallel imaging technique that does not require a separated calibration series to acquire a coil sensitivity map. It simplifies work flow and is extremely powerful against parallel imaging artifacts.

- Parallel imaging represents an important concept for MSK imaging. It allows acceptable acquisition times for several applications like CUBE, MAVRIC SL, PROPELLER, and others.

Fat Suppression

Spectral Selective Fat Saturation

- Spectral selective fat saturation is a method that applies a frequency-selective saturation pulse at the frequency of fat before the imaging excitation pulse with the result being a signal measurement primarily from water. Because the fat and water frequency separation depends on the magnetic field strength (220Hz at 1.5T/440Hz at 3.0T), fat saturation techniques based on this method are more effective at higher field strengths because the saturation can more effectively distinguish fat from water.

- The disadvantage of this method is the dependency on the homogeneity of the B_0 field. Poor field homogeneity may cause the frequency-selective pulse to saturate water, instead resulting in regions where water rather than fat will be saturated. Alternately, because of poor B_0 homogeneity (often caused by magnetic susceptibility artifacts), the frequency-selective pulse may not saturate any signal at all.

STIR (Short TI Inversion Recovery)

- STIR is an inversion recovery method that takes advantage of the T1 difference between water and fat to allow selection of the signal to suppress. In order to eliminate the signal from tissues, the TI time must match exactly the null point of the tissue that needs to be suppressed. The TI time is approximately 69% of the T1 relaxation time of the tissue. Because this is an inversion recovery technique, the resulting image will be inherently T1 weighted, but at short TI time, T1 contrast will be inverted. It is also possible to acquire T2 contrast by using a long TE; T2 contrast will not be inverted.

- STIR is very effective at suppressing fat signal because it can be made less dependent on field homogeneity by proper design of RF pulses and is less dependent on the magnetic field homogeneity. The disadvantage of this sequence is longer acquisition time because inversion recovery techniques need longer TR times to give the spins enough time to recover.

SPIR (Spectral Presaturation with Inversion Recovery)

- SPIR is a technique that uses both STIR and selective excitation of the fat signal. The TI value for the null point of a tissue follows the same rules as the STIR sequence. There will be no inherent T1-weighted contrast because only the fat signal is excited and water is not affected.

- The disadvantages include increase on scan acquisition times; it is also sensitive to B_1 uniformity and requires good separation of fat and water. SPIR can be improved by incorporation of an adiabatic pulse because adiabatic pulses are insensitive to B_1 nonuniformity. The result, SPAIR or ASPIR, is a fat suppression technique that is relatively insensitive to both B_0 and B_1 inhomogeneity.

SPAIR (Spectral Selective Adiabatic Inversion Recovery) or ASPIR (Adiabatic Spectral Selective Inversion Recovery)

- SPAIR or ASPIR method is a solution for poor fat suppression due to B_1 inhomogeneity. It is based on the frequency and the relaxation fat behaviors.

- It applies a spectrally selective adiabatic inversion pulse to excite the fat spins; imaging pulses are then applied after TI null time when longitudinal magnetization of fat crosses zero. The disadvantages include sensitivity to B_0 and longer scan times.

Dixon

- The two-point Dixon technique is based on the difference between fat and water resonance frequencies; therefore, they have different precession rates. With this method, two images are acquired, one with fat and water spins in phase and the other with them out of phase. When these images are added pixel by pixel, the result is a fat-suppressed image, and their subtraction results in a water-suppressed image.

- The three-point Dixon method is similar to the two-point technique, except that one extra image is acquired to correct phase effects like susceptibility or eddy currents. Dixon is a very robust fat suppression technique, but scan times are longer because extra images are acquired. The final result is four images with four different contrasts: fat only, water only, in phase, and out of phase. The out-of-phase contrast is mostly used for abdominal imaging to evaluate the border between fatty and nonfatty tissues.

Uniformity Corrections: Image Enhancement Filters

- Signal intensity is most efficiently collected in the areas of the anatomy that are closest to the coil. This characteristic may cause nonuniformity of signal: the image will be brighter in the periphery close to the coil and relatively darker in the center away from the coil.

- Intensity correction algorithms can be applied to the images to minimize the nonuniformity.

- Phased Array Uniformity Enhancement (PURE) and Surface Coil Intensity Correction (SCIC) (GE Healthcare) are two techniques designed to normalize the surface coil intensity variations. PURE or SCIC can be used with compatible surface coils. PURE corrects field inhomogeneity using a low-resolution PD-weighted calibration scan, whereas SCIC uses statistics from the actual image for inhomogeneity correction and does not require a calibration scan.

PURE: Phased Array Uniformity Enhancement

- PURE corrects the field inhomogeneity by collecting a calibration scan from the (uniform) body coil and the (nonuniform) surface coil and calculating maps that relate the intensity correction values to the images. The correction is therefore stable across many image contrasts but is limited to the RF fields of the surface and body coil. It cannot correct for fat saturation uniformity.

- Pure data can be automatically acquired during the exam acquisition or applied afterward by postprocessing if a calibration series was acquired. PURE postprocessing will be available only for the series acquired after the calibration. Images are corrected by intensifying the signal. Areas of lower SNR will intensify the noise as well as signal, so the corrected images may appear "noisier" after correction on those areas. That is, both the detail and noise are amplified together in the process of making the average tissue intensity more uniform. To avoid the increased intensity of noise, prescribe your FOV in an area with proper coil coverage.

SCIC: Surface Coil Intensity Correction

- SCIC is a method that uses statistics from the actual image for inhomogeneity correction. It uses an optimized set of parameters for tuning that are defined according to the different anatomies and coils. Because SCIC does not use an acquired reference image, the correction results will make the image contrast appear flatter when compared to images corrected by PURE. It compensates for smooth variations arising from any source, and its performance can vary depending on the contrast of the image to be corrected.

- SCIC can also be applied automatically during acquisition or during postprocessing. The low SNR areas will appear slightly darker, and noise enhancement is less noticeable than in images corrected with PURE.

- SCIC and PURE methods are dependent on coil compatibility.

Segmentation

- Segmentation is the process by which regions of interest in an image, typically anatomic structures, are separated from the rest of the image.

- Accurate segmentation requires correct identification of structural boundaries in each slice of the acquired image volume. In its most simple form, delineating structural boundaries is done manually, by tracing or drawing a line on the structure boundary, to separate it from the rest of the image data. This is tedious and exacting work that must be performed repeatedly for each image slice in which the segmented structure is visible.

- Software tools can assist with the segmentation process by "finding" structure boundaries based on signal contrast at the structure's border or by automatically adding adjacent voxels to a structure based on the signal similarity of the voxels.

- Advanced segmentation methods can segment structures based on factors including the three-dimensional morphology of the structure, the signal properties of voxels contained within, and the relationship of the structure with other anatomic features. This information can be captured in anatomic atlases, which can be used by mathematically driven processes to provide time savings and precision to the segmentation process via automation.

- Once segmented, anatomic structures can be reconstructed as three-dimensional shapes or surfaces, enabling precise quantification of morphology, or constraint of signal data sampling (e.g., anatomic masks for T2 relaxation time assessment).

FIGURE 1.10 Segmentation example. Raw and segmented knee image slice, with corresponding 3D surface reconstructions of femoral and tibial cartilage, colorized by cartilage thickness at each location (0 to 4mm). (Courtesy of Jose Tamez-Peña, Qmetrics Technologies.)

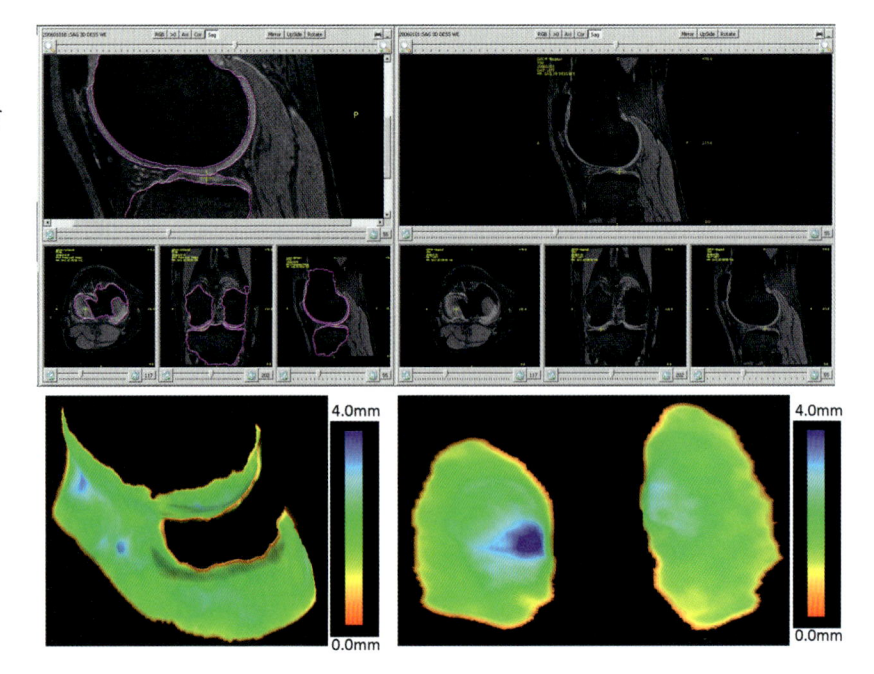

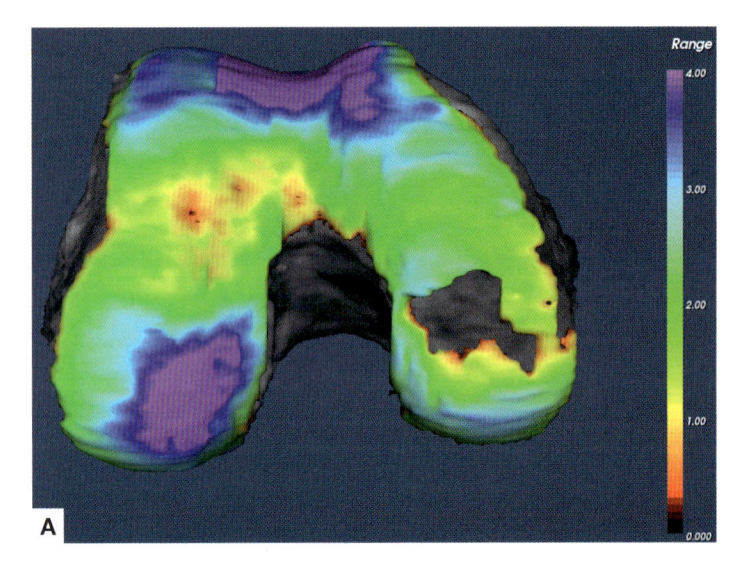

FIGURE 1.11 Full thickness chondral defect. (**A**) 3D reconstruction of a subject with a full thickness defect in the femoral condyle. The defect is irregular, and typical 2D assessment would be limited to in-plane (anterior-posterior) measurement and number of slices (medial-lateral); this defect has a significant oblique dimension that would be difficult to quantify. (**B**) Raw and segmented MRI corresponding to the 3D reconstruction of a subject with a defect in the femoral condyle. (Courtesy of Jose Tamez-Peña, Qmetrics Technologies.)

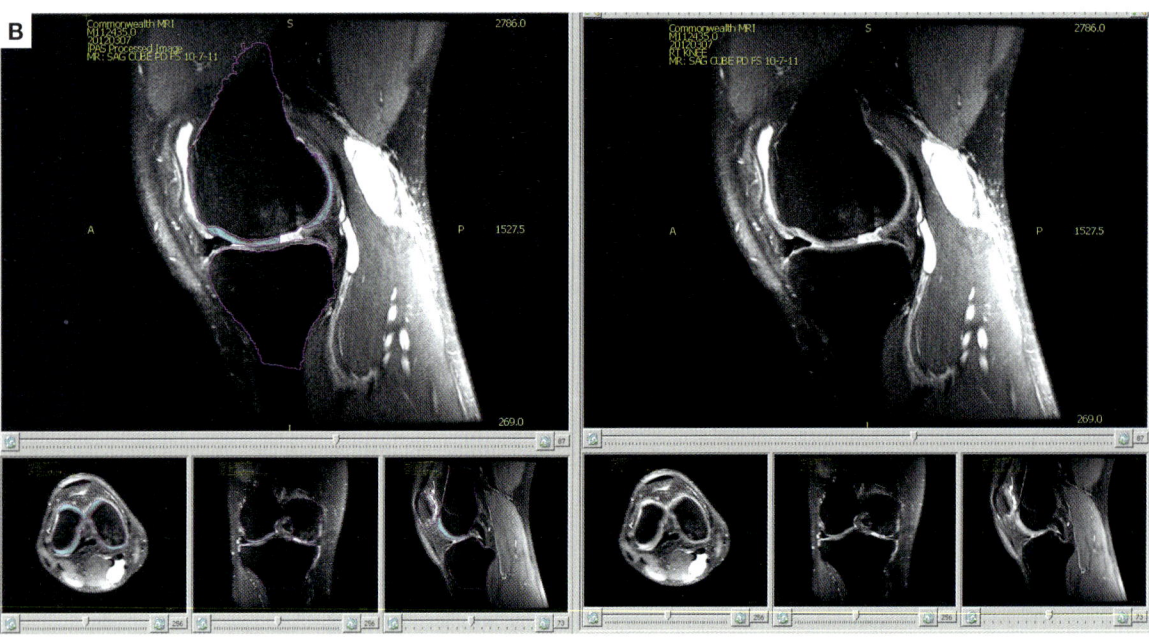

Sequence and Parameter Acronyms

The technical information provided in this chapter uses GE Healthcare sequence and parameter nomenclature as reference. The tables below provide the list of acronyms from Siemens and Philips.

Pulse Sequences		
GE	Siemens	Philips
FSE (Fast Spin Echo)	TSE (Turbo Spin Echo)	TSE (Turbo Spin Echo)
GRE	GRE	FFE
STIR	STIR	STIR
CUBE	SPACE	VISTA
PROPELLER	Blade	MultiVane
IDEAL	DIXON	mDIXON
MAVRIC SL	syngoWARP	SEMAC
MERGE	MEDIC	MFFE

Parameters		
GE	Siemens	Philips
Bandwidth (BW [kHz]; $BW_{GE} = BW_{SIE}/2 \times Nb\_points$)	Bandwidth BW ([Hz/pixel]; $BW_{SIE} = 2 \times BW_{GE}/Nb\_points$)	WFS/BW Hz; Water Fat Shift (WFS) & (Hz/Pixel)
FR (Fast Recovery)	RST (Restore)	DV (Driven Equilibrium)
ETL (Echo Train Length)	TF (Turbo Factor)	ES (Echo Spacing)
ARC/ASSET	GRAPPA/mSENSE	SENSE
SCIC/PURE	Normalize/Prescan Normalize	CLEAR (Constant Level Appearance)
NPW (no phase wrap)	Phase Oversampling	FO (Fold Over Suppression)
NEX	Average	NSA
FOV cm	FOV mm	FOV mm
ASPIR	SPAIR	SPAIR

2
Knee Anatomy

MR Normal Anatomy (pages 31-62)

Knee and Related Muscles (pages 63-94)

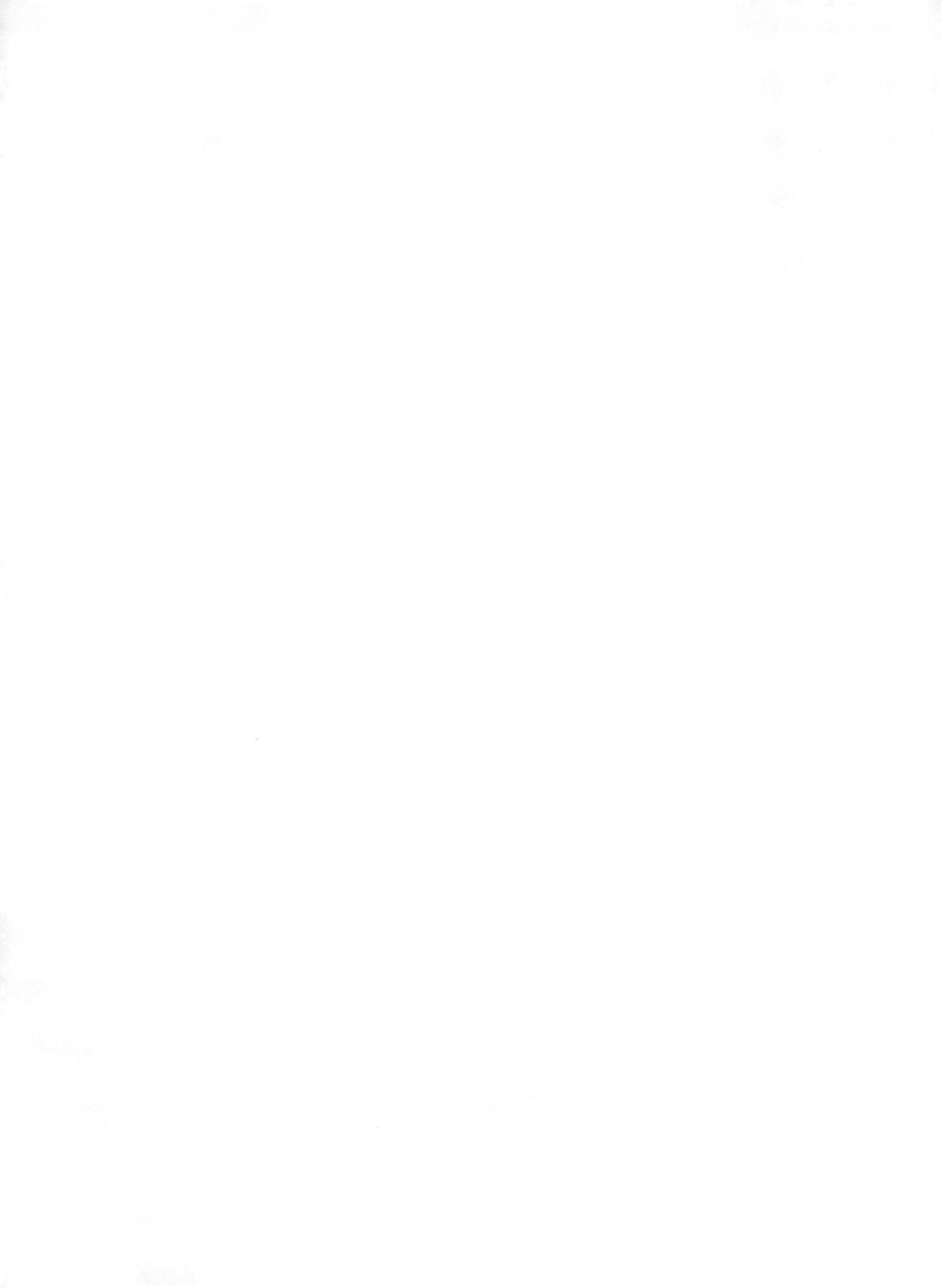

The Knee
MR Normal Anatomy

Axial
Figures 2.1A to 2.1L

Sagittal
Figures 2.2A to 2.2N

Coronal
Figures 2.3A to 2.3L

Knee MR Normal Anatomy

Axial Images

- Used as localizers to determine sagittal and coronal coverage

- Used to confirm circumferential meniscal tear patterns by directly displaying the entire surface and free edge of the meniscus on one or two axial image locations

- The medial and lateral patellar facets and the articular cartilage are demonstrated on axial images through the patellofemoral joint.

- Patellofemoral disease (i.e., chondromalacia) may be over- or underestimated on sagittal images alone.

- Routine axial images at 4 or 5mm are too thick to be sensitive to meniscal pathology.

- Sagittal images provide the best demonstration of internal meniscal anatomy and pathology because they section the meniscus perpendicular to its surface.

- Axial joint dissection displays the osseous relations among the patella, femur, and tibia.

- The following anatomic features contribute to the superolateral movement of the patella in full knee extension:
    - The medial femoral condyle is longer than the lateral condyle and is oriented toward the lateral aspect of the knee as it extends from the posterior to anterior.[225]
        - The medial tibial articular facet has a greater anterior-to-posterior dimension than the lateral tibial articular facet.
        - Both tibial plateau articular facets have a mild concavity in the coronal plane.
        - The lateral facet displays a convexity in the sagittal plane.

- The osseous contribution to the screw-home mechanism causes the tibia to undergo external rotation during the last degrees of full extension as it rolls anteriorly.
    - The trochlear groove or surface is continuous inferiorly and posteriorly with the intercondylar notch.
- The two patellar facets are divided by a median ridge.
    - The lateral facet is usually larger than the medial facet.
    - The supratrochlear tubercle represents the nonarticular area of the anterior distal femur, in which the patella rests in full extension.
- Outerbridge's ridge describes the sharp or distinct drop-off between the distal femur articular cartilage and the supratrochlear tubercle.

- The circumferential surface anatomy of the menisci and attachments of the cruciate and collateral ligaments:
    - Shown by disarticulation of the femur from the tibia
    - Directly visualized on corresponding axial plane images
    - The anterior and posterior horns of the lateral meniscus are attached to the nonarticular area of the tibial plateau, contributing to its relatively circular appearance.[225]
    - The anterior and posterior horns of the C-shaped medial meniscus are attached forward on the anterior aspect of the proximal tibia and on the posterior tibia above the posterior cruciate attachment, respectively.
    - The transverse ligament is a fibrous band that connects the anterior horns of the medial and lateral menisci.
    - The ligament of Wrisberg and the ligament of Humphrey (the posterior and anterior meniscofemoral ligaments, respectively) are variably present and pass from the posterior horn of the lateral meniscus to the medial aspect of the intercondylar notch.
        - The ligament of Wrisberg passes posterior to the posterior

cruciate ligament (PCL), and the ligament of Humphrey passes anterior to the PCL.

- The tibial plateau is visualized on inferior axial images.
    - The posterior cruciate insertion is displayed on the posterior tibial surface and demonstrates low signal intensity on cross-section.
- The popliteus muscle is visualized posterior to the tibia at the level of the superior tibiofibular joint.
- The medial and lateral menisci are seen with uniform low signal intensity at the midjoint level.
    - The medial meniscus has an open C-shaped configuration with a narrow anterior horn and wider posterior horn.
    - The lateral meniscus has a more circular shape and consistent width. Sections that are 3mm or less in thickness display both menisci on axial images.
- The transverse ligament is a band of low signal intensity connecting the anterior horn of the lateral and medial menisci.
    - The ligament can be identified where it transverses Hoffa's infrapatellar fat pad.
- The semimembranosus and semitendinosus tendons:
    - Circular structures of low signal intensity located lateral to the medial head of the gastrocnemius muscle and posterior to the medial tibial plateau
    - The semimembranosus tendon appears larger than the semitendinosus tendon.
- The elliptical sartorius muscle and the circular gracilis tendon are located more medial and posterior than the semimembranosus and semitendinosus tendons, and are in line with the medial collateral ligament (MCL).
- Proximal to its insertion on the fibular head, the biceps femoris tendon is positioned anterolateral to the lateral head of the gastrocnemius muscle.

- ■ The popliteal artery is found anterior to the popliteal vein, anterior to and between the two heads of the gastrocnemius muscle.
    - ■ Potentially at risk for injury during meniscal repair because it is located posterior to the posterior horn of the lateral meniscus
- ■ In cross-section, the low-signal-intensity lateral collateral ligament (LCL), or fibular collateral ligament, may be surrounded by high-signal-intensity fat.
    - ■ The anterior cruciate ligament (ACL) and PCL insertions are within the intercondylar notch.
        - The ACL can be identified superior to the joint line, 15 to 20 degrees off axis, in an anteromedial orientation.[280]
        - The origin of the ACL is on the medial aspect of the lateral femoral condyle.
        - The PCL is circular in cross-section.
        - The origin of the PCL is on the lateral aspect of the medial femoral condyle.
- ■ Hoffa's infrapatellar fat pad is bordered by the low-signal-intensity iliotibial band (ITB) laterally, the medial retinaculum medially, and the thick patellar tendon anteriorly.
- ■ The peroneal nerve is located lateral to the plantaris muscle, demonstrates low to intermediate signal intensity, and is encased in fat.
- ■ At the level of the femoral condyles, the tibial nerve is located posterior to the popliteal vein and demonstrates intermediate signal intensity.
- ■ The large lateral patellar facet and the oblique medial patellar facet are also seen in the axial plane.
- ■ The thick articular cartilage surfaces of the patella show intermediate signal intensity on T1- and T2-weighted images.
- ■ The medial and lateral patellar retinacular attachments are seen at the level of the patellofemoral joint and are of low signal intensity.
- ■ Medial and lateral reflections of the suprapatellar bursa should not be mistaken for retinacular attachments or plicae.

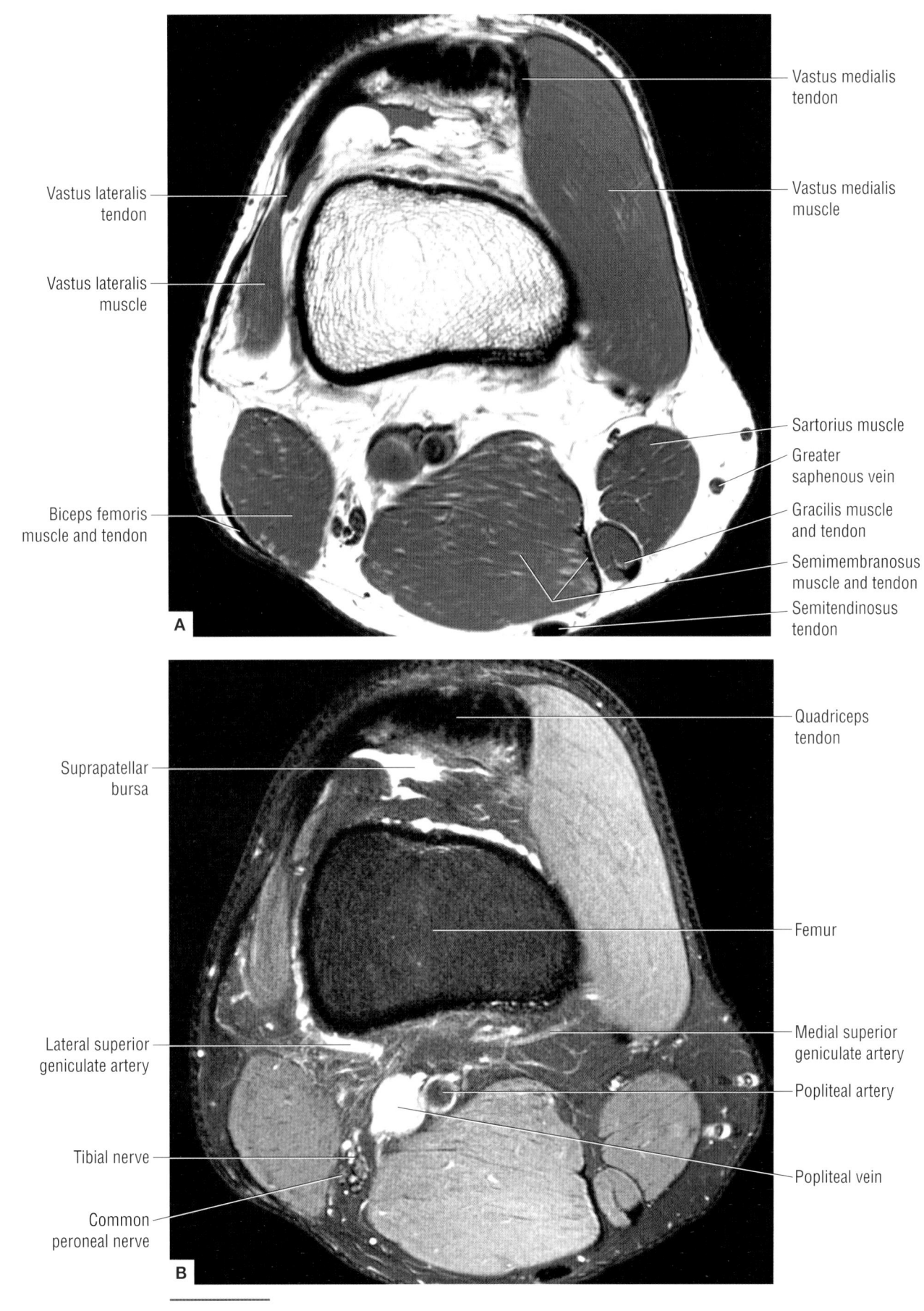

FIGURE 2.1 A, B

Knee Anatomy

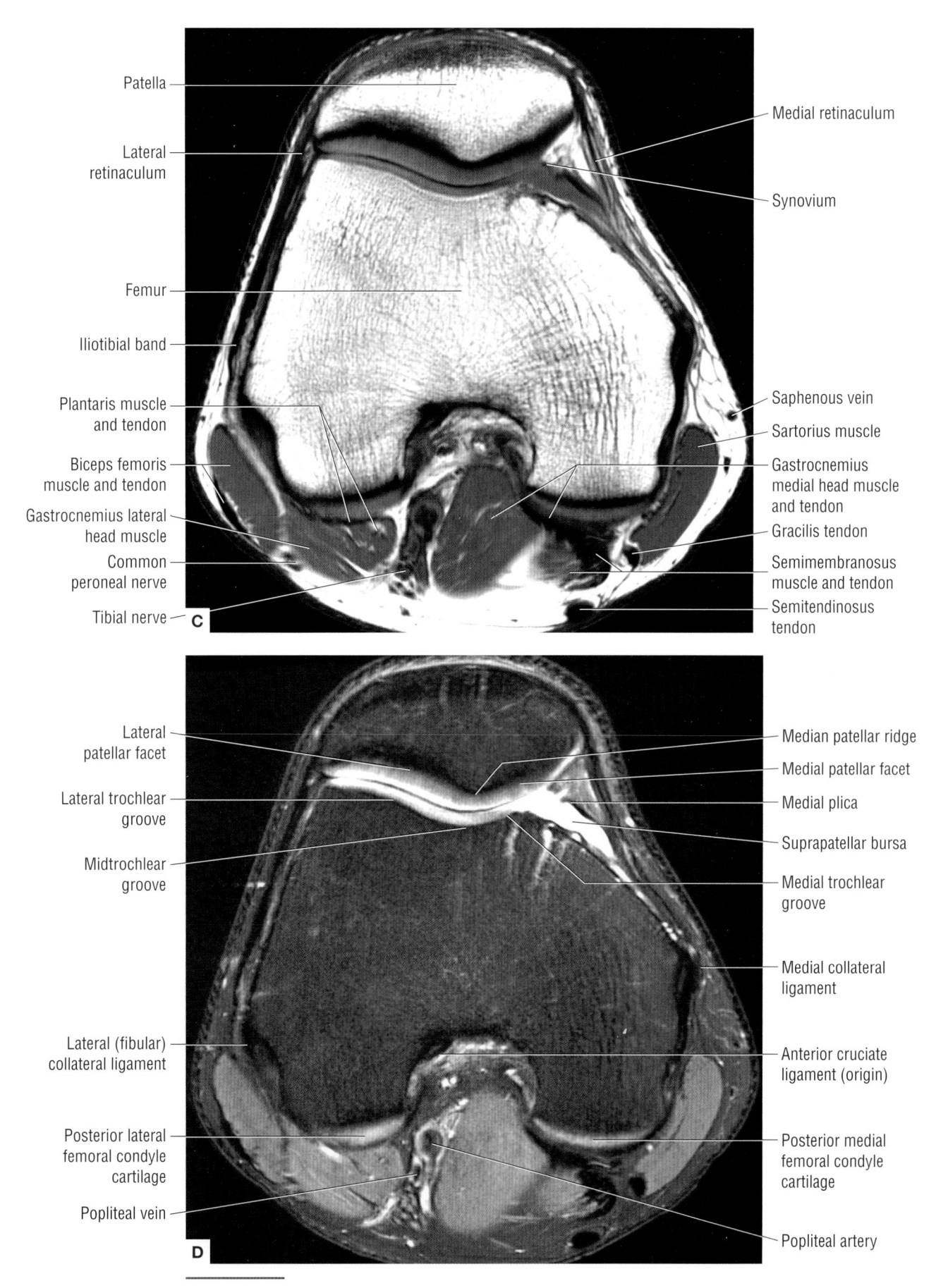

FIGURE 2.1 C, D

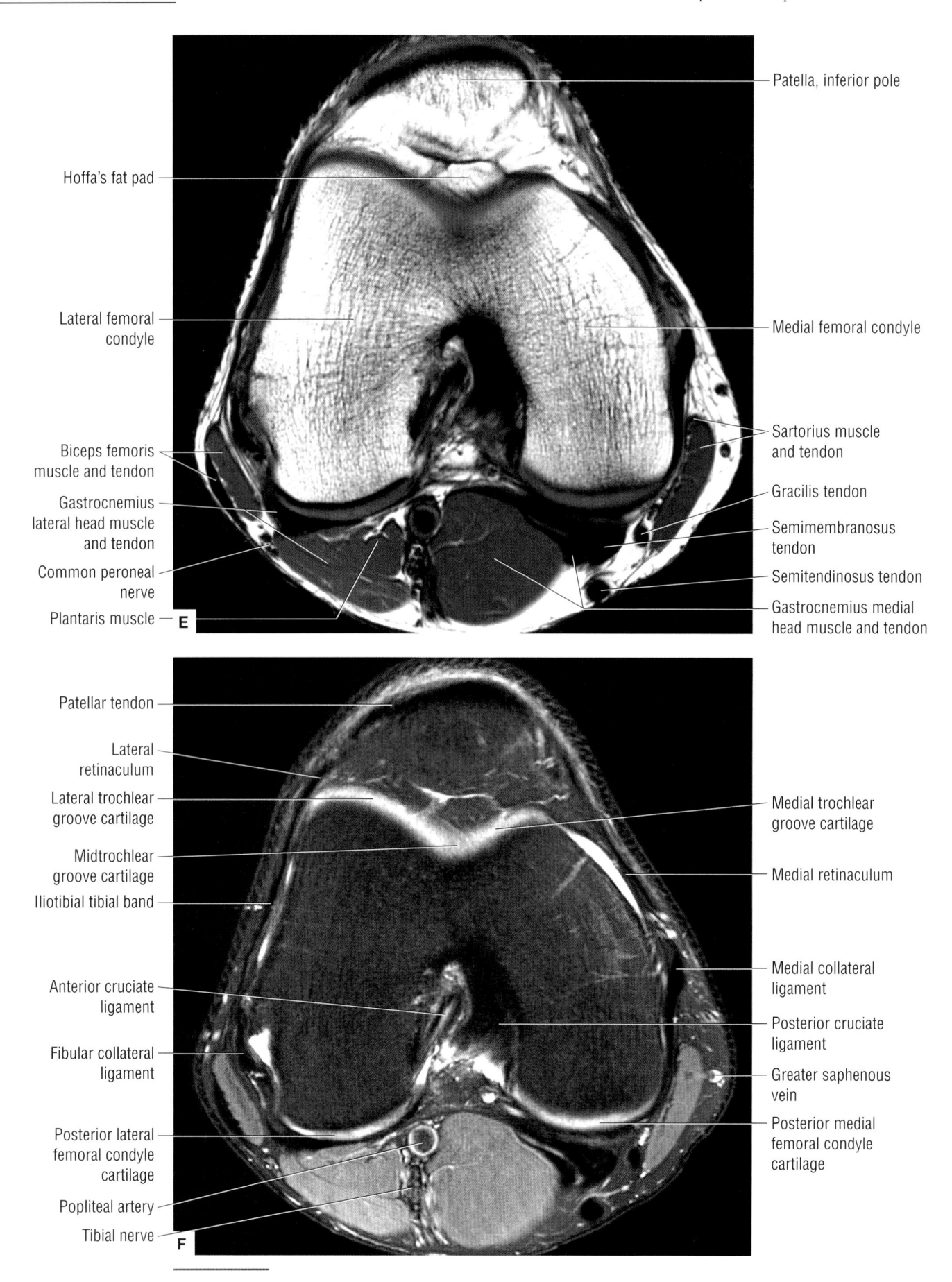

FIGURE 2.1 E, F

Knee Anatomy

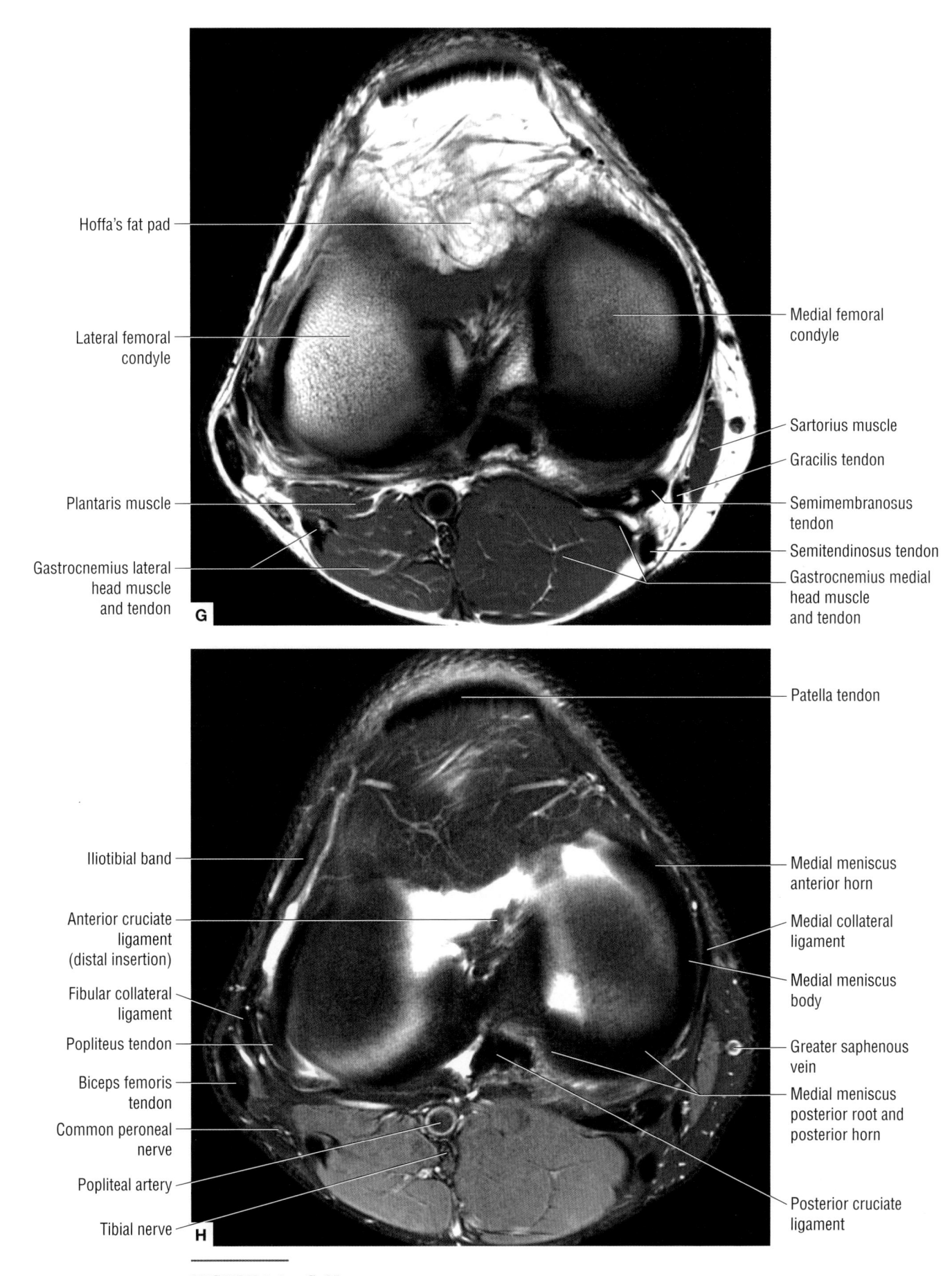

FIGURE 2.1 G, H

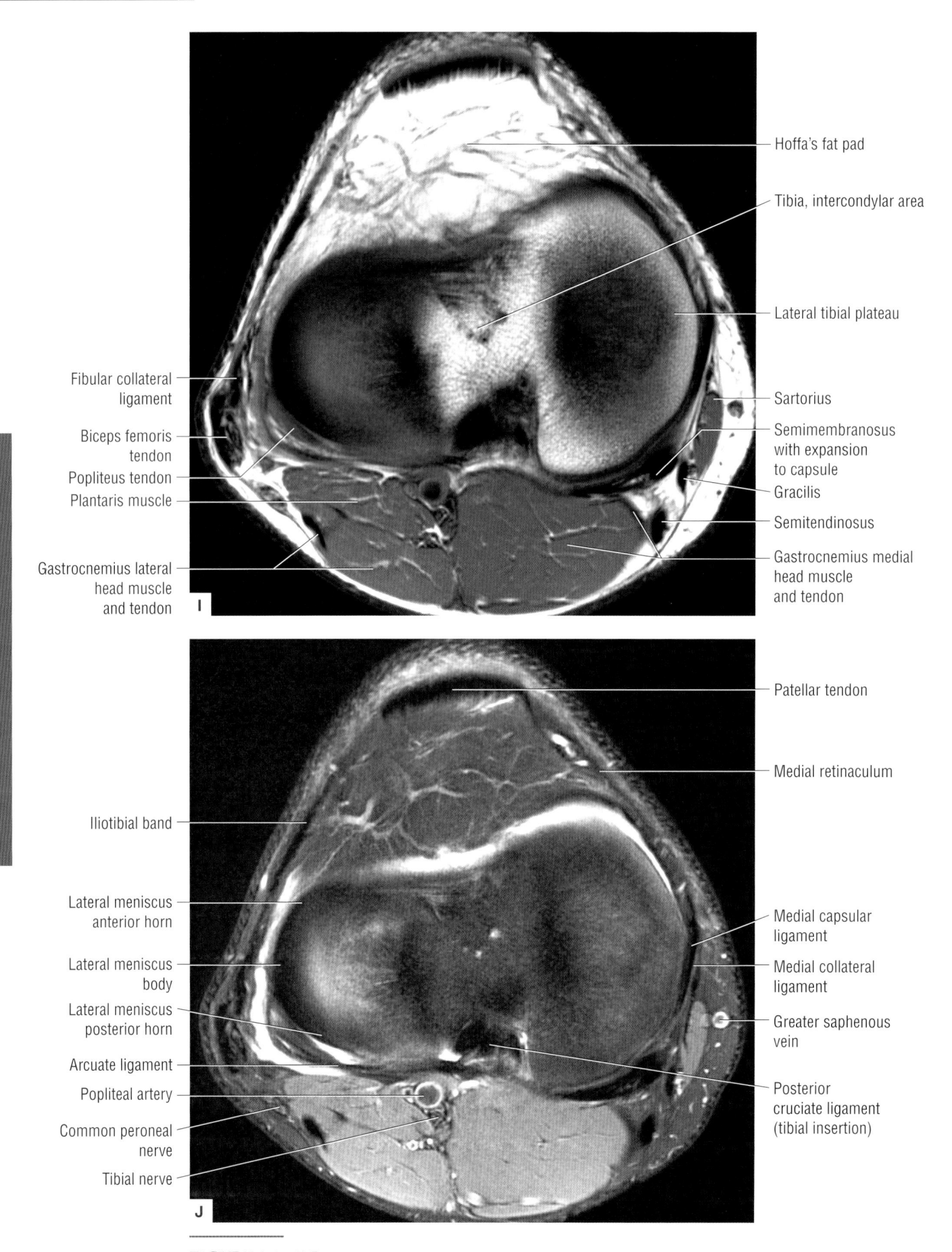

FIGURE 2.1 I, J

Knee Anatomy

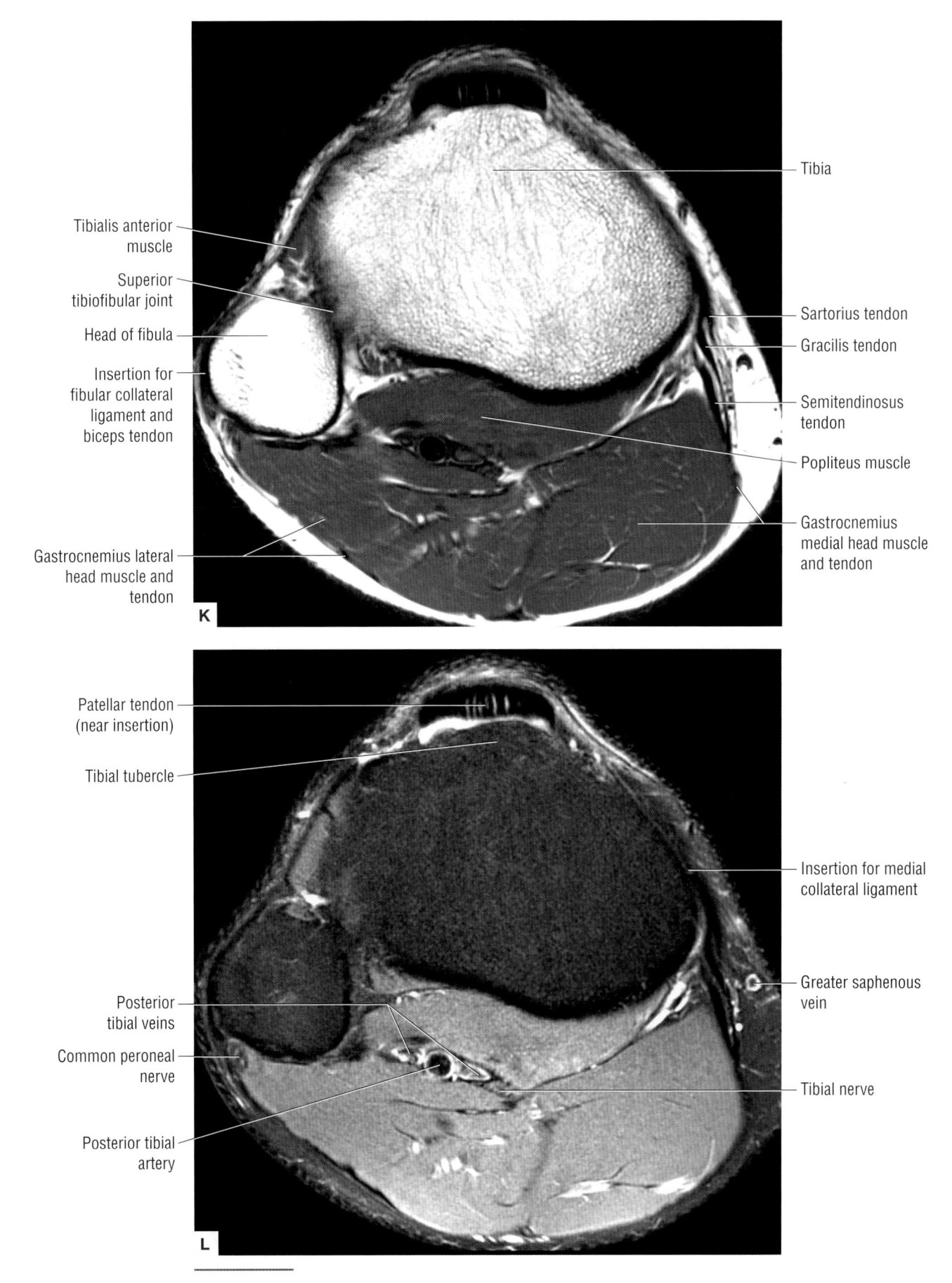

FIGURE 2.1 K, L

Sagittal Images

- Sagittal plane dissection displays the components of the MCL and LCL and the adjacent capsule:
    - The patellofemoral compartment, quadriceps, and patellar tendon are demonstrated on midsagittal dissections.
        - The suprapatellar bursa (pouch) extends 5 to 7cm proximal to the superior pole of the patella.[225]
        - Superficial medial dissection displays the conjoined pes anserinus tendons (semitendinosus, gracilis, and sartorius) as they course along the posteromedial aspect of the knee.
        - The pes anserinus runs superficial to the distal MCL and inserts into the anteromedial tibial crest distal to the joint line.
        - On the lateral aspect of the knee, the LCL and the more posteriorly located fabellofibular ligament (structures of the posterolateral corner of the knee) can be seen.
        - The fabellofibular and arcuate ligaments have insertions on the posterior aspect of the fibular styloid, posterior and deep to the LCL.
        - These ligaments course superficially and posteriorly, blending with the origin of the lateral head of the gastrocnemius and the oblique popliteal ligament.
        - The arcuate ligament extends toward the popliteus capsular hiatus.
    - The ACL and PCL are best displayed on sagittal images.
        - The LCL, or fibular collateral ligament, and the biceps femoris tendon also may be seen on peripheral sagittal sections.
        - Images in the sagittal plane are key in evaluating anatomy for meniscal degenerations and tears.
        - The MCL is partially defined in the sagittal plane on peripheral

medial sagittal images.

- Complex meniscal and bucket-handle tears may require coronal images to identify displaced meniscal tissue or fragments.

■ On medial sagittal images, the low-signal-intensity semimembranosus tendon and intermediate-signal-intensity muscle are seen posteriorly.

- The vastus medialis muscle makes up the bulk of the musculature anterior to the medial femoral condyle.
- On T1-weighted images, fatty (i.e., yellow) marrow demonstrates bright signal intensity, whereas adjacent cortical bone demonstrates uniform low signal intensity.
- Femoral and tibial hyaline articular cartilage demonstrates intermediate signal intensity on T1- and conventional T2-weighted images, bright signal intensity on T2*-weighted images, and low to intermediate signal intensity on FS PD FSE images. The anterolateral femoral articular cartilage, which is particularly thick, is frequently the site of early erosions or attenuation in osteoarthritis (trochlear groove chondromalacia).
- The tibial cortex appears thicker than the femoral cortical bone because of a chemical-shift artifact.

■ The medial meniscus:
- Composed of fibrocartilage
- Demonstrates uniform low signal intensity
- The body of the medial meniscus has a continuous bowtie shape on at least one or two consecutive sagittal images taken in 4- to 5-mm sections.
- In medial compartment images approaching the intercondylar notch, the separate anterior and posterior horns of the medial meniscus can be seen.
- The meniscal horns appear as opposing triangles on a minimum of two or three consecutive sagittal images.

- The posterior horn root attachment of both menisci should always be identified adjacent to the intercondylar notch.

- The posterior horn of the medial meniscus is larger than the opposing anterior horn. The medial head of the gastrocnemius muscle sweeps posteriorly from its origin along the distal femur.

- A small band of high-signal-intensity fat (the bursa) is seen between the posterior horn of the medial meniscus and the posterior capsule.

■ When sagittal images are viewed in the medial to lateral direction, the PCL is seen before the ACL.

- The thick, uniform, low-signal-intensity PCL arcs from its anterolateral origin on the medial femoral condyle to its insertion on the posterior inferior tibial surface.

- With partial knee flexion, the convex curve of the PCL becomes taut as the anterolateral band or bundle of the PCL is lax in extension.

- The anterior and posterior meniscofemoral ligaments (the ligaments of Humphrey and Wrisberg, respectively) are seen individually or together on either side of the PCL.

■ In the lateral portion of the intercondylar notch, the ACL extends obliquely from its semicircular origin on the posteromedial aspect of the lateral femoral condyle to its insertion.

- Its insertion starts 15mm from the anterior border of the tibial articular surface (between the tibial spines).

- On average, it is 30mm in length through the anterior intercondylar area.[30,162]

■ The ACL is composed of two functional bands of fibers (the anteromedial and posterolateral bundles).

- The anteromedial and posterolateral bundles of the ACL cannot be differentiated on sagittal images.

- ACL fibers may display minimally higher signal intensity than those of the PCL, and this difference is seen independent of a partial-volume effect with the lateral femoral condyle.

- Normally, the ACL is seen on at least one sagittal image when the knee is properly positioned or when proper sagittal oblique images are prescribed.

- Fiber-bundle striations of the ACL are prominent at femoral and tibial attachments, especially when oblique sagittal images are performed to display attachment sites.

■ Portions of both cruciate ligaments may be observed on the same sagittal section.

- Excessive external rotation of the knee causes elongation of the anterior-to-posterior dimensions of the femoral condyles.

- Excessive internal rotation also prevents adequate visualization of the ACL unless sagittal oblique images are used to compensate for redirecting the ACL away from the orthogonal sagittal plane.

■ On midsagittal sections, the quadriceps and patellar tendons are seen at their anterior attachments to the superior and inferior patellar poles, respectively.

- Hoffa's infrapatellar fat pad is directly posterior to the patellar tendon and demonstrates bright signal intensity.

- The posterior patellar articular cartilage displays a smooth or a convex arc on sections through the medial and lateral patellar facets.

- In the absence of joint fluid, the collapsed patellar bursa is not seen proximal to the superior pole of the patella.

■ On intercondylar sagittal images, the popliteal vessels are seen in long axis.

- The artery is in an anterior position and the vein in a posterior position.

- On extreme sagittal sections, the conjoined insertion of the LCL and the biceps femoris tendon on the fibular head can be identified.
    - The lateral head of the gastrocnemius muscle is seen posterior to the fibula and follows an inferior course from the distal lateral femoral condyle behind the popliteus muscle.
    - The low-signal-intensity popliteus tendon and its intermediate-signal-intensity sheath are seen in their expected anatomic location, between the capsule and the periphery of the lateral meniscus.
    - Separate synovium-lined fascicles, or struts, of the menisci allow intraarticular passage of the popliteus tendon.
    - In its middle third (i.e., body), the C-shaped lateral meniscus also demonstrates a bowtie shape.
    - On more medial sections through the lateral compartment, the separate triangular shapes of the anterior and posterior horn, which are oriented toward each other and are nearly symmetric in size and shape, can be distinguished.
    - The popliteofibular ligament is identified in the sagittal plane posterior to the lateral tibial plateau and distal to the course of the popliteus tendon.
    - The medial limb of the arcuate ligament is posterior to the popliteus tendon usually seen in the same sagittal image location as the posterior horn of the lateral meniscus and the superior popliteomeniscal fascicle.
    - The normal deficiency of the inferior popliteomeniscal fascicle (to accommodate the passage of the popliteus tendon) occurs at the location medial to the body of the lateral meniscus.

Knee Anatomy

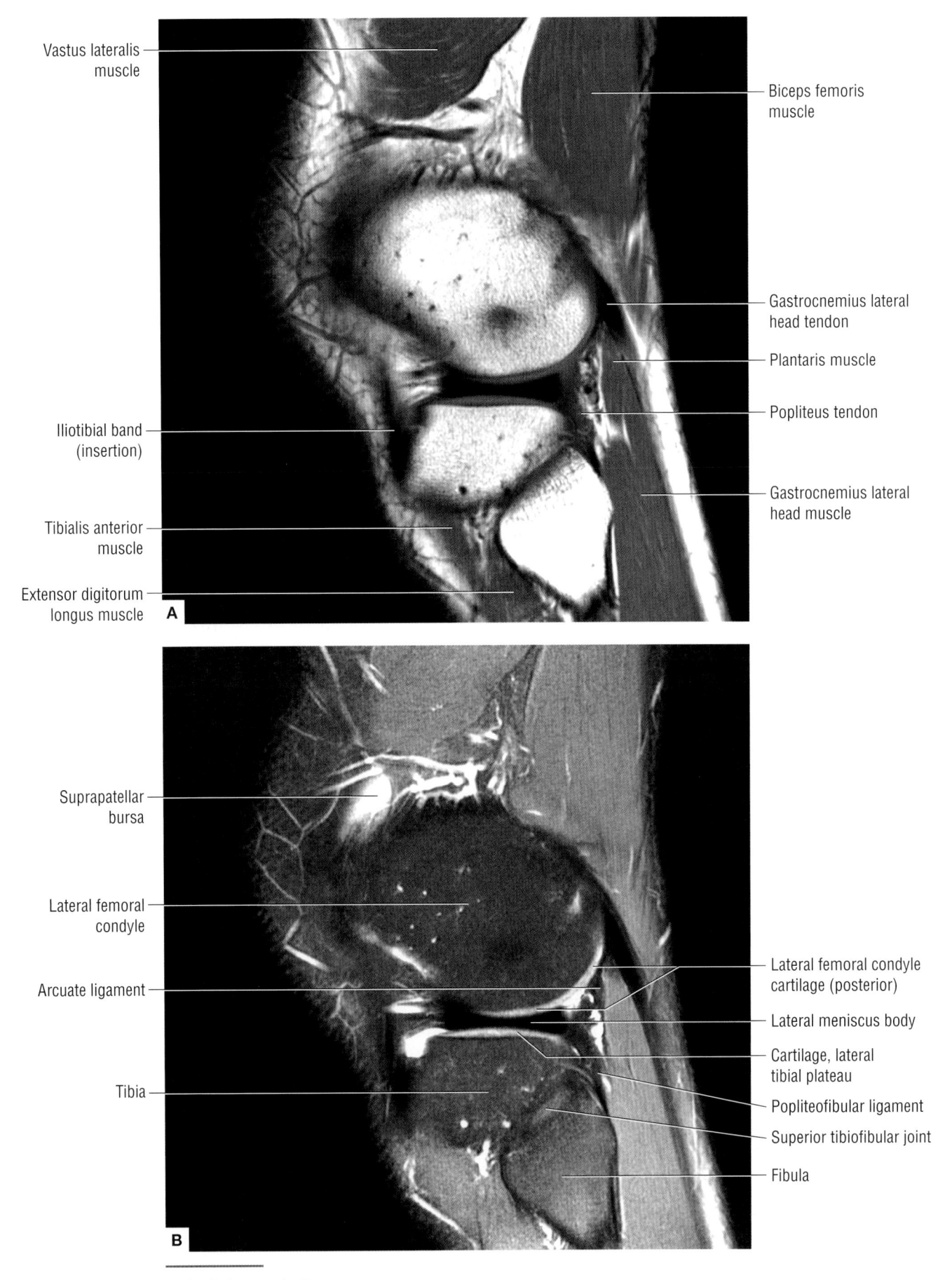

FIGURE 2.2 A, B

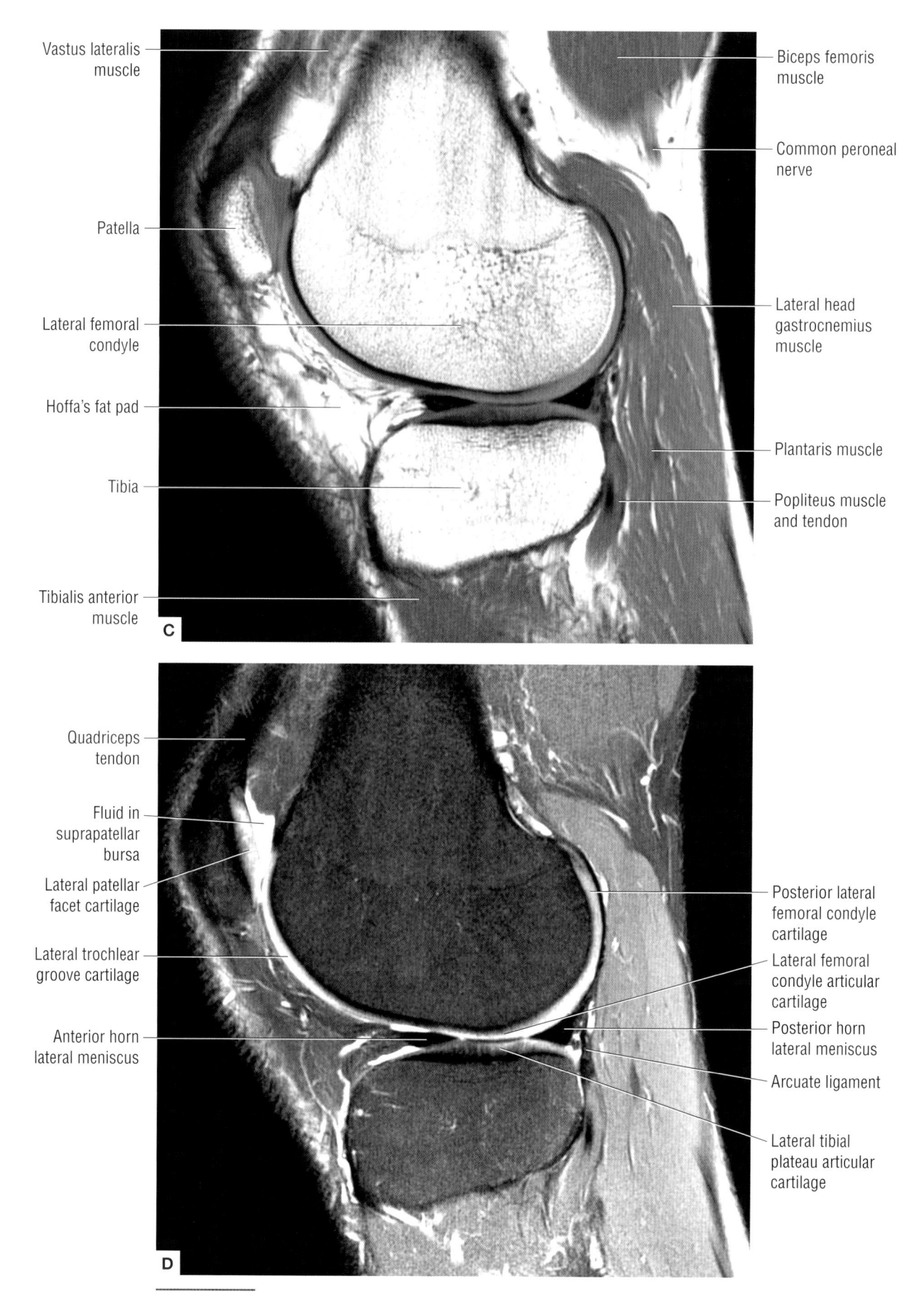

FIGURE 2.2 C, D

Knee Anatomy

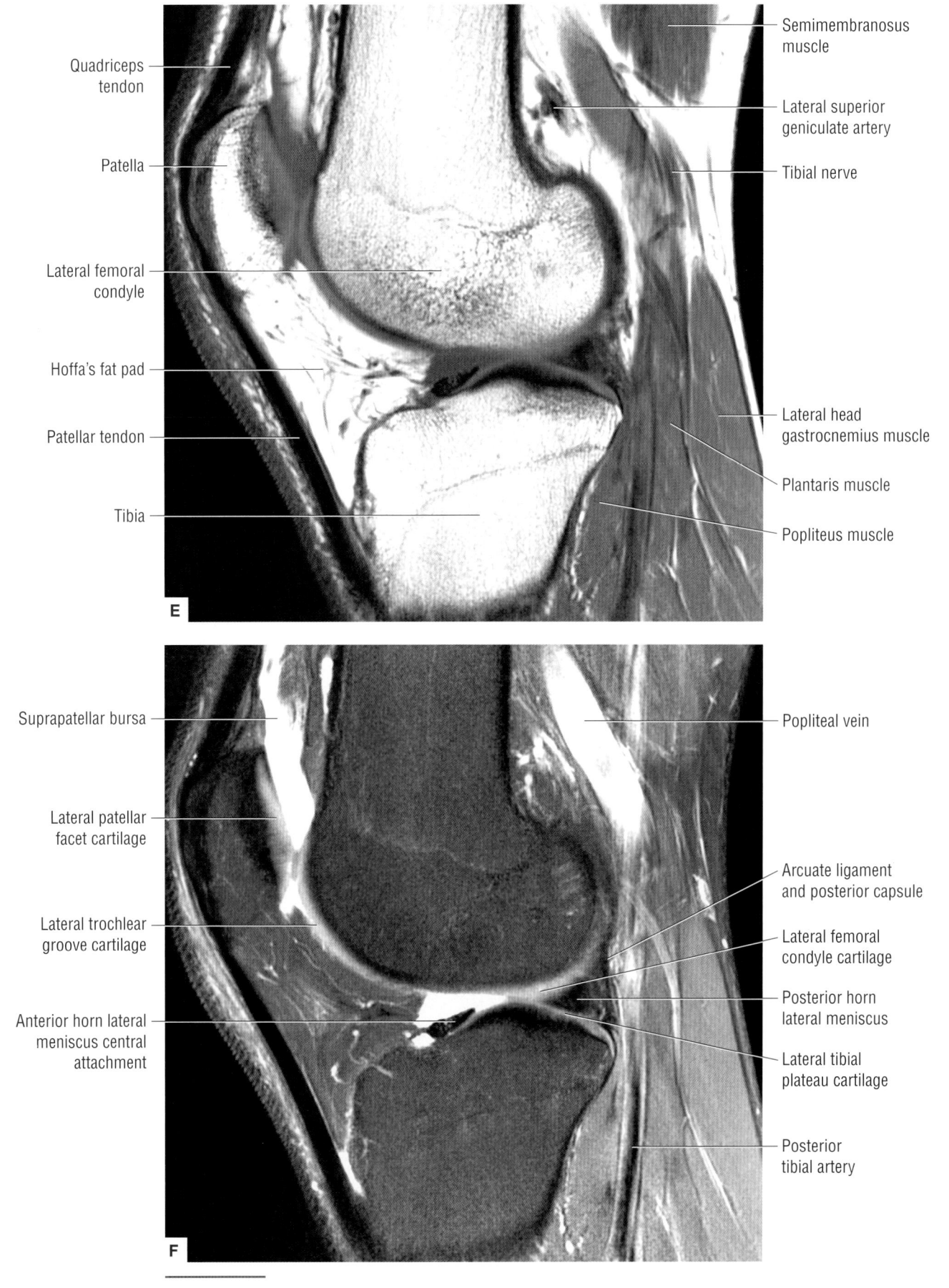

FIGURE 2.2 E, F

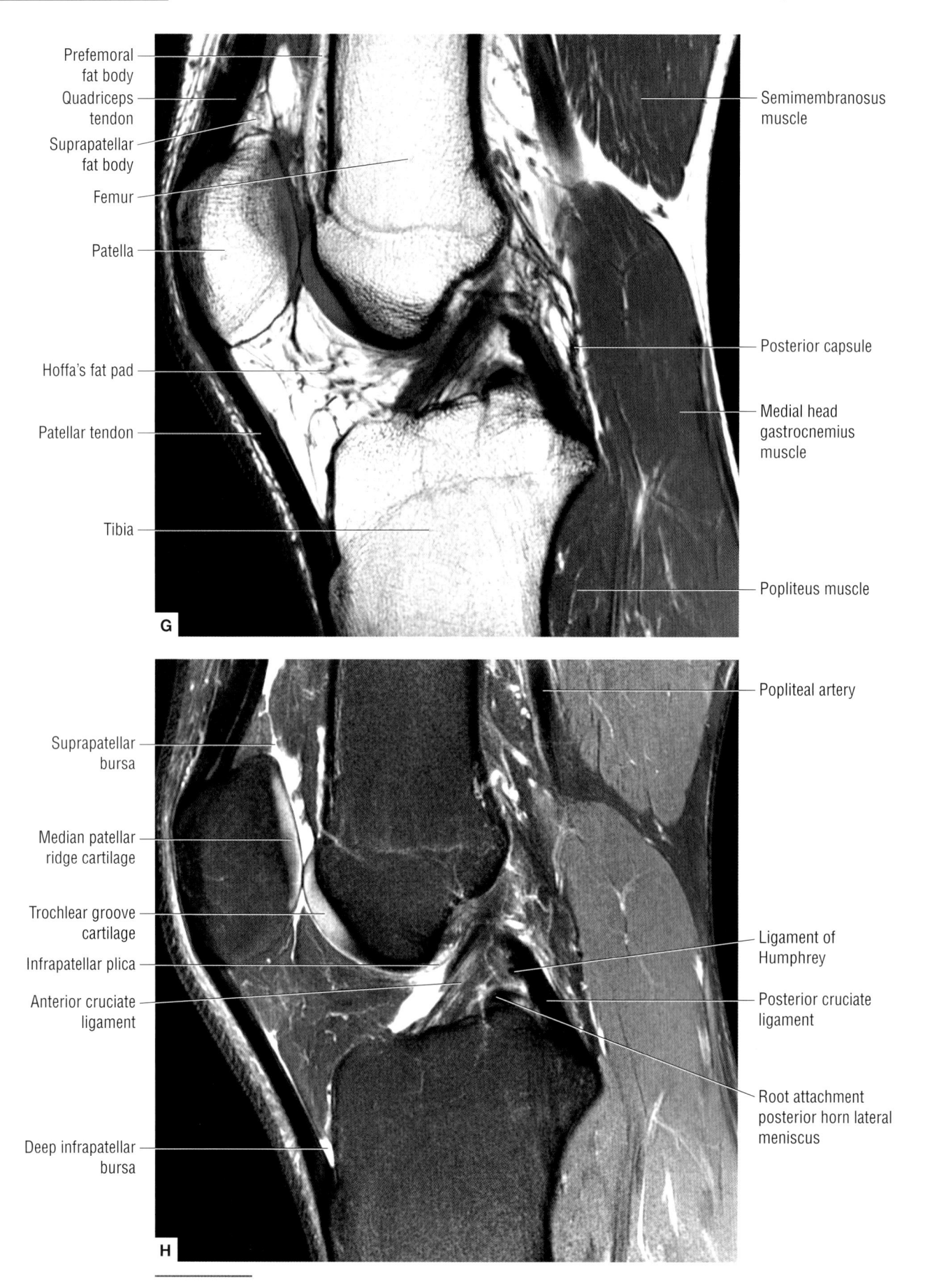

FIGURE 2.2 G, H

Knee Anatomy

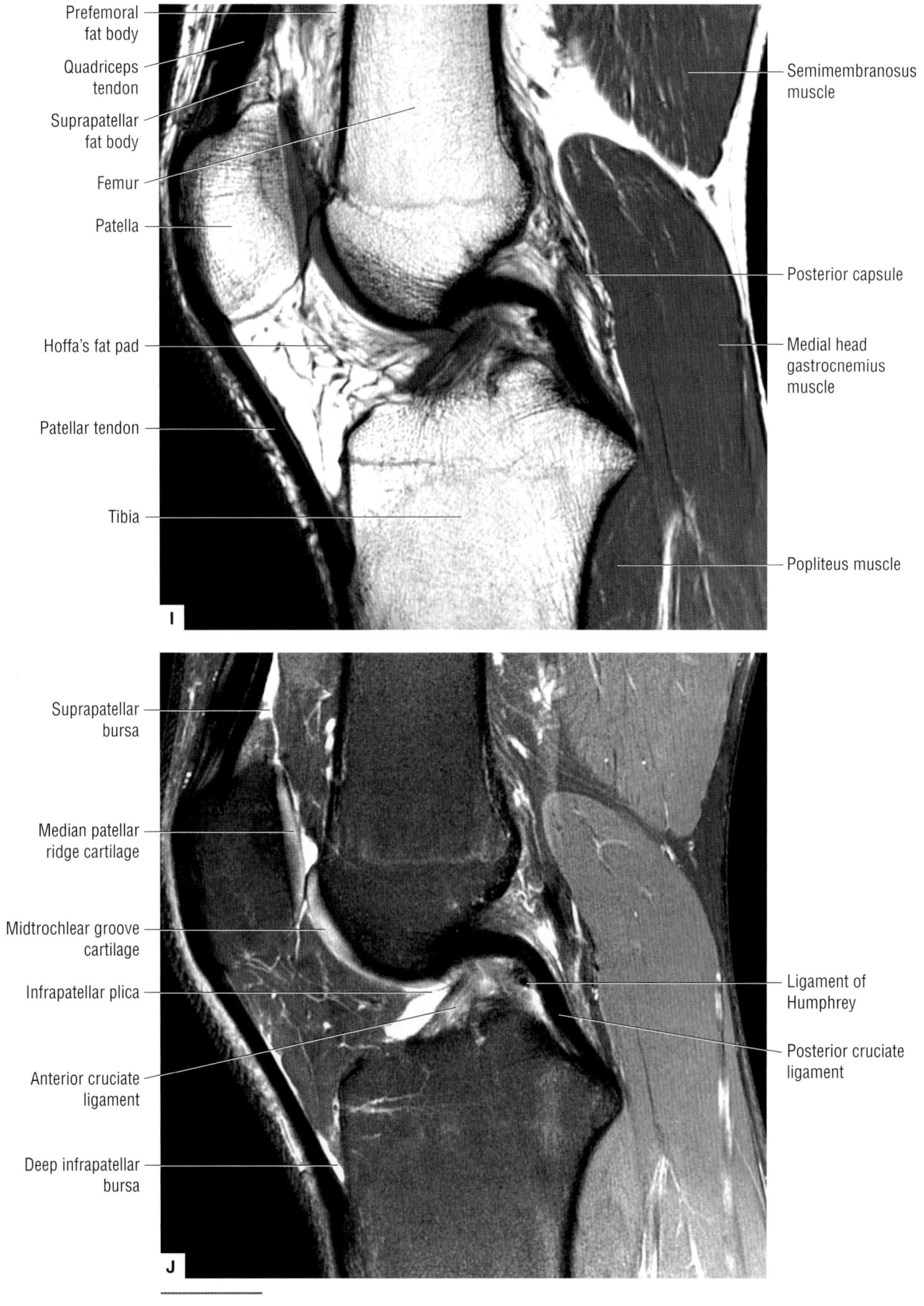

FIGURE 2.2 I, J

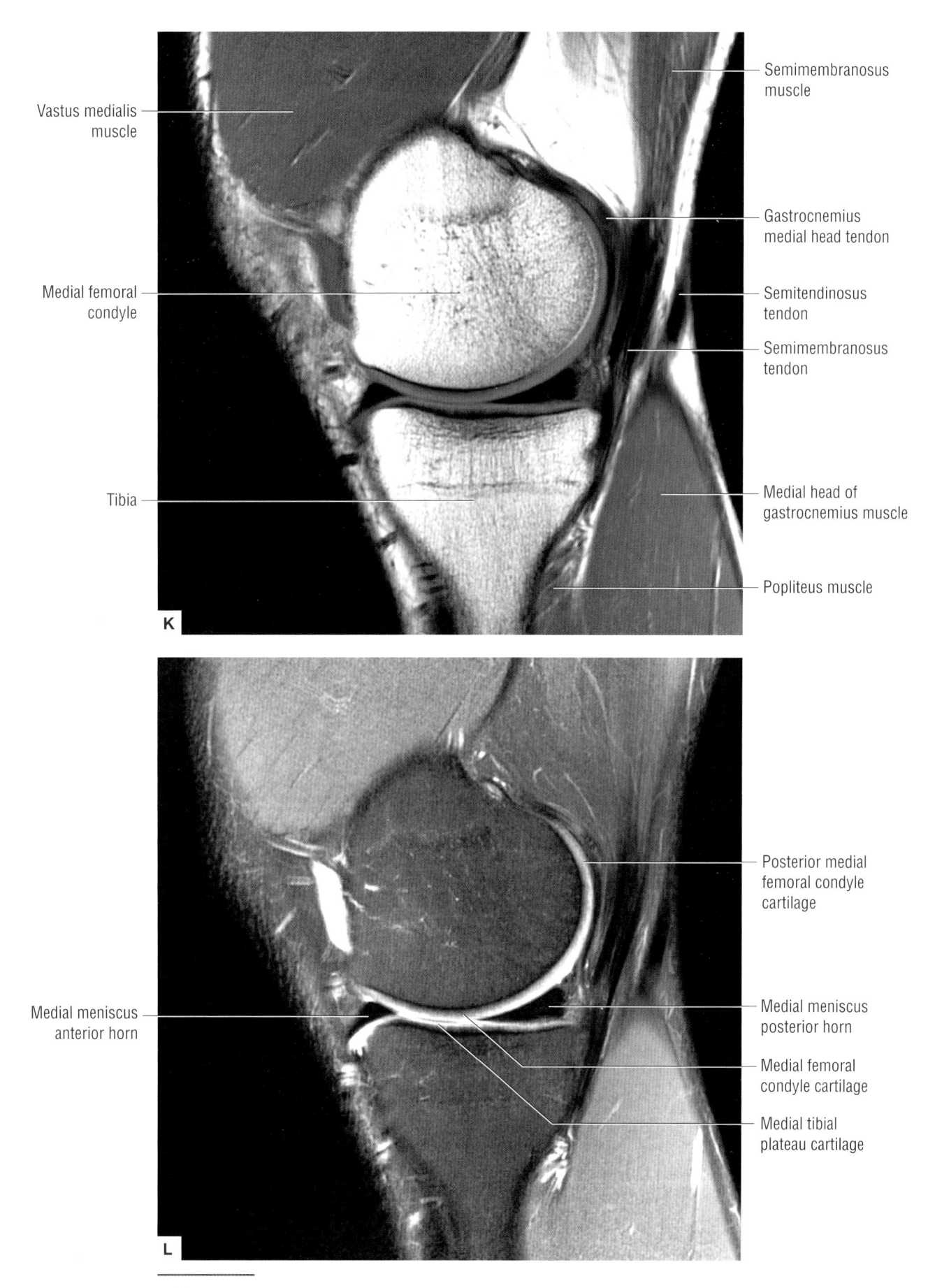

FIGURE 2.2 K, L

Knee Anatomy

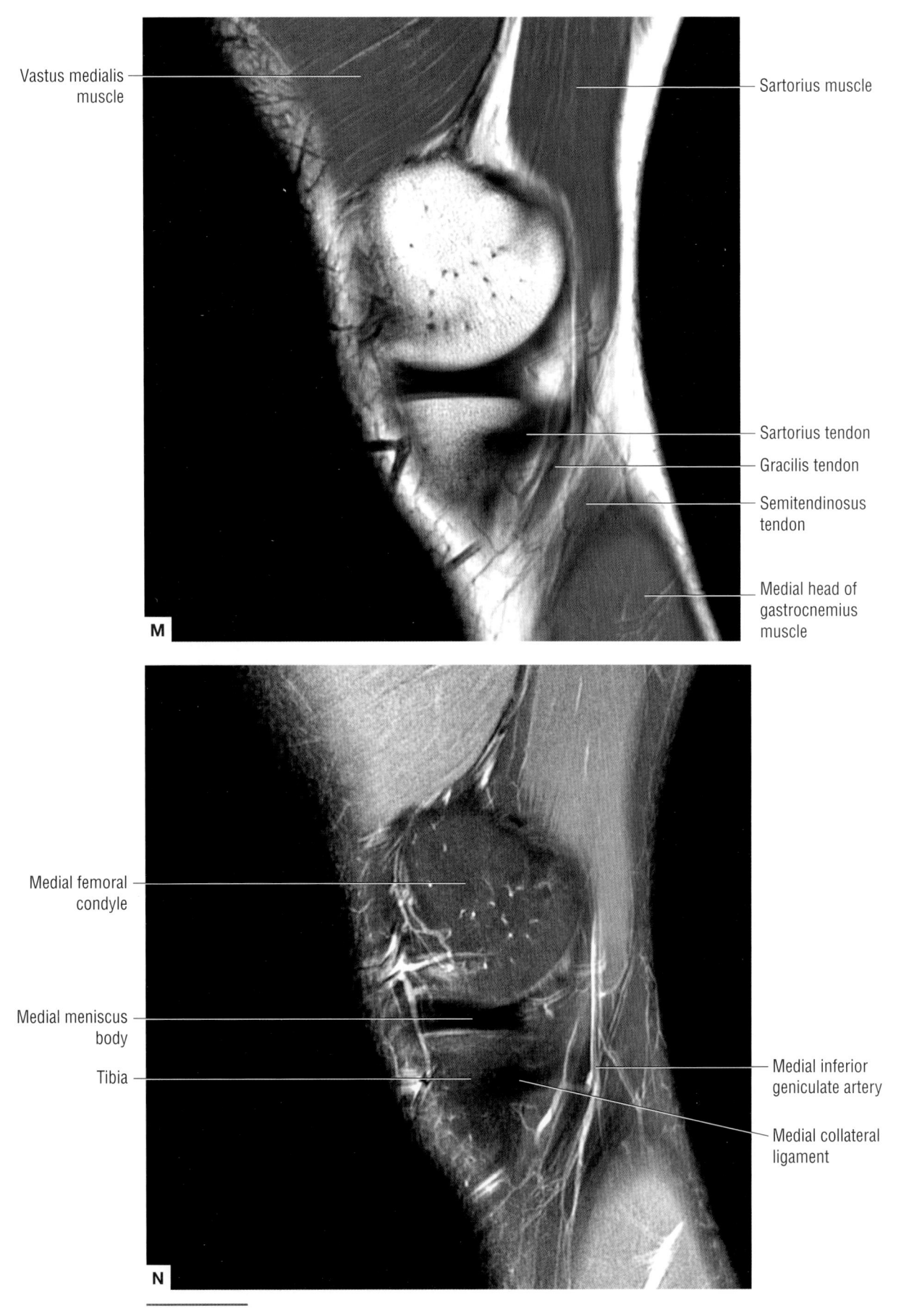

FIGURE 2.2 M, N

Coronal Images

- Posterior-to-anterior coronal anatomic dissection demonstrates the posterior capsule, the popliteus tendon, the cruciate ligaments and menisci, the collateral ligaments, and the extensor mechanism.

- Coronal images:
    - Used to identify collateral ligament anatomy
    - Display the posterior femoral condyles, which are common sites of articular erosions

- The oblique popliteal ligament and arcuate popliteal ligament define the posterior capsule.

- Low-signal-intensity popliteal vessels are also identified on posterior coronal images:
    - The LCL (fibular collateral ligament) is seen as a low-signal-intensity cord stretching from its insertion on the fibular head to the lateral epicondyle of the femur.
        - It is separated from the lateral meniscus by the thickness of the popliteus tendon.
    - At the level of the femoral condyles, the meniscofemoral ligaments (the ligaments of Wrisberg and Humphrey) may be observed as thin, low-signal-intensity bands extending from the posterior horn of the lateral meniscus to the lateral surface of the medial femoral condyle.
        - The ligament of Humphrey is variable in size.
        - Although one or the other of the branches of the meniscofemoral ligament may be identified on one third of knee studies, the coexistence of the two is seen in only 3% of examinations.[510]
    - The functional location of the anteromedial and posterolateral bundles of the ACL may be discerned on anterior and posterior coronal images, respectively.
        - The PCL is circular and of uniform low signal intensity on anterior and mid-coronal sections.

- On posterior coronal images, the triangular attachment of the PCL can be differentiated as it fans out from the lateral aspect of the medial femoral condyle.
- The MCL, or tibial collateral ligament, is identified on mid-coronal sections, anterior to sections in which the femoral condyles appear to fuse together with the distal metaphysis.
  - The MCL is seen as a band of low signal intensity extending from its femoral epicondylar attachment to the medial tibial condyle.
  - It consists of superficial and deep layers attached to the periphery of the medial meniscus.
  - The femoral and tibial attachments of the intact MCL are uniformly dark (low signal intensity) and are indistinguishable from underlying cortical bone.
  - From the plane of the posterior femoral condyle, the MCL can be seen on at least two or three coronal images if they are acquired with 4-mm sections and no interslice gap.
  - A line of intermediate signal intensity separating the medial meniscus from the deep layer of the MCL represents a small bursa.
- The body and the anterior and posterior horns of the medial and lateral menisci are seen as distinct segments and not as opposing triangles as on sagittal images.
  - On posterior coronal images, the plane of section is parallel with the posterior curve of the C-shaped menisci, and the posterior horn may be seen as a continuous band of low signal intensity.
  - The root attachments of both meniscal fibrocartilages are visualized in the same posterior coronal plane image as the PCL in its distal tibial insertion.
- Mid-coronal sections display the anterior tibial spine, whereas anterior images are marked by the high signal intensity of Hoffa's infrapatellar fat pad

- anterior to the lateral knee compartment.
- Anteriorly, the ITB blends with the lateral patellar retinaculum, and the vastus medialis is in continuity with its medial retinacular patellar attachment.
- The low-signal-intensity fibers of the quadriceps and patellar tendons can be identified on most anterior sections in the same plane as the patella.
- Coronal oblique images are obtained when evaluating tears of the quadriceps tendon.
    - The correct orientation of the quadriceps tendon plane is prescribed from sagittal images.
        - Reference the correct angle to optimize the coronal oblique plane to follow the course of the quadriceps tendon.
    - The normal quadriceps tendon has a trilaminar morphology.
        - Superficial
        - Intermediate
        - Deep layer fibers
    - The display of the quadriceps on coronal oblique images improves the conspicuity of the tear propagation from medial or lateral.
    - Improved visualization of anterior rectus femoris, intermediate layer vastus medialis/lateralis muscle and tendon contributions, and deep layer vastus intermedius fibers
    - A dedicated quadriceps evaluation requires additional images and coil repositioning to follow the course of more proximal pathology.

Knee Anatomy

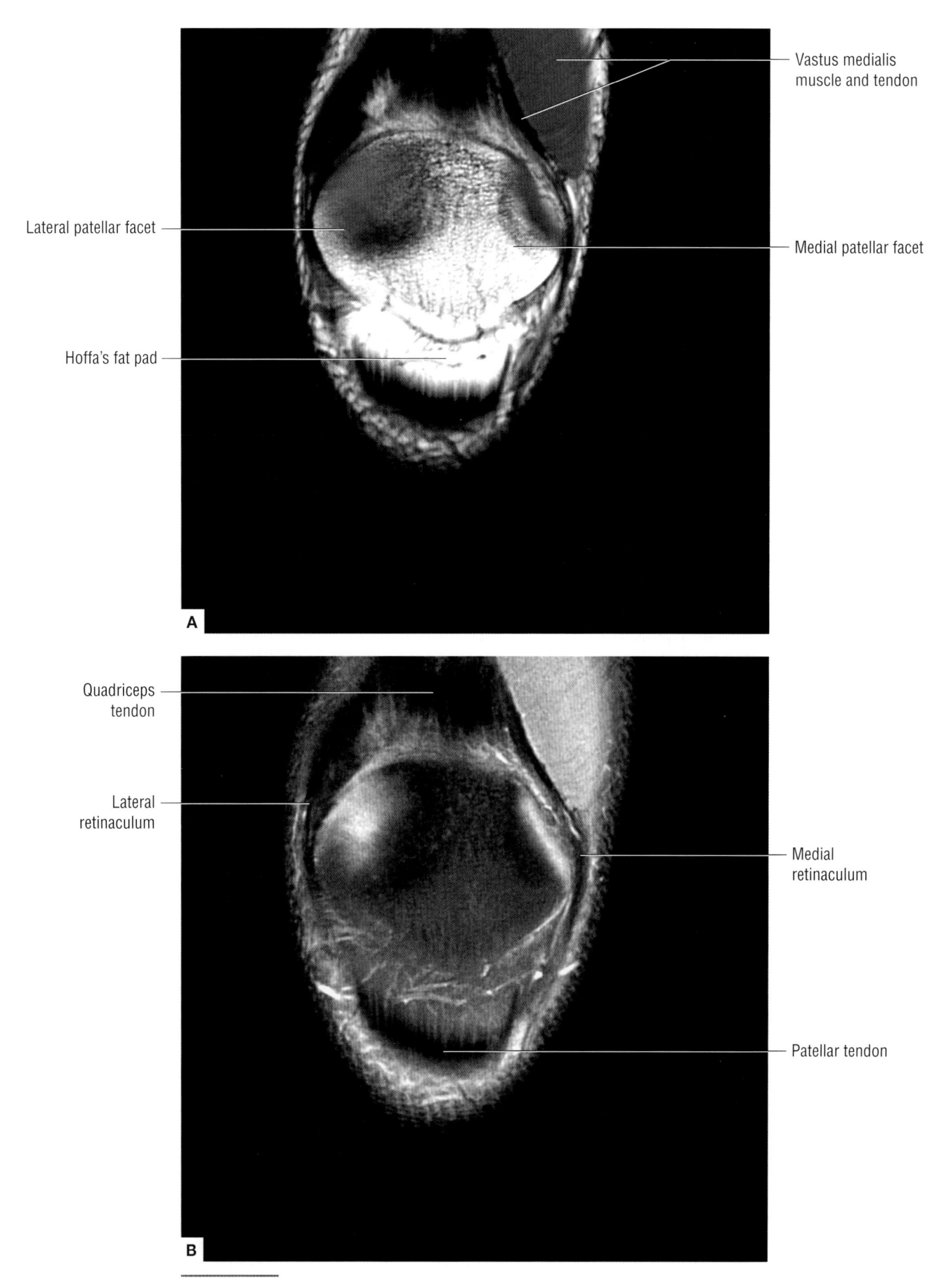

FIGURE 2.3 A, B

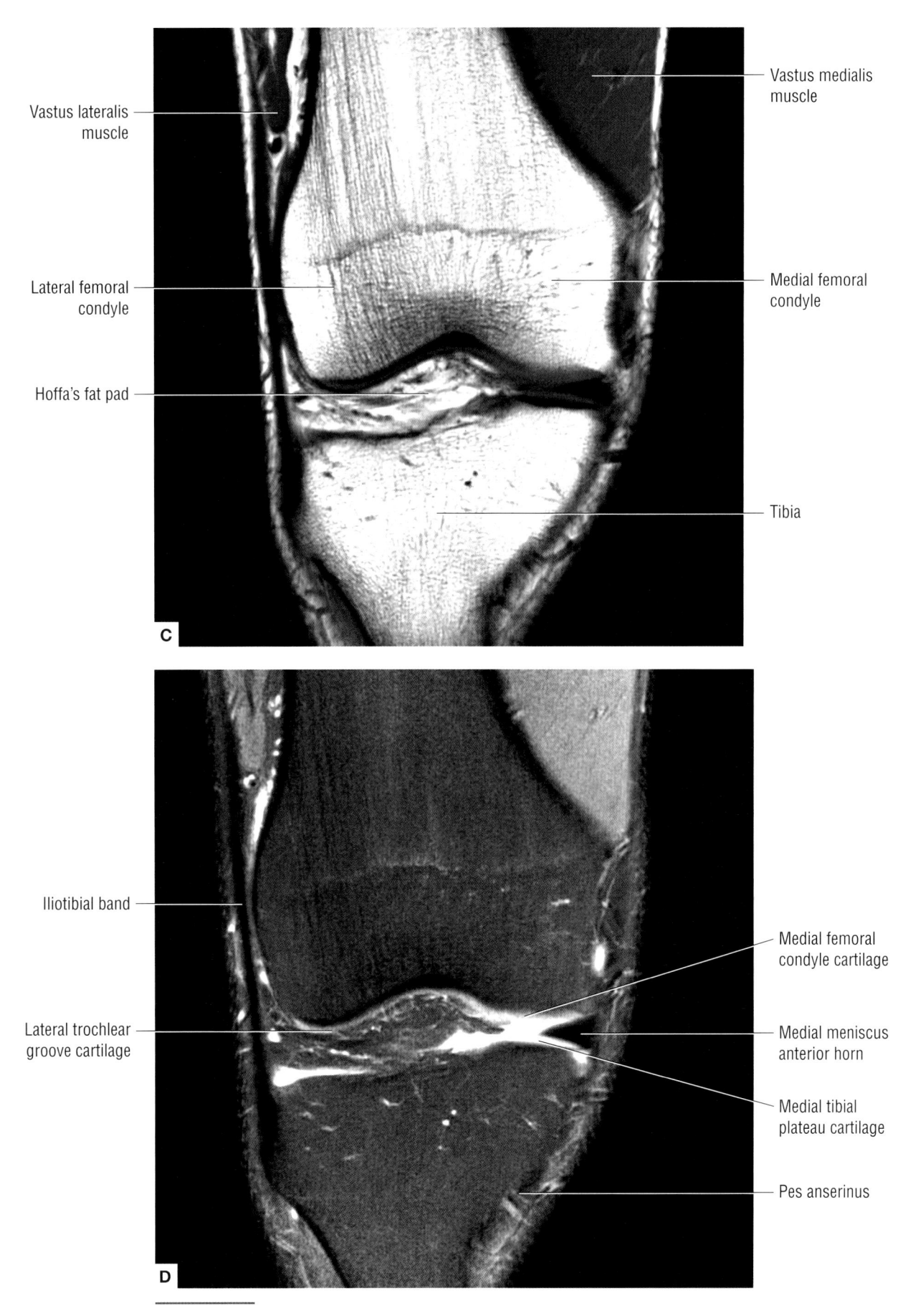

FIGURE 2.3 C, D

Knee Anatomy

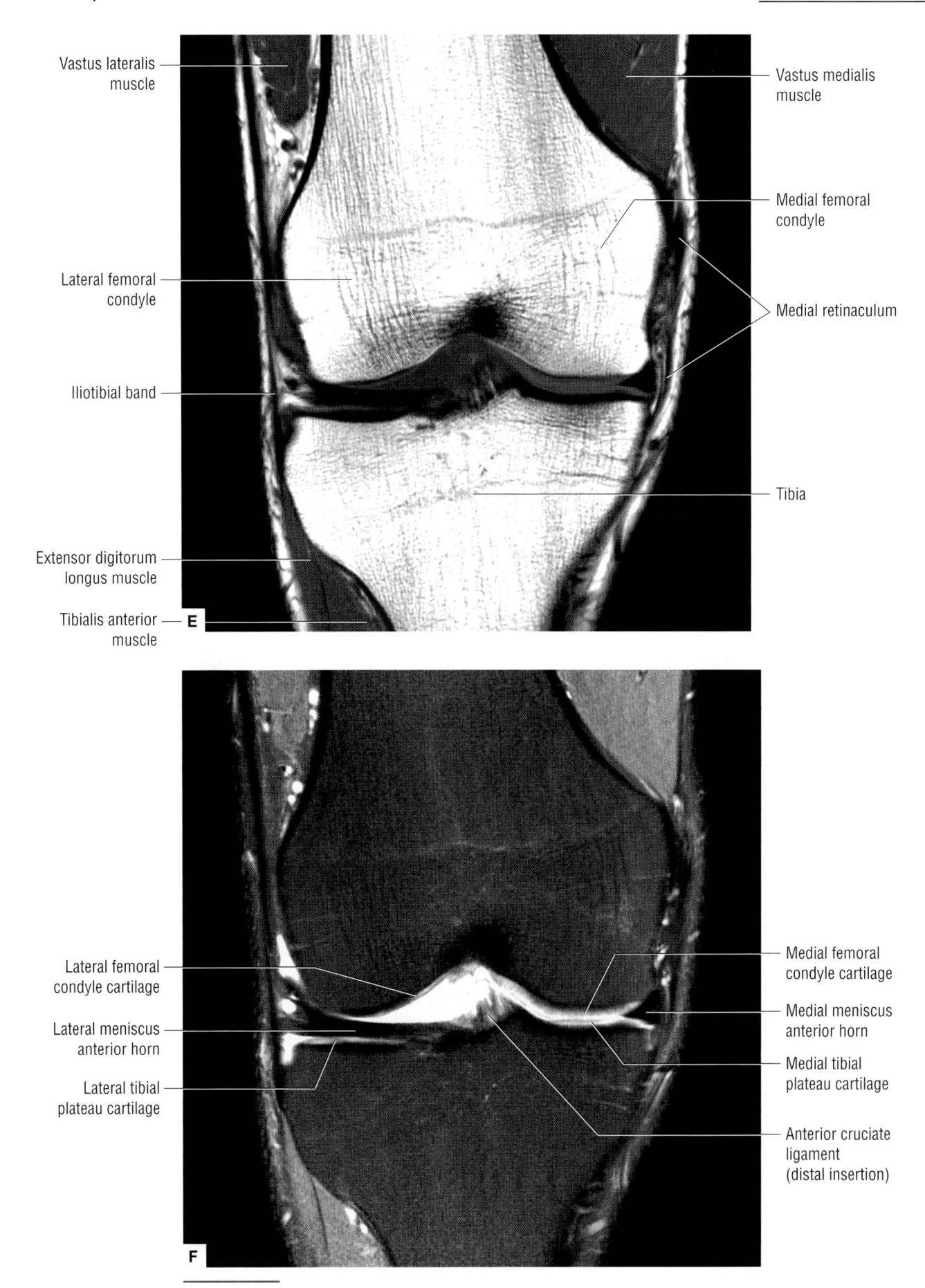

Vastus lateralis muscle — Vastus medialis muscle — Medial femoral condyle — Lateral femoral condyle — Medial retinaculum — Iliotibial band — Tibia — Extensor digitorum longus muscle — Tibialis anterior muscle

E

Lateral femoral condyle cartilage — Medial femoral condyle cartilage — Lateral meniscus anterior horn — Medial meniscus anterior horn — Lateral tibial plateau cartilage — Medial tibial plateau cartilage — Anterior cruciate ligament (distal insertion)

F

FIGURE 2.3   E, F

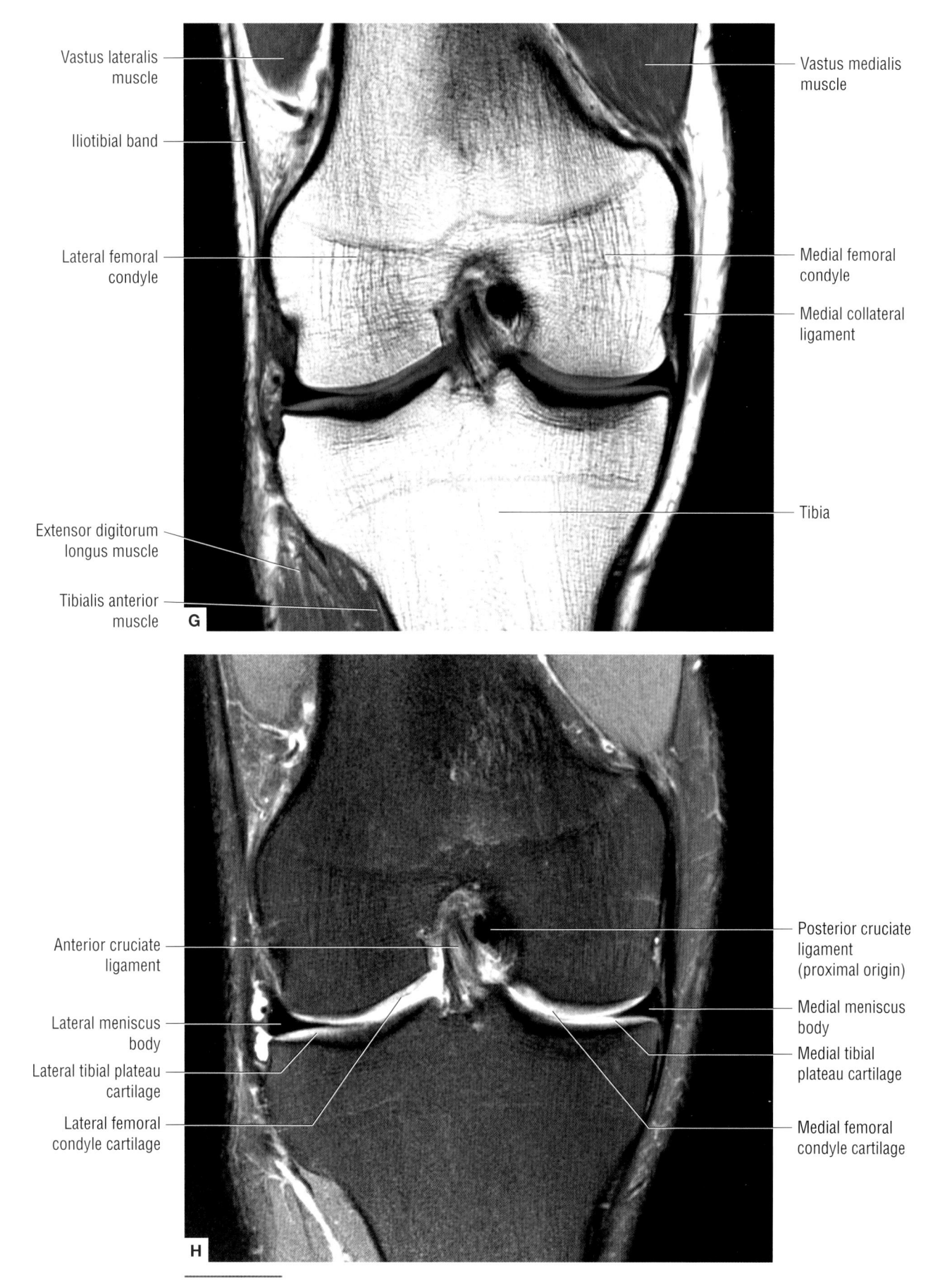

FIGURE 2.3 G, H

Knee Anatomy

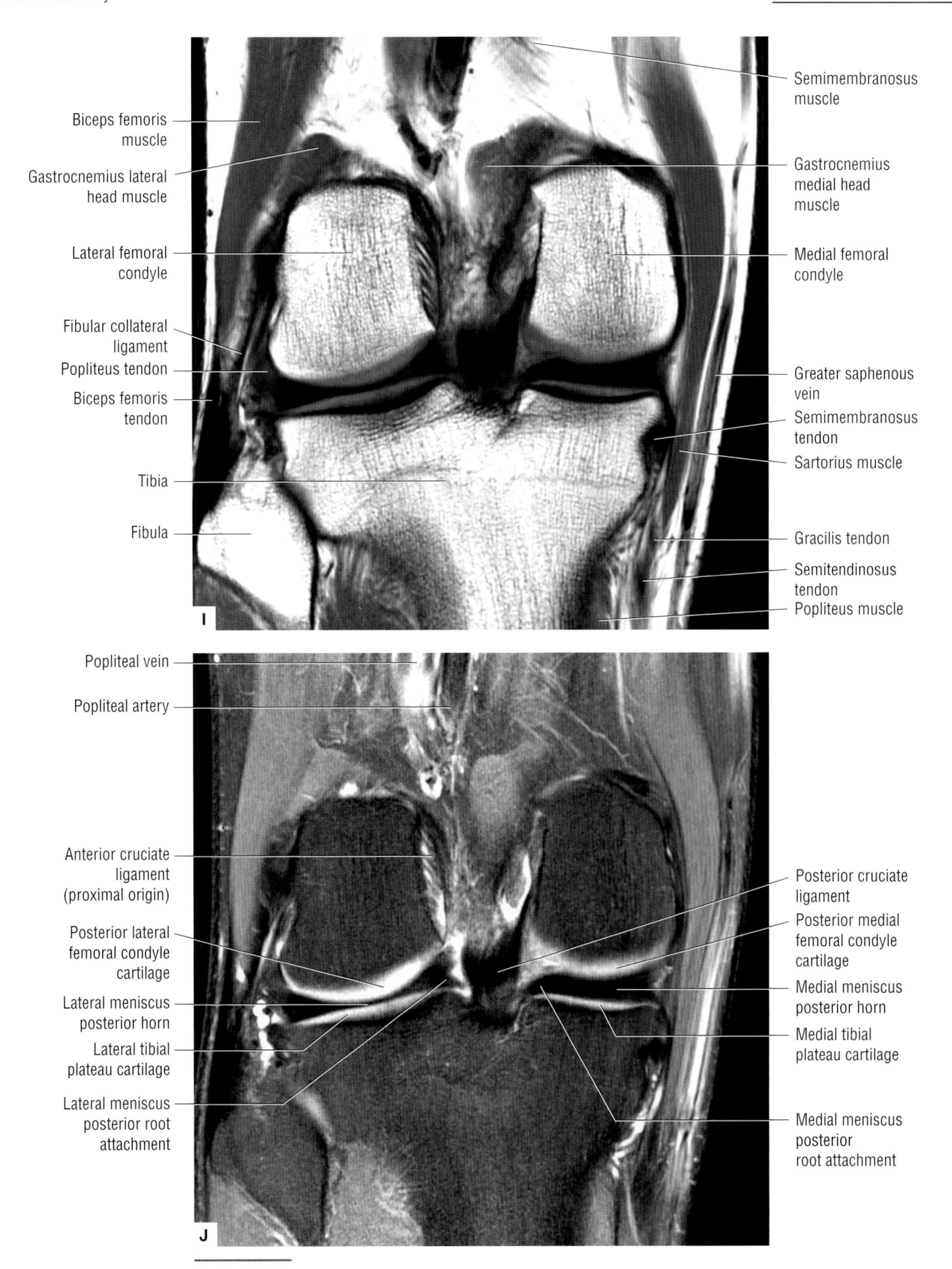

FIGURE 2.3 I, J

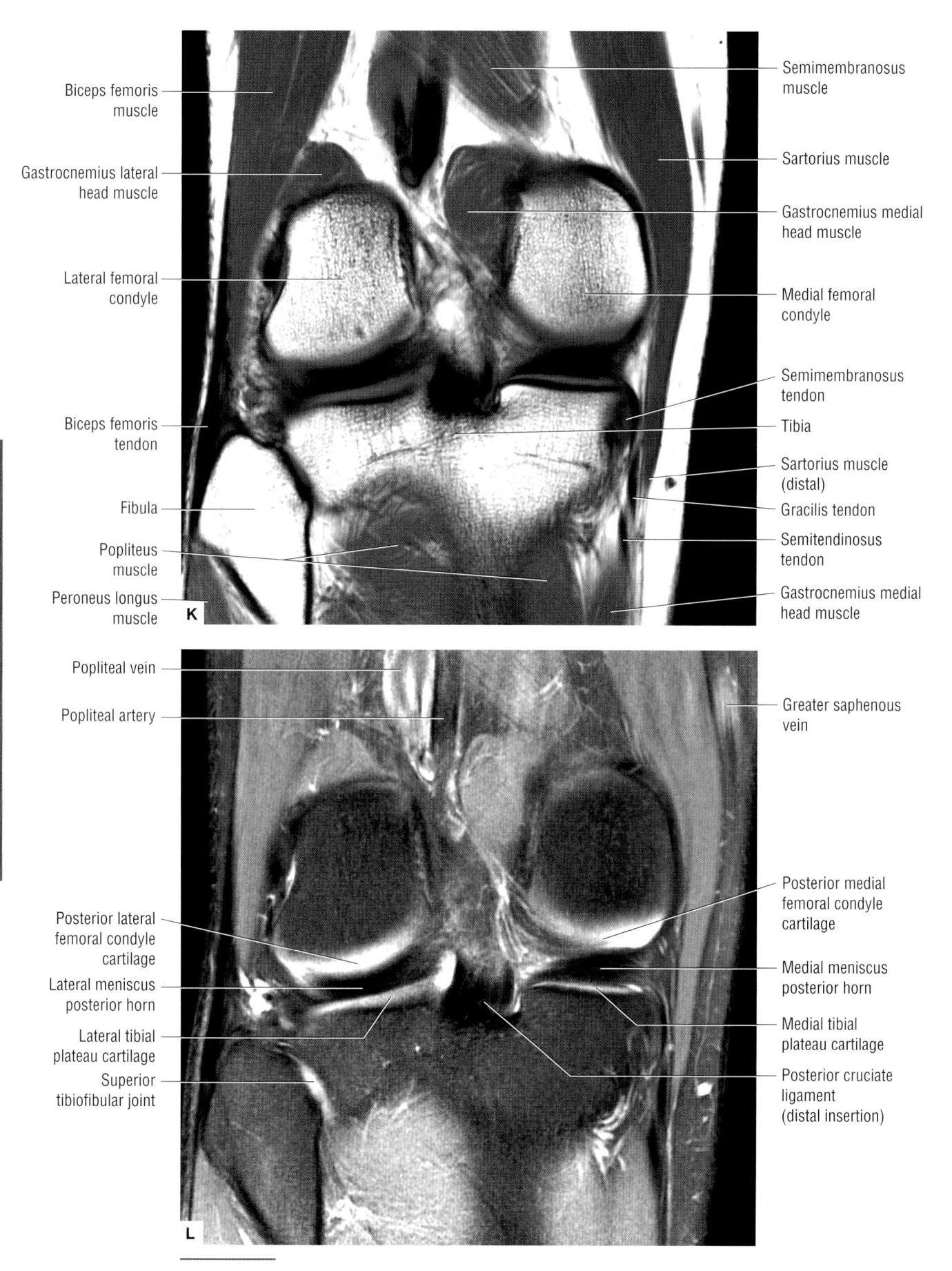

FIGURE 2.3 K, L

Knee Anatomy

Knee and Related Muscles
Thigh Muscle Innervation

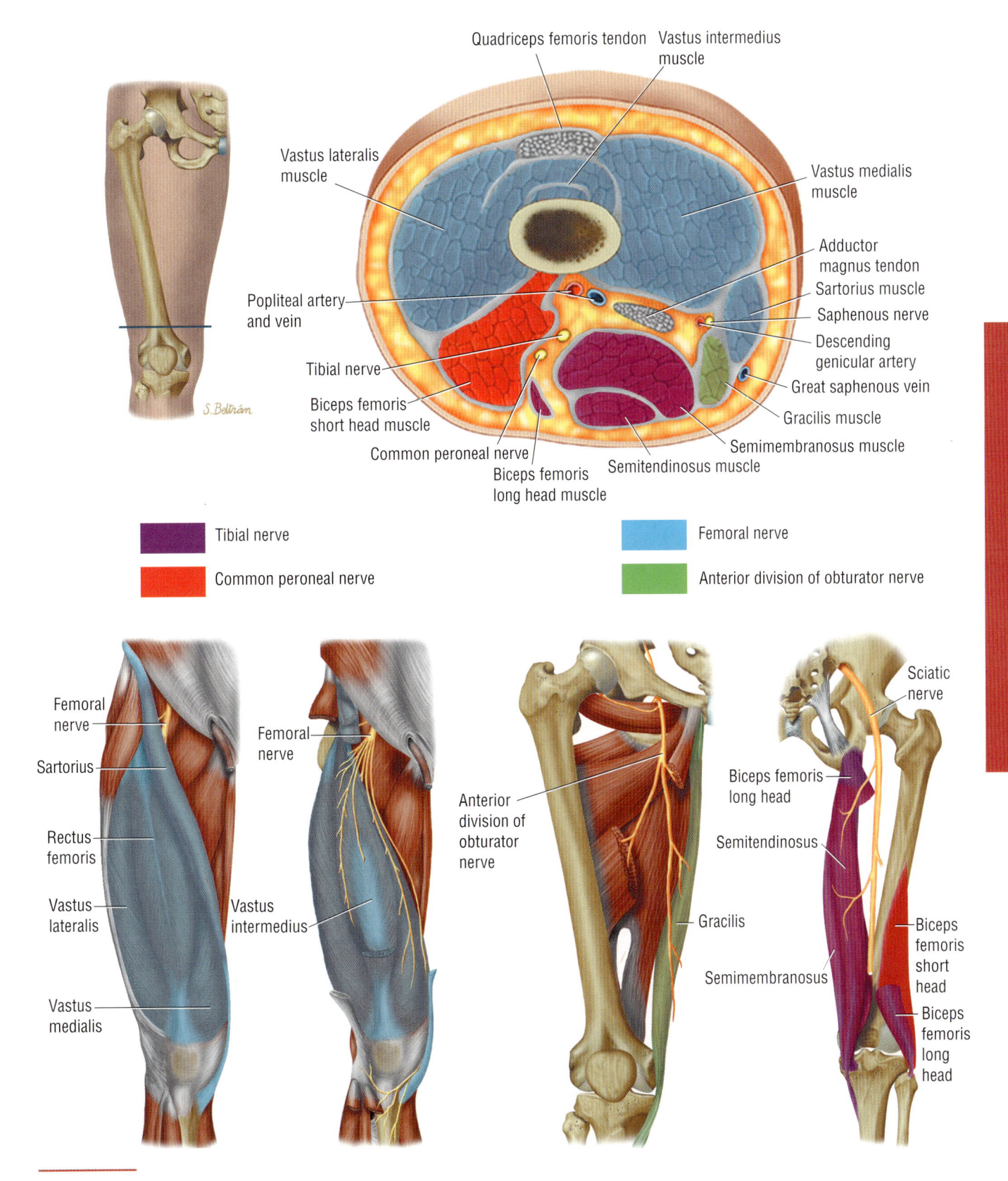

FIGURE 2.4 Distal thigh muscle innervation.

Leg Muscle Innervation

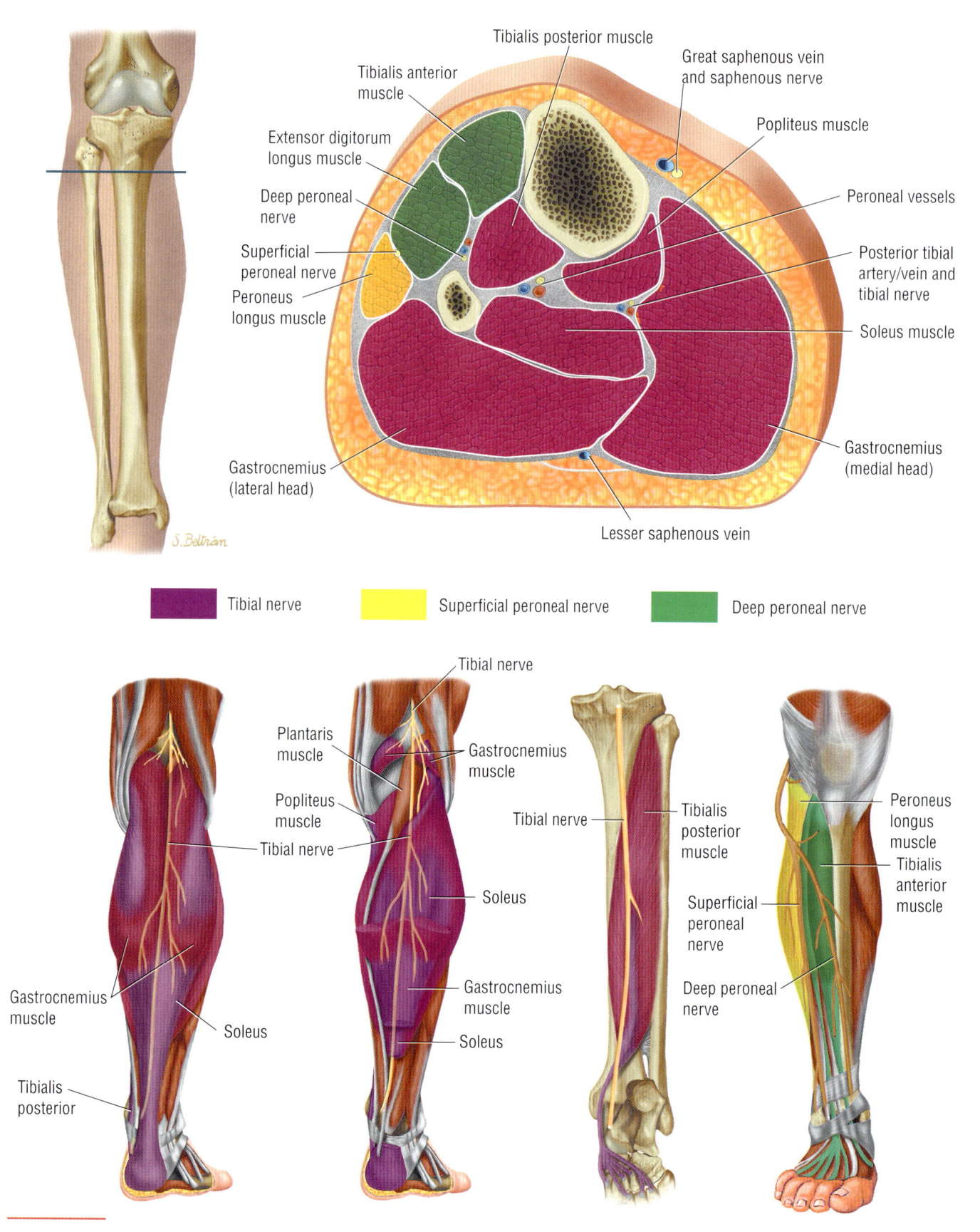

FIGURE 2.5 Proximal leg muscle innervation.

Vastus Lateralis

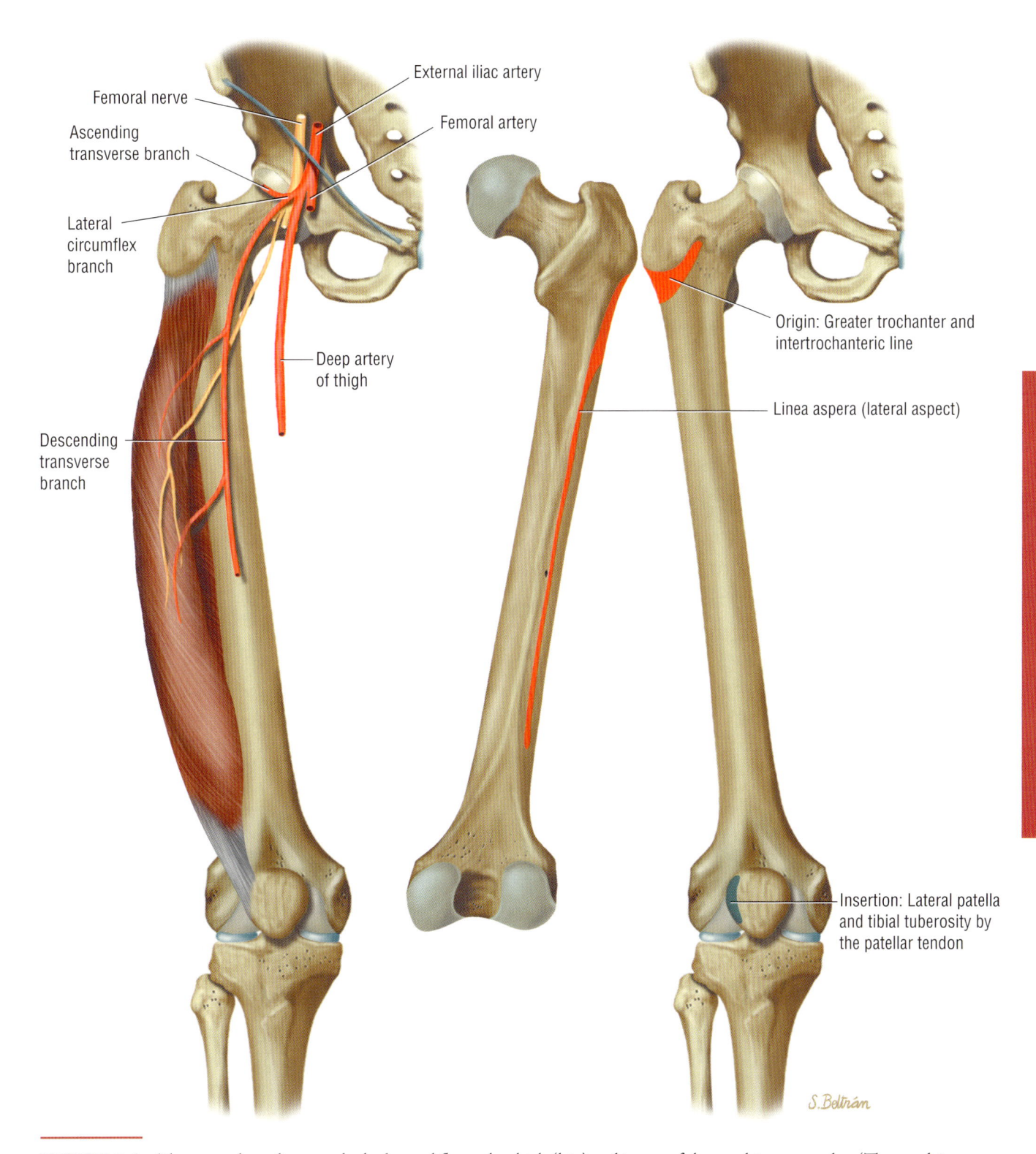

FIGURE 2.6 The vastus lateralis extends the leg and flexes the thigh (hip) and is one of the quadriceps muscles. (The quadriceps group includes the vastus lateralis, vastus medialis, vastus intermedius, and rectus femoris.) Quadriceps muscle fibers are predominantly type II, adapted for rapid forceful activity. The vastus lateralis obliquus (VLO) fibers of the vastus lateralis muscle interdigitate with the lateral intermuscular septum and insert onto the patella. The VLO may be selectively sectioned in a lateral retinacular release without involving the main vastus lateralis tendon proper.

Vastus Medialis

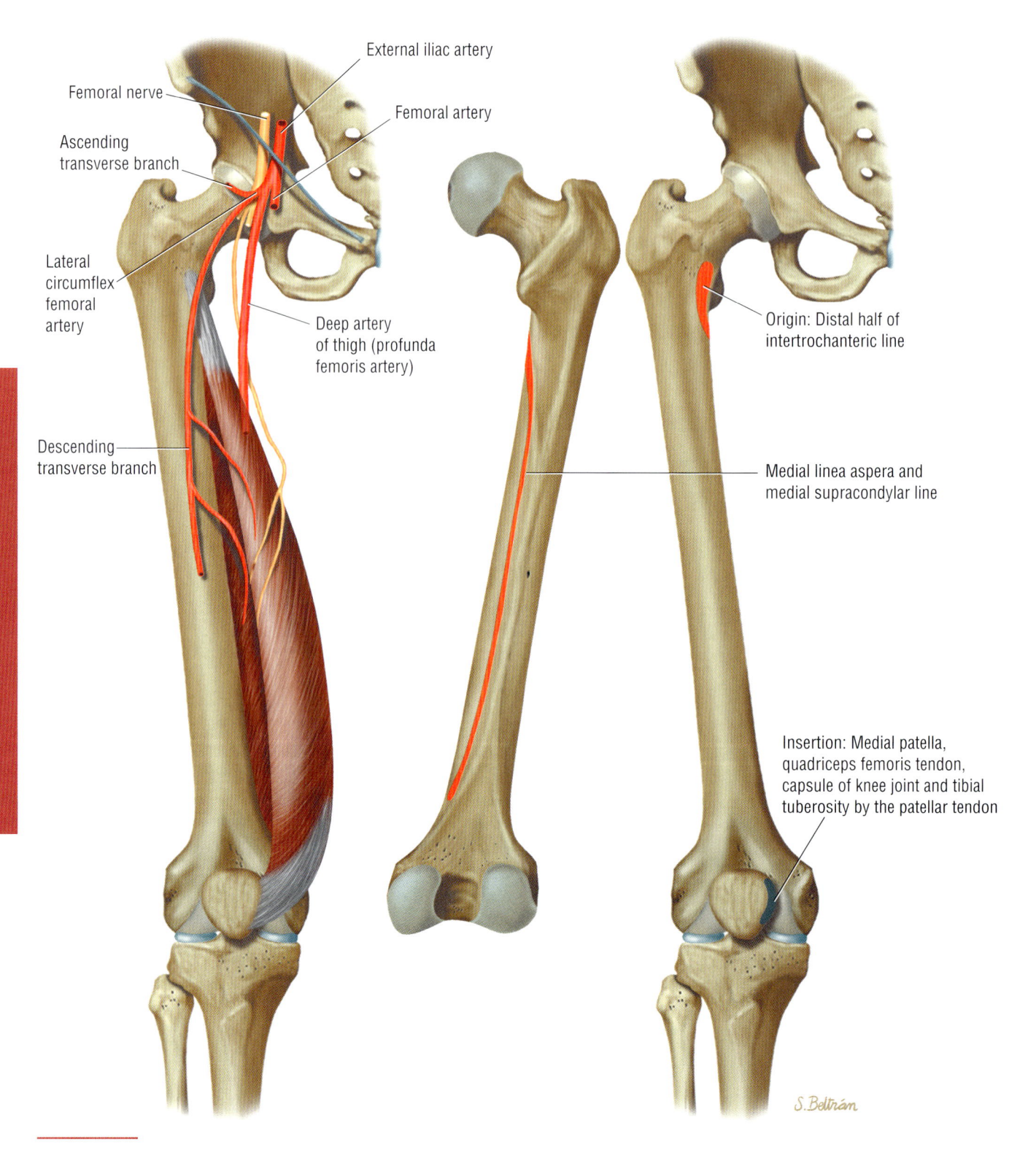

FIGURE 2.7 The vastus medialis extends the leg and pulls the patella medially. The quadriceps muscles, which include the vastus lateralis, the vastus medialis, the vastus intermedius, and the rectus femoris, converge distally, forming the quadriceps tendon, which inserts onto the proximal pole of the patella. The vastus medialis assists in preventing patellar dislocation and may be weakened in patellofemoral disorders. Vastus medialis obliquus injuries are associated with transient patellar dislocation.

Vastus Intermedius

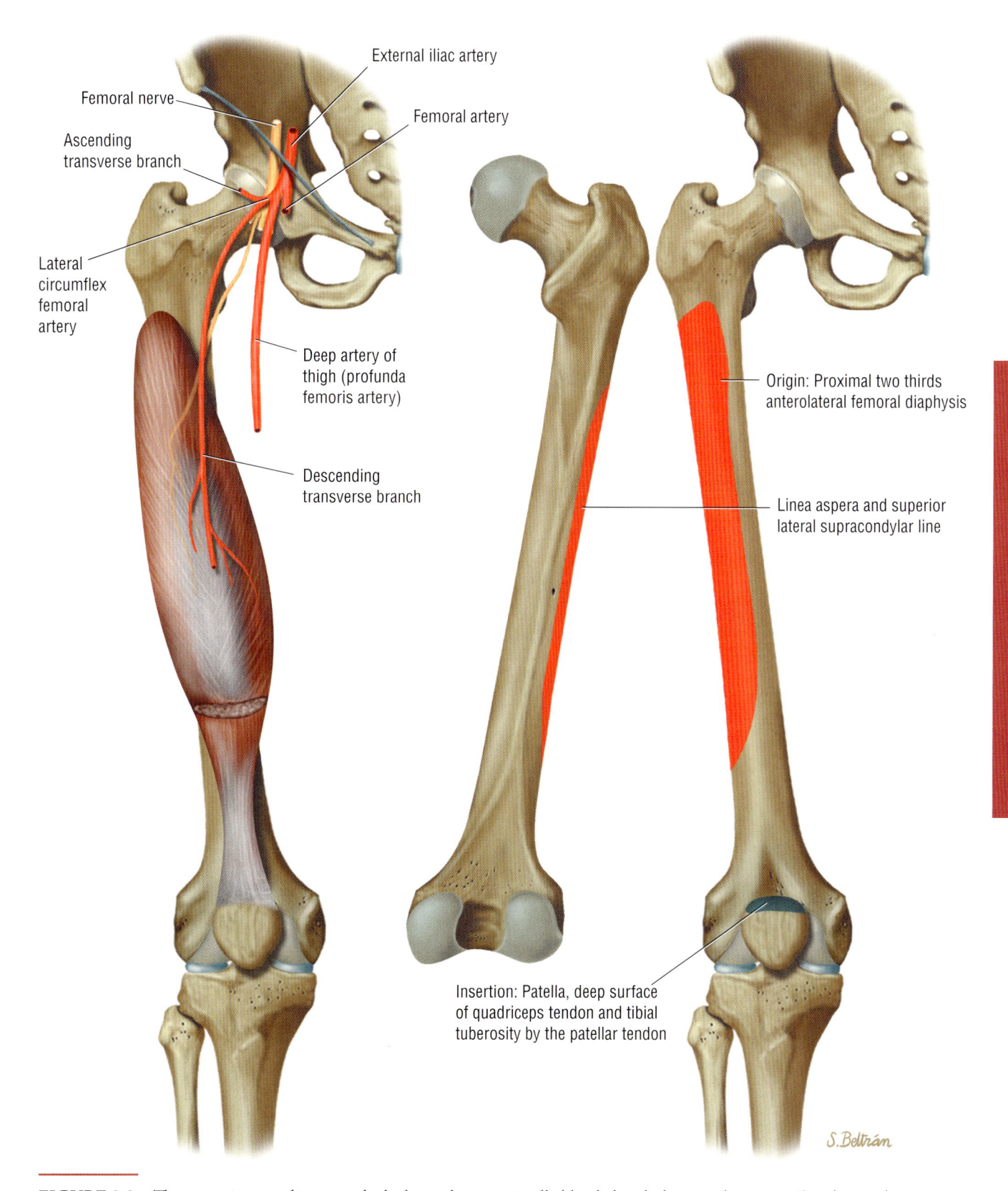

FIGURE 2.8 The vastus intermedius extends the leg and is occasionally blended with the articularis genu. Quadriceps (vastus lateralis, vastus medialis, vastus intermedius, and rectus femoris) injuries, including strains and tendon ruptures, result from eccentric muscle contractions. The articularis genu muscle is responsible for retracting the knee joint capsule superiorly in extension.

Rectus Femoris

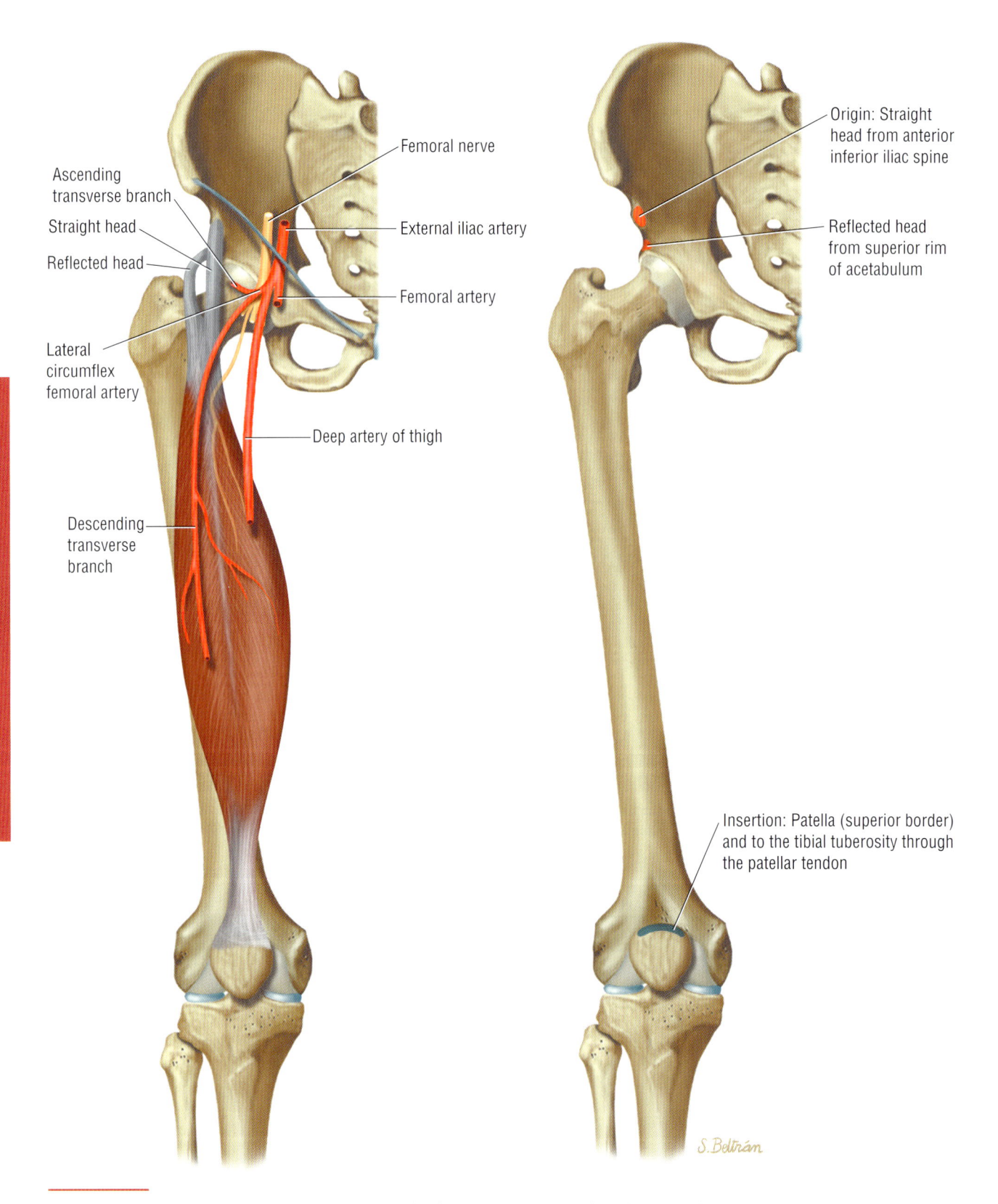

FIGURE 2.9 The rectus femoris flexes the thigh (hip) and extends the leg (knee). Of the four quadriceps muscles, only the rectus femoris has an origin that crosses the hip joint. Soccer, football, basketball, and track and field athletes are at risk for distal musculotendinous junction injuries and for proximal intrasubstance tears of the musculotendinous junction of the indirect head of the rectus femoris.

Knee Anatomy

Biceps Femoris

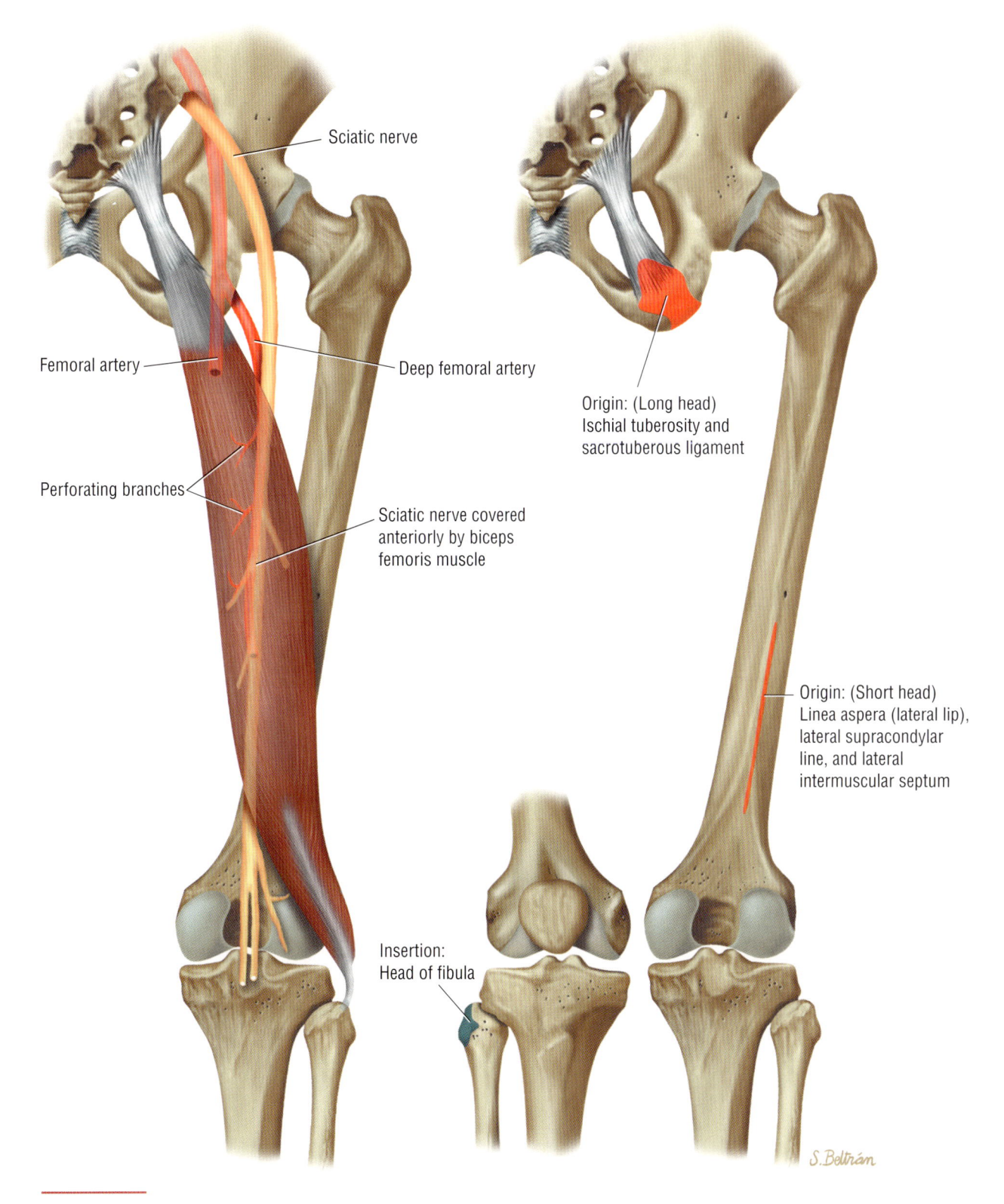

FIGURE 2.10 The biceps femoris extends the thigh, flexes the leg, and contributes to the lateral stability of the knee as an external rotation of the tibia. The muscles of the hamstring group (which include the biceps femoris and the semimembranosus and semitendinosus muscles) all cross the hip and the knee joint, except for the short head of the biceps femoris. Musculotendinous junctions extend the entire length of the muscle and serve as potential sites for strains. The short head of the biceps femoris is innervated by the peroneal branch of the sciatic nerve. The other hamstring muscles are supplied by the tibial branch of the sciatic nerve.

Semimembranosus

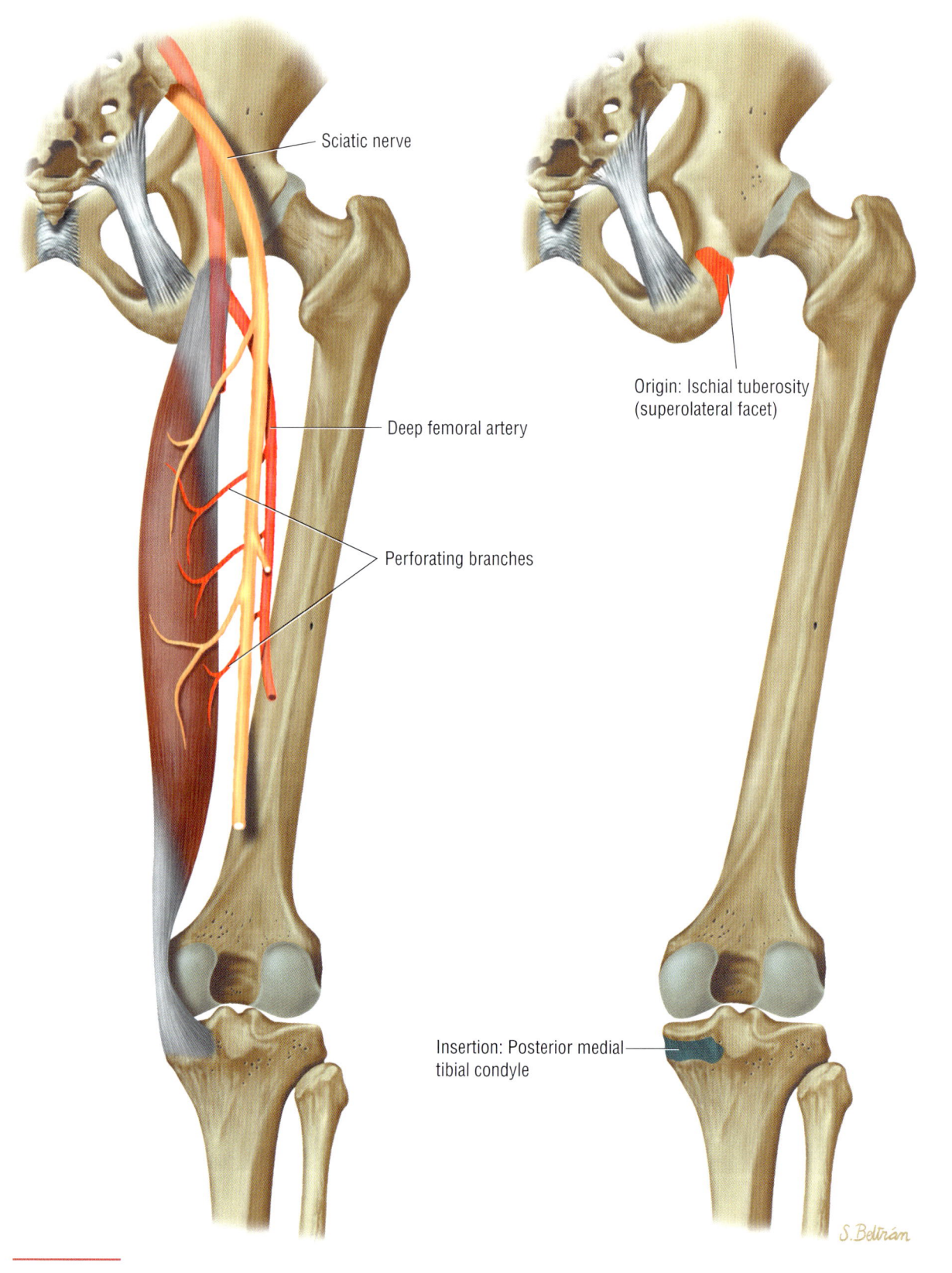

FIGURE 2.11 The semimembranosus extends the thigh and flexes the leg. As a group, the hamstring muscles (biceps femoris, semimembranosus, semitendinosus) make up the posterior thigh. Except for the short head of the biceps femoris, the hamstrings arise from the ischial tuberosity and are responsible for ischial avulsion fractures in the young athlete.

Semitendinosus

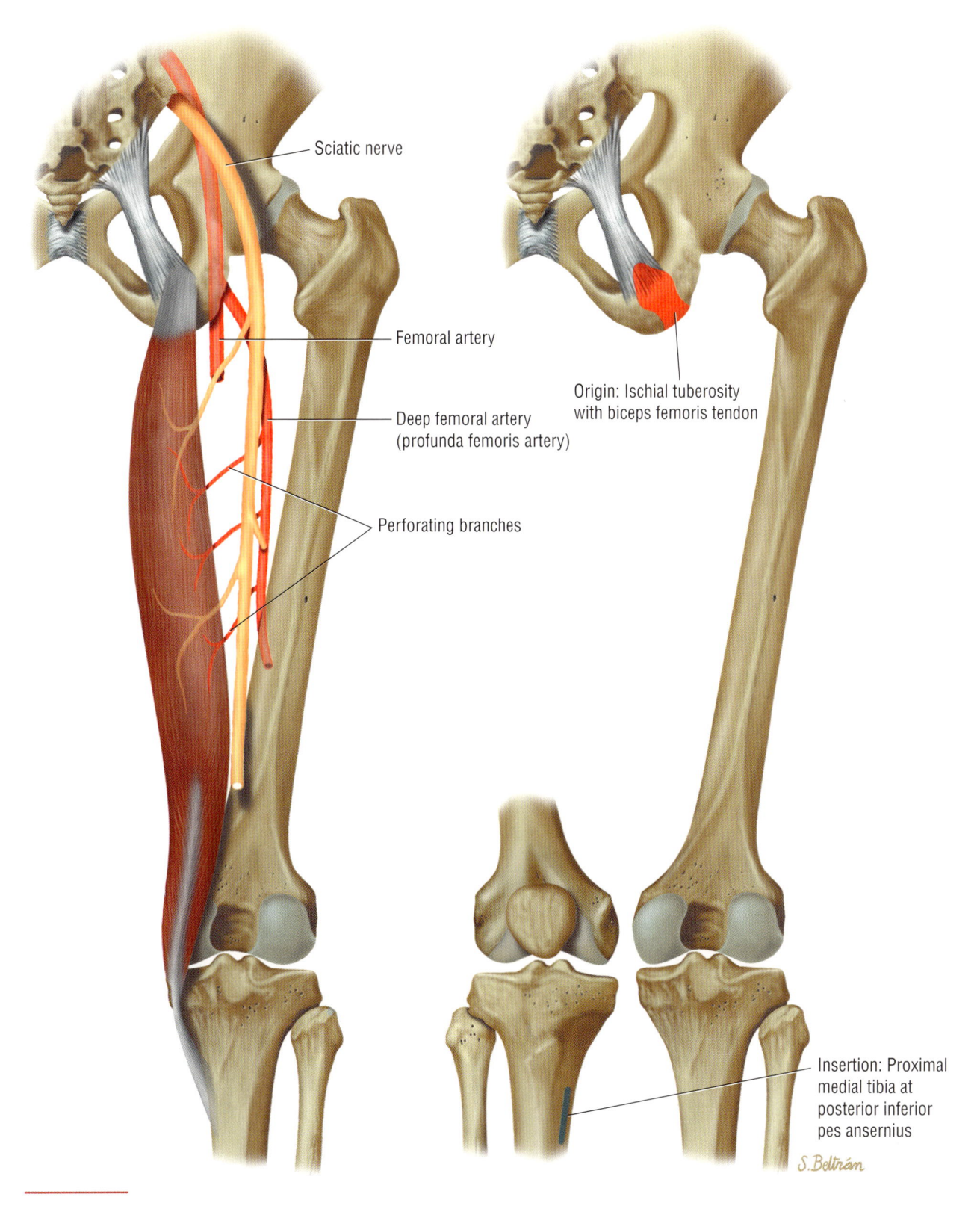

FIGURE 2.12 The semitendinosus (part of hamstring muscle group) extends the thigh and flexes the leg. The hamstring muscles are important in anterior cruciate ligament reconstructions, in posterolateral knee reconstructions, and in tenodesis for patellar subluxation. The posteromedial tendons are seen on axial knee images at the joint line. Hip hyperflexion with simultaneous knee extension is a mechanism of injury for proximal hamstring injuries in adults and apophyseal avulsions in young skeletally immature athletes.

Sartorius

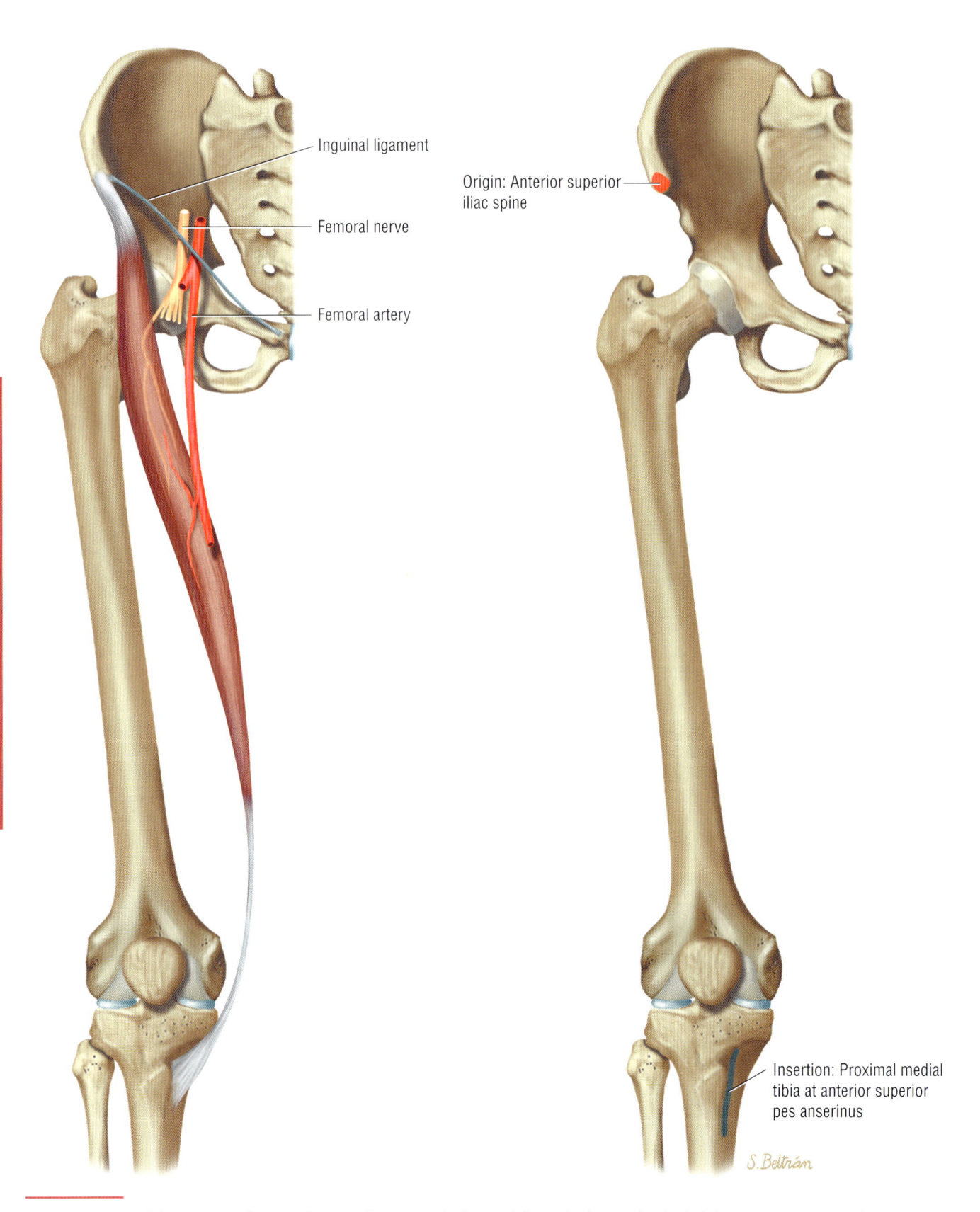

FIGURE 2.13   The sartorius flexes and externally rotates the hip and flexes the leg on the thigh. The anterior superior iliac spine at the origin of the sartorius is a common location for an avulsion fracture. These injuries are seen in sprinters, jumpers, and soccer and football players.

Knee Anatomy

Gracilis

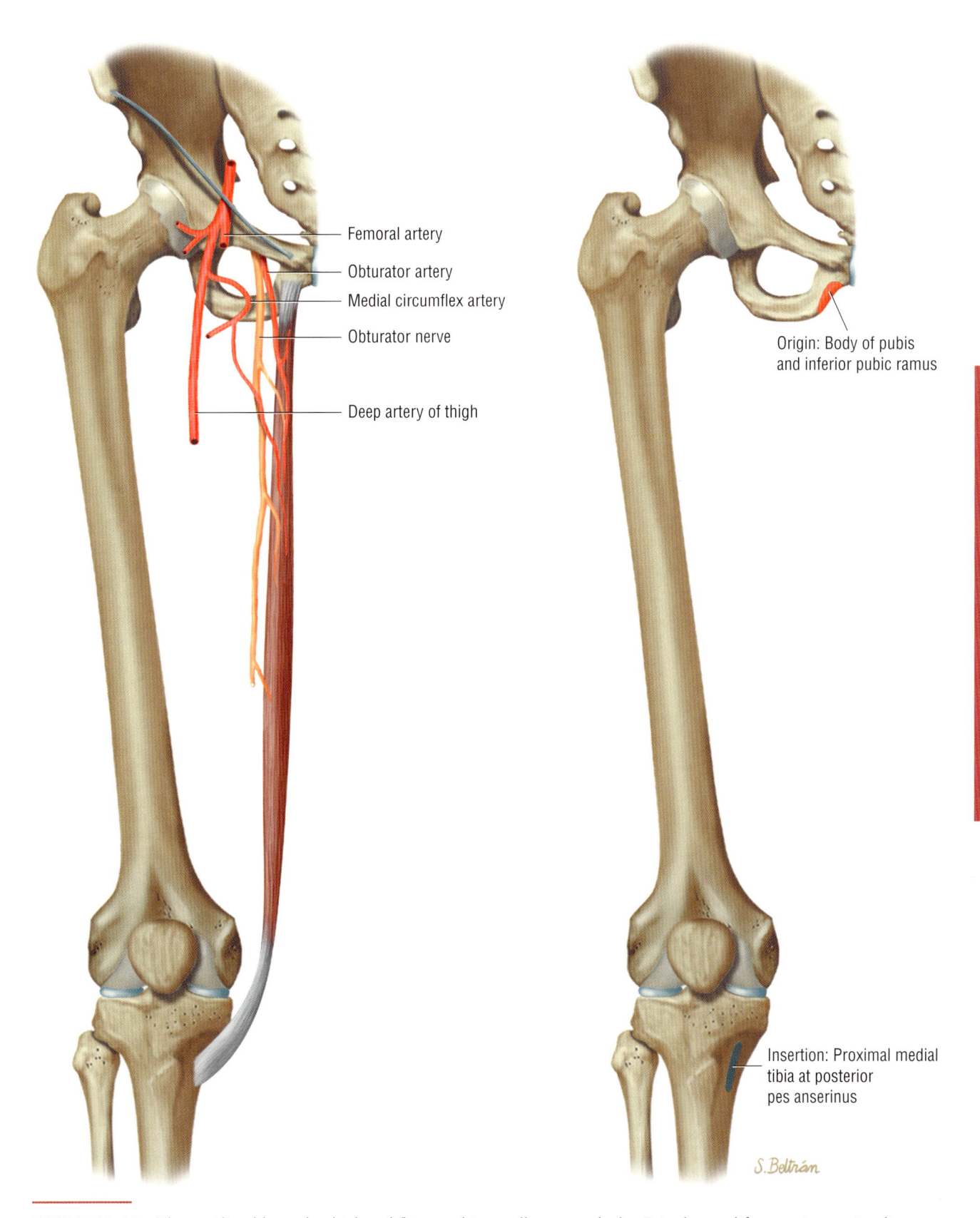

FIGURE 2.14 The gracilis adducts the thigh and flexes and internally rotates the leg. It is also used for anterior cruciate ligament reconstructions. The gracilis is the one muscle of the medial aspect adductors of the thigh (the others being the adductor longus, magnus, and brevis and the pectineus) that does not attach to the linear aspect of the femur.

Popliteus

Tibial nerve

Popliteal artery

Origin: Lateral femoral condyle

Insertion: Proximal posterior tibia (proximal to soleal line)

S. Beltrán

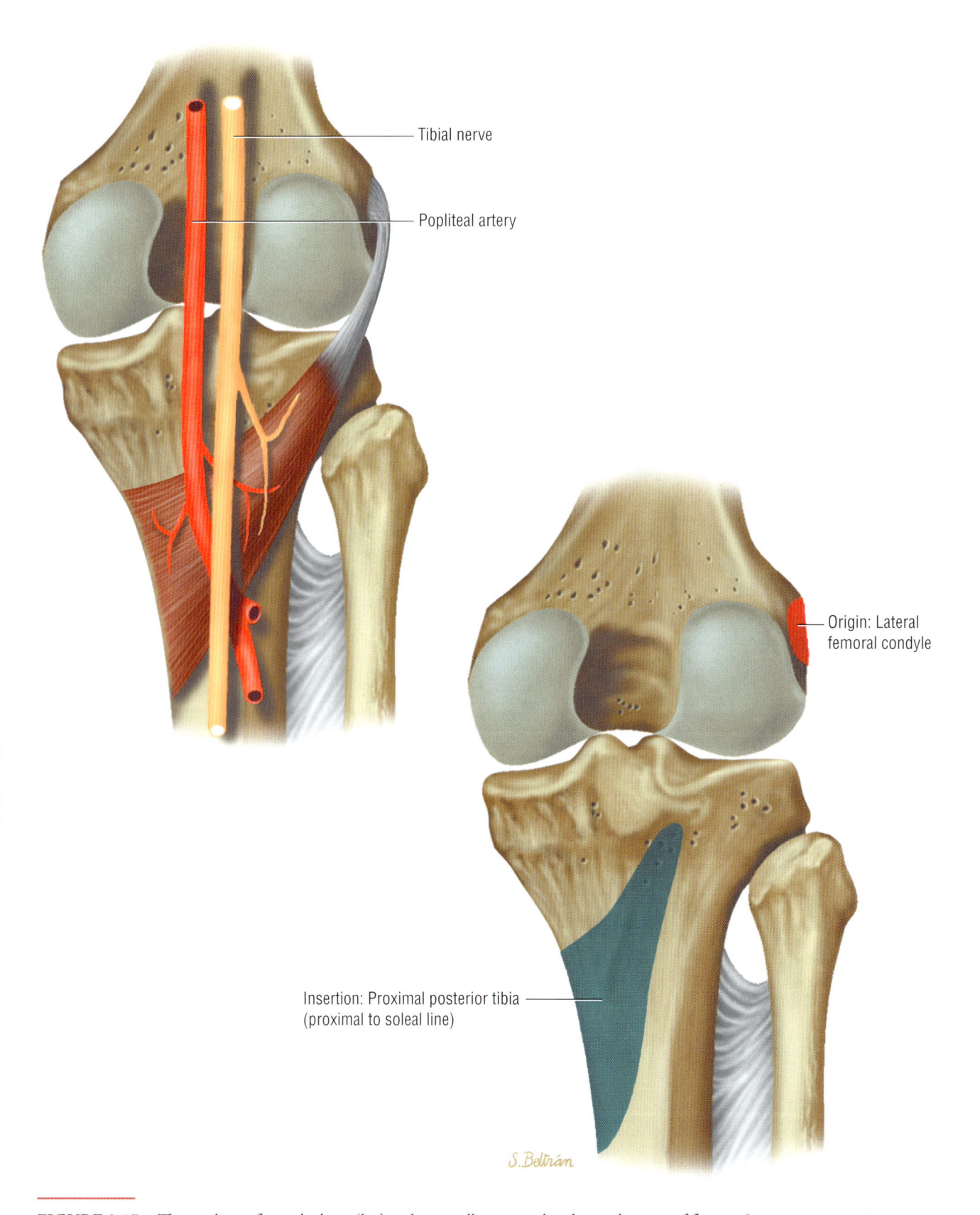

FIGURE 2.15 The popliteus flexes the knee (leg) and internally rotates the tibia at the start of flexion. It is important in injuries to the posterolateral structures. A hiatus in the coronary ligament allows passage of the popliteus tendon to its insertion on the lateral femoral epicondyle. Posterosuperior and posteroinferior popliteomeniscal fascicles attach the popliteus to the lateral meniscus.

Knee Anatomy

Gastrocnemius

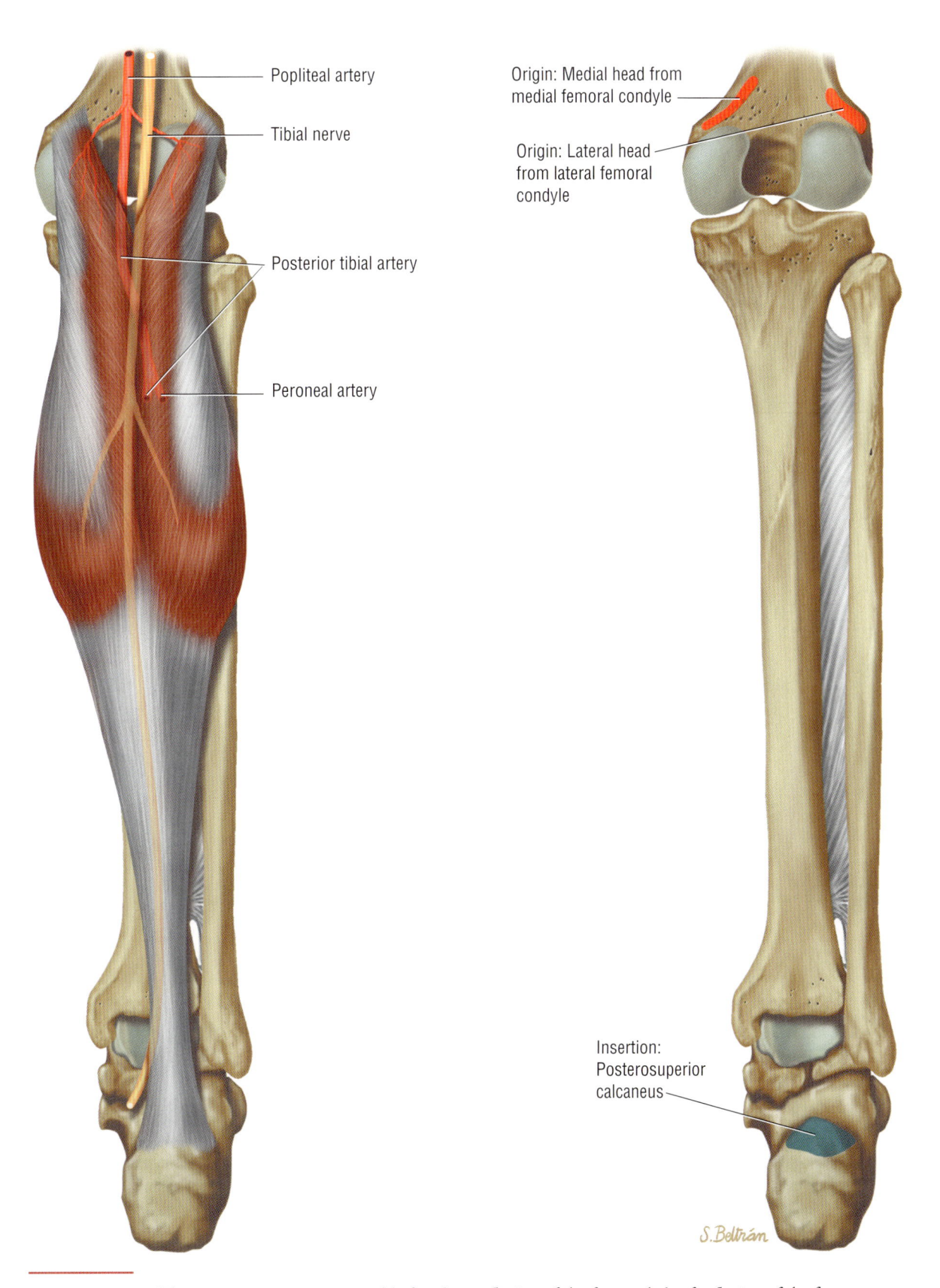

- Popliteal artery
- Tibial nerve
- Posterior tibial artery
- Peroneal artery

- Origin: Medial head from medial femoral condyle
- Origin: Lateral head from lateral femoral condyle
- Insertion: Posterosuperior calcaneus

FIGURE 2.16 The gastrocnemius is responsible for plantar flexion of the foot and also for flexion of the femur on the tibia. Medial head strains are frequently seen in tennis leg. Gastrocnemius fascia is used in augmentation of Achilles tendon repairs.

Plantaris

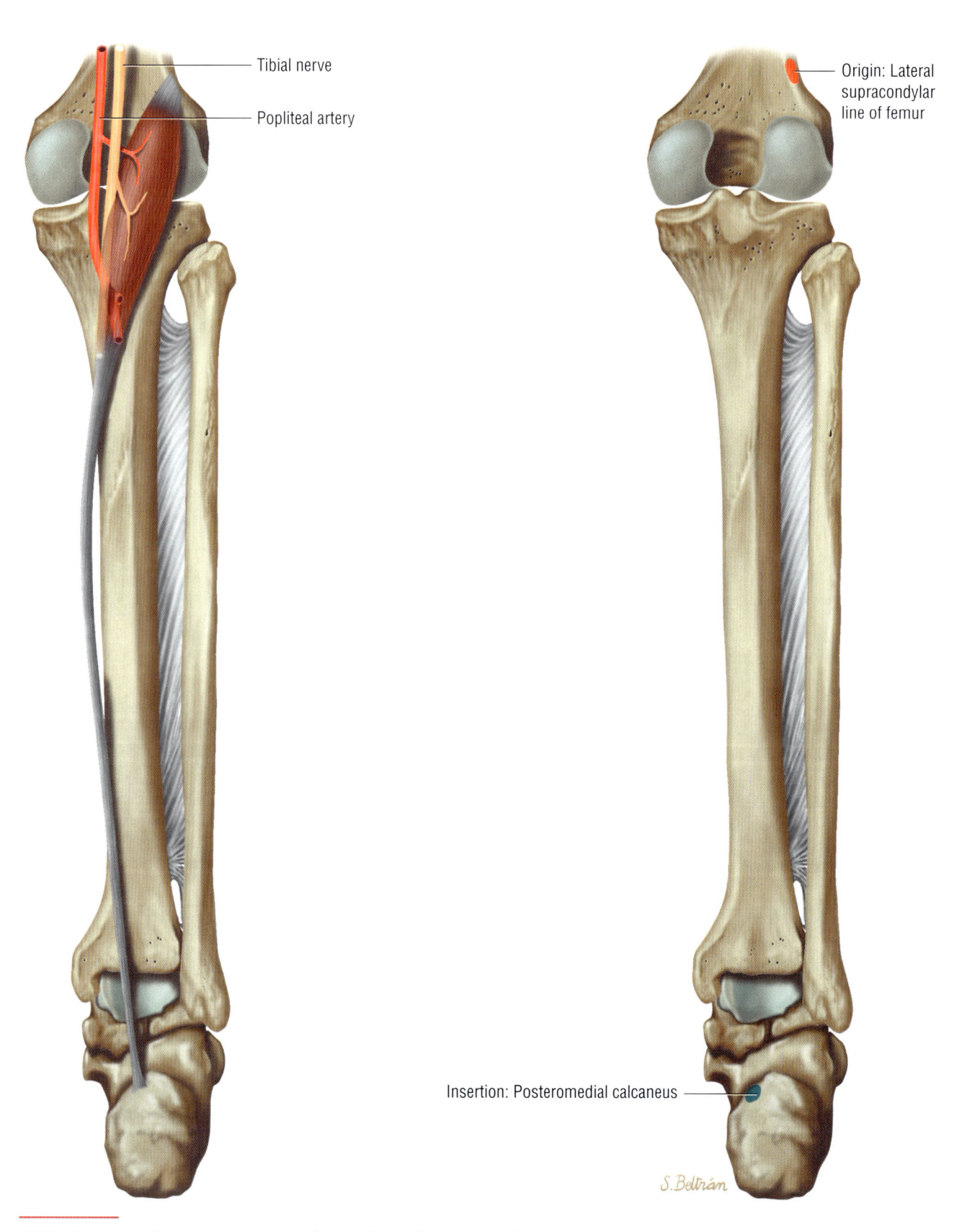

FIGURE 2.17　The plantaris is responsible for plantar flexion of the foot. The short muscle belly is posterolateral at the level of the knee joint, and its long tendon courses between the soleus and medial head of the gastrocnemius medially.

Knee Anatomy

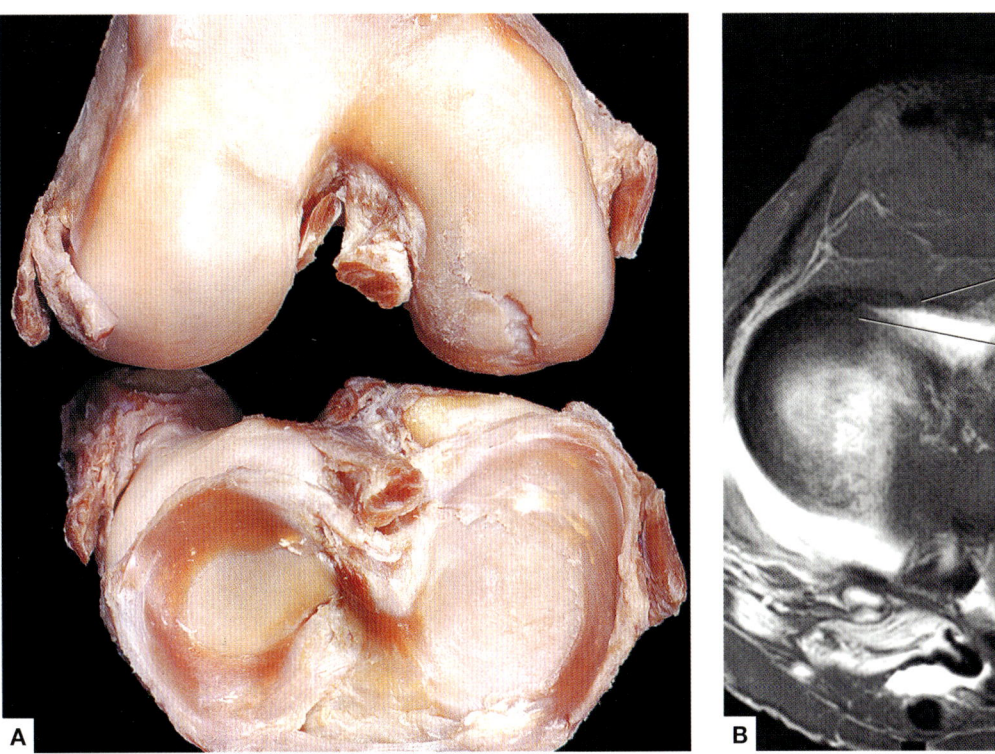

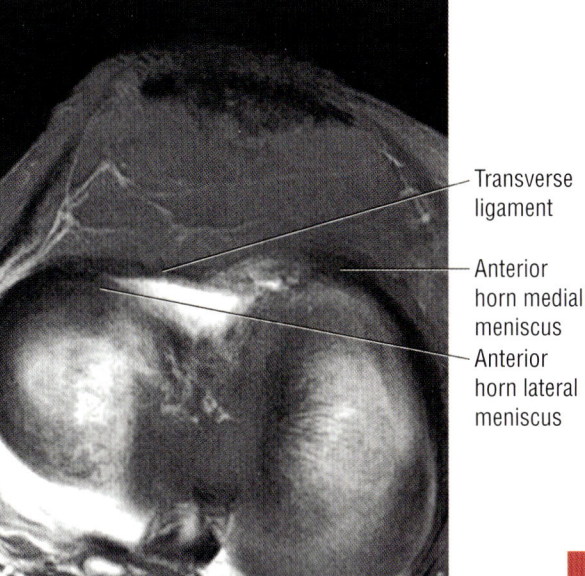

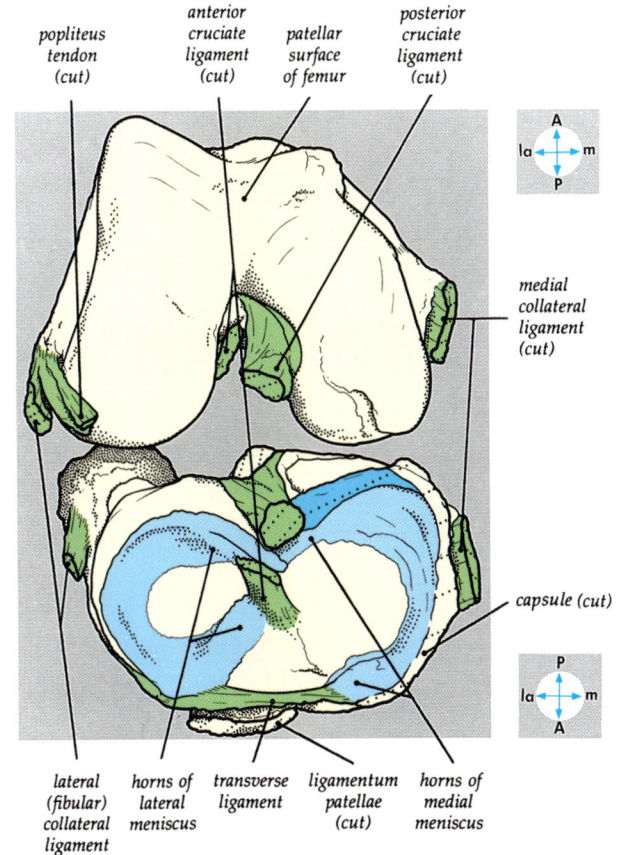

FIGURE 2.18 (**A**) The attachments of the cruciate ligaments and the shape and attachments of the menisci. Sectioning of the cruciate and collateral ligaments allows the femur to be separated from the tibia. (**B**) Axial FS PD FSE image showing the transverse ligament coursing from the anterior horn of the lateral meniscus to the anterior horn of the medial meniscus.

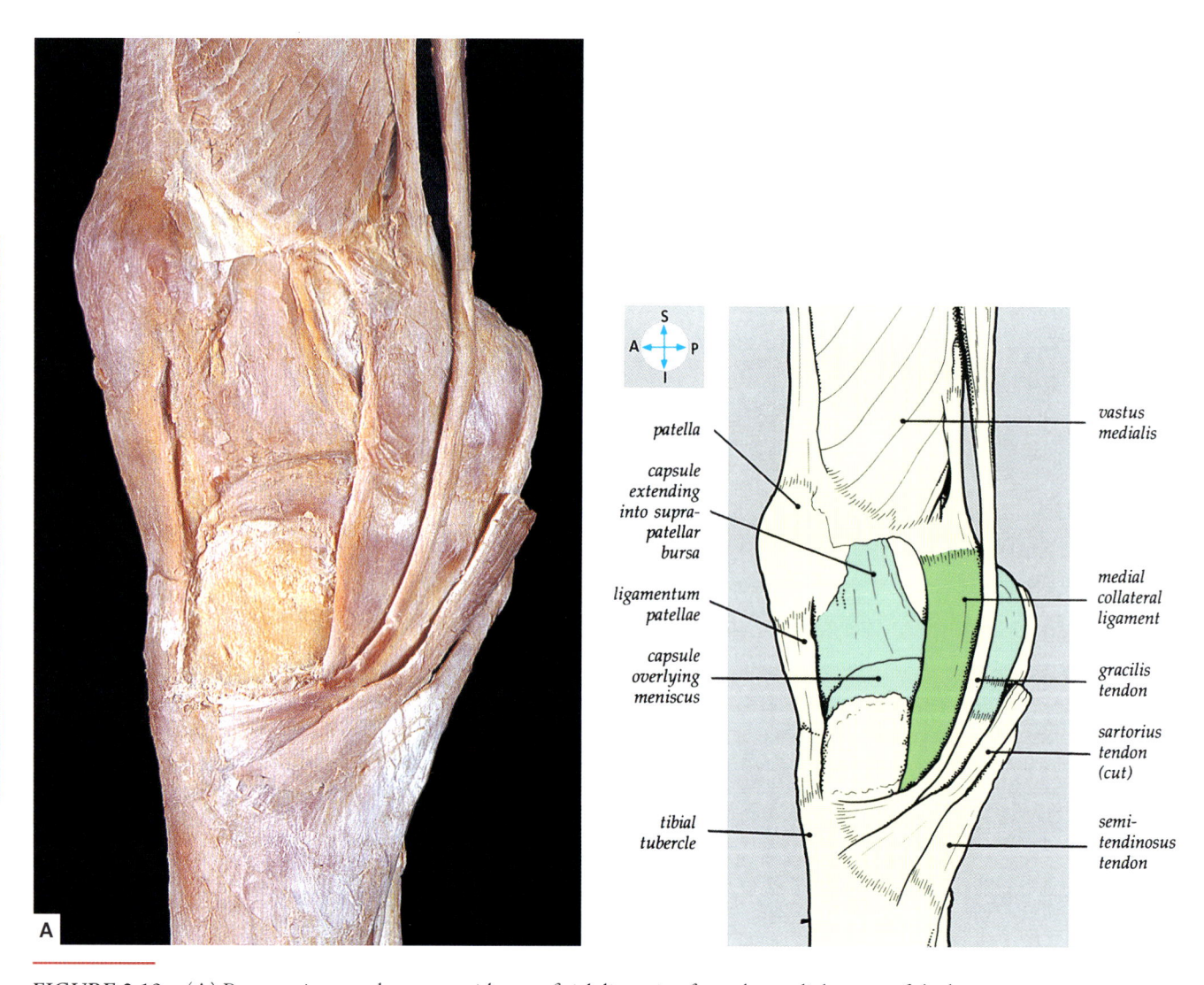

FIGURE 2.19 (**A**) Pes anserinus tendons seen with superficial dissection from the medial aspect of the knee.

Knee Anatomy

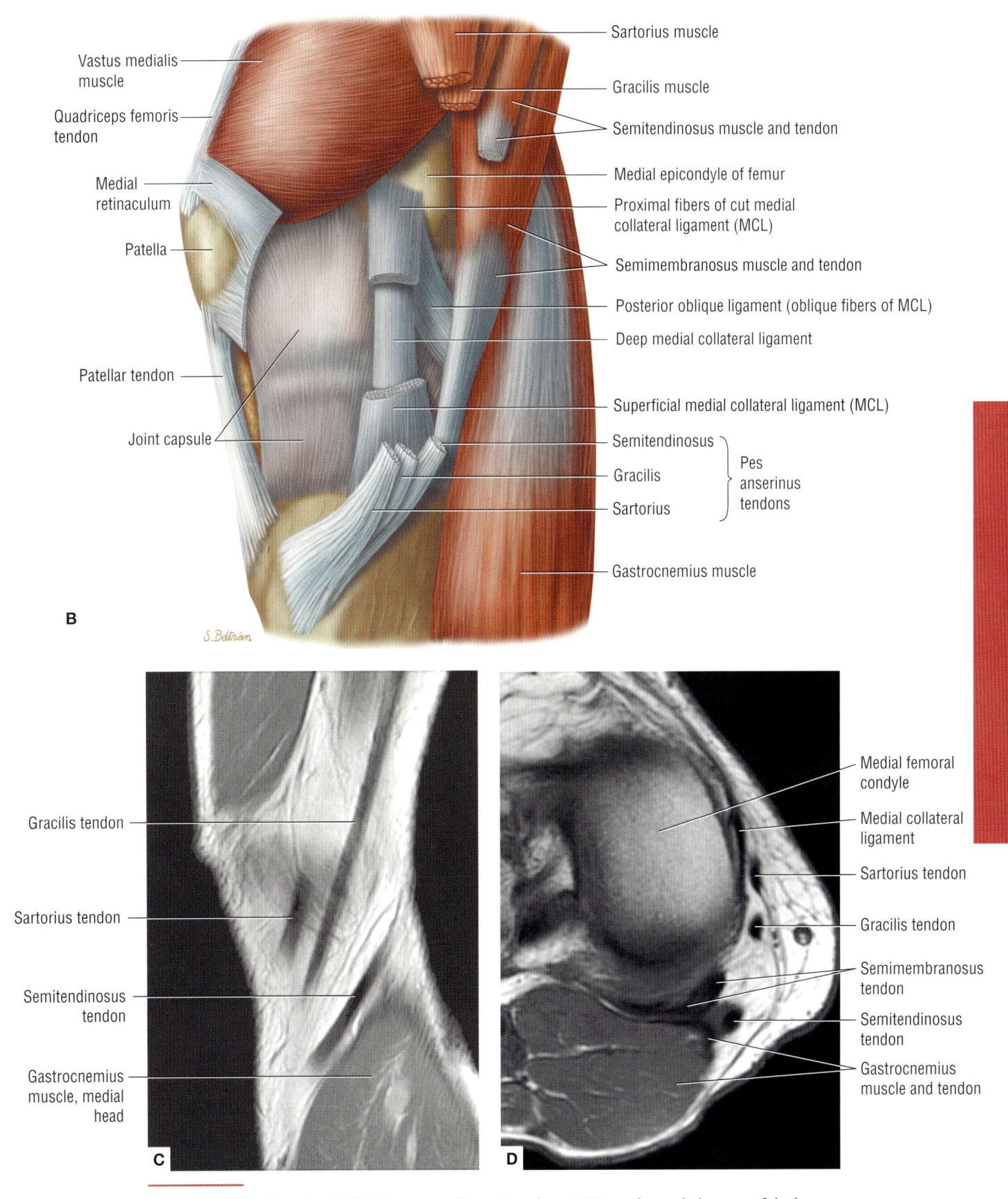

FIGURE 2.19 *(Continued)* (**B**) Exposure of layer 3 or deep MCL on the medial aspect of the knee. Pes tendons are sectioned and shown on sagittal (**C**) and axial (**D**) PD FSE images.

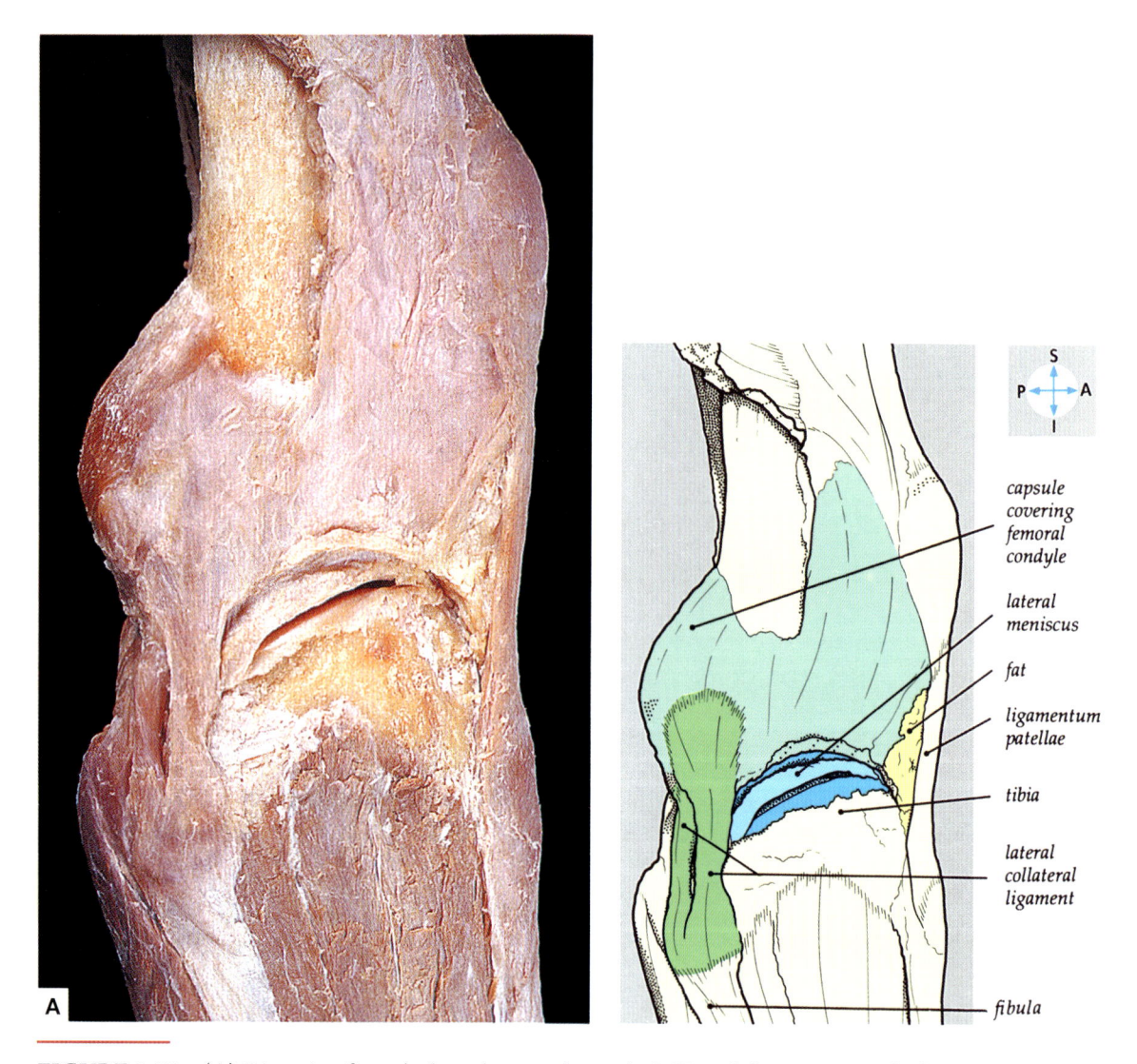

FIGURE 2.20 (**A**) Dissection from the lateral aspect shows the LCL and the meniscus, which are revealed by removing part of the capsule.

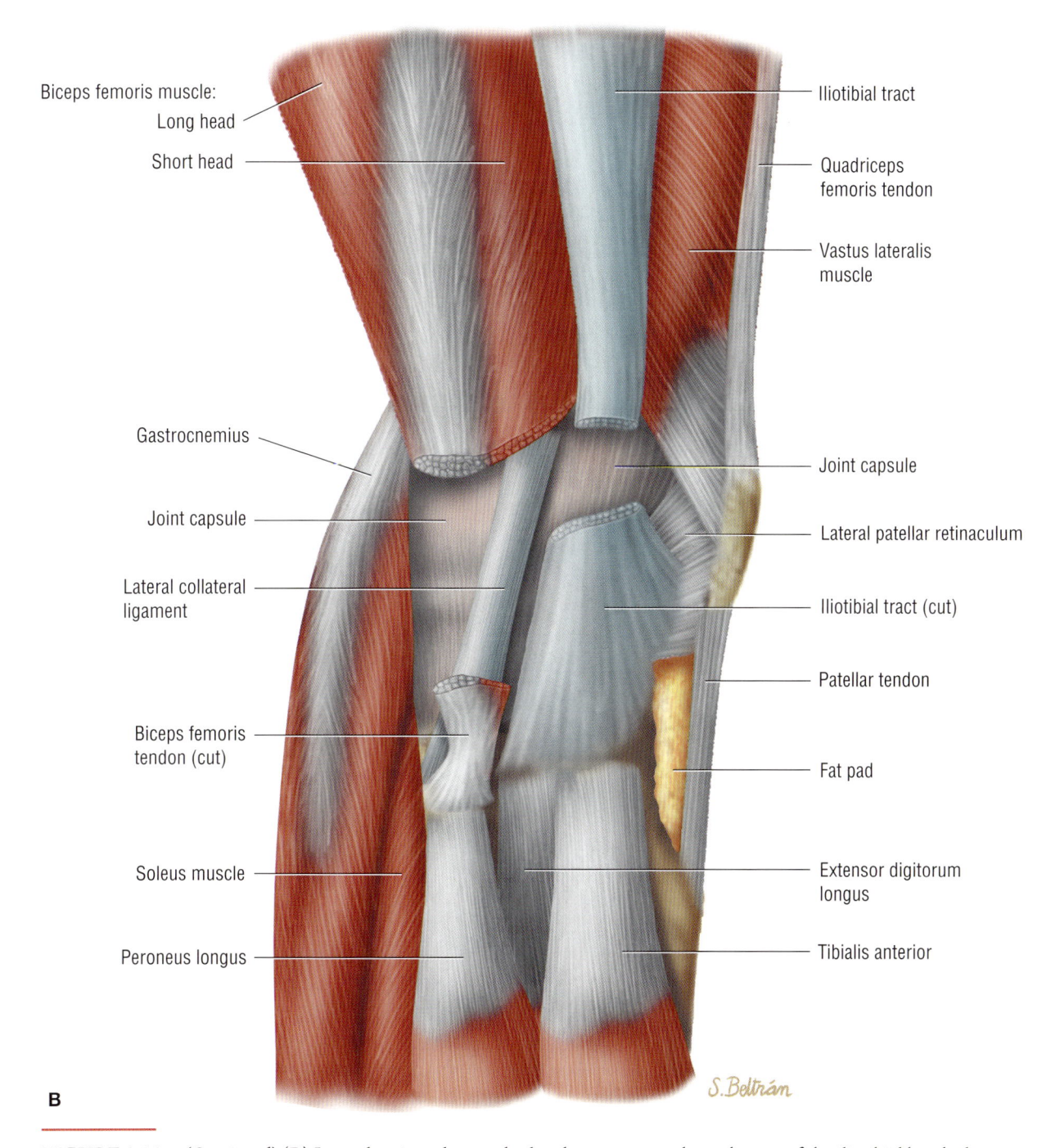

FIGURE 2.20 *(Continued)* (**B**) Lateral retinaculum and related structures and attachment of the iliotibial band, also referred to as the iliotibial tract, to Gerdy's tubercle. The thickened fascia lata forms a longitudinal fiber band referred to as the iliotibial tract. The iliotibial tract and tensor fasciae latae originate from the anterior superior iliac spine. The distal iliotibial tract divides into anterior intermediate and posterior fibers. Strong "Kaplan fibers" bind the iliotibial tract to the femoral diaphysis.

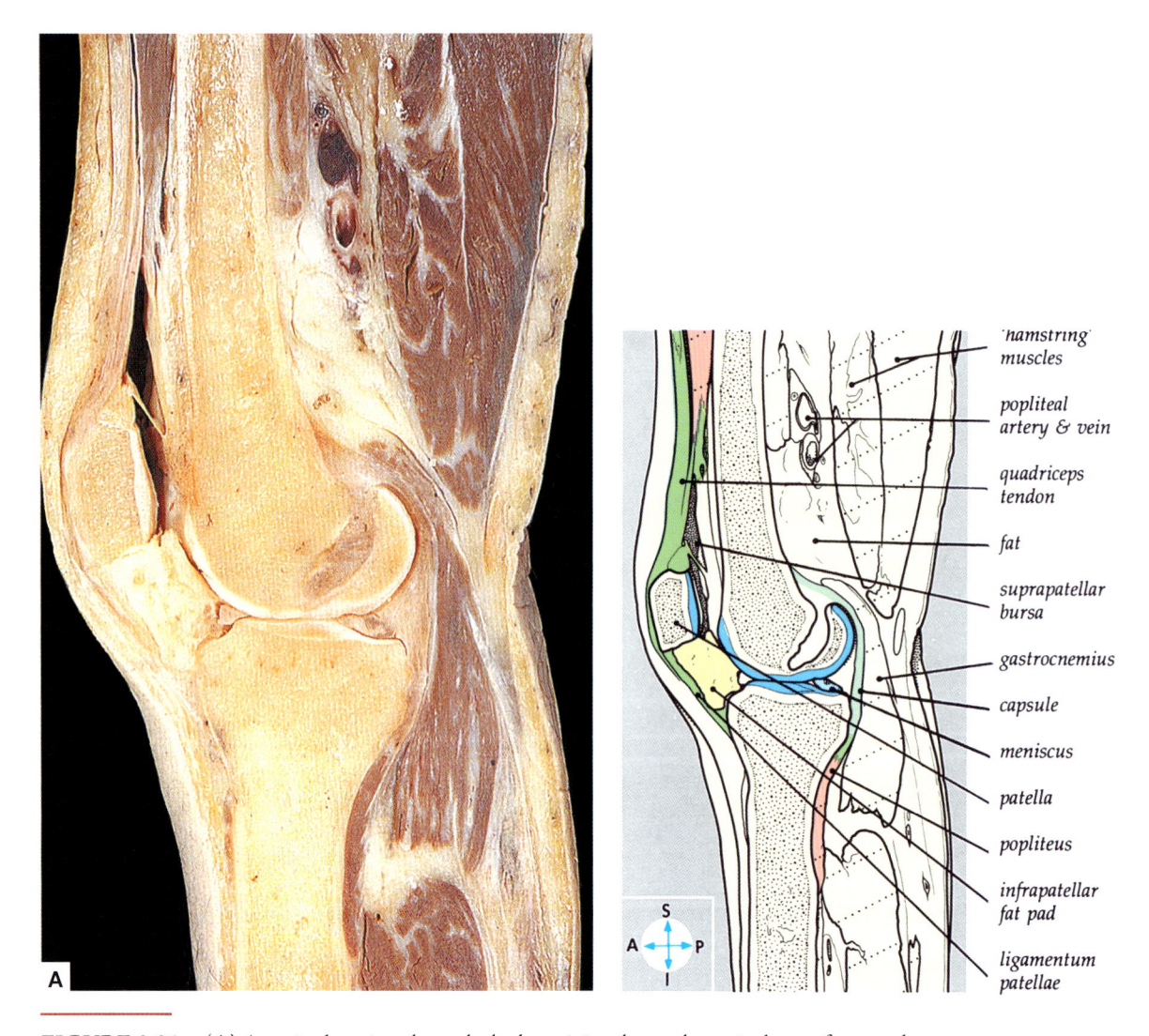

FIGURE 2.21 (**A**) A sagittal section through the knee joint shows the articular surfaces and suprapatellar pouch.

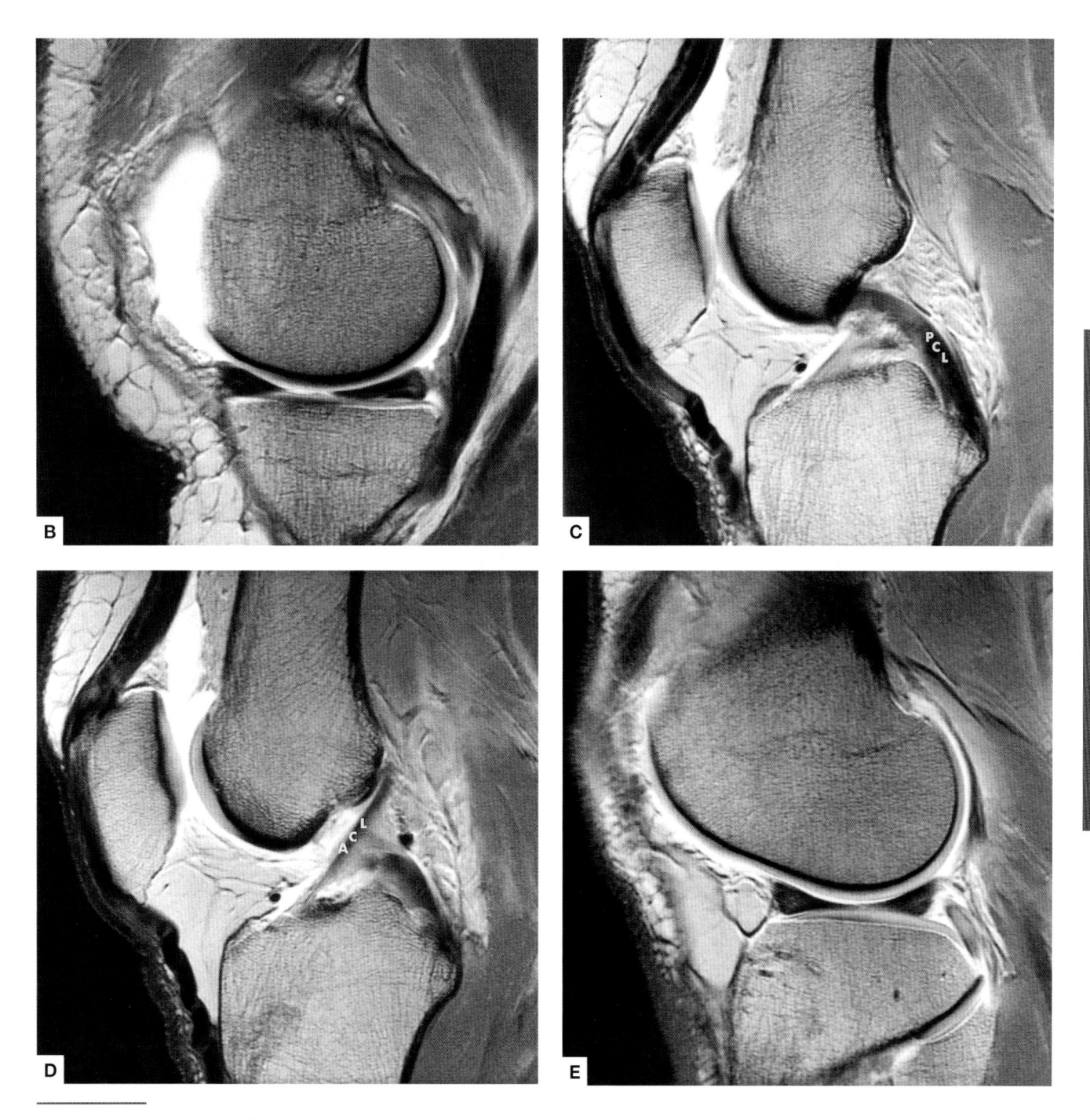

FIGURE 2.21 *(Continued)* Representative sagittal MR arthrographic images through the medial compartment (**B**), PCL (**C**), ACL (**D**), and lateral compartment (**E**).

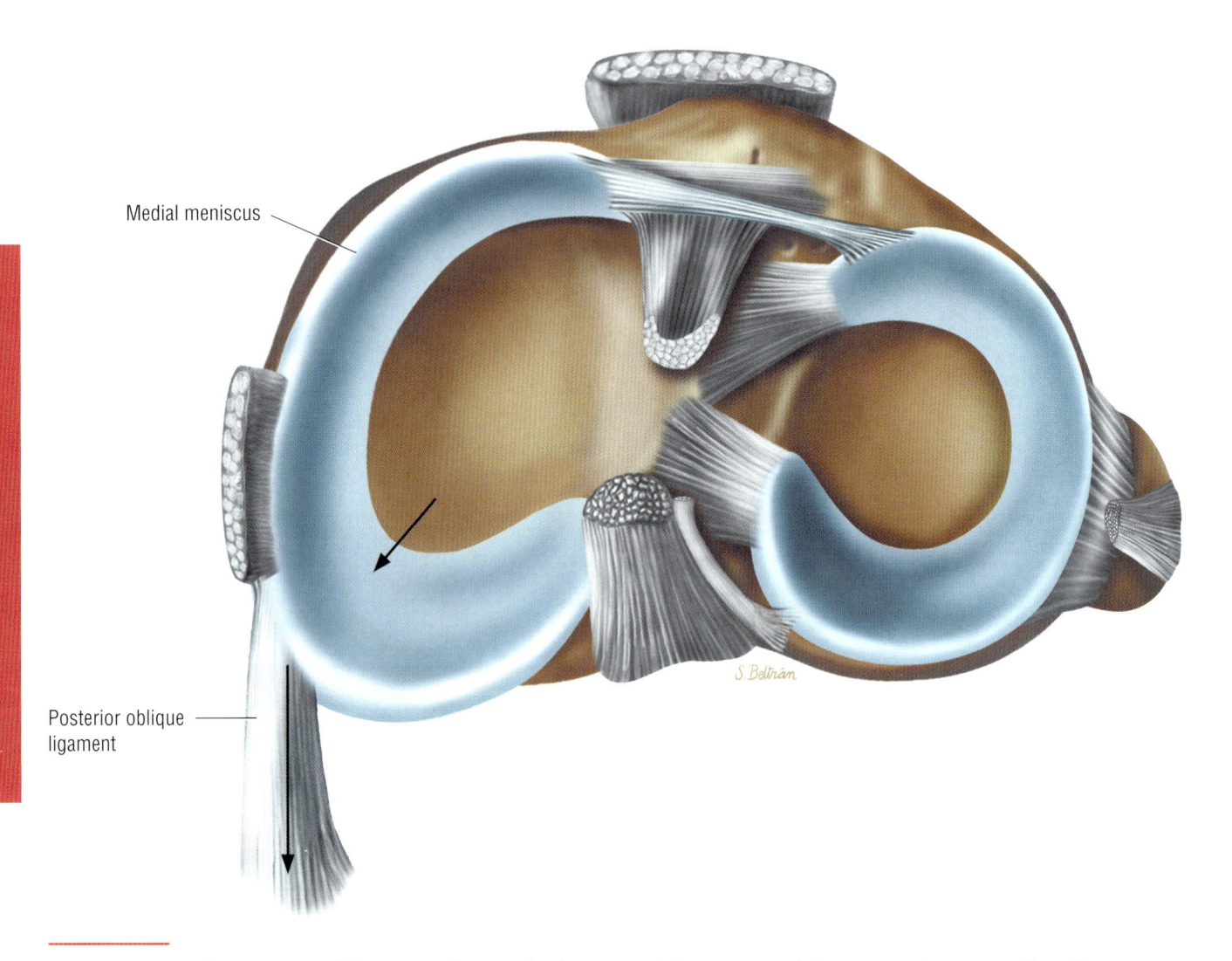

FIGURE 2.22 Superior view of the menisci showing the dynamic stabilizing action of the semimembranosus pull on the posterior oblique ligament. Tension of the posterior oblique ligament assists in posterior medial retraction.

Knee Anatomy

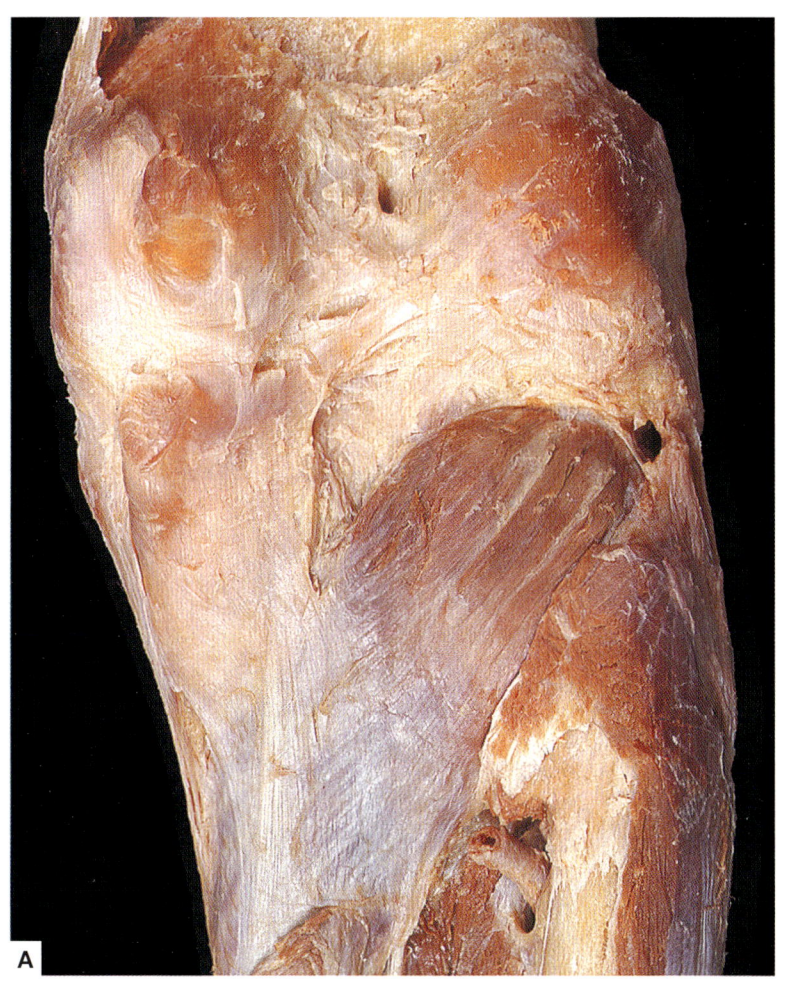

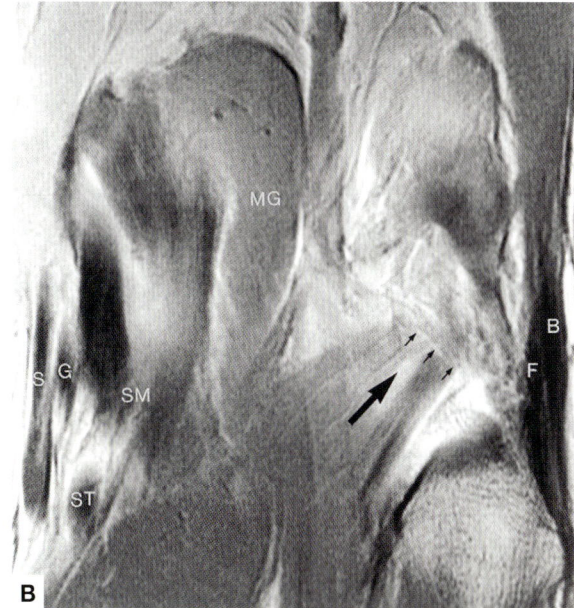

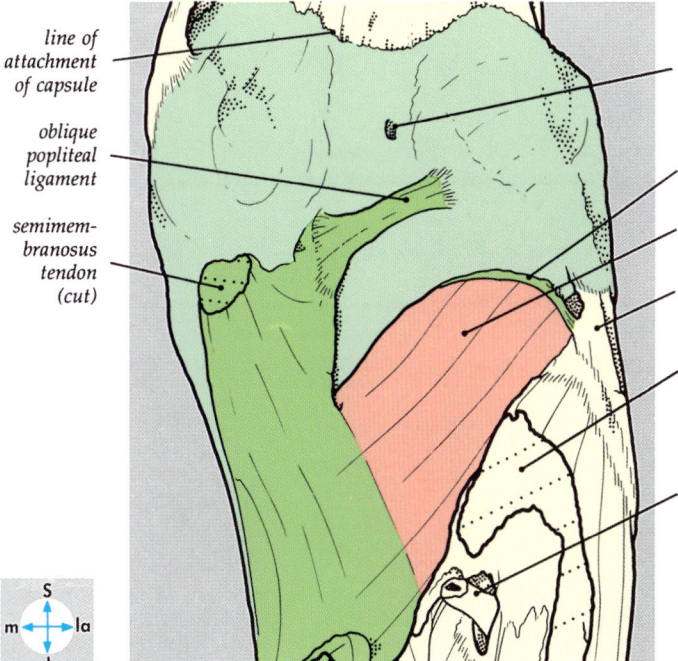

FIGURE 2.23 (**A**) Superficial dissection from the posterior aspect reveals the capsule, semimembranosus insertion, oblique popliteal ligament, popliteus tendon, and arcuate ligament. The oblique popliteal ligament is a tendinous expansion of the semimembranosus muscle. The arcuate ligament arches over the popliteus muscle. (**B**) Posterior coronal image identifying the location of the arcuate ligament (*small arrows*) and popliteus muscle (*large arrow*). B, biceps femoris tendon; F, fibular collateral ligament; G, gracilis tendon; MG, medial head gastrocnemius muscle; S, sartorius tendon; SM, semimembranosus tendon; ST, semitendinosus tendon. (*Continued*)

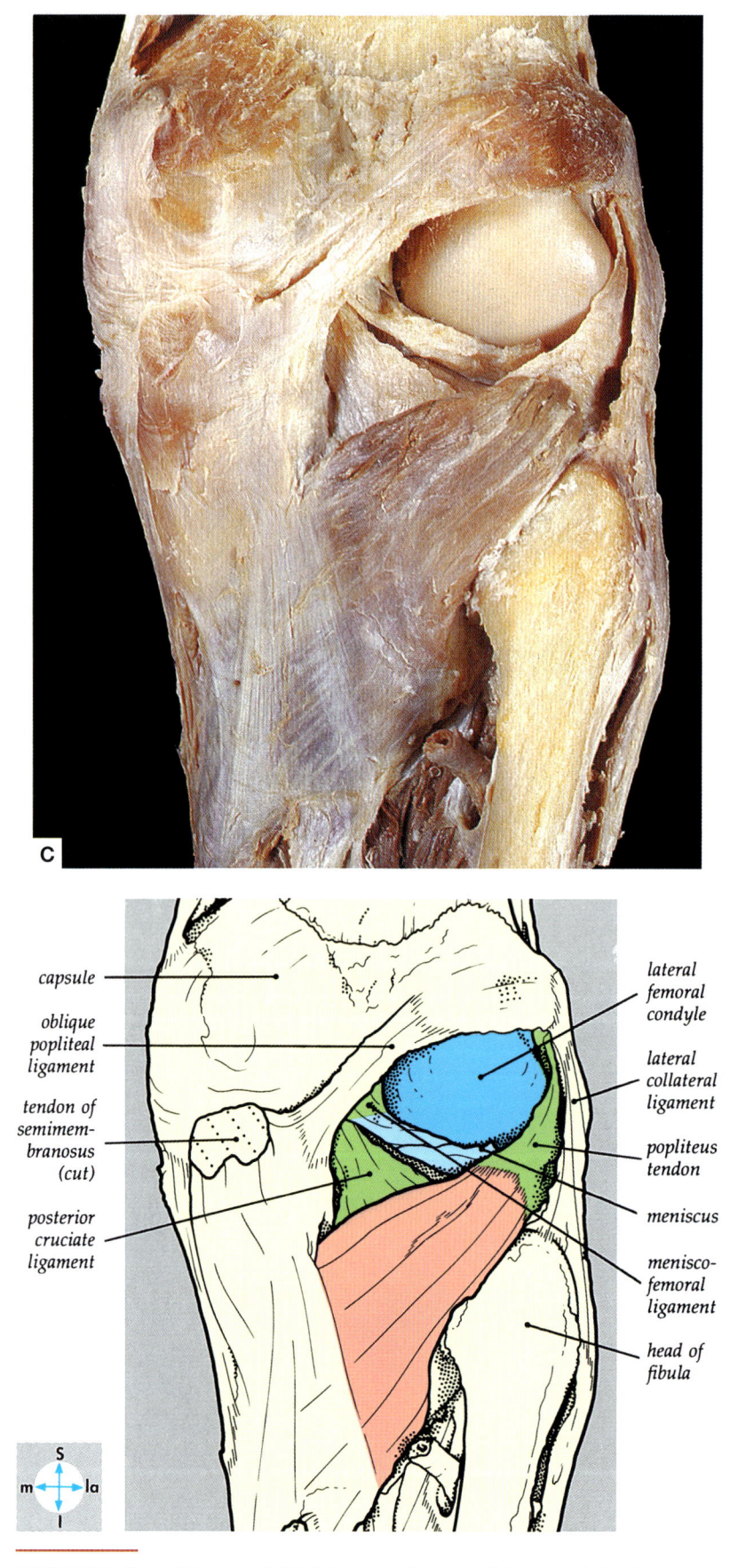

FIGURE 2.23 *(Continued)* (**C**) The posterior part of the capsule has been removed to reveal the meniscofemoral ligament, the PCL, and the popliteus tendon.

Knee Anatomy

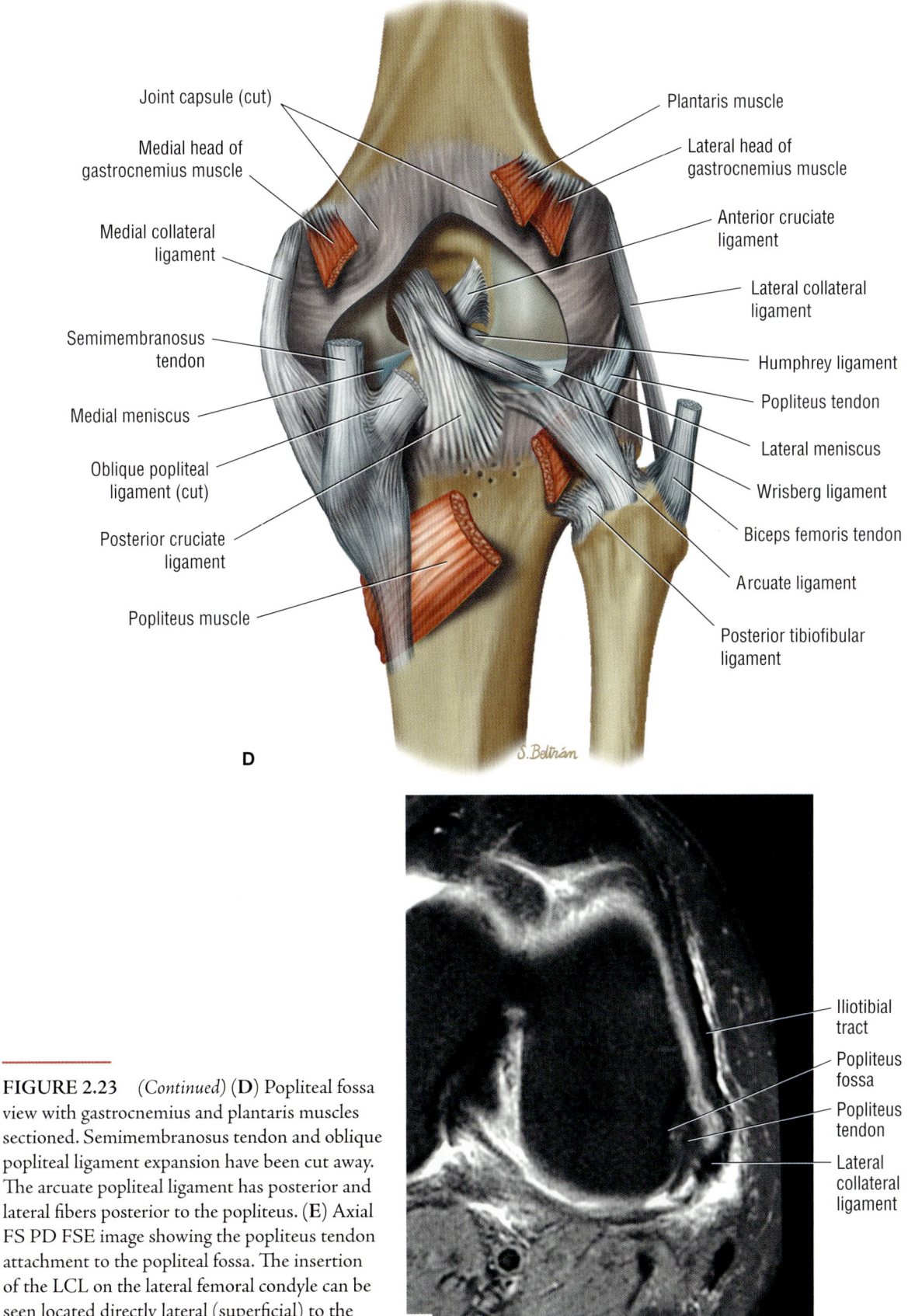

FIGURE 2.23 *(Continued)* **(D)** Popliteal fossa view with gastrocnemius and plantaris muscles sectioned. Semimembranosus tendon and oblique popliteal ligament expansion have been cut away. The arcuate popliteal ligament has posterior and lateral fibers posterior to the popliteus. **(E)** Axial FS PD FSE image showing the popliteus tendon attachment to the popliteal fossa. The insertion of the LCL on the lateral femoral condyle can be seen located directly lateral (superficial) to the popliteus tendon.

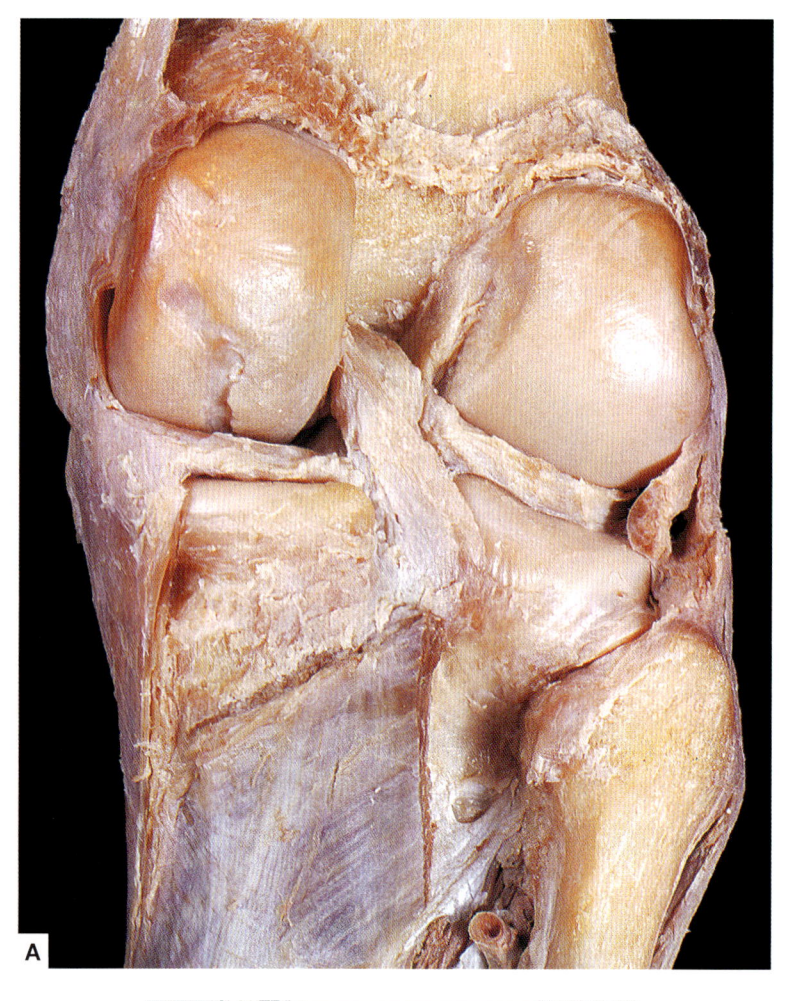

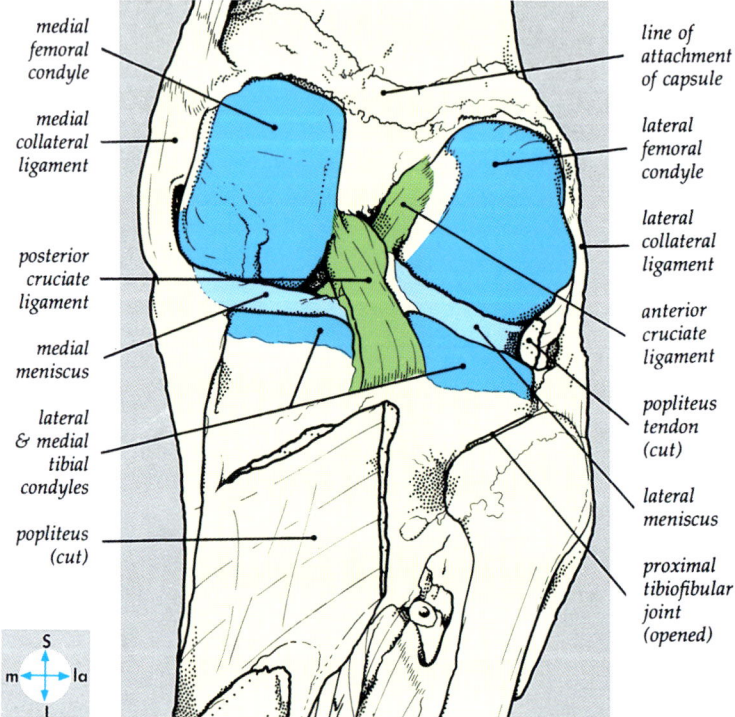

FIGURE 2.24 (**A**) The posterior part of the capsule has been removed to reveal the ACL, PCL, and menisci.

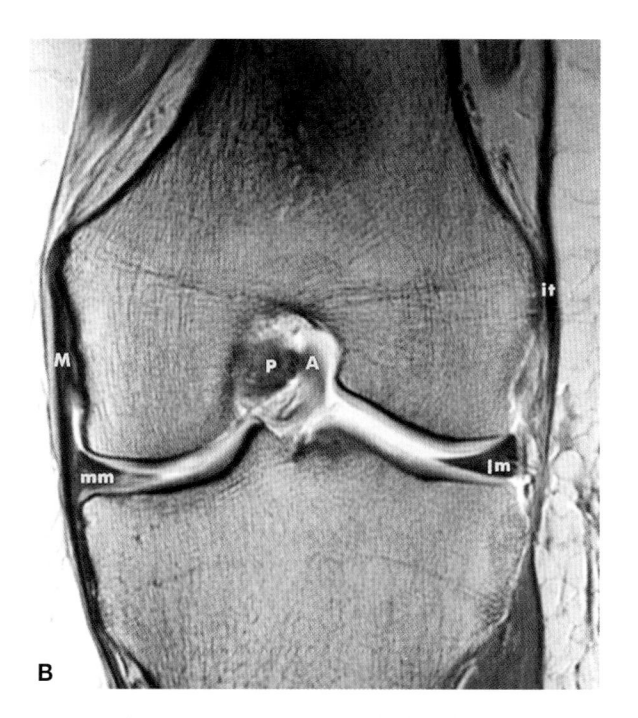

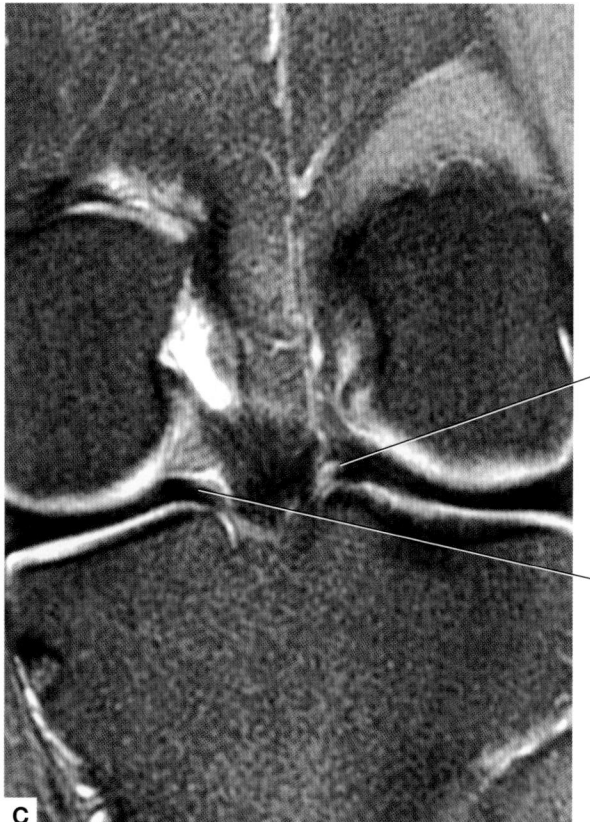

FIGURE 2.24 *(Continued)* (**B**) Coronal image obtained more anteriorly in the plane of the MCL (M) and iliotibial tract (it). A, ACL; lm, lateral meniscus; mm, medial meniscus; P, PCL. (**C**) Root attachment of the posterior horn of the medial and lateral menisci.

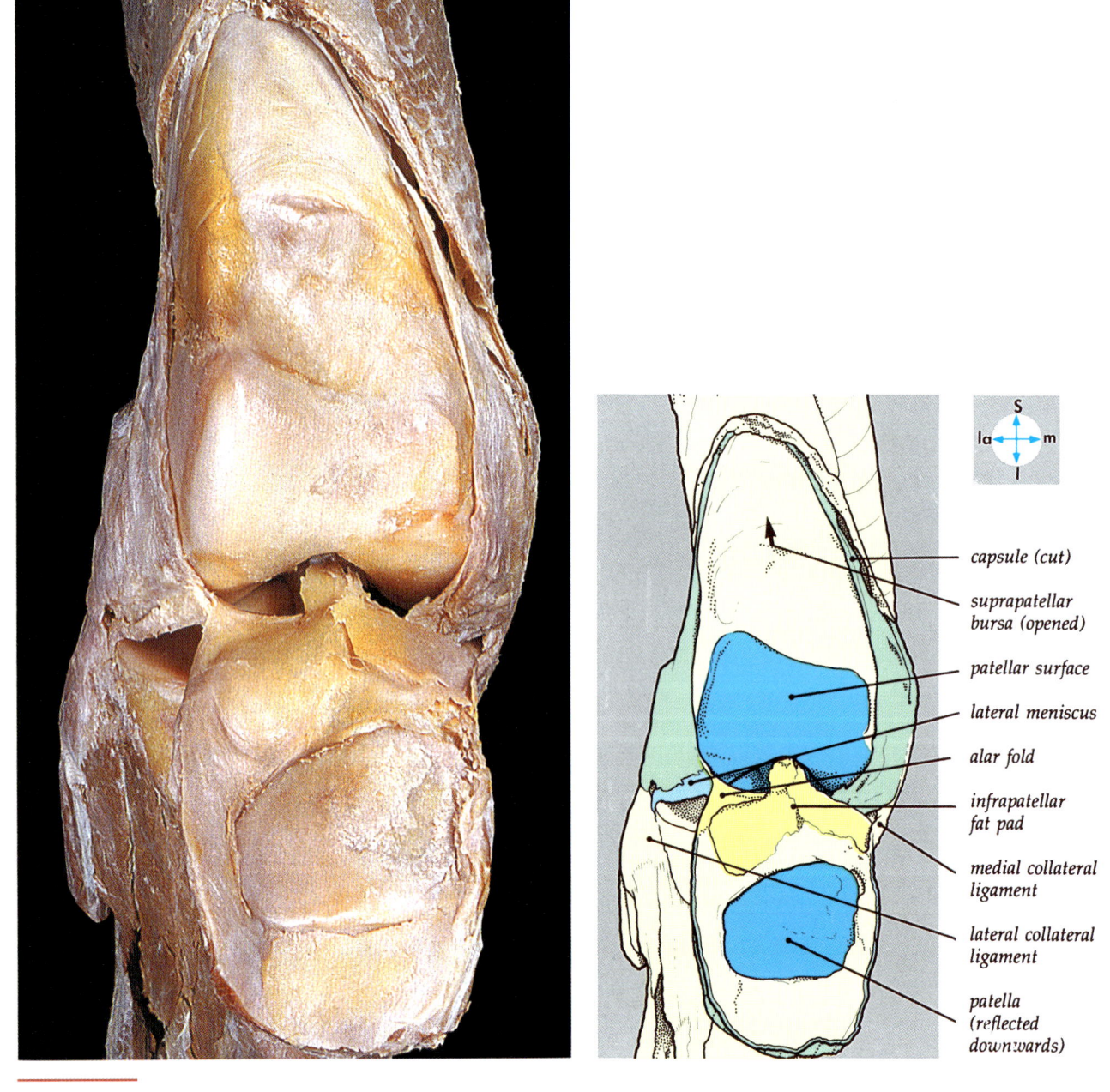

FIGURE 2.25 The interior of the joint and the suprapatellar pouch are exposed by opening the capsule anteriorly and reflecting the patella downward.

Knee Anatomy

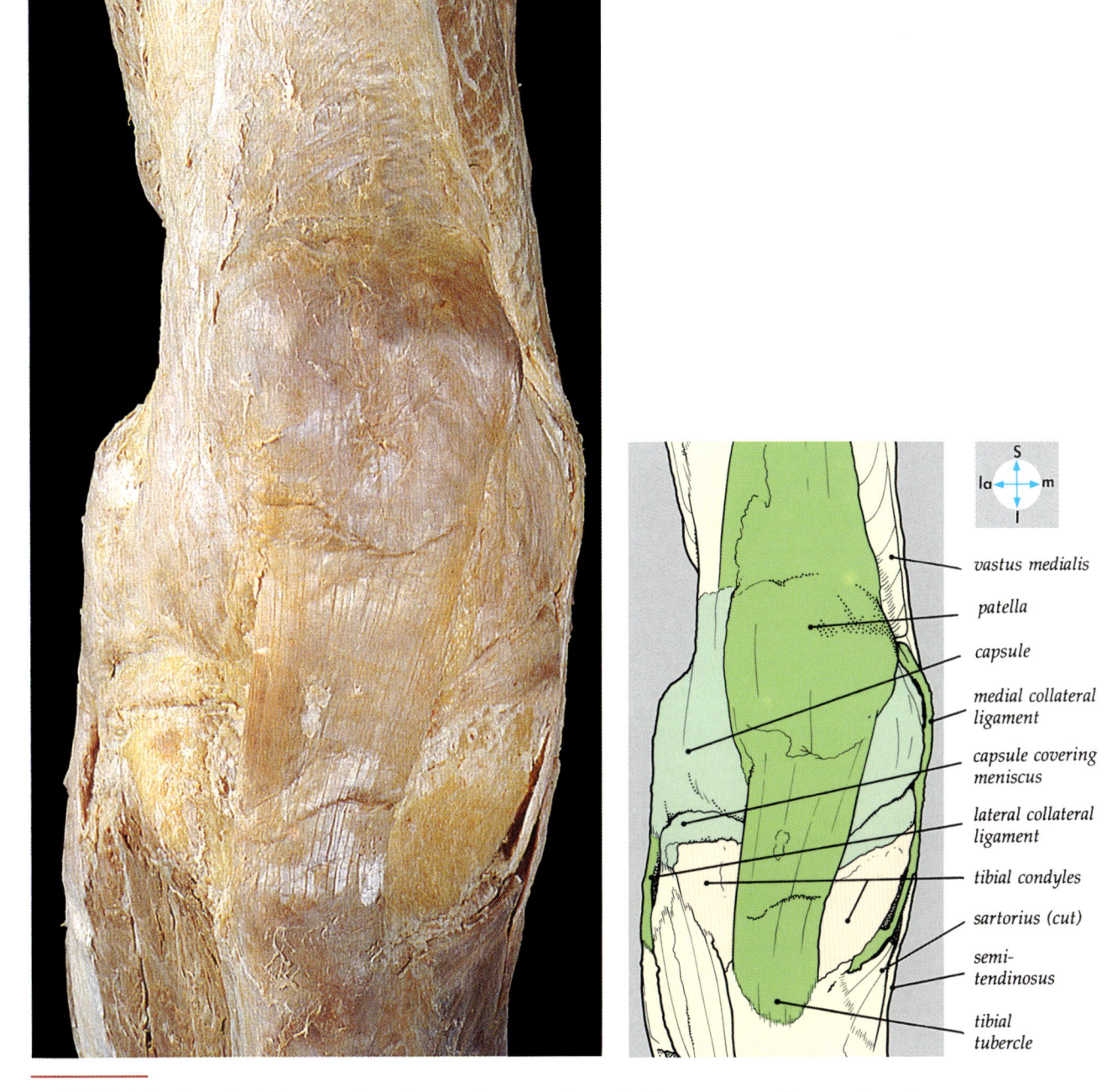

FIGURE 2.26 Superficial dissection from the anterior aspect shows the ligamentum patellae, capsule, and MCL and LCL.

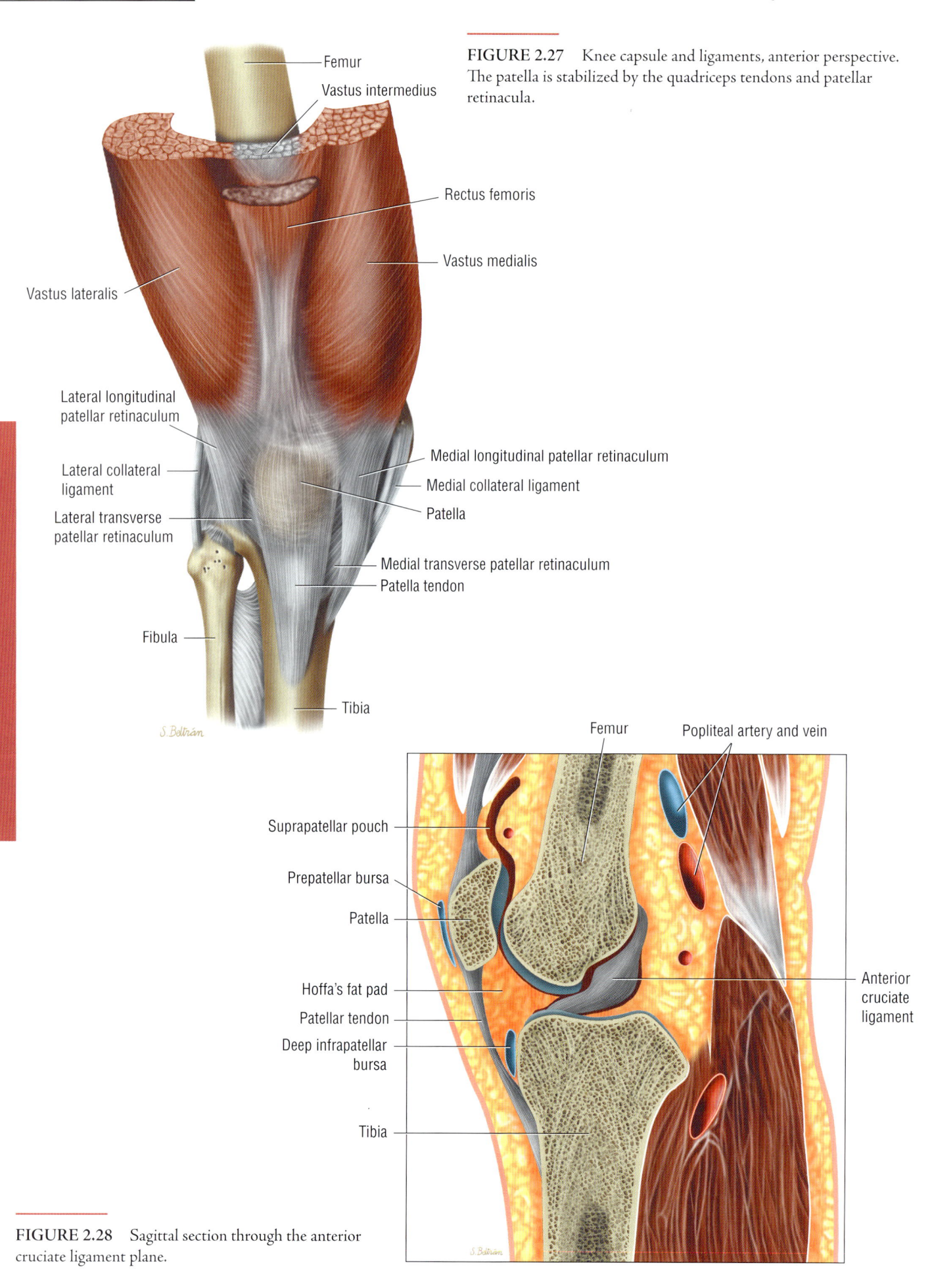

FIGURE 2.27 Knee capsule and ligaments, anterior perspective. The patella is stabilized by the quadriceps tendons and patellar retinacula.

FIGURE 2.28 Sagittal section through the anterior cruciate ligament plane.

Knee Anatomy

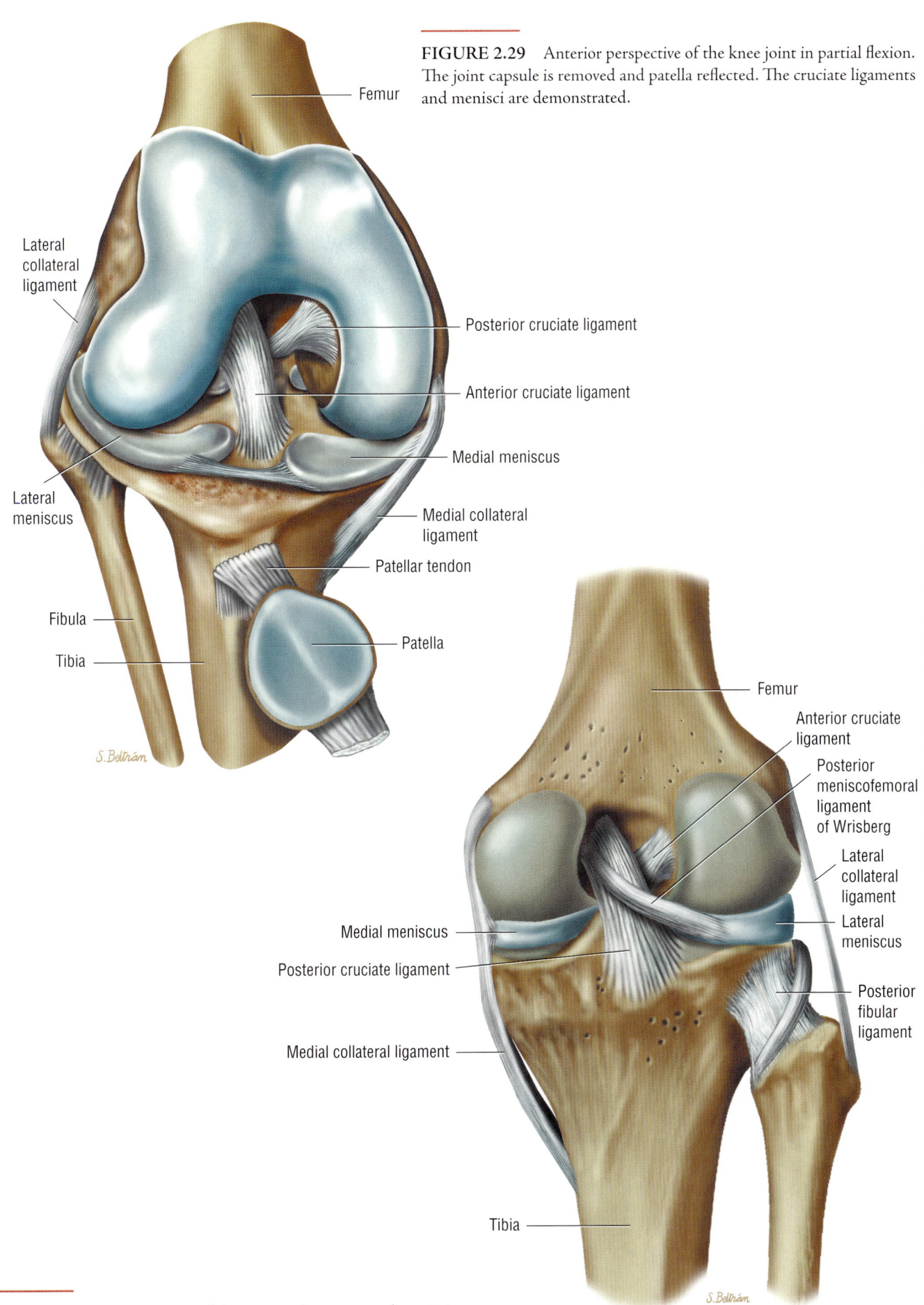

FIGURE 2.29 Anterior perspective of the knee joint in partial flexion. The joint capsule is removed and patella reflected. The cruciate ligaments and menisci are demonstrated.

FIGURE 2.30 Posterior view of the cruciate ligaments and menisci.

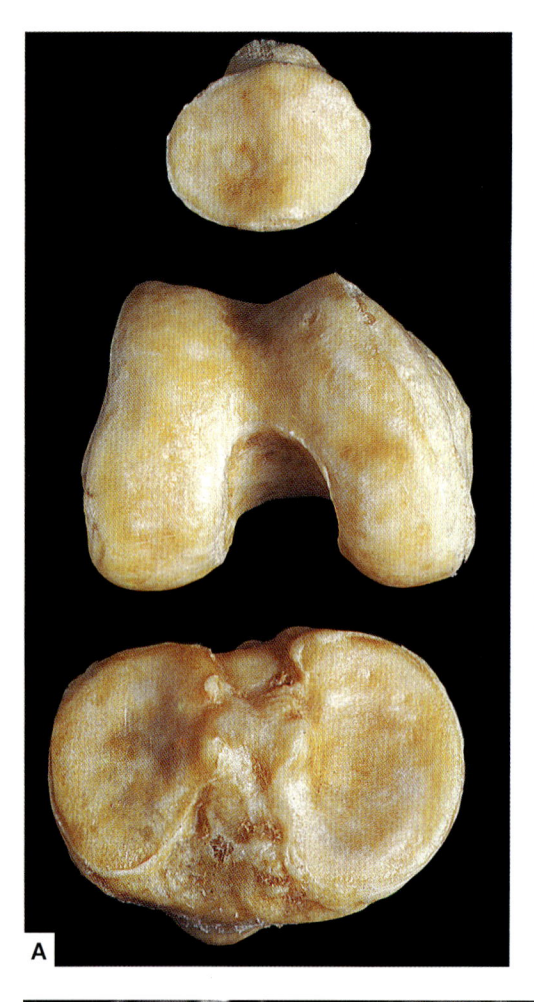

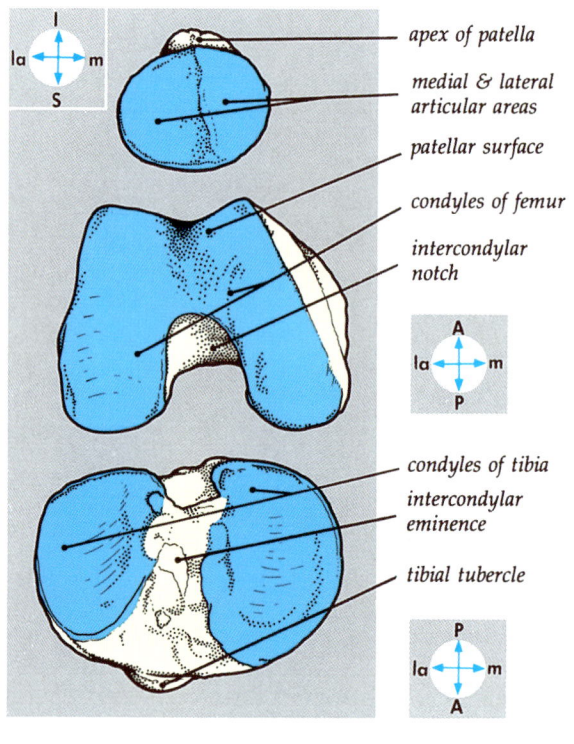

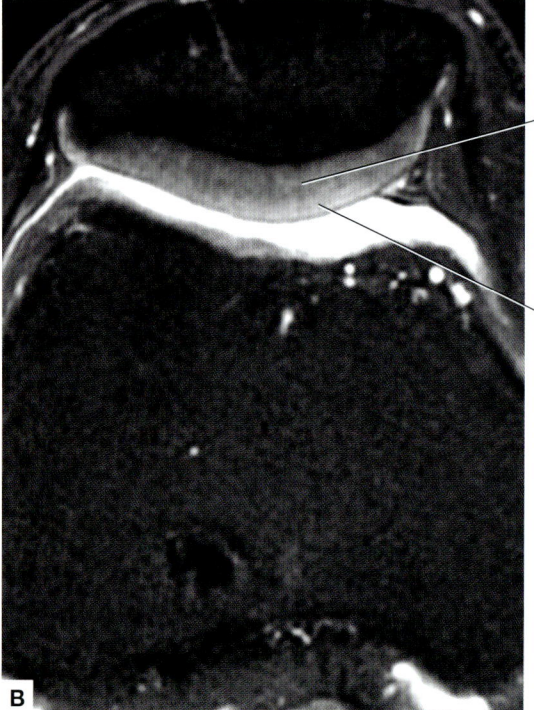

FIGURE 2.31 **(A)** Articular cartilage covers the posterior surface of the patella to the apex. The posterior surface of the patella demonstrates a smaller convex medial facet and larger concave lateral facet. When present, a secondary retropatellar crest subdivides the medial facet into the medial facet proper and an odd facet located between the medial facet proper and the lateral facet. The condylopatellar limiting grooves separate the tibial surfaces of the femoral condyles from the more anterosuperior femoral patellar surface, where the condyles fuse. The medial tibial plateau is concave, whereas the lateral plateau is convex on corresponding sagittal sections. **(B)** Axial FS PD FSE image showing the laminar display of patellar facet articular cartilage.

3
Stoller's Knee Checklist and Protocols

Coronal Plane Checklist (pages 98–102)

Sagittal Plane Checklist (pages 103–111)

Axial Plane Checklist (pages 112–116)

Protocols for Evaluation of the Meniscus (pages 146–148)

Application and Techniques for Routine Protocols (pages 149–150)

Stoller's Knee Checklist

Coronal

Medial Collateral Ligament
Lateral Collateral Ligament
Anterior Cruciate Ligament
Posterior Cruciate Ligament
Menisci
Articular Cartilage
Osseous and Marrow
Iliotibial Tract

Sagittal

Medial Meniscus
Lateral Meniscus and Posterolateral Corner
Articular Cartilage
Trochlear Groove
Anterior Cruciate Ligament
Posterior Cruciate Ligament
Posteromedial Corner
Patellar and Quadriceps Tendons
Subchondral Bone and Marrow
Hoffa's Fat Pad
Joint Effusion
Plicae

Axial

Patellar Facets and Trochlear Groove
Quadriceps and Patellar Tendon
Retinaculum
Cruciate Ligaments
Menisci
Medial Collateral Ligament
Lateral Collateral Ligament
Joint Fluid
Iliotibial Band and Posterolateral Corner

Stoller's Knee Checklist

Coronal Plane Checklist

Collateral Ligaments

- Medial Collateral Ligament (MCL)
    - The MCL is initially located on the image that demonstrates fusion of the medial and lateral femoral condyles.
    - On this image, the posterior aspect of the MCL is seen as a hypointense band of fibers extending along the peripheral aspect of the medial femoral condyle and medial tibial plateau.
    - Proceeding in an anterior direction, the entire posterior-to-anterior extent of the MCL is demonstrated over the next one or two images.
    - A coronal image through the intact posterior fibers of the MCL may not demonstrate a partial thickness tear, since these injuries preferentially involve the anterior fibers.
    - It is important to examine the entire course of the MCL from its origin on the medial femoral condyle to its distal insertion on the proximal tibial metaphysis, as tears can occur anywhere along this course.
- Lateral Collateral Ligament (LCL)
    - Identification of the LCL also starts with the image on which the femoral condyles fuse.
    - The origin of the LCL from the lateral femoral condyle is visualized on either this image or one image posterior to it.
    - Unlike the MCL, which has a nearly straight vertical course, the LCL runs posteriorly in an oblique inferior direction.
    - Proceeding in a posterior direction, it is demonstrated in its entire course, to the attachment of the LCL at the tip of the fibular head, over two images.

Cruciate Ligaments

- Anterior Cruciate Ligament (ACL)
    - Identification of the ACL starts with the image that demonstrates the femoral condyles fusing.
    - Proceeding for two or three images in a posterior direction, the origin of the ACL is identified along the medial margin of the lateral femoral condyle.
    - From this image location, proceeding in an anterior direction, the entire posterior-to-anterior course of the ACL is demonstrated over the next five or six images.
    - The ACL follows an inferior oblique course to its insertion on the anterior tibia. Individual fibers of the normal ACL can be distinguished (taut and dark), separated by bands of intermediate- to high-signal-intensity normal synovium.
        - ACL is composed of an anteromedial (AM) and posterolateral (PL) bundle
    - Scarred, degenerated, or sprained ACL fibers are indistinct, thickened, or increased in signal intensity.
    - At the site of an acute tear, the fibers are replaced by edema, hemorrhage, or synovitis.
    - Fibers proximal and distal to the tear appear wavy, lax, and edematous.
- Posterior Cruciate Ligament (PCL)
    - The origin of the PCL, at the anterior lateral aspect of the medial femoral condyle, can be identified on or near the same image as the distal insertion of the ACL.
    - On coronal images, proximal PCL fibers are in cross-section.
    - Progressing in a posterior direction for four or five images, the PCL fibers can be seen to gradually turn 90 degrees and course vertically downward to their insertion on the posterior tibia.
    - Enclosed in its own synovial sheath
    - Always supplement coronal image evaluation by identifying PCL integrity on sagittal images in three separate locations:
        - Femoral attachment
        - Central or middle third
        - Tibial attachment

Menisci

- The posterior horns of the menisci are identified on the coronal image on which the fibula first comes into view.

- The meniscal root ligaments:
    - Thin, short, hypointense fibrous bands
    - Extend from the inner margins of the posterior horns to where they attach centrally near the tibial spines

- The root is a frequent location for radial tears.
    - Disrupt the root attachment
    - Undermine the meniscal hoop containment fibers, which keep the meniscus from extruding peripherally with joint loading

- The body segments of the menisci are demonstrated on coronal images anterior to the level of the fibula.

- Continuing in an anterior direction, the anterior horns can be seen at the margins of the anterior edge of the tibia.

- Normal anterior horn and body segments appear on coronal images as black triangles with sharp tips, which represent the inner free edge.

- There is no increased signal interrupting either the superior or inferior articular surface of the meniscus.

- On coronal images, displaced flaps of meniscal tissue are seen as meniscal tissue protruding either from the body segment into the coronary or meniscofemoral recesses or from the posterior horn toward the tibial spines.

- A triangle of missing tissue near the free edge on the undersurface or inferior leaflet of the meniscus is characteristic of a flap tear.

- If seen, the coronary recess, meniscofemoral recess, and intercondylar notch should be carefully examined to identify a displaced flap of meniscal tissue corresponding to the area of deficient meniscal fibrocartilage.

- Arthroscopic probing determines location, size, and stability of a meniscal tear.
    - Meniscal extrusion in the coronal plane is associated with an unstable meniscal tear (e.g., root tear, radial tear from free edge to periphery with circumferential zone involvement).
    - Meniscal extrusion also seen with articular cartilage loss in the absence of a meniscal tear

Articular Cartilage

- Cartilage can be seen covering the medial and lateral tibial plateau and distal femur.
- The anterior horns of the menisci are the landmarks for demarcating cartilage compartments on coronal images.
- Cartilage that covers the femoral condyle and tibial plateau is classified as medial or lateral compartment cartilage located posterior to the anterior horns.
- Cartilage that covers the distal anterior femur (i.e., the trochlear groove) on images anterior to the anterior horns is referred to as "trochlear groove" cartilage and is part of the patellofemoral compartment.
- In the medial and lateral compartments, cartilage covers the mid-weight-bearing surfaces of both the tibial plateau and femoral condyle, which contact each other in extension.
- The cartilage surface continues posteriorly along the posterior surface of the femoral condyle, which contacts the tibia in flexion.
  - It is necessary to examine the entire cartilage surface from anterior to posterior.
- Chondral abnormalities of the posterior femoral condyle are easily overlooked if the posterior cartilage surfaces are not carefully evaluated.
- Cartilage is inspected for chondral fissures, erosions, fibrillation, thinning, defects, and flap formation.
- The underlying subchondral bone is also examined to identify reactive bone marrow edema or cystic change subjacent to areas of chondral erosion.
- Evaluation of the articular cartilage surfaces includes examination of the joint spaces for loose bodies originating from sites of chondral defects or erosions.
- Chondral degeneration commonly located posteromedial aspect of the lateral tibial plateau and lateral aspect of the medial femoral condyle.
  - Articular cartilage lesions can be intrasubstance, partial or full thickness injuries.
  - Chondral surface area of involvement is focal or diffuse.

- Loose bodies vary in appearance and can manifest as tiny spots of debris; free-floating thin, elongated, intermediate intensity cartilage fragments; cartilage bodies with varying amounts of subchondral bone attached; or predominantly osseous fragments of varying sizes and shapes.

- On coronal images, loose bodies are often identified along the posterior joint line posterior to the PCL and menisci, along the anterior joint line anterior to the ACL, and within the patellofemoral recesses between the patella and distal femur.

Osseous Structures

- The cortical, subchondral, and trabecular bone are examined for the presence of fractures, contusions, stress-related edema, infection, osteonecrosis, or neoplasms.
    - Evaluate fat marrow on either a T1-weighted or PD-weighted image (adjust contrast and density to stimulate T1-weighting) when interpreting PD- or intermediate weighted images.

Iliotibial Tract

- The distal attachment of the iliotibial tract (ITT or ITB) is visualized at the anterolateral margin of the tibial plateau (called Gerdy's tubercle).
    - The tendon is identified on at least four or five consecutive coronal images.
    - Origin at iliac crest (fascial components of gluteus maximus, gluteus medius, and tensor fasciae latae)
    - Fibrous connection between ITB and intermuscular septum; continuous with lateral patellar retinaculum
    - The lateral synovial and vascularized fatty tissue occupies the space between the femur and the ITB.
    - ITB functions as a lateral hip stabilizer resisting hip adduction.

- The normal iliotibial tract should appear taut and thin. Focal thickening suggests scarring, and in the proper clinical setting, high-signal-intensity edema and synovitis deep to the tendon is associated with iliotibial band (ITB) friction syndrome.

Sagittal Plane Checklist

Medial and Lateral Menisci

- The body of the meniscus is identified between the femoral condyle and tibial plateau on peripheral images through the medial or lateral compartment.

- The body segment is bow tie–shaped.

- A small gap in the middle portion of the bow tie indicates a free edge radial tear of the body segment.

- An eccentric gap, off to one side of the bow tie, indicates a free edge radial tear involving the junction of the body with the anterior or posterior horn.

- In meniscal flap tears, the first sagittal image on which the peripheral aspect of the body segment is seen is useful for visualizing flaps of meniscal tissue displaced either into the coronary or meniscofemoral recess.

- The anterior and posterior horns of the meniscus appear as black triangles with a sharp inner free edge.

- The root of the posterior horn can be identified in the peripheral aspect of the medial or lateral compartment, approaching the intercondylar notch.

- A radial tear through the root of the posterior horn appears as a "ghost meniscus," with absence of meniscal signal in the expected location of the posterior horn root.

- The "ghost meniscus" appearance is due to localization of the sagittal image in a plane directly through the gap in the posterior horn meniscal tissue caused by the radial tear.

- Zone description of meniscal anatomic location includes:
    - Anterior (anterior horn)
    - Body
    - Posterior (posterior horn)
    - Peripheral
    - Middle
    - Central (free edge)

Medial and Lateral Compartment Articular Cartilage

- Cartilage covers the medial and lateral femoral condyles from anterior to posterior.

- The anterior meniscal horn demarcates the division between the trochlear groove cartilage (located anterior to the anterior horn) and the femoral condyle cartilage (located at and posterior to the anterior horn).

- Covering the mid-weight-bearing surfaces of the femoral condyles, the cartilage extends posteriorly past the level of the posterior horn of the meniscus and posterosuperiorly to cover the extreme posterior aspect of the femoral condyle subjacent to the gastrocnemius tendon origins.

- The extreme posterior part of the femoral condyle becomes the weight-bearing surface when the knee is in flexion.

- Chondral abnormalities may be seen anywhere along the articular surface. Cartilage also covers the articular surfaces of the medial and lateral tibial plateau.

- After examination of the cartilage for chondral abnormalities, the underlying subchondral bone is inspected for reactive bone marrow edema and cystic change, and the joint recesses are evaluated for the presence of loose bodies.

- Chondral lesions are associated with joint synovitis.
    - Irregular contour of Hoffa's fat pad
    - Intermediate-weighted synovial thickening surrounded by hyperintense joint fluid on fluid sensitive images

- Outerbridge classification
    - Grade 0 (normal cartilage) to Grade 4 (exposed subchondral bone)

- International Cartilage Repair Society (ICRS) articular cartilage classification
    - Grade 0: normal
    - Grade 1: softening or blisters with focal convexity
    - Grade 2: less than 50% depth of cartilage layers
    - Grade 3: more than 50% depth of cartilage layers
    - Grade 4: full depth with extension to subchondral bone

Trochlear Groove Cartilage

- The trochlear groove is a V-shaped concave notch formed by the inward sloping contour of the anterior-inferior medial and lateral femoral condyles.

- The concave surfaces of the trochlear groove articulates with the convex surfaces of the patella.

- On sagittal images, any cartilage covering the femoral condyles anterior to the anterior horns of the menisci is considered trochlear groove cartilage.

- Anatomically, the trochlear groove comprises medial, mid, and lateral articular surfaces.

- The entire extent of the trochlear groove chondral surface from medial to lateral can be examined on sagittal images.

- Cartilage covers three anatomic regions of the patella.
    - The lateral articular surface of the patella is called the lateral patellar facet, the central portion is called the median ridge, and the medial articular surface is referred to as the medial facet.

- As a rule, the median ridge cartilage is identified on midline sagittal images, the medial facet cartilage is visualized medial to the midline, and the lateral facet cartilage is seen lateral to the midline.
    - This rule does not apply in cases of patellar subluxation.

- The median ridge cartilage can also be identified by finding the sagittal image through the thickest portion of the patella in the anteroposterior dimension.

- Patella is engaged in the trochlea at about 40 degrees of knee flexion.

- Proximal lateral portal used at arthroscopy for visualization of the patellofemoral joint

- More accurate to evaluate trochlear groove first on sagittal images and then secondarily on axial images because of issues of partial volume effect of mistaking normal suprapatellar fat for an area of chondral erosion.

Anterior and Posterior Cruciate Ligaments

- The entire course of the ACL and PCL can be seen on two or three midline sagittal images.

- Complete acute tears are characterized with respect to involvement of:
  - The origin
  - Proximal third
  - Middle third
  - Distal attachment

- Full thickness tears present as complete discontinuity of ACL or PCL fibers.

- Sprains are characterized by continuous fibers traversing the entire length of the notch.

- In the case of ACL scarring, fibers also appear lax or indistinct.

- Sagittal images should also be examined for anterior translation of the tibia beneath the femur, since this presentation indicates ACL insufficiency from previous injury or scarring.

- ACL insufficiency can exist even though the ACL appears continuous on magnetic resonance (MR) images, due to laxity of scarred fibers or scarring of a previously torn ACL to the PCL mimicking an intact ACL appearance.
  - The anterior leading edge of the ACL represents the anteromedial bundle on sagittal images when the knee is positioned in extension.

- Since sagittal images section the ACL in an oblique plane, ACL fibers should always be assessed first in the coronal plane.

- The two separate anteromedial and posterolateral bundles are often more difficult to discern on sagittal compared to coronal images.

- Meniscofemoral ligaments include the ligament of Humphrey (anterior to the PCL) and the ligament of Wrisberg (posterior to the PCL). These meniscofemoral ligaments course from the posterior horn of the lateral meniscus to the respective portions of the PCL insertion.

Posteromedial and Posterolateral Corners

- Sagittal imaging is used to assess the structures of the posteromedial corner, including:
    - Tendons
    - Ligaments
    - Capsular structures that traverse the posterior medial quadrant of the knee
- Individual tendons are not always depicted on each MR image. The *MCL* is seen on the most peripheral sagittal image.
- The origin of the *semimembranosus* is at the posteromedial margin of the medial tibial plateau.
- The origin of the medial head of the *gastrocnemius* is at the posteromedial margin of the medial femoral condyle metaphysis.
- The *meniscotibial* and *meniscofemoral ligaments* (aka *meniscocapsular ligaments*) are seen along the entire course of the posteromedial corner, fanning out and away from the posterior edge of the posterior horn of the medial meniscus.
- The meniscocapsular ligaments are also visualized extending along the anteromedial quadrant to form a full arc around the entire course of the meniscus.
- Meniscocapsular separation and tears:
    - Characterized by fluid signal interrupting the normally dark to intermediate strands of meniscocapsular ligament
    - Can occur at any point along the course of the ligaments
- MCL exists in two layers:
    - Deep MCL (dMCL)
    - Superficial MCL (sMCL)
- Three principal structures of the posteromedial corner:
    - dMCL, sMCL, and the posteromedial capsule (PMC)
- Dynamic stabilization of the medial aspect of the knee includes the hamstring muscles.
    - Semimembranosus and semitendinosus

- **Posterolateral Corner:** The most peripheral image through the posterolateral corner demonstrates the V-shaped convergence of the *fibular collateral ligament* (anterior limb of the "V") and the distal *biceps femoris tendon* fibula.
    - On the next image, the origin of the *popliteus tendon* along the posterolateral aspect of the lateral femoral condyle is displayed.
    - The *popliteofibular ligament* may be displayed on this same image.
- The arcuate ligament is posterior to the popliteus tendon.
    - Medial limb of the arcuate ligament
- The lateral meniscocapsular ligaments extend from the peripheral edge of the lateral meniscus.
    - Mid-third lateral capsular ligament
- Iliotibial band or tract is a consistent landmark over the posterolateral corner.
- Long head of the biceps femoris
    - Direct and anterior arms
- Short head of the biceps femoris
    - Direct arm, capsular arm (distal capsular arm = fabellofibular ligament), and anterior arm (attaches to posterior aspect meniscotibial portion of the mid-third lateral capsular ligament)
    - Short head avulsed with osseous or soft tissue Segond fractures of the tibia
- Lateral gastrocnemius tendon
    - Blends into meniscofemoral portion of the posterolateral capsule
- Popliteus complex (posterolateral rotary stabilizer)
    - Three popliteomeniscal fascicles:
        - Anteroinferior (strongest)
        - Posterosuperior
        - Posteroinferior
- Coronary ligament to the lateral meniscus
    - Meniscotibial portion of the posterior capsule from the popliteomeniscal fascicles to the root attachment of the posterior horn

Patellar and Quadriceps Tendons

- The distal quadriceps tendon and the entire course of the patellar tendon can be seen on five or six consecutive sagittal images through the patella.

- All sagittal images displaying tendon tissue should be examined carefully, since partial tears and tendinosis occasionally involve only the peripheral margin of the tendons.

- Distal quadriceps tendinosis is characterized by thickening and increased signal intensity at the distal quadriceps insertion on the superior pole of the patella.

- Patellar tendinosis commonly occurs at the proximal origin of the patellar tendon on the inferior pole of the patella.

- Patellar tendon inflammation:
  - Associated with Osgood-Schlatter disease
  - Displayed on sagittal images at the distal insertion of the patellar tendon on the tibial tubercle

- Patella baja and patella alta are diagnosed on sagittal images based on the relative position of the patella (and length of the patellar tendon) with respect to the femur.

Subchondral Bone and Marrow

- The subchondral bone surfaces and marrow of the femoral condyles, tibial plateau, and patella are examined for the presence of edema, fractures, or masses.

- In chondromalacia, reactive bone marrow edema can be seen in the subchondral bone directly underlying the areas of significant chondral abnormality.
  - Subchondral edema may be associated with either basilar degeneration or with full thickness grade 4 chondral loss.

- In fractures, the degree of displacement or depression of the subchondral plate is quantified, and injuries to the overlying cartilage are documented.
  - Posttraumatic chondral hyperintensity may develop into articular cartilage breakdown and fragmentation.

Joint Fluid/Effusion

- On sagittal images, joint effusions are most prominently displayed:
  - Anterior to the medial and lateral femoral condyles (in the medial and lateral patellofemoral recesses, respectively)
  - In the midline between and above the patella and femur (suprapatellar bursa)
- Smaller collections of joint fluid can be seen in the recesses around the menisci and in the intercondylar notch around the cruciate ligaments.
  - Joint effusions extending just posterior to Hoffa's fat pad are classified as small.
- Large joint effusions extend superiorly into the suprapatellar bursa, above the patella.
- Simple joint effusions are surrounded by normal, thin, well-defined synovium.
- Circumscribed by thickened, shaggy, often frond-like inflamed synovium in the presence of synovitis
- A small amount of joint fluid can be physiologic.
- All joint effusions should be examined for loose osseous or chondral bodies and debris.
- An irregular free edge contour of Hoffa's fat pad is associated with inflammation of the overlying synovial reflection and is a secondary sign of synovitis.
  - Primary sign of synovial thickening visualized as intermediate signal in thickened synovium adjacent to hyperintense fluid on a fluid sensitive sequence
- Classify popliteal cysts as typical (adjacent to medial head gastrocnemius) or atypical (lateral or other location without apparent communication with the knee joint).
  - Use intravenous contrast to show peripheral and not central enhancement if the atypical cyst contains fluid.
  - Central enhancement of an atypical cyst requires further investigation to exclude a more aggressive process (e.g., sarcoma)

Hoffa's Fat Pad

- On sagittal images, Hoffa's fat pad appears as a triangle of fat bounded:
  - Superiorly by the patella
  - Inferiorly by the tibial tubercle
  - Posteriorly by the anterior horns of the menisci
- Irregularity of the posterior margin of Hoffa's fat pad, with strands of joint fluid extending into its posterior aspect, indicates synovitis.
- Focal fat pad edema is indicative of a tight lateral retinaculum.
  - Causes painful entrapment of the fat pad between the lateral patellar facet and lateral trochlear groove
- The posterior aspect of Hoffa's fat pad is a typical location for localized pigmented villonodular synovitis.
  - This should not be mistaken for a sarcoma.
- Postoperatively, the fat pad should be inspected for scarring.
- Mass-like scarring suggests arthrofibrosis, a painful postoperative condition that can cause limited range of motion.

Plicae

- Three varieties of plicae are common, but not present in all patients.
- The infrapatellar plica:
  - Depicted on midline sagittal images and appears as a U-shaped band of intermediate or dark fibers originating from the anterior intercondylar notch (anterior to the ACL), extending downward and anteriorly into Hoffa's fat pad
  - May be associated with trochlear groove chondromalacia and, in such instances, may be resected
- The suprapatellar plica is located at the superior aspect of the suprapatellar bursa on midline sagittal images.
  - May be visualized merging imperceptibly with a *medial plica* that traverses the medial patellofemoral recess

Axial Plane Checklist

Patellofemoral Compartment

- The primary structures reviewed on axial images are in the patellofemoral compartment.

- The medial patellar facet, median ridge, and lateral patellar facet cartilages are clearly demonstrated.

- The full superior–inferior extent of the patellar cartilage is demonstrated on consecutive axial images.

- It is more difficult to distinguish trochlear groove cartilage from adjacent synovium and Hoffa's fat pad on axial images.

- Overlap with adjacent synovium may produce false-positive trochlear groove fissuring on axial images.

- The medial plica, extending from the medial capsule toward the medial patellar facet, may be seen on axial plane images.

- The patellar and quadriceps tendons are evaluated by examining consecutive superior-to-inferior images above and below the patella.
    - The patellar and quadriceps tendon fibers are oriented nearly 90 degrees to the axial plane.

- On superior axial images above the level of the patella, the tendons for the vastus medialis and lateralis are seen just medial and lateral to the distal quadriceps tendon.

- As the superior aspect of the patella comes into view, the medial and lateral retinacula are depicted, originating on the medial and lateral aspect of the patella and extending peripherally to insert on the medial and lateral femoral condyles, respectively.

- In transient lateral subluxation of the patella, tears of the medial retinaculum are often identified at the patellar origin or the medial femoral condyle insertion.

- If transient lateral subluxation is identified, there may be associated osteochondral defects and associated loose bodies.

Intercondylar Notch

- On superior images through the femoral condyles, the posterior intercondylar notch is:
    - A U-shaped, wide, concave groove
    - Located between the posterior medial and lateral femoral condyles
- The origin of the ACL is:
    - A thin, obliquely oriented band of fibers
    - Located along the anterolateral aspect of the "U"
    - Formed by the posterior intercondylar notch
- It is important to identify a normal ACL origin in the axial plane, since tears commonly occur at or near the ACL origin.
- Tears are seen as ill-defined high-intensity signal that replaces the normal thin hypointense band of ACL origin fibers.
- Moving in an inferior direction through the notch, as the intercondylar notch opens anteriorly, consecutive axial images depict the ACL origin fanning out into multiple distinct dark ACL fibers that course medially and inferiorly through the intercondylar notch.
- The ACL ends distally as a foot-shaped insertion upon the anterolateral tibia.
- The PCL origin:
    - Can be seen two images inferior to the axial image displaying the ACL origin
    - Depicted as a broad band of fibers occupying the medial half of the "U" formed by the posterior intercondylar notch
    - Located parallel to the axial plane, accounting for its broad appearance on these images. Proceeding in an inferior direction from the origin, the PCL can be seen to make a 90-degree turn on the next one or two images.

- At this point, it becomes perpendicular to the axial plane and descends in the mid-posterior notch to insert on the posterior tibia.

- Pathologic changes in the cruciate ligaments should first be identified on axial plane images and confirmed by triangulating on images of the cruciate ligaments in the coronal and sagittal planes.

Menisci

- An axial image between the femur and tibia often displays the medial and lateral menisci.

- The lateral meniscus is the smaller of the two C-shaped structures along the rim of the tibial plateau.

- Meniscal tears found on images in other planes are confirmed on axial plane images.

- Meniscal tears are:
  - Horizontal cleavage
  - Flap
  - Radial tear (vertical by definition)
    - Includes root
    - Includes free edge and extensive radial tears from free edge to periphery (involving circumferential fibers)
  - Longitudinal
  - Bucket-handle
    - Medial meniscus with double PCL sign and double delta sign
  - Lateral meniscus with deficient posterior horn resulting from displaced meniscal tissue anteriorly

- Correlation of tear patterns increases the degree of confidence in characterizing morphologic changes.

- Displaced meniscal flap fragments may be seen protruding into the coronary recess or toward the tibial spines into the intercondylar notch.
  - Flap tears may present with meniscal tissue displaced deep to the meniscofemoral or meniscotibial ligament

Collateral Ligaments

- Three tissue layers over the medial aspect of the knee:
    - Superficial MCL (sMCL) part of layer 2
    - Deep MCL (dMCL) part of layer 3
    - Posteromedial capsule (PMC)
        - Includes posterior oblique ligament (POL) from distal/posterior to the adductor tubercle to the rim of the posterior medial tibial plateau; visualized posterior to the sMCL on corresponding coronal images
- The MCL and fibular collateral ligament are oriented at a 90-degree angle to the axial plane.
- At the medial margin of the medial femoral condyle, the origin of the MCL can be seen as a thin short band of fibers that course along the medial joint line to insert on the proximal tibia, anterior to the pes anserinus tendons.
- The LCL:
    - Depicted at the lateral margin of the lateral femoral condyle
    - Courses inferiorly to insert on the lateral tip of the fibula
- Complete rupture of the collateral ligaments is seen as a "ghost ligament."
    - Caused by the absence of ligament fibers on the axial image directly through the level of the tear
    - Often accompanied by prominent surrounding edema and synovitis
- Synovitis and edema subjacent to the ITB is caused by the ITB friction syndrome and can also be appreciated on axial plane images.
- The posterolateral corner structures adjacent to the LCL are identified on axial images.
- The popliteus tendon origin is just posterior and deep to the LCL origin along the lateral femoral condyle.
    - On more inferior images, the popliteus tendon swings medially to course posterior to the posterior lateral tibial plateau.
- The arcuate ligament and popliteofibular ligament are seen posterior to the popliteus tendon on images above the level of the fibula.

Joint Fluid/Effusion

- Joint effusions are evaluated on axial images to determine the size of the effusion and the character of its contents.

- In chondromalacia or osteochondral lesions, associated loose bodies may be present within the effusion.
    - Loose bodies may be osseous, chondral, or osteochondral in nature.
    - Location common in the medial and lateral patellofemoral recesses, the suprapatellar bursa, the popliteus tendon sheath, the posterior intercondylar notch, and within popliteal cysts
    - Frequently requires use of both T1/PD and fluid-sensitive sequence to appreciate cartilaginous or osteocartilaginous composition

- Popliteal cysts may also be found between the semimembranosus tendon and the tendon for the medial head of the gastrocnemius.
    - Classified as typical popliteal cysts
    - Associated with internal knee degeneration in adults

- Bursitis in multiple locations, including prepatellar bursitis, pes anserinus bursitis, and tibial collateral ligament bursitis, may also be depicted.
    - Anterior knee bursae
        - Prepatellar
        - Deep infrapatellar
        - Superficial infrapatellar
        - Suprapatellar in communication with the knee (not a true bursae)

- Morel-Lavallée lesion of the knee distinct from prepatellar bursitis
    - Internal degloving injury of prepatellar soft tissues
    - Seen in professional football players
    - Shearing trauma with disruption of perforating vessels

Stoller's Knee Checklist

CORONAL

Medial Collateral Ligament

Posterior Coronal
- Image location where condyles transition to intercondylar roof
- Anterior to posterior oblique ligament location

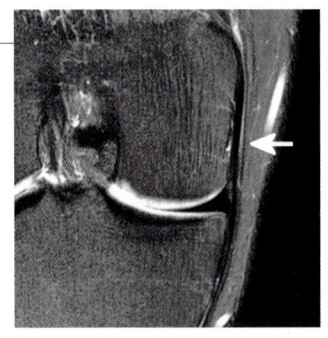

Posterior

Mid Coronal
- The deep MCL is visualized deep to the superficial MCL.

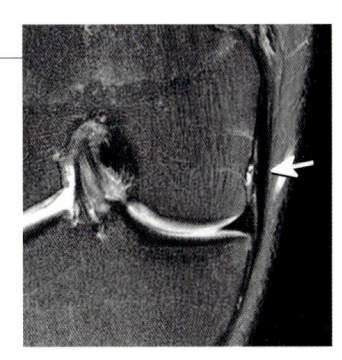

Mid

Anterior Coronal
- Not an accurate location to assess distal MCL continuity
- The anterior third of layer 3 (joint capsule) is reinforced by the medial retinaculum.

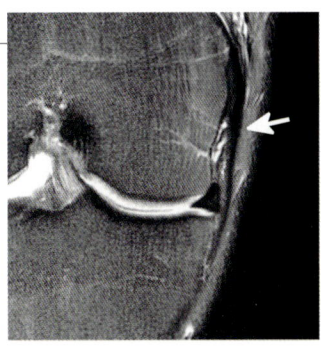

Anterior

MCL Pathology

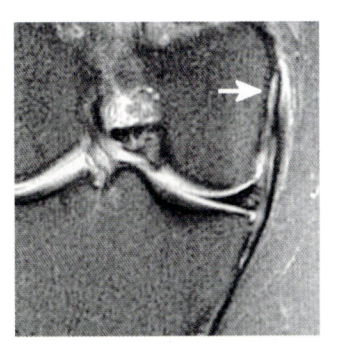

Grade 1 Sprain 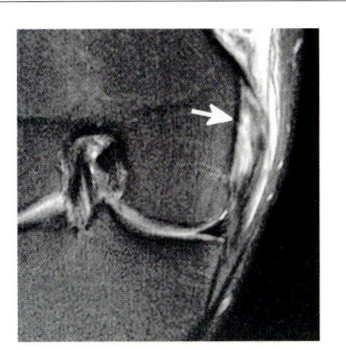   Grade 2 Sprain (Partial Tear) 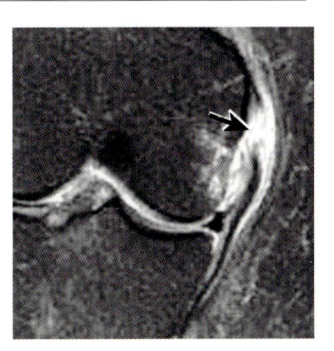   Grade 3 Sprain (Proximal Rupture)

Lateral Collateral Ligament

Proximal LCL

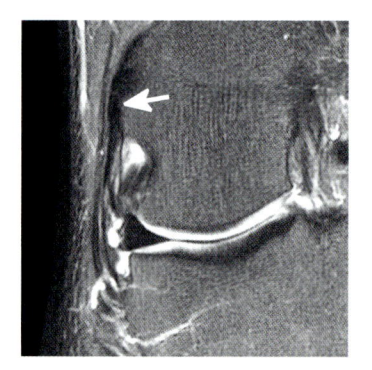

- Identify on image where femoral condyles fuse on one image posterior to the plane of the MCL.

Origin LCL on Lateral Femoral Condyle

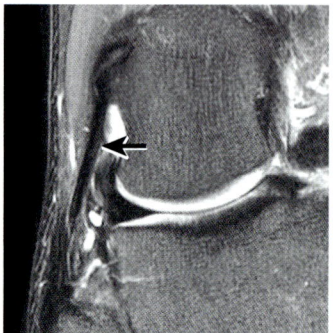

Mid LCL

- Oblique course shows segmental visualization unless there is anterior translation of the tibia, in which case the LCL may be seen in a single coronal image in its entirety.

Mid LCL

Distal LCL

- Conjoined attachment with the biceps femoris tendon on the fibular head

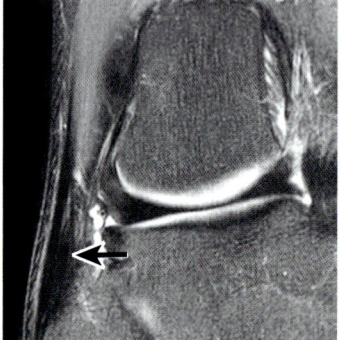

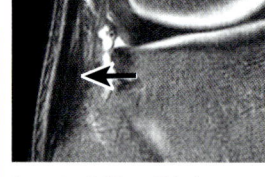

Insertion LCL on Fibula

LCL Pathology

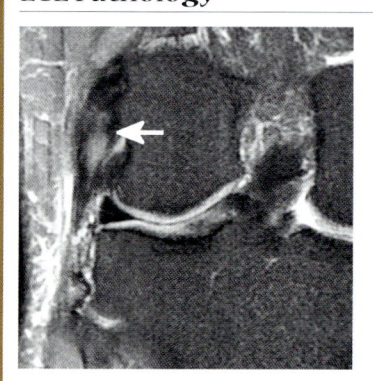

Grade 2 Sprain Proximal LCL

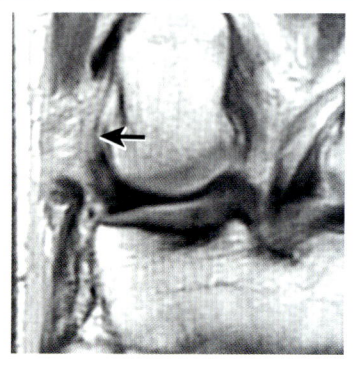

Grade 3 Tear Mid LCL

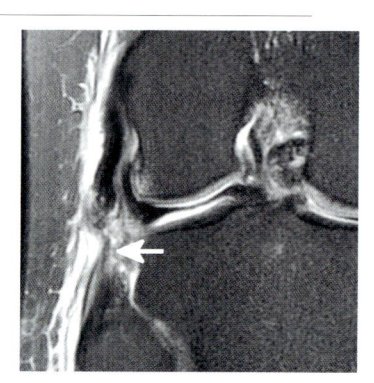

Grade 3 Tear Mid to Distal LCL

CORONAL

Anterior Cruciate Ligament

Anterior Cruciate Ligament

- First identify ACL in the same image location as the MCL (where the femoral condyles first fuse when viewing from posterior to anterior).
- The proximal ACL is identified on either two or three images posterior to the plane of the MCL.
- Use T1 or PD to identify normal hypointense proximal fibers.
- Use fluid-sensitive sequences to document continuity of ACL if T1 or PD images demonstrate intermediate ACL signal intensity.
- Identify anteromedial (AM) and posterolateral (PL) bundles of the ACL.
- Always follow distal ACL course to tibial eminence.

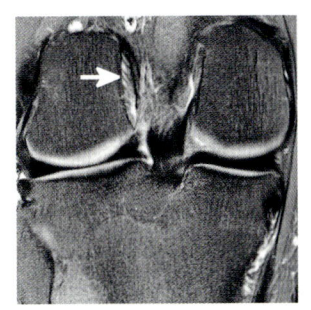

ACL Origin 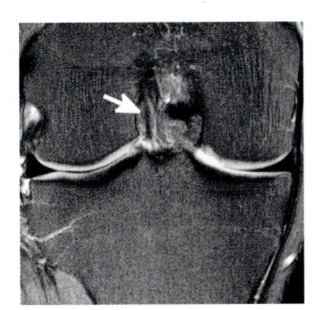 | ACL Proximal Fibers 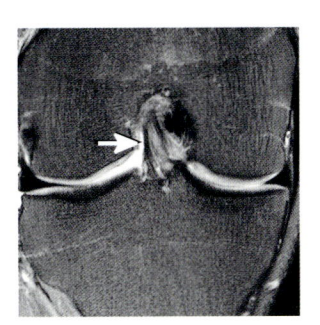 | ACL Mid Fibers 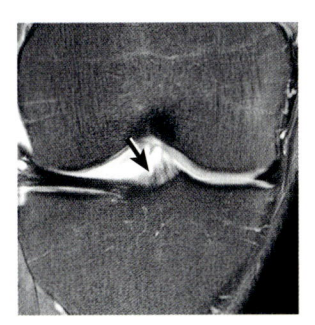 | ACL Distal Insertion

Anterior Cruciate Ligament Pathology

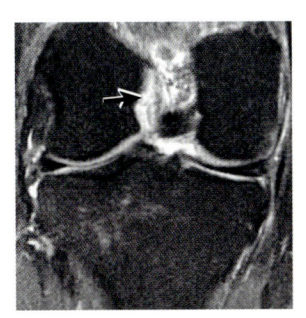

Tear Origin ACL 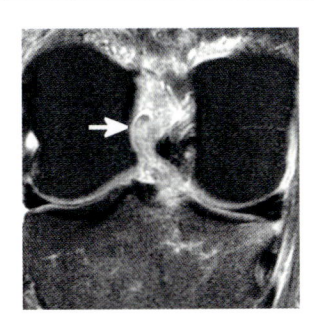 | Tear Proximal ACL 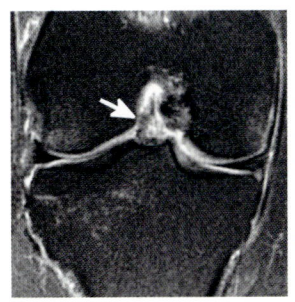 | Moderate Sprain Mid ACL 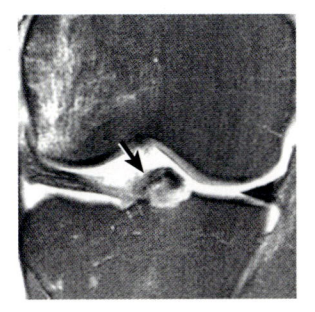 | Avulsion Distal ACL from Tibia

- Proper use of the coronal plane in ACL assessment obviates the need to prescribe oblique sagittal images parallel to the ACL fibers as an additional sequence to supplement the routine sagittal oblique plane.
- Oblique coronal images parallel to the longitudinal axis of the ACL are not routinely performed but have been used to improve visualization of the AM and PL bundles.

CORONAL

Posterior Cruciate Ligament

Posterior Cruciate Ligament

- PCL is hypointense throughout its course.
- Posterior coronal images parallel to the distal fibers; otherwise, the PCL is seen in cross-section on anterior and mid-coronal images
- Always confirm intact femoral and tibial attachments on sagittal images.

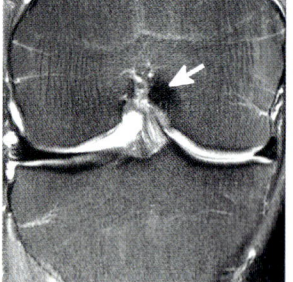

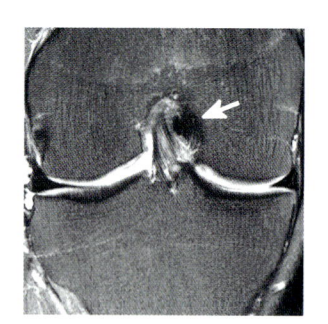

PCL Origin

PCL Proximal Fibers

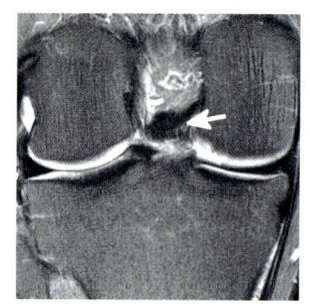

PCL Distal Fibers

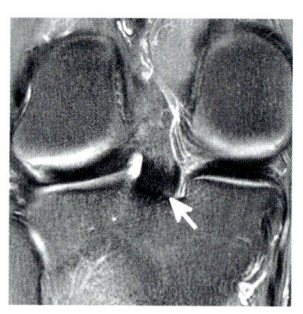

PCL Distal Insertion

Posterior Cruciate Ligament Pathology

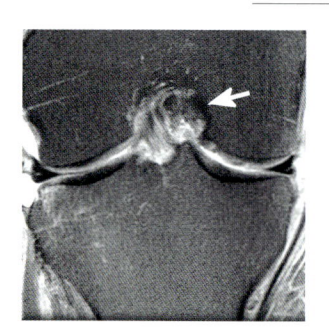

Moderate Sprain PCL Origin

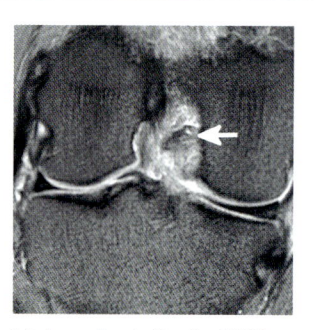

Moderate Sprain Proximal PCL Fibers

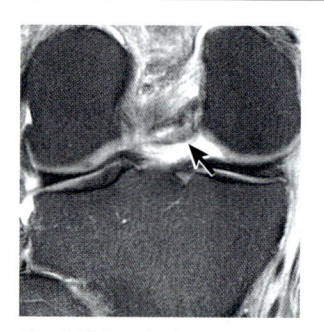

Tear PCL Distal Fibers

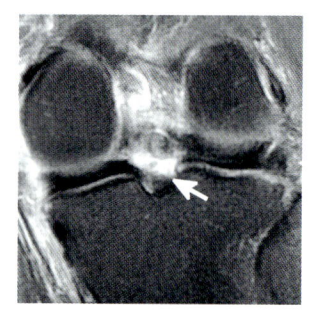

Tear PCL Insertion

- PCL consist of an ALB and PMB.
- Coronal images best suited to visualize the more horizontal component of the curved PCL
- Always confirm an intact femoral and tibial attachment and continuity of central third ligament on corresponding sagittal images.
- Identify the more anterior proximal fibers of the ALB from the lateral aspect of the medial femoral condyle anterior to the femoral footprint of the PMB.
- The two PCL bundles insert onto the posterior aspect of the proximal tibia about 1cm distal (inferior) to the articular surface.

CORONAL

Menisci

Menisci

- First document intact root attachments.
- The menisci should have a well-defined tapered and sharp free edge on mid-coronal images; otherwise, there may be a radial tear.
- Flap tears may be associated with displaced tissue in the meniscofemoral or meniscotibial recess.
- Exclude a meniscal fragment in the anterior notch as would be seen in a classic bucket-handle tear.

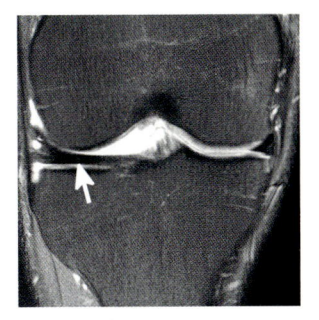

Anterior Horn 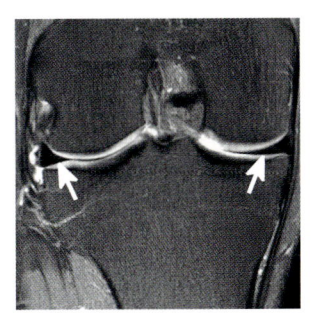 | Body 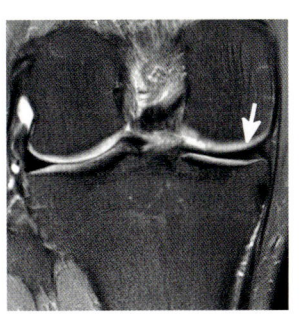 | Posterior Horn 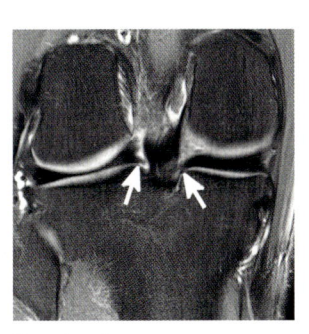 | Root Attachments

Meniscal Pathology

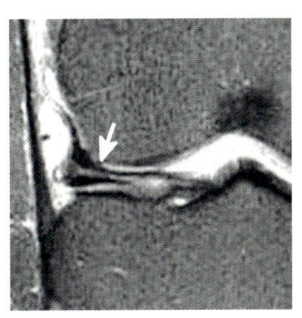

Horizontal Tear Anterior Horn 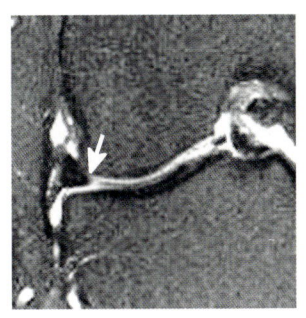 | Radial Tear Free Edge Body 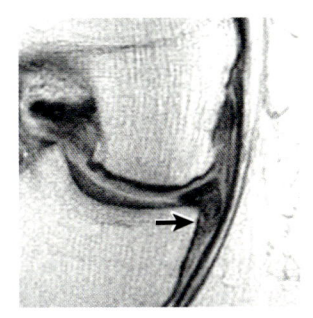 | Displaced Flap Tear Body 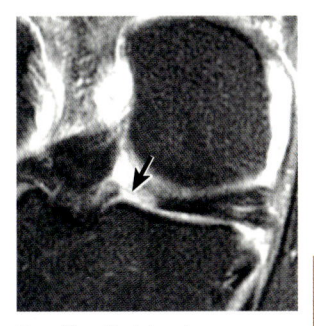 | Root Tear, Peripheral Subluxation

- Root tears may involve the meniscotibial ligament attachment directly or occur with a fragment of meniscus attachment to the root ligament.
- Central or free edge radial tears are associated with a blunted or truncated free edge of the meniscus unless the coronal images are too thick and failure to section the meniscus in the tear plane.
- Flap tears are secondarily visualized on posterior coronal images.

CORONAL

Articular Cartilage

Articular Cartilage

- Chondral lesions are commonly seen in the lateral aspect of the medial femoral condyle and posteromedial aspect of the lateral tibial plateau.
- Identify associated marrow changes of edema or sclerosis in the posterior femoral condyle.

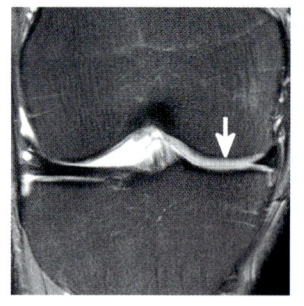

Normal Cartilage—Anterior

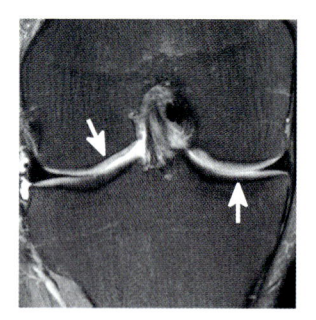

Normal Cartilage—Mid

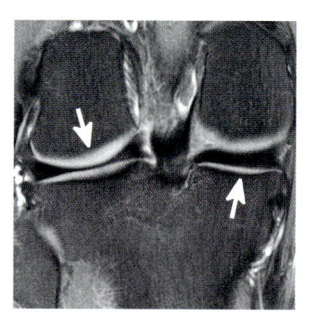

Normal Cartilage—Posterior

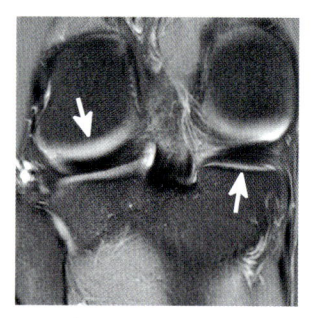

Normal Cartilage—Posterior

Articular Cartilage Pathology

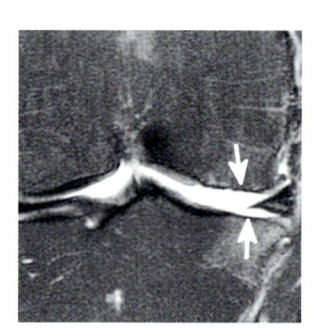

Cartilage Loss to Bone

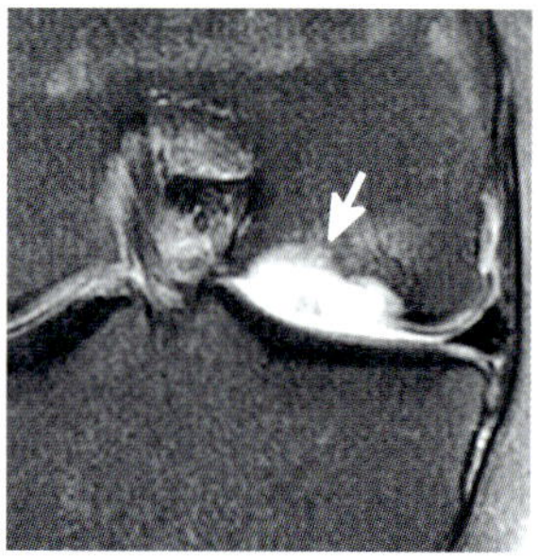

Grade 4 OCL

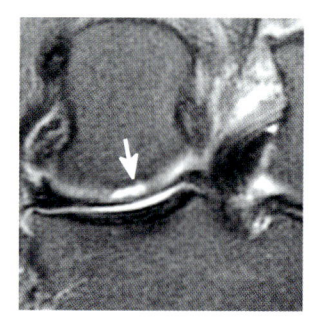

Chondral Defect

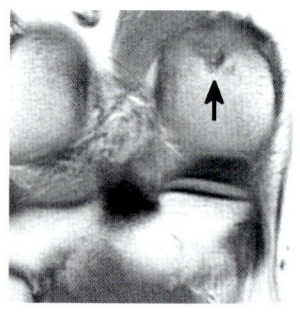

Posterior Femoral Condyle Erosion

- Areas susceptible to early chondral lesions include the lateral aspect of the medial femoral condyle (posterior coronal images) and posteromedial aspect of the lateral tibial plateau (posterior coronal images).
- Subchondral marrow sclerosis, cysts, or erosions should be triangulated to the corresponding chondral fissures on sagittal images to optimize visualization of the articular cartilage and subchondral plate.

CORONAL

Osseous and Marrow

Subchondral
- Use T1 or PD to assess hypointense sclerosis or hyperintense edema (degenerative or posttraumatic).

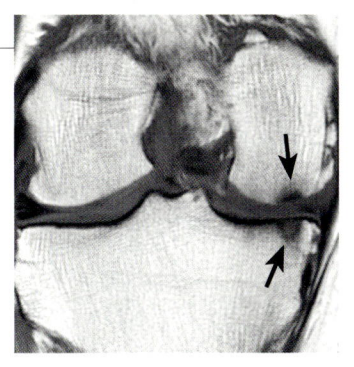

Subchondral Sclerosis

Tibial Eminence
- Identify involvement in distal ACL avulsions.

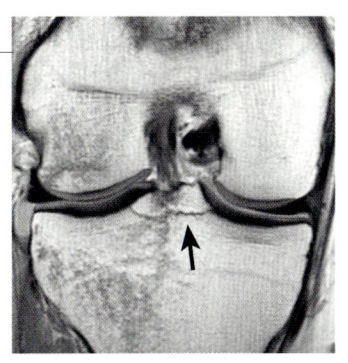

Tibial Spine Avulsion and Bone Contusions

Osseous Lesion
- Determine if trabecular architecture is destroyed or altered.
- Use two planes to show cortical transgression.
- Evaluate associated soft tissue mass and perilesional edema.

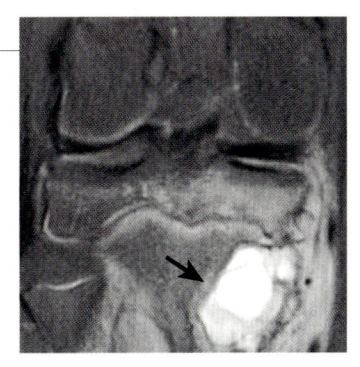

ABC with Pathologic Fracture

Fracture
- Discrete hypointense fracture (acute phase) or hyperintense fracture (subacute)
- Stress or insufficiency fracture may only be associated with subchondral plate thickening.

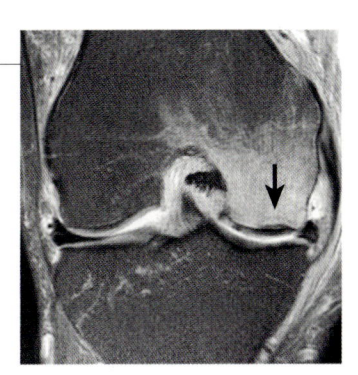

Insufficiency Fracture Medial Femoral Condyle

CORONAL

Iliotibial Tract

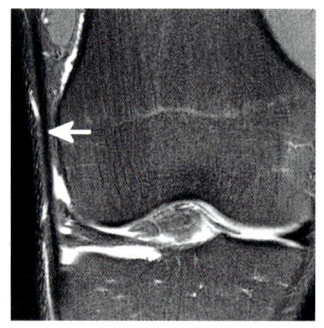

Normal Iliotibial Band

Iliotibial Tract

- Taut structure courses to Gerdy's tubercle
- Iliotibial tract = Iliotibial band

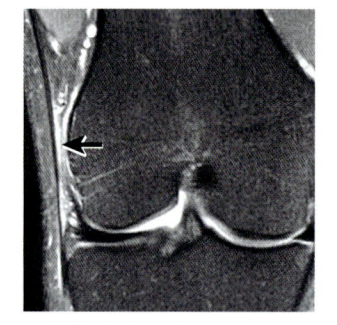

Mild Iliotibial Band Friction Syndrome

- Fluid-sensitive sequences to identify hyperintense edema fluid or synovium deep to ITB

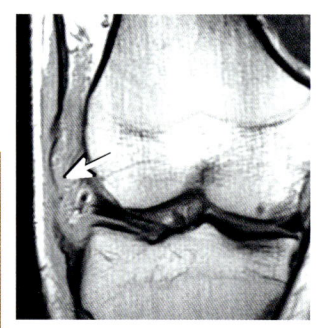

Tear Iliotibial Tract

- ITB tear may be associated with a severe posterolateral corner injury.

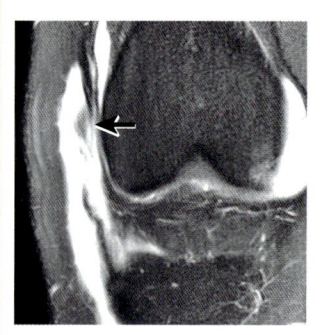

Tear Iliotibial Tract

- Overlying the lateral epicondyle (originates from tensor fasciae latae and gluteus maximus)
- Edema may be superficial and deep to ITB.
- Less common presentation involves distal attachment to Gerdy's tubercle.

SAGITTAL

Medial Meniscus

Body
- Flap tears may involve body or central third.

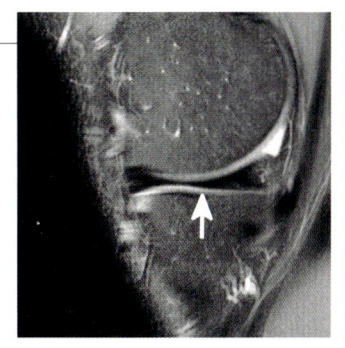

Body

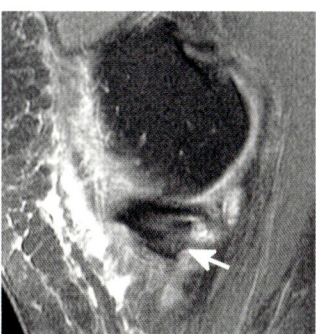

Flap Tear Displaced Inferiorly (Body)

Anterior and Posterior Horn
- Posterior horn is larger than anterior horn.
- A radial tear involves either the body or anterior horn body or posterior horn body junction.
- A displaced flap tear may be part of a bucket-handle tear if meniscal tissue is displaced toward the notch.

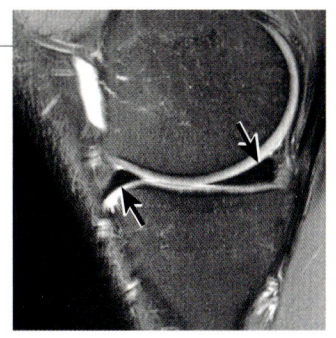

Anterior and Posterior Horn

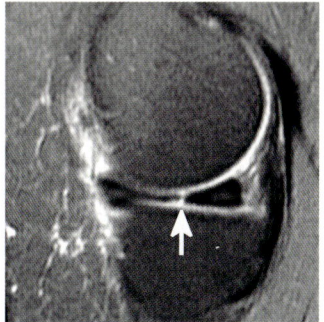

Radial Tear PH-Body Junction

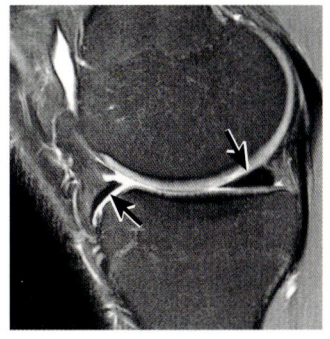

Anterior and Posterior Horn

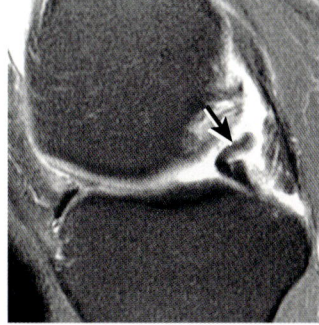

Displaced Flap Tear (Posterior Horn)

Root
- The absence of posterior horn tissue seen in a displaced root tear.
- The root attachment may be degenerative and associated with an adjacent cystic fluid collection.

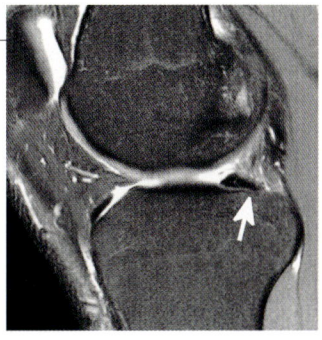

Root Posterior Horn

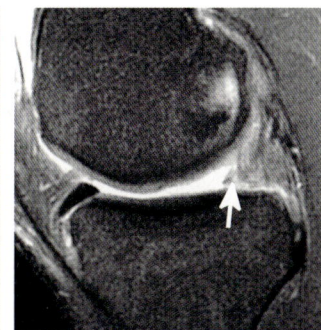

Root Tear PH (Ghost Meniscus)

SAGITTAL
Lateral Meniscus and Posterolateral Corner

Lateral Meniscus and Posterolateral Corner
- The LCL and biceps femoris are lateral to the popliteus tendon.

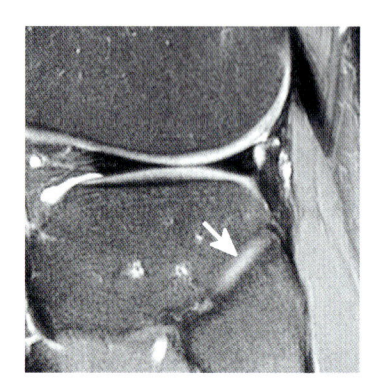

LCL and Biceps Femoris

- The lateral aspect of the tibiofibular joint corresponds to the fibular styloid attachment of the popliteofibular ligament.

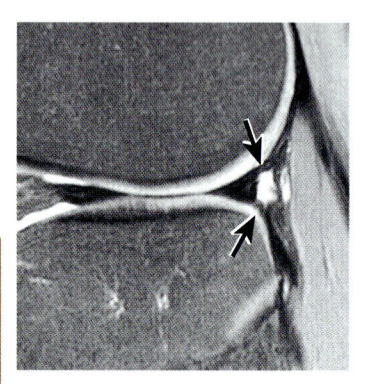

Tibiofibular Joint

- The popliteal hiatus shows relatively symmetric superior and inferior popliteomeniscal fascicles.
- Identify the presence and passage of the popliteus tendon through the hiatus in all cases of posterolateral corner injuries.

Meniscal Fascicles

- The popliteofibular ligament attaches to the upper facet of the apex of the fibular head (directly medial to the attachment of the arcuate ligaments).

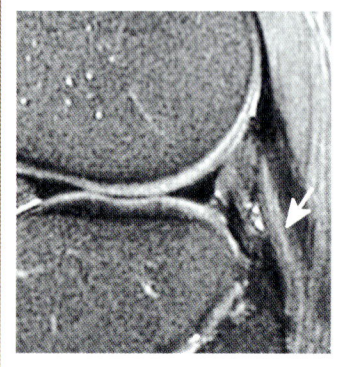

Arcuate and Popliteofibular Ligaments

SAGITTAL

Articular Cartilage

Articular Cartilage

- Evaluate posterior femoral condyles, which are weight-bearing surfaces in flexion.

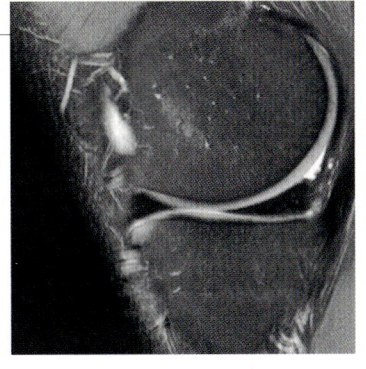

Medial Cartilage—Peripheral

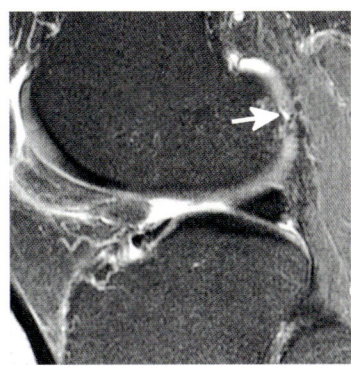

Chondral Fissure Posterior Lateral Femoral Condyle

- Describe areas of basilar degeneration.

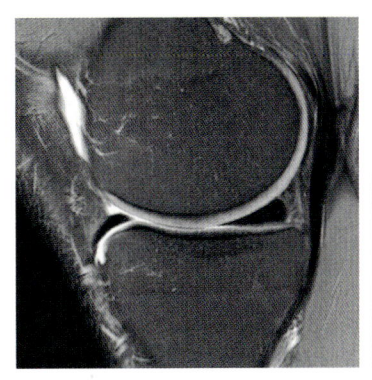

Medial Cartilage—Mid

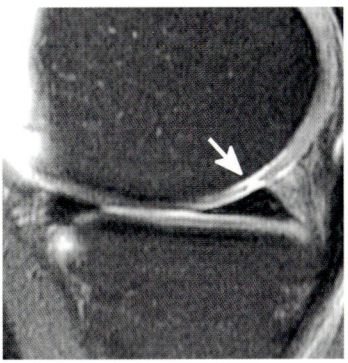

Unstable Chondral Flap Mid Medial Femoral Condyle

- Identify the thickness and extent of cartilage involvement (anterior to posterior and medial to lateral).

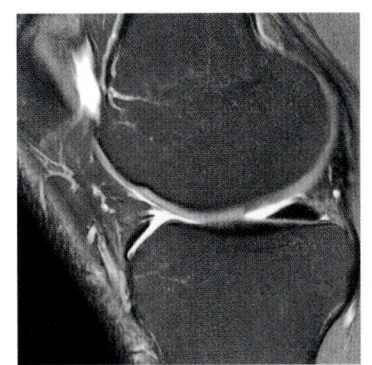

Medial Cartilage—Mid Central

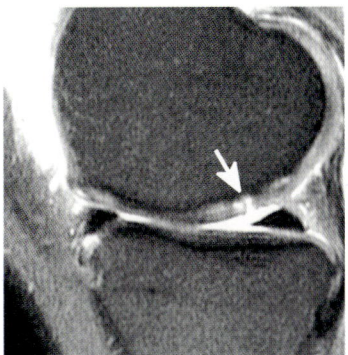

Chondral Fissure Mid Medial Femoral Condyle

- Correlate sagittal extent of chondral degeneration with coronal plane images.
- Evaluate for chondral involvement on both opposing surfaces of the femur and tibia.

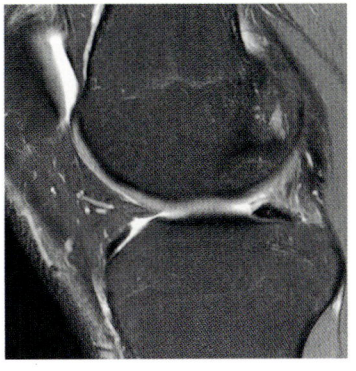

Medial Cartilage—Central

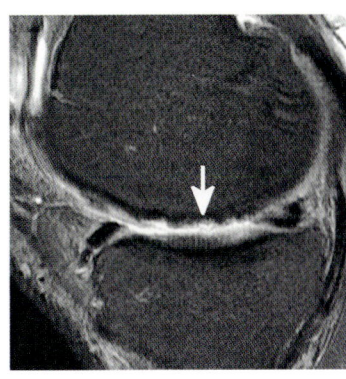

Chondral Fibrillation Medial Femoral Condyle

SAGITTAL
Trochlear Groove

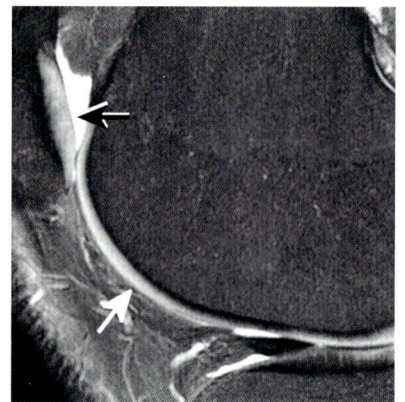

Lateral Trochlear and Lateral Facet Cartilage

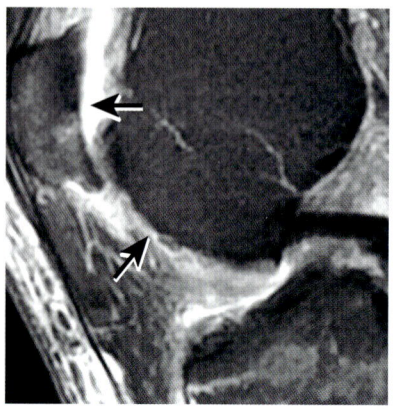

Grade 4 Chondromalacia Medial Patellofemoral Compartment

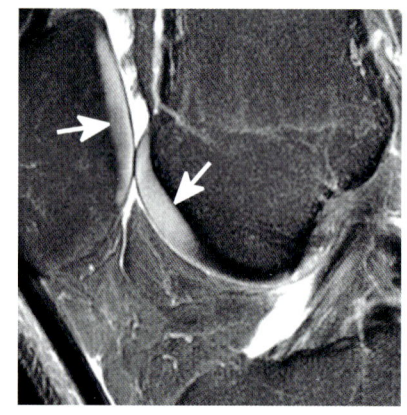

Mid-Trochlear and Median Ridge Cartilage

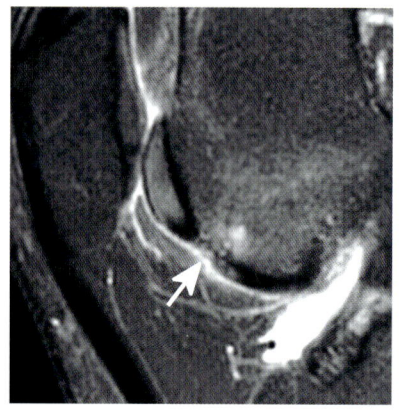

Chondral Erosion Mid Trochlea

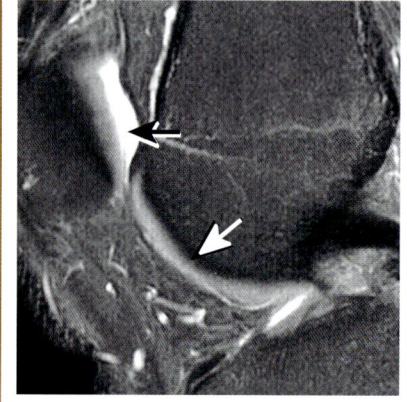

Medial Trochlear and Medial Facet Cartilage

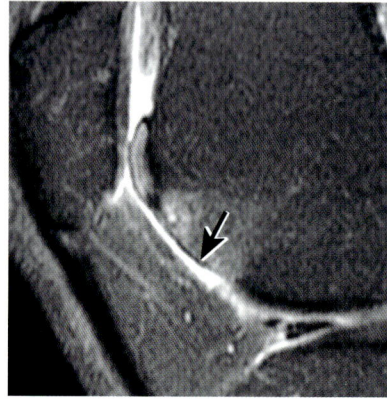

Grade 4 Chondromalacia Lateral Trochlea

Trochlear Groove

- The sagittal plane is the primary plane to evaluate trochlear groove chondral pathology (axial is the secondary plane of assessment).

- Lateral patellar facet also visualized in the sagittal plane (medial facet of patellar requires axial images because of its oblique orientation)
- Evaluate subchondral plate.

- Medial patellar facet suboptimally visualized in the sagittal plane
- Evaluate associated subchondral edema in grade 4 lesions.

SAGITTAL

Anterior Cruciate Ligament

Anterior Cruciate Ligament
- Anterior leading edge of ACL is parallel to intercondylar roof.

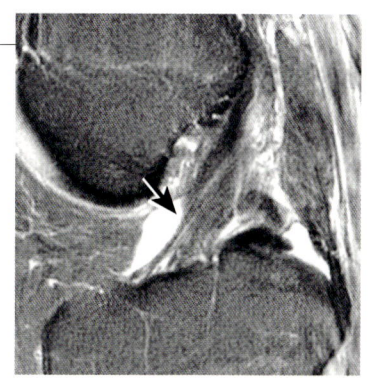

ACL

- Distal ACL avulsions are confirmed on coronal plane images.
- The ACL should maintain parallel fiber striation.

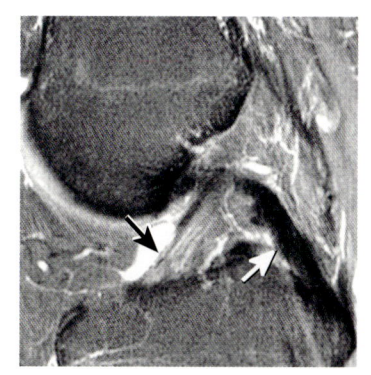

Distal ACL and PCL

- Most grade 3 ACL tears are proximal.
- Confirm discontinuity from lateral femoral condyle (LFC) on coronal images.

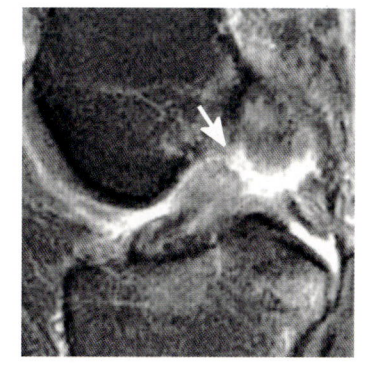

ACL Tear

- Mucoid ACL not associated with lateral compartment contusions or anterior tibial translation.

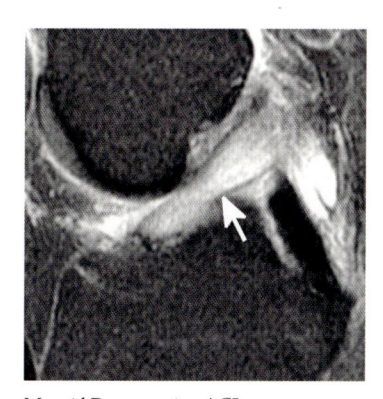

Mucoid Degeneration ACL

Posterior Cruciate Ligament

SAGITTAL

Posterior Cruciate Ligament

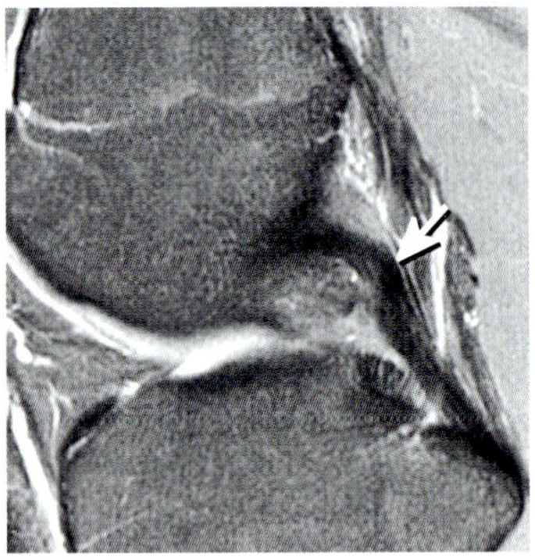

- Identify intact femoral attachment.

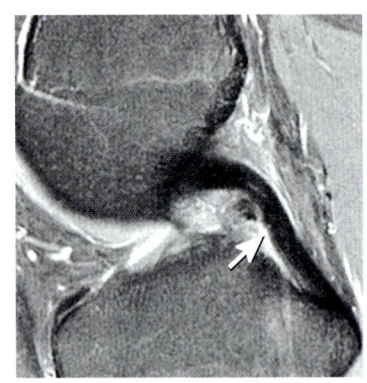

PCL

- Continuity of middle third of PCL and follow course to tibial attachment

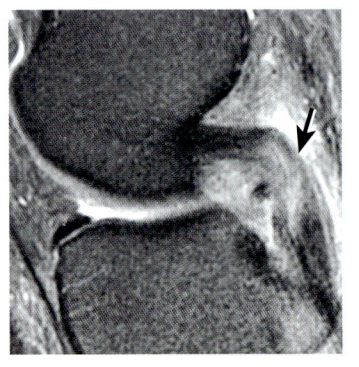

PCL

- Partial disruption of PCL fibers
- Always locate meniscofemoral ligaments, which may be mistaken for intact PCL fibers.

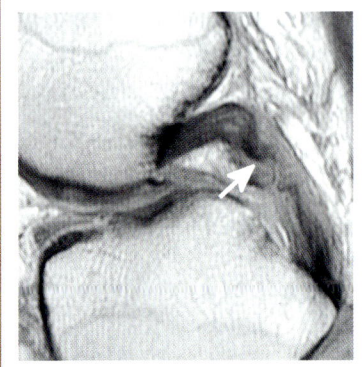

PCL Grade 2 Sprain

- Chronic PCL tears may contain intermediate-signal synovium or granulation tissue.

PCL Tear

SAGITTAL

Posteromedial Corner

Posteromedial Corner

- Sagittal plane is of secondary value in evaluating MCL.
- MCL visualized as taut on MR

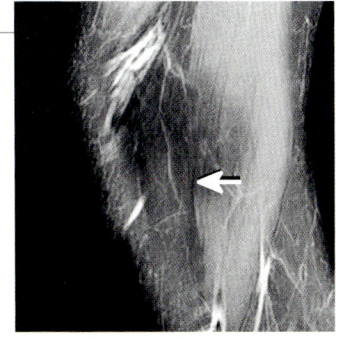

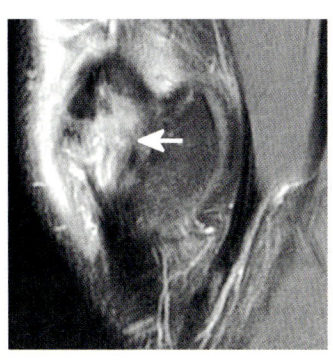

Normal MCL

MCL Tear (proximal)

- Insertion of the MCL is covered by pes anserinus tendons.

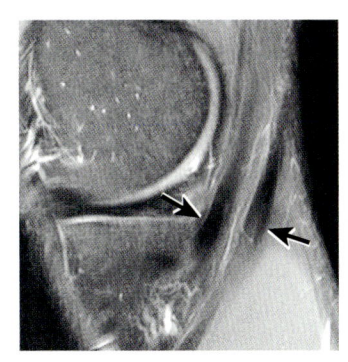

Normal Gracilis and Semitendinosus

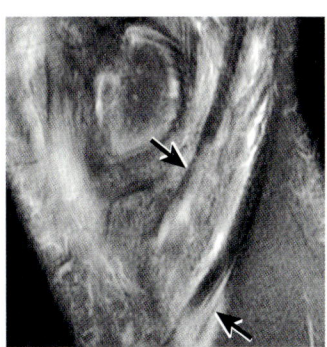

Distal Gracilis and Semitendinosus Strain

- Posteromedial corner receives contribution from semimembranosus tendon.
- Posterior oblique ligament represents connection between capsular attachment of the semimembranosus and oblique fibers of superficial MCL.

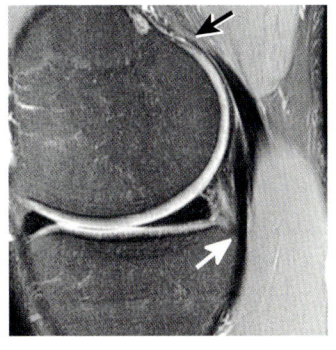

Normal Medial Gastrocnemius Origin and Semimembranosus Insertion

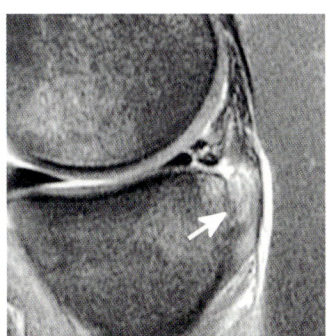

Semimembranosus Distal Strain

- Normal meniscocapsular connection with intermediate-signal-intensity capsular tissue preventing the influx of fluid posterior to posterior horn.

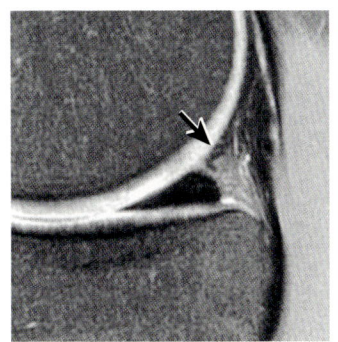

Normal Meniscocapsular Ligaments

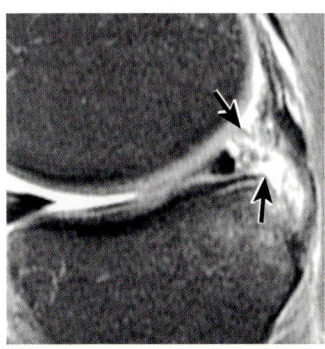

Meniscocapsular Injury

SAGITTAL

Patellar and Quadriceps Tendons

Patellar and Quadriceps Tendons

- Gradient echo is sensitive to patellar tendon degeneration.
- FS PD FSE is sensitive to inferior pole edema and hyperintensity of the supralateral portion of Hoffa's fat pad.

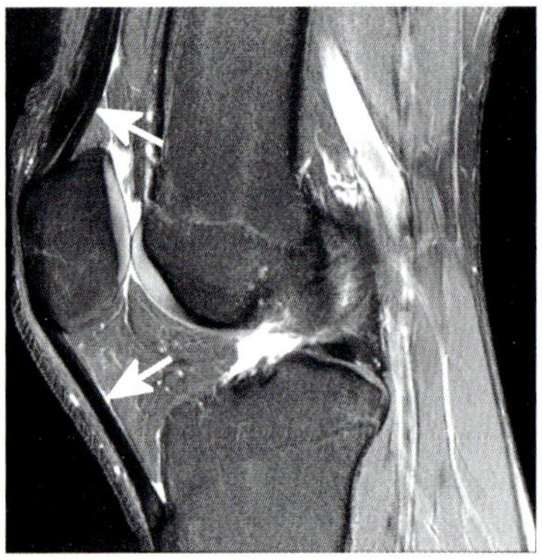

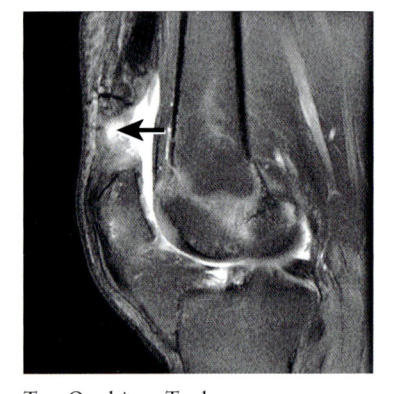

Normal Patellar and Quadriceps Tendon

- Quadriceps tendon tears can be further evaluated on coronal oblique images parallel to the sagittal course of the quadriceps tendon.

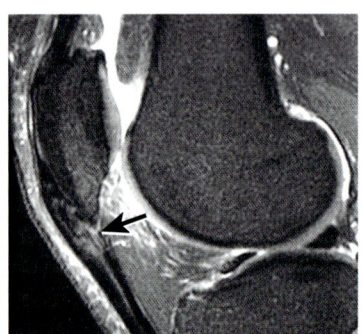

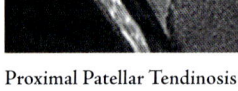

Torn Quadriceps Tendon

- Patellar tendon thickening of the anterior-to-posterior and intermediate-weighted signal specific for degeneration
- Linear hyperintense fluid in interstitial partial tears

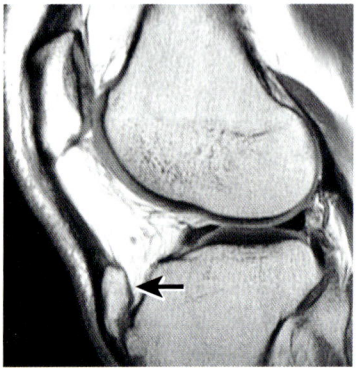

Proximal Patellar Tendinosis

- Acute Osgood-Schlatter with patellar tendinosis, fragmentation, and edema of tibial tubercle and reactive fluid/edema of Hoffa's fat pad and/or deep infrapatellar bursa

Osgood-Schlatter Distal Patellar Tendon

SAGITTAL

Subchondral Bone and Marrow

Subchondral Bone and Marrow

- Subchondral edema associated with full thickness chondral defects

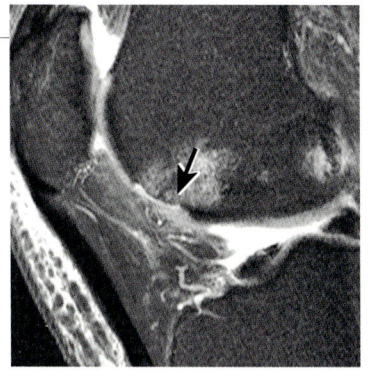

Subchondral Marrow Edema with Overlying Chondral Defect

- Assess chondral surface and subchondral plate.

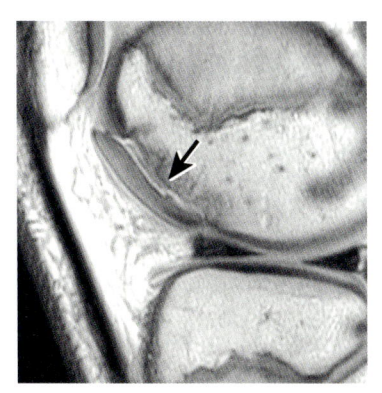

Osteochondral Defect Trochlear Groove

- Lateral compartment contusions are frequently nondisplaced subchondral fractures.

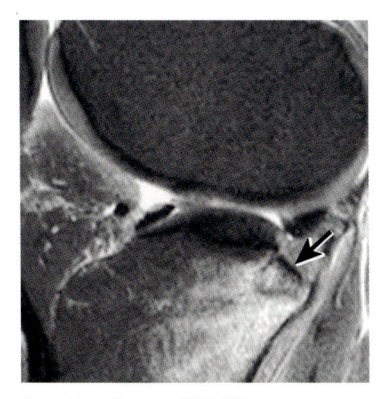

Impaction Fracture Tibial Plateau

- Thickening of the subchondral plate is associated with a stress or insufficiency fracture. The marrow edema is most hyperintense adjacent to the fracture site.

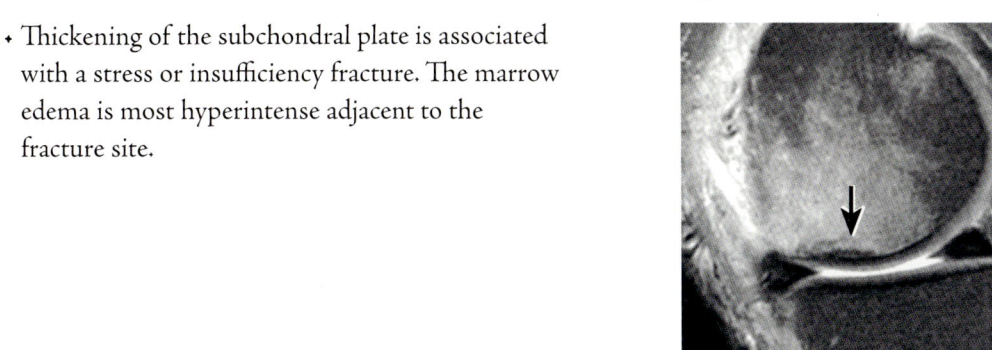

Subchondral Fracture Femoral Condyle

SAGITTAL

Hoffa's Fat Pad

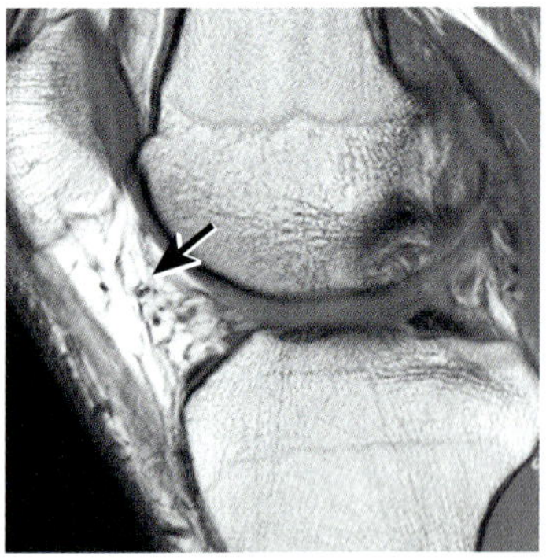

Hoffa's Fat Pad

- Normal fat pad has a smooth free concave edge.

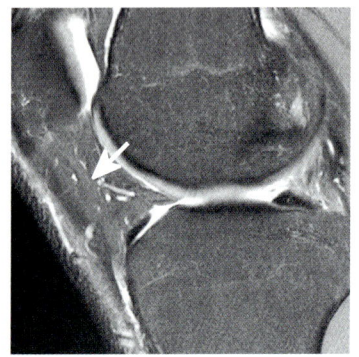

Medial Hoffa's Fat Pad T1

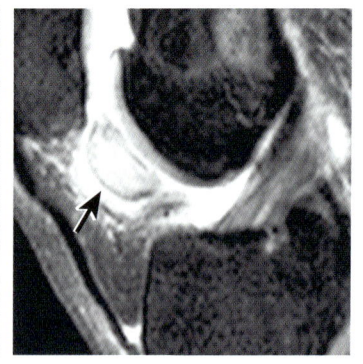

Localized PVNS

- Synovial reaction/inflammation in the knee is associated with an irregular contour of the free edge of Hoffa's fat pad or the direct visualization of intermediate signal in thickened synovium.

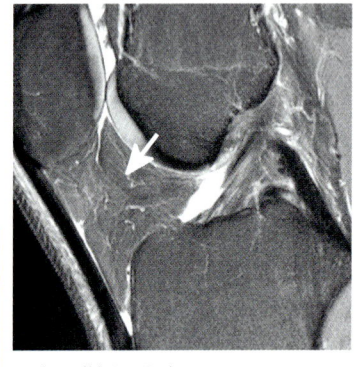

Medial Hoffa's Fat Pad FS PD

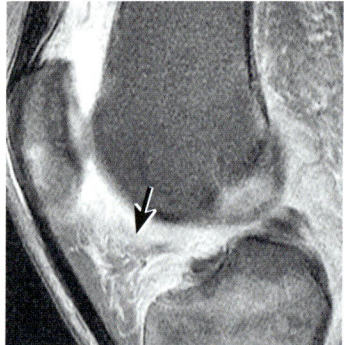

Severe Synovitis

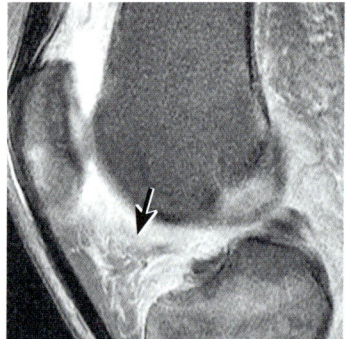

- Hypointense scarring in postoperative knee
- Identify extension of scar to posterior patellar tendon (tethering).
- Intermediate signal of cyclops nodule

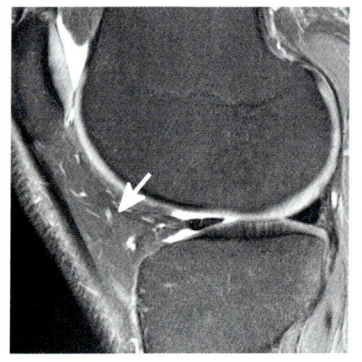

Mid Hoffa's Fat Pad

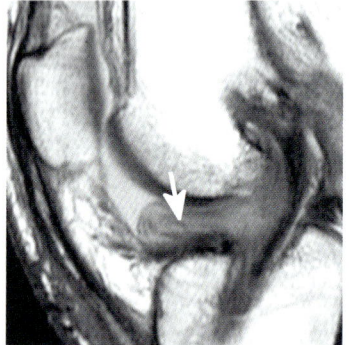

Scarring Posterior Hoffa's with Cyclops

- Patellar multitracking associated with edema of superolateral aspect of Hoffa's fat pad

Lateral Hoffa's Fat Pad

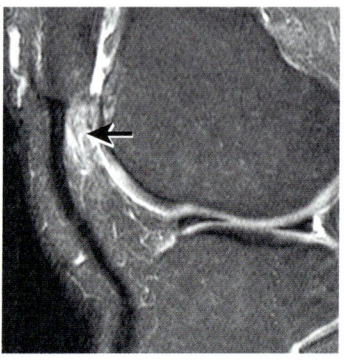

Fat Pad Impingement Syndrome (Superolateral Hoffa's)

SAGITTAL

Joint Effusion

Joint Effusion
- Evaluate for synovial thickening by areas of intermediate signal.

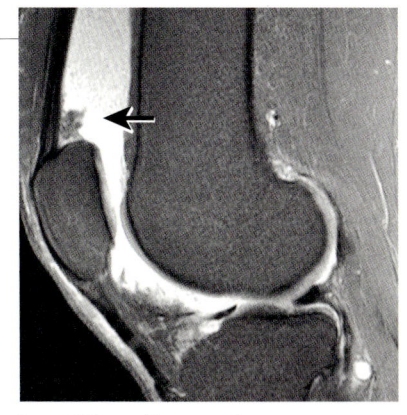

Large Effusion (Suprapatellar Bursa)

- Characterize the contour of Hoffa's fat pad.

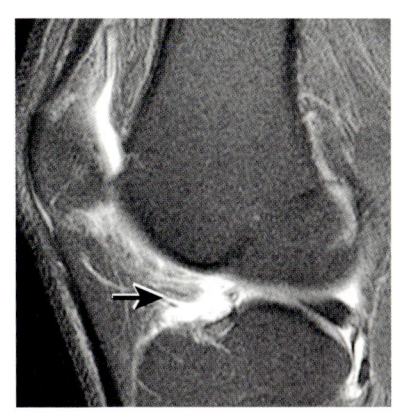

Small Effusion (Posterior to Hoffa's)

- Synovial thickening occurs along lining of joint capsule.
- Pannus tissue is defined by a thick rind of synovium that develops into mass-like thickening or extension into the adjacent joint fluid.

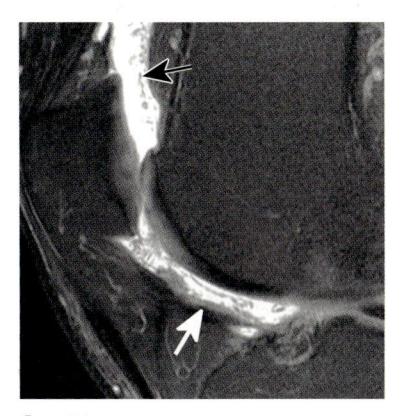

Synovitis

SAGITTAL
Plicae

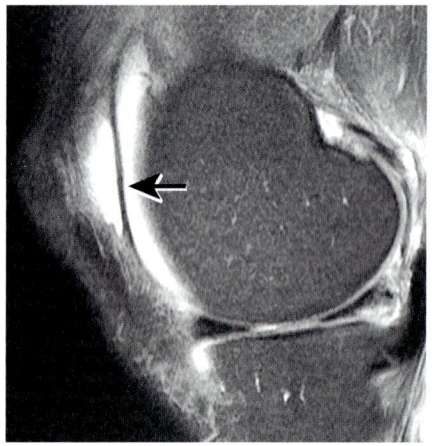

Medial Plica

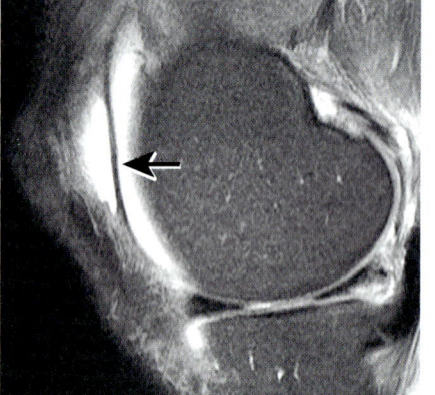

Medial
- Medial plica on medial sagittal images
- Correlate with axial plane for shelf-like extension anterior to medial femoral condyle (MFC).
- Evaluate as normal plica or thickened.

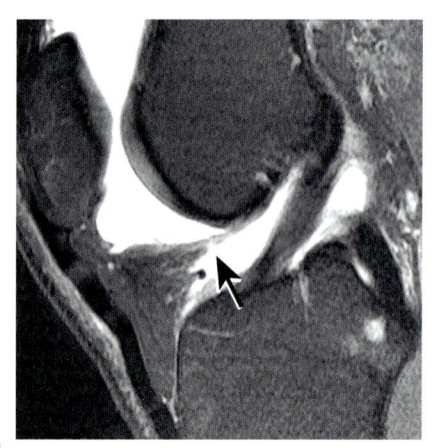

Infrapatellar Plica

Infrapatellar
- Anterior to ACL with extension to Hoffa's fat pad and inferior pole
- Not to be mistaken for the anterior meniscofemoral ligament, which attaches to the anterior horn

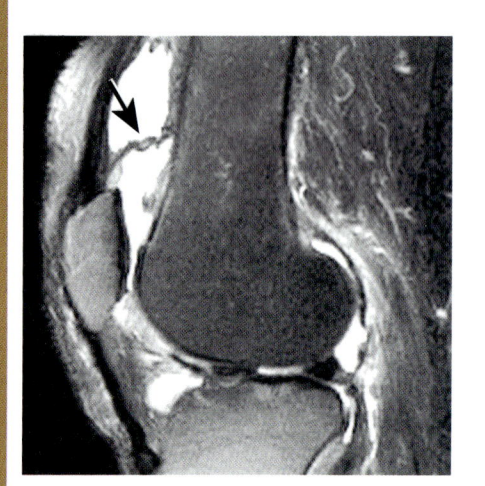

Suprapatellar Plica

Suprapatellar
- If complete, may create a one-way valve for the accumulation of fluid that does not drain

AXIAL

Patellar Facets and Trochlear Groove

Patellar Facets and Trochlear Groove

- Axial plane best to evaluate medial and lateral facets and chondral stratification

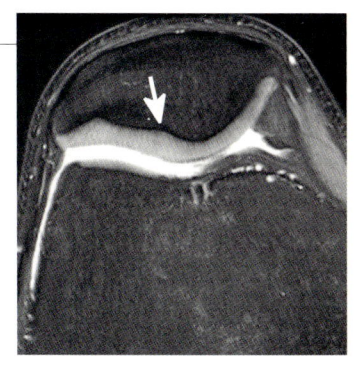

Patellar Cartilage

- Trochlear groove secondarily assessed on axial images after sagittal review

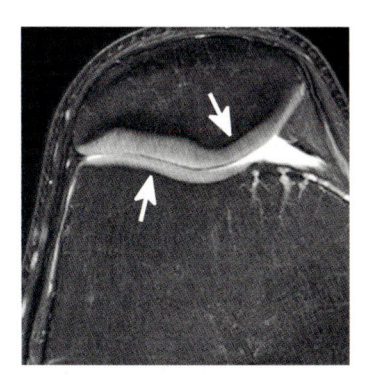

Patellar and Trochlear Cartilage

- Axial evaluation of trochlear groove may result in overestimation of chondral degeneration if region of interest includes adjacent fat that mimics chondral surface on fluid-sensitive sequence.

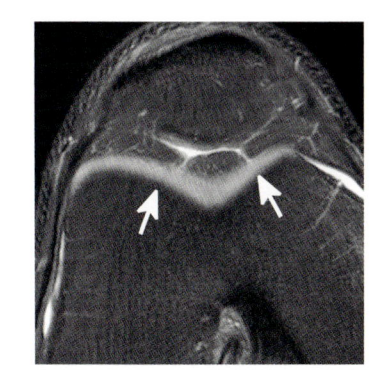

Trochlear Groove Cartilage

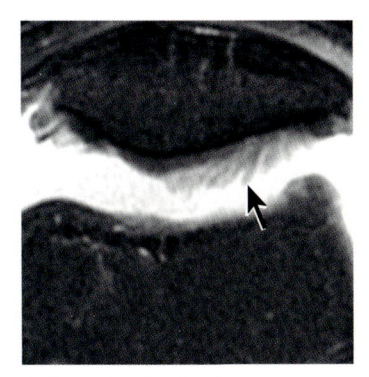

Crabmeat Patellar Cartilage
Lateral Facet

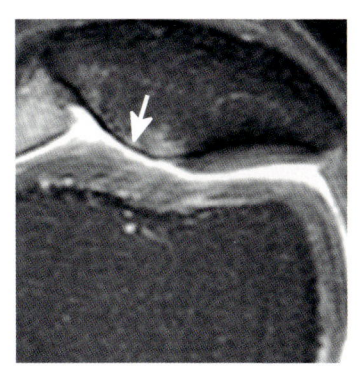

Full Thickness Chondral Loss
Medial Facet

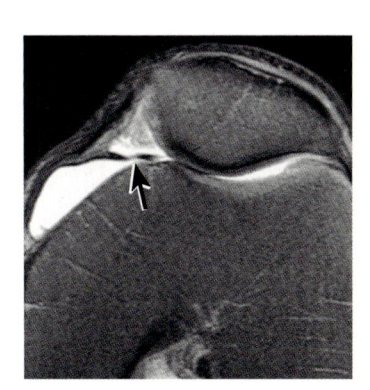

Medial Plica

138   Stoller's Orthopaedics and Sports Medicine: The Knee

AXIAL

Quadriceps and Patellar Tendon

Quadriceps and Patellar Tendon

- Normal striations of distal quadriceps tendon

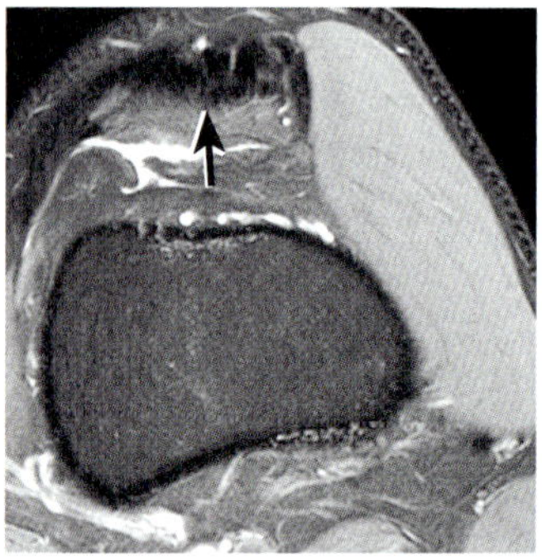

Distal Quadriceps Insertion

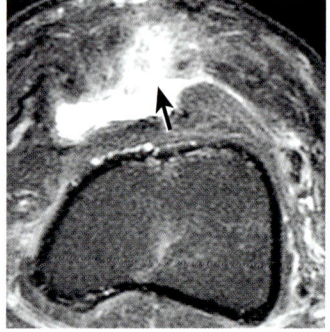

Tear Distal Quadriceps Tendon

- Patellar tendinosis preferential involvement of central to medial fibers

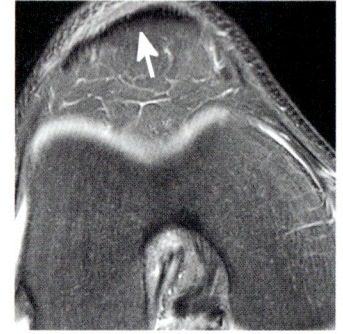

Proximal Patellar Tendon Origin

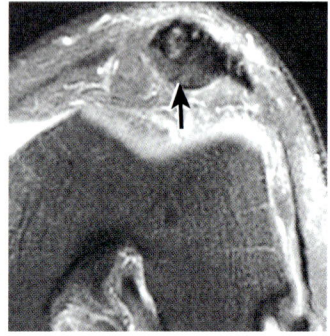

Proximal Patellar Tendinosis

- T1 PD images for heterotopic bone

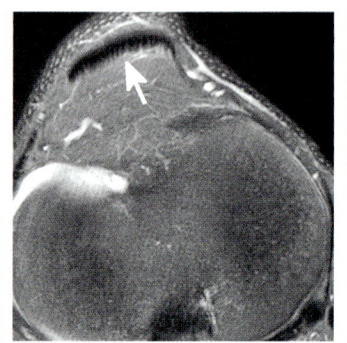

Mid Patellar Tendon

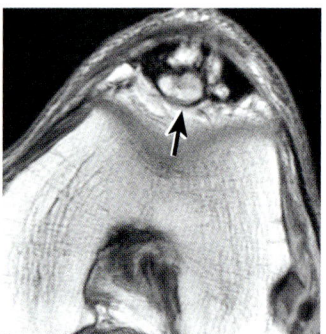

Heterotopic Ossification Proximal Patellar Tendon

- Correlate with anterior and posterior tendon contour on sagittal images.

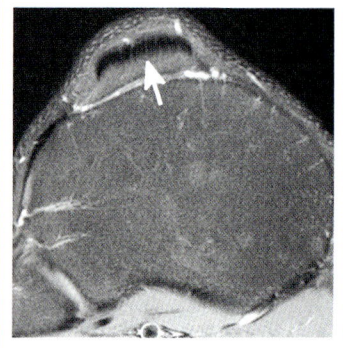

Distal Patellar Tendon

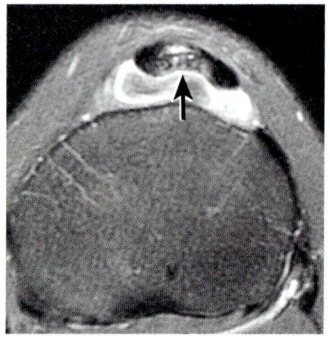

Tendinosis and Interstitial Tear Distal Patellar Tendon

AXIAL

Retinaculum

Retinaculum

- Fascial extensions of vastus medialis and lateralis muscles

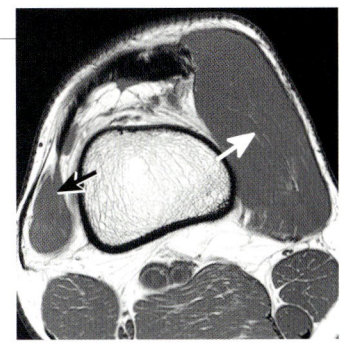

Vastus Lateralis and Medialis

- Lateral retinaculum composed of two layers (superficial and deep layer)
- A lateral release best seen using T1/PD contrast

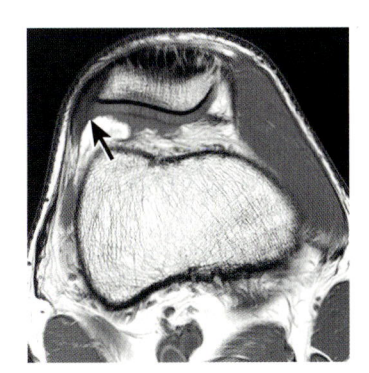

Lateral Retinaculum (Patellar Attachment)

- Normal retinacula linear and hypointense

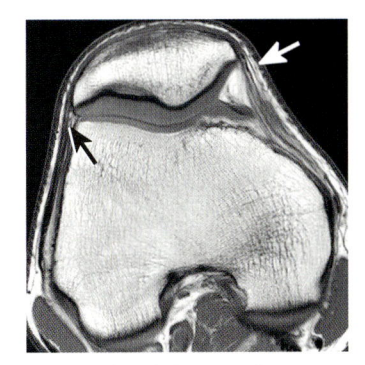

Lateral and Medial Retinacula

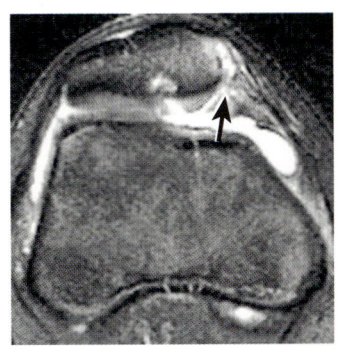

Tear Medial Retinaculum (Patellar Insertion)

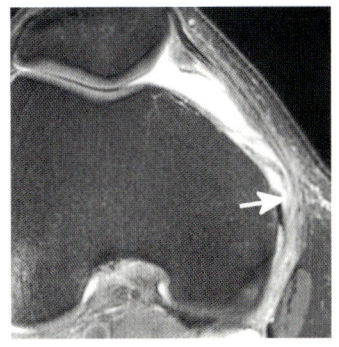

Tear Medial Retinaculum Patellofemoral Ligament (Femoral Attachment)

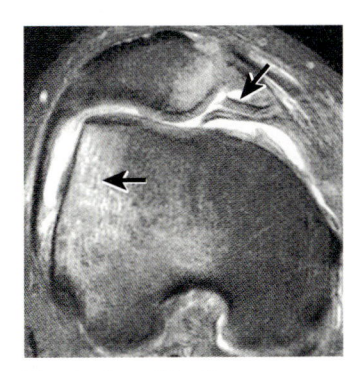

Transient Lateral Patellar Dislocation with Loose Body

AXIAL

Cruciate Ligaments

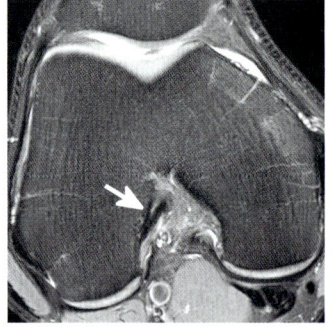

ACL Origin

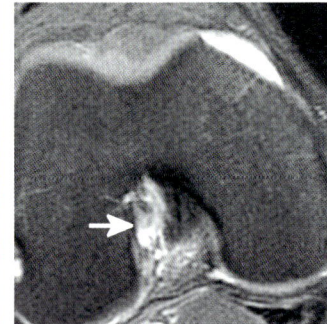

Tear ACL Origin

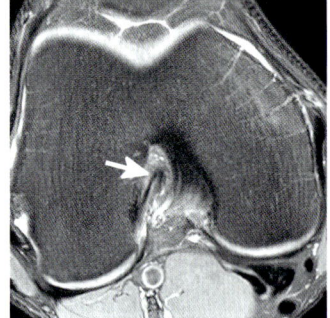

PCL Origin; Proximal ACL

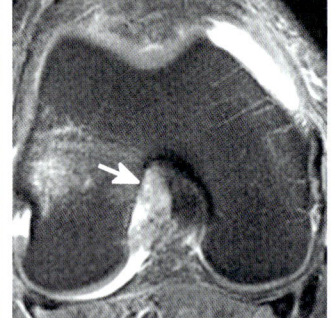

Tear Proximal ACL

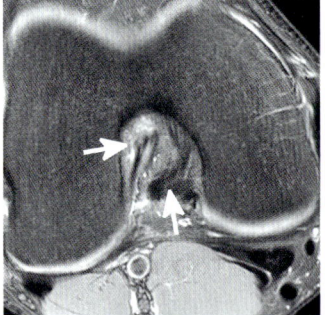

Mid ACL; Mid PCL

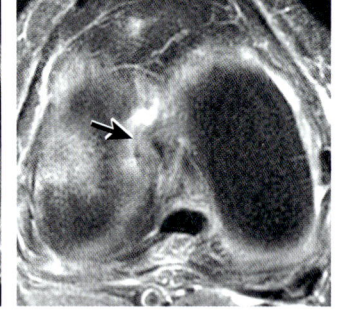

Moderate Sprain Mid ACL

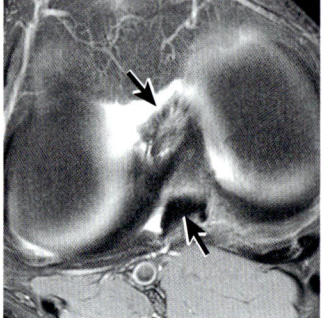

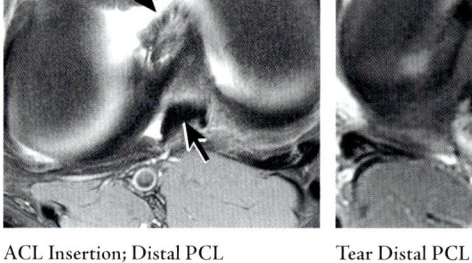

ACL Insertion; Distal PCL

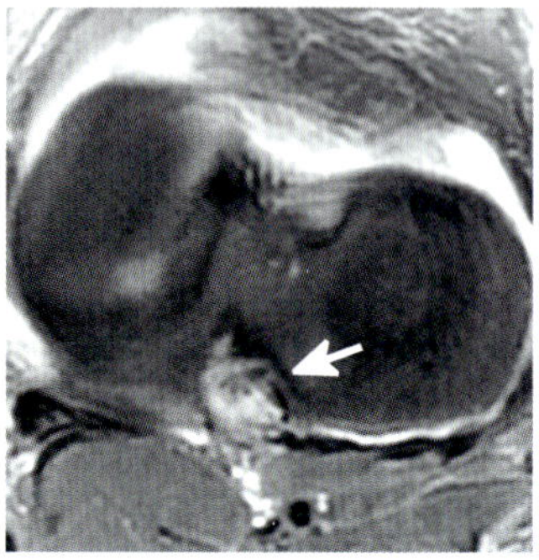

Tear Distal PCL

Cruciate Ligaments

- Origin best assessed on coronal images

- Fluid should not replace proximal fibers or be interposed between the LFC and ACL origin in a normal ligament.

- ACL sprains, especially grade 2, are associated with loss of fiber striation or involve a selective bundle rupture.

- Distal ACL assessment best on coronal images, while distal PCL best on sagittal images; secondary documentation of morphology in the axial plane

AXIAL

Menisci

Menisci

- Axial image prescriptions are performed parallel to the medial compartment to show the entire medial meniscus on a single image.

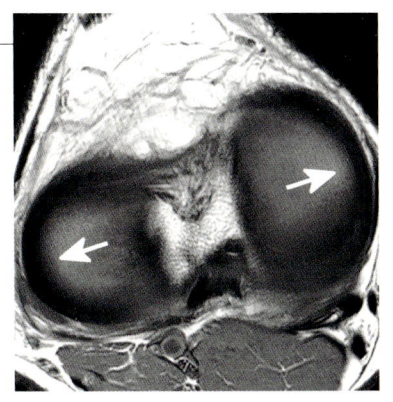

Normal Lateral and Medial Meniscus

- Meniscal tear patterns can be correlated with axial images to appreciate surface tear morphology as a radial, flap, longitudinal, or horizontal tear.

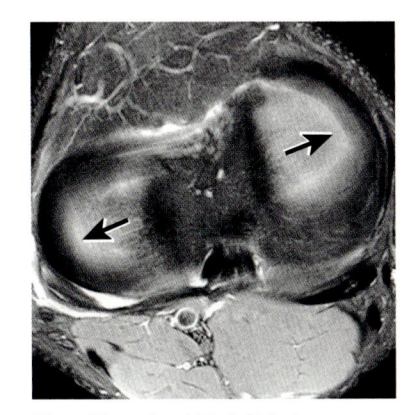

Normal Lateral and Medial Meniscus

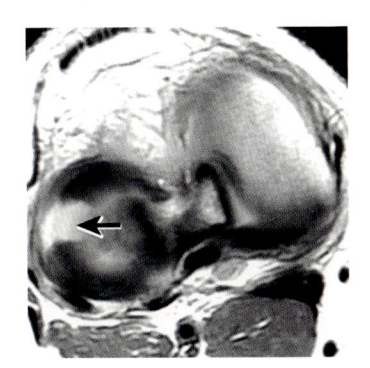

Large Radial Tear (Full Thickness) Body Lateral Meniscus

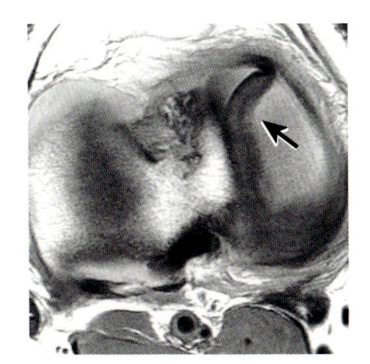

Bucket-Handle Tear Medial Meniscus

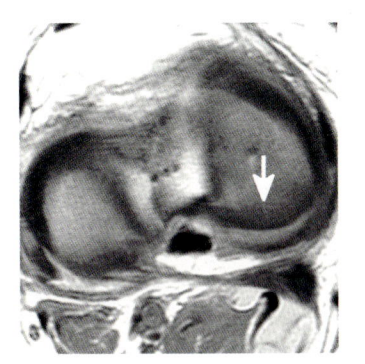

Longitudinal Vertical Tear Posterior Horn Medial Meniscus

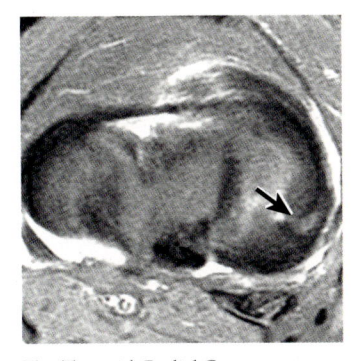

Flap Tear with Radial Component Medial Meniscus

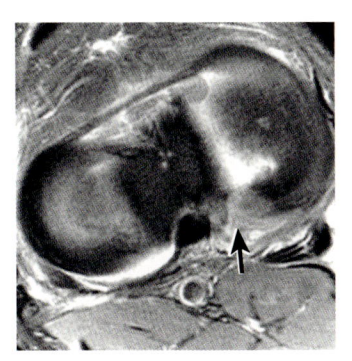

Radial Root Tear Medial Meniscus

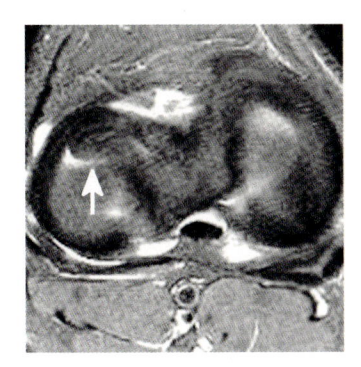

Anterior Flipped Lateral Meniscus

AXIAL

Medial Collateral Ligament

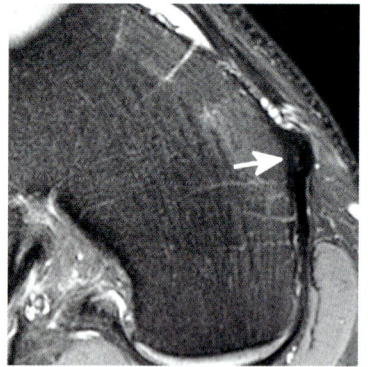

Proximal MCL

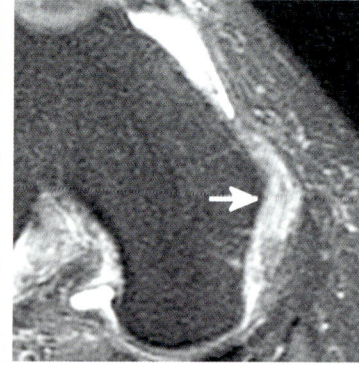

Absent Proximal MCL (Grade 3 Tear)

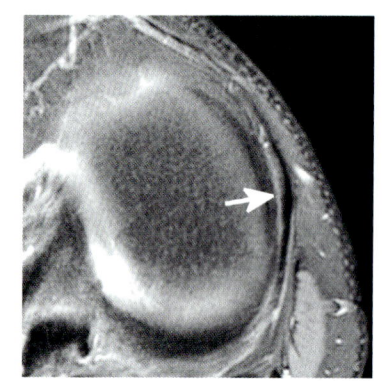

Mid MCL

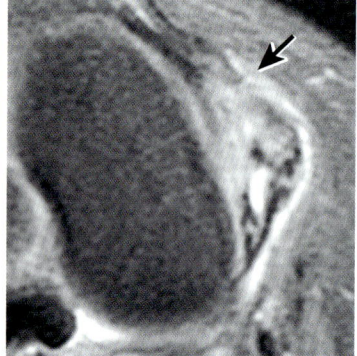

Mid MCL Tear (Grade 2–3)

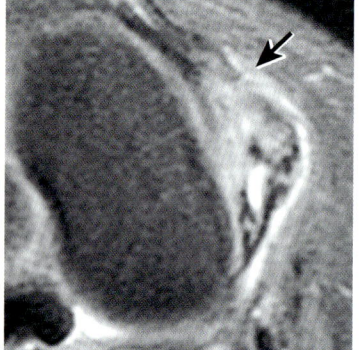

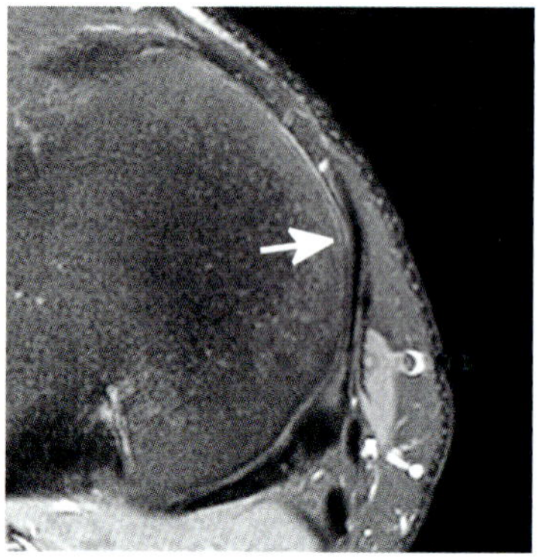

Distal MCL

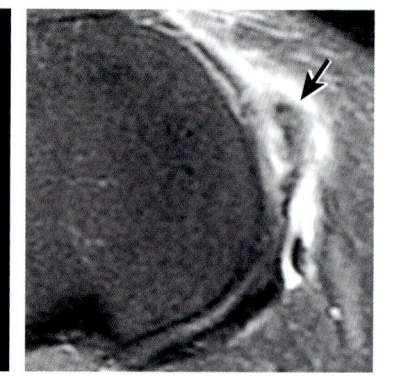

Distal Grade 2 MCL Sprain

Medial Collateral Ligament

- Extends from medial epicondyle (adductor tubercle)

- Layer 3 (meniscofemoral and meniscotibial attachments) is deep to the superficial MCL (layer 2) at the joint line.

- Grade 3 MCL represents ligament discontinuity.
- MCL laxity with an intact epicondylar attachment is associated with a distal tear.

Stoller's Knee Checklist

AXIAL

Lateral Collateral Ligament

Lateral Collateral Ligament

- Locate the LCL lateral to the popliteus tendon at the joint line before following its superior and inferior course.

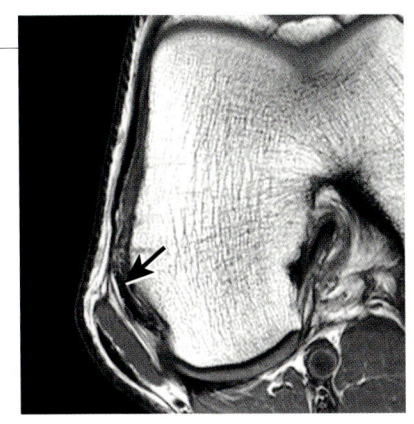

Proximal LCL

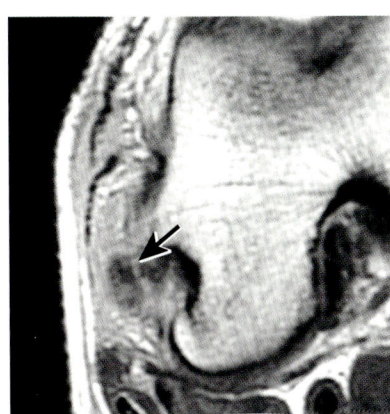

Proximal LCL Tear

- Correlative coronal changes in ligament morphology with axial images

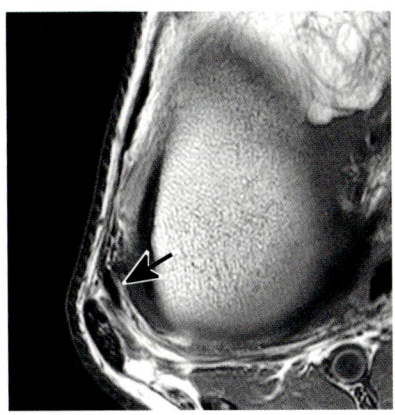

Mid LCL

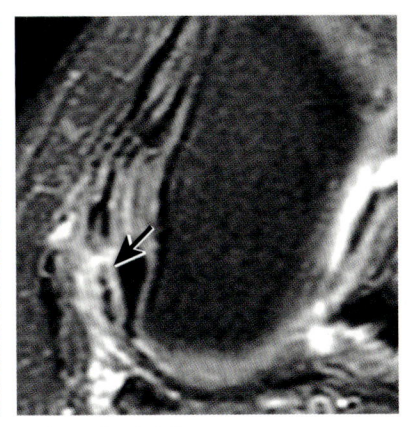

Mid LCL Grade 2 Sprain

- The distal LCL is traced along with the biceps femoris tendon to the lateral margin at the fibular head and not the styloid.

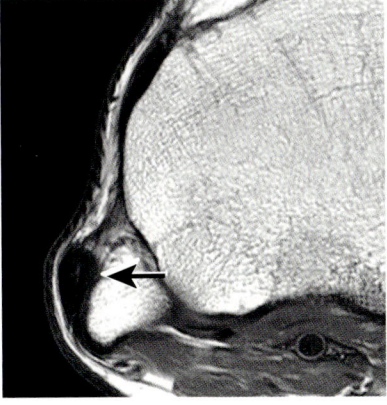

Distal LCL

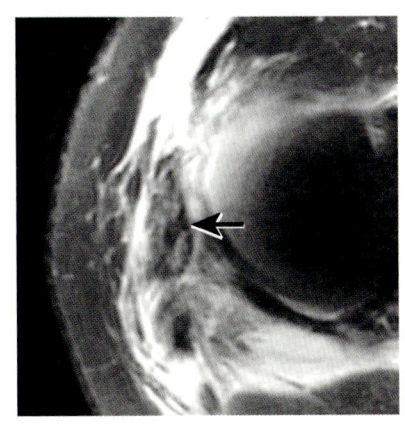

Distal LCL Tear

143

AXIAL

Joint Fluid

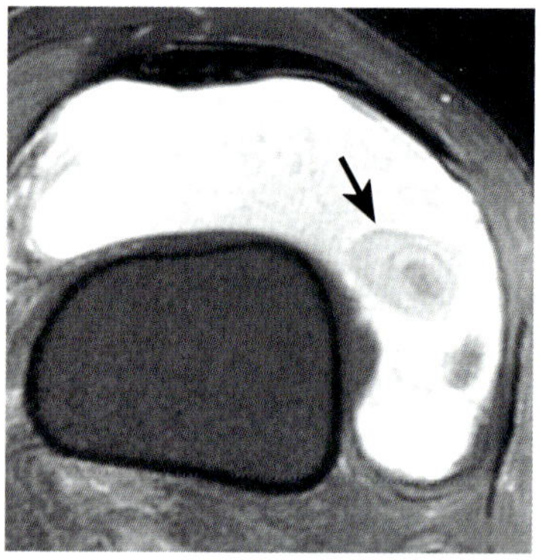

Joint Fluid

- Use PD and fluid-sensitive sequences to characterize cartilage or osseous characteristics of loose bodies.

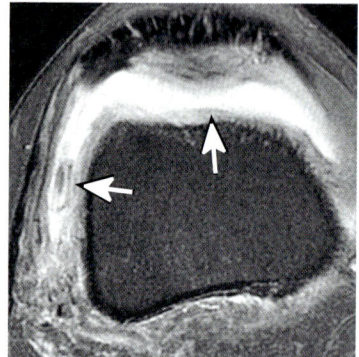

Large Effusion with Loose Bodies

- Intermediate thickened synovium following the capsular contours

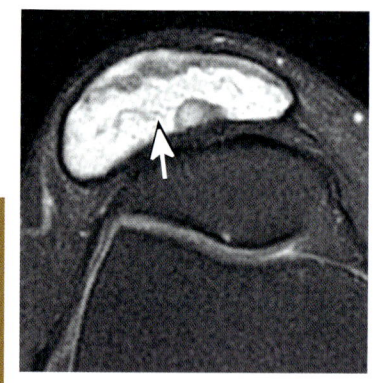

Severe Synovitis

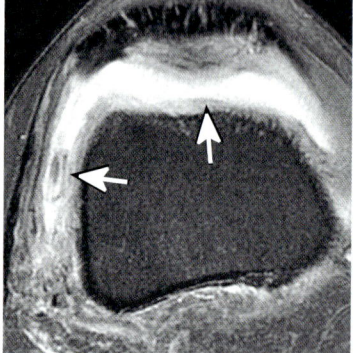

- Describe the homogeneity of bursal fluid distension.

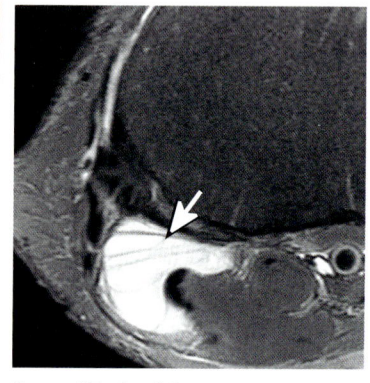

Prepatellar Bursitis

- Distinguish between medial popliteal cysts and atypical cysts in other locations that may not communicate with joint.

Septated Popliteal Cyst

AXIAL
Iliotibial Band and Posterolateral Corner

Iliotibial Band and Posterolateral Corner

- Localized hypointense thickening of iliotibial band in cross-section

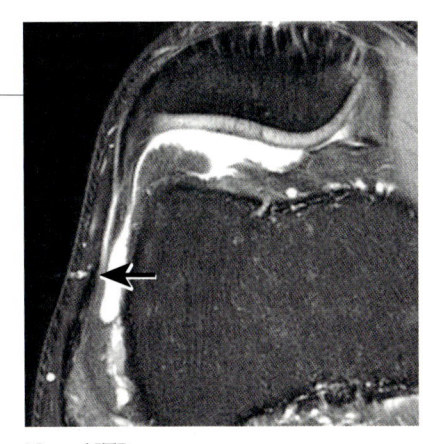

Normal ITB

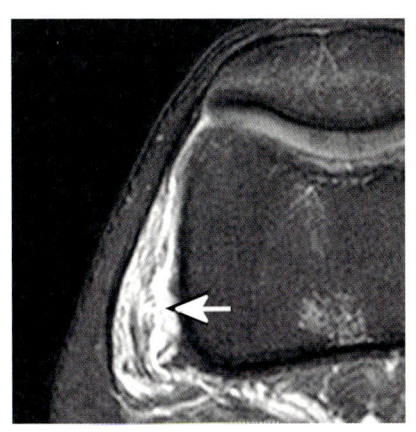

Severe Iliotibial Band Friction Syndrome

- Popliteus tendon is identified at its femoral attachments, the hiatus, and below the joint line.

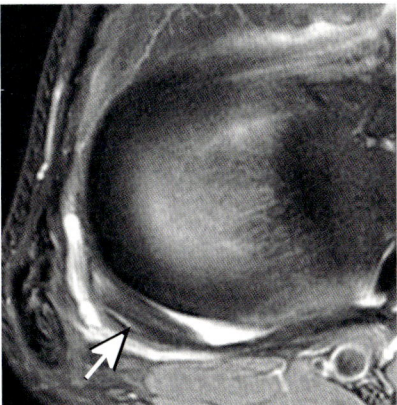

Normal Popliteus Tendon

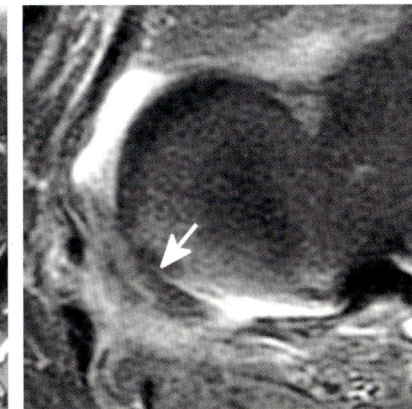

Popliteus Tendon Strain

- Posterior fibular styloid edema (upper facet) or fracture of the posterior fibular head is associated with injury to the popliteofibular and arcuate ligaments.
- Best assessment of popliteofibular ligament is on coronal and sagittal images.

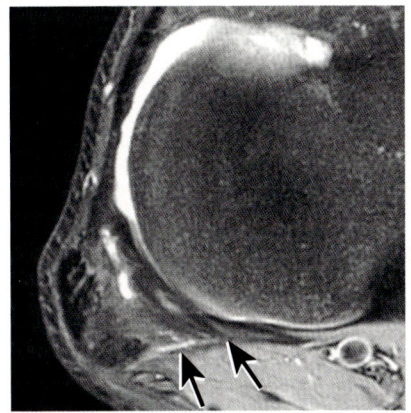

Normal Arcuate and Popliteofibular Ligaments

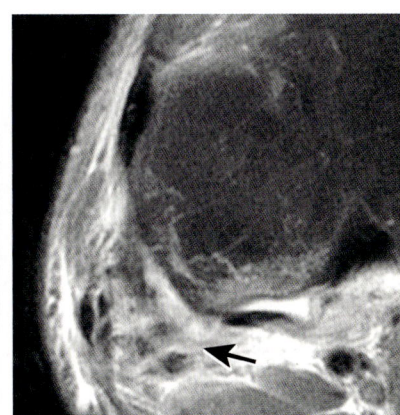

Arcuate and Popliteal Ligament Tear

Protocols for Evaluation of the Meniscus

- T1-weighted images and intermediate PD-weighted images are considered optimal protocols for detecting meniscal lesions.
    - Meniscal lesions are sensitive to the T1 shortening of imbibed synovial fluid in tears and mucinous degenerations.
- Images acquired with a short TE are more sensitive than images with a longer TE in the detection of meniscal degenerations and tears.
- GRE T2*-weighted images are sensitive to grade 1 (focal) and 2 (linear) intrasubstance degenerations and meniscal tears.
    - GRE T2* -weighted images do not rely on contrast window and level manipulation.
- In the presence of an osseous contusion, T1-weighted, STIR, or FS PD-weighted FSE sequences are more sensitive than T2*-weighted images to subchondral marrow edema.
- The chronic subchondral sclerosis seen in degenerative arthrosis and chondromalacia is better visualized on T1- than T2*-weighted images.
- Marrow fat (yellow marrow) signal is best visualized on T1-weighted images.
    - The rate of false-positive results is lower with GRE sequences than with conventional two-dimensional (2D) spin-echo sequences in the detection of meniscal pathology.
- An FS PD conventional spin-echo sequence can also be used to characterize meniscal signal and avoids the potential for false-negative results inherent in relying solely on FSE sequences.
- FSE images offer faster data acquisition but are less sensitive to meniscal pathology than conventional T2 spin-echo pulse sequences.
    - With a shorter ETL to reduce image blurring, the sensitivity (65%) and specificity (96%) for meniscal pathology are decreased with FSE techniques.

- Long-TE FSE sequences may be used to partially reduce blurring and loss of meniscal signal intensity.
- Although useful for the evaluation of the morphology of the meniscus (especially in complex tears, postoperative partial meniscectomies, and primary repairs), reliance on FSE images alone is not recommended for the primary diagnosis of meniscal degenerations or tears.
- A grade 3 meniscal signal may be falsely interpreted as grade 2 signal on a PD FSE or FS PD FSE image.

- Three approaches to sagittal protocols for evaluation of the meniscus:
  - The first echo of a conventional T2-weighted pulse sequence is used to produce intermediate-contrast images for the identification of meniscal lesions.
    - A sagittal FS PD conventional spin-echo sequence generates higher signal intensity within suspected meniscal tears.
  - A second approach is the use of either 2D or three-dimensional (3D) FT T2* sagittal images to demonstrate increased signal intensities in grade 1, 2, and 3 meniscal injuries.
  - The third approach is to use PD FSE images to identify meniscal tears.
    - Many protocols use a combination of PD and FS PD FSE images.
    - Image blurring may result in an underestimation of meniscal signal extension to an articular surface.
    - Adjustments in bandwidth, resolution (matrix), and ETL can partially compensate for this limitation.
- Intravenous gadolinium aids in identification of the postoperative meniscus interface of meniscal implants functioning as artificial menisci.
- Intraarticular gadolinium is used to differentiate healing from repeated injury after primary meniscal repair or partial meniscectomy.
- A fluid-sensitive sequence is used to identify a meniscal cyst associated with a meniscal remnant.

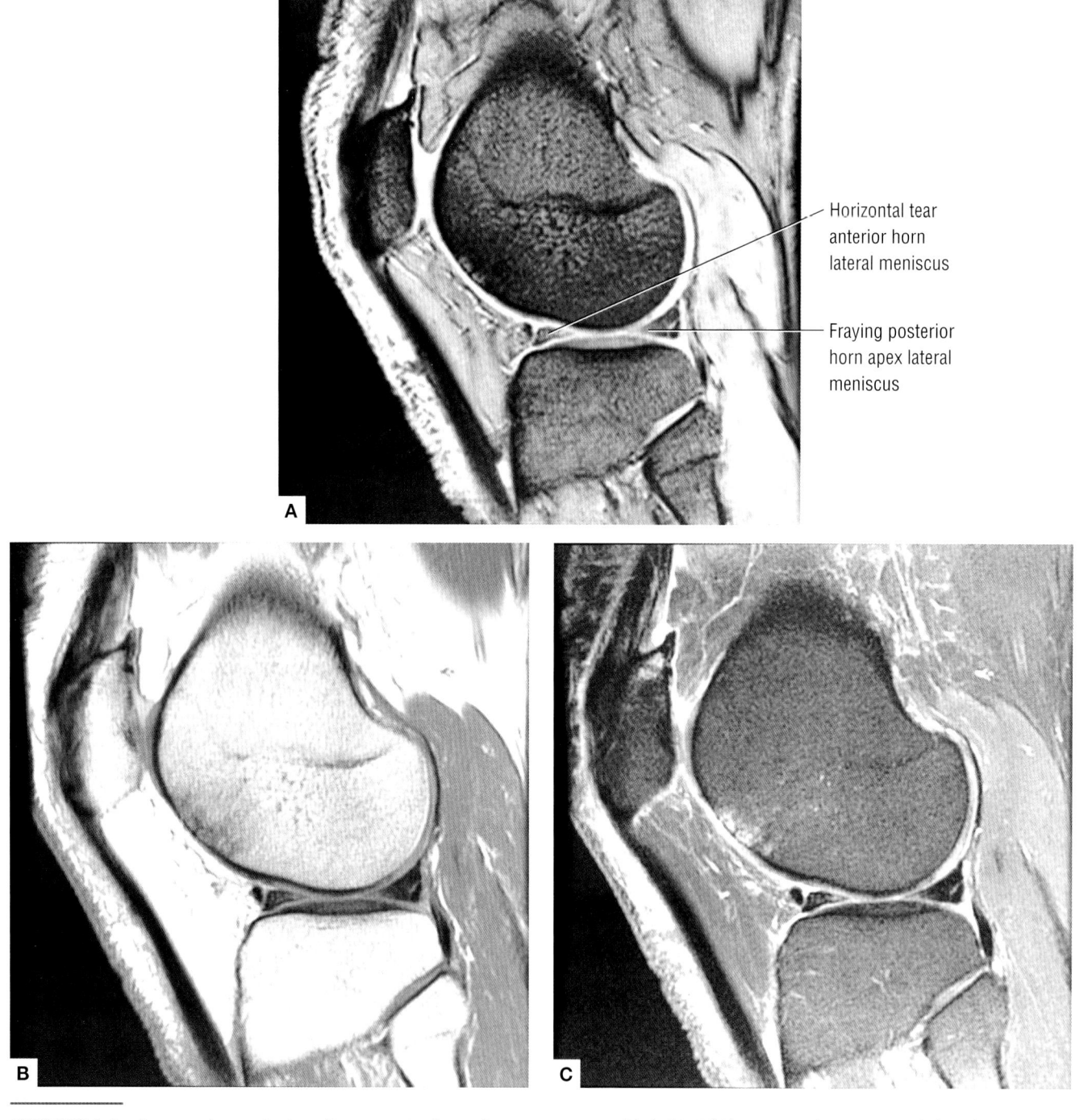

FIGURE 3.1 Increased conspicuity of intrameniscal signal intensity tear on T2* GRE (**A**) compared to PD FSE (**B**) and FSE PD FSE (**C**) sagittal images.

Application and Techniques for Routine Protocols

- Echo Time (TE)
    - Time at which receiver "listens" for signal (sampling)
    - Dephasing after the RF pulse ends represents T2 effect.
    - Increased TE—increased dephasing (increased T2 effects)
    - Increasing the TE decreases SNR. However, resolution increases because the center of k-space is moved to later echoes. Early echoes exhibit dephasing at a faster rate, which results in increased blurring of the image.
    - Fat saturation decreases the overall SNR of the image by suppressing the signal contribution from fat (FS PD FSE images should not use long TE values [e.g., >50msec]; otherwise the SNR decreases).

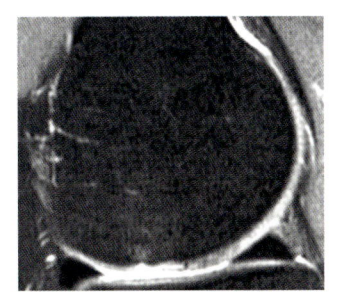

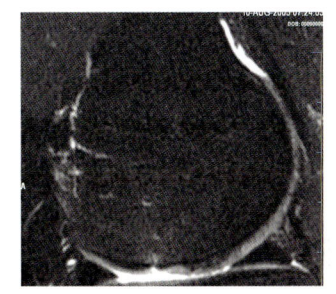

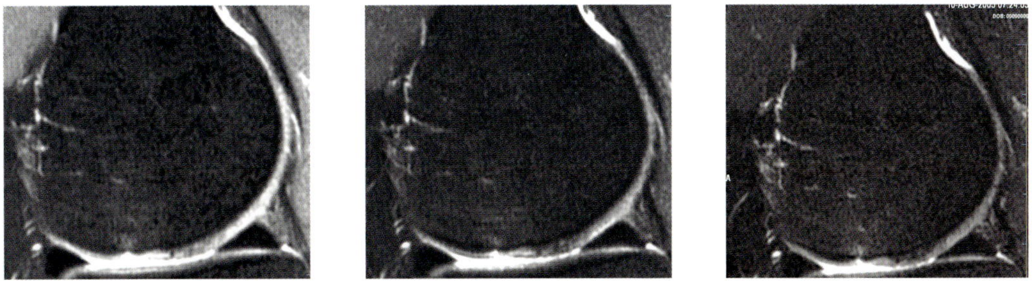

TE 31msec   TE 47msec   TE 78msec
Fat suppressed PD FSE with TE 31, 47, 78msec. BW, TR, FOV, Matrix unchanged.

- Repetition Time (TR)
    - TR controls the amount of saturation (T1 effects).
    - In PD and T2-weighted imaging, the TR must be at least three (and preferably five) times as long as the longest T1 of the tissue being imaged; otherwise, T1 contribution will change the overall image contrast.
    - TR values <3000msec on FS PD FSE images may result in decreased contrast and signal between fluid and articular cartilage.

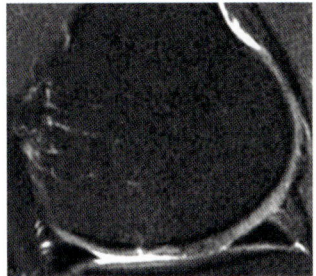

TR 2500msec   TR 3000msec   TR 3500msec
TR 2500, 3000, 3500msec, respectively. BW, TE, FOV, Matrix unchanged.

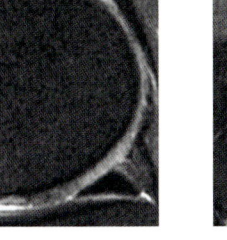

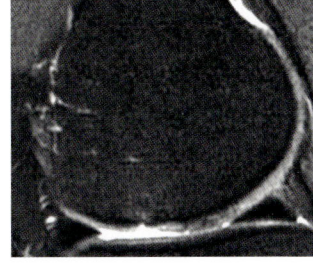

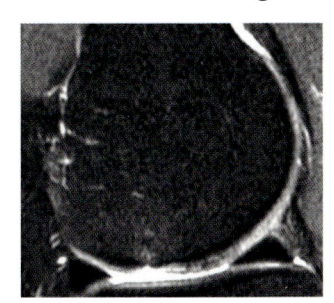

- Receiver Bandwidth (RBW)

    - RBW increases SNR since the amplitude of the readout gradient is reduced. However, it can also result in blurring, increased flow pulsation, and decreased number of slices. Date sampling takes longer with lower RBWs.

    - Blurring in FSE images occurs with lower bandwidth values because of the increase in space between echoes in the echo train length (ETL).

    - Chemical shift increases with shorter RBWs because of a similar range of frequencies sampled across the field of view.

    - To minimize image blurring, recommended bandwidths for PD FSE images are 15 to 30kHz. With bandwidths of 15 to 20kHz, there is greater SNR.

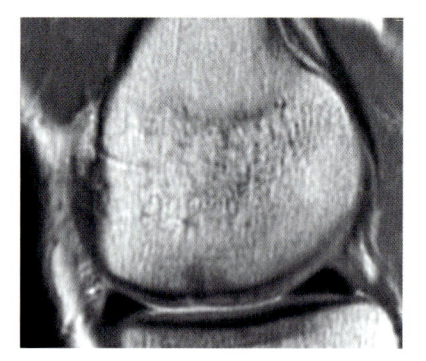

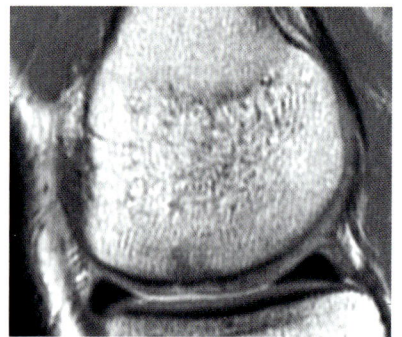

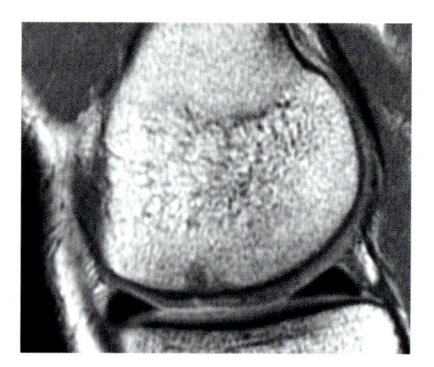

BW 10kHz   BW 15kHz   BW 30kHz
BW 10, 15, 30kHz. TR, TE, FOV, and Matrix unchanged.

- Fluid-sensitive pulse sequences

    - Optimized TR values ≥3200msec

    - Optimized TE values ≥40msec but ≤50msec

- Matrix resolution and ETL (echo train length) will influence image blurring potentially problematic when assessing chondral surfaces.

- Motion correction pulse sequences may blur detail of articular cartilage surfaces and deeper zones.

4
The Meniscus

Normal Anatomy and MR Imaging of the Meniscus (pages 153–155)

Medial Meniscus (page 156)

Lateral Meniscus (pages 157–158)

Microstructure of the Meniscus (pages 159–161)

Vascular Supply of the Meniscus (pages 162–171)

Meniscal Degenerations and Tears (pages 172–332)

Postoperative Appearance of the Meniscus (pages 333–364)

Miscellaneous Meniscal Pathology Including Meniscocapsular Separations, Meniscal Cysts, CPPD, and Meniscal Ossicle (pages 365–393)

The Meniscus

Normal Anatomy and MR Imaging of the Meniscus

- The fibrocartilaginous menisci/semilunar cartilages:
  - C-shaped
  - Attach to the condylar surface of the tibia
  - Provide added mechanical stability for femorotibial gliding
  - The integrity of the peripheral one third of the meniscus is essential for both load transmission and stability.
    - The inner two thirds of the meniscus is also important, but secondary compared to the peripheral one third in maximizing joint contact area.[40]
- The meniscus:
  - Has a bowtie appearance peripherally
  - Tapers to a thin, free edge facing the intercondylar notch
  - Protects the articular cartilage by acting as a buffer between femoral and tibial surfaces with loading
  - Provides joint lubrication
  - Increases joint stability by providing congruence between femoral and tibial articular surfaces
    - This congruence is assisted by deepening of the articular surface of the tibial plateaus to accommodate the articulation between the femoral condyles.[90]
- The proximal/superior meniscal surface:
  - Smooth and concave in shape
  - Produces greater contact with the femoral condyles
- The inferior meniscal surface:
  - Flat in shape
  - Location rests on the opposing surface of the tibia.
- The peripheral aspects of the menisci:
  - Thick and convex in shape
  - Attach to the inside of the joint capsule

- Tibial attachments to the meniscus are made through the meniscofemoral, meniscotibial, or coronary ligaments of the joint capsule.
- The meniscus is relatively avascular in adults, except for the peripheral 10% to 25% of the meniscus supplied by the perimeniscal capillary plexus.[16,17]
- In children, vascularity is restricted to the peripheral third of the meniscus, and the inner two thirds are relatively avascular.
- Intact menisci:
    - Demonstrate uniform low signal intensity on T1-, T2-, and T2*-weighted images
    - Triangular in cross-section with an outer convex curve
    - Apex is directed toward the intercondylar notch.
- The meniscus is divided into thirds:
    - The anterior horn
    - The body
    - The posterior horn
- On sagittal images, the meniscus is visualized with opposing triangular shapes close to the intercondylar notch.
    - These opposing triangular shapes represent the anterior and posterior horns.
- Functions of the menisci include[525]:
    - Transmission of axial and torsional forces across the joint
    - Joint stability
        - Medial meniscectomy has minimal effect on anteroposterior motion in the stable knee.
        - In the anterior cruciate ligament (ACL)-deficient knee, meniscectomy results in increased anterior tibial translation of up to 58% at 90 degrees of flexion.
    - Cushioning of mechanical loading
        - The meniscus is one half as stiff as articular cartilage and thus plays a role in shock absorption.
    - Protection from arthritic changes in an ACL-deficient knee
    - Limitation of comprehensive displacement
    - Distribution of synovial fluid

The Meniscus

- Increasing the surface area for femoral condylar motion
- Prevention of synovial impingement
- Proprioception

■ The stabilizing effect and vascularization of the peripheral third of the meniscus form the basis for attempts to preserve tissue in partial meniscectomies.

- However, preservation may not protect the joint from degenerative changes.[16,532]

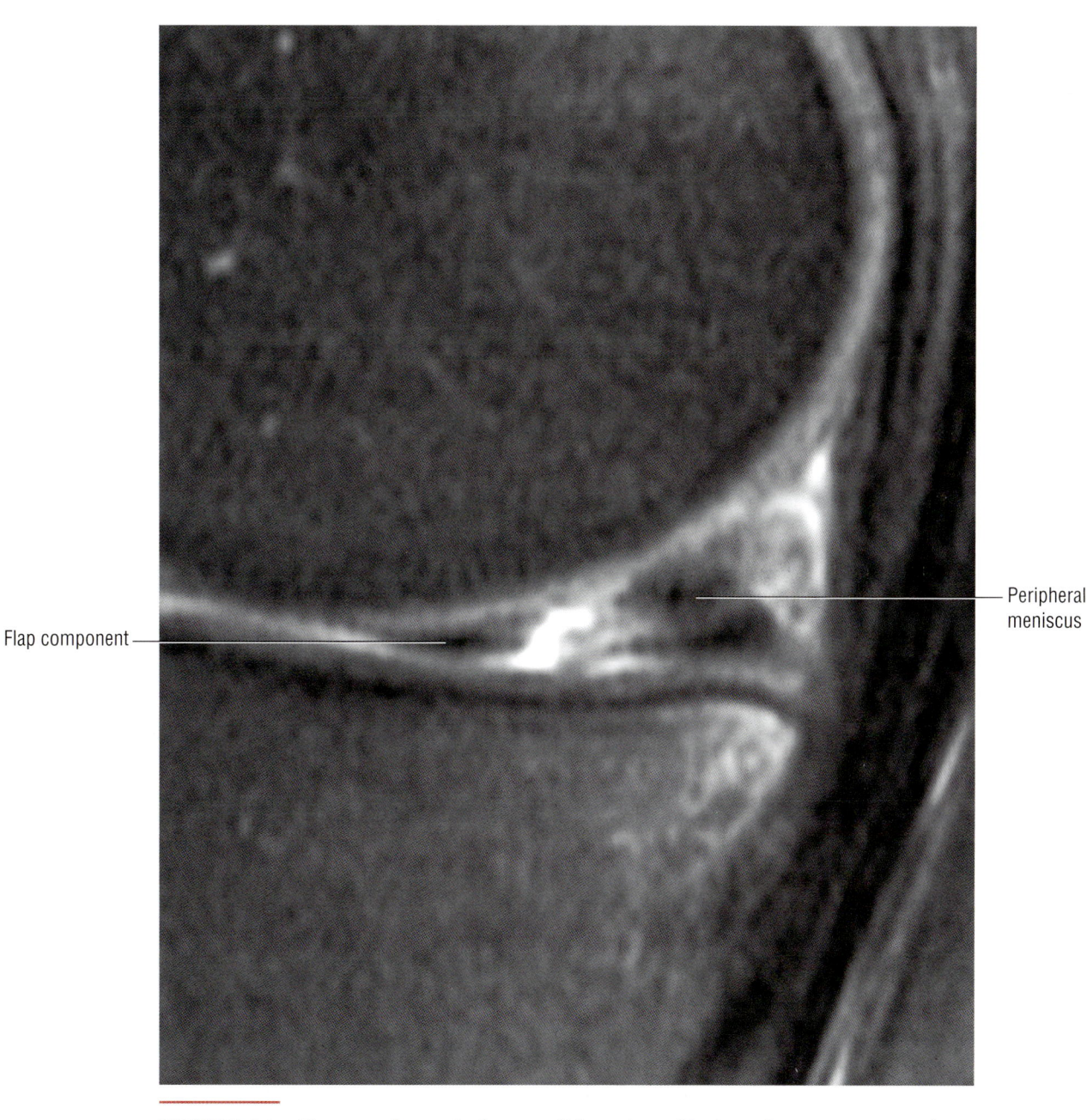

FIGURE 4.1 Flap tear of posterior horn medial meniscus. The inner flap component involves the avascular portion of the meniscus. Sagittal FS PD FSE image.

Medial Meniscus

- The medial meniscus:
    - Semicircular in shape
        - Has a more open C-shaped configuration than the more circular lateral meniscus
    - Has a wide posterior horn
    - Narrows anteriorly
    - Attaches to the joint capsule along its entire peripheral circumference
- The anterior horn of the medial meniscus:
    - Attachment is variable.
    - Attaches to the area of the intercondylar fossa of the tibia anterior to the tibial attachment of the ACL
        - Has largest insertion area of $61.4mm^2$ on the tibial surface[40]
    - Posterior fibers of the anterior horn attachment of the medial meniscus attach to the transverse ligament.
        - The transverse ligament of the knee connects the anterior horns of the medial and lateral menisci.
- The posterior horn of the medial meniscus:
    - Primary restraint against an applied anterior tibial force in an ACL-deficient knee
    - Attachment located at the posterior intercondylar fossa of the tibia
        - Identified between the attachment of the posterior horn of the lateral meniscus and the posterior cruciate ligament (PCL).
    - Medial meniscus posterior root attaches anterior to the insertion of the PCL and posterior to the medial tibial spine.
- Limited mobility of the medial meniscal attachment to the deep layer of the medial collateral ligament (MCL) and capsule renders the medial meniscus susceptible to injury.
    - The coronary ligament is the capsular attachment or meniscotibial component of the deep capsular ligament or deep tibial component of the deep MCL.
    - The meniscofemoral ligament component of the deep MCL spans the meniscus to the femur.
- A small intermediate-signal-intensity bursa separates the posterior horn of the medial meniscus from the joint capsule.

Lateral Meniscus

- The lateral meniscus:
    - Forms a tight C shape (more circular than the medial meniscus)
        - Covers a larger portion of the tibial articular surface area than the medial meniscus[388]
        - Anterior and posterior horns attach closer to each other compared to the medial meniscus.
    - Relatively symmetric in width from anterior to posterior
    - Accommodates the popliteus tendon posteriorly
    - Separated from the lateral collateral (extracapsular) ligament
    - Has posterior horn attachments to the PCL and medial femoral condyle through the ligaments of Wrisberg (posterior to the PCL) and Humphrey (anterior to the PCL)
        - The ligaments of Wrisberg and Humphrey represent branches of the meniscofemoral ligament attaching the posterior horn of the lateral meniscus to the lateral aspect of the medial femoral condyle.
    - Relatively mobile (allowing for greater rollback on the lateral tibial plateau)
    - Covers two thirds of the tibial articular surface
    - Has a loose peripheral attachment to the joint capsule (except for the passage of the popliteus tendon)
    - No direct attachment of the lateral meniscus to the fibular collateral ligament or lateral collateral ligament (LCL)
- The anterior horn of the lateral meniscus attaches between the tibial intercondylar eminence and the anterior attachment of the ACL.[90,222,254]
- The posterior horn of the lateral meniscus is attached between the tibial intercondylar eminence and the posterior medial meniscus.
- The posterior root is posterior to the lateral tibial eminence.
- The popliteus recess allows passage to the popliteus tendon through a 1-cm hiatus in the posterolateral attachment of the lateral meniscus.
    - Meniscal tears near the popliteus hiatus area are less likely to heal.
- The superior fascicle (posterosuperior popliteomeniscal fascicle) is visualized medial to the inferior fascicle (anteroinferior popliteomeniscal fascicle) as the popliteus tendon penetrates the meniscocapsular junction.

- The function of the popliteal tendon attachments to the lateral meniscus is to pull the lateral meniscus posterior when the knee is flexed.[40,227,462]
    - Disruption of the popliteomeniscal fascicles may result in increased meniscal motion at the hiatus with hypermobility of the posterior horn of the lateral meniscus. A disrupted posterosuperior fascicle is thus associated with a tear of the posterior horn of the lateral meniscus.
    - This unlocking of the knee from full extension is the reverse of the screw-home mechanism of the knee.
        - The screw-home mechanism functions to lock the knee in extension with internal rotation of the femur relative to the tibia.
- Greater mobility and thus excursion of the lateral meniscus compared to the medial meniscus[40]
    - Less rigorous attachments of the lateral meniscus to the articular capsule

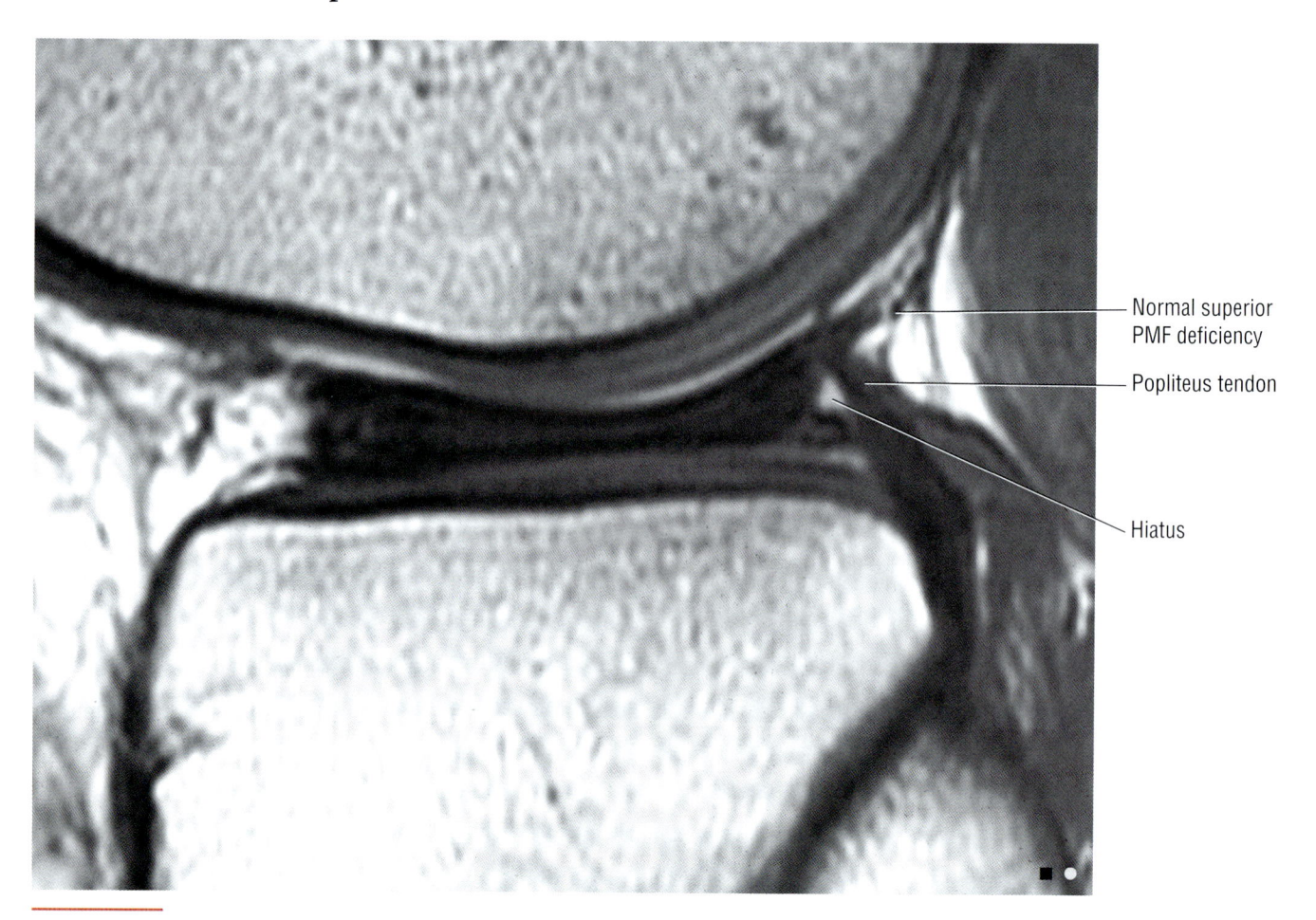

FIGURE 4.2 Normal deficiency of the superior (posterosuperior) popliteomeniscal fascicle (PMF) in a partial discoid lateral meniscus. Sagittal PD FSE image.

Microstructure of the Meniscus

Key Concepts

- Meniscal Microstructure
    - Circumferential collagen fibers create normal meniscal hoop tension.
    - Radial (radial tie) fibers stabilize longitudinally oriented circumferential collagen fibers and also help resist meniscal extrusion.
    - Middle perforating collagen fibers represent a concentration of radially oriented collagen fibers in the central plane of the meniscus.

Collagen Bundle Zones

- Meniscus is composed of fibrochondrocytes within the extracellular matrix.[40]
    - The extracellular matrix is composed of collagen and proteoglycans and allows for load-bearing function.
    - The fibrochondrocytes synthesize the fibrocartilaginous matrix.
        - Superficial oval and deeper rounded cells
        - Fibrochondrocytes are rich in endoplasmic retinaculum and Golgi complexes with few mitochondria.
- The microstructure of the fibrocartilaginous meniscus is organized so that the collagen bundles form two distinct zones:
    - Circumferential zone
        - Circumferential fibers or bundles are concentrated in the peripheral third of the meniscus.
        - Their function is to resist longitudinal loading by absorbing compressive forces.[69]
        - The meniscocapsular junction is peripheral to the circumferential zone.

- Transverse zone
    - Radial collagen fibers bridge the circumferential zone of the meniscus peripherally toward the free edge.
    - Radial fibers at the surface and in the midsubstance of the meniscus contribute to structural rigidity and provide resistance to longitudinal splitting.[90]
    - On cross-section, the transverse zone is divided into superior and inferior leaves by the middle perforating collagen bundle made up of a high concentration of radially oriented fibers.
    - Middle perforating collagen fibers normally cannot be distinguished from adjacent meniscal tissue on magnetic resonance (MR) images.
    - Secondary vertical collagen fibers, which function as secondary stabilizers, also may be present within the transverse zone.
    - In internal degenerations, the middle perforating collagen bundle corresponds to the location of the predominantly horizontal signal intensity seen in grade 2 menisci.

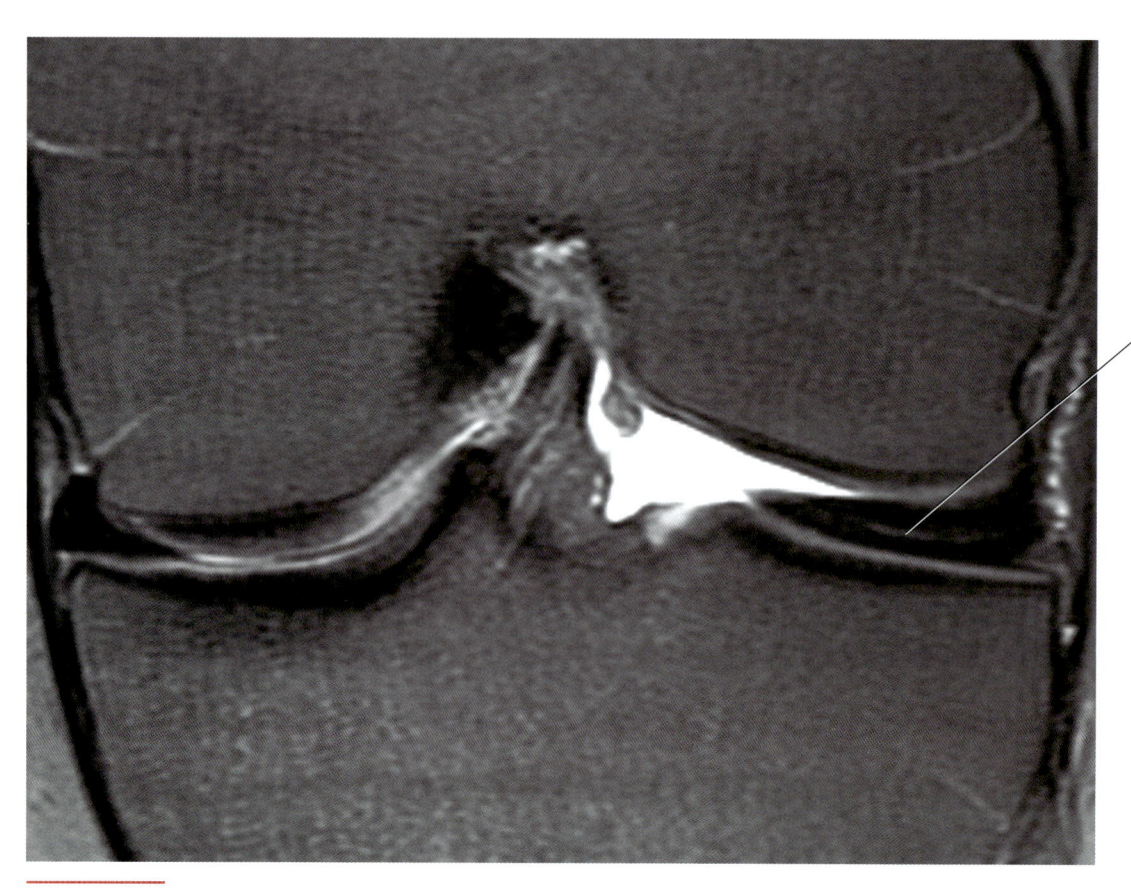

FIGURE 4.3   Horizontally oriented intrasubstance degeneration along the middle perforating collagen bundle (shear plane of the meniscus). Coronal FS PD FSE image.

Structural Layers of the Meniscus

- The collagen fibers of the meniscus exist in layers.[40]
    - Most collagen fibers are directed along the longitudinal axis of the meniscus.
    - Oblique and radial fibers reinforce the structural integrity of the meniscus.
- The meniscus is characterized by three structurally distinct layers:
    - A superficial layer with fine fibrils woven into a mesh-like pattern
        - Important in the disruption of shear stress
    - A surface layer deep to the superficial layer with randomly oriented collagen fibers
    - A middle layer with a circumferential pattern of collagen fibers[91]
- Radial fibers extend from the periphery of the middle layer into the inner rim.
    - Radial fibers function as tie fibers to resist longitudinal tearing.
    - The unique framework of the middle layer allows the meniscus to resist tensile forces by converting axial loads to circumferential stresses.
    - Circumferential fibers resist resultant hoop stresses, which are transmitted to the tibia through strong anterior and posterior meniscal attachments.[122]
        - Compressive loads are dispersed by circumferential fibers.
    - Normal hoop tension is reduced by a radial tear that extends to the capsular margin of the meniscus.
- Ninety percent of collagen in the meniscus is type I.
    - The remainder of meniscal collagen is composed of types II, III, V, and VI.
- Elastin and noncollagenous proteins are present in the meniscal fibrocartilage.[40]

Vascular Supply of the Meniscus

- The entire meniscus is vascularized at birth.

- The inner one third of the meniscus is avascular by 9 months.

- The adult vascular pattern is reached by age 10 years as the meniscal vascularity decreases after birth.[40]

- The perimeniscal capillary plexus[90,209]:
    - Originates from branches of the lateral and medial geniculate arteries
    - Supplies the periphery of the meniscus throughout its attachment to the joint capsule
    - Penetrates the peripheral border of the meniscus with a circumferential network and radial branches oriented toward the center of the joint

- In the adult meniscus, vascular penetrations may extend to 15% of the width of the meniscus.
    - Because of the relative avascular quality of the inner portion of the meniscus as cell nutrition occurs primarily through the diffusion of synovial fluid

- The lateral meniscus is relatively avascular at the popliteal hiatus.

- The meniscus can be divided into red-red, red-white, and white-white zones.[40]
    - The red-red zone is the outer third of the meniscus and is vascular.
    - The red-white zone is the mid-third of the meniscus and receives nourishment from both blood supply and synovial fluid.
    - The white-white zone is avascular and receives its nutrition by the diffusion of synovial fluid.

- The vascular/red zone is represented by a band of peripheral hypointensity on MR images.[360]
    - Fat and vascularized connective tissue located between the meniscus and capsule should not be mistaken for the red zone of the meniscal fibrocartilage.

- Peripheral meniscal vascularity does not show intravenous (IV) contrast enhancement.
    - Perimeniscal soft tissue shows enhancement adjacent to the meniscus.

The Meniscus

- A vascularized synovial fringe adherent to the articular surfaces of the menisci is demonstrated throughout the peripheral attachment of the medial and lateral meniscus.
  - This synovial reflection does not directly contribute vessels to the meniscus but may be surgically stimulated to facilitate a reparative response.
- Neuroanatomy is similar to the pattern of the meniscus vascular supply.
  - Meniscal roots are richly innervated.
  - The body of the meniscus is innervated peripherally.
  - At the extremes of flexion and extension, the horns of the meniscus are compressed with neural cell stimulation occurring.
  - Peripheral meniscal tissue is more sensitive than more central fibrocartilage.[40,147]

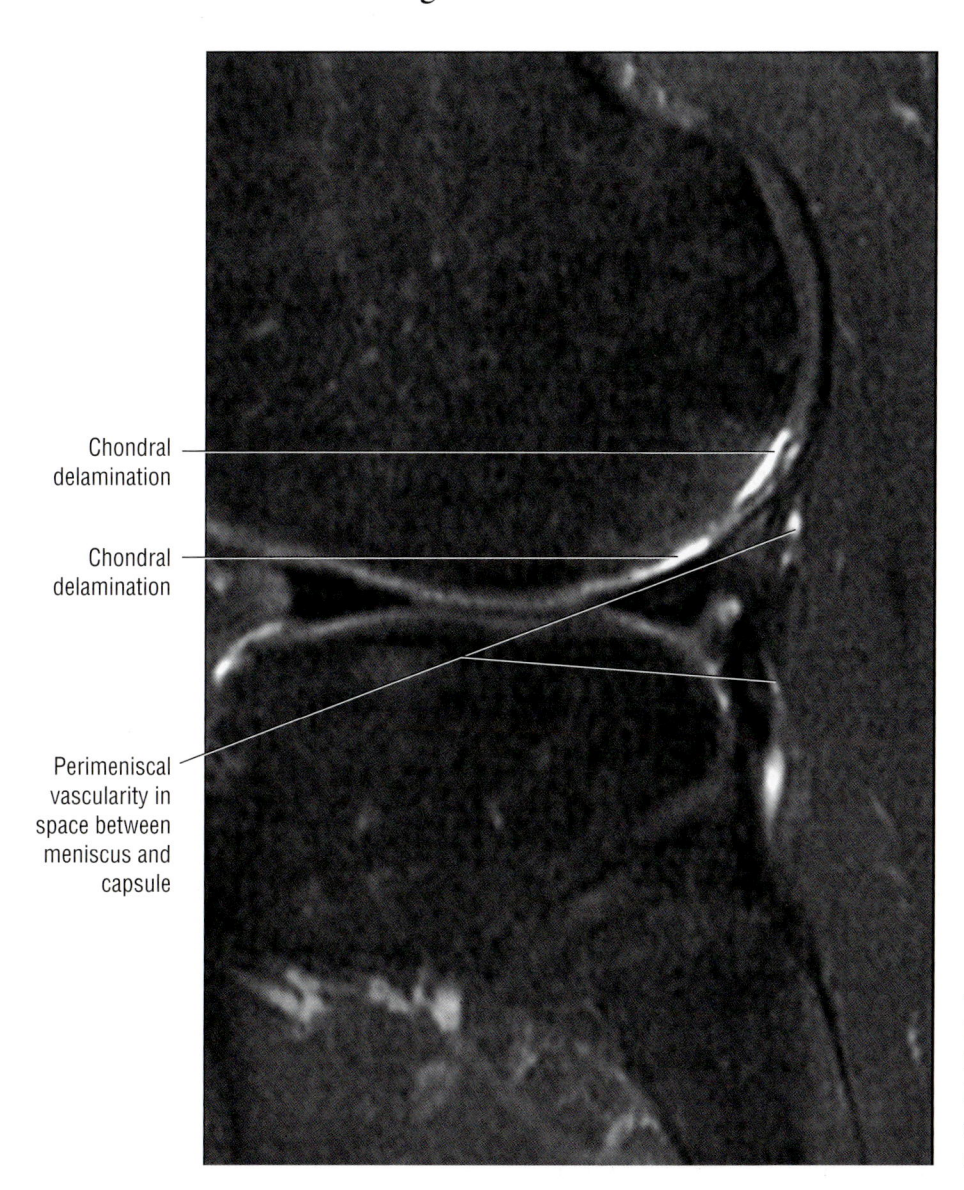

FIGURE 4.4 Chondral delamination of the lateral femoral condyle shown on sagittal FS PD FSE image. Vascularity associated with the posterior capsule. This is peripheral to the red-red zone of the meniscal fibrocartilage.

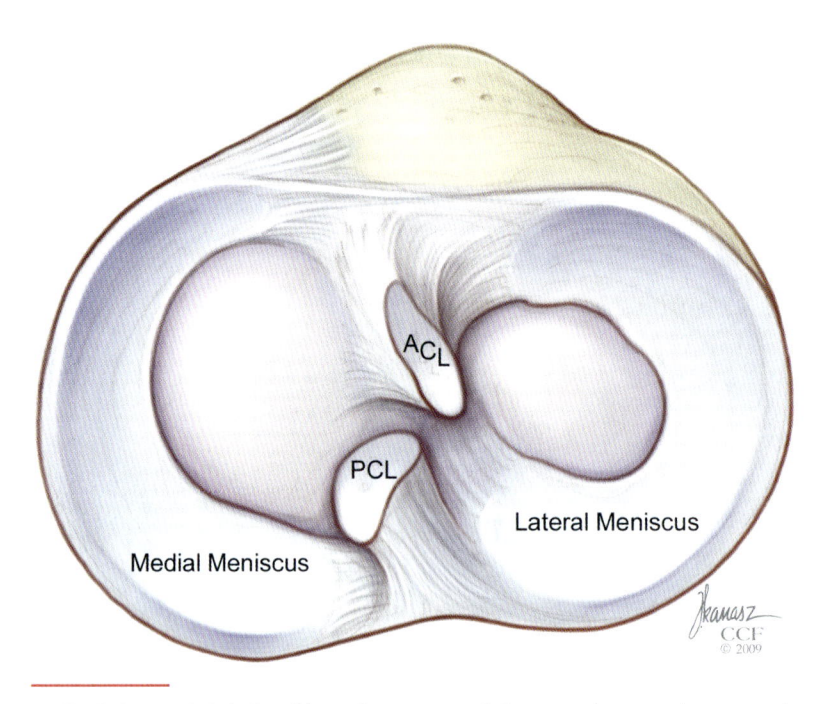

FIGURE 4.5 Medial and lateral menisci and their attachments. (Reprinted from Fu FH. *Master Techniques in Orthopaedic Surgery: Sports Medicine*. Philadelphia, PA: Lippincott Williams & Wilkins; 2010, with permission.)

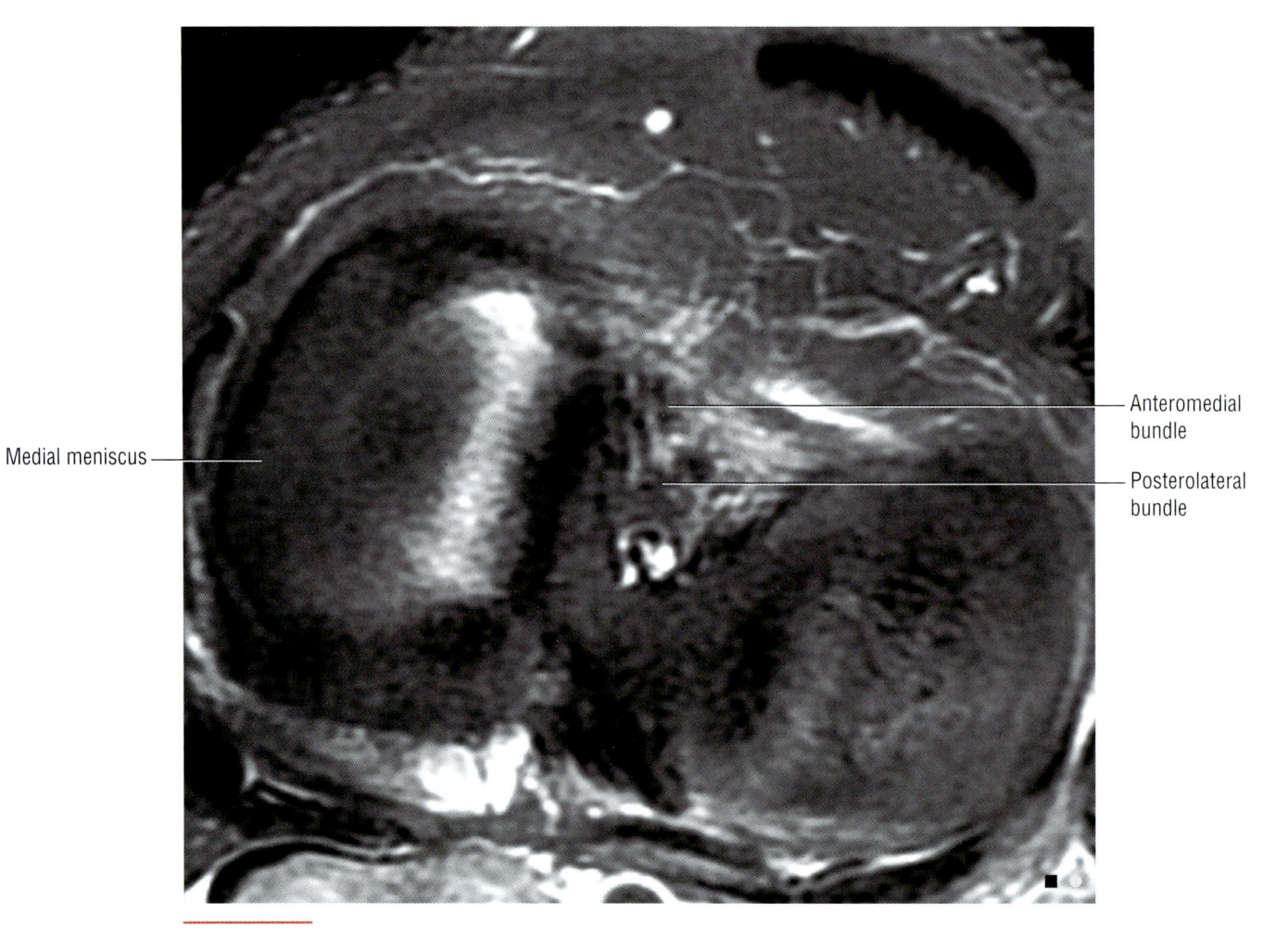

FIGURE 4.6 Medial meniscus tibial attachments and double bundle ACL distal insertions, axial image.

The Meniscus

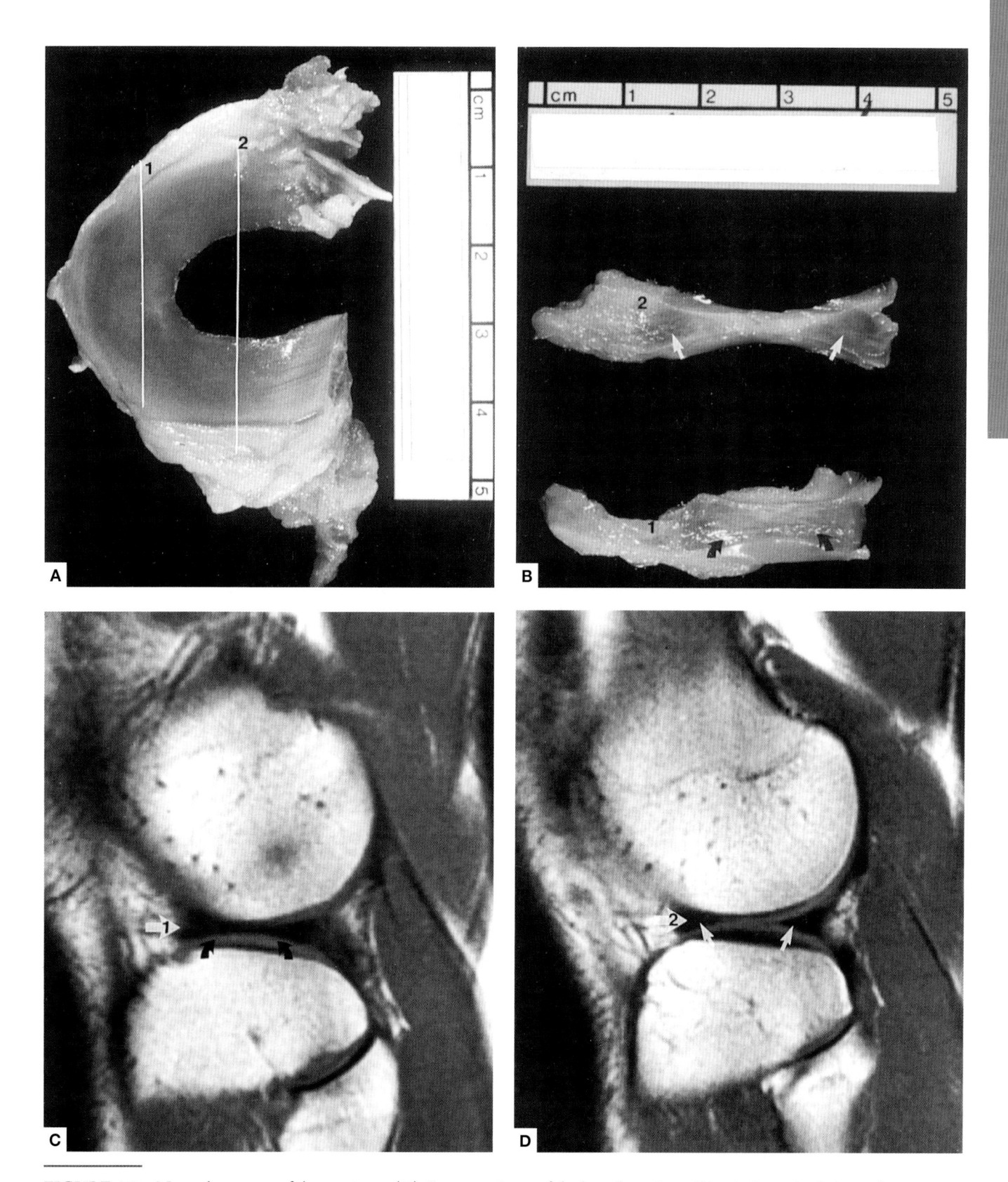

FIGURE 4.7 Normal anatomy of the meniscus. (**A**) Gross specimen of the lateral meniscus. Line 1, the sagittal plane of section through the body of the lateral meniscus; line 2, the sagittal plane of section through the anterior and body of the lateral meniscus. (**B**) The corresponding gross sagittal sections (1 and 2) are seen through the body (*curved black arrows*) and anterior and posterior horns (*straight white arrows*) of the lateral meniscus. The periphery or body of the meniscus has a continuous bowtie appearance. The anterior and posterior horns are oriented as opposing triangles of fibrocartilage. (**C, D**) The corresponding sagittal plane images (1 and 2) demonstrate the low-signal-intensity body (*curved black arrows*) and anterior and posterior horns (*straight white arrows*) of the lateral meniscus.

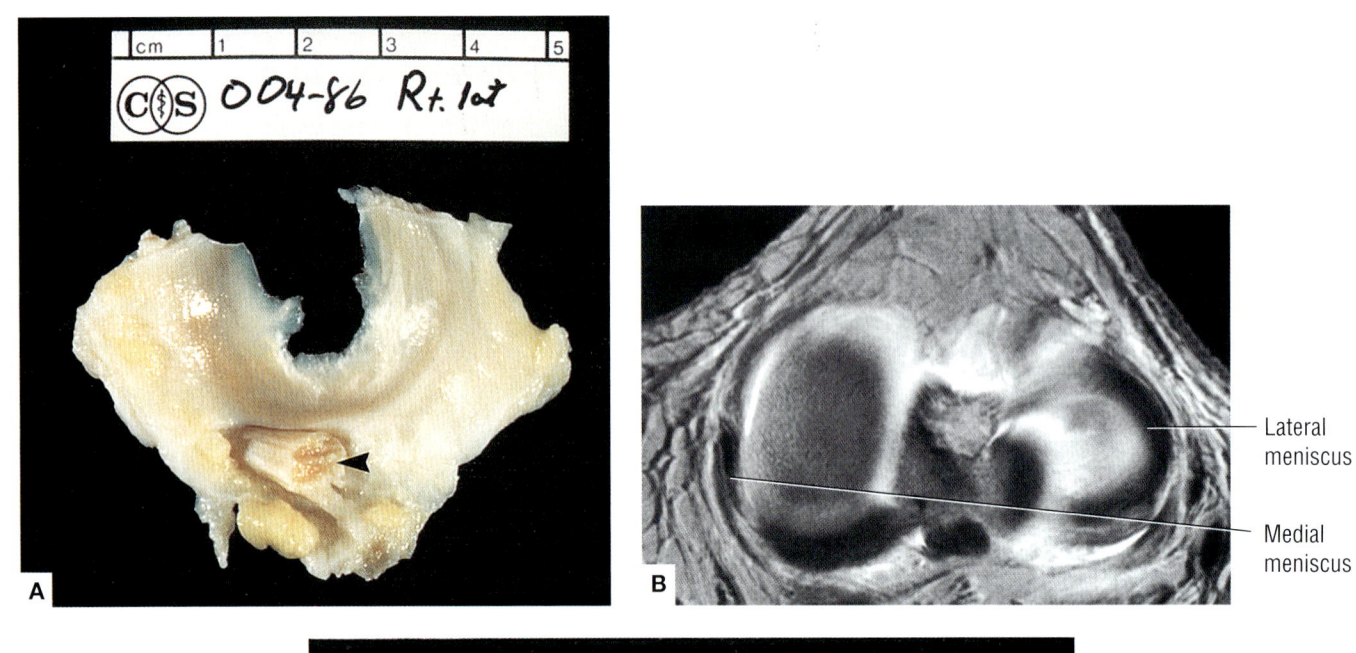

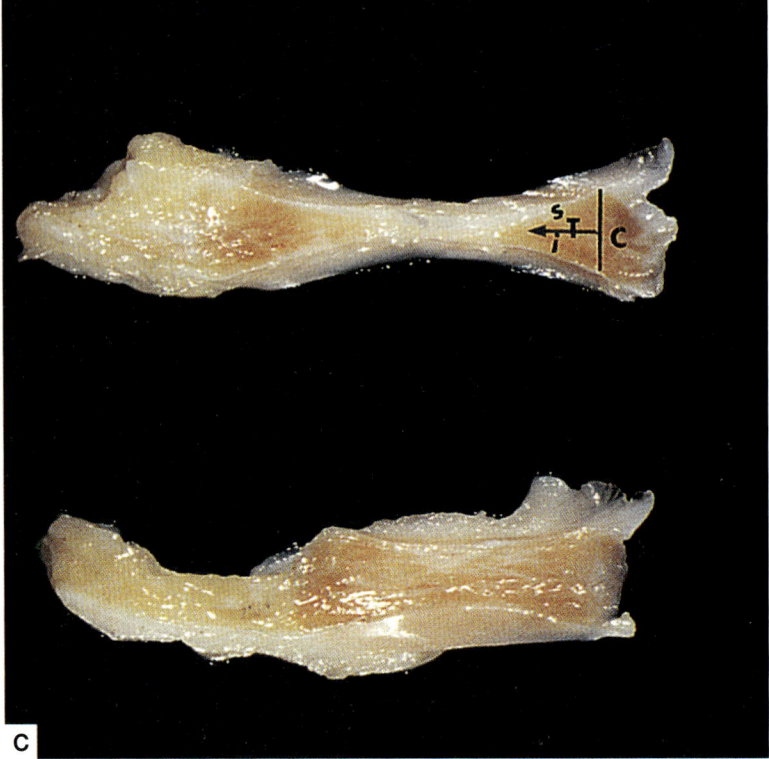

FIGURE 4.8 (**A**) Gross anatomy of the lateral meniscus and associated popliteus tendon (*arrowhead*). (**B**) Corresponding MR axial image demonstrates the C-shaped medial meniscus and the more O-shaped lateral meniscus. The medial meniscus is more constrained, which helps to explain its greater susceptibility to tearing in an ACL-deficient knee. (**C**) The circumferential (C) and transverse (T) zones of the meniscus. The middle perforating collagen bundle (*arrow*) divides the transverse zone into superior (s) and inferior (i) leaves.

The Meniscus 167

Perforating collagen fibers

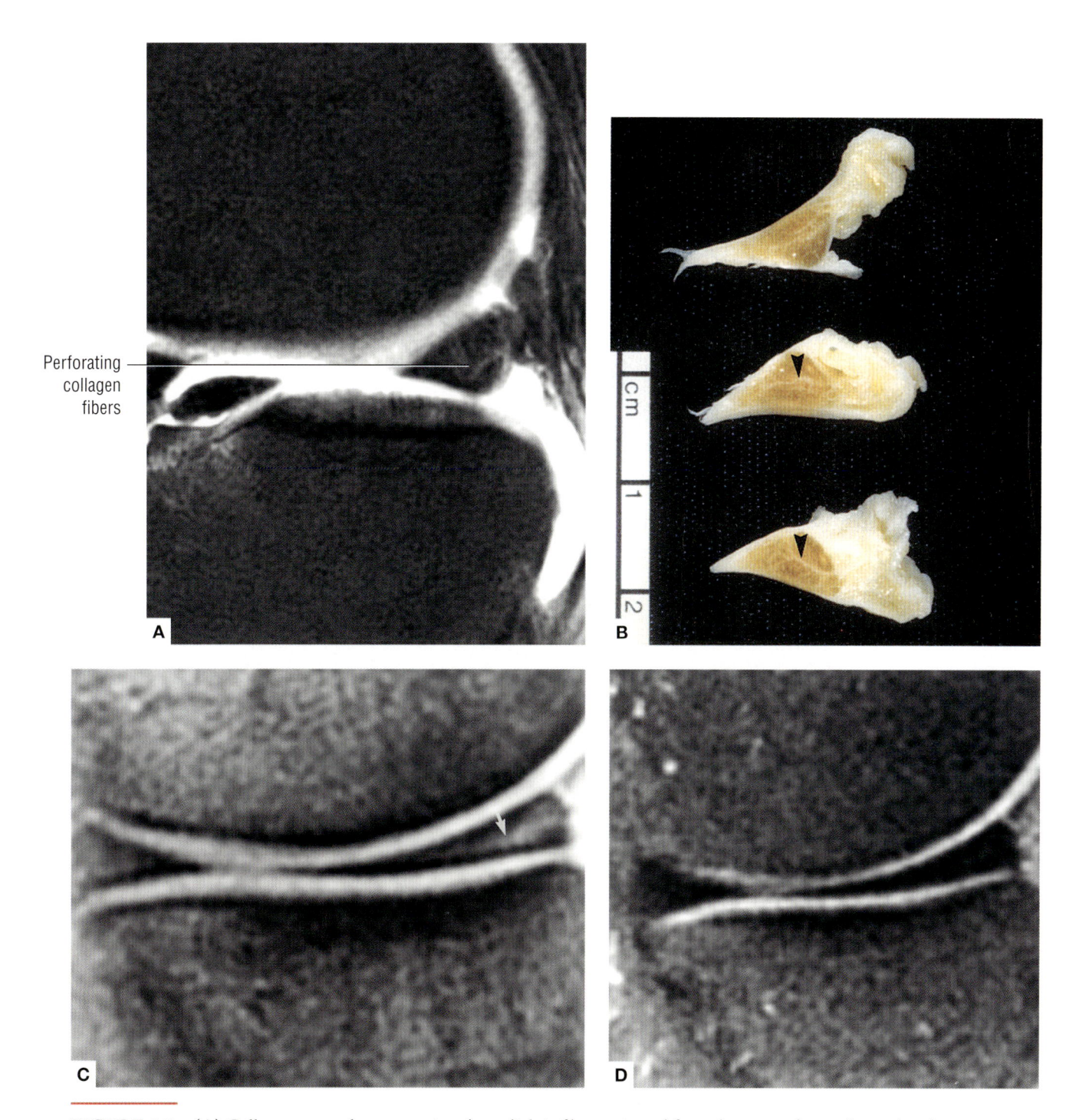

FIGURE 4.9 (**A**) Collagen network representing the radial tie fibers oriented from the circumferential peripheral zone. (**B**) Gross meniscal sections identify the location of the middle perforating collagen bundle and the site of preferential horizontal mucinous degeneration (*arrowheads*). (**C**) Grade 2 signal intensity (*arrow*) is seen in the posterior horn of the medial meniscus on a T2*-weighted image. (**D**) Grade 2 signal seen in **C** is not apparent on the corresponding FS T2-weighted FSE image.

Meniscal Fibrocartilage Structure

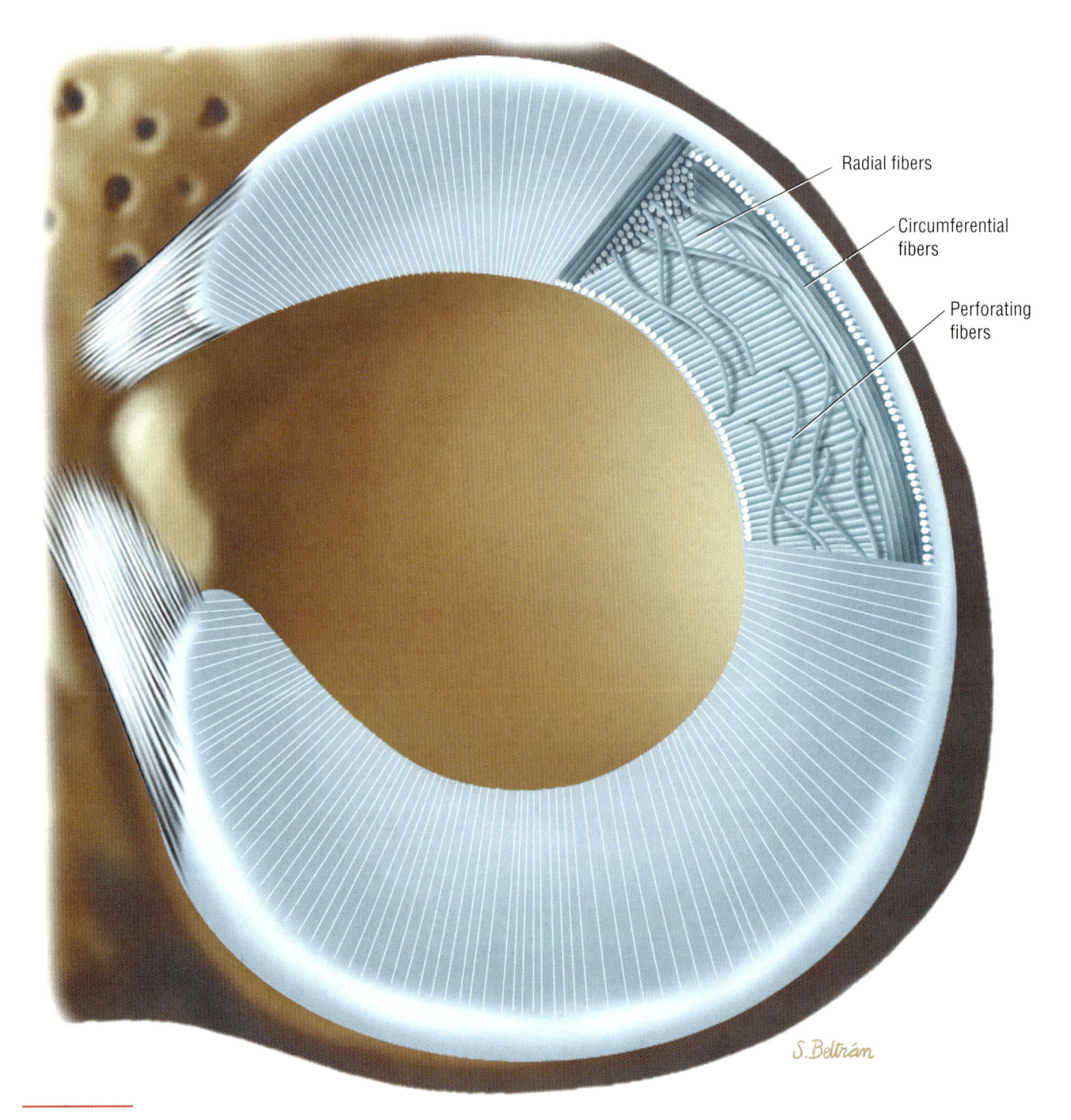

FIGURE 4.10 Idealized structure of meniscal fibrocartilage with peripheral circumferential fibers and perforating fibers. The middle layer of the meniscus functions in load transmission across the knee joint. Prominent and coarse collagen fibers directed in a parallel and circumferential direction to the meniscal periphery allow this middle layer to resist tensile forces. (Based on Miller RH. Knee injuries. In: Canale ST, ed. *Operative Orthopaedics*, 10th ed. Philadelphia: Mosby, 2003; 2184.)

Geniculate Artery and Perimeniscal Capillary Plexus

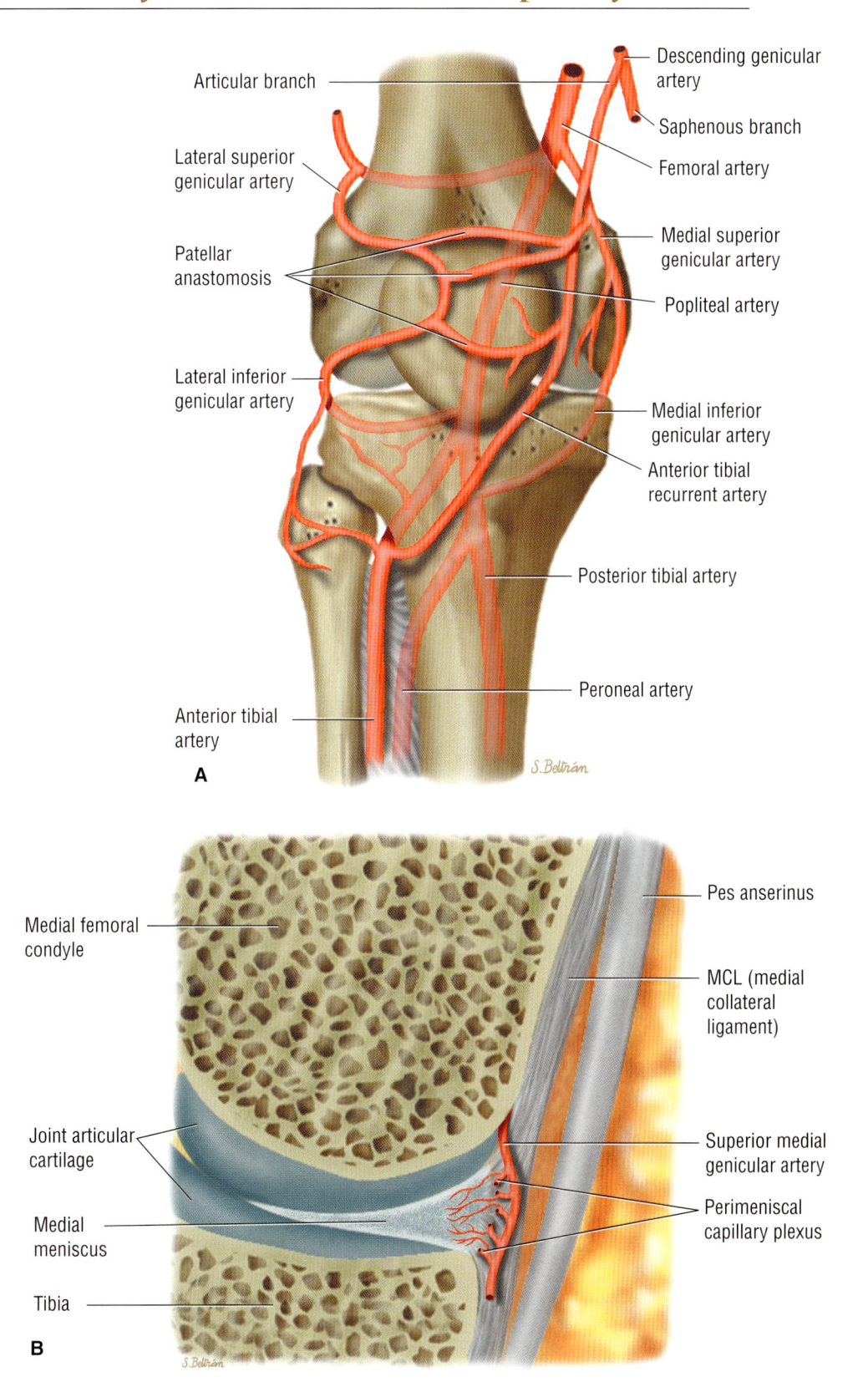

FIGURE 4.11 (**A**) The geniculate (genicular) artery anatomy, anterior anastomosis, and branches of the popliteal artery (in transparency). The vascular circle of the patellar anastomosis supplies the patella through nutrient arteries that enter at the inferior pole. The menisci receive their vascular supply primarily from the medial and lateral geniculate arteries, with the inferior and superior branches forming the perimeniscal capillary plexus within the synovium and capsular tissues. (**B**) Peripheral blood supply to the meniscus through vascular branches of the perimeniscal capillary plexus. This plexus receives terminal branches of all four medial and lateral geniculate arteries.

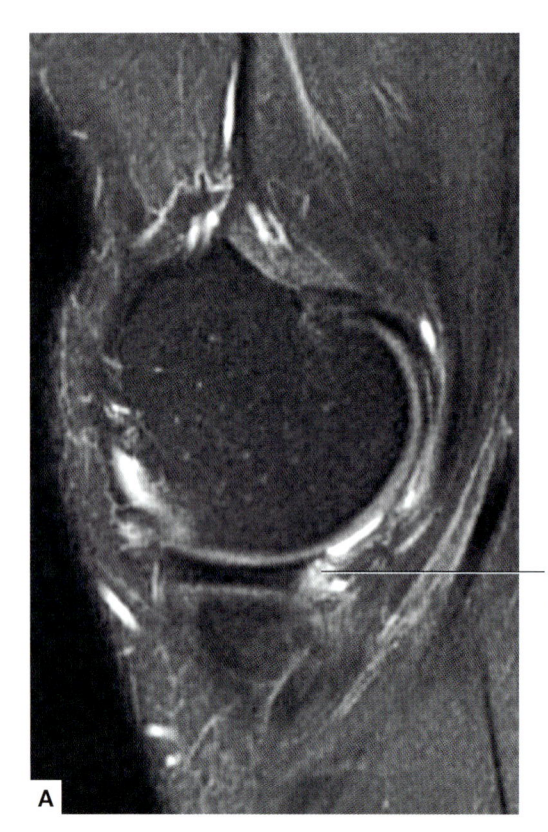

Perimeniscal capillary plexus

FIGURE 4.12 (**A**) Sagittal FS PD FSE image displays the hyperintense perimeniscal capillary plexus posterior to the body segment or central third of the meniscus. (**B**) Color illustration shows peripheral perimeniscal capillary plexus.

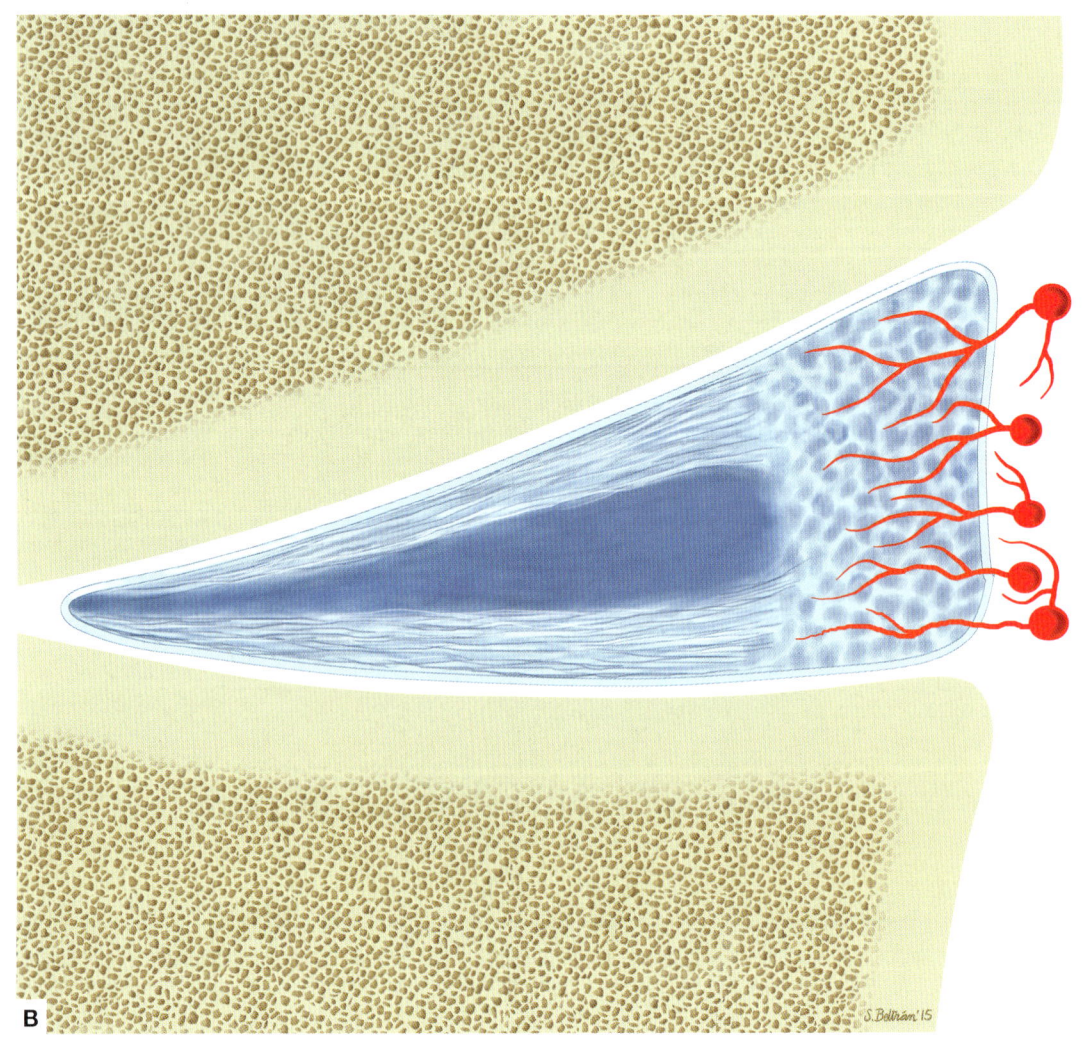

Meniscus Vascular Zones and Perimeniscal Plexus

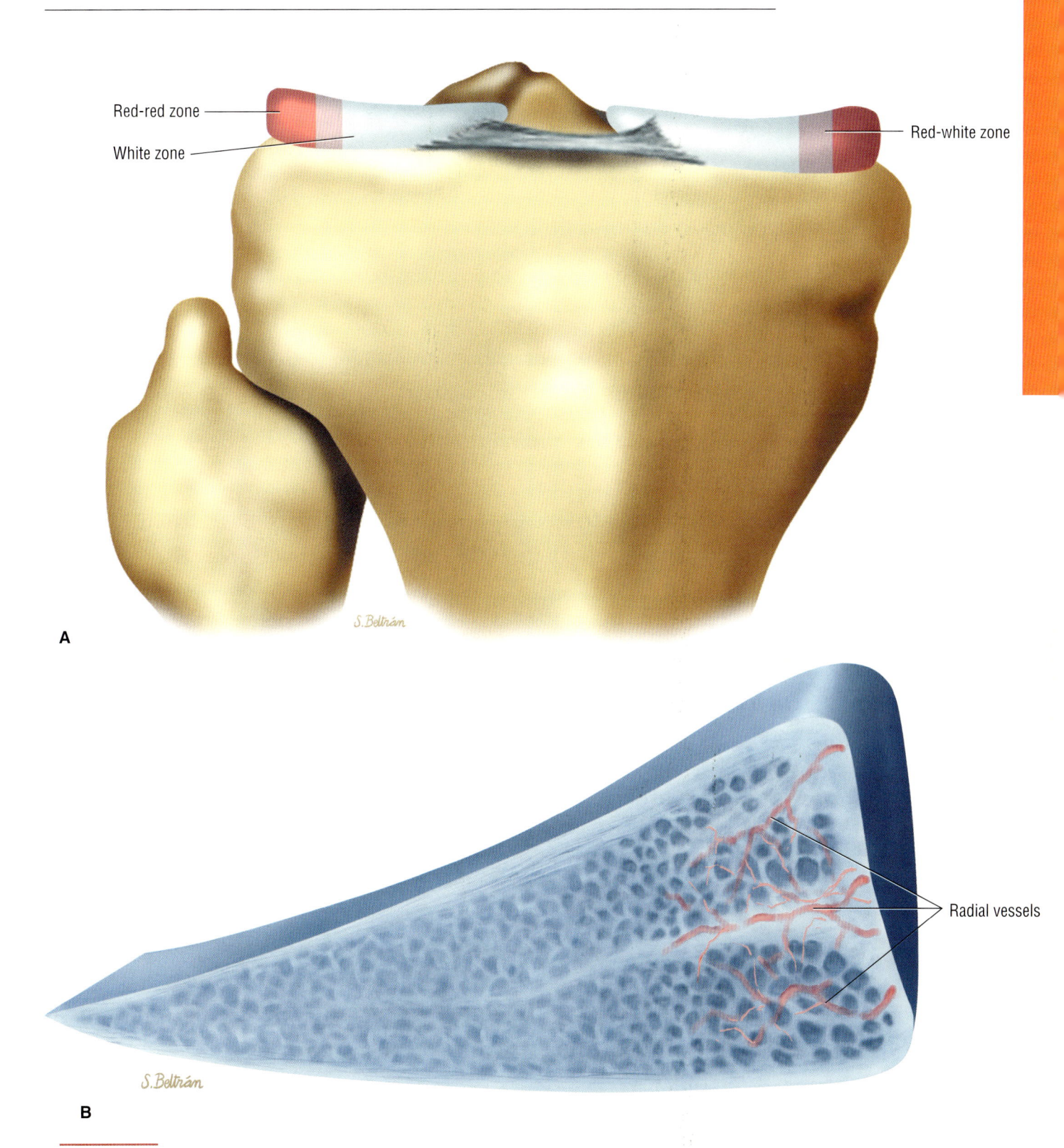

FIGURE 4.13 (**A**) The meniscal vascular supply is divided into zones of vascularity to help determine feasibility or success of repair. The red-red zone, the peripheral 3mm of the meniscus, maintains an excellent blood supply. The centrally located red-white zone demonstrates variable vascularity. The white-white zone extends beyond 5mm from the periphery and represents the avascular inner portion (including the free edge) of the meniscus. (**B**) Corresponding sagittal cross-section of the meniscus. The perimeniscal capillary plexus supplies the branching radial vessels, which penetrate the peripheral or outer border of the meniscus. A circumferential pattern of perimeniscal vessels is formed with the radial branches directed centrally. Peripheral vascular penetration is 10% to 30% of the width of the medial meniscus, and 10% to 25% of the width of the lateral meniscus.

Meniscal Degenerations and Tears

Pathogenesis and Clinical Presentation

- The meniscal fibrocartilage supports 50% of load transmission in the medial compartment and more than 50% in the lateral compartment.[75]
    - In knee extension, the medial meniscus transmits 50% and the lateral meniscus 70% of the load.
    - In knee flexion (90 degrees), the transmitted load to the menisci increases to 85%.[40,147]

- The menisci are important in joint stabilization and in reduction of compressive forces acting on articular cartilage.

- Conservation of meniscal tissue minimizes the development of degenerative joint changes.[293]
    - Resection of the medial meniscus leads to a 50% to 70% reduction in femoral contact area and a 100% increase in contact stress.
    - Removal of the lateral meniscus (total meniscectomy) results in a 40% to 50% decrease in contact area and increases contact stress in the lateral compartment to 200% to 300% of normal.[40,147]
        - The lateral compartment is more meniscus dependent than the medial compartment.

- The rotation of the femur against a fixed tibia during flexion and extension places the menisci at risk for injury.[394]

- Tears involving the medial meniscus usually start on the inferior surface of the posterior horn.

- The lateral meniscus is more prone to transverse or oblique tears.

- Related hemorrhage and tearing of peripheral meniscal attachments may contribute to the pain perceived in meniscal tears.

- Meniscal injury may be associated with a history of twisting, squatting, or cutting.[509]

- Tears of the meniscus may occur from an acute traumatic event or be associated with chronic degeneration.

- Abnormal shear forces generated during compression and rotation at the knee lead to meniscal damage.

- Clinical signs of meniscal pathology include:
    - Joint pain (at the joint line)
        - Increased in position of deep flexion or squatting
        - Joint line tenderness corresponding to the involved meniscus[379]
    - Giving way
    - Clicking
    - Effusions[360]
    - Locking in fixed flexion (which may occur immediately after displacement of a meniscal fragment)
    - Pseudo-locking (secondary to hamstring muscle spasms)[61]
    - Positive McMurray test with a palpable clunk is very specific for a meniscal tear (98% specificity), but has a sensitivity of only 15%.[379]
    - Positive Apley grinding test has a specificity of 70% and sensitivity of 60% for meniscal tears.
- The differential diagnosis of a meniscal tear includes:
    - Osseous bone contusions (occult bony injuries)
    - Plica syndromes
    - Popliteal tendinitis
    - Osteochondritis and chondral lesions
    - Loose bodies
    - Patellofemoral pain and instability
    - Fat-pad impingement syndrome
    - Inflammatory arthritis
    - Physeal or tibial spine fractures
    - Meniscotibial ligament sprain
    - Synovial lesions or tumors
    - Discoid menisci[61]

- ■ Sequelae of complete meniscectomy include degenerative joint disease as well as increased instability, especially in the ACL-deficient knee.[69,258,532]

    - ■ These changes are less likely to occur with partial meniscectomy and are minimized with primary meniscal repair.

    - ■ The increase in contact stresses in the knee joint is proportional to the amount of meniscal tissue removed, especially when excision extends into the more peripheral portions of the meniscus.

    - ■ When hoop tension is compromised in segmental meniscectomy, the result is equivalent to total meniscectomy in the load-bearing position.[40,147]

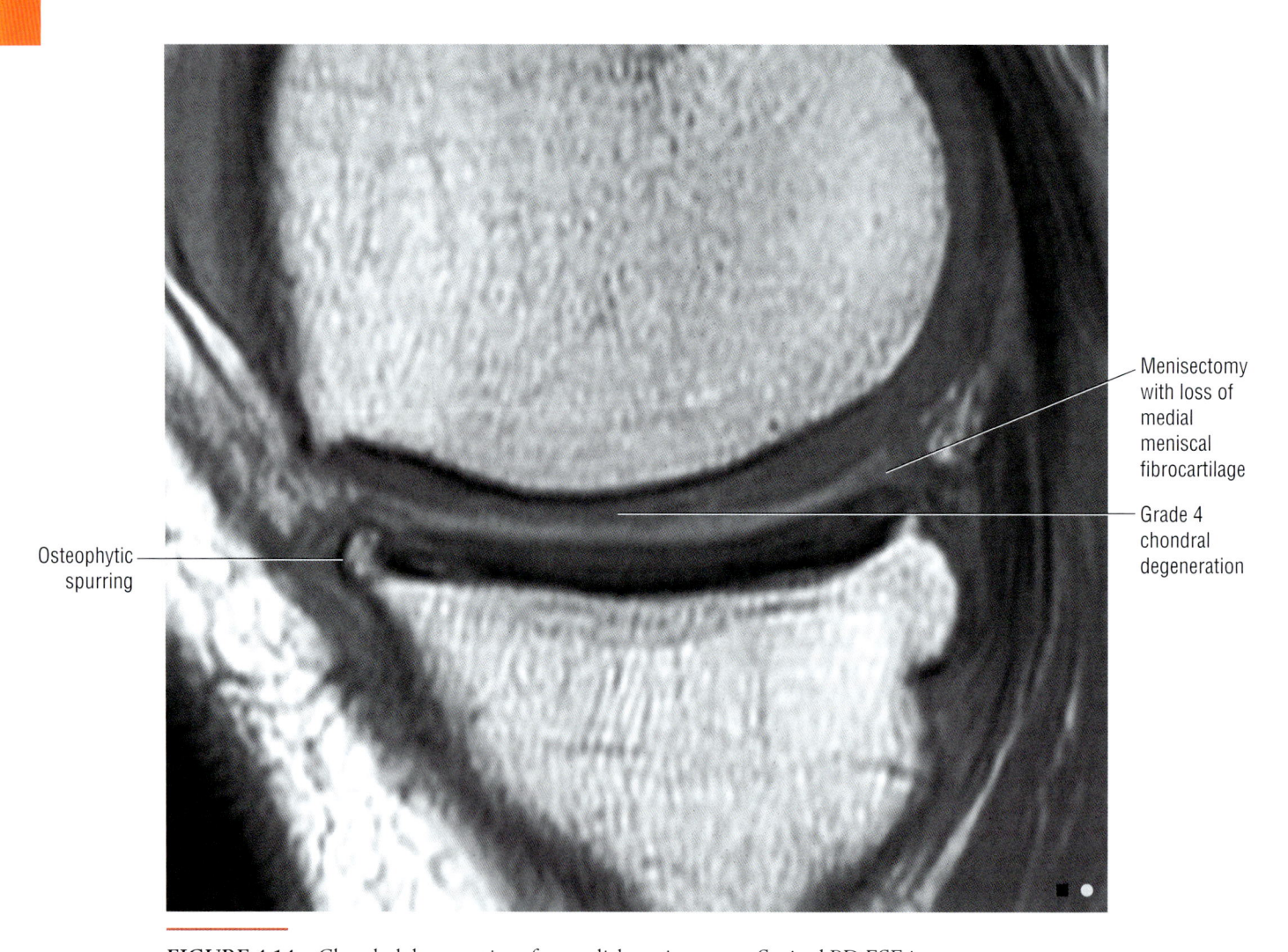

FIGURE 4.14 Chondral degeneration after medial meniscectomy. Sagittal PD FSE image.

MR Findings of Meniscal Degenerations and Tears

- Meniscal Degenerations and Tears
    - Grade 1 and grade 2 signal intensity represent intrasubstance degeneration.
    - Grade 3 signal intensity represents a meniscal tear.
        - The term "degeneration" (not "tear") should be used to describe grade 1 or grade 2 signal.
    - A closed meniscal tear is characterized by grade 3 signal intensity that weakens or attenuates as it approaches the articular surface of the meniscus.
        - The articular surface of the meniscus is defined as an inferior or superior surface or the free edge apex of the meniscal fibrocartilage.
- The normal meniscus demonstrates homogeneous low signal intensity on T1-weighted, PD, T2-weighted (conventional and FSE), gradient echo (GRE), and short tau inversion recovery (STIR)-weighted images.
- The low signal intensity of the intact meniscus is attributed to the lack of mobile protons (water molecules within the meniscus are closely related to or absorbed within larger collagen macromolecules).[88]
- Dephasing of hydrogen nuclei results in shortening of T2 time, contributing to the low signal intensity of meniscal tissue on all pulse sequences.
- In degenerations and tears of the meniscus, imbibed synovial fluid results in increased signal intensity:[468]
    - As synovial fluid diffuses through the meniscus, areas of degeneration and tears trap water molecules onto surface boundary layers, increasing the local spin density.
        - This interaction of synovial fluid with large macromolecules in the meniscus slows the rotational rates of protons and shortens T1 and T2 values.[468]
        - This phenomenon explains the sensitivity of T1-weighted and intermediate-weighted (i.e., PD-weighted images) in revealing meniscal degenerations and tears.

- Degenerative changes and tears result in local increases in the freedom of trapped water molecules.
    - An increase in T2 times allows detection of increased signal intensity on short–echo time (TE) sequences.
- The increased intrameniscal signal intensity seen in degeneration and tears is best visualized on short-TE images using T1, intermediate-weighted (PD), or GRE sequences.
    - Increased signal intensity in synovial fluid gaps has been confirmed in surgically induced tears in animal models.[25]
- Meniscal degenerations and tears may decrease in signal intensity on T2-weighted images in the absence of a joint effusion.
    - On T2*-weighted GRE images, intrasubstance degeneration and tears generate increased signal intensities.
    - GRE sequences are extremely sensitive to the spectrum of meniscal degenerations and tears.
- FSE sequences are not as useful in the evaluation of intrasubstance meniscal signal intensity and tears.
    - FSE images may underestimate the extent of MR signal intensity and/or mask the presence of a tear.
    - Blurring, which limits the usefulness of FSE images, is more pronounced with the use of a shorter effective TE, a longer echo train, and a smaller acquisition matrix.
        - Rubin et al.[409] have attributed this blurring to a ghosting artifact or an increase in magnetization transfer.
    - Short effective TE-related blurring occurs secondary to attenuation by T2 decay of later echoes (high-spatial-frequency data) at the edges of k-space.
- To understand the significance of increased signal intensity in meniscal abnormalities, an MR grading system has been developed and correlated with a pathologic model.[468]
- Areas of degeneration demonstrate increased signal intensity in a spectrum of patterns or grades based on the morphology of signal distribution relative to an articular meniscal surface or meniscal apex.

- The articular meniscal surfaces include the superior and inferior aspects of the meniscus opposite the distal femoral and proximal tibial articular cartilage surfaces.

- The extent of signal intensity changes include:
    - MR grade 1:
        - A nonarticular focal or globular intrasubstance increased signal intensity is seen.
        - Grade 1 signal intensity correlates with foci of early mucinous degeneration and chondrocyte-deficient or hypocellular regions that are pale-staining on hematoxylin and eosin preparations.
        - The terms "mucinous," "myxoid," and "hyaline" degeneration can be used interchangeably to describe the accumulation of increased production of mucopolysaccharide ground substance in stressed or strained areas of the meniscal fibrocartilage.
            - These changes usually occur in response to mechanical loading and degeneration.
        - Grade 1 signal intensity is not clinically significant, but may be seen in asymptomatic athletes and normal volunteers.
    - MR grade 2:
        - A horizontal, linear intrasubstance increased signal intensity extends from the capsular periphery of the meniscus without involving an articular meniscal surface.
        - Areas and bands of mucinous degeneration are more extensive in MR grade 2 than in MR grade 1.
        - No distinct cleavage plane or tear is observed in grade 2 menisci.
            - Microscopic clefting and collagen fragmentation may be seen in hypocellular regions of the fibrocartilaginous matrix.

- The low-spin-density meniscus and the middle collagen perforating bundle:
    - Divide the meniscus horizontally into superior and inferior leaves
    - Demonstrate low signal intensity
    - Cannot be differentiated in the normal knee
- The middle perforating collagen bundle:
    - Creates a neutral or buffer plane for the superior femoral and inferior tibial frictional forces
    - Site for preferential accumulation of mucinous ground substance that displays grade 2 signal intensity
    - Represents the shear plane of the meniscus and often is the site of horizontal degenerative tears of the meniscus
- Grade 2 signal intensity is a continuation of progressive degeneration from grade 1 and is not a discrete isolated histologic occurrence.
- Patients with images of grade 2 signal intensity are usually asymptomatic.
- The posterior horn of the medial meniscus is the most common location of grade 2 signal intensity.
- Grade 2 signal intensity cannot be used as a prognostic indicator for development of grade 3 signal intensity.
- The presence of mucinous degeneration is thought to represent potential structural weakening within collagen fibers.
- Grade 3 signal intensity tears develop adjacent to areas of grade 2 meniscal degenerations.

- The increased prevalence of grade 2 signal intensity in the posterior horn of the medial meniscus is consistent with the increased frequency of grade 2 findings in this location found in cadaver menisci.
- Grade 2 signal intensity and discoid menisci may represent cystic areas or cavities of mucinous degeneration.
    - These areas may be symptomatic and require treatment with partial meniscectomy.
- It is not common practice (even in symptomatic patients) to treat menisci with grade 2 intrasubstance signal intensity surgically.
    - The exception is discoid menisci, which should be treated surgically.
- In the immature meniscus of a child, primarily reabsorbed vascular ingrowth cannot fully explain grade 2 signal intensity without associated fibrocartilaginous degeneration.
- In adults, increased signal intensity distinctly correlates with areas of mucinous degeneration.

- **MR grade 3**
    - The area of increased signal intensity communicates or extends to at least one articular surface.
    - A meniscus may contain multiple areas of grade 3 signal intensity, or the entire meniscal segment may be involved.
    - Fibrocartilaginous separation or tears can be found in all menisci with grade 3 signal intensity.
    - Closed meniscal tears:
        - Diagnosis requires arthroscopy and can be missed on a routine arthroscopic examination if surface extension is not identified.
        - Attenuation of grade 3 meniscal signal intensity as it approaches an articular surface is characteristic of closed tears.

- May represent some of the false-positive interpretations of grade 3 signal intensity when correlated with arthroscopy
  - Intrasubstance tears may present with pain in rheologically abnormal menisci.
- False-negative correlations with arthroscopy may be related to spurious interpretation of areas of fraying or fibrillation as meniscal tears.
- Meniscal tears frequently occur adjacent to areas of intrasubstance degeneration.

- The morphology (i.e., size and shape) of the meniscus should be assessed when evaluating meniscal lesions.
  - The normal meniscus measures 3 to 5mm in height.
  - The medial meniscus varies in width from 6mm at the anterior horn to 12mm at the posterior horn.
  - The lateral meniscus is approximately 10mm in width.
- Regenerative chondrocytes and synovium represent attempts at meniscus healing along the tear–meniscus interface.
- Arthroscopic rasping is performed to induce a neovascular response by abrading synovium and creating a blood supply.
- Synovial ingrowth in degenerative tears contributes to the development of acute and chronic pain.
- Hypertrophy of the synovium occurs, secondary to joint debris in degenerative osteoarthritis, and must be arthroscopically resected.
- Peripheral perimeniscal capillary ingrowth may be seen perforating areas of degeneration and fibrocartilaginous separation, supporting preferential healing in this location.
- Acute traumatic tears have less predictable orientations and smaller areas of associated mucinous degeneration than degenerative tears (horizontal, cleavage, or flap tears).

The Meniscus

- Grade 3 signal intensity is most frequent in the posterior horn of the medial meniscus.

- Arthrographic and arthroscopic surface evaluations are insensitive to grade 1 and 2 intrasubstance degenerations.

- MR detects multiple meniscal tears that may be overlooked on arthrography.

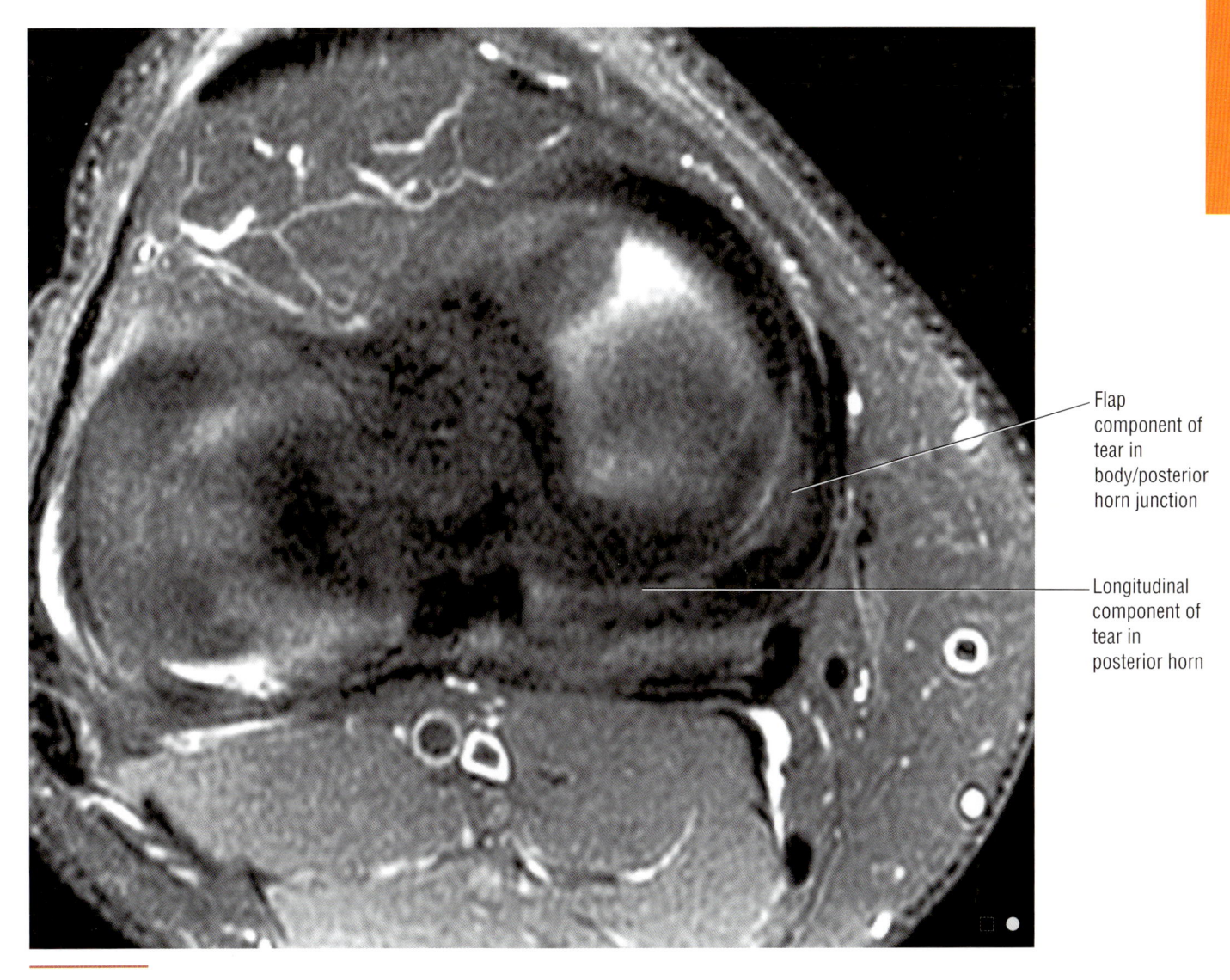

FIGURE 4.15 The identification of both flap and longitudinal surface tear patterns by visualization of the entire meniscal surface on axial FS PD FSE image.

Classification of Meniscal Tears

Key Concepts

- **Classification of Meniscal Tears**
    - Based on MR sagittal sections:
        - Vertical
        - Horizontal
    - Based on circumferential or surface anatomy:
        - Longitudinal (vertical or horizontal on corresponding meniscal sections)
        - Flap (vertical or horizontal)
        - Radial (vertical)
    - Longitudinal and flap tears have either a primary vertical or horizontal tear pattern on corresponding sagittal images.
    - Longitudinal and flap tears have been previously classified only as vertical tear types (historic classification prior to use of MR).
    - Radial tears are vertical tears.

Cross-Sectional Patterns: Vertical and Horizontal Tears

- Classifying meniscal tears as grade 3 signal intensity relative to a meniscal articular surface does not address the anatomy of various horizontal and vertical tear patterns identified during arthroscopic surgery of the knee.[29]

- Meniscal tears can be classified into two primary tear planes using the cross-sectional anatomy of the meniscus seen on sagittal images.
    - Vertical tears
    - Horizontal tears

- Most meniscal tears are not exclusively perpendicular or parallel with the tibial plateau surface.

- Tears classified as either vertical or horizontal may have secondary tear patterns.
    - Most horizontal tears extend to the inferior surface of the meniscus.
- An accurate description of the morphology and location of the tear is useful in choosing between primary meniscal repair and partial meniscectomy.[220]
- Meniscal tear patterns may be identified using axial images through the menisci.[479]
- A pure horizontal cleavage tear only extends to the meniscal apex and does not demonstrate superior or inferior articular surface disruption.
- Vertical tears extend to the meniscal surface as longitudinal, radial, or oblique tears.
- Noncleavage horizontal tears display either longitudinal or flap surface tear patterns.
- Horizontal tears are sometimes referred to as "fish-mouth" tears.
- Horizontal cleavage tears or flap tears with horizontal components are most frequently associated with meniscal cysts.
- Complex tears:
    - Display combinations of vertical and horizontal and/or surface tear patterns
    - May demonstrate more than one circumferential or surface tear pattern in the same meniscus[209]
        - A radial and flap tear, a radial and horizontal tear, or a horizontal and flap tear may exist in different locations (e.g., body vs. posterior horn) in the meniscus.
    - May result from meniscal degeneration or be caused by significant trauma

Horizontal Tears

- A pure horizontal cleavage tear:
  - Extends to the apex of the meniscus
  - Results from excessive shear stress
  - May be difficult to appreciate on axial images because of a partial volume effect
  - Should demonstrate apex extension on either coronal or sagittal images
  - Less common than flap tears

- The term "horizontal tear" is used to describe a horizontal cleavage tear that extends to the free edge of the meniscus in the plane of the middle collagen fibers with peripheral signal degeneration that may extend to the capsular periphery.

- Horizontal tears:
  - Occur in the horizontal plane and dissect circumferential collagen fibers
  - Location most common within the posterior horn of the medial meniscus
  - Demonstrate linear hyperintensity that extends to the free edge of the meniscus on MR images
  - Commonly associated with meniscal cysts
  - Involve the free edge and progress transversely to involve the more peripheral aspects of the meniscus
    - Approximately parallel to the tibial articular surface
  - Usually result from excessive shear forces between the femoral condyle and the tibial plateau[209]

- Flap tears and longitudinal tears may have a relative horizontal tear vector or may demonstrate obliquely oriented grade 3 signal intensity on cross-section of the meniscus in the sagittal plane.
  - These tears should not be classified as horizontal or pure cleavage tears.

- Horizontally oriented linear grade 2 signal intensity may be mistaken for a complete horizontal tear.

The Meniscus

- A flap tear results when there is superior or inferior extension resulting in a change of direction of the meniscal tear pattern.

- Flap tears may also develop from a radial tear with a secondary longitudinal component.

- If the tear reaches the peripheral portion of the meniscus, the innervated vascular region, tenderness is typically noted at the joint line.

- Horizontal tears that are restricted to the free edge of the meniscus may be asymptomatic.[538]

- Horizontal tears are treated by trimming back to a stable rim.
    - The more degenerated or smaller leaf is resected, and the other leaf is preserved.

- In the presence of a meniscal cyst, the meniscus can be trimmed and the cyst decompressed arthroscopically.

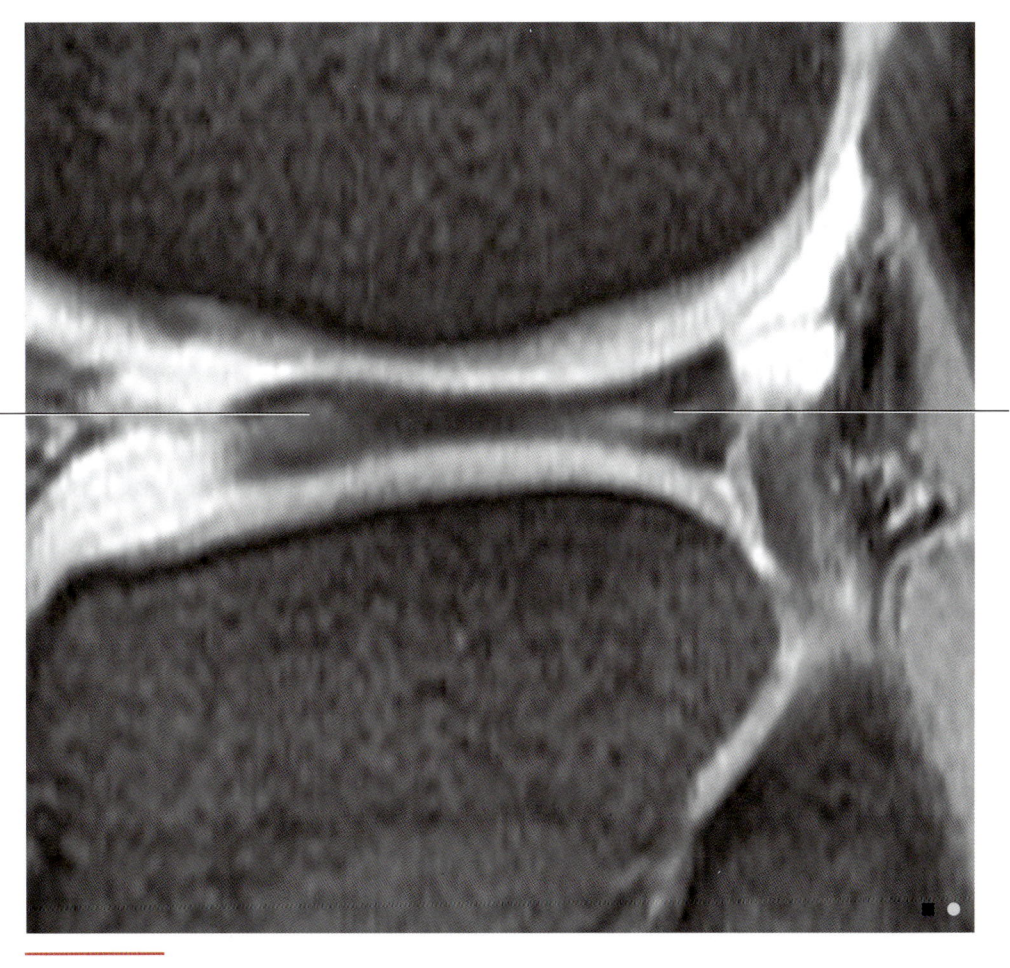

Intrasubstance degeneration

Closed meniscal tear discoid-like (incomplete discoid) posterior horn/body

FIGURE 4.16 Horizontal tear in a partial discoid lateral meniscus. Without direct extension to the free edge (apex), secondary signs of meniscal cyst formation may be necessary to distinguish between a closed horizontal tear and a cleavage tear that communicated with the periphery or free edge. Sagittal FS PD FSE.

Circumferential or Surface Patterns: Longitudinal, Radial, and Flap Tears

- Surface tear patterns are created by the extension of vertical or horizontal tear planes to the articular surface of the meniscus.
    - Surface tear types can be prospectively identified based on MR signal orientation and location as well as changes in meniscal morphology.
    - Three tear patterns can be identified from the surface of the meniscus at arthroscopy:
        - Longitudinal
        - Radial or transverse
        - Flap or oblique[69]

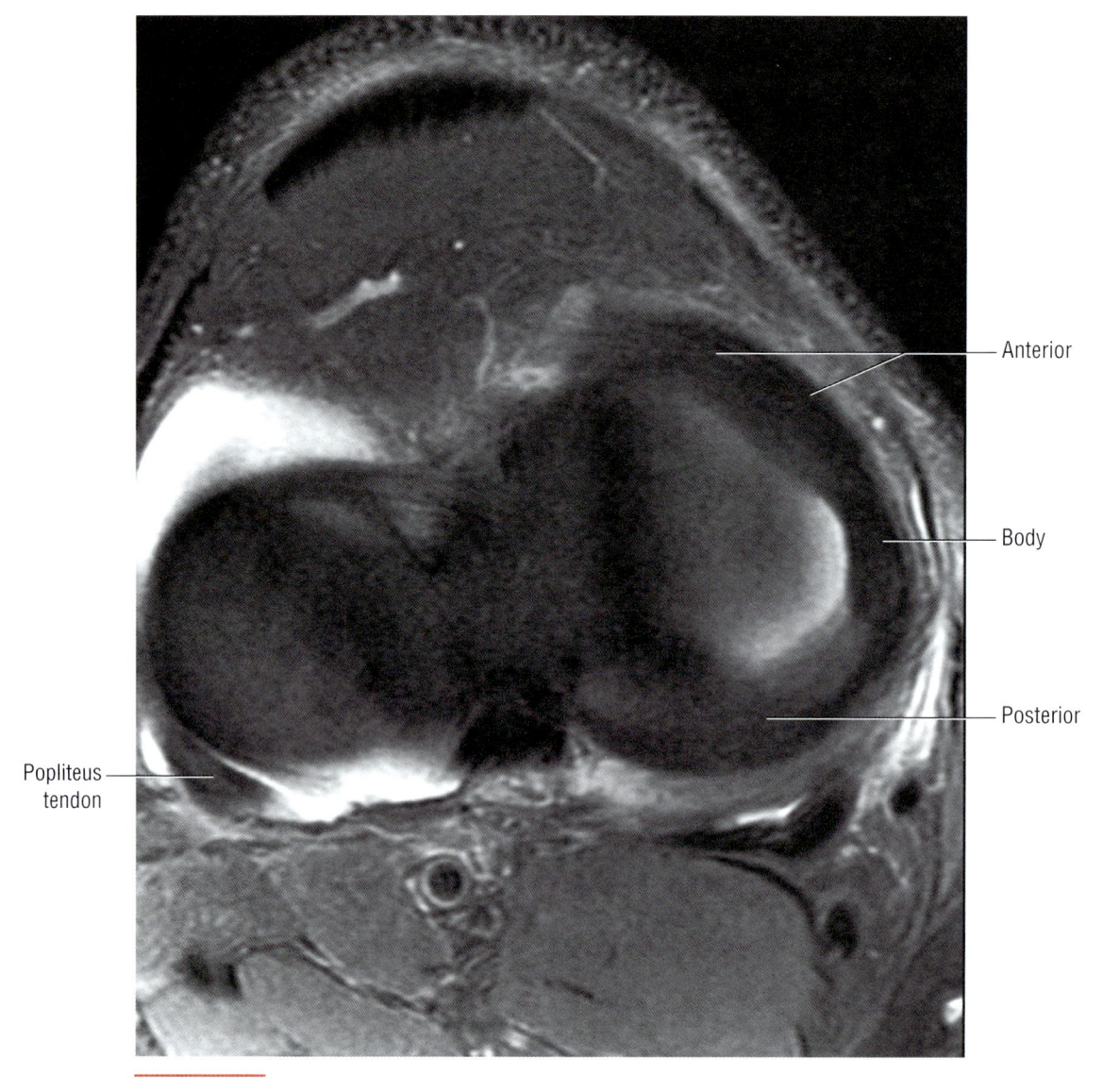

FIGURE 4.17 Division of the medial meniscus in anterior third (anterior horn), middle third (body), and posterior horn (posterior third). The popliteus tendon laterally is a useful landmark to identify the joint line quickly. Axial FS PD FSE image.

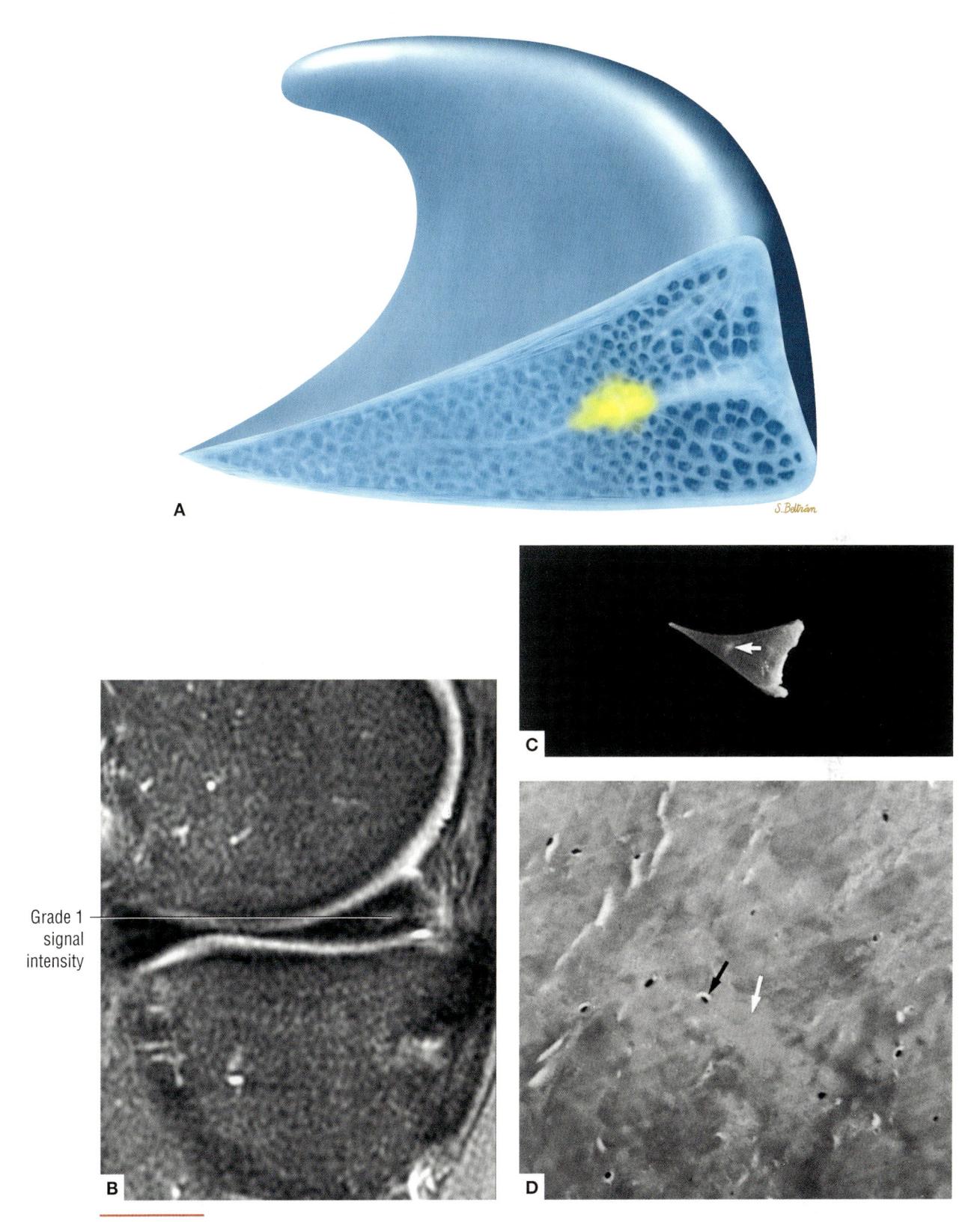

FIGURE 4.18 (**A**) Focal or globular intrameniscal degeneration (*yellow*) within the central shear plane of the middle collagen fibers. (**B**) Corresponding grade 1 signal intensity within the posterior horn of the medial meniscus on an FS PD FSE sagittal image. (**C**) On a cut gross section, a focus of meniscal degeneration (*arrow*) can be seen. (**D**) The corresponding photomicrograph shows hypocellularity, with decreased numbers of chondrocytes (*black arrow*) in pale-staining areas (*white arrow*). (Hematoxylin and eosin stain.)

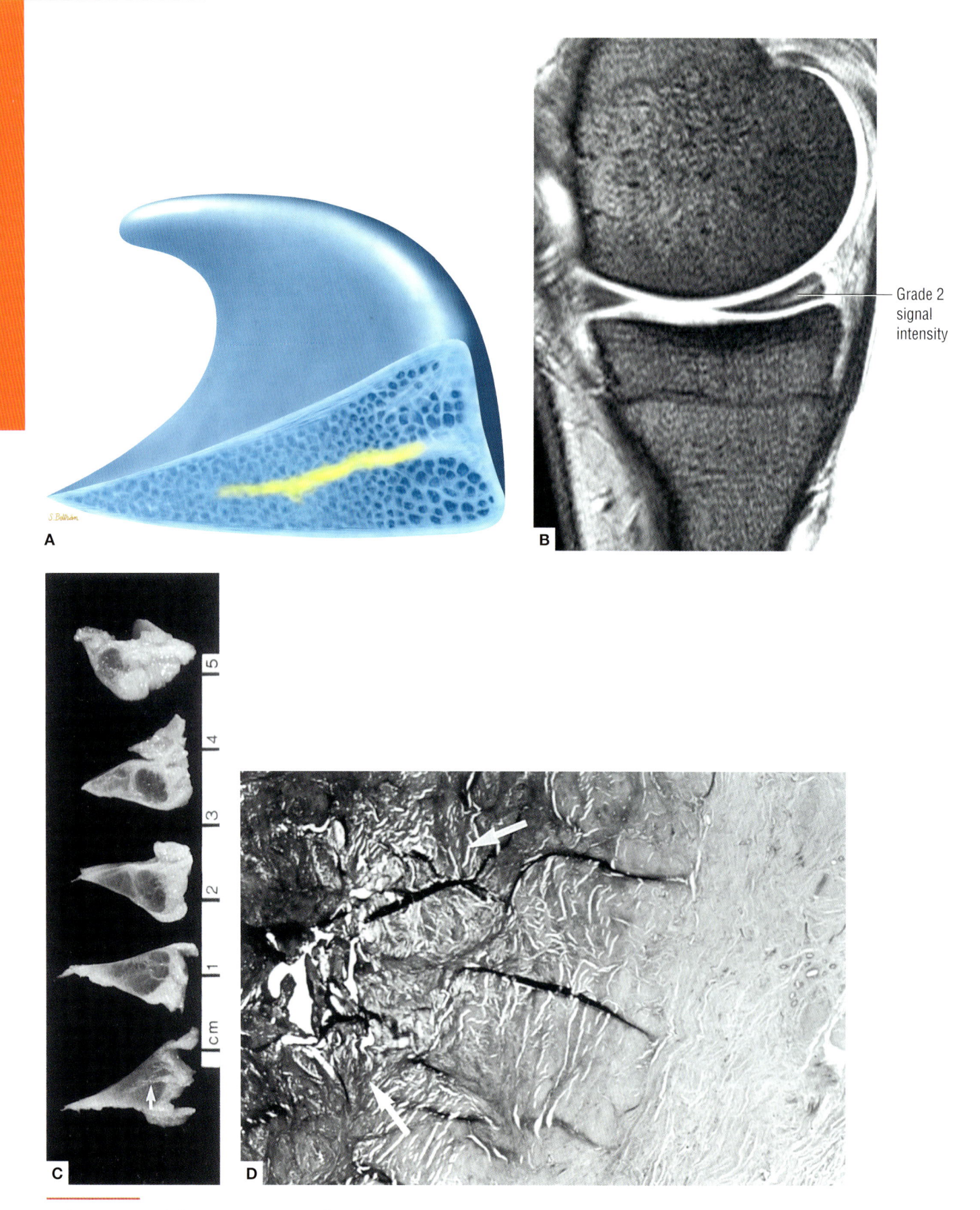

FIGURE 4.19 (**A**) Linear orientation of grade 2 intrasubstance degeneration (*yellow*) in the middle layer of the meniscal fibrocartilage. (**B**) Corresponding linear grade 2 signal intensity located in the central shear plane of the meniscus between the superior and inferior leaves of the meniscal fibrocartilage. (**C**) The corresponding gross section demonstrates linear mucinous meniscal degeneration (*arrow*). (**D**) The corresponding histologic study shows a focus of mucinous degeneration within the meniscal fibrocartilage (*arrows*).

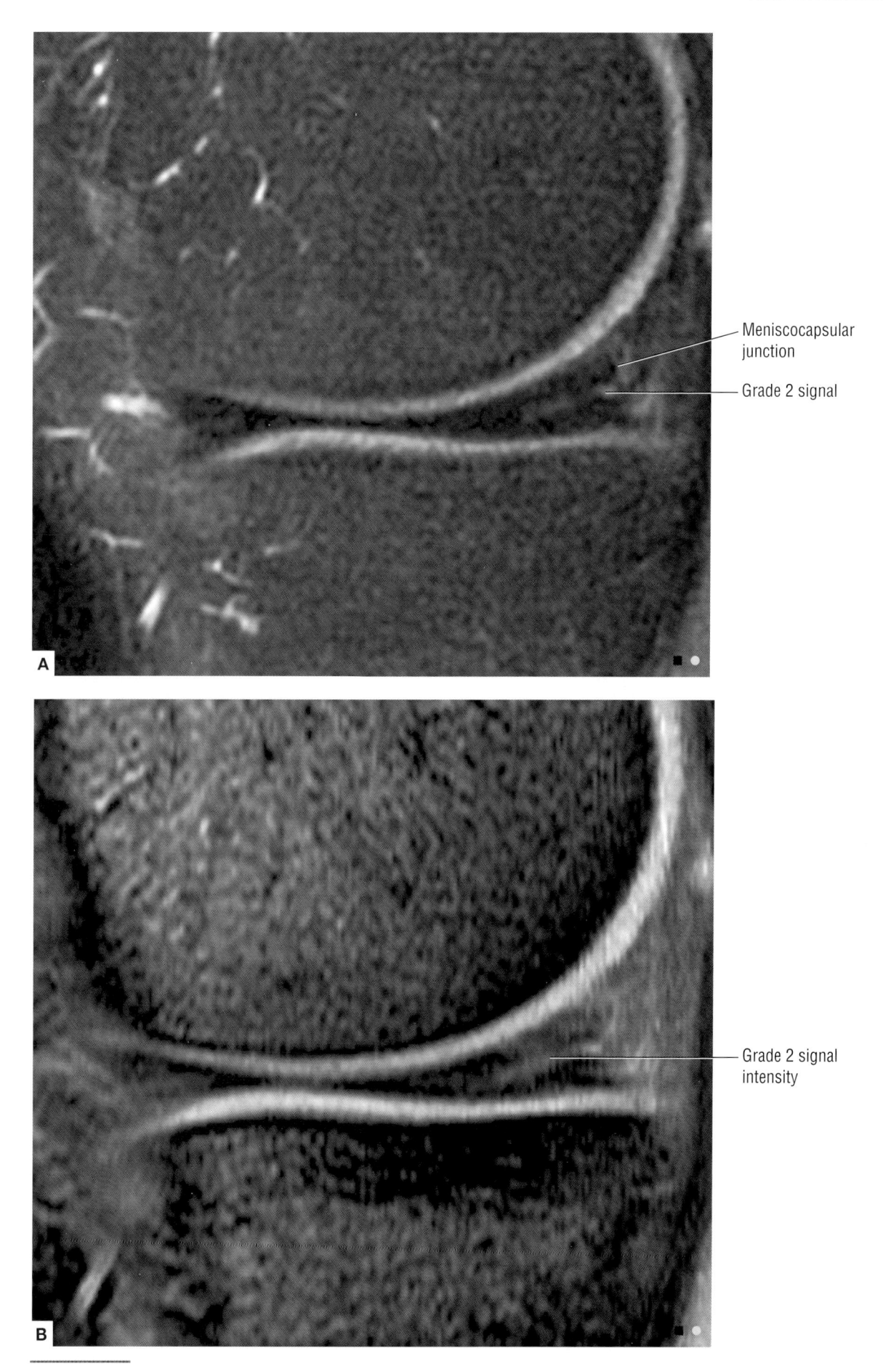

FIGURE 4.20 Increased conspicuity of grade 2 intrasubstance signal comparing sagittal FS PD FSE (**A**) to gradient echo (**B**) image.

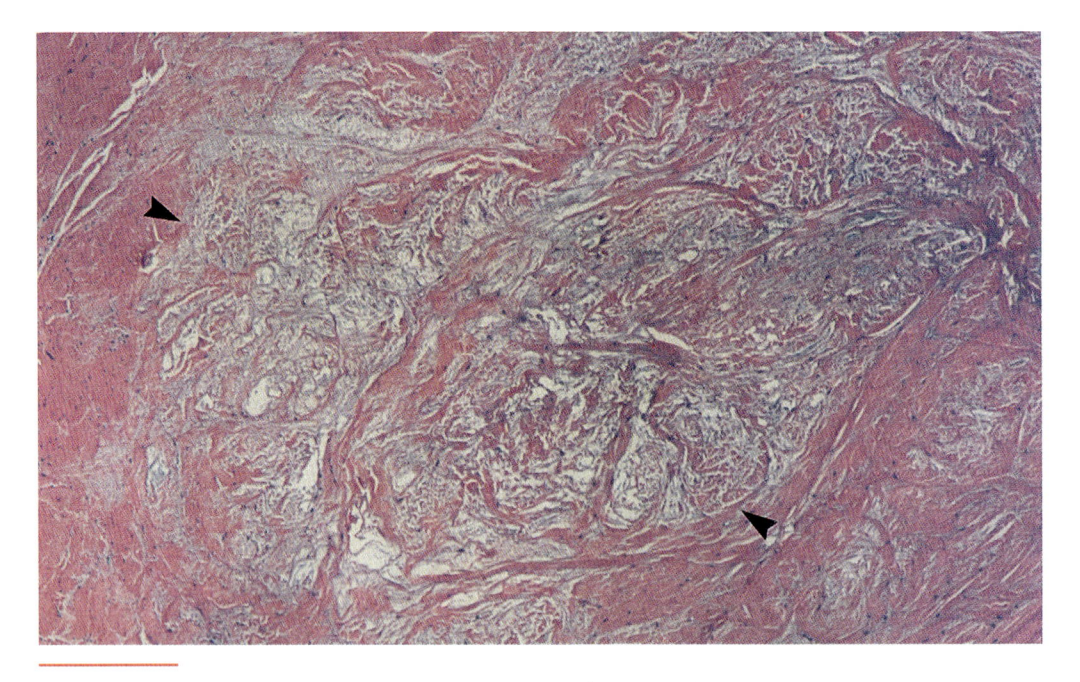

FIGURE 4.21 The region of mucinous degeneration (*arrowheads*) corresponds to grade 2 meniscal intrasubstance degeneration. (Hematoxylin and eosin stain.)

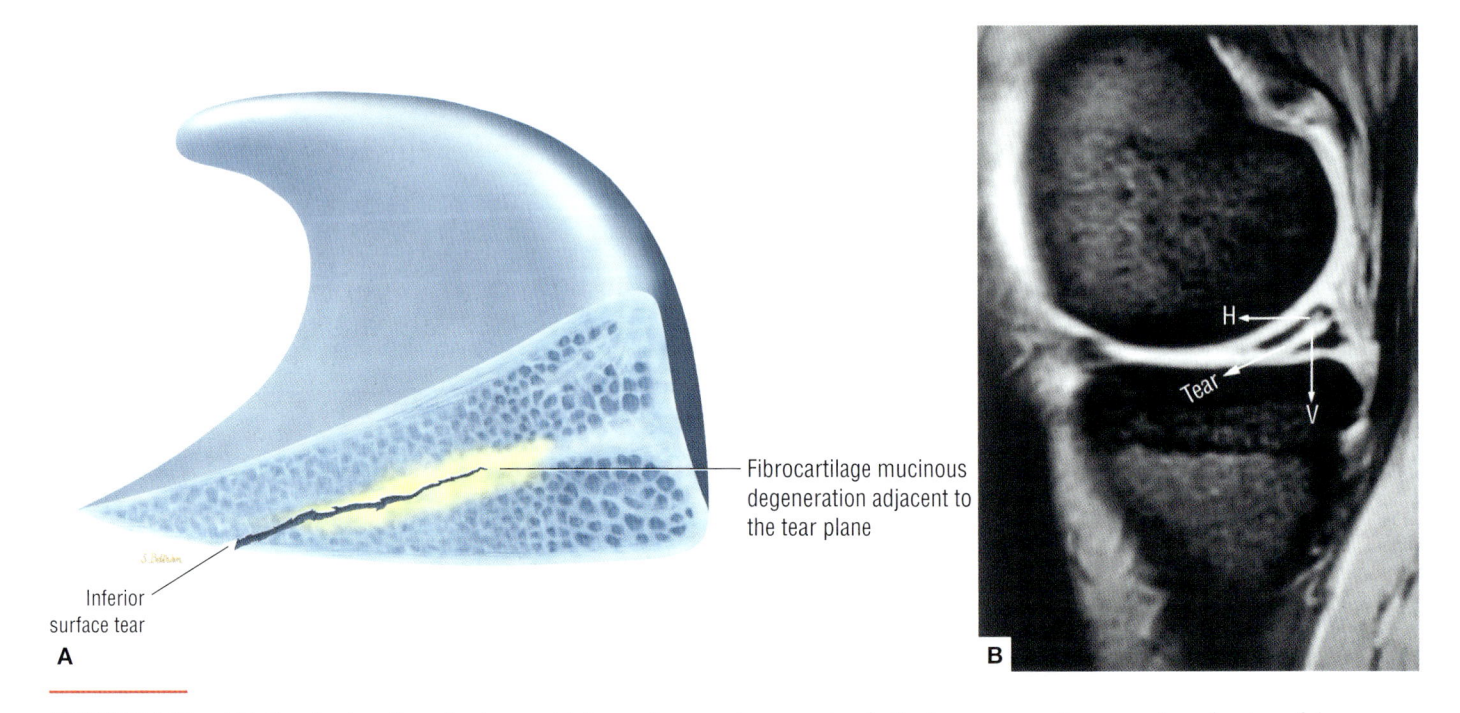

FIGURE 4.22 (**A**) Continuity of meniscal tear with intrasubstance degeneration (*yellow*) as an area of structural weakening of the meniscal fibrocartilage. (**B**) Flap tear inferior surface extension and continuity with peripheral directed meniscal hyperintensity. There are both horizontal (H) and vertical (V) components to this obliquely oriented tear.

The Meniscus

Fibrocartilaginous separation in a closed tear

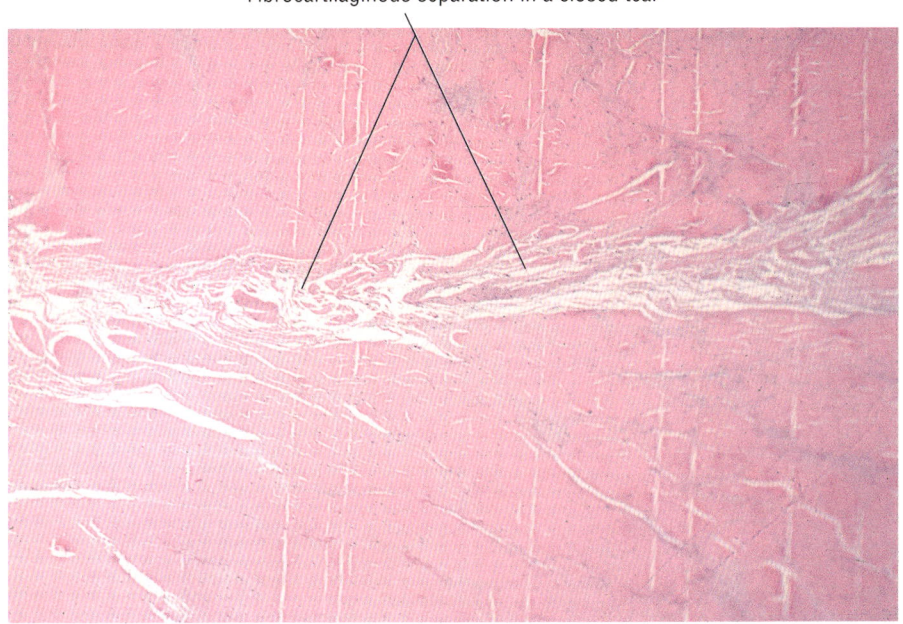

FIGURE 4.23 Photomicrograph demonstrates confined fibrocartilaginous separation in a closed meniscal tear.

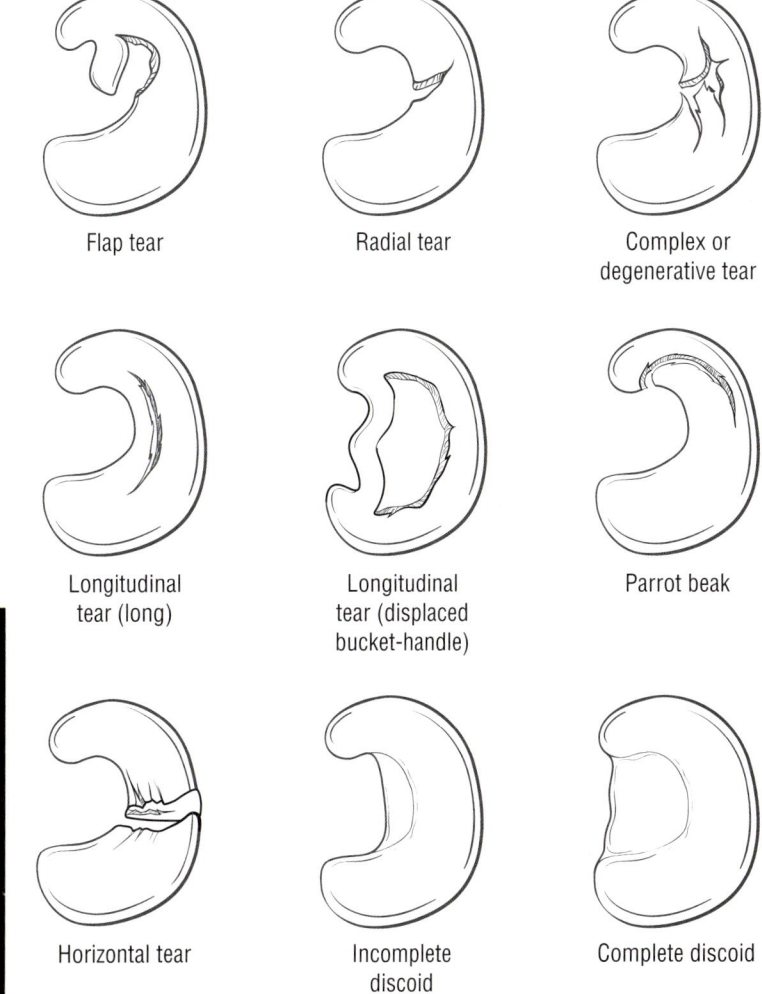

Flap tear

Radial tear

Complex or degenerative tear

Longitudinal tear (long)

Longitudinal tear (displaced bucket-handle)

Parrot beak

Horizontal tear

Incomplete discoid

Complete discoid

FIGURE 4.24 Idealized directions of horizontal (H, *white arrow*) and vertical (V, *black arrows*) tear patterns in a gross cross-section of the meniscus.

FIGURE 4.25 Common meniscal tear patterns. The term parrot beak is equivalent to a nondisplaced flap tear. (Reprinted from Fu FH. *Master Techniques in Orthopaedic Surgery: Sports Medicine*. Philadelphia, PA: Lippincott Williams & Wilkins; 2010, with permission.)

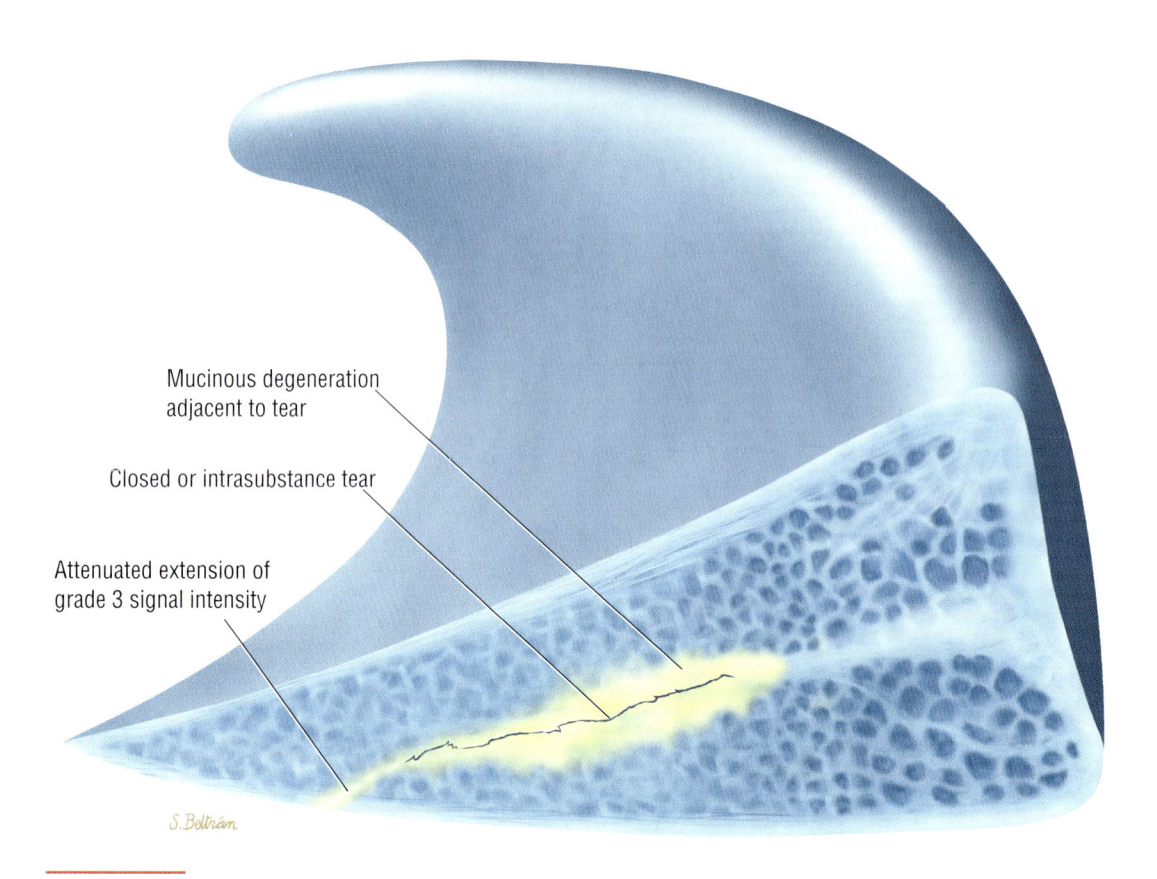

FIGURE 4.26 Attenuated grade 3 signal intensity that weakens toward the inferior articular surface of the meniscus in a closed tear (sagittal perspective).

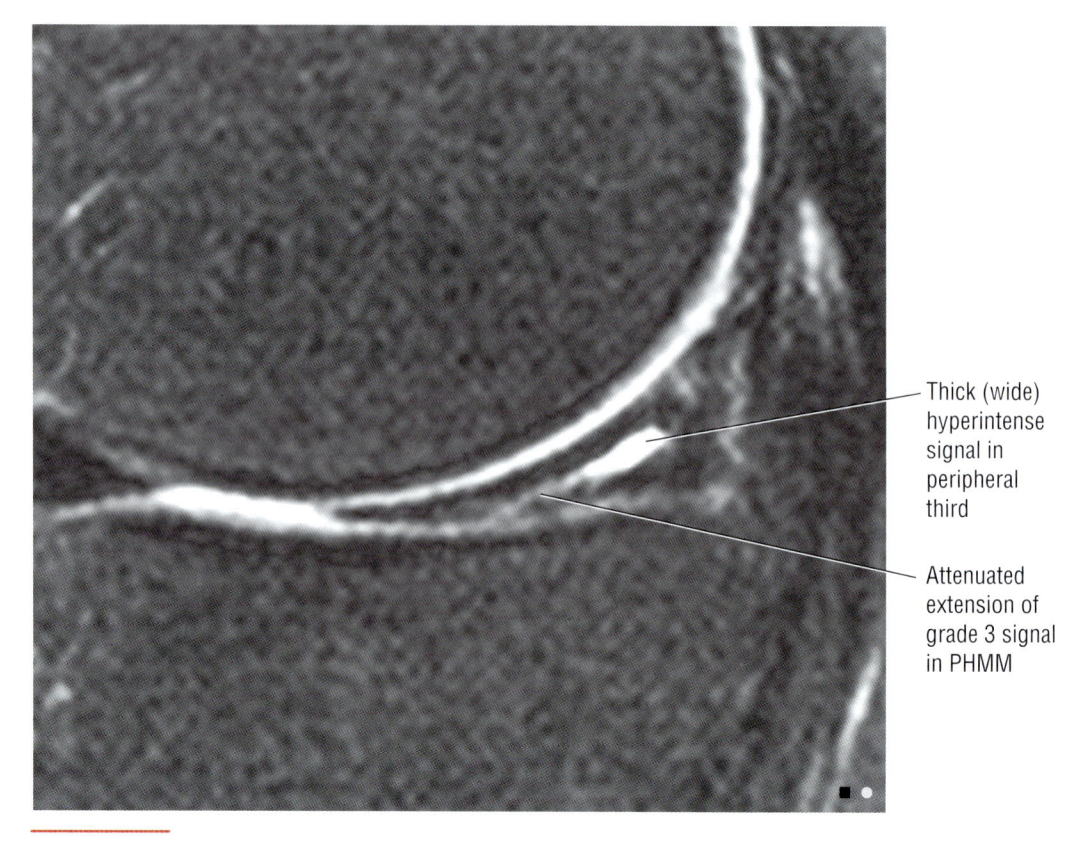

FIGURE 4.27 Closed meniscal tear with attenuation of grade 3 signal intensity as the tear approximates the inferior surface. FS PD FSE sagittal image.

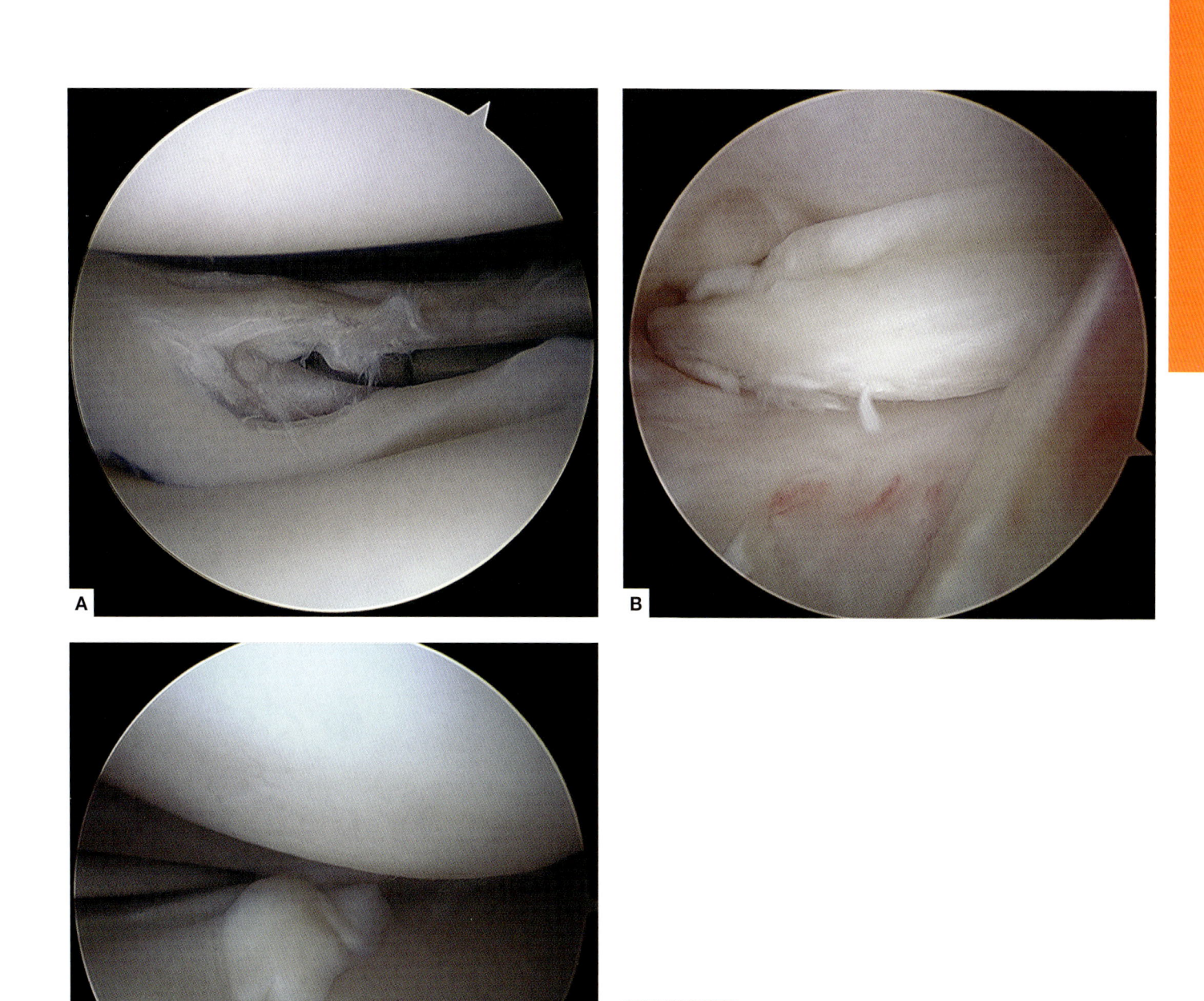

FIGURE 4.28 Arthroscopic images of meniscal tears. (**A**) Complex meniscal tear. (**B**) Displaced bucket-handle meniscal tear within the notch. (**C**) An undersurface tear discovered upon inspection of the inferior meniscal surface. (Reprinted from Fu FH. *Master Techniques in Orthopaedic Surgery: Sports Medicine*. Philadelphia, PA: Lippincott Williams & Wilkins; 2010, with permission.)

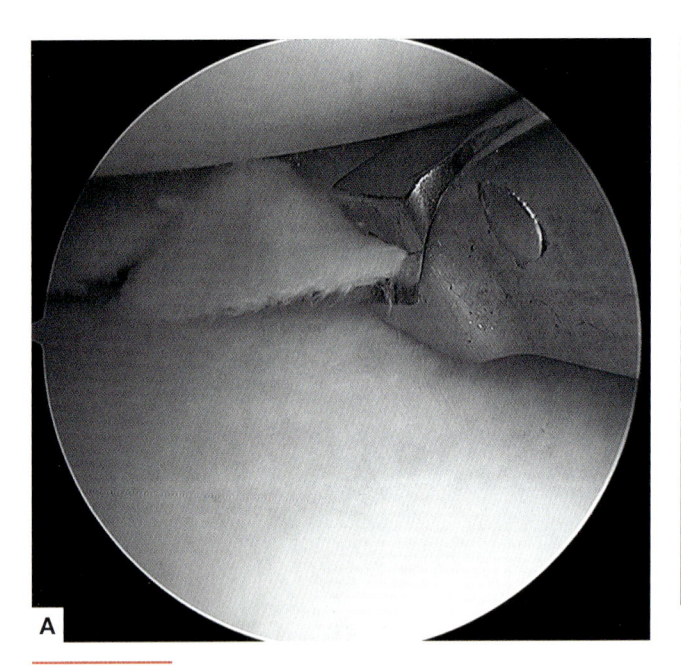

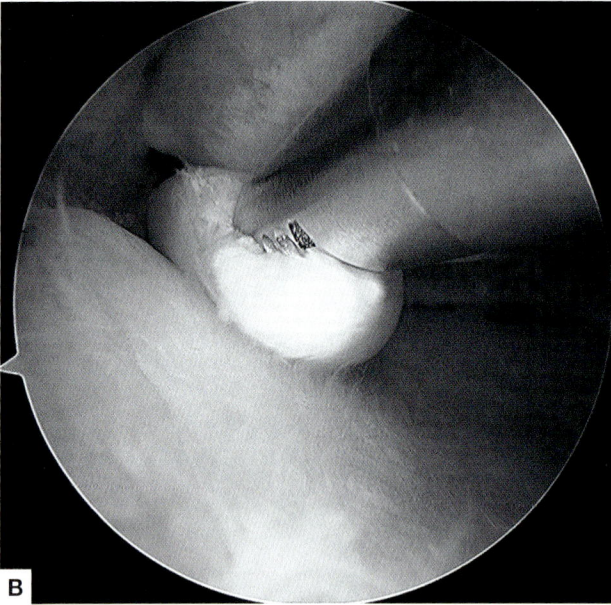

FIGURE 4.29 Arthroscopic instruments. (**A**) Utilization of the biter during meniscal debridement. (**B**) Use of a shaver during meniscal debridement. (Reprinted from Fu FH. *Master Techniques in Orthopaedic Surgery: Sports Medicine*. Philadelphia, PA: Lippincott Williams & Wilkins; 2010, with permission.)

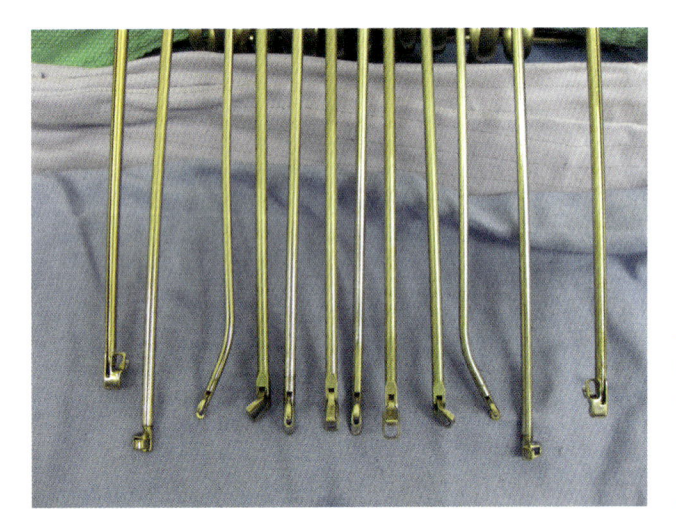

FIGURE 4.30 A variety of biters are available for resecting meniscal tears based on tear location. (Reprinted from Fu FH. *Master Techniques in Orthopaedic Surgery: Sports Medicine*. Philadelphia, PA: Lippincott Williams & Wilkins; 2010, with permission.)

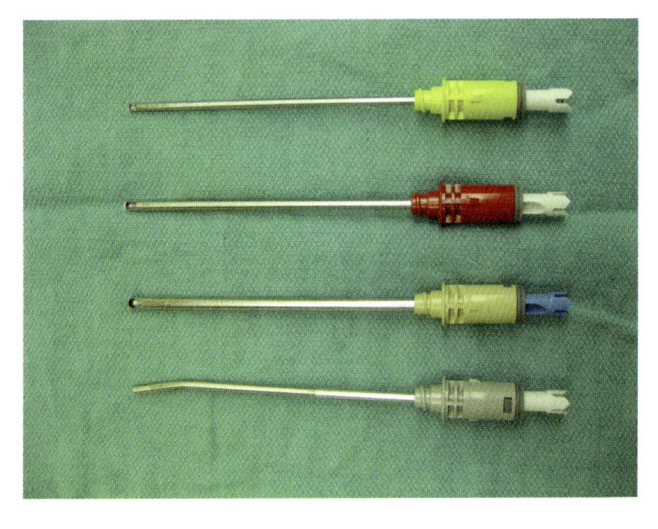

FIGURE 4.31 Shavers of various size and angle are available. (Reprinted from Fu FH. *Master Techniques in Orthopaedic Surgery: Sports Medicine*. Philadelphia, PA: Lippincott Williams & Wilkins; 2010, with permission.)

Meniscal Tear Patterns

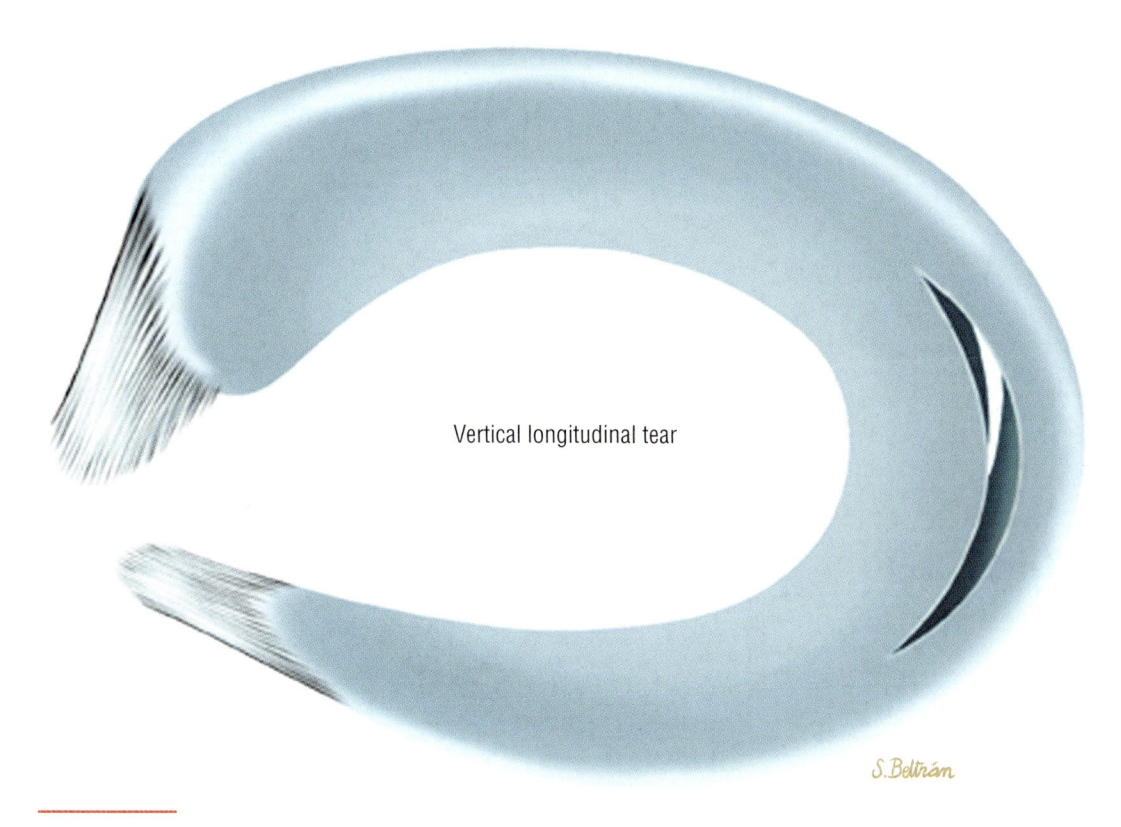

FIGURE 4.32 Circumferential surface tear pattern of a longitudinal tear.

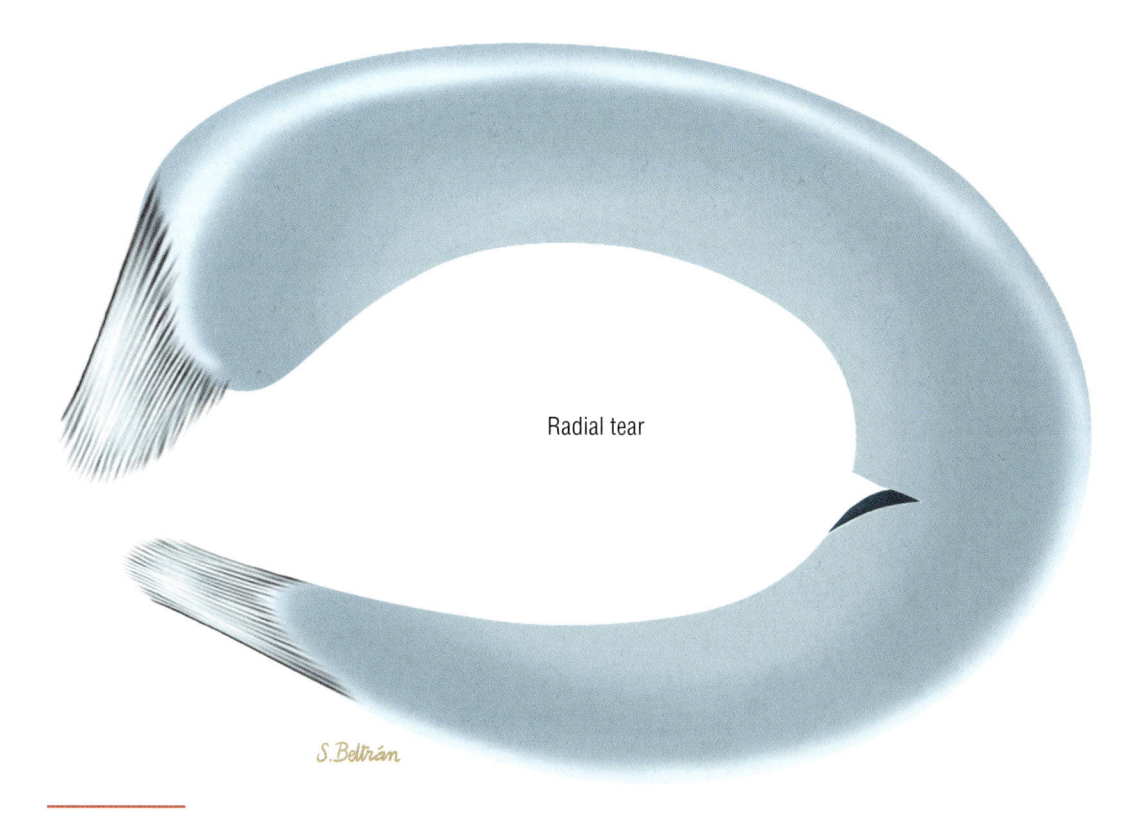

FIGURE 4.33 Free edge radial tear.

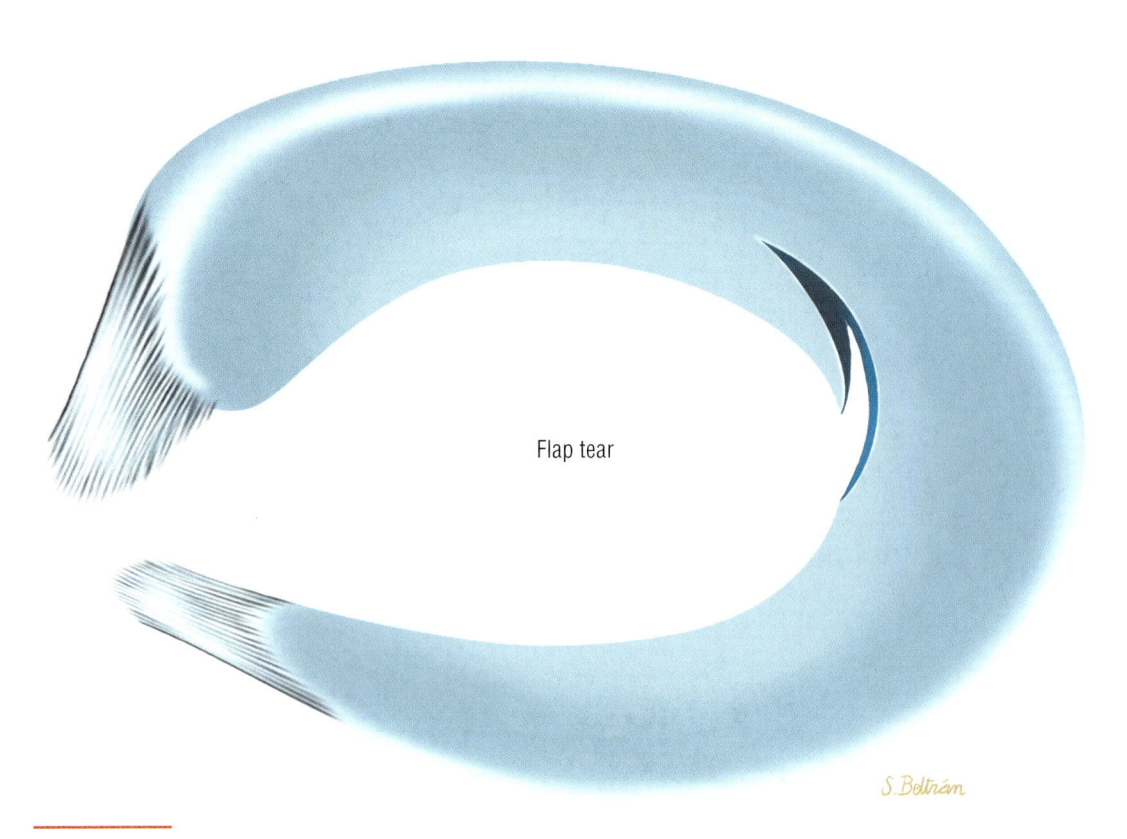

FIGURE 4.34 The flap tear demonstrates features of a radial tear that changes direction to a longitudinal path.

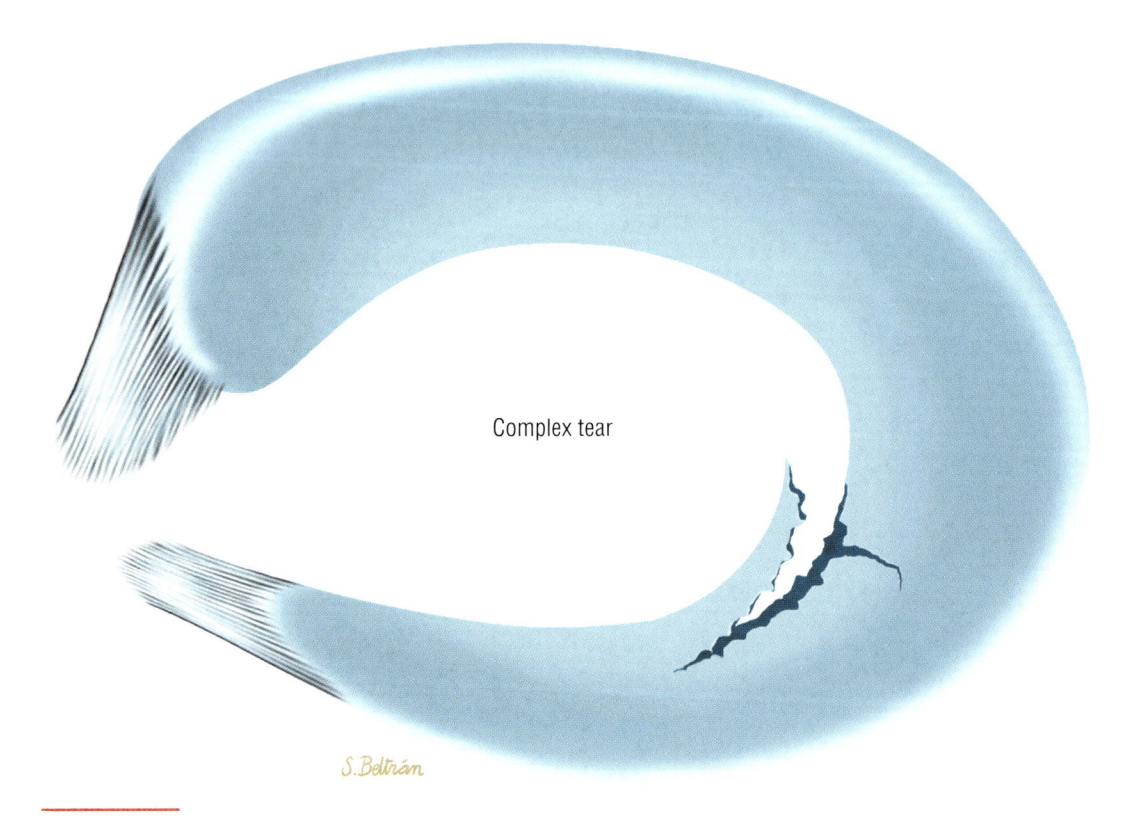

FIGURE 4.35 Complex meniscal tear with radial and flap components.

Horizontal Cleavage Tear

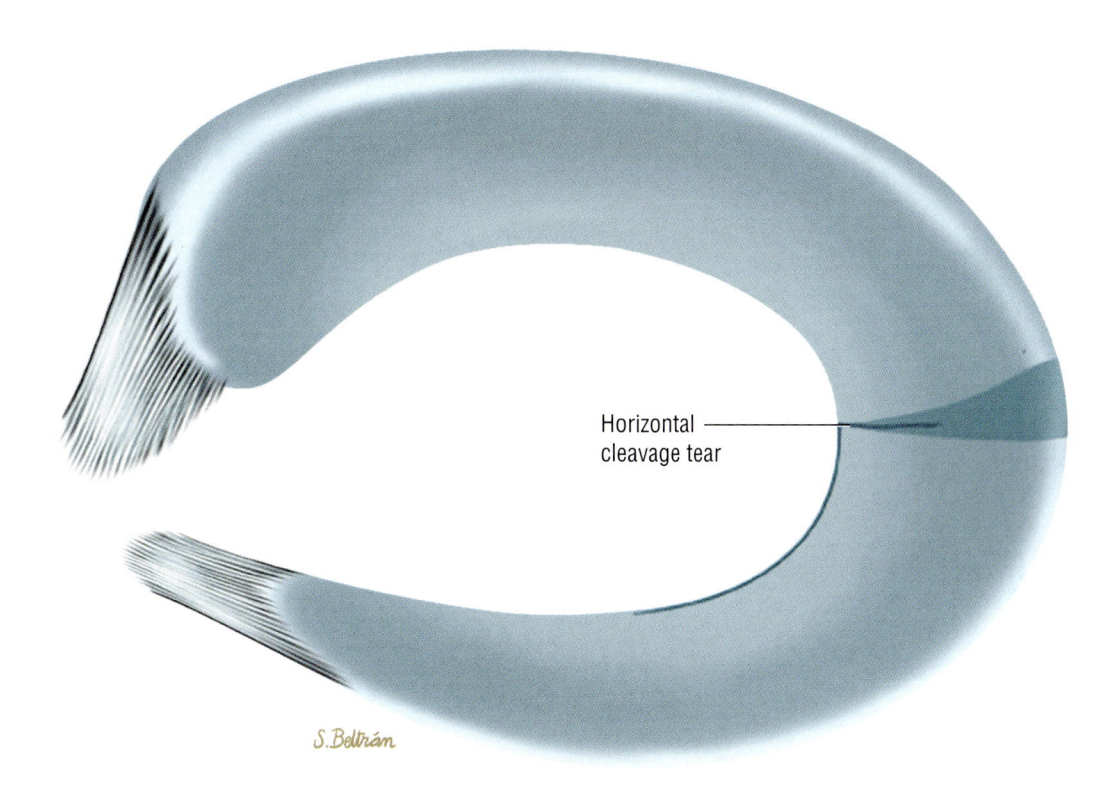

FIGURE 4.36 Horizontal cleavage tear extending to the meniscal apex and parallel to the tibial plateau. These tears result from excessive shear stress between femoral condylar and tibial plateau forces.

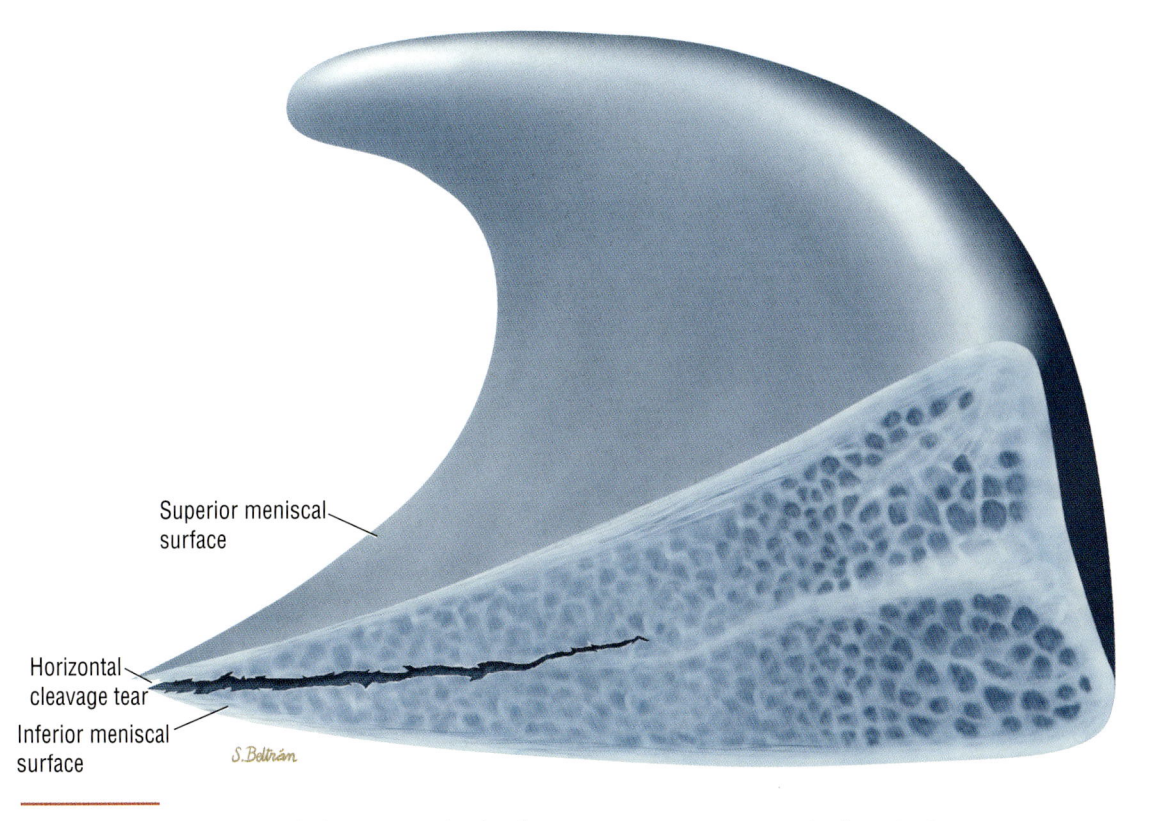

FIGURE 4.37 Horizontal cleavage tear divides the meniscus into superior and inferior leaflets.

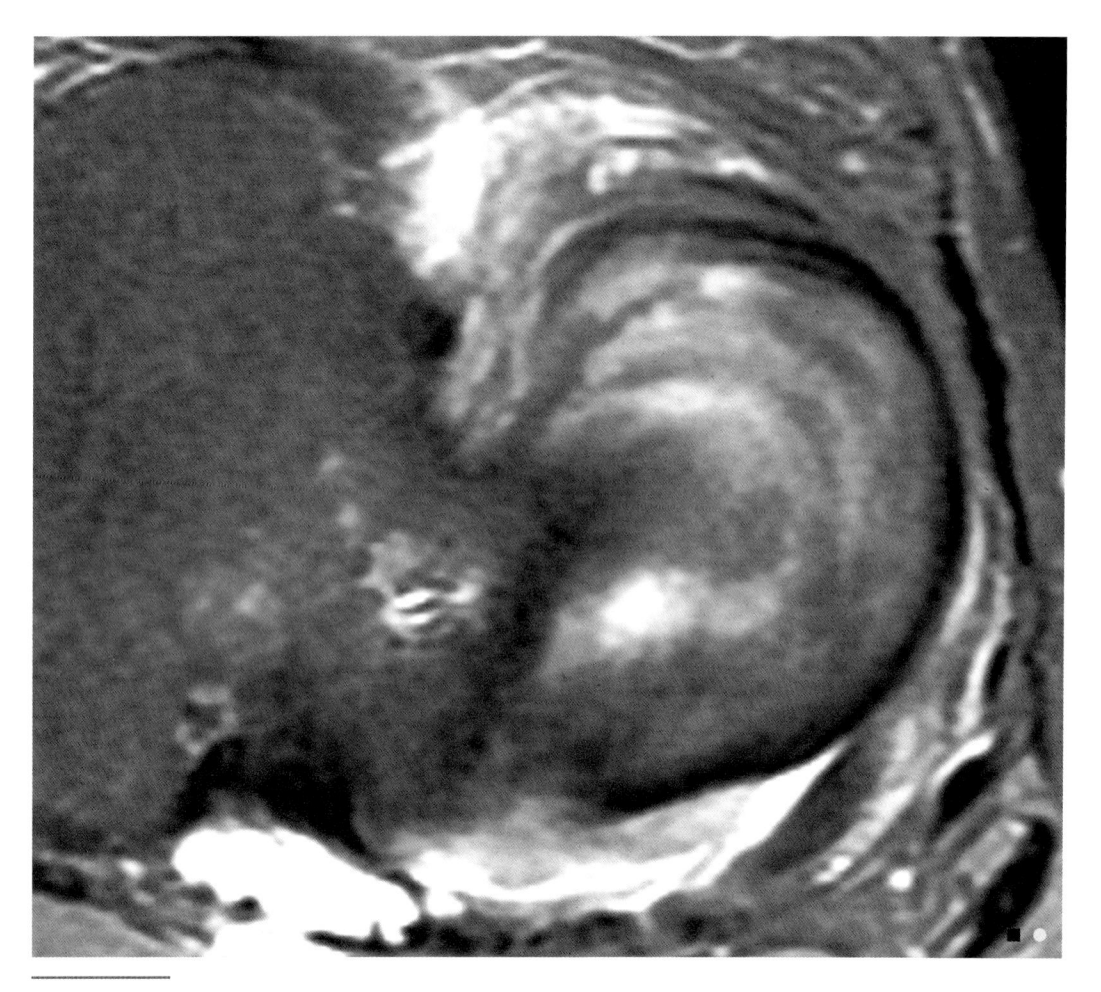

FIGURE 4.38 Horizontal tear of the lateral meniscus visualized as diffuse hyperintensity as the axial image is precisely parallel to the tear plane in this degenerative tear. Axial FS PD FSE image.

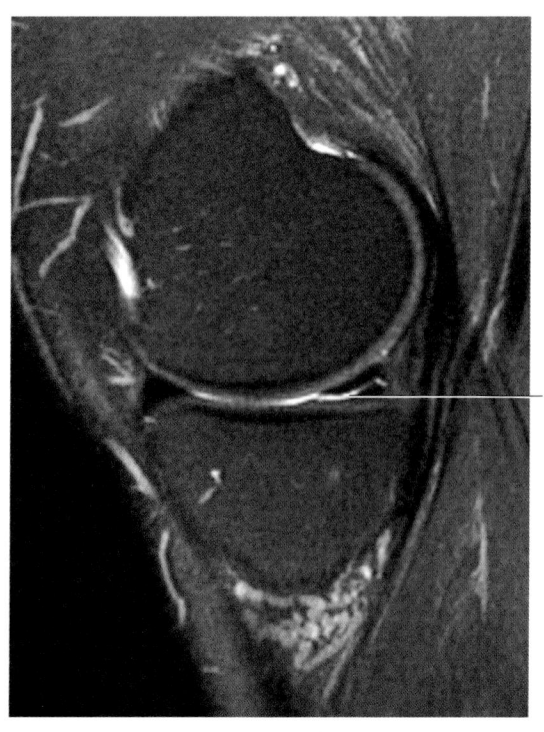

Horizontal tear posterior horn medial meniscus

FIGURE 4.39 Free extension of hyperintense joint fluid within the horizontal plane of a horizontal cleavage tear parallel to the tibial plateau. The term "fish-mouth" tear describes the equal separation of the meniscal leaves (leaflets) at the inner free edge or apex of the meniscus.

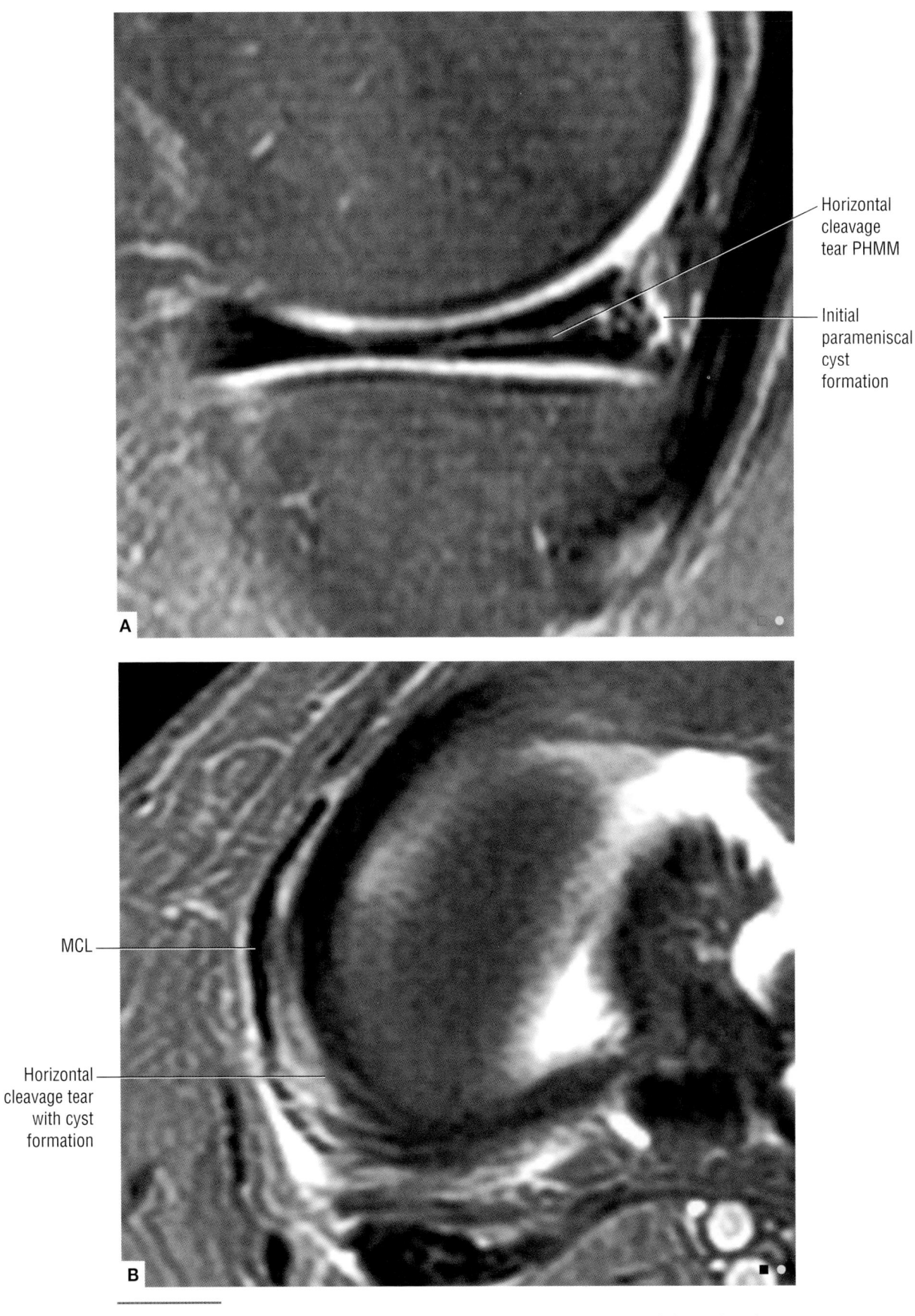

FIGURE 4.40 Horizontal cleavage tear parallel to the tibial plateau and directed to the apex region of the posterior horn (PHMM) and body of the medial meniscus. FS PD FSE sagittal (**A**) and axial (**B**) images.

Horizontal tear medial meniscus

Meniscal cyst
Horizontal tear medial meniscus

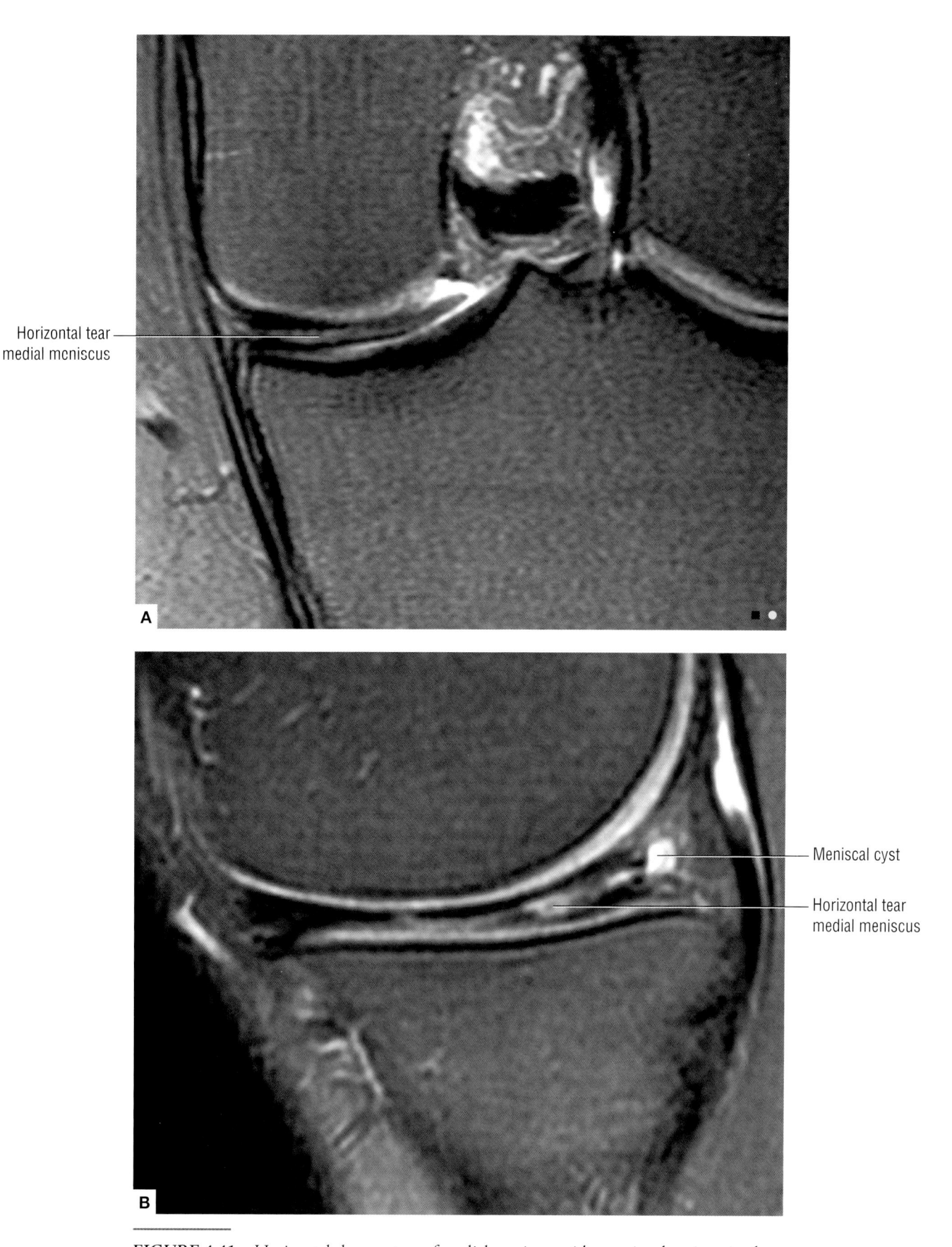

FIGURE 4.41 Horizontal cleavage tear of medial meniscus with associated perimeniscal cyst. FS PD FSE coronal (**A**) and sagittal (**B**) images. Meniscal cysts occur adjacent to the peripheral extension of the horizontal tear or peripheral degeneration in continuity with the tear.

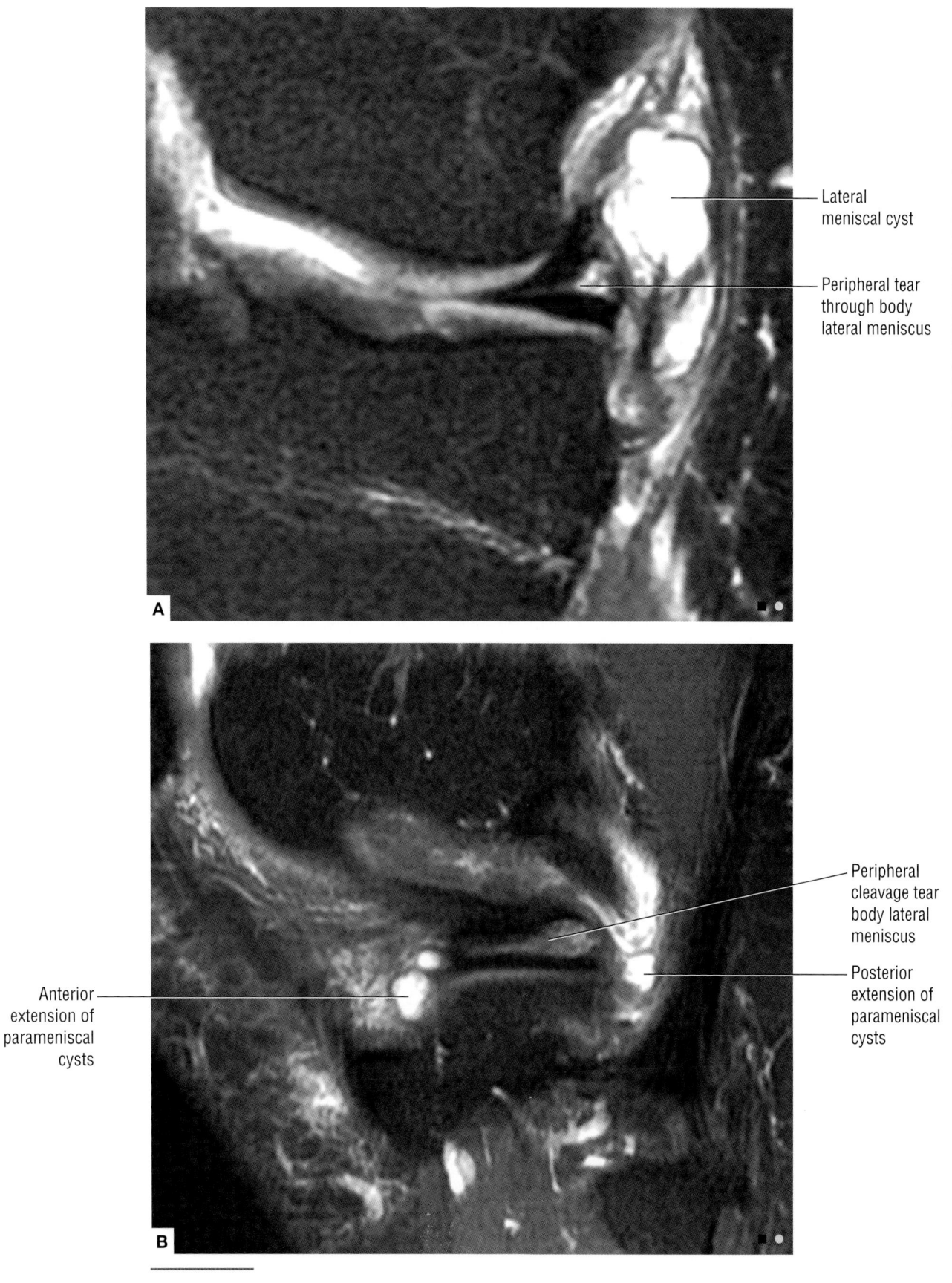

FIGURE 4.42 Peripheral horizontal tear evident because of the decompression of synovial fluid into a peripheral meniscal cyst. Without the meniscal cyst, the sagittal image would be interpreted as a closed peripheral horizontal cleavage tear. FS PD FSE coronal (**A**) and sagittal (**B**) images.

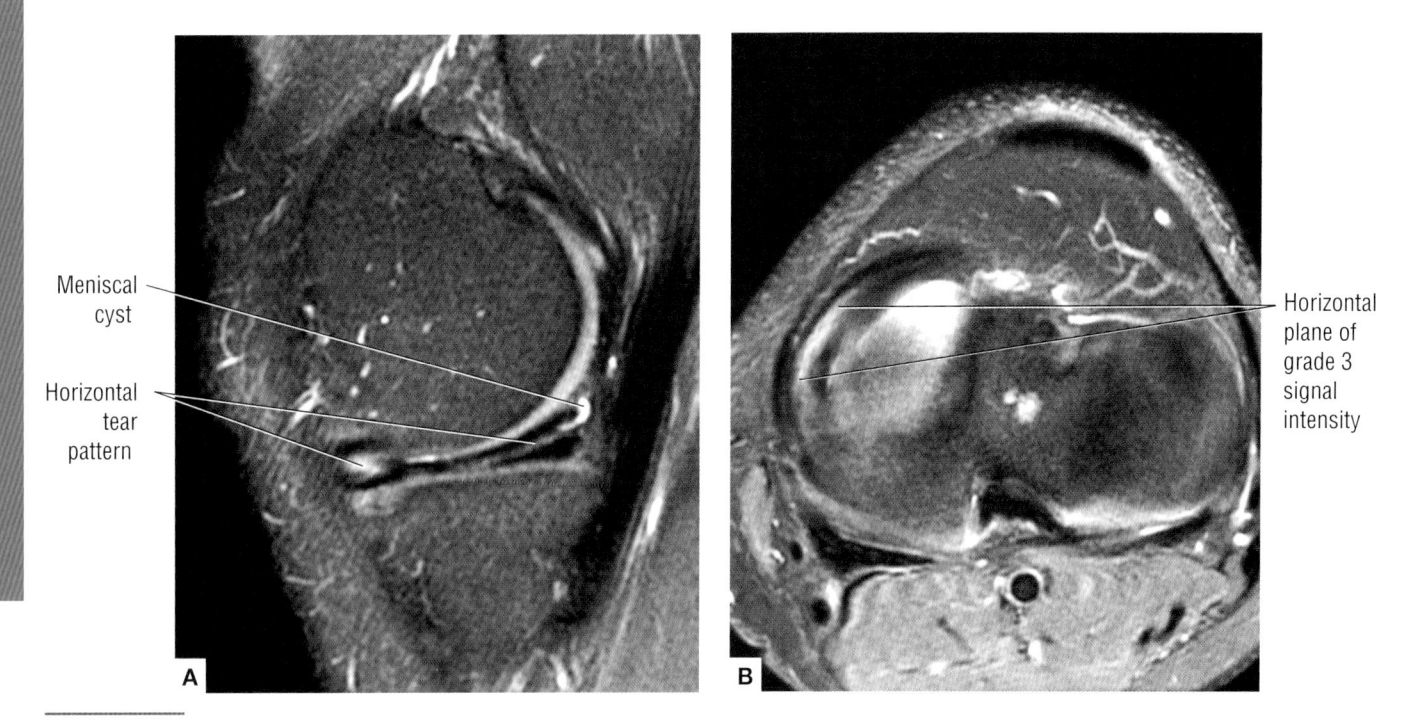

FIGURE 4.43 Horizontal tear with extension from the anterior horn to the posterior horn. Grade 3 signal intensity is identified within the central third or body of the medial meniscus on FS PD FSE sagittal (**A**) and axial (**B**) images. A small meniscal cyst has developed in posterior capsular tissues in continuity with the posterior horn of the medial meniscus (**A**). The corresponding axial image of the horizontal tear (**B**) demonstrates a wide area of grade 3 signal intensity within the central or middle plane of the meniscus. Because a longitudinal tear with a horizontal component would be directed to either the superior or inferior articular surface, it would not display a wide area of grade 3 signal intensity restricted to the middle or central plane extending to the meniscal apex.

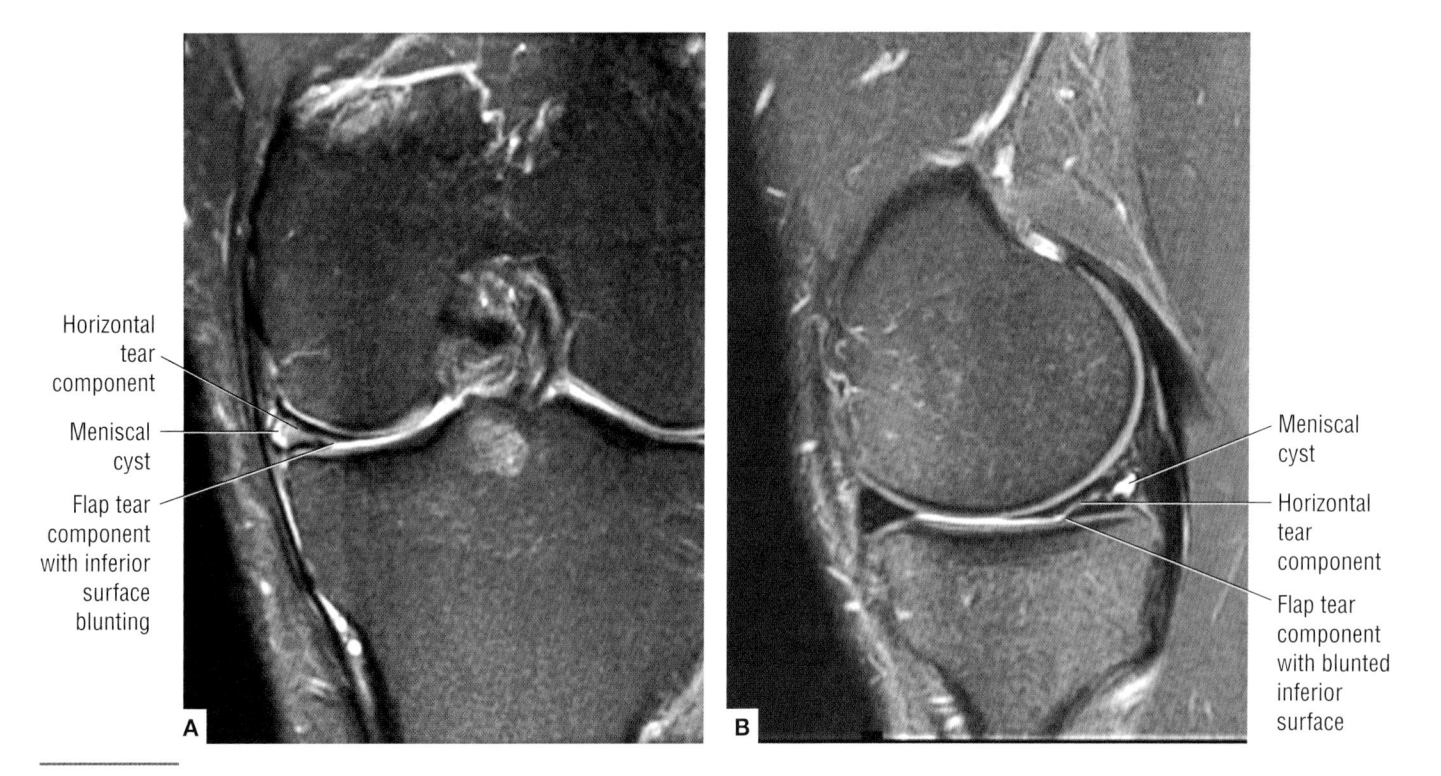

FIGURE 4.44 Coexistence of horizontal and flap tear patterns in the posterior horn of the medial meniscus on FS PD FSE coronal (**A**) and sagittal (**B**) images. The blunting of the inferior leaf of the meniscus with articular surface extension represents flap tear morphology. The peripheral meniscal tear pattern is primarily horizontal and is associated with a small meniscal cyst. Flap tears, however, may be characterized by either horizontal or vertical tear patterns on corresponding sagittal images.

Longitudinal Tears

- Vertical peripheral tears occurring along the longitudinal axis of the meniscus (viewed on axial images)
- Occur in the peripheral aspect of the meniscus
  - Tear pattern begins in the posterior horn and advances in the direction of the circumferential collagen fibers.
  - Extend circumferentially along the anteroposterior extent of the meniscus (parallel to the meniscal margin in the long axis)
- Identified on either coronal or sagittal images by peripheral grade 3 signal intensity
- Correspond to the long or longitudinal axis of the meniscus in the axial plane
- Not restricted to vertical tear patterns on sagittal images
- May present with oblique or horizontally oriented signal (not parallel to the tibial plateau) that extends to an articular surface
- May not extend through both meniscal leaflets
- Commonly associated with ACL and/or MCL tears
- Orientation confirmed at arthroscopy
- Visualized only on an inferior or superior articular surface
- Usually occur in younger patients in an acute traumatic setting
- Thin-section axial images demonstrate linear signal intensity parallel to the long axis of the meniscus.
- If vertical signal intensity is located in the inner third of the meniscus, it is considered a flap tear.
- Location common in the peripheral aspect of the meniscus, where there is an increased concentration of circumferential collagen fibers adjacent to the meniscal peripheral attachment

- Normal anatomic structures that may be mistaken for a longitudinal tear include:
    - The insertion of the transverse intermeniscal ligament
    - The insertion of the meniscofemoral (Humphrey's and Wrisberg's) ligaments to the posterior horn of the lateral meniscus.
- Vertical longitudinal tears can occur parallel to the popliteus tendon sheath.
- Increased axial load (compressive force) results in radial strain and splitting of the meniscus longitudinally (between circumferential collagen fibers).
    - The tear originates as a small longitudinal split that disrupts the posterior horn and then advances along the plane of the circumferential collagen fibers, which are split along their long axis.
- Multiple longitudinal tears may occur within the same meniscus.
- A bucket-handle or flap tear results when there is inner fragment displacement.
- Joint locking is usually related to pain and spasm associated with tension on the abnormally mobile fragments.
- Peripheral vertical tears are treated with primary meniscal repair.
- Horizontal tears that extend into avascular fibrocartilage are treated with partial meniscectomy.
- The peripheral extension of MR grade 3 signal intensity to the stable meniscal rim may assist the arthroscopist in performing a partial meniscectomy but may not be appreciated at arthroscopy.
    - Consistent with the frequent appearance of grade 3 signal intensity in an asymptomatic partial meniscectomy meniscal remnant on MR.

Longitudinal Meniscal Tear

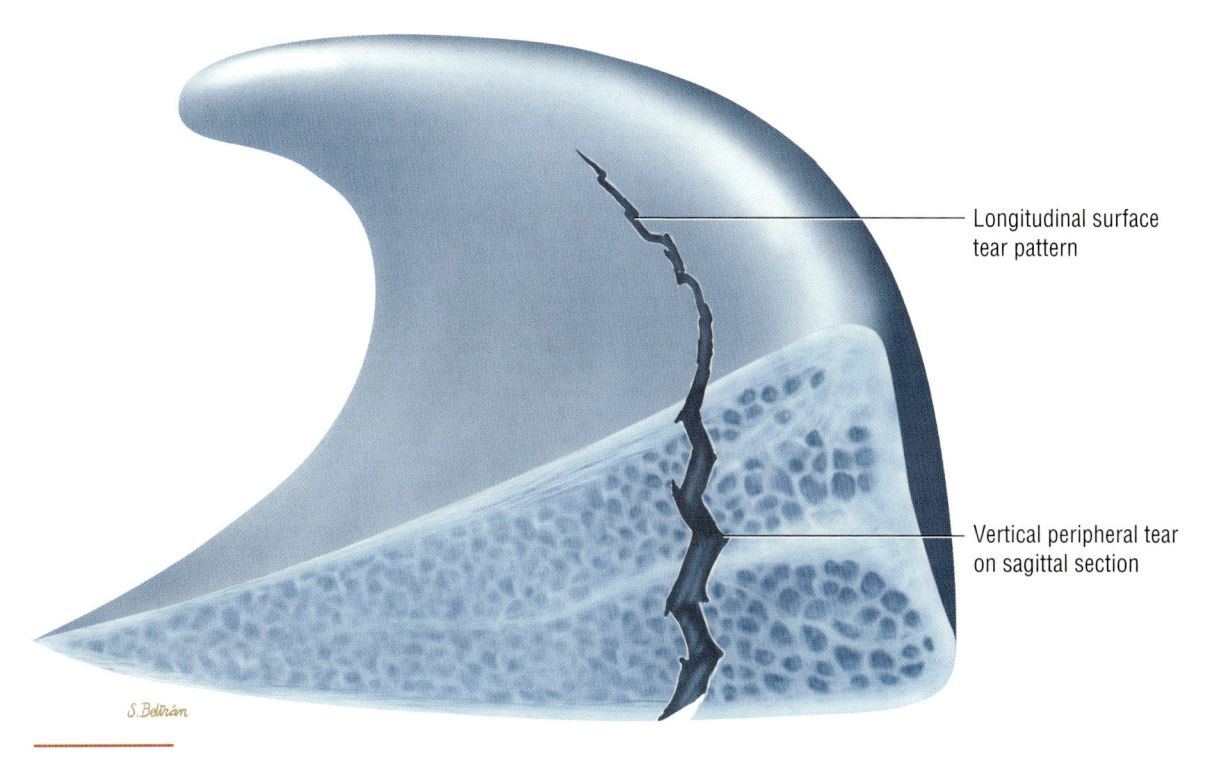

FIGURE 4.45 Longitudinal tear with peripheral vertical orientation through the circumferential collagen fibers. These tears result from excessive axial loads that produce radial strain that exceeds the capacity of the radial tie fibers to resist plastic deformation. Longitudinal tears are associated with ACL injuries because the meniscus may become trapped between the distal femoral condyle and the tibial plateau.

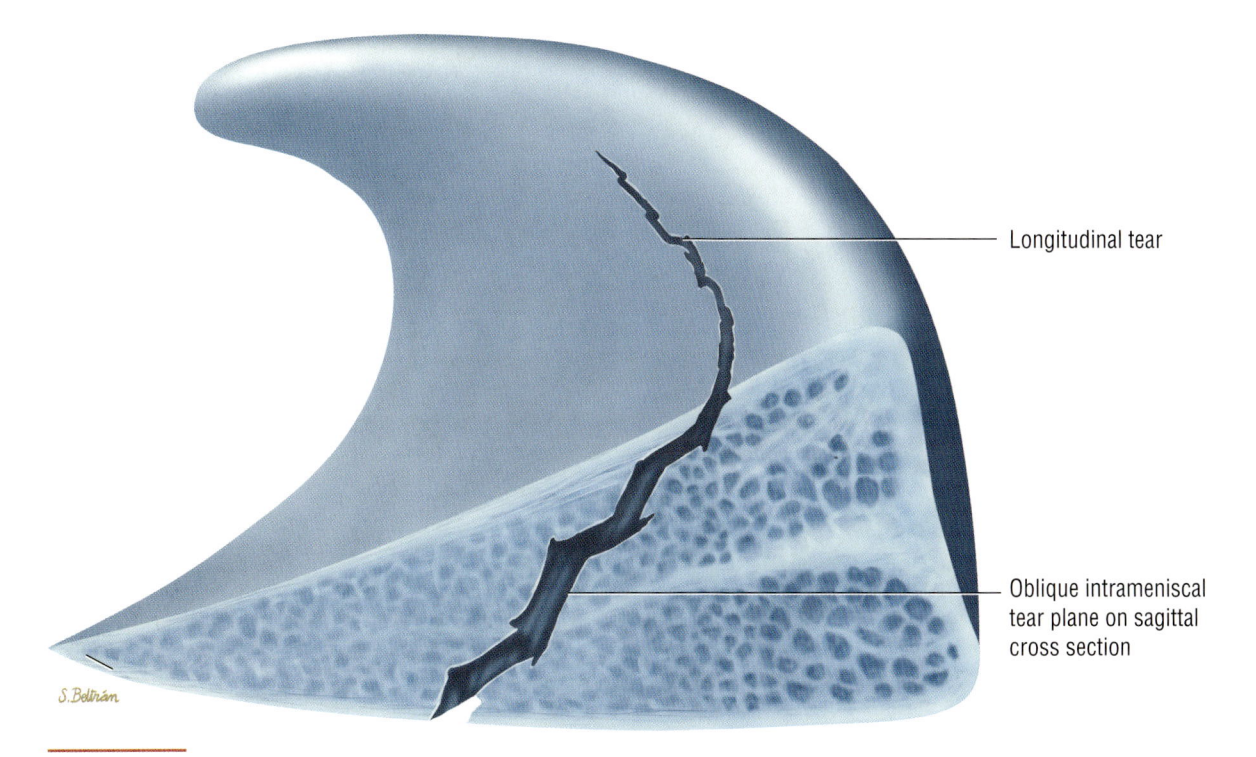

FIGURE 4.46 Surface longitudinal tear created by a cross-sectional pattern of both vertical and horizontal forces producing an oblique tear plane.

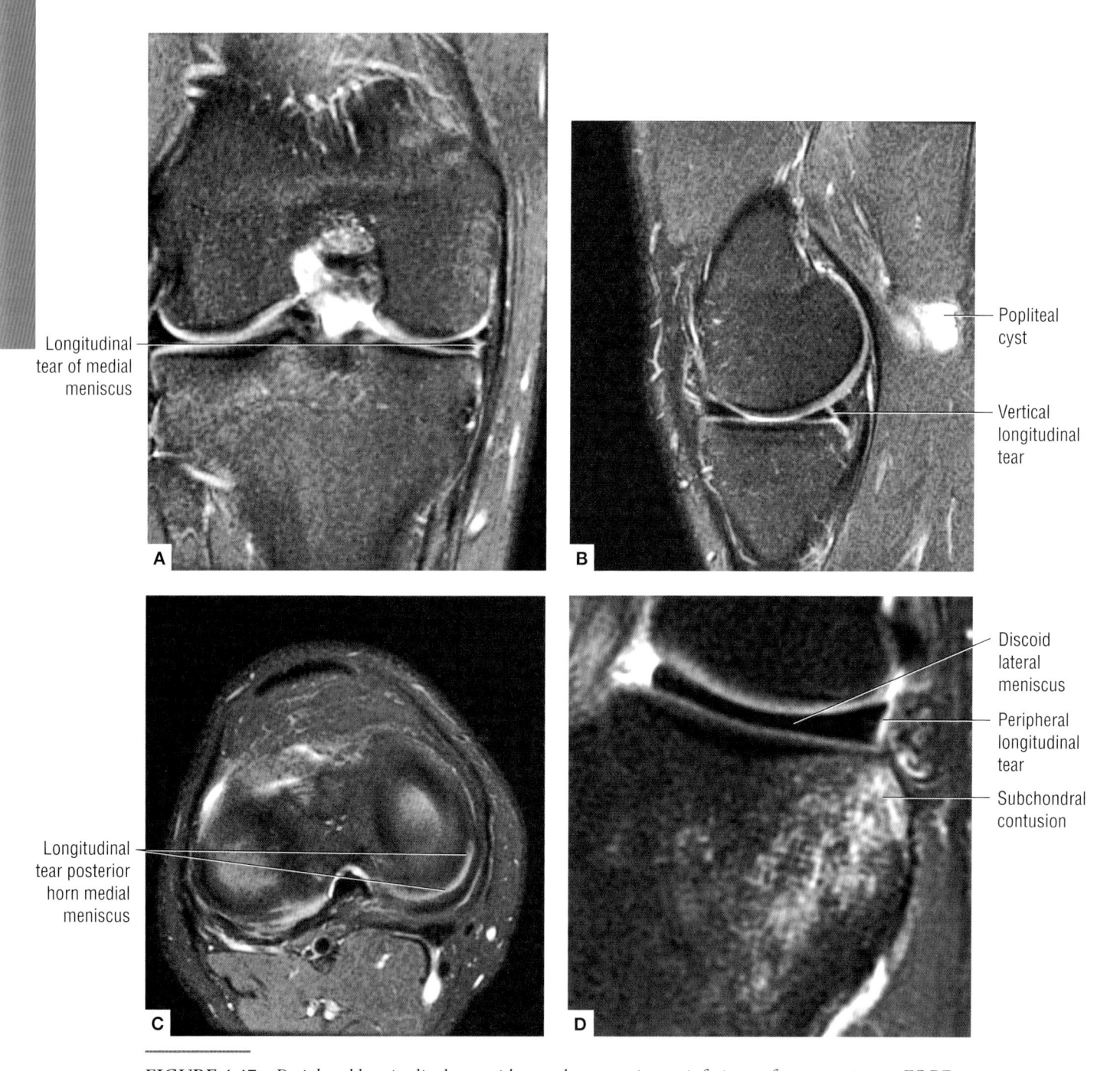

FIGURE 4.47 Peripheral longitudinal tear with complete superior-to-inferior surface extension on FS PD FSE coronal (**A**) and sagittal (**B**) images. (**C**) On an axial FS PD FSE image, the longitudinal tear can be seen coursing through the circumferential zone and following the contour of the meniscus. (**D**) Coronal FS PD FSE image showing a peripheral longitudinal tear in a discoid lateral meniscus.

The Meniscus

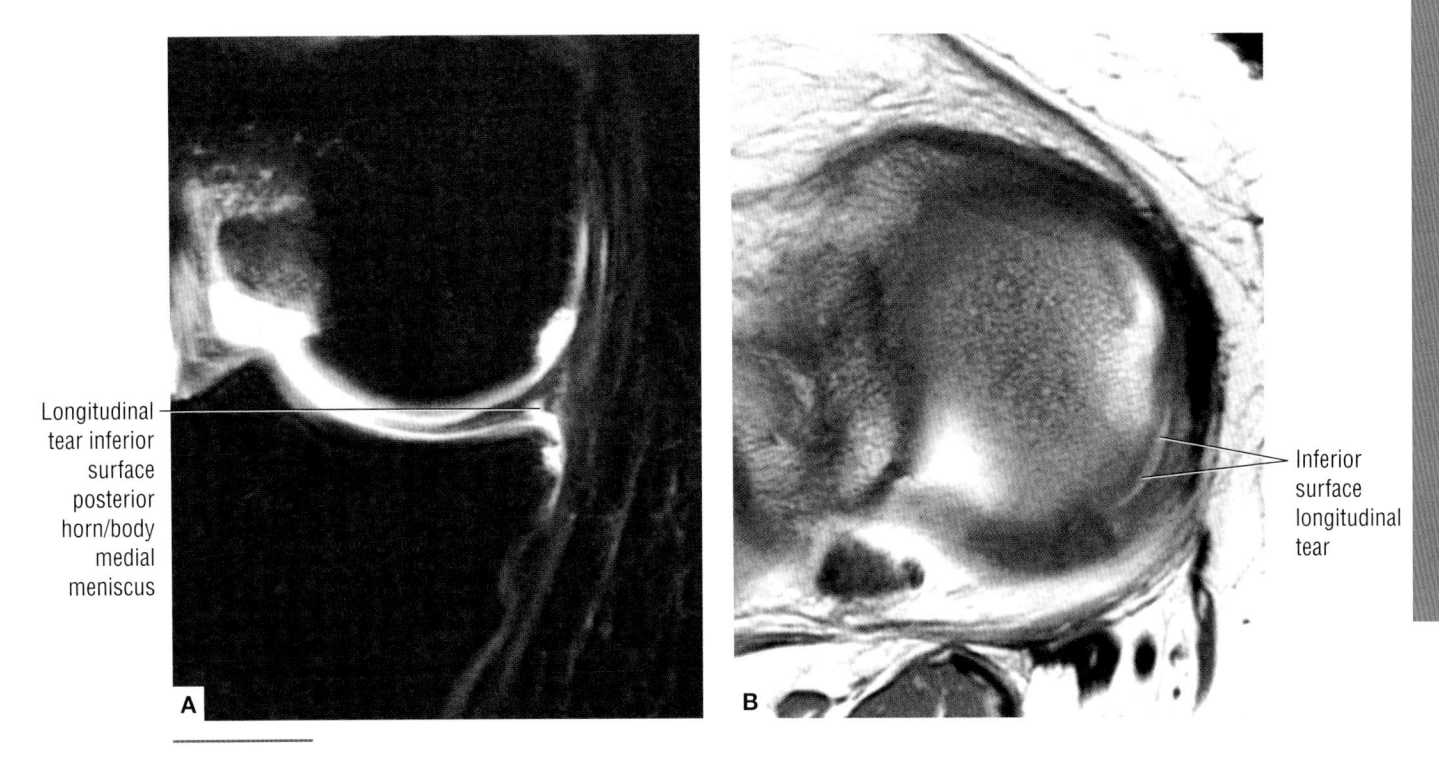

FIGURE 4.48 (**A**) Longitudinal tear with vertical peripheral morphology on FS PD FSE coronal image. (**B**) The longitudinal tear extends to the inferior meniscal surface and courses parallel to the long axis of the meniscus on corresponding PD FSE axial image.

Labels (A): Longitudinal tear inferior surface posterior horn/body medial meniscus
Labels (B): Inferior surface longitudinal tear

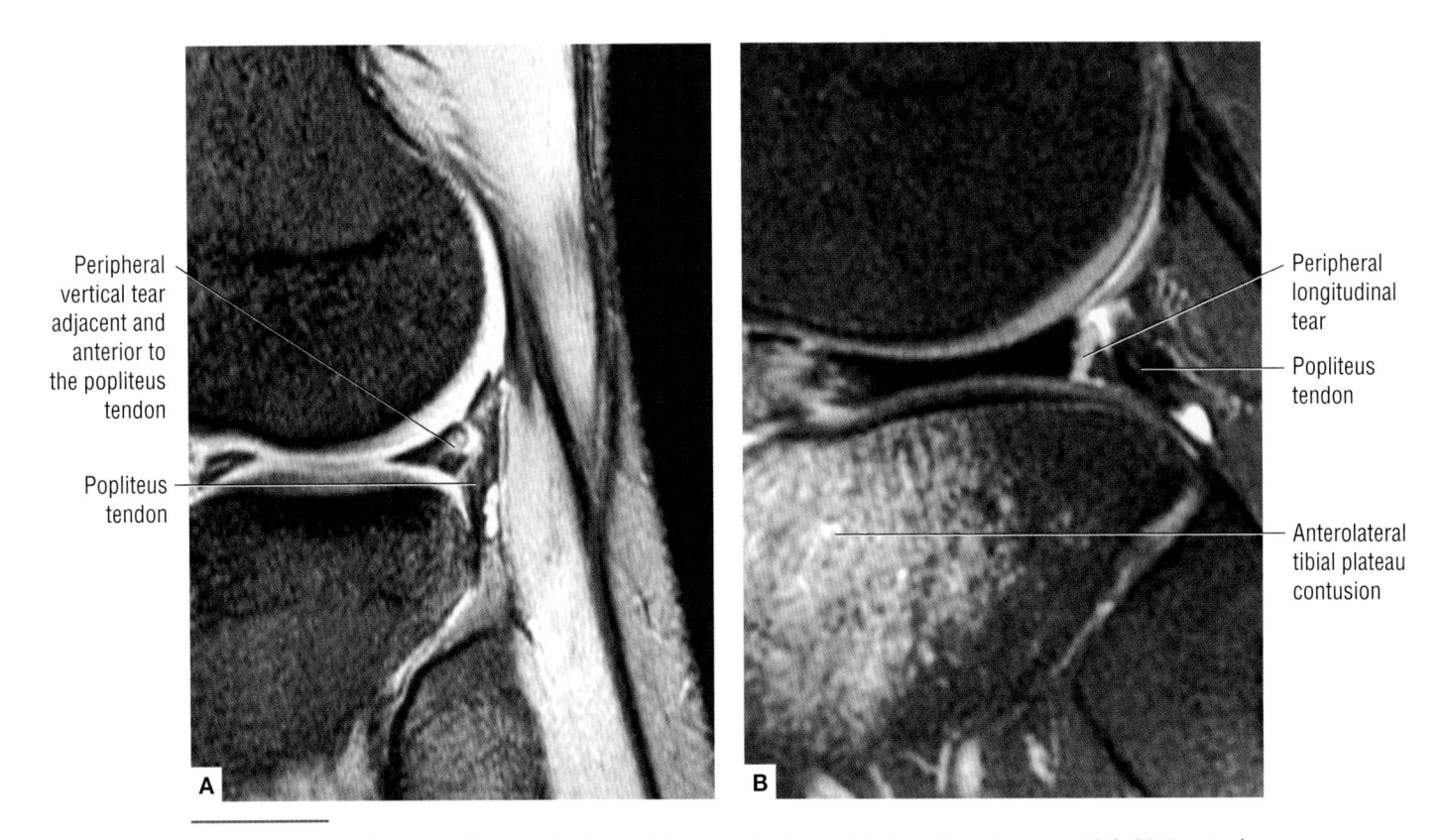

FIGURE 4.49 (**A**) Vertical longitudinal tear of the posterior horn of the lateral meniscus on a T2* GRE sagittal image. The tear is parallel and adjacent to the popliteus tendon sheath. (**B**) Peripheral vertical longitudinal tear of the lateral meniscus anterior to the popliteus tendon sheath on a sagittal FS PD FSE image.

Labels (A): Peripheral vertical tear adjacent and anterior to the popliteus tendon; Popliteus tendon
Labels (B): Peripheral longitudinal tear; Popliteus tendon; Anterolateral tibial plateau contusion

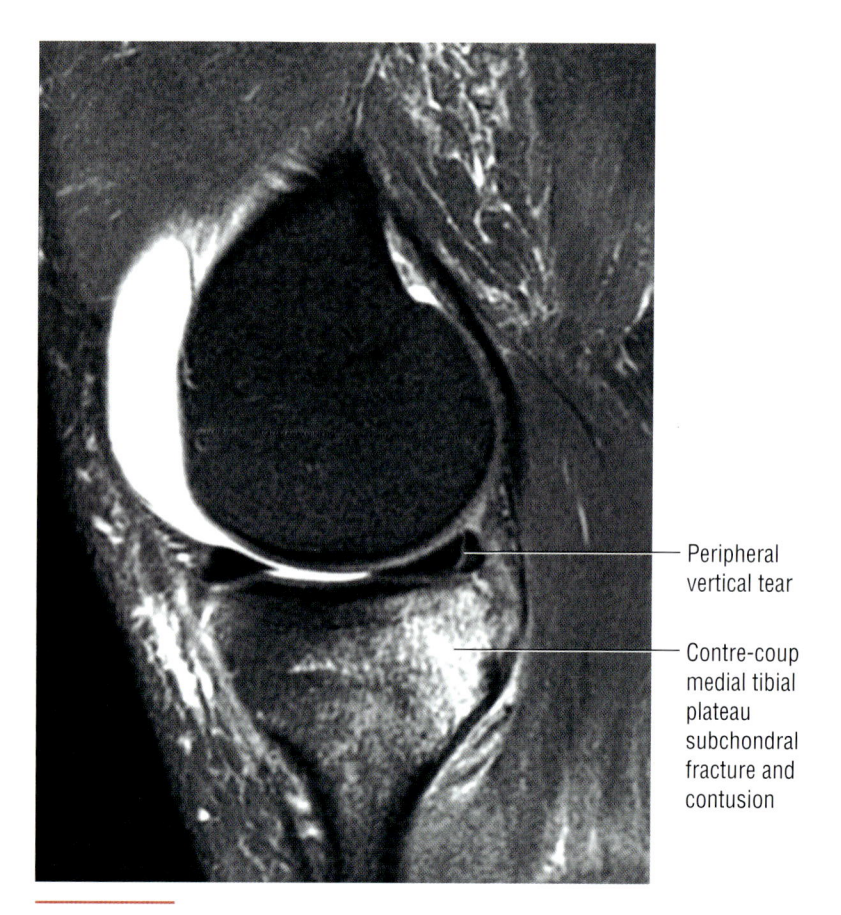

FIGURE 4.50 Characteristic peripheral vertical tear of the medial meniscus associated with a contrecoup medial tibial plateau fracture in an acute ACL tear (FS PD sagittal image).

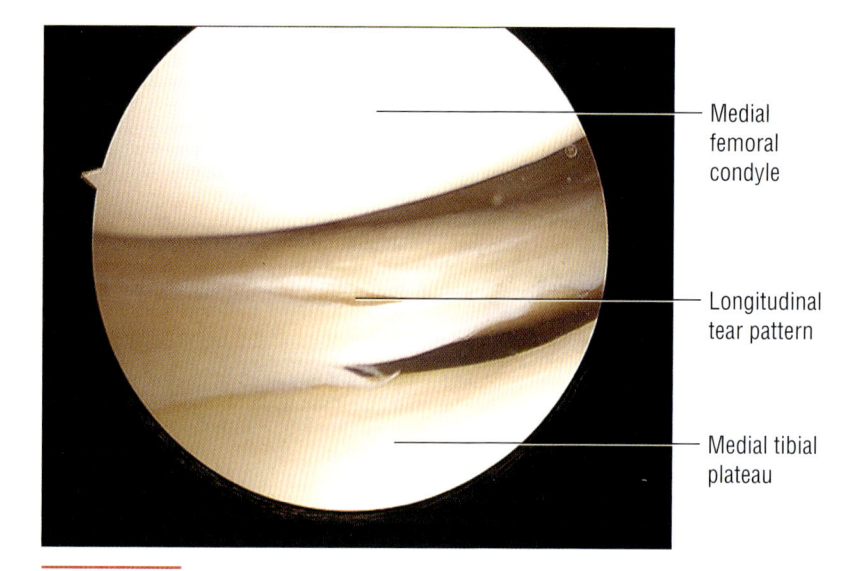

FIGURE 4.51 Arthroscopic view of a medial meniscus longitudinal tear.

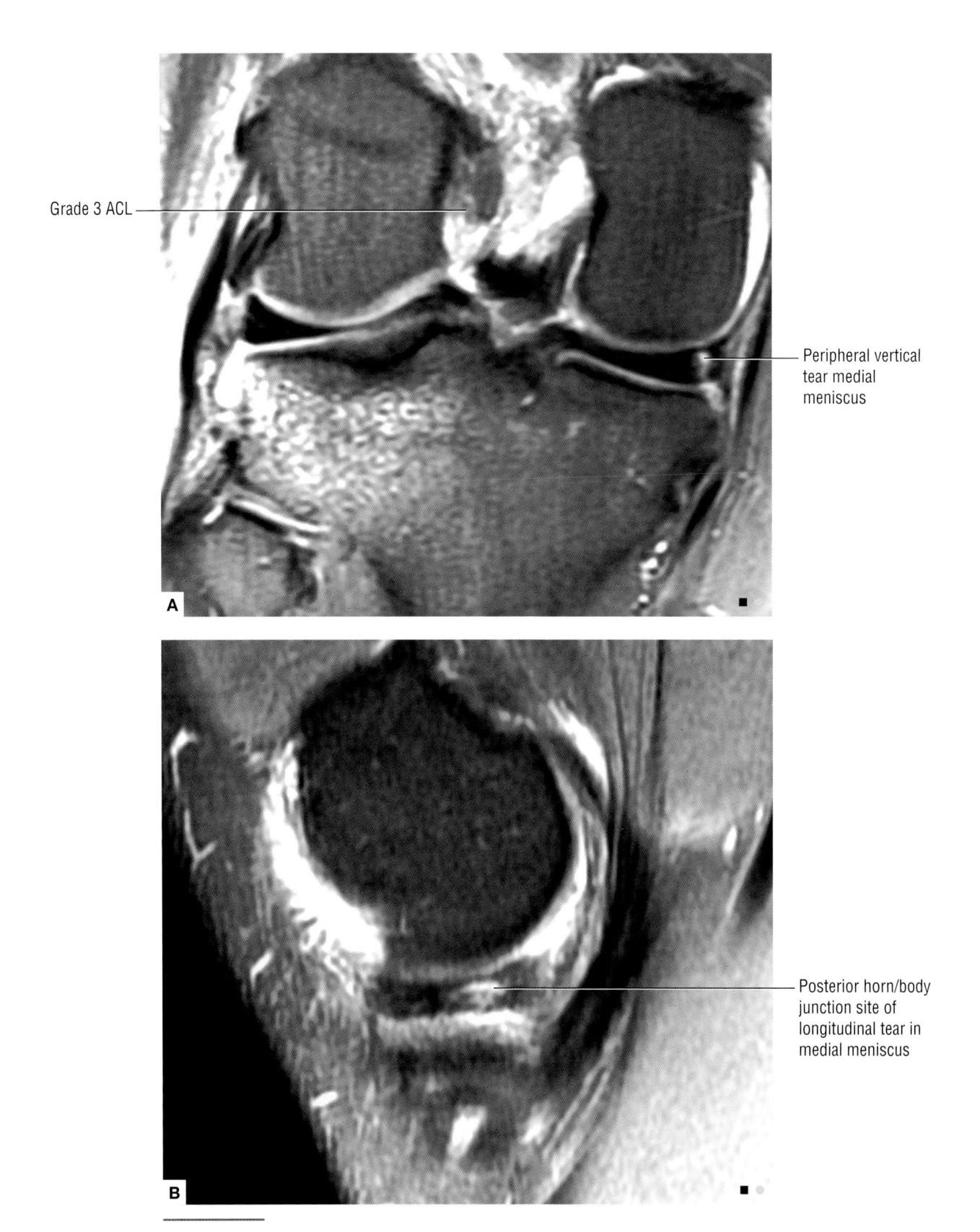

FIGURE 4.52 Peripheral vertical longitudinal tear of the medial meniscus associated with a grade 3 ACL tear. The orientation of the tear is perpendicular to the medial tibial plateau. The tear involves the outer third or circumferential zone of the meniscus. FS PD FSE coronal (**A**) and sagittal (**B**) images.

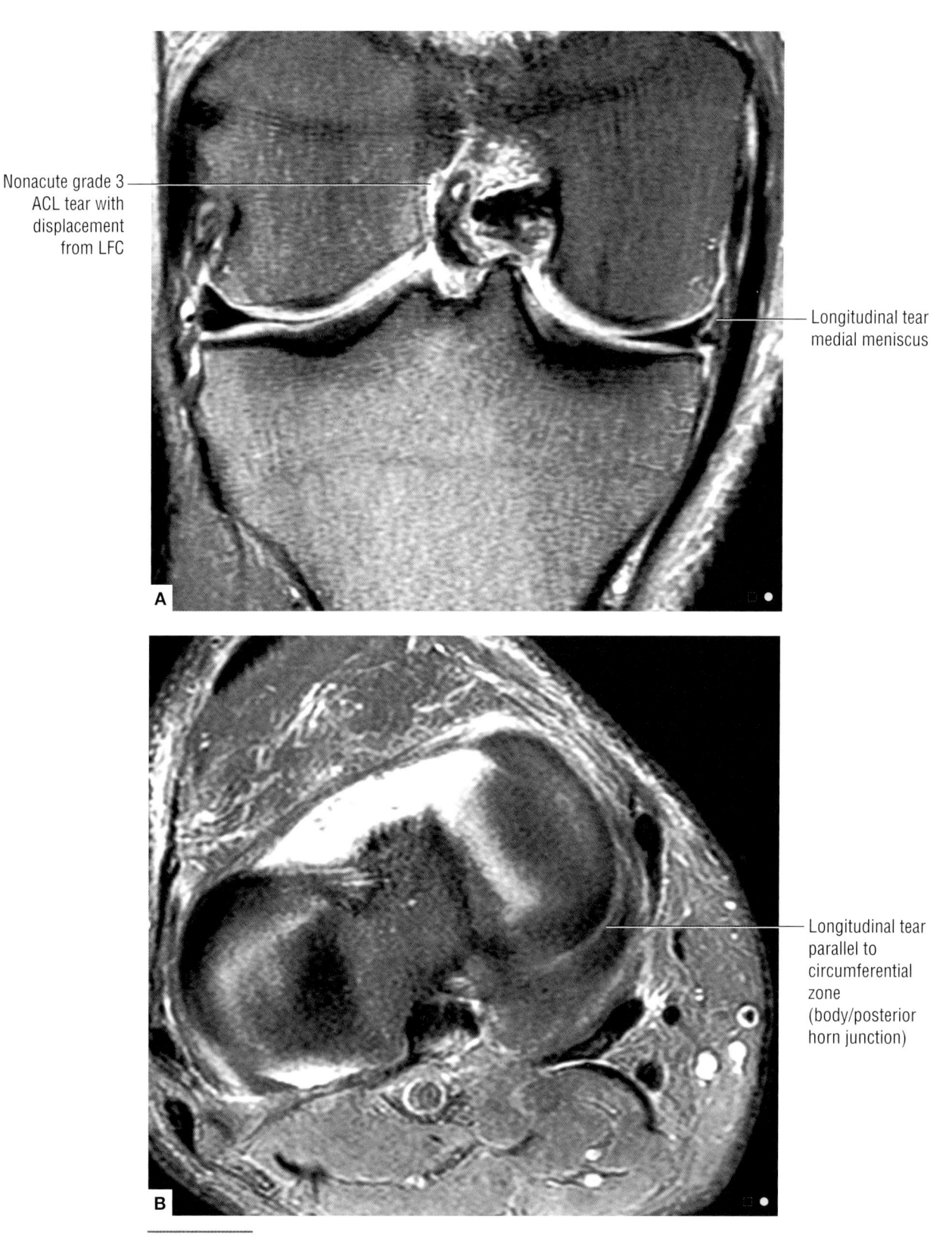

FIGURE 4.53 Longitudinal vertical tear on FS PD FSE coronal (**A**) and sagittal (**B**) images. Medial meniscus tears associated with ACL tears commonly involve the meniscocapsular junction, posterior inferior corner, or are parallel to the periphery.

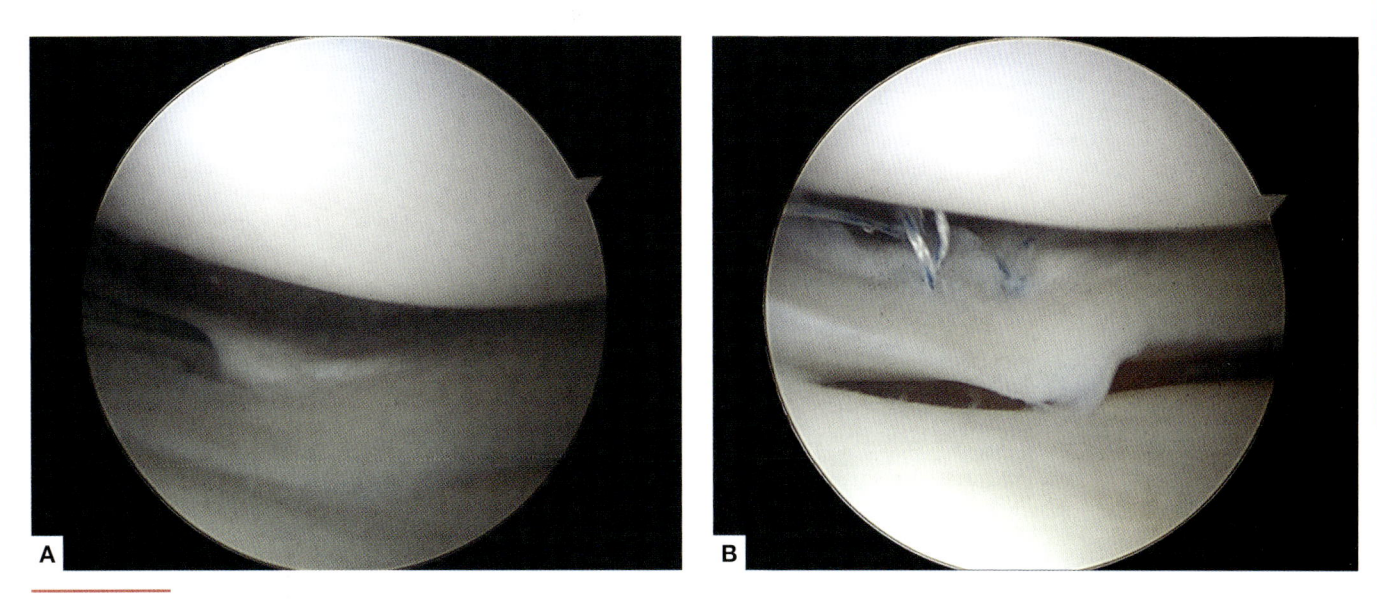

FIGURE 4.54 (**A**) Arthroscopic view of a longitudinal tear of the lateral meniscus in a left knee from the lateral portal. (**B**) Arthroscopic view of an all-inside meniscus repair of the lateral meniscus using two FasT Fix devices. (Reprinted from Fu FH. *Master Techniques in Orthopaedic Surgery: Sports Medicine*. Philadelphia, PA: Lippincott Williams & Wilkins; 2010, with permission.)

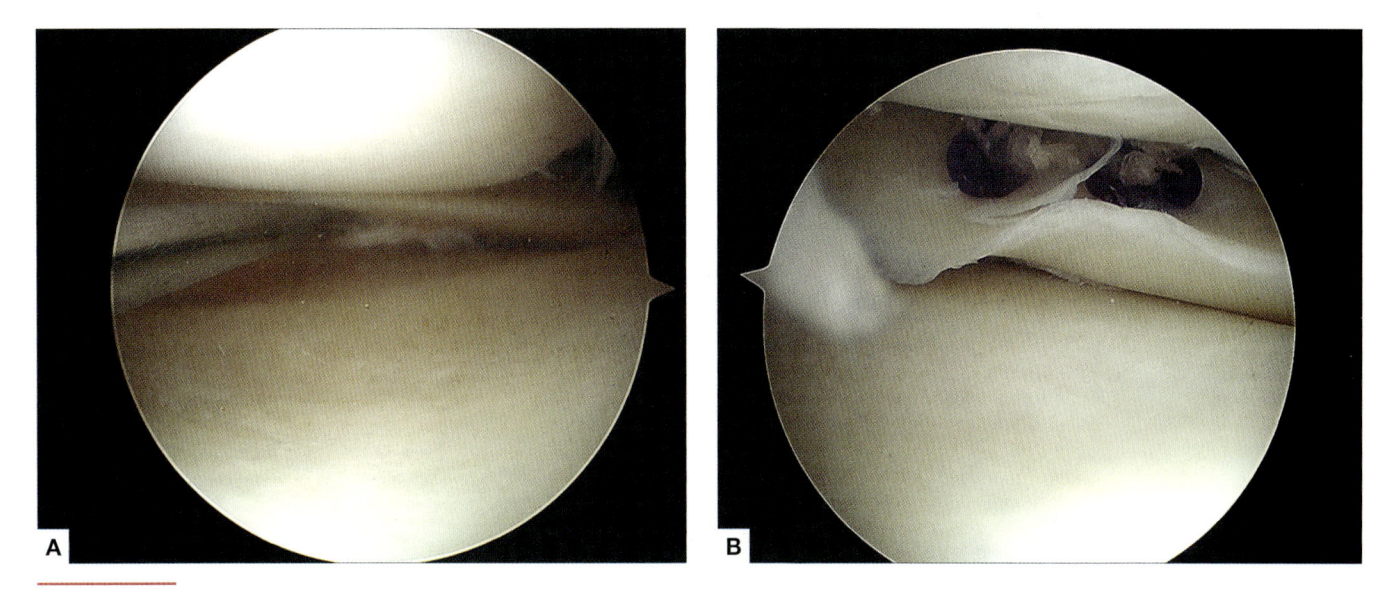

FIGURE 4.55 (**A**) Arthroscopic view of an undersurface longitudinal medial meniscus tear in a left knee from the lateral portal. (**B**) Arthroscopic view of an all-inside meniscus repair of the medial meniscus using two RapidLoc devices. (Reprinted from Fu FH. *Master Techniques in Orthopaedic Surgery: Sports Medicine*. Philadelphia, PA: Lippincott Williams & Wilkins; 2010, with permission.)

Longitudinal tear PHMM with vertical morphology

Longitudinal tear PHMM

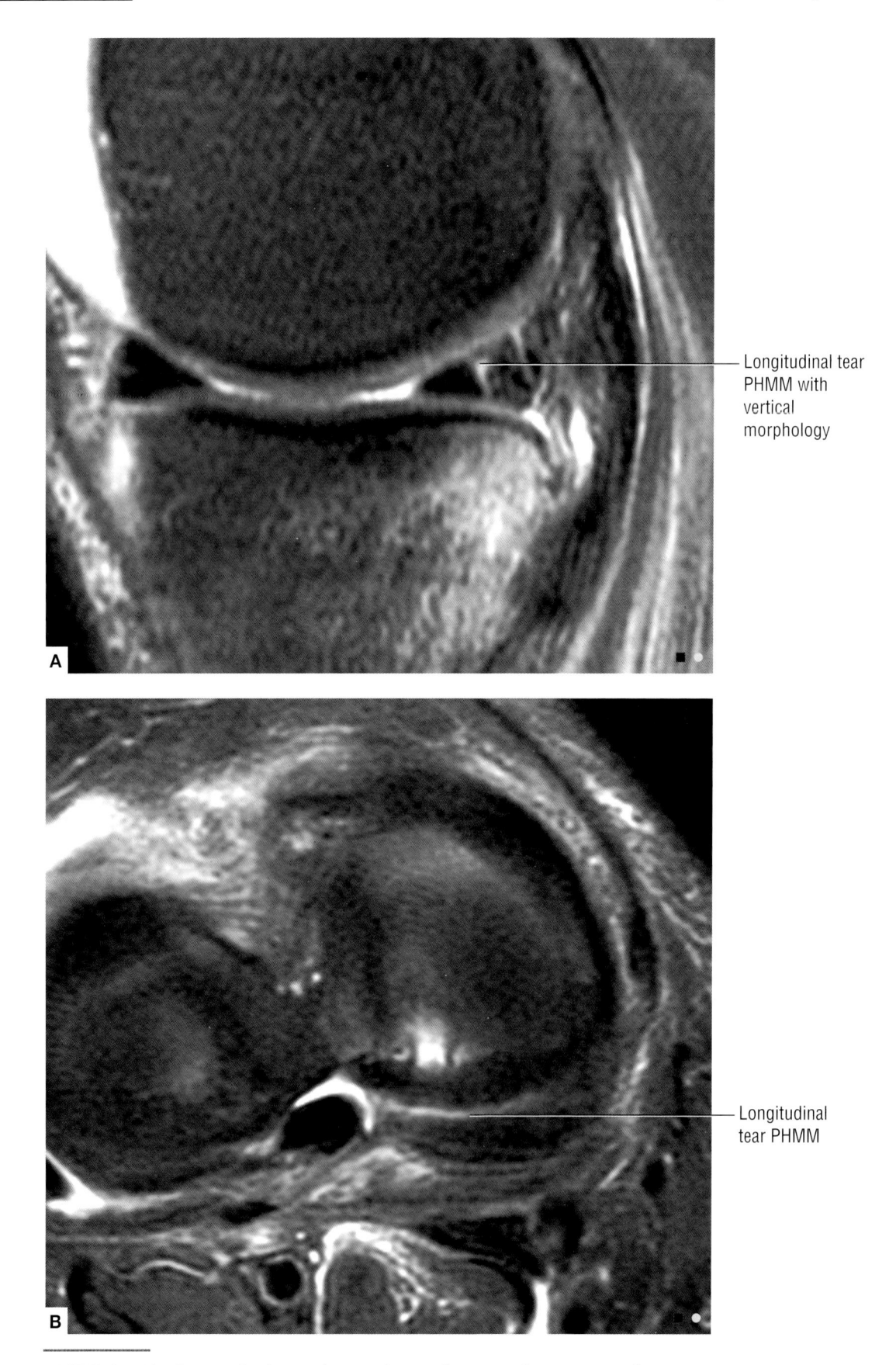

FIGURE 4.56 Longitudinal vertical tear with secondary vertical tear on sagittal section associated with an ACL-related medial tibial plateau contrecoup trabecular contusion. FS PD FSE sagittal (**A**) and axial (**B**) images. Posterior horn medial meniscus (PHMM)

Bucket-Handle Tears

- A displaced longitudinal tear of the meniscus (usually the medial meniscus)
    - The separated central fragment resembles the handle of a bucket.[468]
    - The remaining larger peripheral section of the meniscus is the bucket.
- An unstable meniscal fragment locks into the intercondylar notch and involves at least two thirds of the meniscal circumference.
- Common in young patients secondary to significant trauma[404]
- Frequently associated with ACL injury
- May originate from either primary vertical or horizontal longitudinal tear patterns
- Diagnosis of a bucket-handle tear requires identification of displaced meniscal tissue from posterior to a relative anterior coronal location.
    - If displaced meniscal tissue is restricted to posterior coronal images, consider a displaced flap tear pattern.
- Sagittal MR findings include:
    - Double delta sign
    - Double PCL sign
- Vertical longitudinal tears are further classified:
    - *Single vertical longitudinal tears*
    - *Displaced bucket-handle type tears*
    - *Broken bucket-handle tears*
    - *Double and triple vertical longitudinal bucket-handle tears*[62]
- **Medial Meniscus Bucket-Handle Tears**
    - The central fragment of a bucket-handle tear may be completely or partially displaced into the intercondylar notch.
    - May occur with a shorter tear of the posterior meniscus
    - Three times more frequent than bucket-handle tears involving the lateral meniscus

- A bucket-handle tear effectively reduces the width of the meniscus, and peripheral sagittal images fail to demonstrate the normal bowtie configuration of the body of the meniscus.
    - The remaining anterior and posterior horns are often hypoplastic or truncated.
- The posterior horn is wider and has greater height than the anterior horn in the normal medial meniscus (without tear).
- Foreshortening of the posterior horn of the medial meniscus without previous partial meniscectomy is associated with bucket-handle morphology.
- A displaced meniscal fragment can frequently be identified within the intercondylar notch on coronal images.[443]
- The displaced fragment of a bucket-handle tear is seen as a low-signal-intensity band parallel and anterior to the PCL on sagittal images.[516]
- Axial images show the relation of the displaced tear to the remaining meniscus in a single section.
- The *double PCL sign* refers to visualization of the displaced meniscal fragment anterior to the PCL in the intercondylar notch.[57]
- The *double delta sign*:
    - Refers to visualization of flipped inner meniscal fragments adjacent (posterior) to the anterior horn of the donor site
    - Produced by two triangular structures adjacent to each other anteriorly
- The free edge of the native anterior horn is deformed (blunted) at the anterior tear site of the bucket-handle tear.
    - The displaced meniscal tissue has a well-defined free edge and may be mistaken for the native anterior horn meniscus.
- In complex bucket-handle tears, displacement of an anteriorly based flap may widen the gap anterior to the bucket-handle fragment.
    - There is a lack of posterior horn notch fragments as commonly seen in lateral bucket-handle tears.
- A displaced posterior horn or body flap tear may mimic a bucket-handle tear on posterior coronal images.

- A true bucket-handle tear can be seen on multiple cross-sectional coronal images from posterior to anterior.
    - The presence of a third structure (separate from the ACL and PCL) within the intercondylar notch must be documented on more than a single posterior coronal image to fulfill the criteria of a bucket-handle tear.
- Bucket-handle tears in both the medial and lateral compartments are less common.
    - Four meniscal fragments can be seen in the coronal plane.
    - Three separate meniscal fragments can be seen anterior to the PCL on sagittal plane images when the anterior tear site of the bucket-handle tear and the displaced notch fragments are co-linear.

- Lateral Meniscus Bucket-Handle Tears
    - The body of the lateral meniscus is displaced into the intercondylar notch.[529]
    - There may be greater anterior displacement of posterior horn tissue than medial bucket-handle tears.
    - The native anterior horn fragments usually have a blunted free edge.
    - The more posteriorly located (relative to the anterior horn) flipped or displaced fragment may be mistaken for the normal anterior horn segment.
    - To avoid underdiagnosis, the proximity of a lateral meniscus fragment to the ACL should be carefully evaluated on both coronal and sagittal planes.
    - Patients may present with a locked knee or may lack full extension.
    - May also be associated with ACL injuries[404]
    - Single or multiple flaps of meniscal tissue may be generated.

- May start as a longitudinal tear with a primarily horizontal tear pattern
    - A displaced vertical component subsequently generates a bucket-handle morphology.
- Residual peripheral horizontal grade 3 signal intensity may persist after a partial meniscectomy performed to treat a bucket-handle tear.
- More commonly, bucket-handle tears are displaced vertical, longitudinal tears.
- Patients may present with pain as the displaced free edge of the meniscus subluxes between the femoral condyle and tibial plateau into the intercondylar notch.[209]
- Tenderness may be present at the anterior margin of the displaced or mobile meniscus, adjacent to Hoffa's fat pad, because the peripheral meniscal nerve fibers are under tension at the apex of the tear.
- The *posterior spring sign*:
    - Lack of full extension probably secondary to pain and muscle spasm
    - Usually disappears with examination under anesthesia
- Treatment for nonseparated symptomatic tears is a partial meniscectomy.
- Meniscal repair may be undertaken in some double bucket-handle tears.
- Excision of a displaced fragment of a bucket-handle tear is considered in the presence of:
    - A significant radial split tear in the displaced bucket-handle component
    - Meniscal rim size of 5mm or greater, placing the tear clearly in the avascular zone of the meniscus
    - A chronic tear with deformed (twisted) morphology[62]

Bucket-Handle Tear Medial Meniscus

FIGURE 4.57 Displaced fragment of a medial meniscus bucket-handle tear lodged within the intercondylar notch. The intercondylar notch fragments are identified anterior to the PCL.

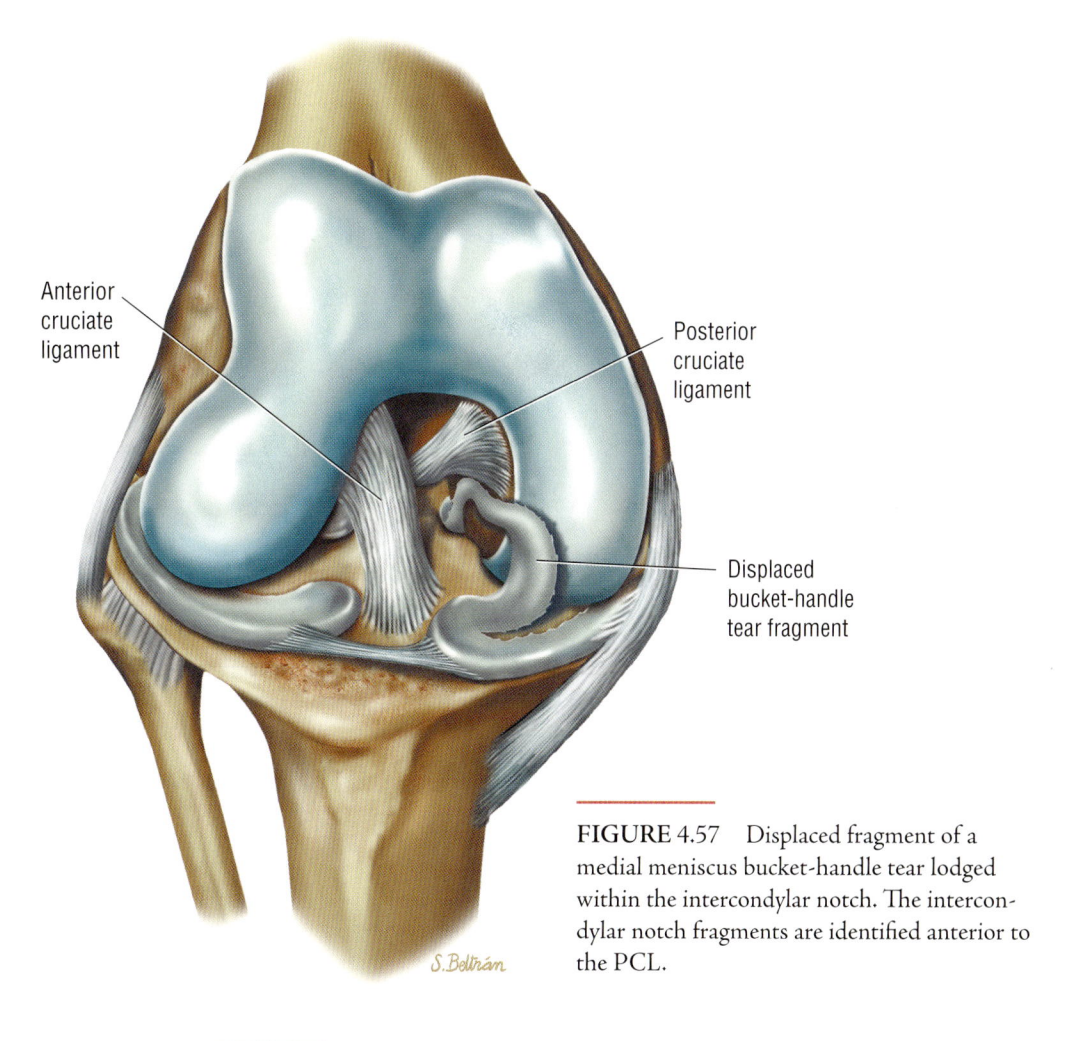

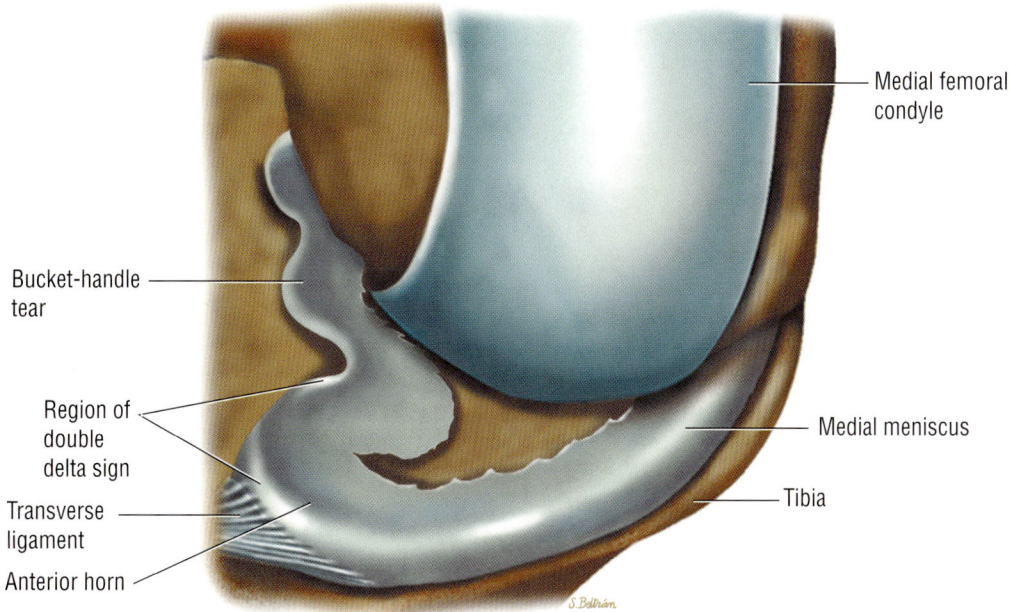

FIGURE 4.58 Bucket-handle tear with the peripheral meniscus shown as the source of the bucket-handle fragment. The anterior double delta sign is created by the location of the anterior portion of the displaced fragment adjacent (posterior) to the native anterior horn of the meniscus.

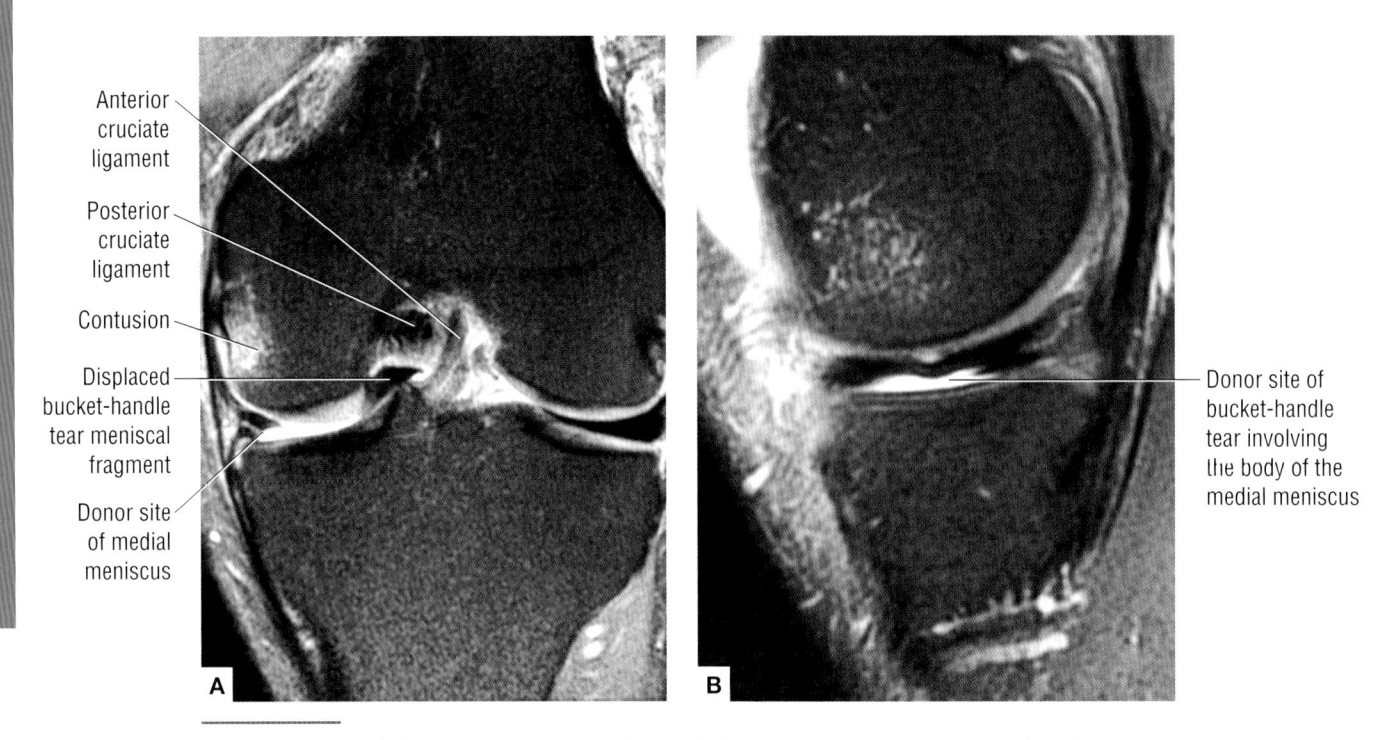

FIGURE 4.59 (**A**) Displaced intercondylar notch fragment representing an extra (in addition to the ACL and PCL) structure within the intercondylar notch. (**B**) Effectively reduced width of the body of the meniscus serving as the donor site for the bucket-handle fragment.

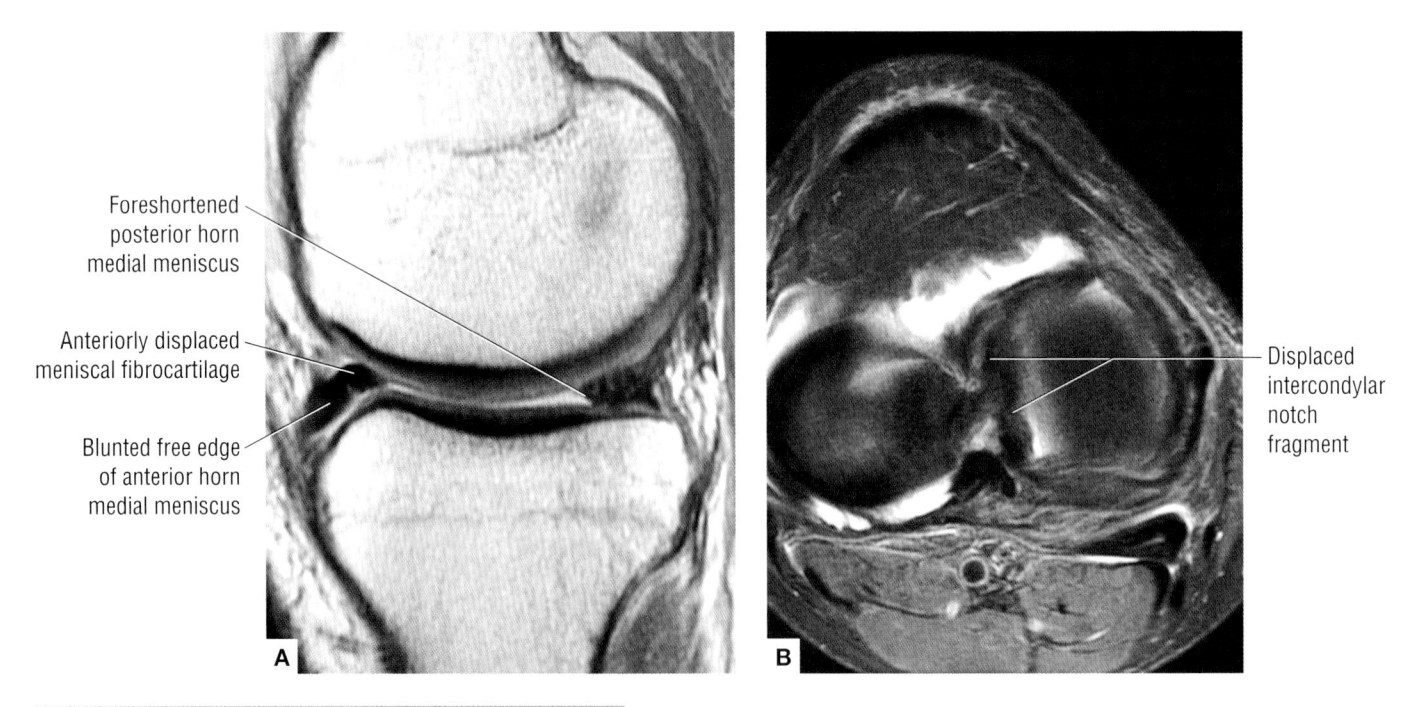

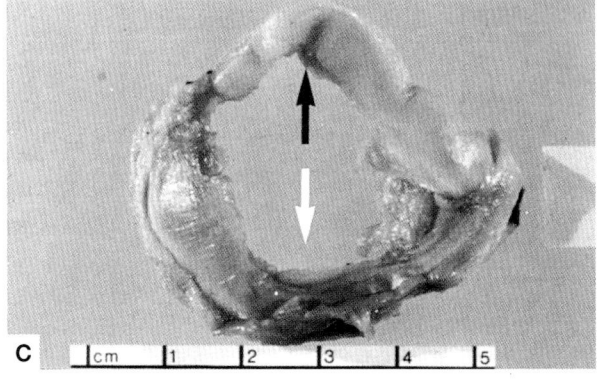

FIGURE 4.60 (**A**) Sagittal PD FSE image showing the anterior double delta sign of a medial meniscus bucket-handle tear. Note the foreshortened posterior horn on this sagittal image. (**B**) An axial FS PD FSE image of the bucket-handle tear. (**C**) A gross specimen demonstrates a displaced longitudinal bucket-handle tear (*black arrows*) from the medial meniscus (*white arrow*).

Bucket-Handle Tear Medial Meniscus

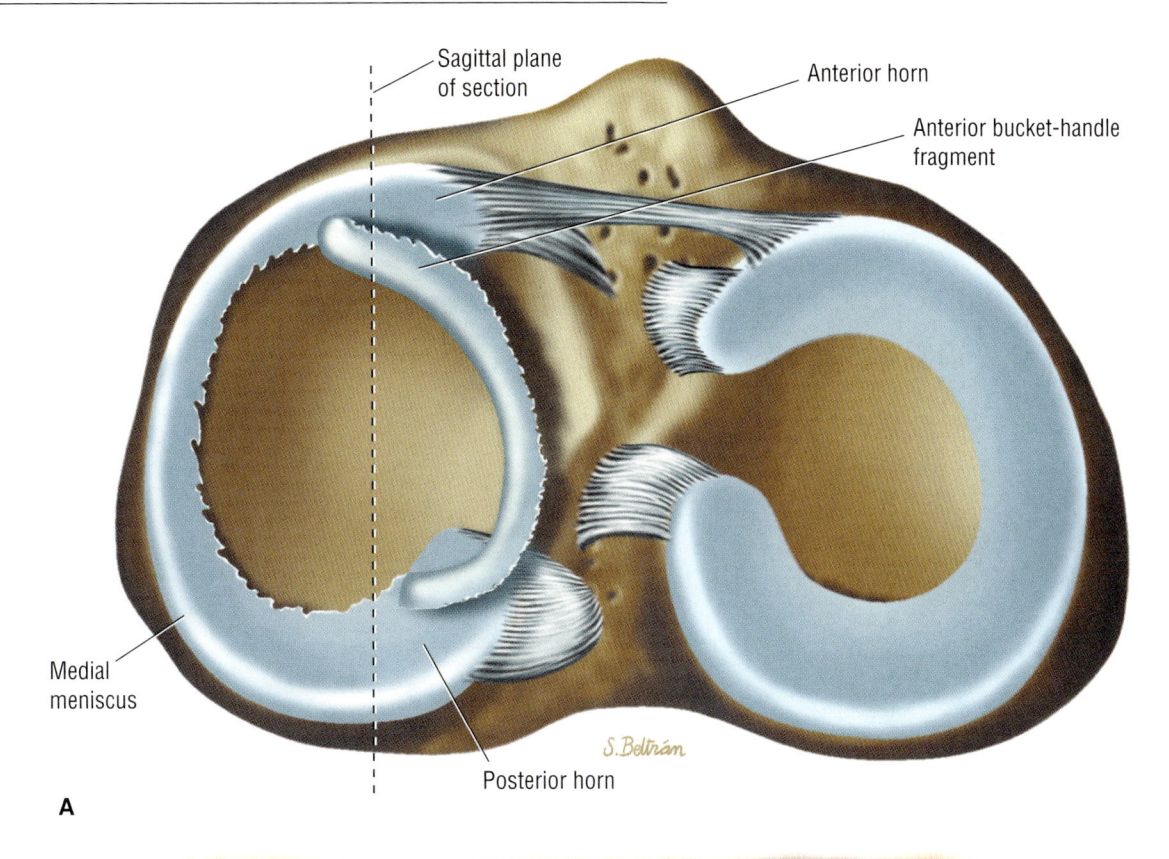

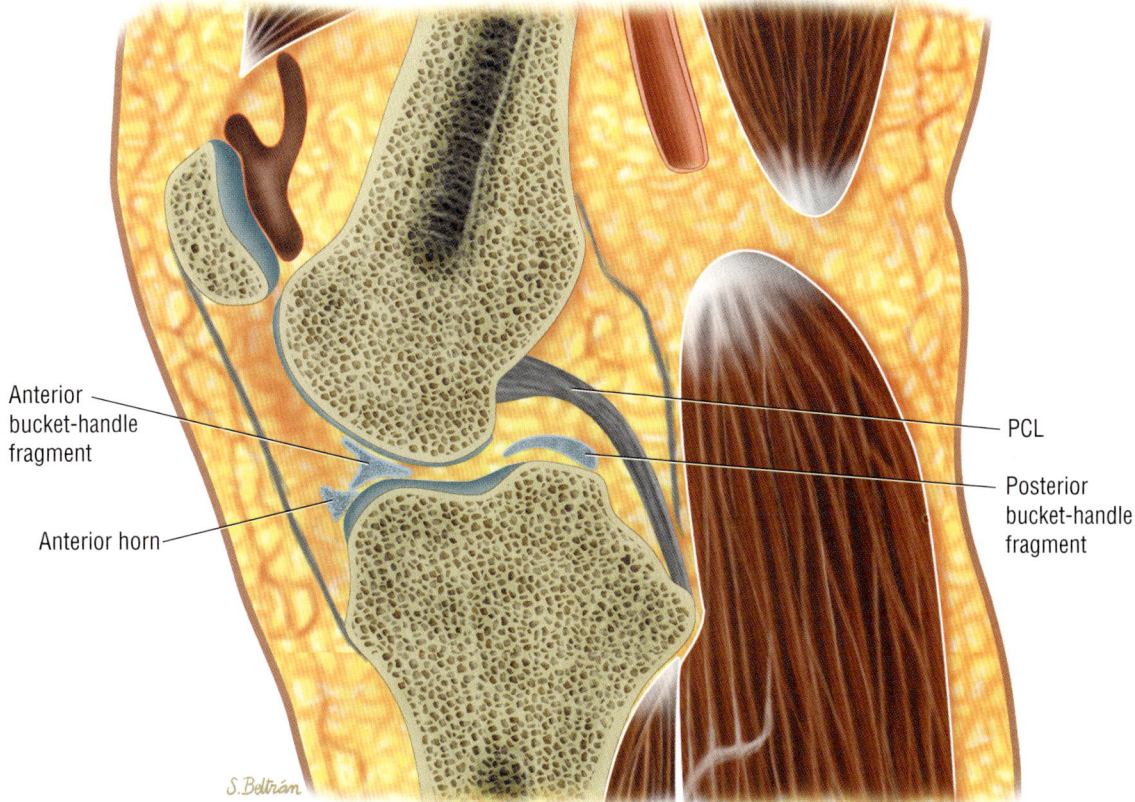

FIGURE 4.61 Double delta and double PCL signs. (**A**) Axial perspective color illustration showing the displaced fragment in proximity and posterior to the anterior horn segment. The central portion of the bucket fragment is responsible for the double PCL sign. (**B**) Corresponding sagittal section with double delta and double PCL fragments. (*Continued*)

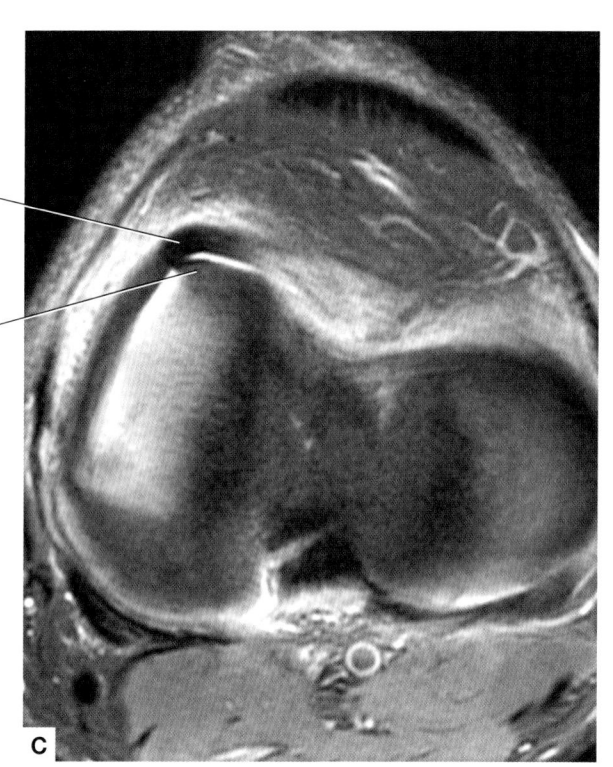

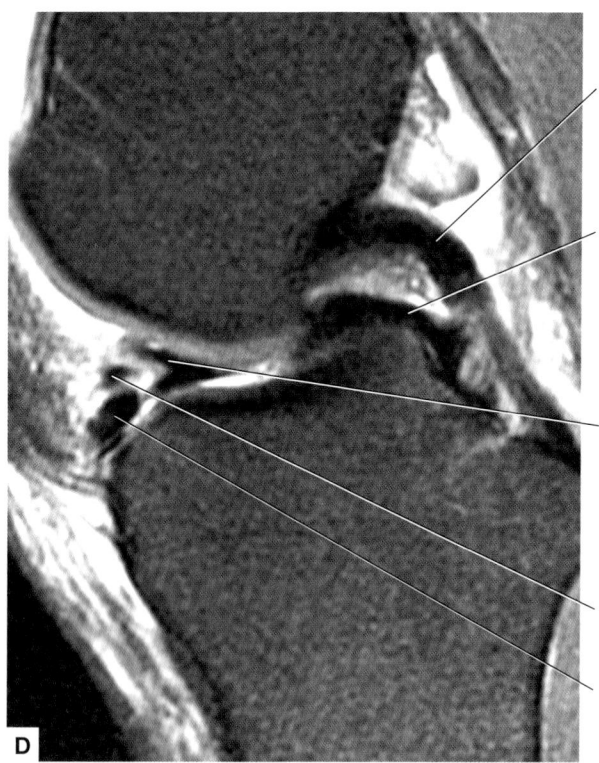

FIGURE 4.61 *(Continued)* **(C)** Effectively reduced width of the body of the meniscus serving as the donor site for the bucket-handle fragment. Native anterior horn of the medial meniscus is characteristically anterior to the displaced notch fragment on direct axial image. **(D)** Double PCL, double delta, and transverse ligament all on one single sagittal image.

The Meniscus 221

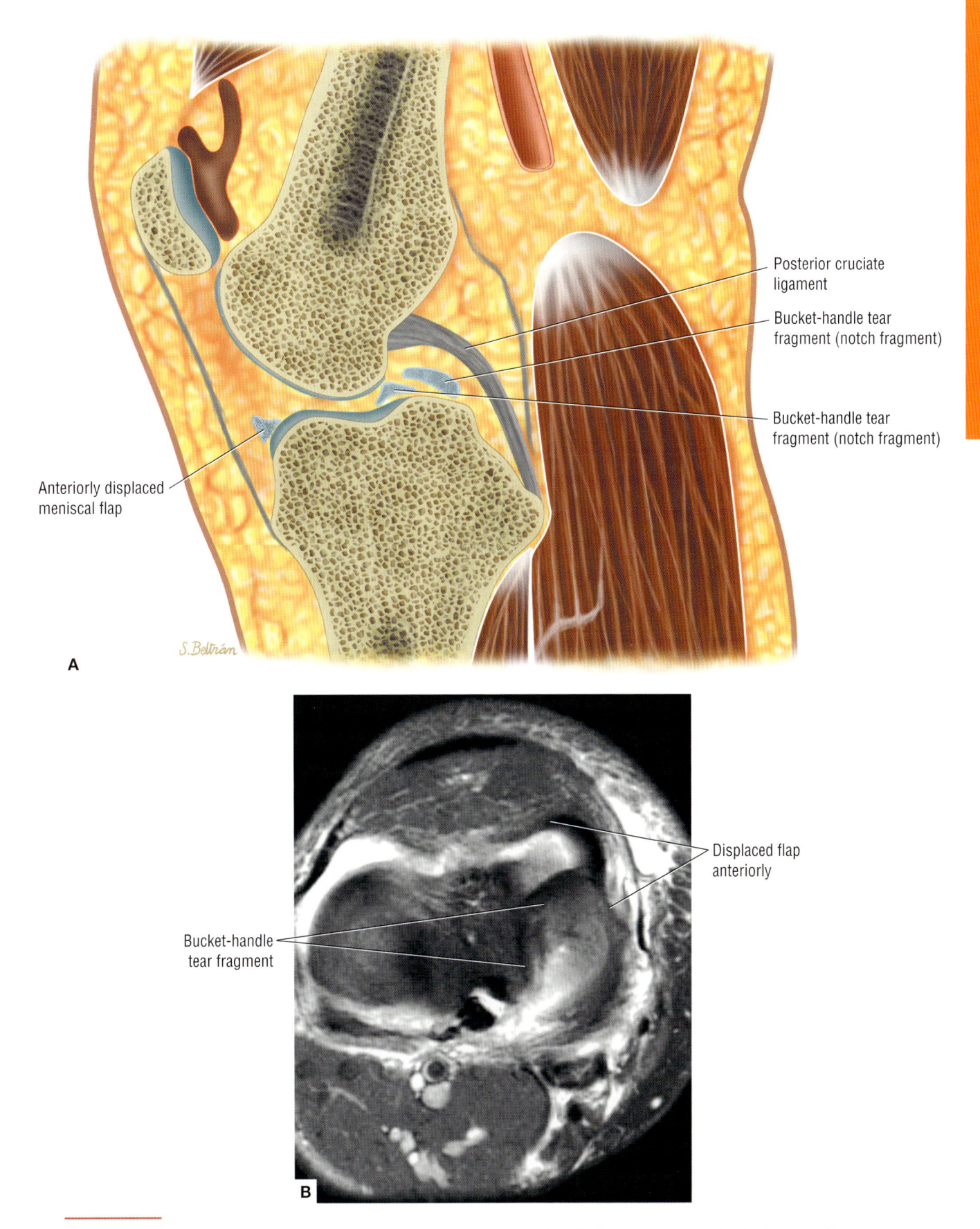

FIGURE 4.62 (**A**) Increased gap between anterior horn and bucket-handle fragments in complex bucket-handle tear. (**B–D**) Complex medial bucket-handle tear with three separate displaced meniscal fragments anterior to the posterior horn (**D**) (**B**, axial FS PD FSE; **C**, sagittal FS PD FSE; **D**, sagittal FS PD FSE). **D** is medial or peripheral to **C**. (*Continued*)

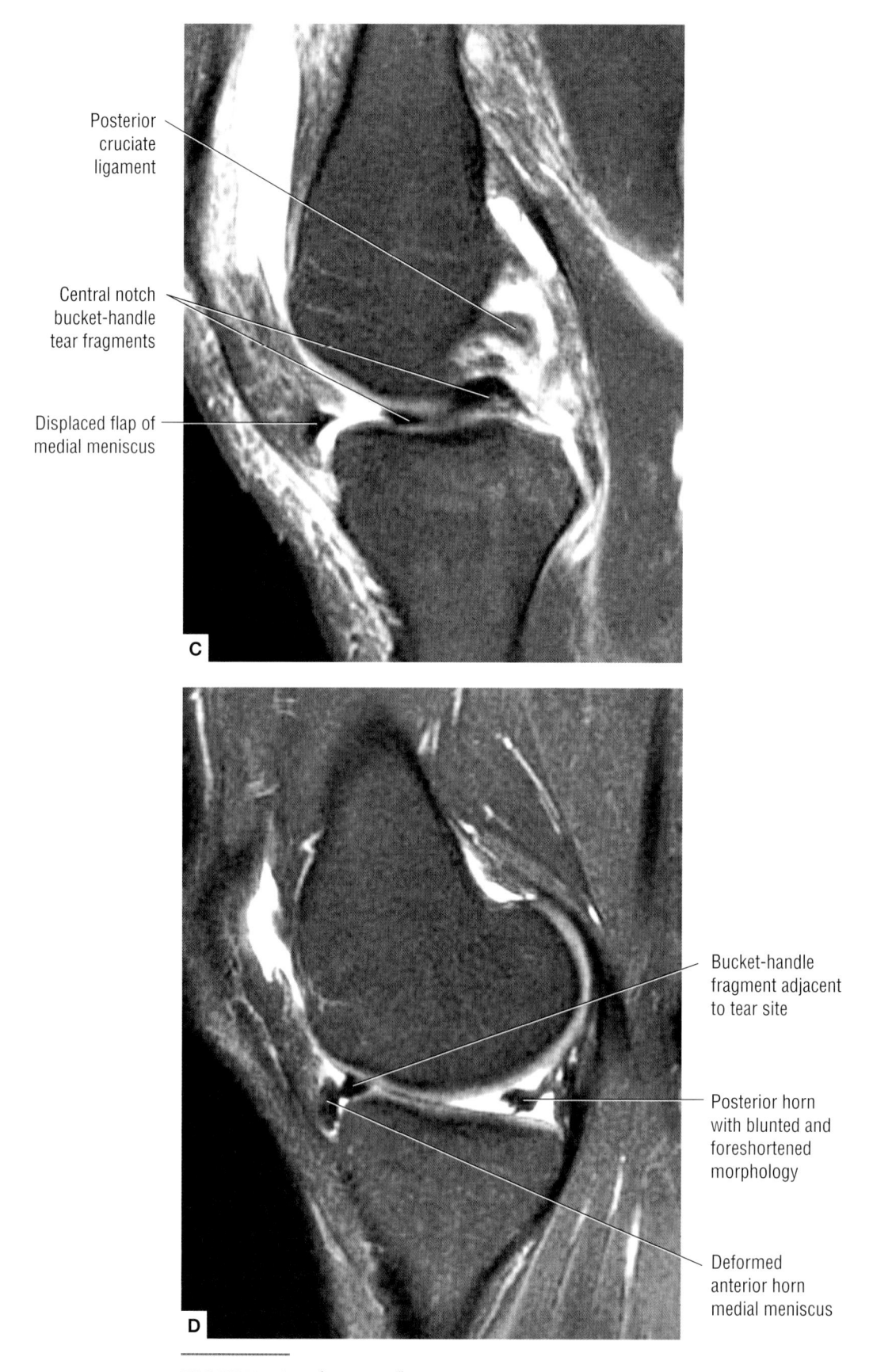

FIGURE 4.62 *(Continued)*

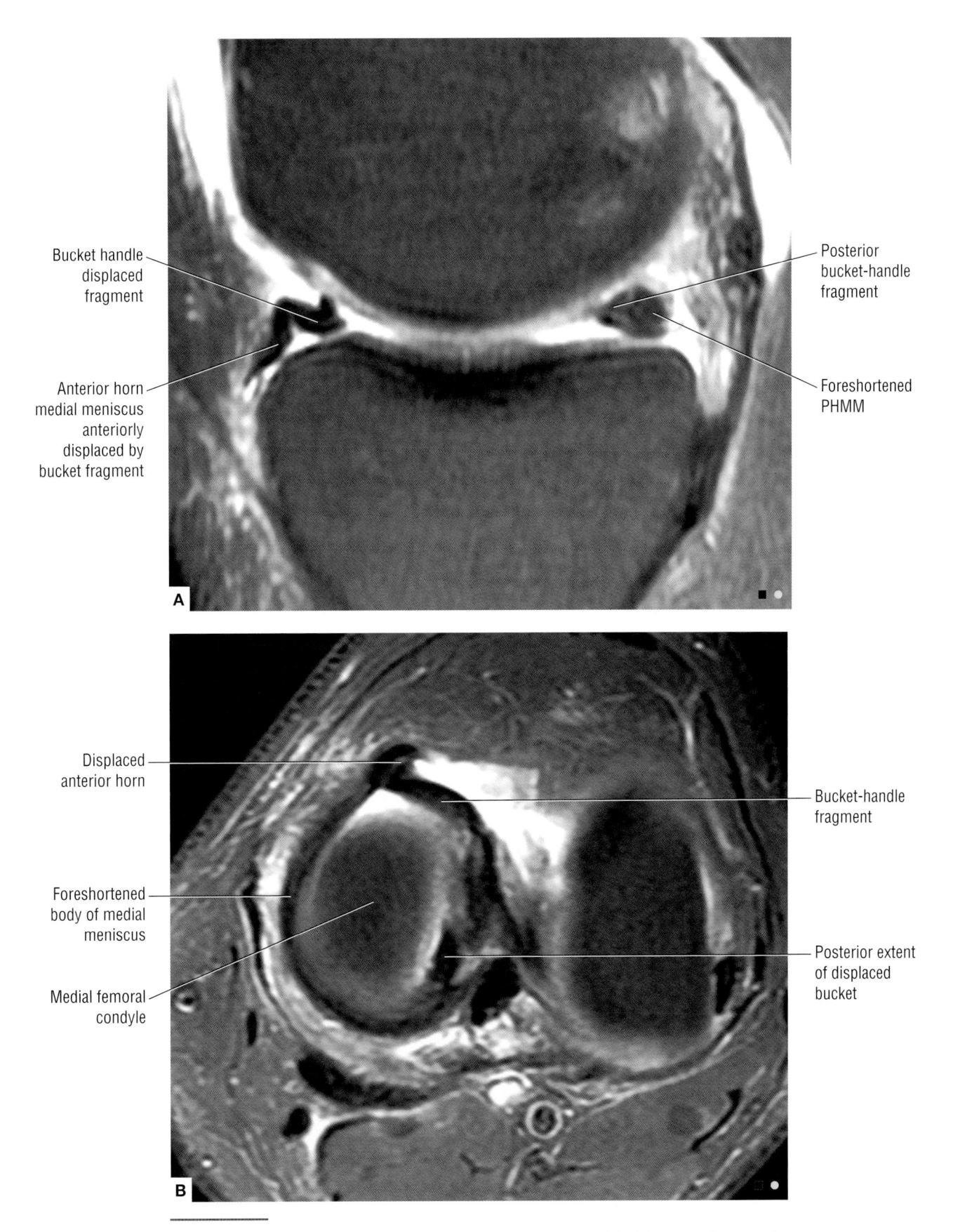

FIGURE 4.63 Bucket-handle tear medial meniscus with double delta sign of anteriorly displaced bucket fragment and foreshortened posterior horn. The central notch fragment is seen in the axial plane. FS PD FSE sagittal (**A**) and axial (**B**) images.

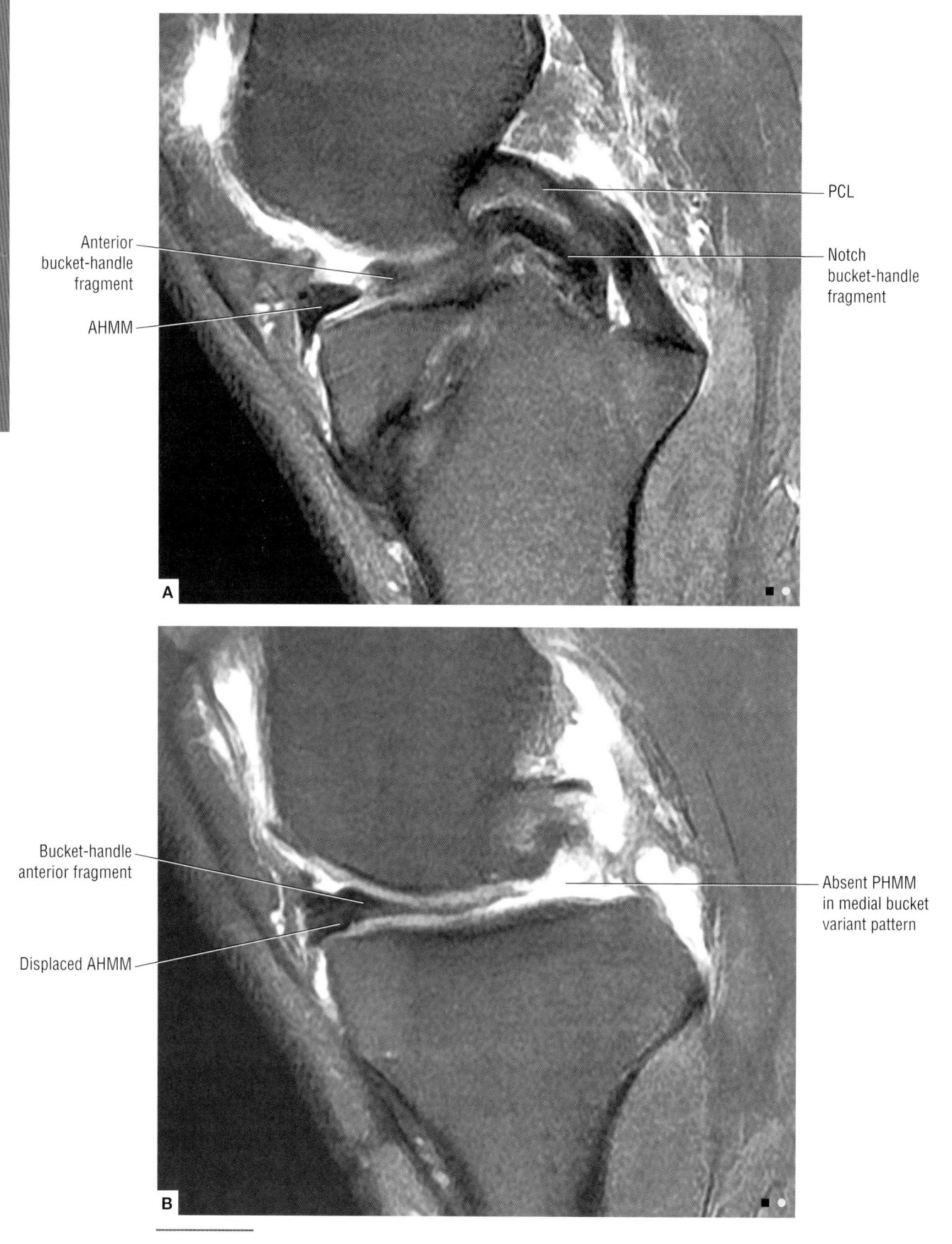

FIGURE 4.64 Double PCL sign from posterior components of displaced notch fragment anterior to the PCL. The posterior horn is absent in this complex bucket-handle variant. (**A**) FS PD FSE sagittal image. (**B**) FS PD FSE sagittal image.

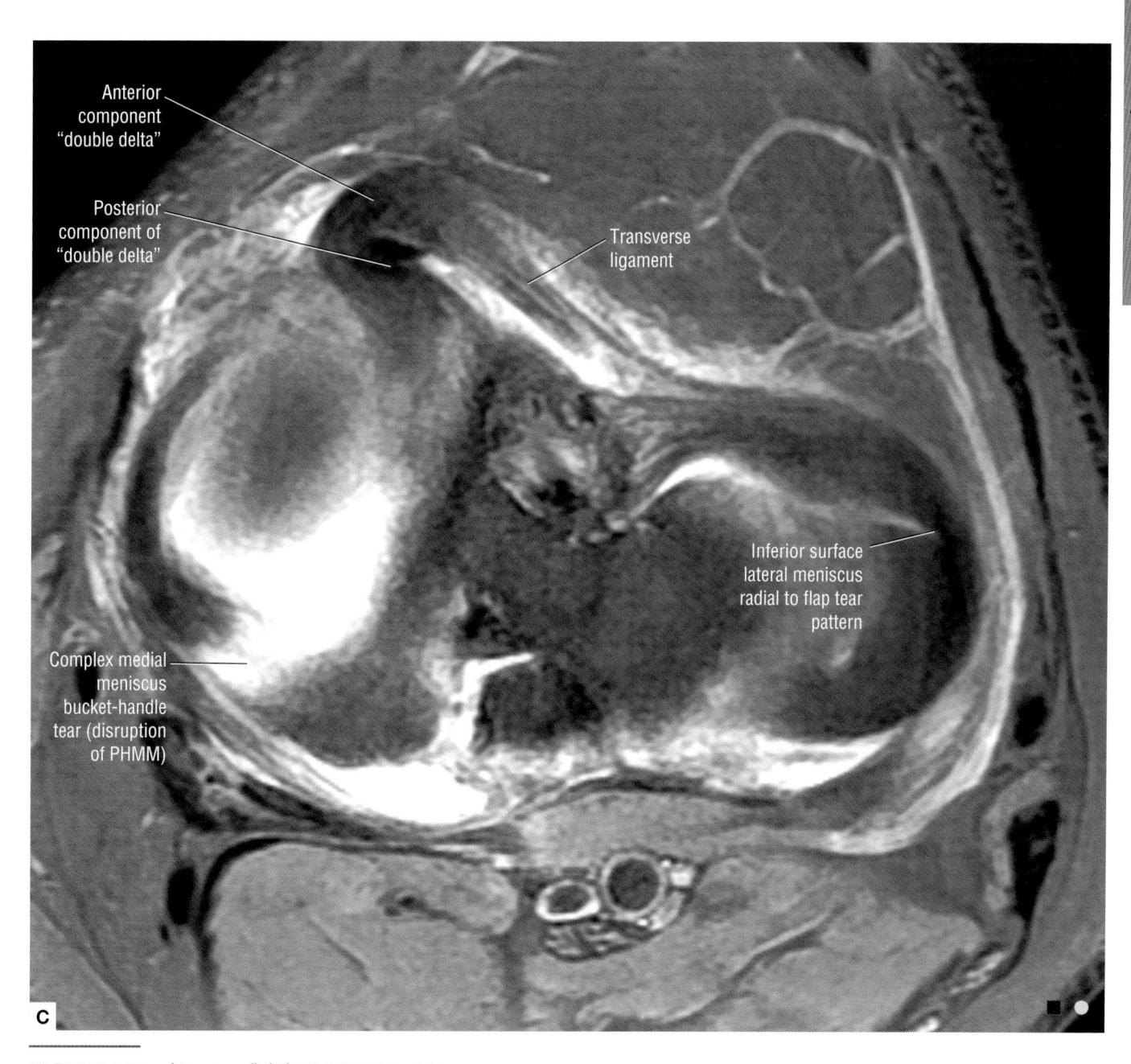

FIGURE 4.64 *(Continued)* (**C**) FS PD FSE axial image.

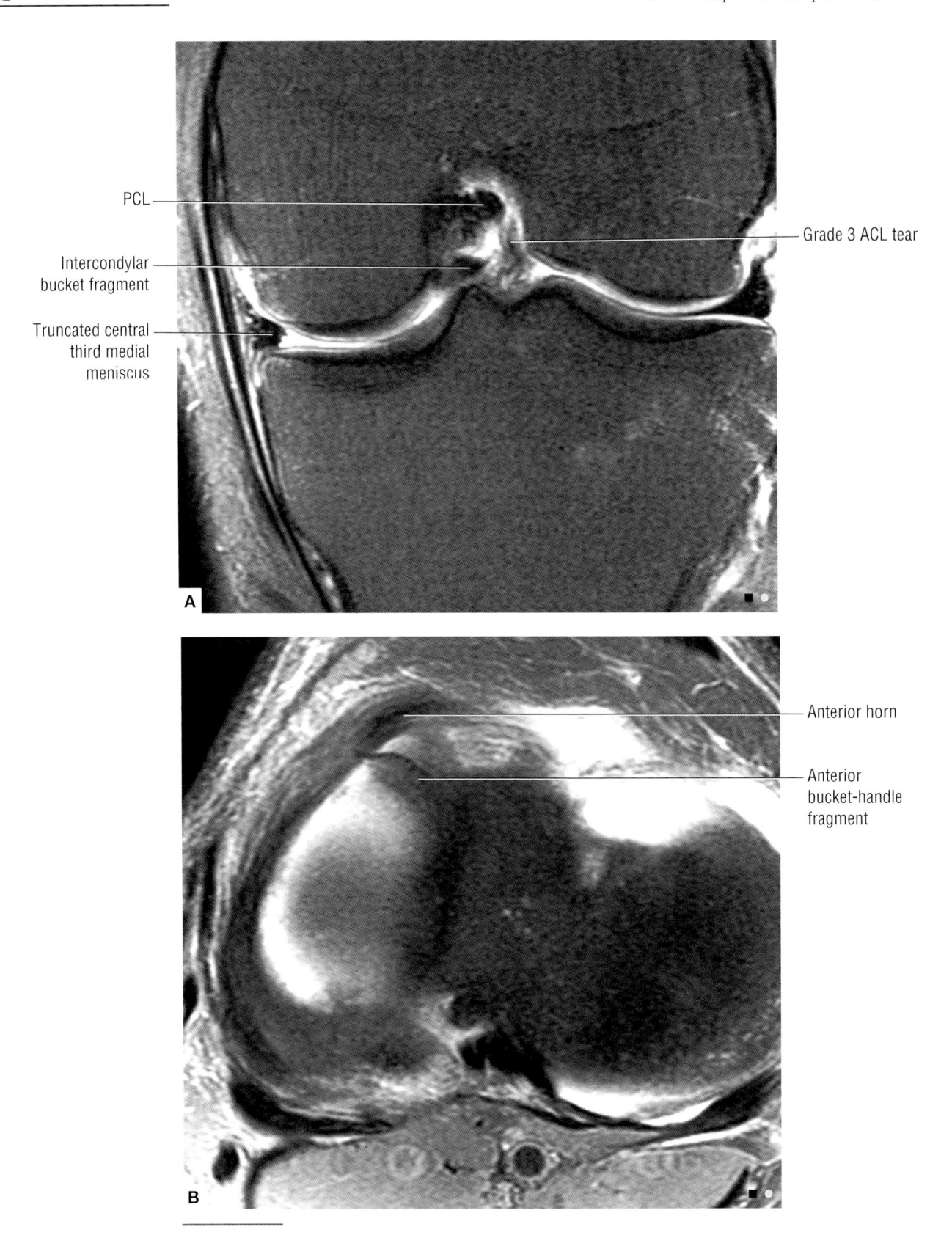

FIGURE 4.65 Bucket-handle tear of the medial meniscus associated with a grade 3 ACL tear. Note the body or central third of the meniscus is truncated on coronal image. The native anterior horn is usually more deformed than the displaced bucket fragment component of the double delta. FS PD FSE coronal (**A**), axial (**B**), and sagittal (**C**) images.

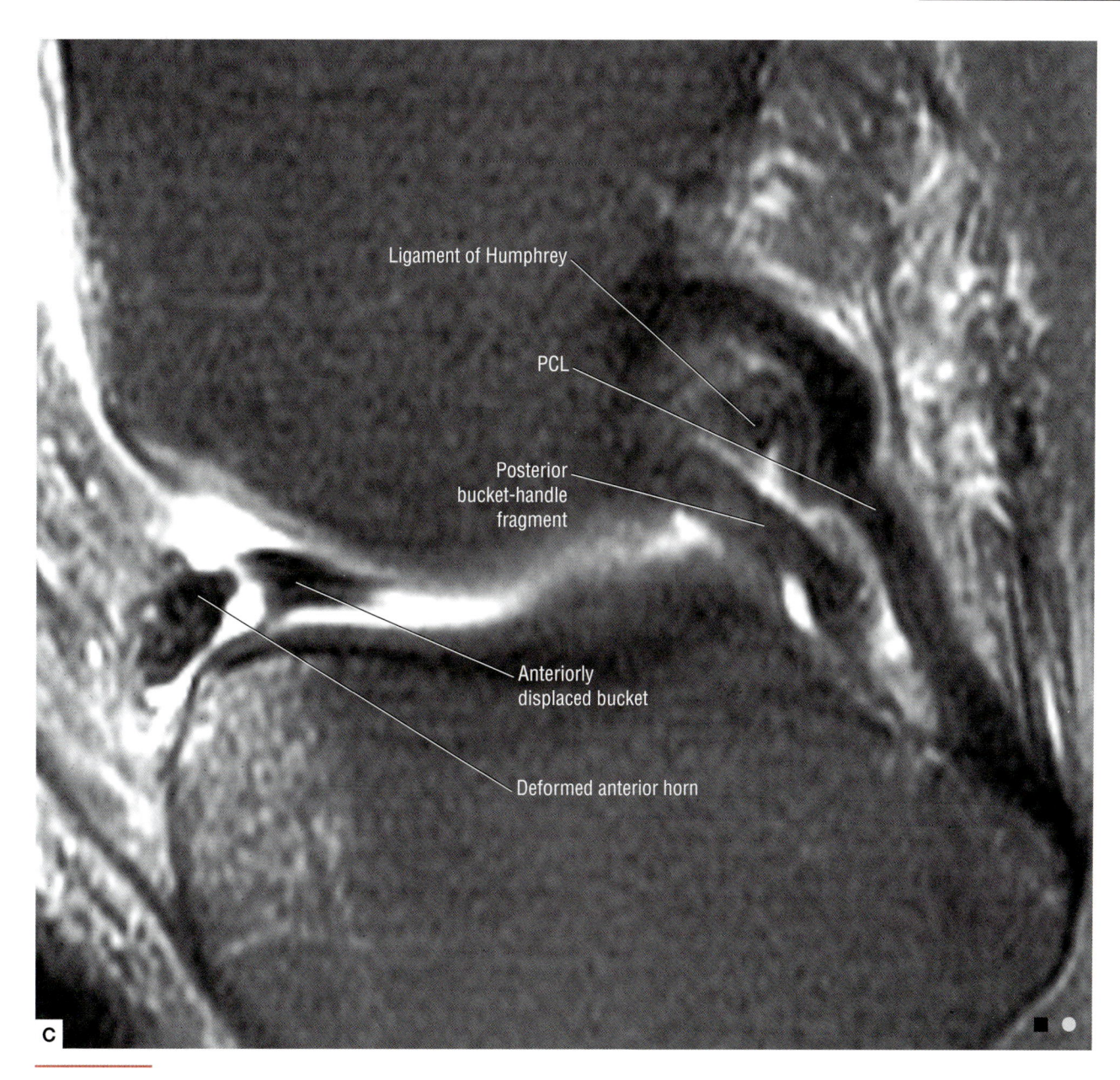

FIGURE 4.65 *(Continued)*

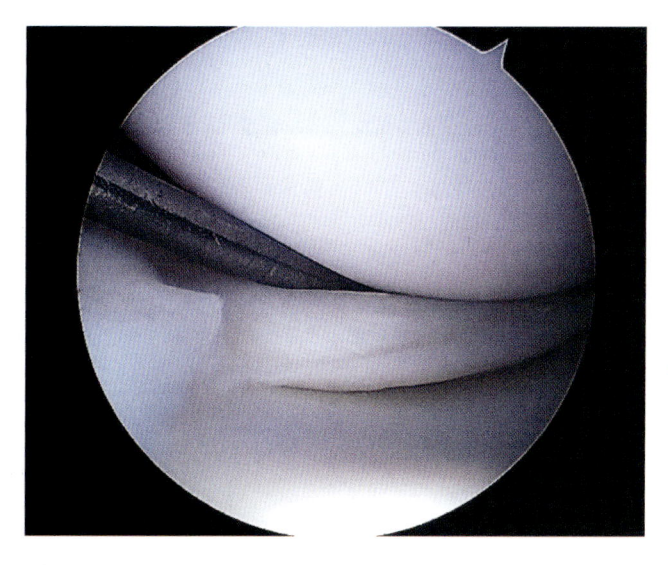

FIGURE 4.66 Unstable longitudinal medial meniscus tear originating near the attachment of the medial collateral ligament. (Reprinted from Fu FH. *Master Techniques in Orthopaedic Surgery: Sports Medicine*. Philadelphia, PA: Lippincott Williams & Wilkins; 2010, with permission.)

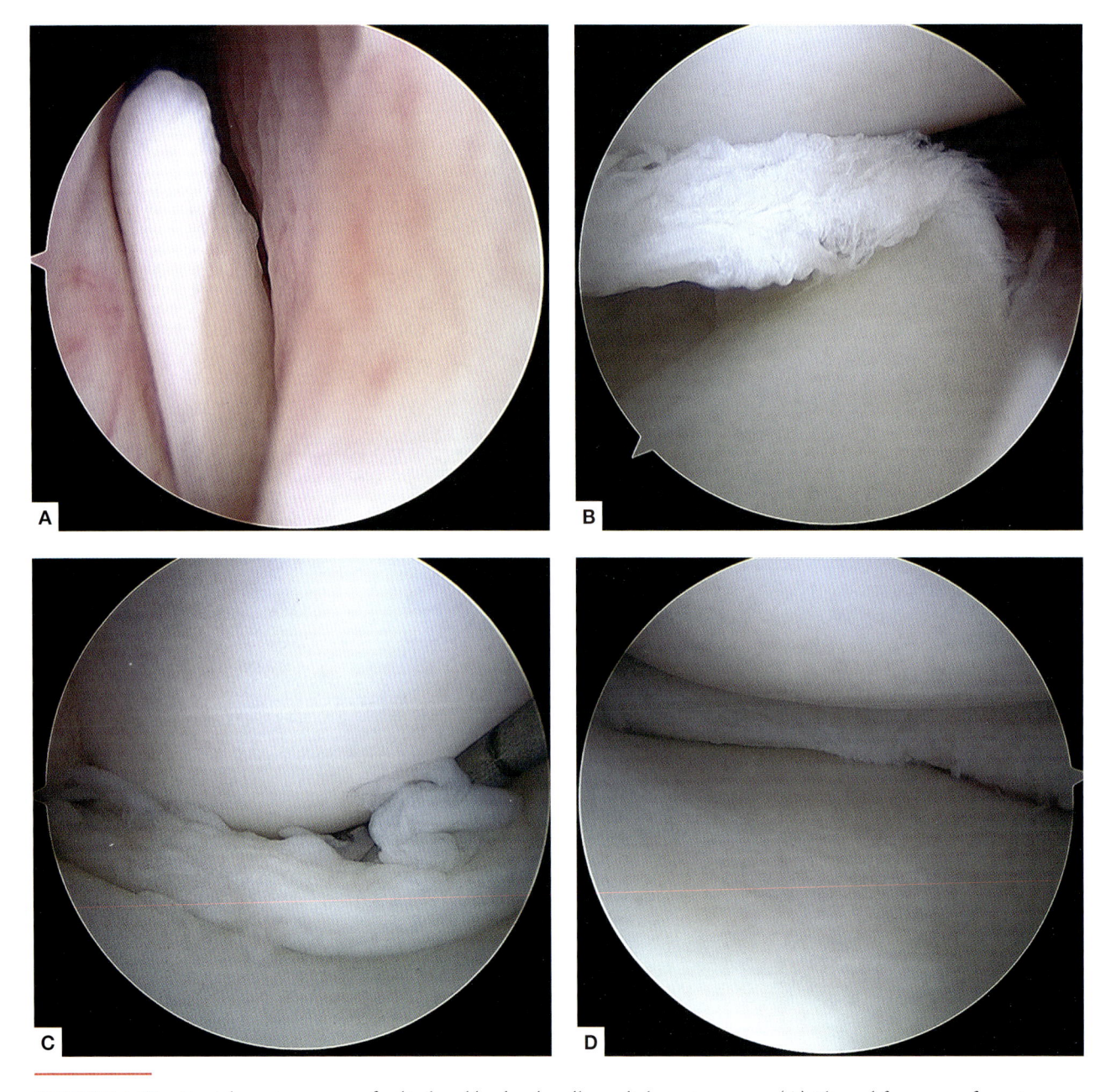

FIGURE 4.67 Partial meniscectomy of a displaced bucket-handle medial meniscus tear. (**A**) Flipped fragment of meniscus in the medial gutter. (**B**) Meniscal flap brought into medial joint. (**C**) Posterior aspect of the complex tear. (**D**) Post partial meniscectomy. (Reprinted from Fu FH. *Master Techniques in Orthopaedic Surgery: Sports Medicine*. Philadelphia, PA: Lippincott Williams & Wilkins; 2010, with permission.)

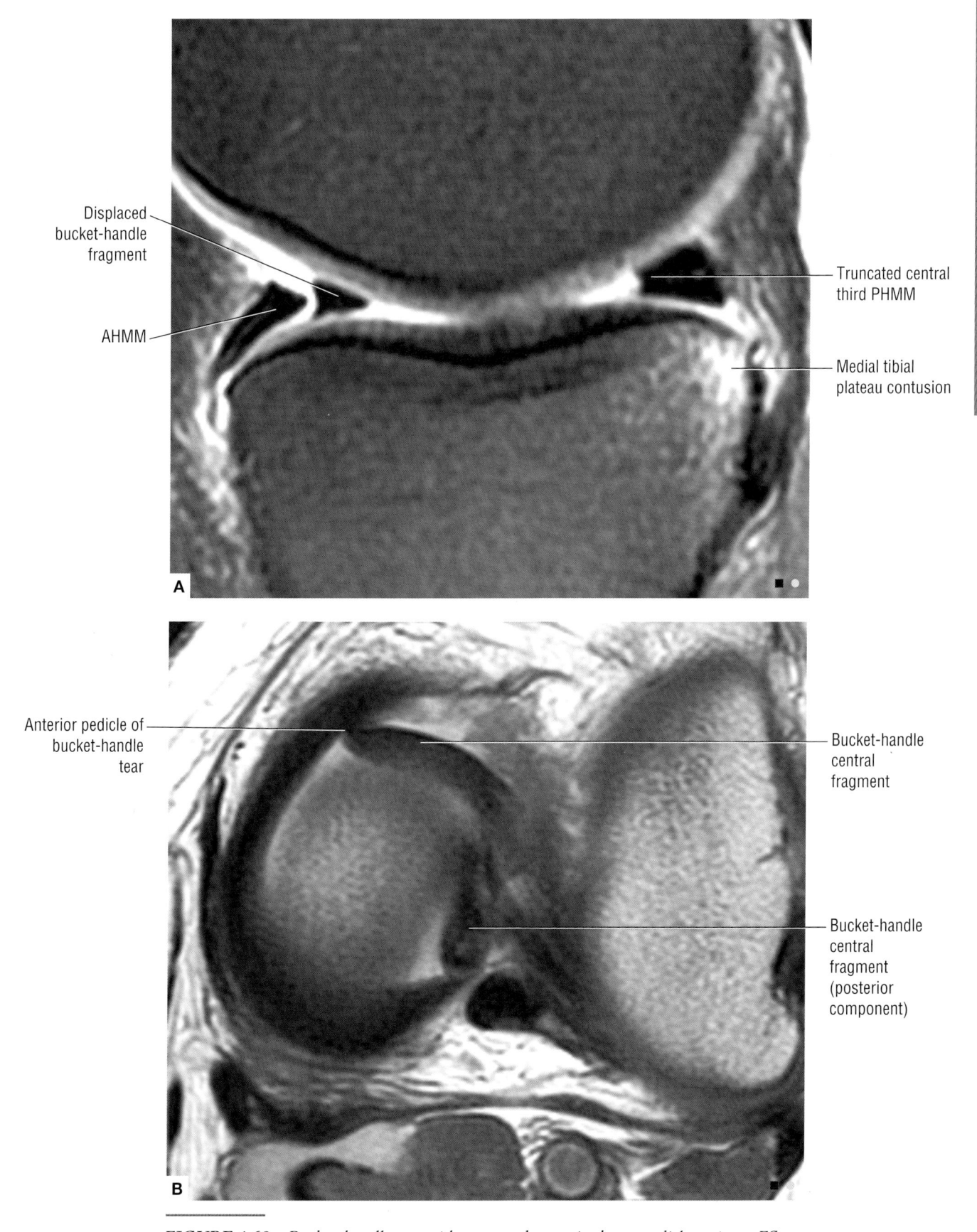

FIGURE 4.68 Bucket-handle tear with truncated posterior horn medial meniscus. FS PD FSE sagittal (**A**) and axial (**B**) images.

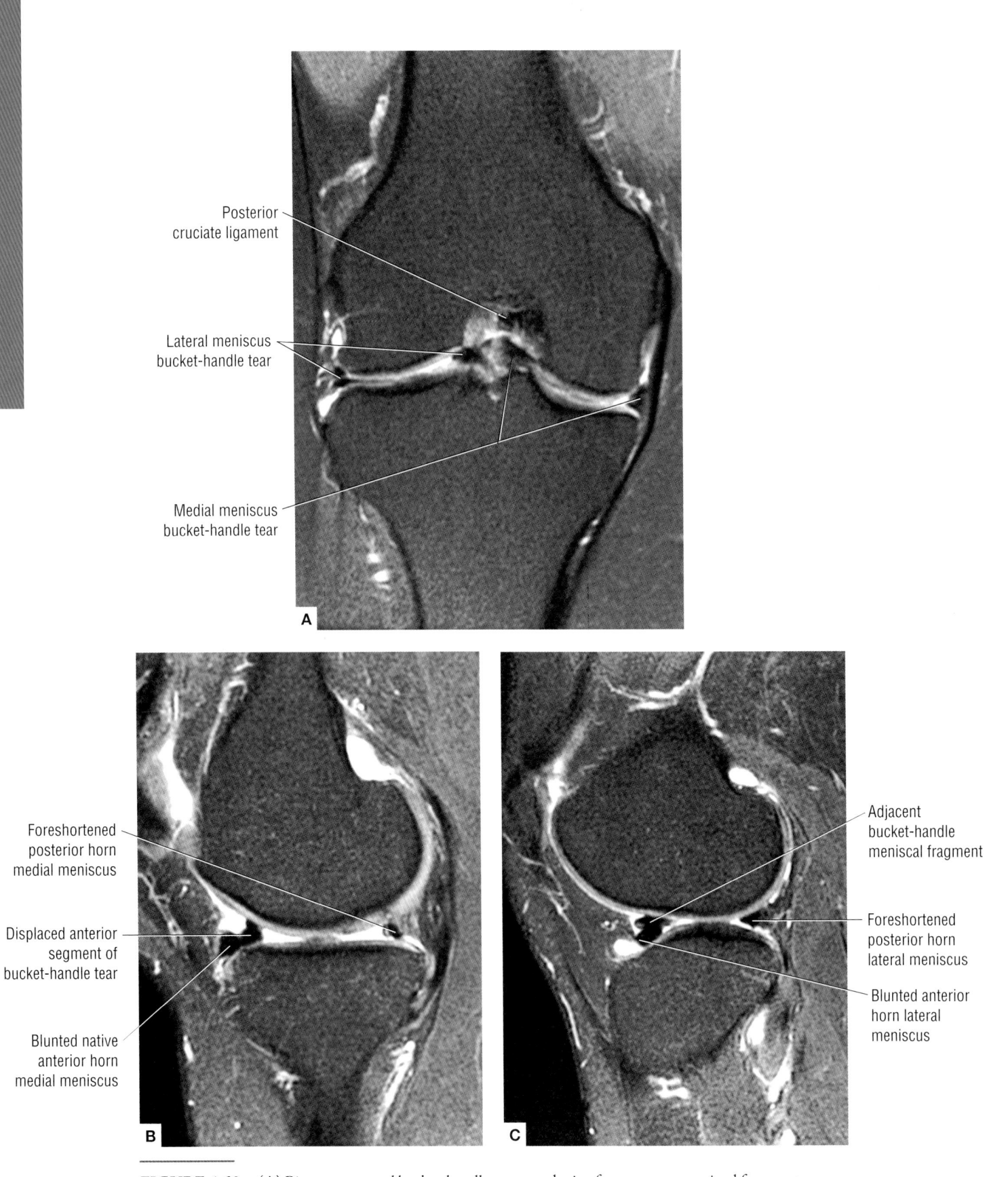

FIGURE 4.69 (**A**) Bicompartmental bucket-handle tears producing four separate meniscal fragments on coronal image. Characteristic double delta sign is demonstrated on corresponding medial (**B**) and lateral (**C**) compartment sagittal images.

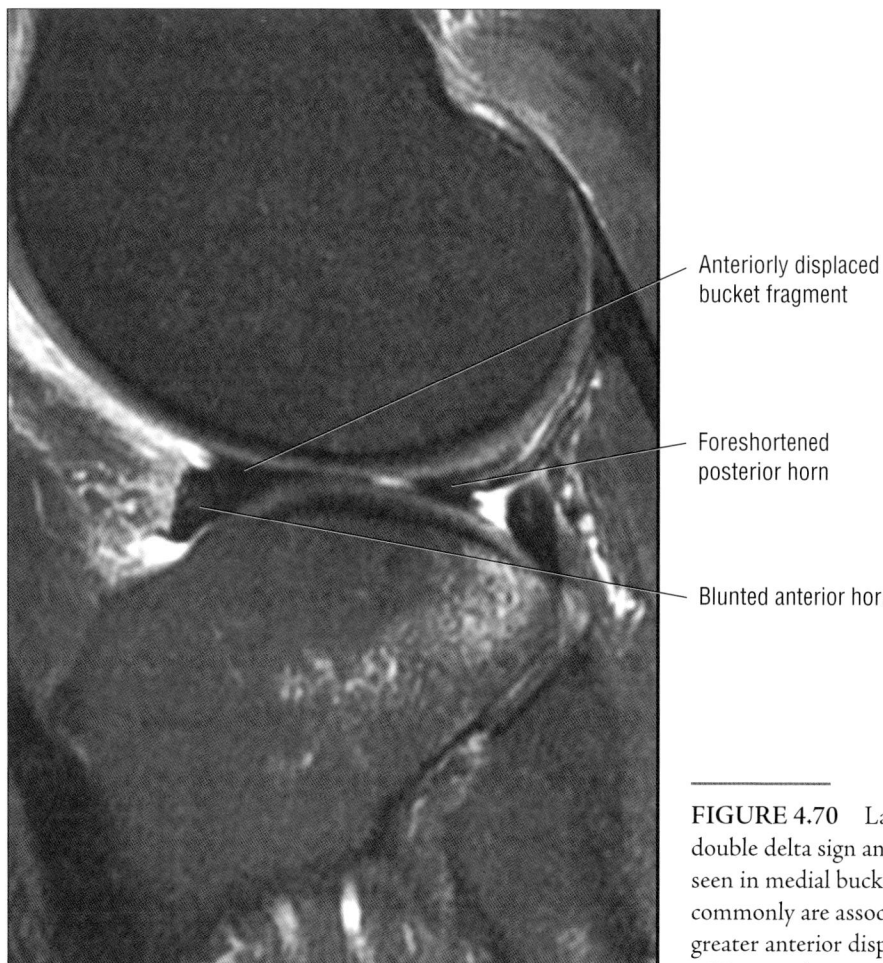

The Meniscus

FIGURE 4.70 Lateral bucket-handle tear demonstrating the same double delta sign and foreshortened posterior horn as commonly seen in medial bucket-handle tears. Lateral bucket-handle tears more commonly are associated with an absent posterior horn as there is greater anterior displacement of the posterior horn complex. FS PD FSE sagittal image.

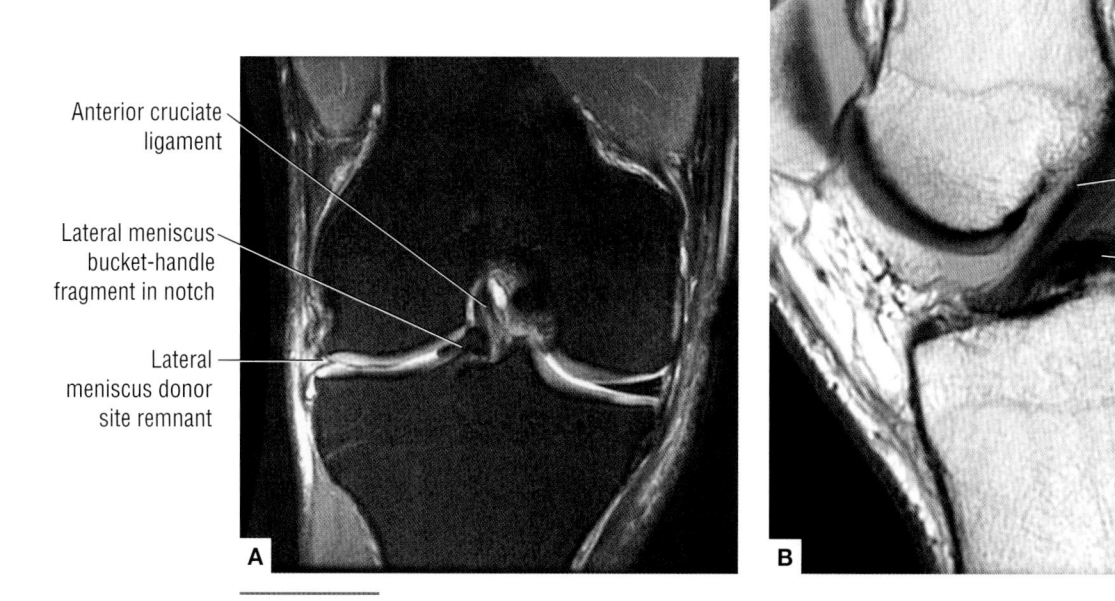

FIGURE 4.71 Coronal FS PD FSE (**A**) and sagittal PD FSE (**B**) images of a lateral bucket-handle tear fragment displacing the ACL from lateral to medial.

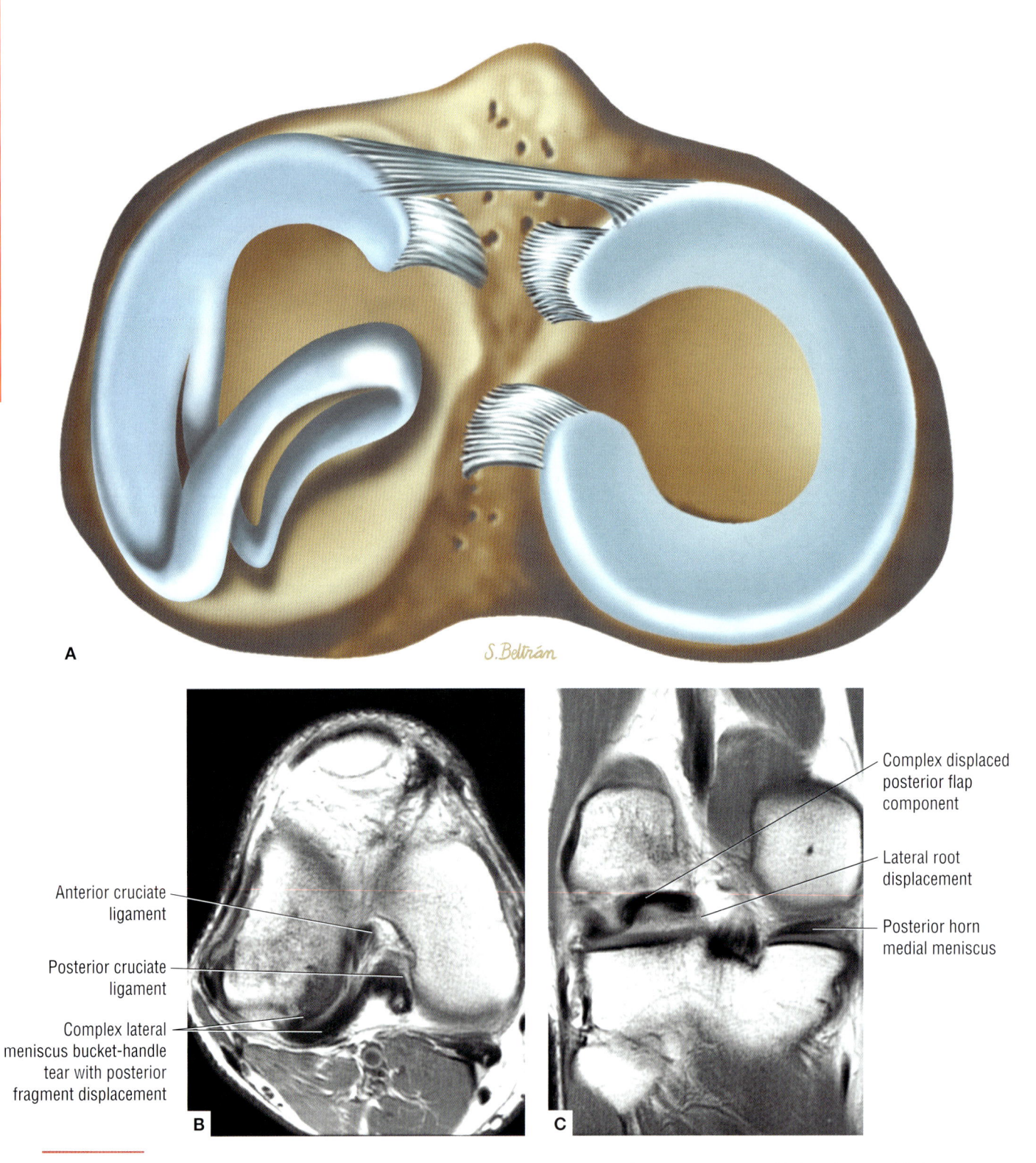

FIGURE 4.72 (**A**) Complex bucket-handle tear with greater posterior horn body involvement. Axial (**B**) and coronal (**C**) PD FSE images show a complex lateral bucket-handle tear with a posterior notch fragment displacement producing redundant folding of the meniscus.

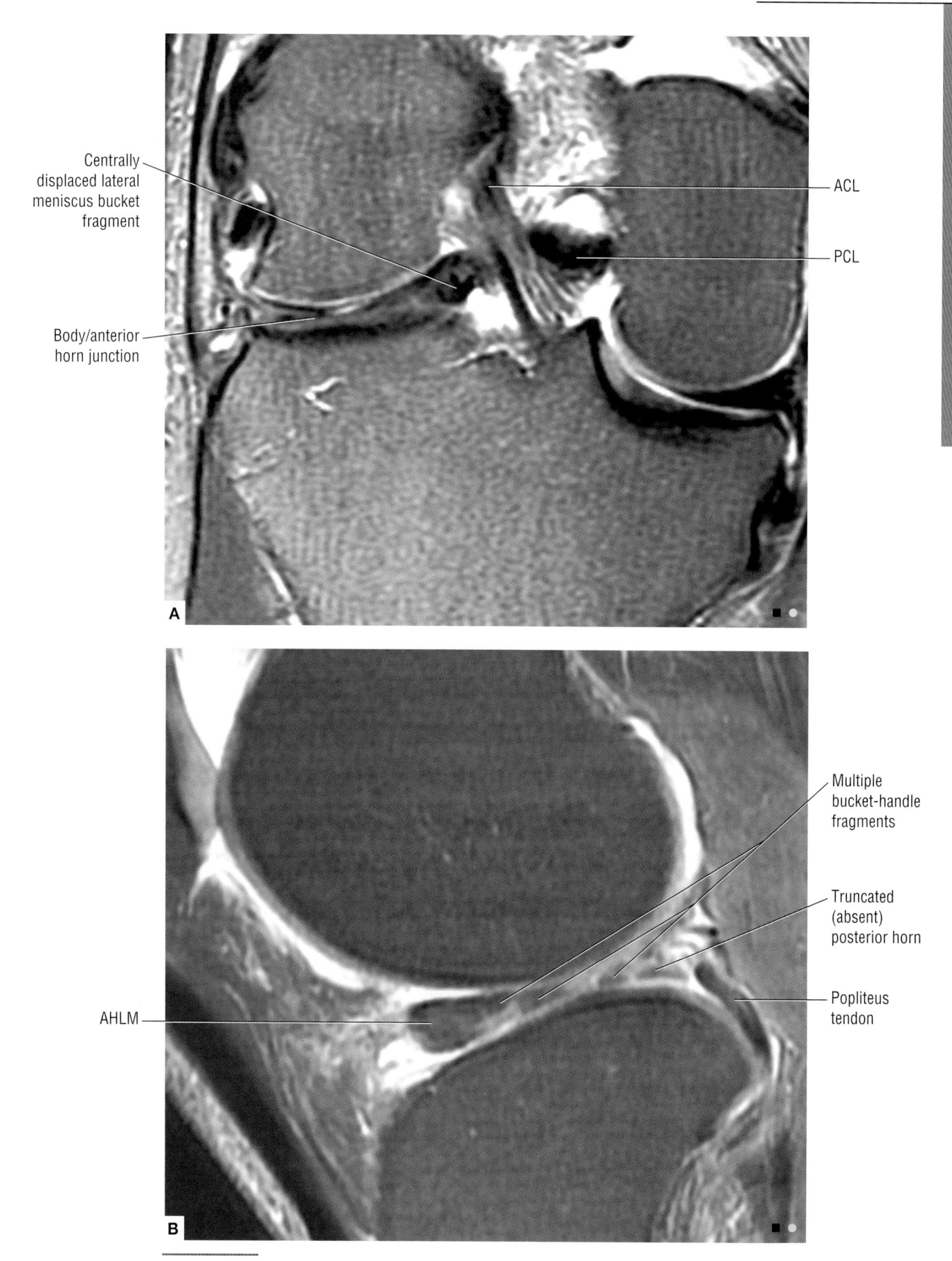

FIGURE 4.73 Characteristic lateral bucket-handle tear with displaced body posterior horn resulting in a truncated or absent posterior horn of the lateral meniscus. FS PD FSE coronal (**A**) and sagittal (**B**) images.

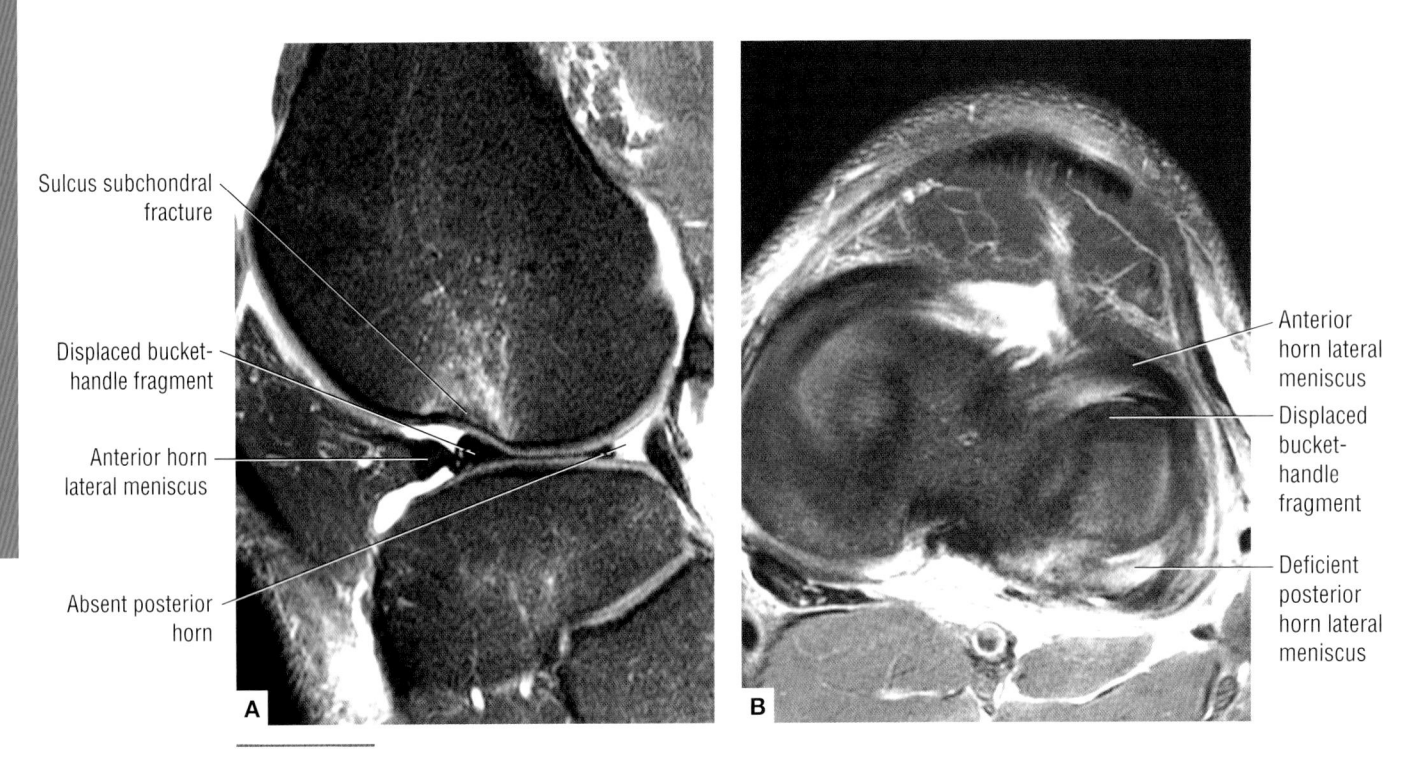

FIGURE 4.74 (**A**) Sagittal FS PD FSE image showing a typical anterior flap lateral meniscus fragment displaced posterior to the native anterior horn. Contusion and deformity of the sulcus resulted from an associated ACL tear. (**B**) Axial FS PD FSE image displaying anterior displacement of a large posterior body fragment in a characteristic lateral meniscus bucket-handle pattern.

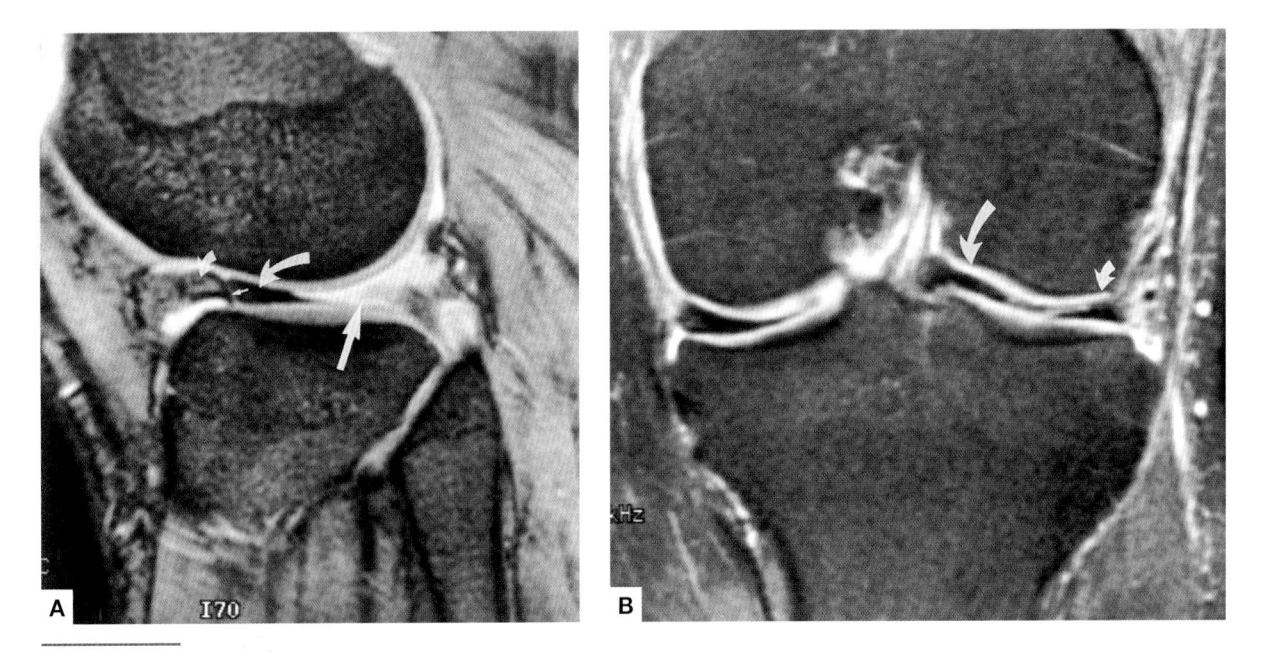

FIGURE 4.75 Bucket-handle tear of the lateral meniscus. (**A**) Sagittal T2*-weighted and (**B**) FS PD-weighted FSE coronal images show an anteriorly displaced posterior horn of the lateral meniscus (*large curved arrow*). Note the absence of meniscal tissue in the expected location (the posterior horn of the lateral meniscus) (*large straight arrow*). This deformity, with blunting of the apex (*small straight arrow*) of the anterior horn segment (*small curved arrow*), is commonly seen as a result of compression by the displaced posterior horn.

The Meniscus

Native anterior horn lateral meniscus

Anteriorly displaced bucket fragment

Foreshortened posterior horn lateral meniscus

Anterior displacement of AHLM

Lateral meniscus version of a double delta sign with anterior displaced fibrocartilage posterior to anterior horn

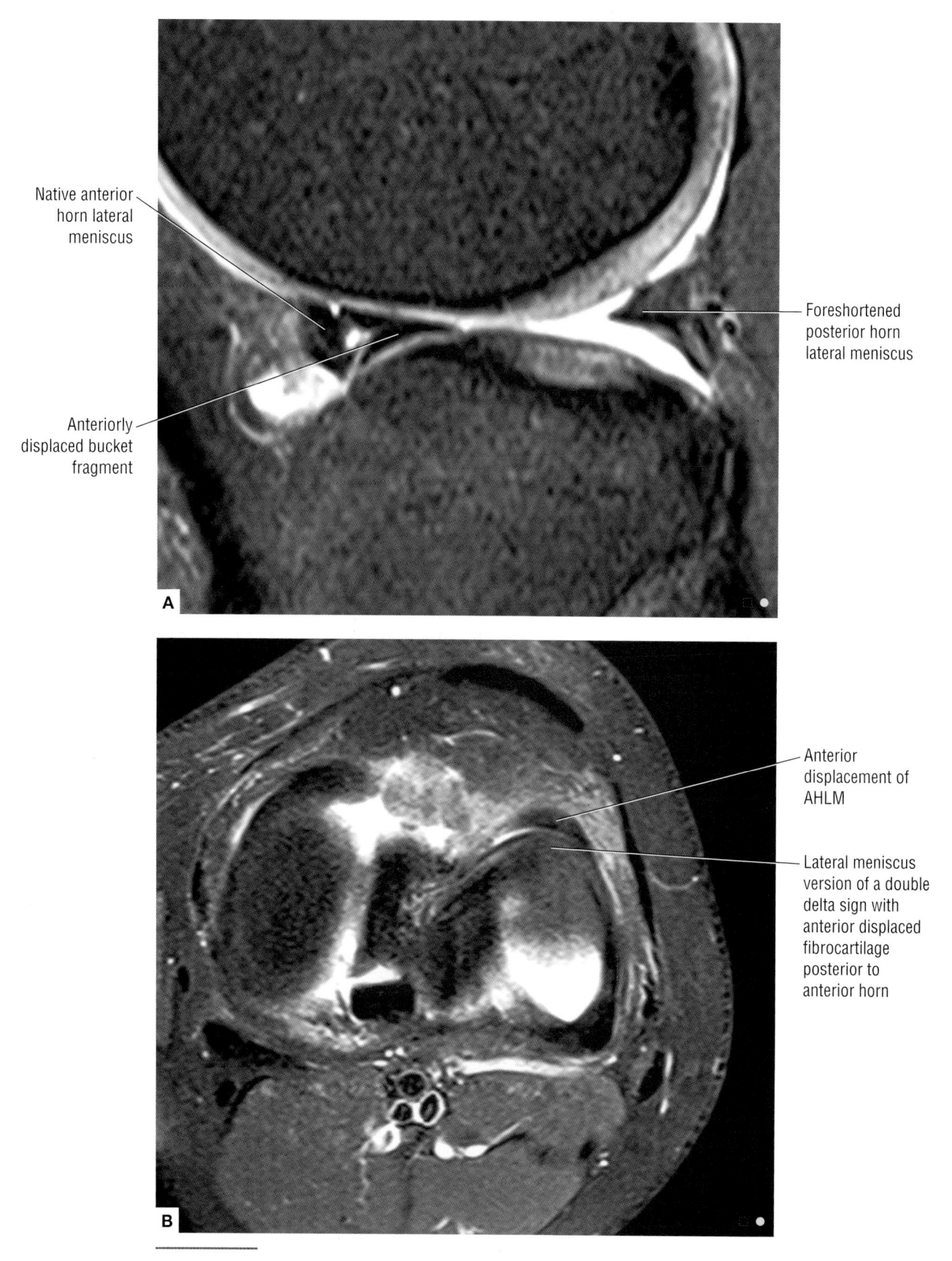

FIGURE 4.76 Double delta pattern of a lateral meniscus bucket-handle tear on FS PD FSE sagittal (**A**) and axial (**B**) images.

Radial Tear

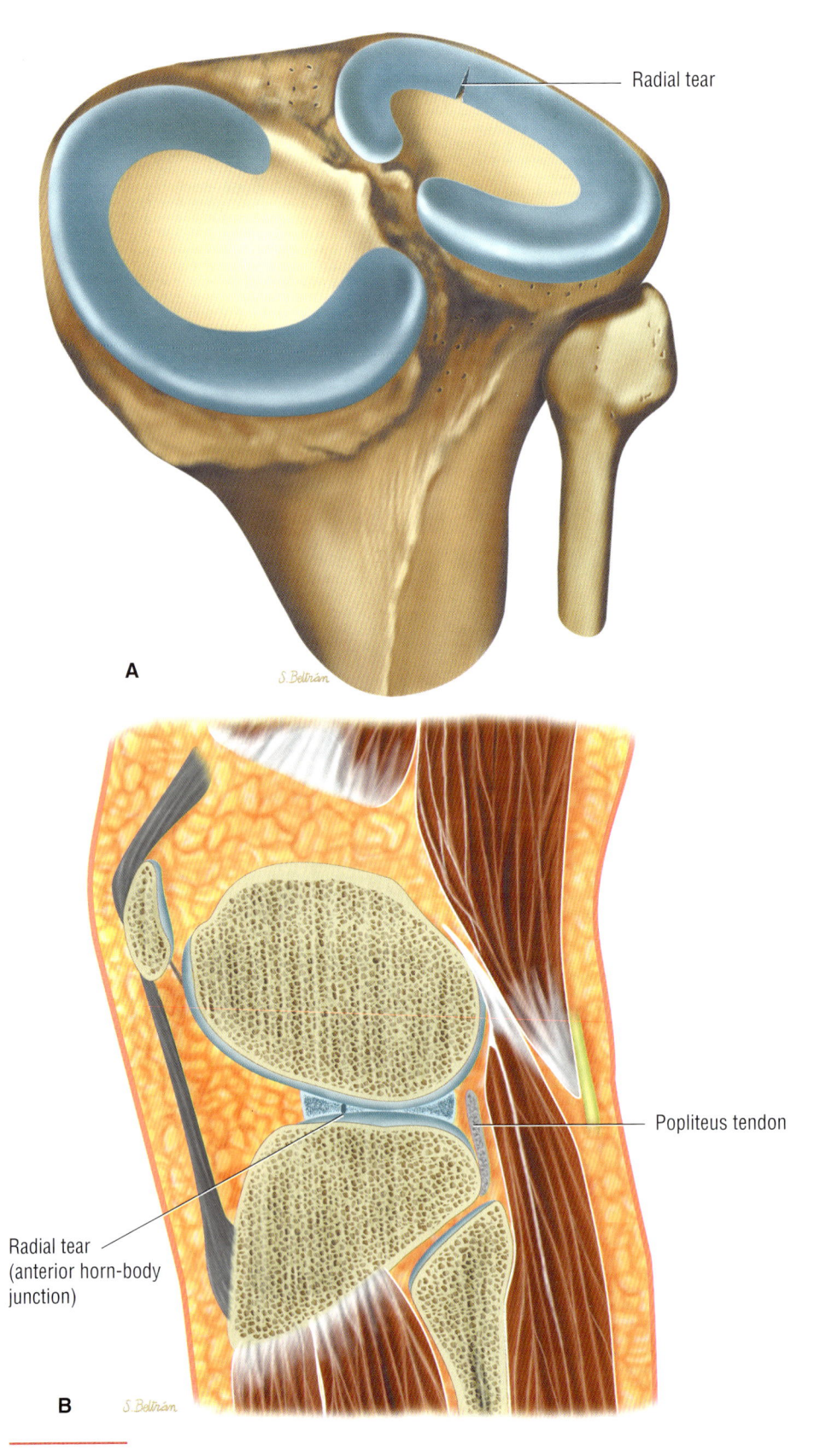

FIGURE 4.77 (**A**) Free edge radial tear at the junction of the anterior horn and body of the lateral meniscus. (**B**) Corresponding sagittal section produces the characteristic blunted foreshortened anterior horn and elongated components of the meniscal body and posterior horn.

Radial or Transverse Tears

- Vertical tears perpendicular to the free edge of the meniscus
- Subdivided into classic radial tears and root tears
    - Classic radial tears are further subdivided into three subtypes by their location within the lateral meniscus:
        - Anterior horn–body junction
        - Body
        - Posterior horn–body junction
- Both classic and root tears may involve either the medial or lateral meniscus.
    - Classic radial tears are more common in the lateral meniscus.
    - Root tears are more common in the posterior horn of the medial meniscus.
- Commonly associated with horizontal tears in the lateral meniscus and flap tears in the medial meniscus
- MR findings in classic radial tears include:
    - A blunted anterior horn and elongated posterior horn body segment
    - A blunted posterior horn in association with an elongated anterior horn body segment
    - Free edge increased signal intensity or blunting restricted to the middle third of the meniscus
        - Does not involve blunting of the anterior or posterior horns or elongation of body segment
- Root tears are defined by abrupt loss or blunting of posterior horn meniscal tissue on posterior coronal images adjacent to the root meniscal insertion.
- A ghost meniscus (relative absence of posterior horn meniscal fibrocartilaginous tissue) is characteristic of root tears on sagittal images located adjacent to the intercondylar notch.

- **Classic Radial Tears**
  - There are three recognized locations of classic radial tears.
    - The most common location involves the anterior horn–body junction of the free edge of the lateral meniscus.
  - There is a higher concentration of radially oriented collagen bundles and thinning out of circumferential longitudinal fibers, increasing the likelihood of tears along the free edge of the meniscus.
  - The position of the lateral aspect of the lateral meniscus contributes to the increased stiffness of radially oriented fibers at the middle perforating collagen bundle and to their susceptibility to shear stresses.
  - Classic radial tears also occur along the middle third of the meniscus (appearing as free edge blunting) or at the posterior horn–body junction of the meniscus (free edge blunting).
  - The sagittal plane sections the meniscus perpendicular to the free edge orientation of the tear.
    - The only evidence of a radial tear on sagittal images may be increased signal intensity (focal grade 3) on one or two peripheral sections.
  - Classic radial tears are characterized by:
    - Blunting anterior horn–body junction (sagittal or coronal)
    - Blunting and elongation posterior horn body segment (sagittal)
  - Tear plane is in the anterior third of the meniscus.
  - The blunted anterior horn:
    - Varies in size relative to the posterior horn body segment, based on the location of the sagittal plane of section
      - The more closely the plane of section approximates the free edge of the meniscus, the more prominent is the blunted anterior horn segment.
  - Sagittal images of a radial tear located at the junction of the posterior horn and body show an anterior horn body segment that is elongated or exaggerated in anterior to posterior length.

- Corresponding coronal images demonstrate the radial tear site in the anterior or posterior horn–body junction without posterior root involvement.

- Radial tears of the middle third of the meniscus are characterized by:
    - Free edge blunting on central coronal images
        - These images may not demonstrate areas of increased signal intensity.
    - Subtle blunting of the apex of the meniscus

- Disruption of hoop containment is associated with extension of radial tears to involve the longitudinal fibers of the circumferential zone.
    - This disruption of the normal hoop tension effect results in peripheral subluxation or partial extrusion of the body of the meniscus.[78]

- The classic radial tear may present as a complex tear in association with a secondary horizontal cleavage tear.
    - The tear propagates anteriorly or posteriorly into the circumferential fibers and results in a split radial variant.
    - These subtypes are more common in the lateral meniscus, but may be seen in the medial meniscus as well.

- Complex radial tears are frequently associated with a flap tear of the posterior horn of the medial meniscus.
    - Characterized by relative deficiency of the free edge of the inferior leaf of the posterior horn

- Classic radial tears are also characterized as:
    - Incomplete (tear is restricted to the free edge of the meniscus)
    - Complete (tear extends peripherally to the meniscal synovial rim)

Radial Tear

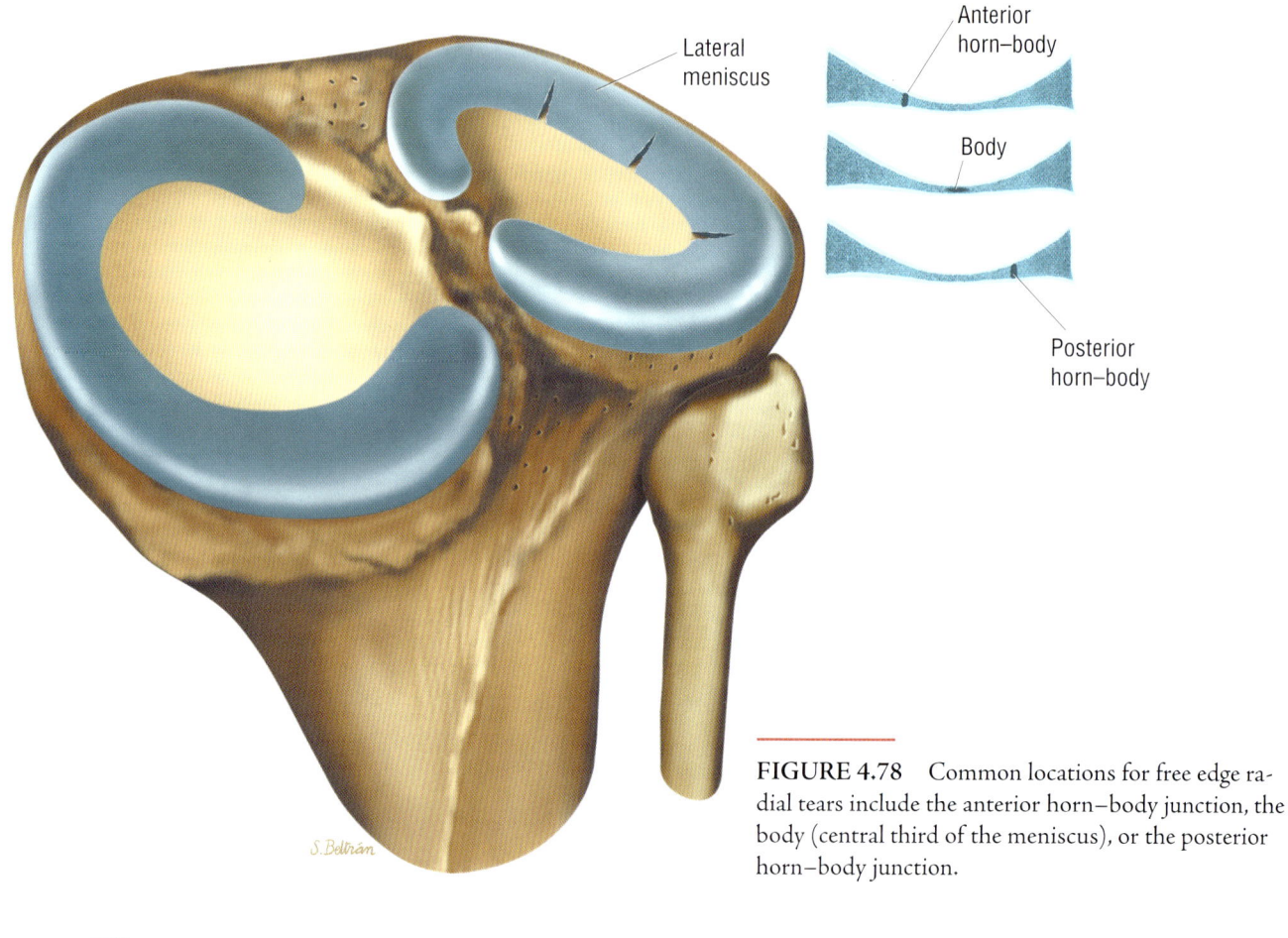

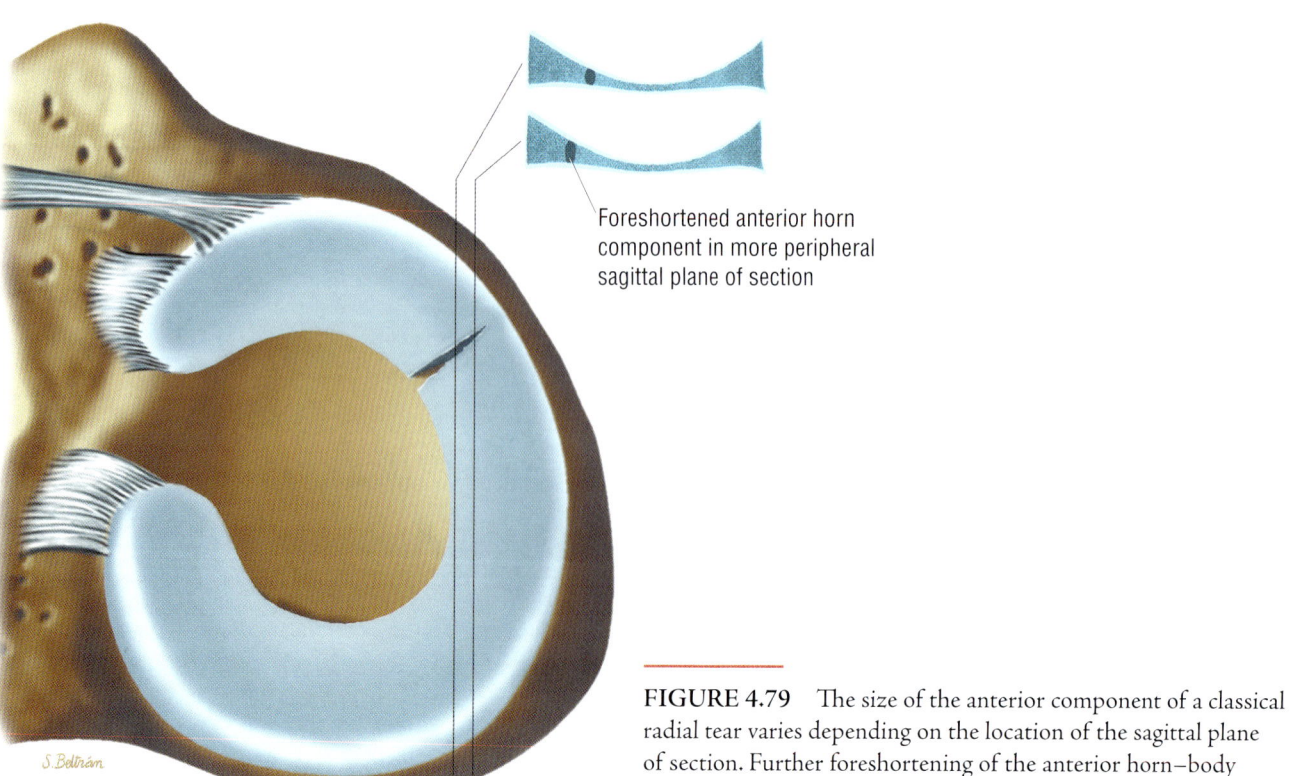

FIGURE 4.78 Common locations for free edge radial tears include the anterior horn–body junction, the body (central third of the meniscus), or the posterior horn–body junction.

FIGURE 4.79 The size of the anterior component of a classical radial tear varies depending on the location of the sagittal plane of section. Further foreshortening of the anterior horn–body junction occurs with a more peripheral plane of section.

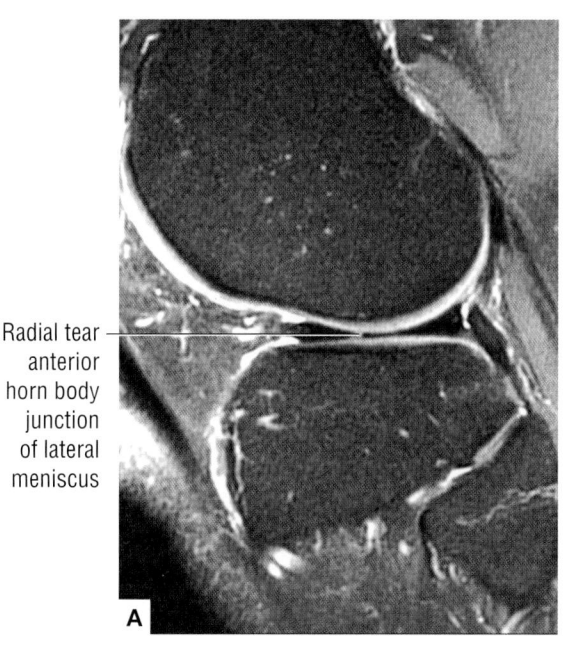

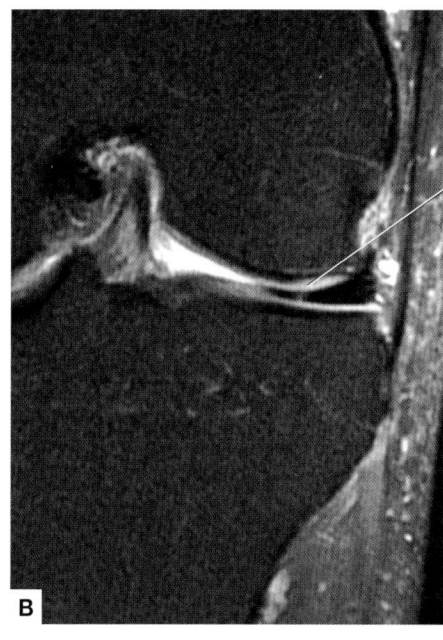

The Meniscus

FIGURE 4.80 (**A**) Classic radial tear involving the anterior horn–body junction of the lateral meniscus. The blunted free edge of the anterior horn and elongated posterior horn are shown on this FS PD FSE sagittal image. (**B**) The corresponding coronal FS PD FSE image at the level where the femoral condyles fuse identifies the radial tear.

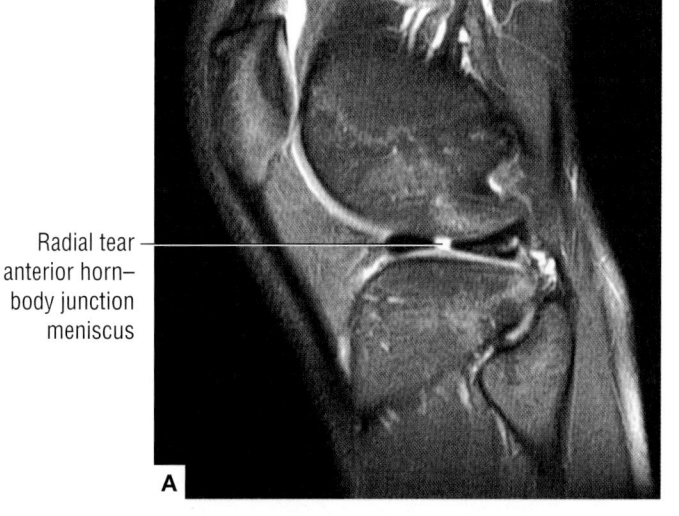

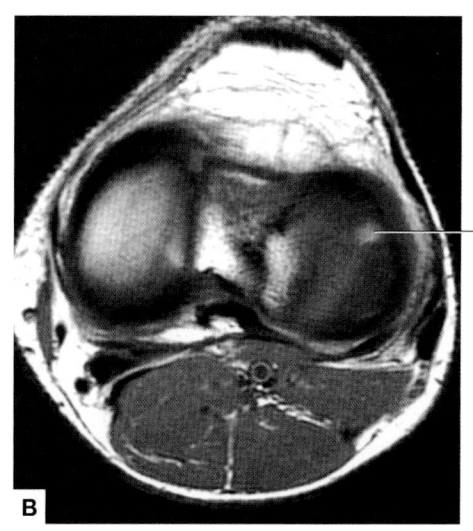

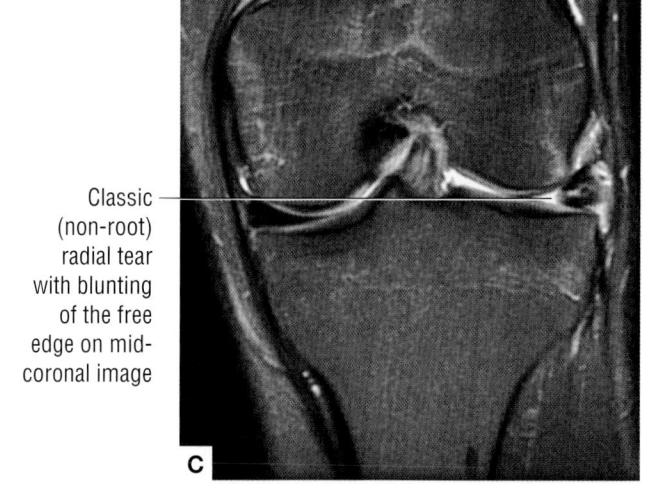

FIGURE 4.81 Classic lateral meniscus radial tear at anterior horn–body junction on an FS PD FSE sagittal image (**A**), a PD FSE axial image (**B**), and an FS PD FSE coronal image (**C**). The resultant blunting of both the anterior and posterior horns with posterior horn elongation is typical of the involvement of the body or middle third of the meniscus in a radial tear. A blunted meniscus on mid-coronal plane images (at or anterior to the plane of the MCL) is also characteristic.

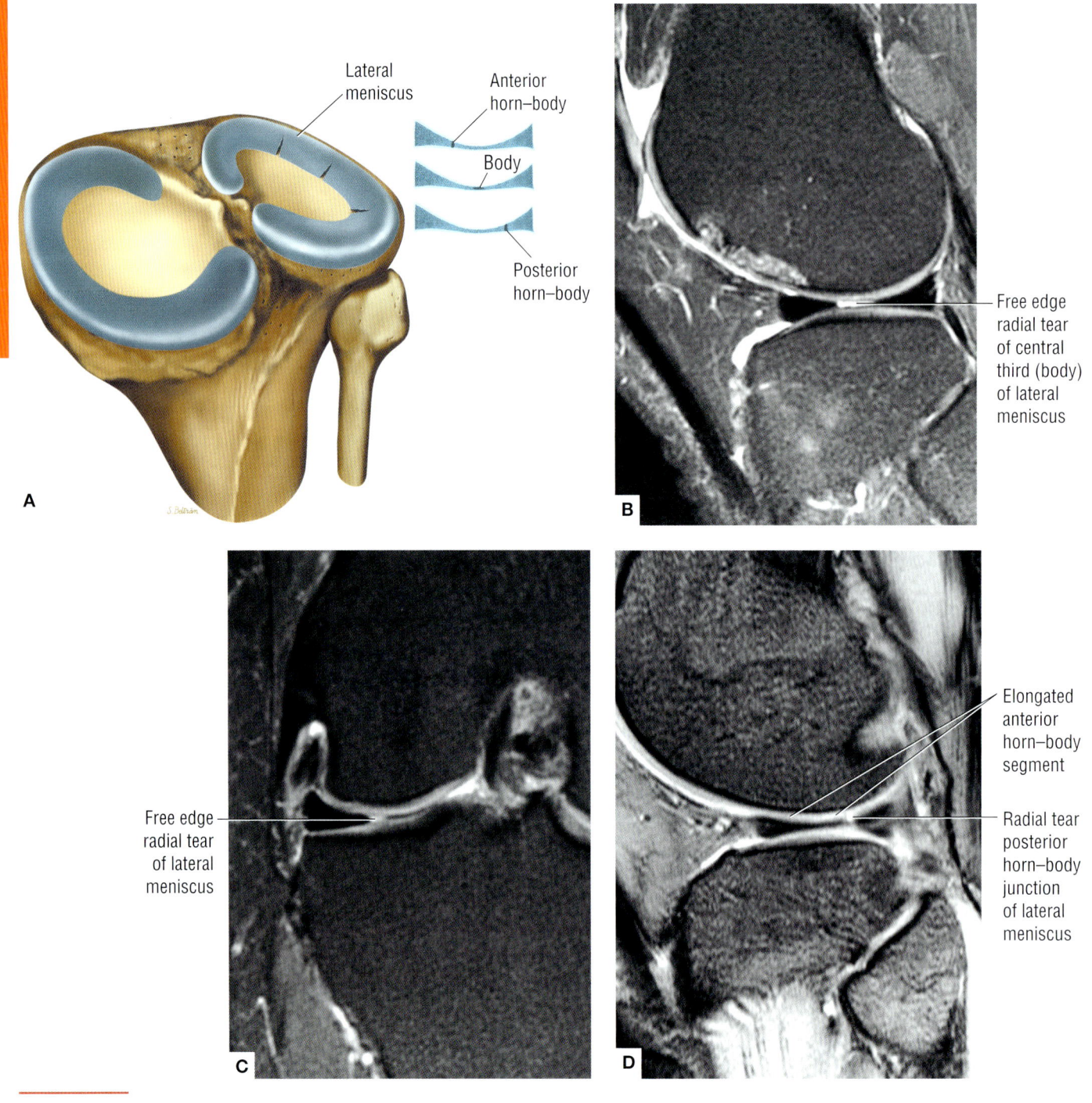

FIGURE 4.82 (**A**) Common locations for free edge radial tears include the anterior horn–body junction, the body (central third of the meniscus), or the posterior horn–body junction. A classic (nonroot) radial tear pattern is located at the free edge of the body of the lateral meniscus on FS PD FSE sagittal (**B**) and coronal (**C**) images. Radial tears are typically visualized on peripheral sagittal images or coronal images through sectioning the body or middle third of the meniscus. Note the characteristic free edge blunting in the coronal plane image. (**D**) Classic (nonroot) radial tear involving the posterior horn–body junction on an FS PD FSE sagittal image. The anterior horn body segment has an elongated morphology as the radial tear involves the posterior horn–body junction.

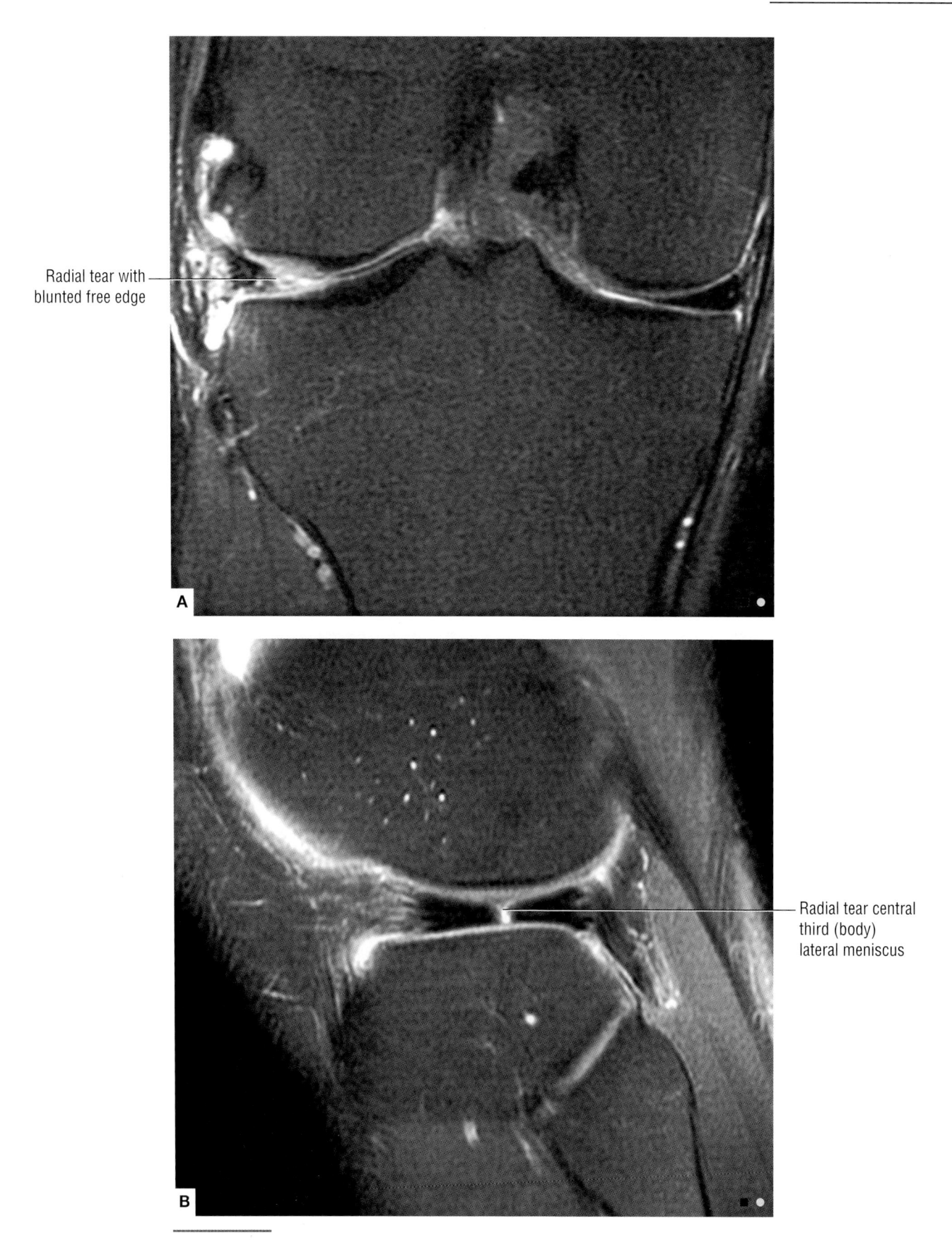

FIGURE 4.83 Radial tear of the lateral meniscus with characteristic blunted free edge of the body of the lateral meniscus on a mid-coronal image (**A**). The radial tear is represented as a single focus of increased signal intensity involving the free edge of the central third of the meniscus on sagittal image (**B**). (**A**) FS PD FSE coronal image. (**B**) FS PD FSE sagittal image.

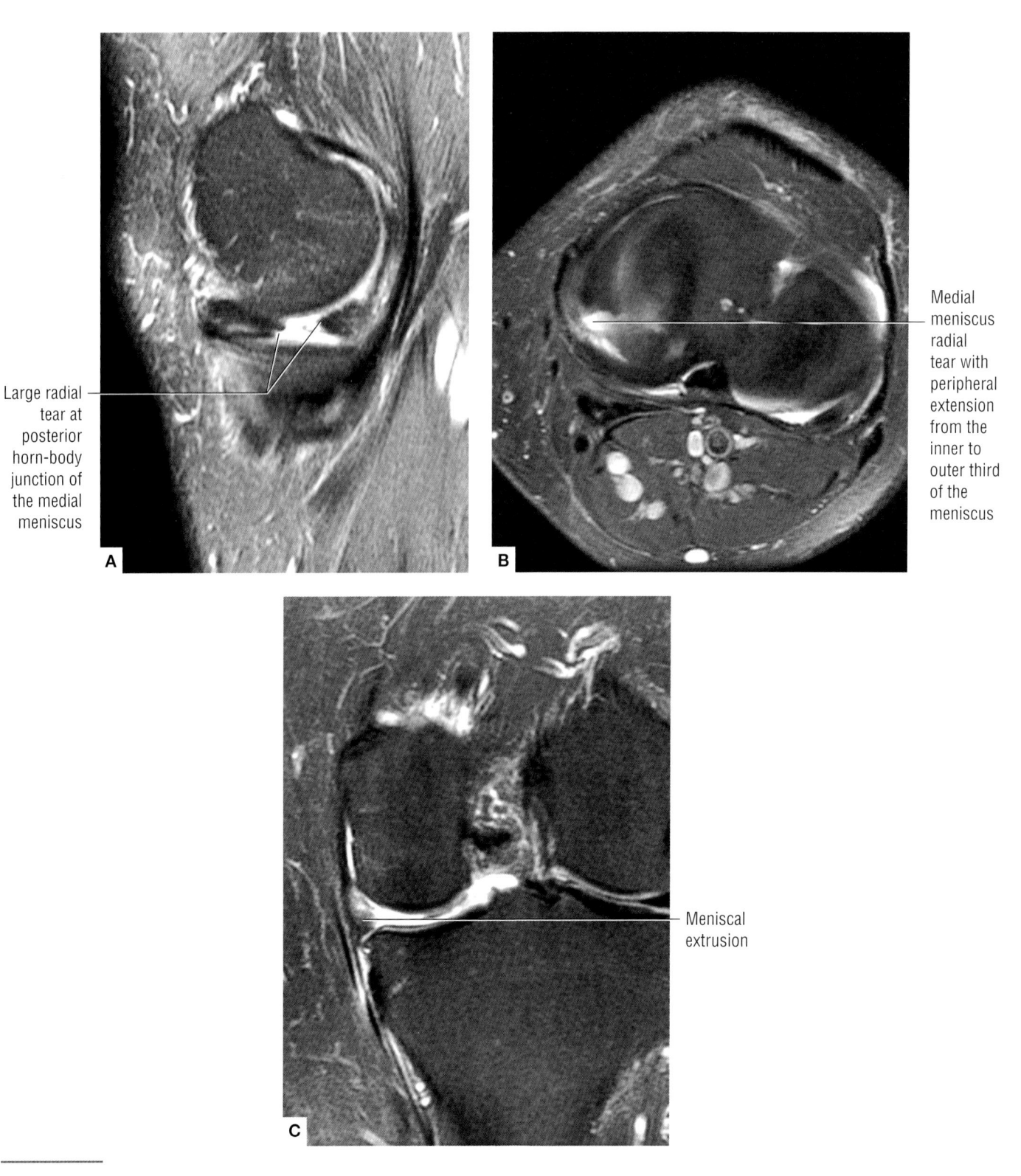

FIGURE 4.84 (**A**) Extensive radial tear of the posterior horn–body junction of the medial meniscus on an FS PD FSE sagittal image. (**B**) Extension of the radial tear into the peripheral circumferential zone on an FS PD FSE axial image. (**C**) Extrusion of the meniscus results from loss of normal meniscal hoop tension.

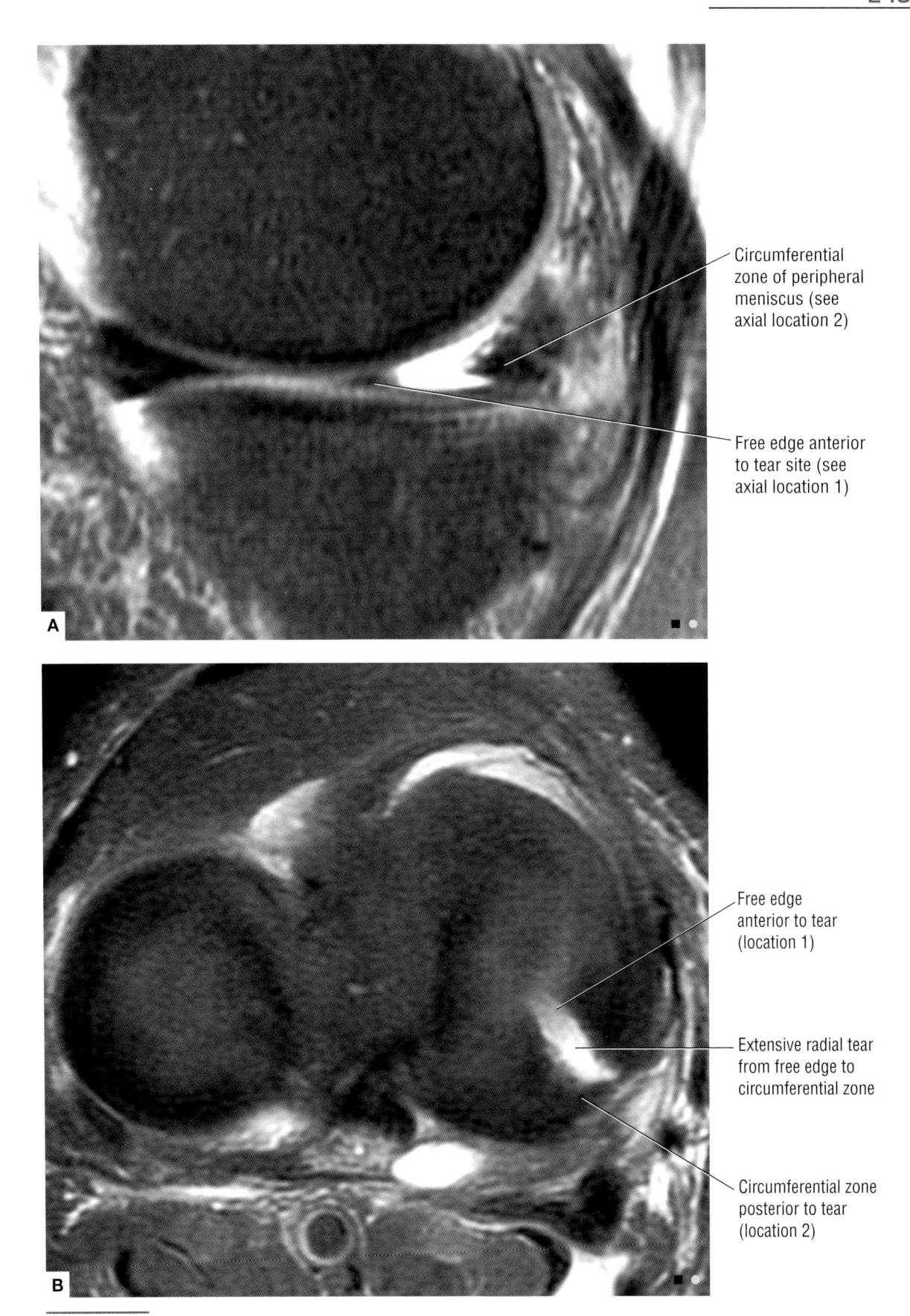

FIGURE 4.85 Extensive radial tear that extends from the free edge to the periphery of the meniscus. Involvement of circumferential fibers results in an unstable tear with associated meniscal extrusion. Location 1 corresponds to free edge anterior to tear. Location 2 corresponds to circumferential zone of meniscus directly posterior to the tear plane. FS PD FSE sagittal (**A**) and axial (**B**) images.

- **Root Tears**
  - Can occur in either the medial or lateral meniscus
    - Occur more commonly in the medial meniscus
  - Typically located at the meniscotibial attachment of the posterior horn or the junction of the meniscus–root interface
  - Displacement of the root tear produces a relative absence of posterior horn meniscal fibrocartilage on sagittal images.
    - Diffuse increased signal intensity seen on sagittal images of displaced root type radial tears represents the *ghost meniscus*.
  - Posterior coronal images demonstrate:
    - Abrupt blunting of the normal meniscotibial attachment
    - Foreshortening of the meniscus toward the posterior aspect of the intercondylar notch
  - Residual meniscofemoral ligament may be mistaken for residual posterior horn tissue in the lateral compartment.
  - Root tears of the posterior aspect of the lateral meniscus may present with:
    - A ghost meniscus appearance of the posterior horn on sagittal images
    - Blunting of the lateral meniscus on posterior coronal images adjacent to the intercondylar notch
  - Lateral meniscus root tears are associated with ACL tears.
    - Displacement of these root tears may result in flipping of meniscal fragments into the posterior aspect of the intercondylar notch.
      - Flipped meniscal fragments are best appreciated on posterior coronal images.

The Meniscus

- Large radial or root tears are:
    - 50% of the meniscal width
    - Associated with significant (>3mm) meniscal extrusion relative to the tibial plateau[78]
- Tears 3mm or less in length are usually asymptomatic.
- Tears greater than 5mm are more likely to produce symptoms.[404]
- Symptomatic tears can be treated by trimming the anterior and posterior leaves adjacent to the tear site.
- Flap tears usually originate from a free edge radial tear that changes direction and creates the meniscal flap.
    - The flap may be displaced toward the notch or become inverted and extruded peripherally.
- Root tears should be repaired unless there is unstable meniscal tissue separated from its peripheral attachment.

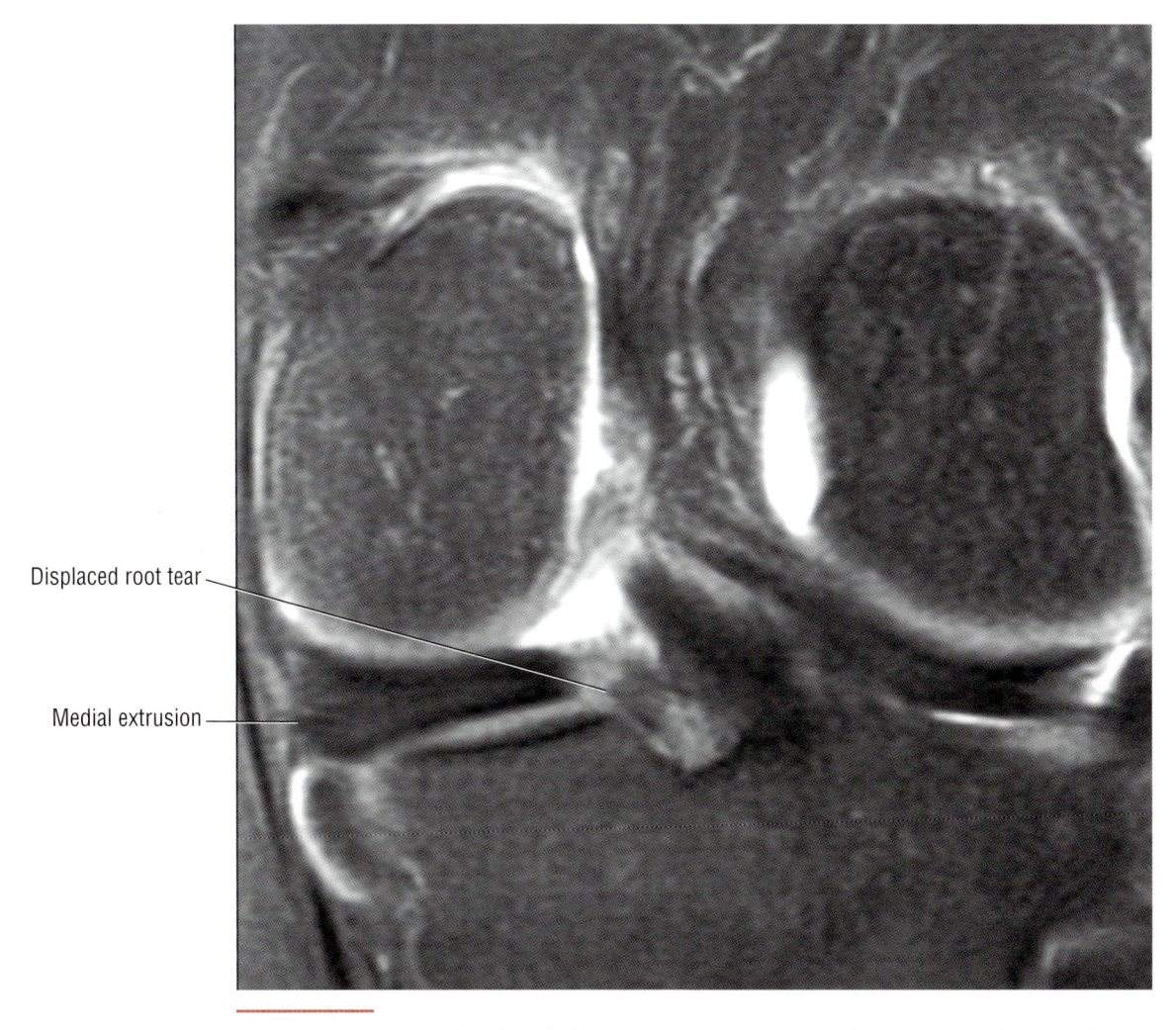

FIGURE 4.86 Displaced medial meniscus root tear with medial extrusion relative to the tibial plateau. Coronal FS PD FSE image.

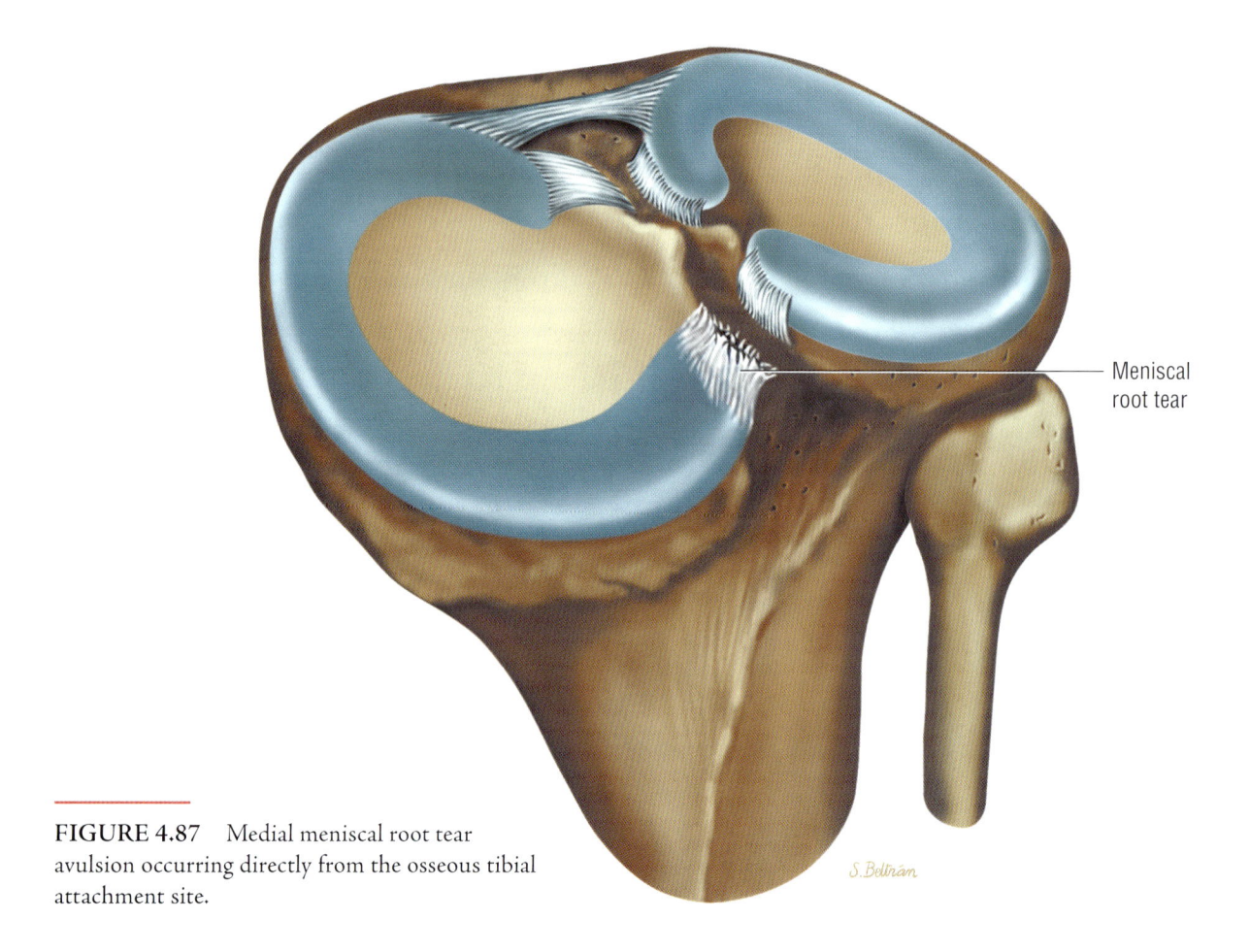

FIGURE 4.87 Medial meniscal root tear avulsion occurring directly from the osseous tibial attachment site.

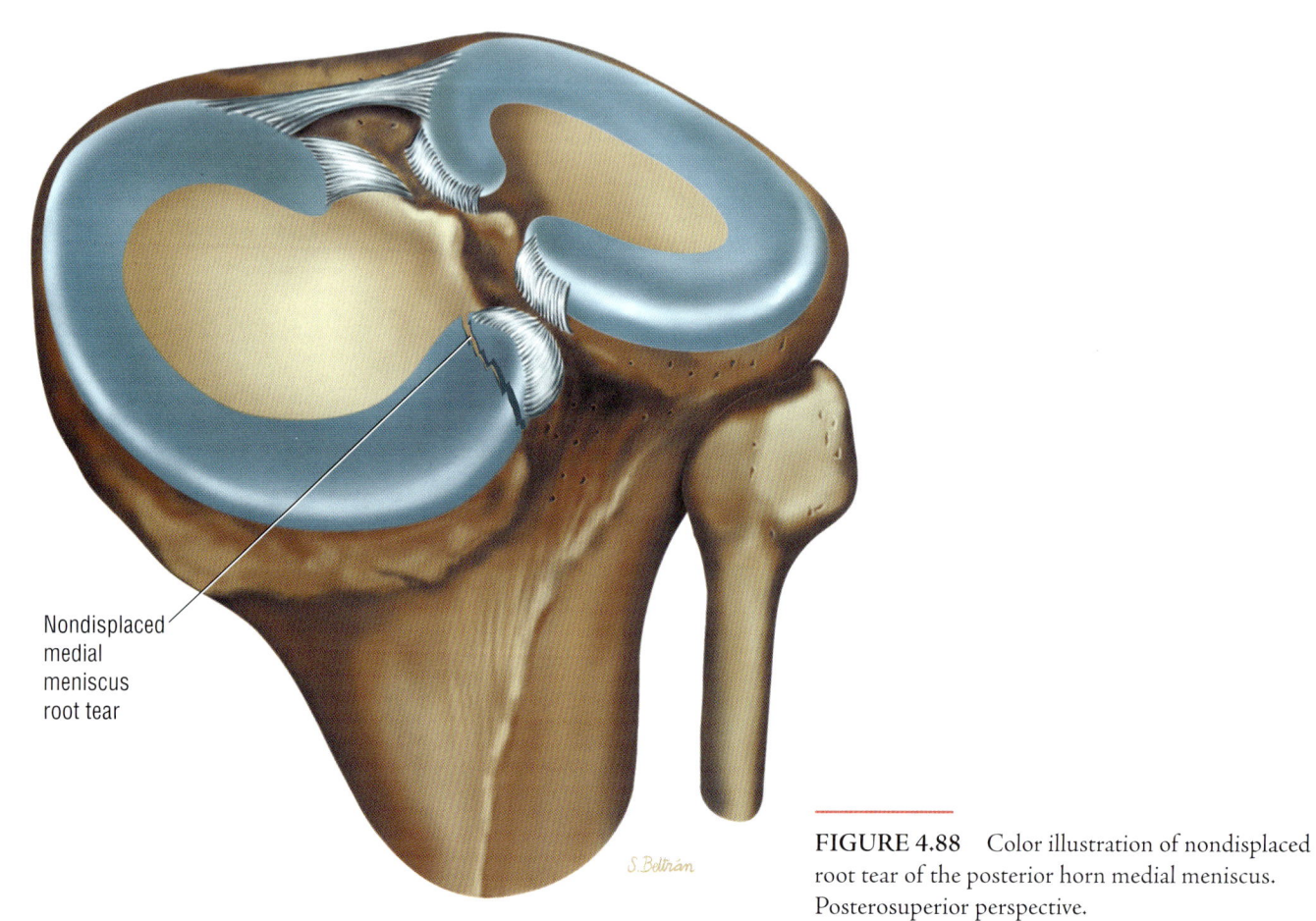

FIGURE 4.88 Color illustration of nondisplaced root tear of the posterior horn medial meniscus. Posterosuperior perspective.

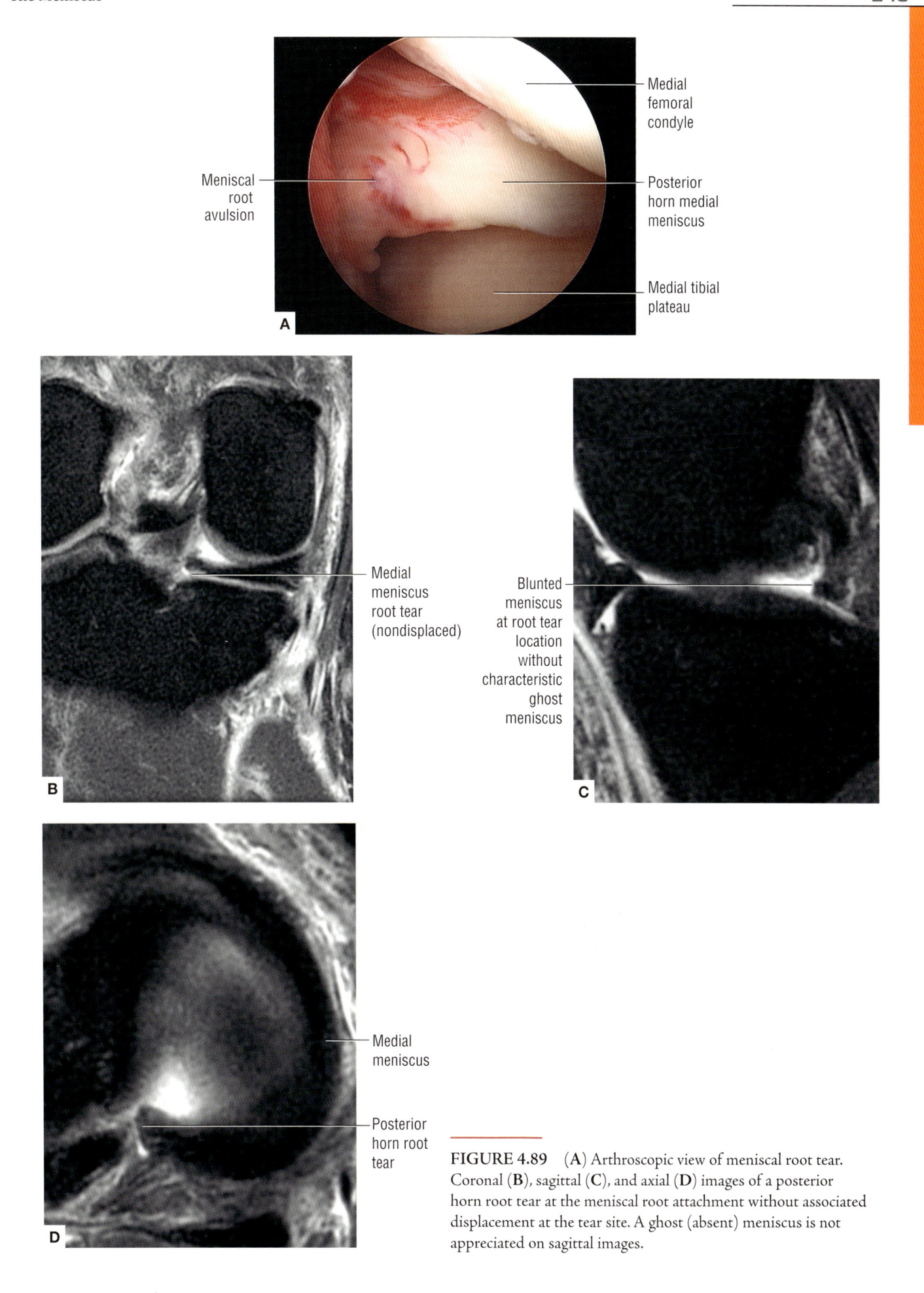

The Meniscus

- Meniscal root avulsion
- Medial femoral condyle
- Posterior horn medial meniscus
- Medial tibial plateau

- Medial meniscus root tear (nondisplaced)

- Blunted meniscus at root tear location without characteristic ghost meniscus

- Medial meniscus
- Posterior horn root tear

FIGURE 4.89 (**A**) Arthroscopic view of meniscal root tear. Coronal (**B**), sagittal (**C**), and axial (**D**) images of a posterior horn root tear at the meniscal root attachment without associated displacement at the tear site. A ghost (absent) meniscus is not appreciated on sagittal images.

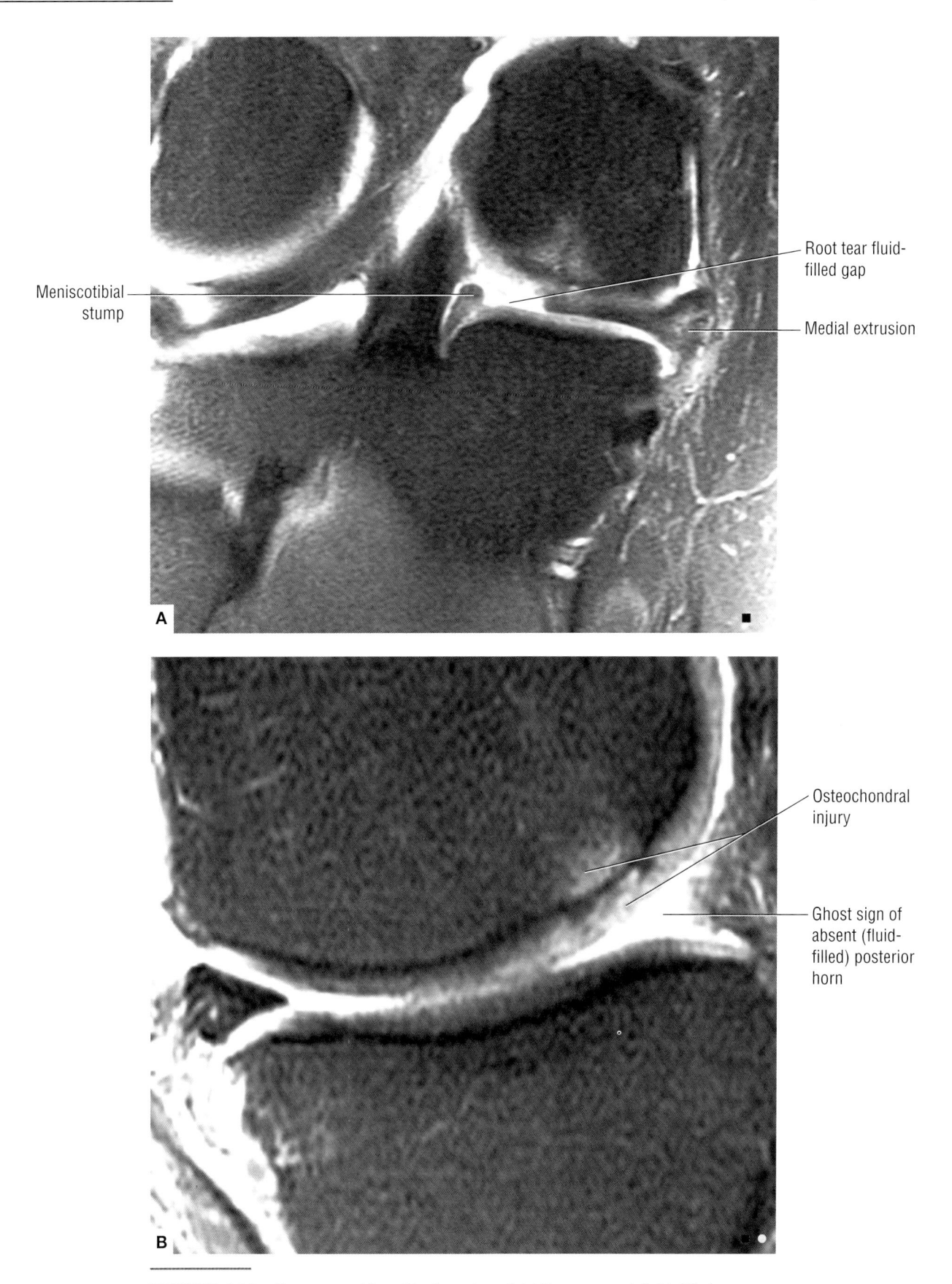

FIGURE 4.90 Root tear with residual meniscotibial ligament and fluid-filled gap at site of meniscal displacement on coronal image (**A**). Ghost meniscus or an apparent absence of the posterior horn is produced on corresponding sagittal image (**B**). FS PD FSE coronal (**A**) and sagittal (**B**) images.

The Meniscus 251

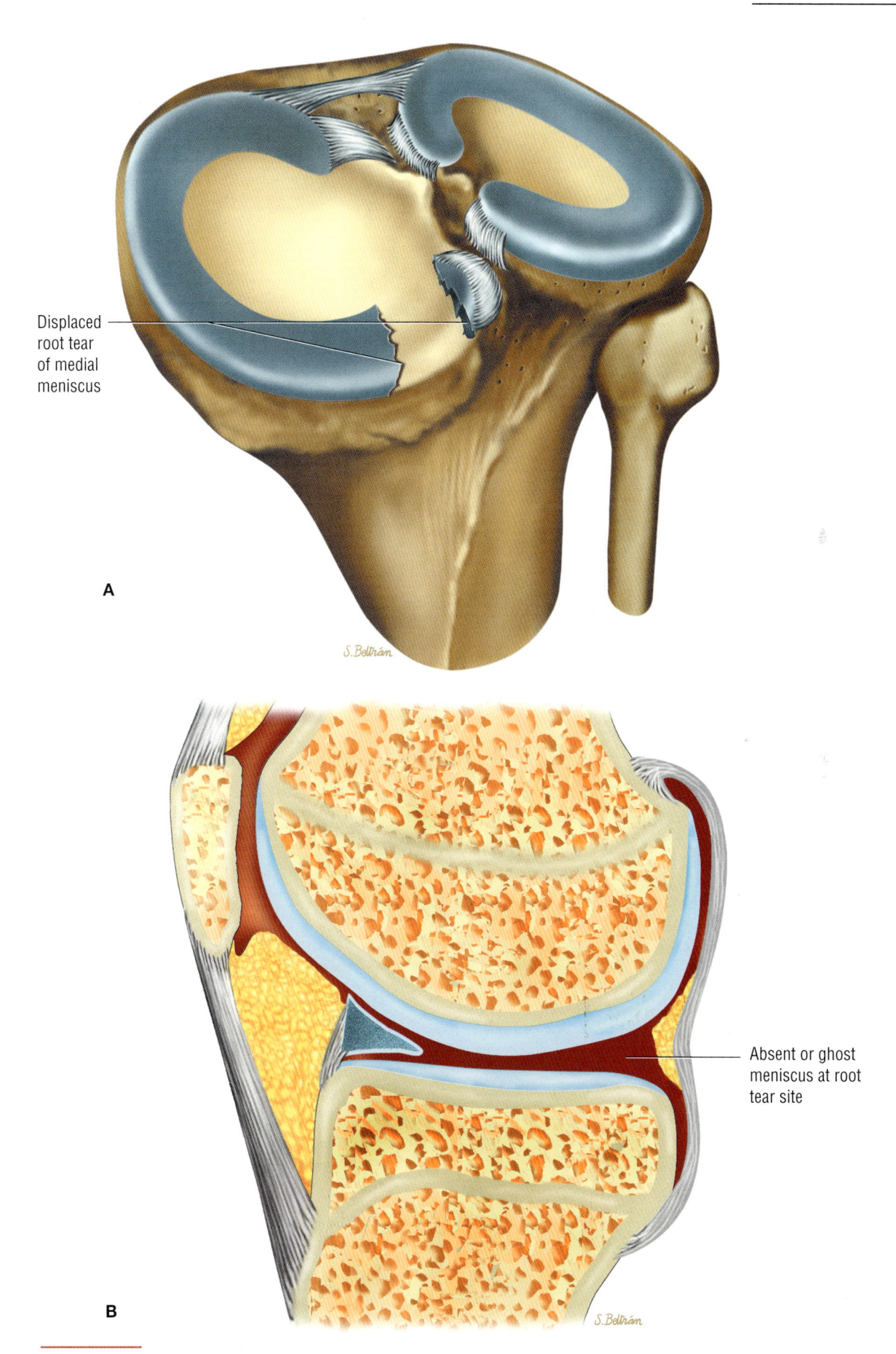

FIGURE 4.91 (**A**) Displaced posterior horn root tear of the medial meniscus on axial illustration. (**B**) "Ghost" meniscus is demonstrated on a sagittal illustration.

Displaced root tear PHMM

Disrupted meniscotibial ligament

Tibial subchondral edema adjacent to root tear

Root tear posterior horn medial meniscus

FIGURE 4.92 Root tear at meniscus connection with meniscotibial ligament. FS PD coronal (**A**) and axial (**B**) images.

Meniscal root

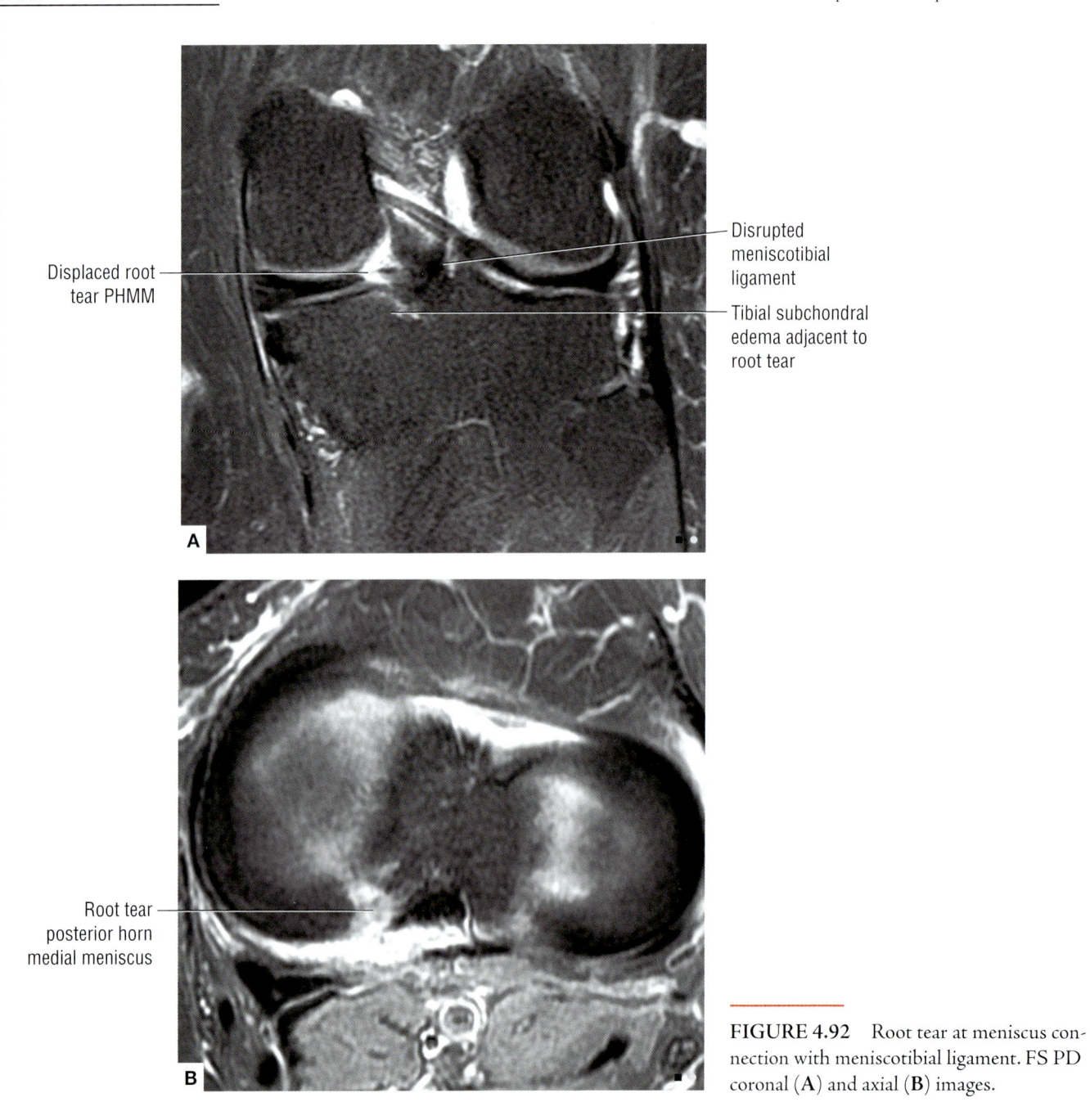

Medial femoral condyle

Root insertion

Medial tibial plateau

FIGURE 4.93 Gillquist view of the posteromedial knee: The arthroscope is passed between the PCL and the medial femoral condyle, allowing direct visualization of the medial meniscal root and the native insertion site. (Reprinted from Fu FH. *Master Techniques in Orthopaedic Surgery: Sports Medicine*. Philadelphia, PA: Lippincott Williams & Wilkins; 2010, with permission.)

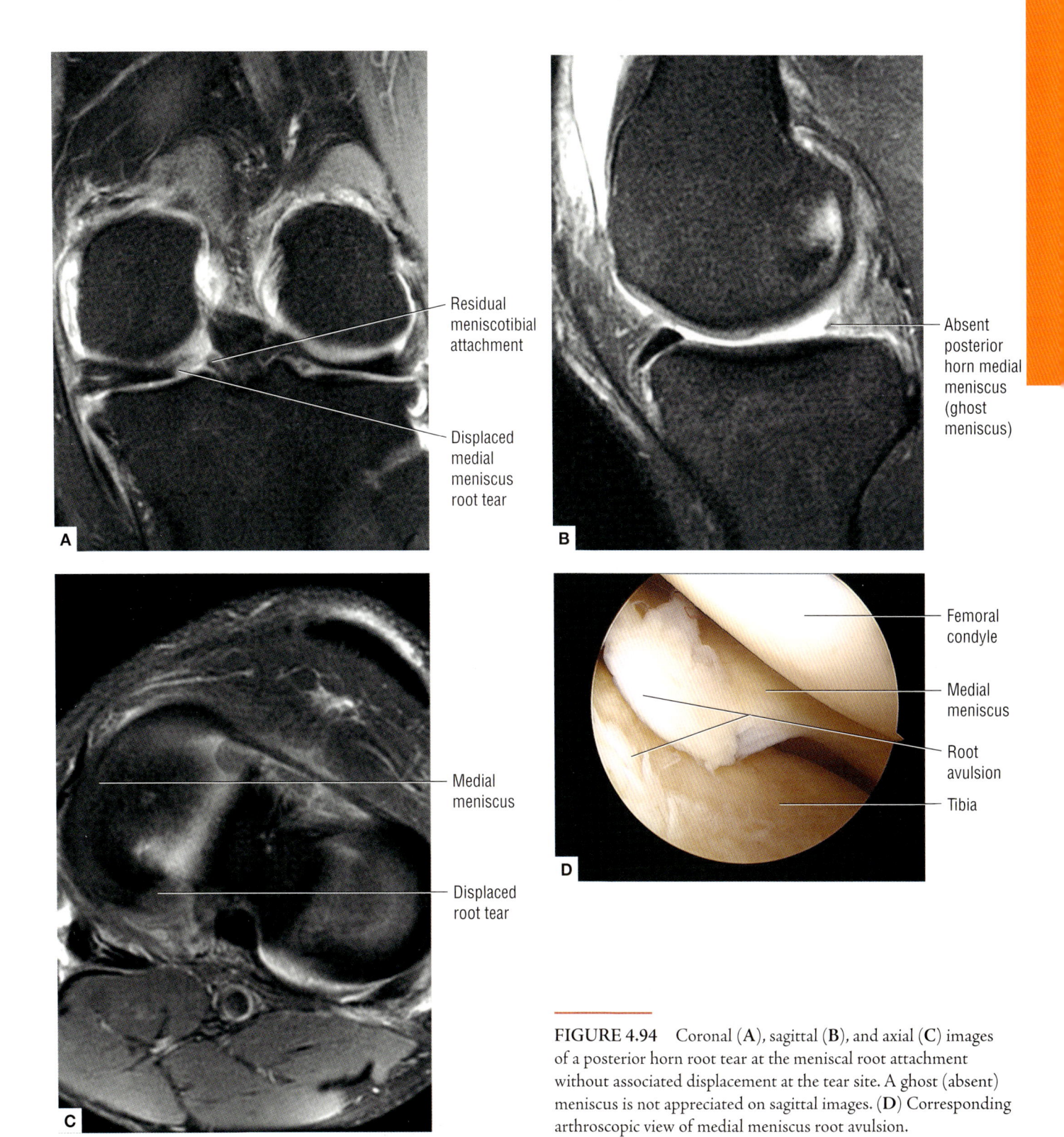

The Meniscus 253

- Residual meniscotibial attachment
- Displaced medial meniscus root tear
- Absent posterior horn medial meniscus (ghost meniscus)
- Medial meniscus
- Displaced root tear
- Femoral condyle
- Medial meniscus
- Root avulsion
- Tibia

FIGURE 4.94 Coronal (**A**), sagittal (**B**), and axial (**C**) images of a posterior horn root tear at the meniscal root attachment without associated displacement at the tear site. A ghost (absent) meniscus is not appreciated on sagittal images. (**D**) Corresponding arthroscopic view of medial meniscus root avulsion.

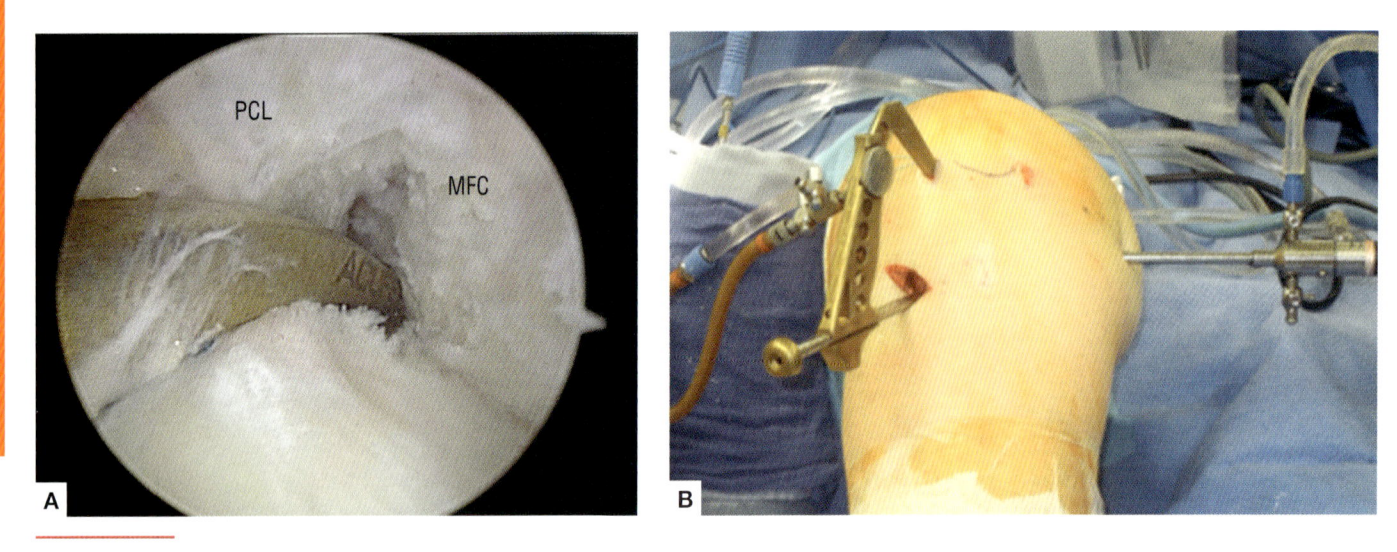

FIGURE 4.95 (**A**) The Acufex ACL tip guide is positioned at the anatomic insertion site of the meniscal root. The correct position is confirmed arthroscopically. (**B**) The guide is then seated on the external tibia just distal to the lateral flare of the tibia. (Reprinted from Fu FH. *Master Techniques in Orthopaedic Surgery: Sports Medicine.* Philadelphia, PA: Lippincott Williams & Wilkins; 2010, with permission.)

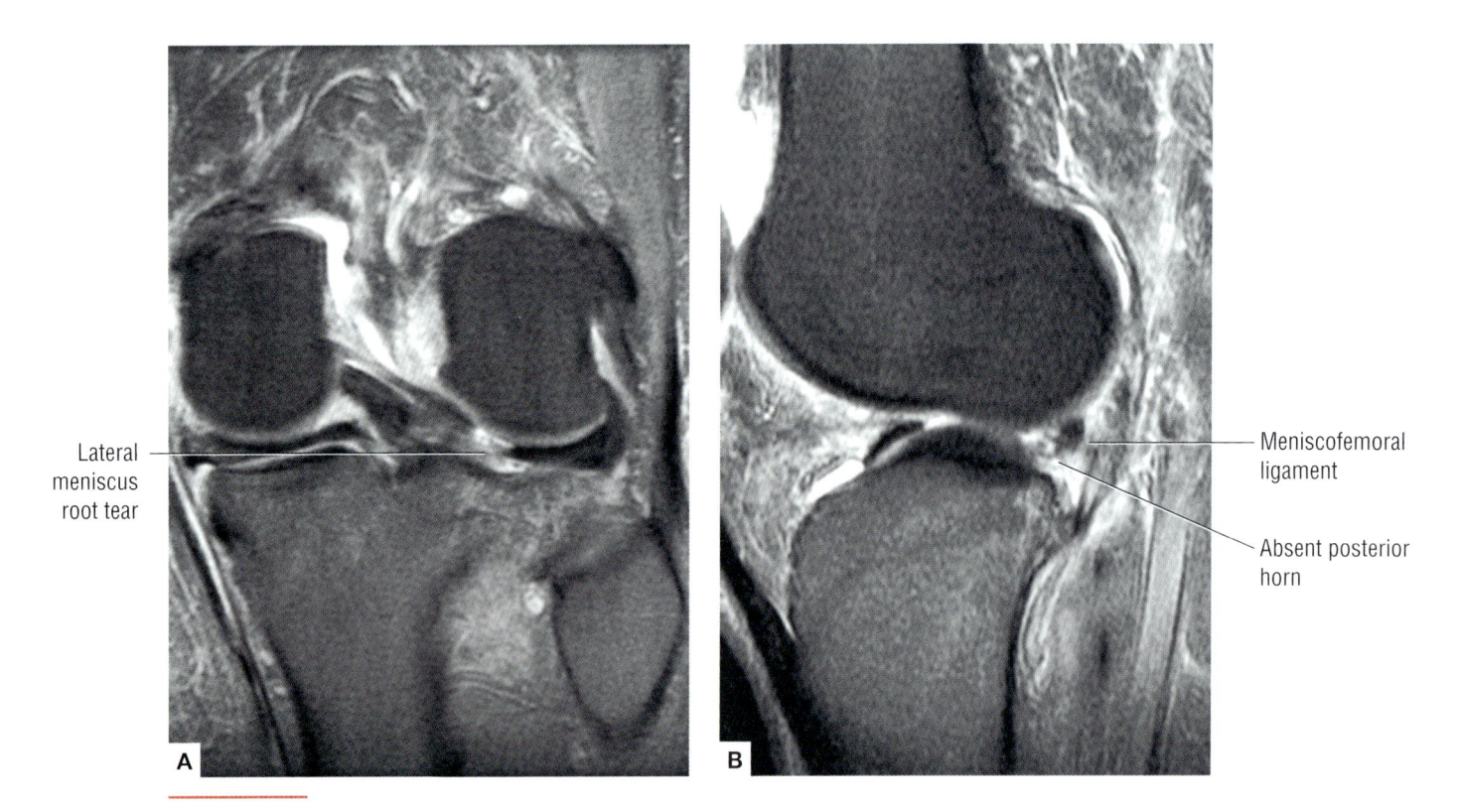

FIGURE 4.96 Lateral meniscal root tear on FS PD FSE coronal (**A**) and sagittal (**B**) images. The hypointense meniscofemoral ligament is identified posterior to the root tear on the sagittal image (**B**).

Flap Tears

- Flap Tears
    - Represent a composite of a longitudinal and a radial tear
    - Start on the free edge of the meniscus and curve obliquely into the meniscal fibrocartilage
    - Also referred to as *oblique tears*
    - Most common meniscal tear pattern
    - Frequently associated with oblique signal intensity on sagittal plane meniscal cross-section (e.g., grade 3 signal intensity commonly extending to the inferior surface of the posterior horn of the medial meniscus)
    - May display either a primary vertical or horizontal tear pattern
    - Can generate an anterior- or posterior-based flap of meniscus[16]
    - Location common at the posterior horn of the medial meniscus, but may also be seen in the lateral meniscus
    - May produce either double-decker or stacked leaflet meniscal morphology or extend into the meniscofemoral or meniscotibial recess as it rotates
    - Frequently develop after minimal meniscal trauma superimposed on a degenerative process resulting from chronic shear forces
    - Are often extensions of radial tears or horizontal cleavage tears
        - Both tear patterns may coexist in the same meniscus and/or in the same meniscal sagittal section or image.
        - The separate features of flap, radial, and longitudinal tears should be described when part of a complex flap tear.
    - Involve the inner one third to one half of the meniscus with superior or inferior leaf extension creating the mobile limb or flap of fibrocartilage
        - Longitudinal tears are more likely to involve the peripheral third of the meniscus where there is a greater concentration of circumferential fibers.

Flap Tear

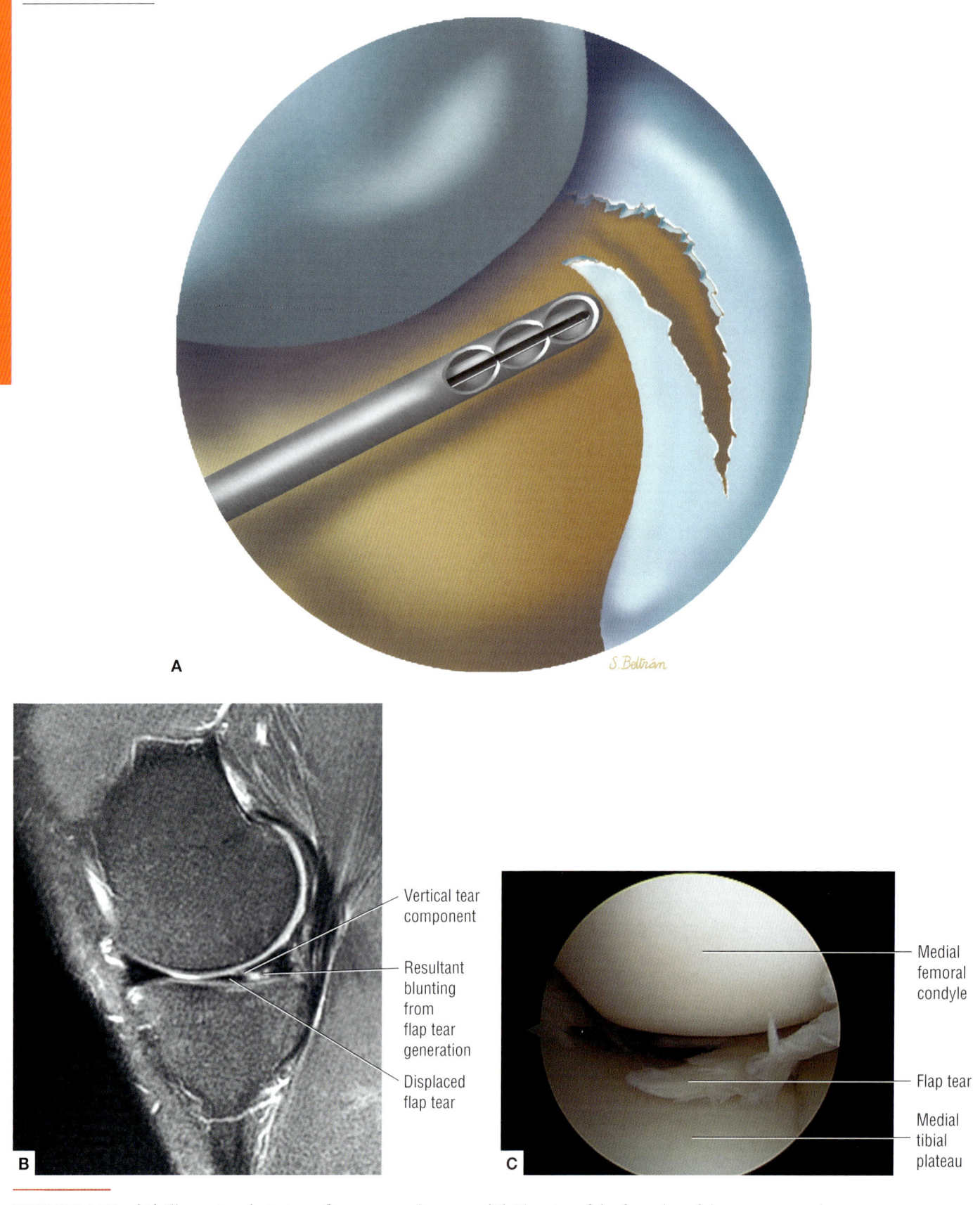

FIGURE 4.97 (**A**) Illustration depicting a flap tear at arthroscopy. (**B**) Blunting of the free edge of the meniscus is shown on a sagittal FS PD FSE image. Sagittal image shows the flap component—fluid interface—peripheral donor site from anterior to posterior. (**C**) Vertical inner third tearing produces an anteriorly displaced meniscal fragment, creating the flap identified at arthroscopy.

- Identification of obliquely oriented grade 3 meniscal signal on sagittal images does not necessarily indicate the presence of a flap or oblique tear.
  - Longitudinal tears may also appear as an oblique course of grade 3 signal intensity extending to the meniscal surface.
- Some classification systems describe a partial cleavage tear with a mobile flap of meniscal tissue as a subtype of horizontal tear.
  - It is more accurate to use the term "flap tear" to describe a distinct tear pattern and not as a subtype of or a synonym for a horizontal tear.
- The terms "flap tear" and "oblique tear patterns" are interchangeable; most orthopaedic surgeons consider "flap tear" to be the proper terminology.
  - Radiologists should avoid using these terms to describe obliquely oriented signal intensity unless a flap tear is directly confirmed and visualized on axial images or is correctly diagnosed using specific criteria for flap tears.
- Criteria for the prospective diagnosis of flap tear patterns:
  - Based on the characteristic morphology of signal intensity and meniscal morphology in the sagittal plane
  - Include coronal images to take into account the characteristic finding of meniscal extrusion into the coronary recess
- Criteria for diagnosis of a flap tear based on sagittal images include:
  - A vertical tear encompassing the inner third of the meniscus, either coapted or noncoapted
  - Relative deficiency of the inner third of the inferior meniscal surface with associated blunting of the remaining inferior leaf
  - A blunted free edge of the meniscus with displaced meniscal tissue inferior to the periphery of the meniscus
  - A change in the slope of the superior surface of the meniscus, indicating a change in the direction of the tear that creates the flap
- Extrusion of a portion of the meniscus into the coronary recess below the joint line is seen on coronal images.

- The displaced flap in the coronary recess is visualized on peripheral sagittal images with hypointense meniscal tissue below the level of the joint line or tibial plateau deep to the MCL on peripheral medial images.[78,274]

- Characteristic findings in flap tears include:
    - Location of vertical signal intensity in the inner one third to one half of the meniscus
    - Relative deficiency of the inner margin of the inferior leaf of the meniscus is a characteristic finding in flap tears.

- When associated with ACL injuries, complex flap tears may displace posteriorly into the intercondylar notch.[496] Complex flap displacement and rotation of the posterior horn of the lateral meniscus may be mistaken for ACL ligamentous tissue (*double ACL sign*).

- Acute tears may occur after sudden impact on the meniscus (usually with a twisting component).

- Degenerative flap tears most commonly involve the inferior leaf.
    - Relative deficiency of the inner margin of the superior surface of the meniscus may also result in a flap tear.
    - Flap tear leaflets may displace anteriorly or posteriorly.

- Flap tears represent a change in the direction of meniscal signal.
    - Morphology can be inferred when grade 3 signal intensity extends to the superior and inferior surfaces of the meniscus on separate sagittal images in different locations.

- The popliteus tendon sheath may serve as a potential space for a displaced lateral meniscus flap tear.

- Reactive plateau edema is frequently associated with displaced flap tears.
    - It is seen more commonly in the medial compartment and is associated with increased load transference to the chondral surface and subchondral bone.
        - This load transference is increased in the presence of meniscal dysfunction.

- Unlike bucket-handle tears, flap tears do not demonstrate complete posterior-to-anterior extension and displacement of the involved meniscal fragment.

- Classic (nonroot) radial tears usually demonstrate normal meniscal morphology on posterior coronal images, but flap tears commonly involve the posterior horn of the meniscus.

- Impingement of the mobile flap fragment results in traction on the innervated peripheral meniscal rim.

- Flap tears that involve the avascular inner edge of the meniscus are irreparable.[62]

- Treatment is partial meniscectomy with transection through the base and contouring of the remaining attachment to a stable rim.[402]

- Residual peripheral horizontal grade 3 signal intensity is often seen after arthroscopic resection of the flap.

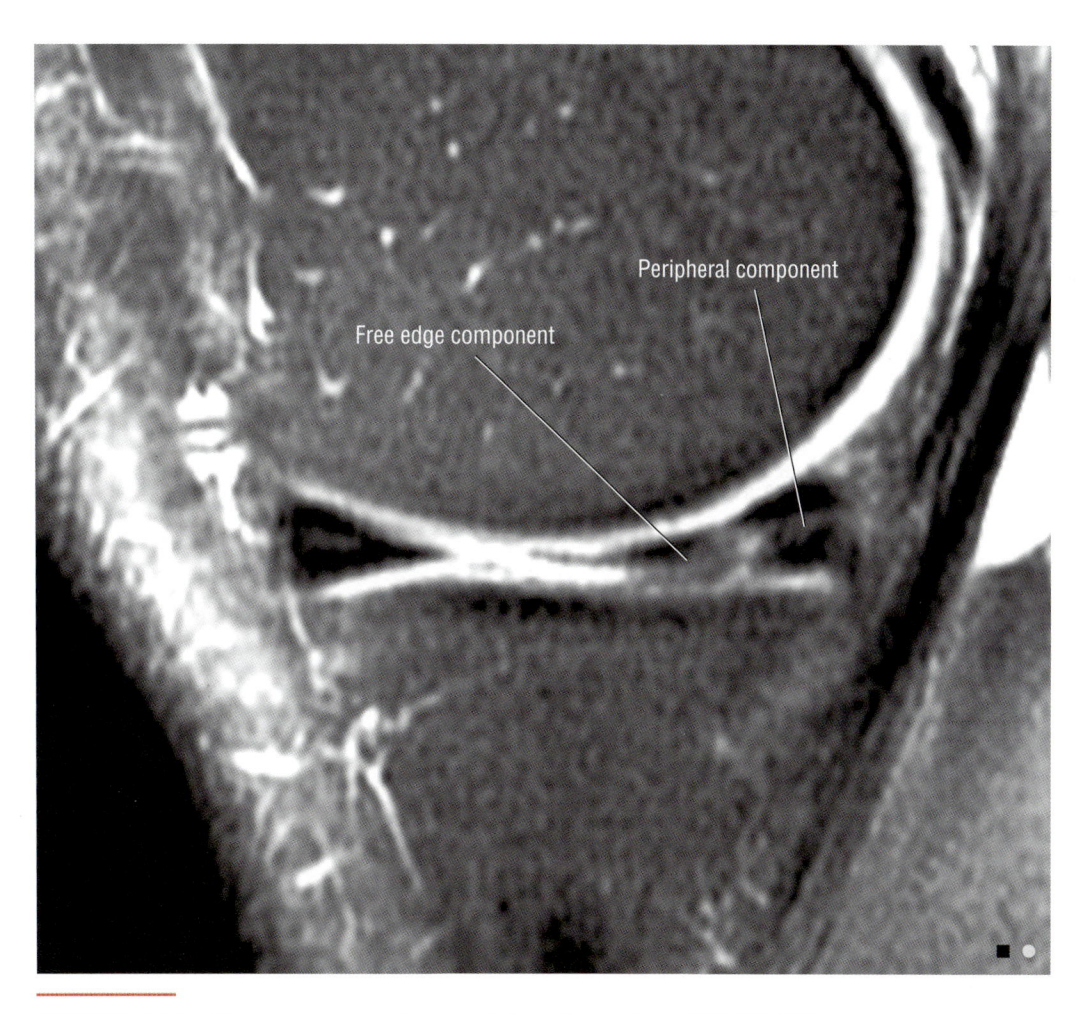

FIGURE 4.98   Flap tear posterior horn medial meniscus. Sagittal FS PD FSE image.

- Posterior horn medial meniscus
- Displaced flap tear generated from the posterior horn body junction of the medial meniscus
- Flap tear medial meniscus
- PHMM

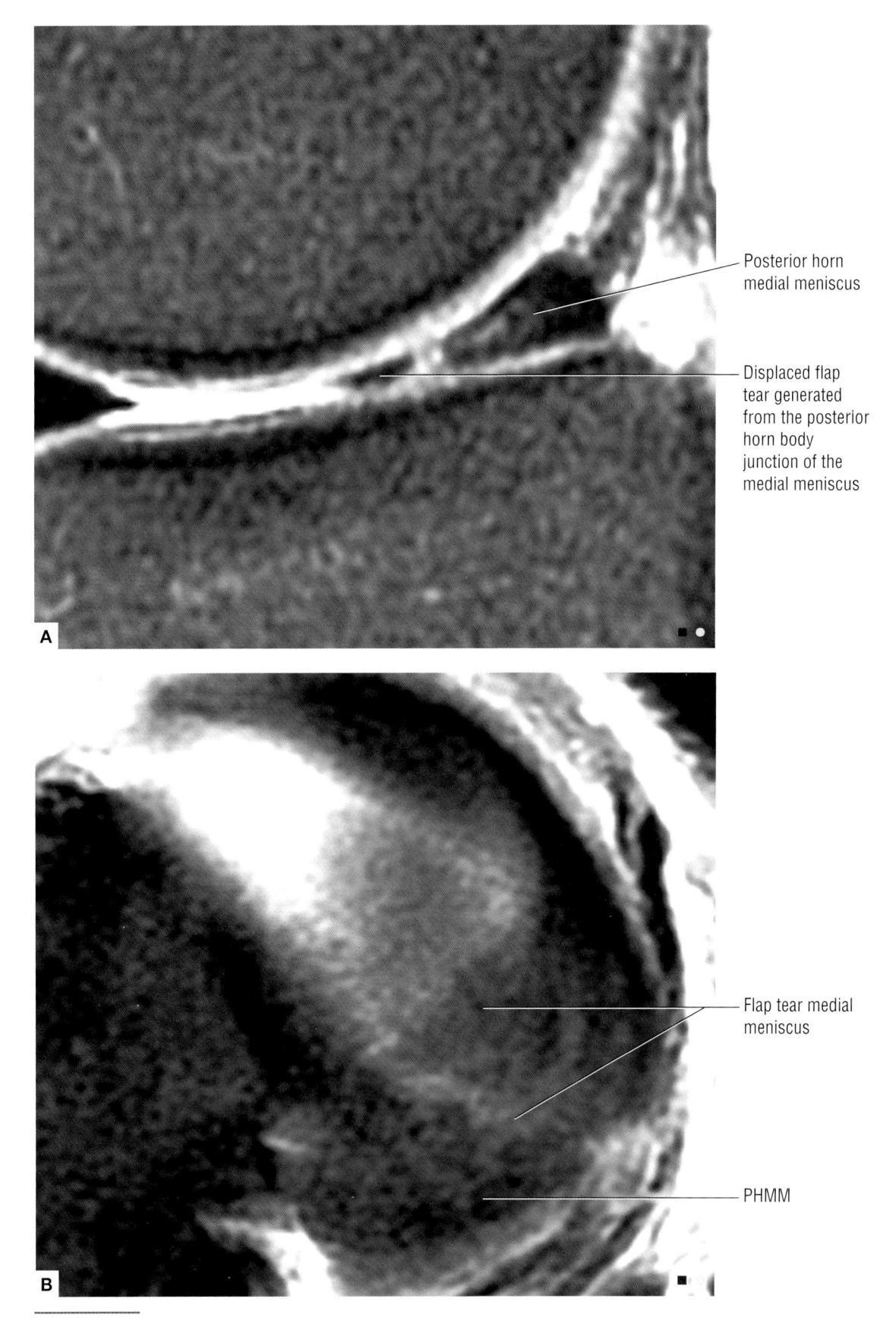

FIGURE 4.99 Flap tear with secondary vertical tear pattern on sagittal image. The tear is prospectively demonstrated on the sagittal image and confirmed with direct visualization of the meniscal surface tear pattern in the axial plane. FS PD FSE sagittal (**A**) and axial (**B**) images.

The Meniscus

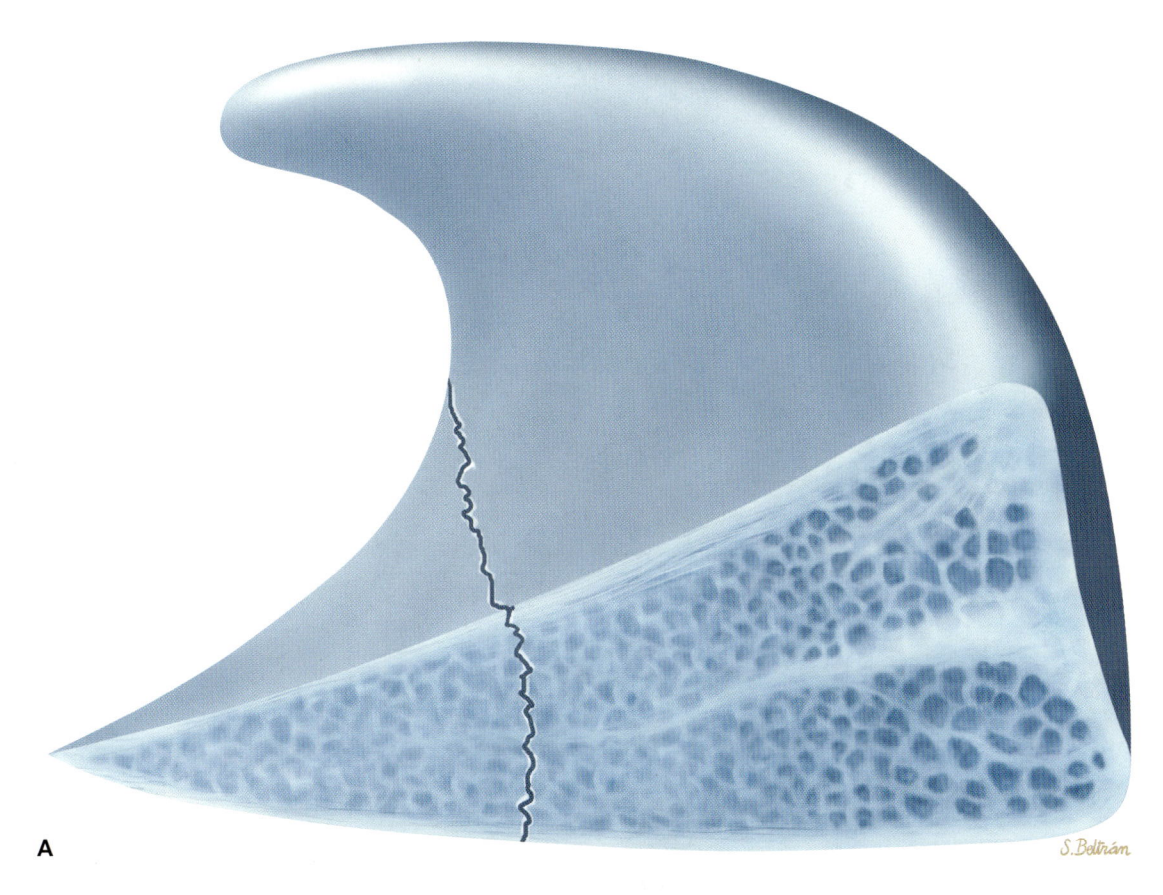

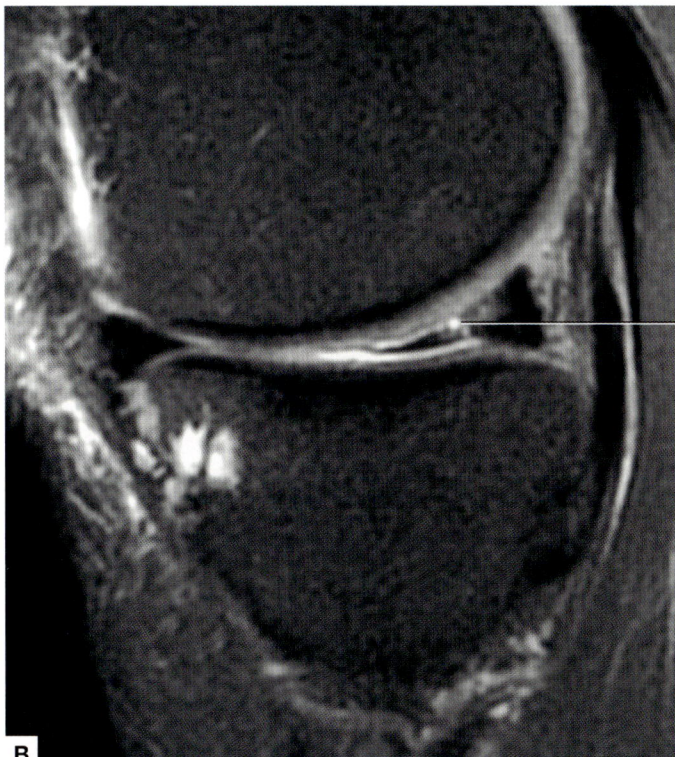

Coapted (nondisplaced) flap tear

FIGURE 4.100 Coapted flap tear with vertical tear morphology involving the inner third of the medial meniscus as seen on a sagittal color illustration with superior and cross-sectional view of the meniscus and flap tear (**A**) and a sagittal FS PD FSE image (**B**).

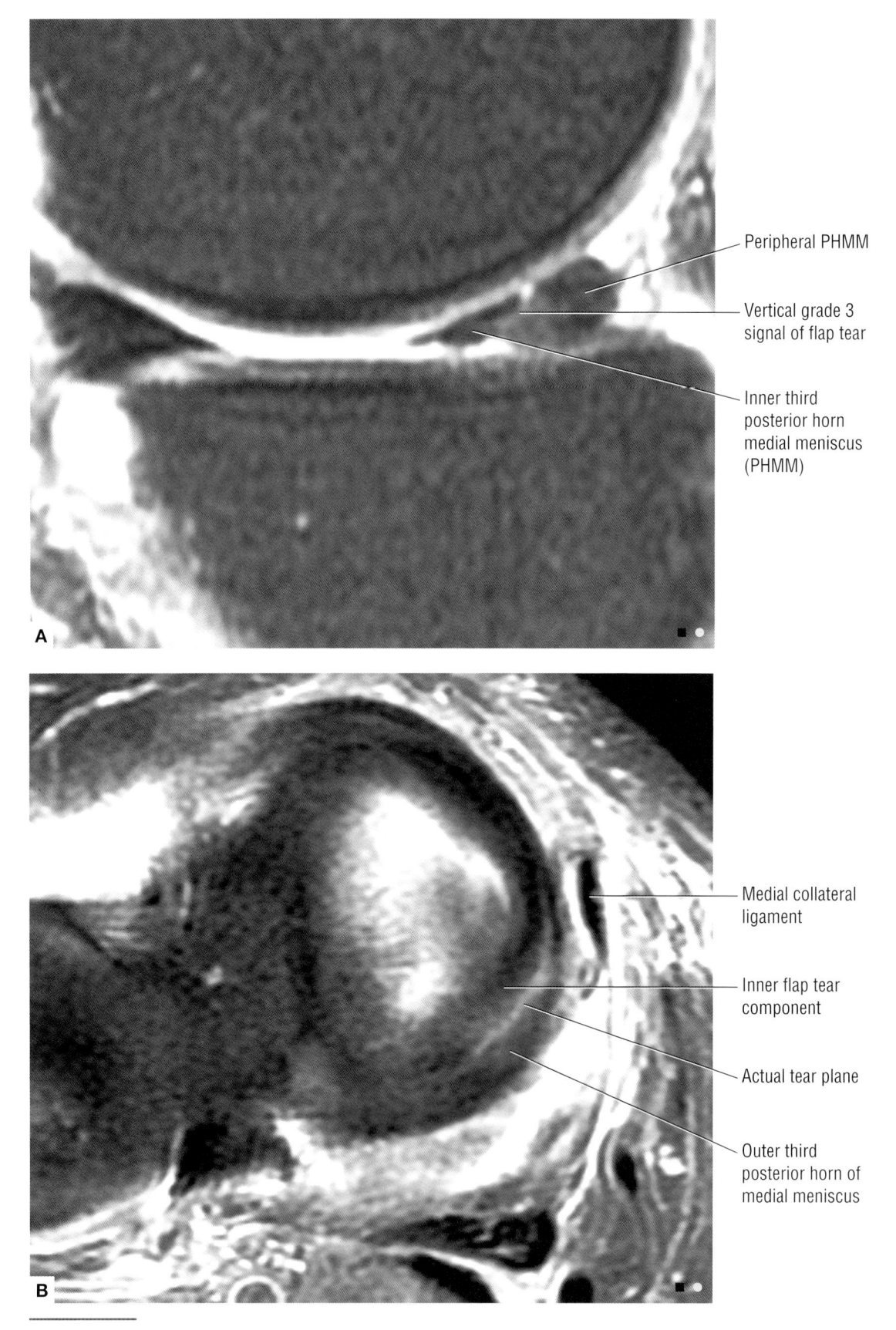

FIGURE 4.101 Flap tear demonstrating relative deficiency of the inner-third inferior surface and secondary vertical component of inner 30% to 40% of the meniscal fibrocartilage. The flap tear always involves the free edge of the meniscus. FS PD FSE sagittal (**A**) and axial images (**B**).

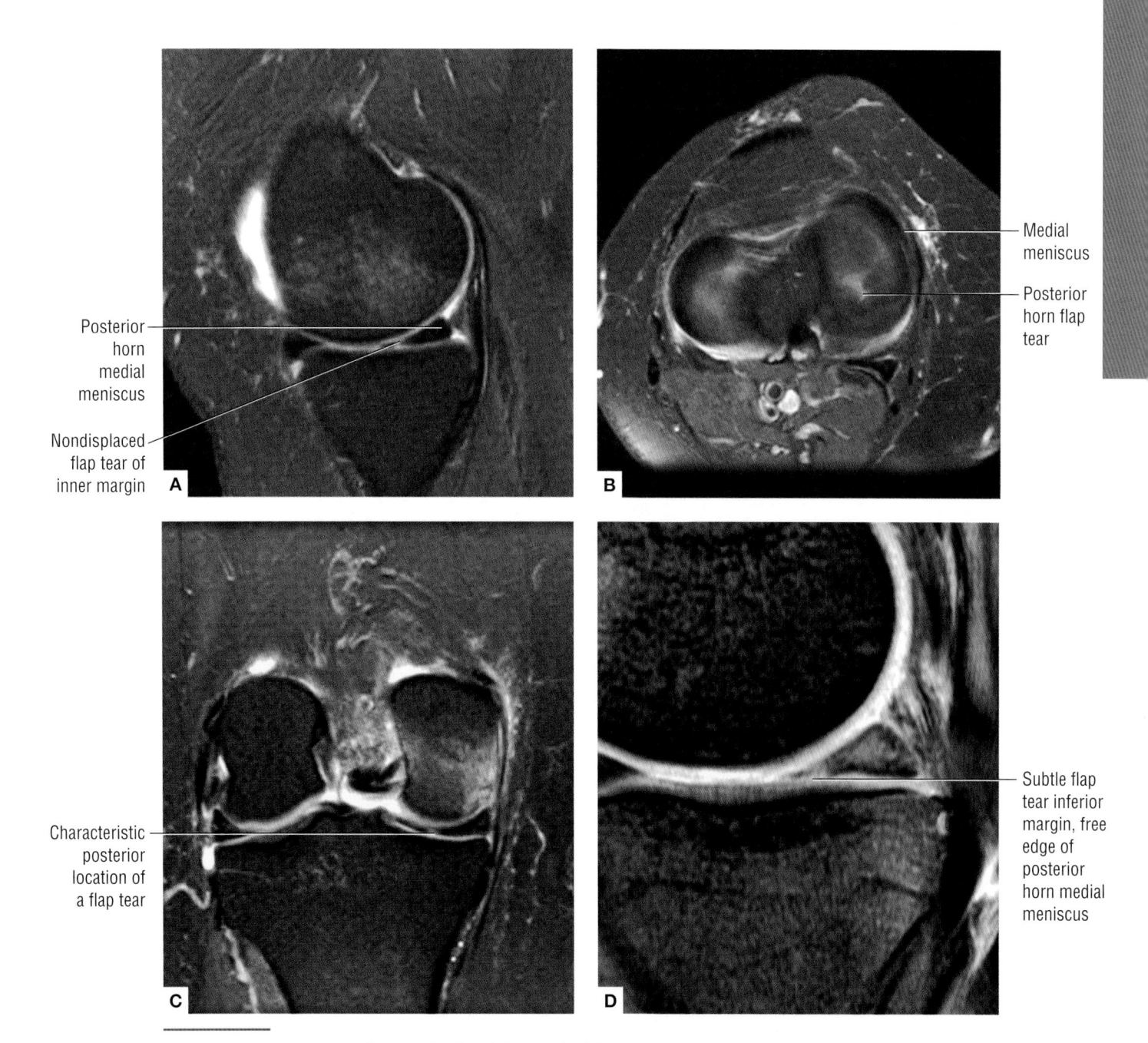

FIGURE 4.102 Coapted or nondisplaced flap tears of the posterior horn medial meniscus. (**A**) Inner margin vertical grade 3 signal intensity is identified in the sagittal plane. (**B**) Direct visualization of flap morphology is demonstrated on this axial image. (**C**) The common location of a flap tear is identified on this posterior coronal image. In comparison, a classic (nonroot) radial tear would be visualized on a more peripheral sagittal image (at the anterior or posterior horn–body junction) and on a coronal image more anterior to the plane of the posterior horn, usually where the condyles fuse. (**D**) Additional flap tear variant limited to the free edge of the meniscus. Although this morphology may be mistaken for meniscal fraying, there is a relative deficiency of the inferior leaf resulting in a small flap tear of the inner margin of the posterior horn.

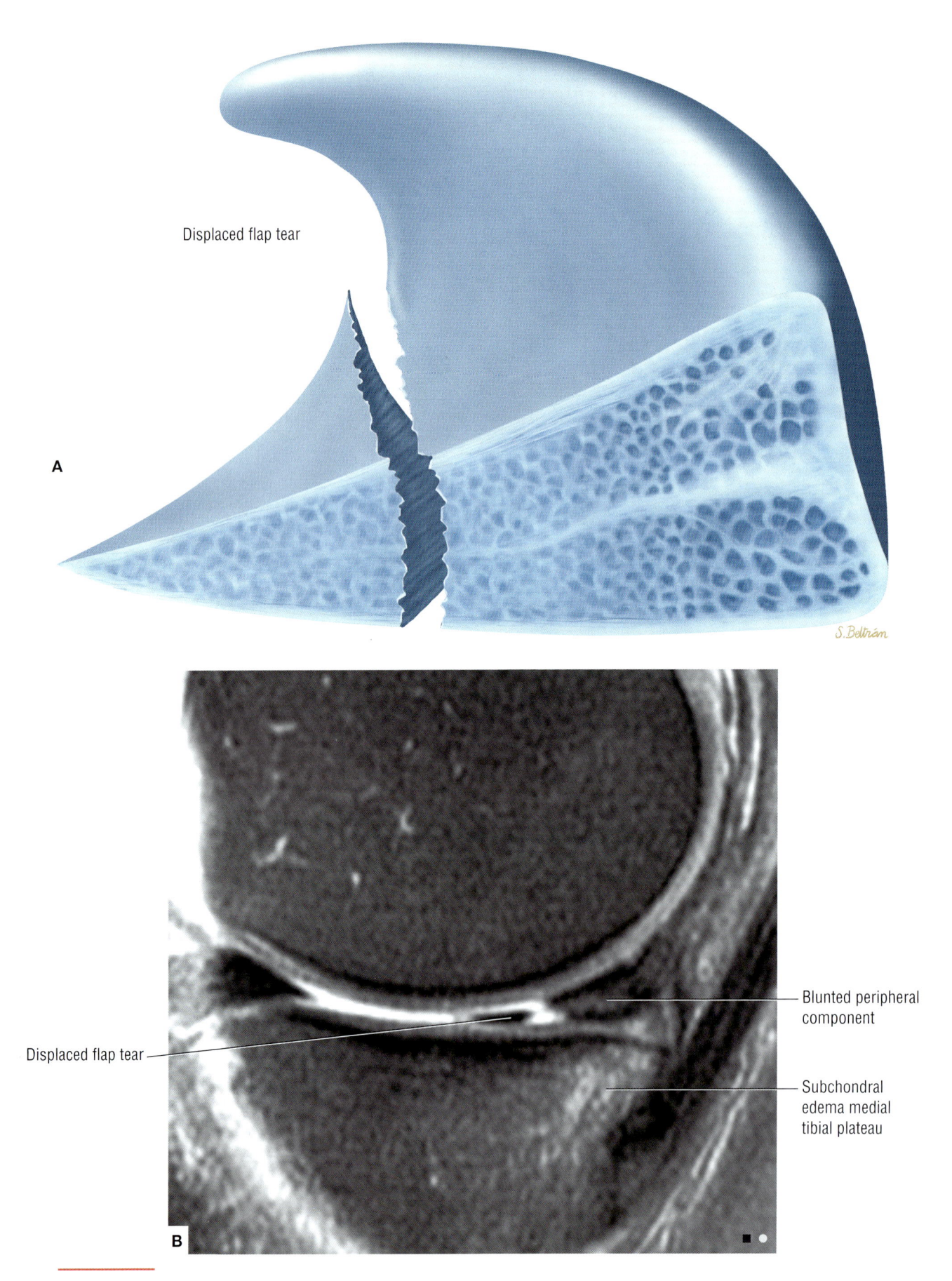

FIGURE 4.103 (**A**) Color sagittal illustration of the superior view of a displaced noncoapted flap tear of the posterior horn of the medial meniscus. (**B**) Displaced flap tear with secondary vertical tear pattern on FS PD FSE sagittal image.

The Meniscus

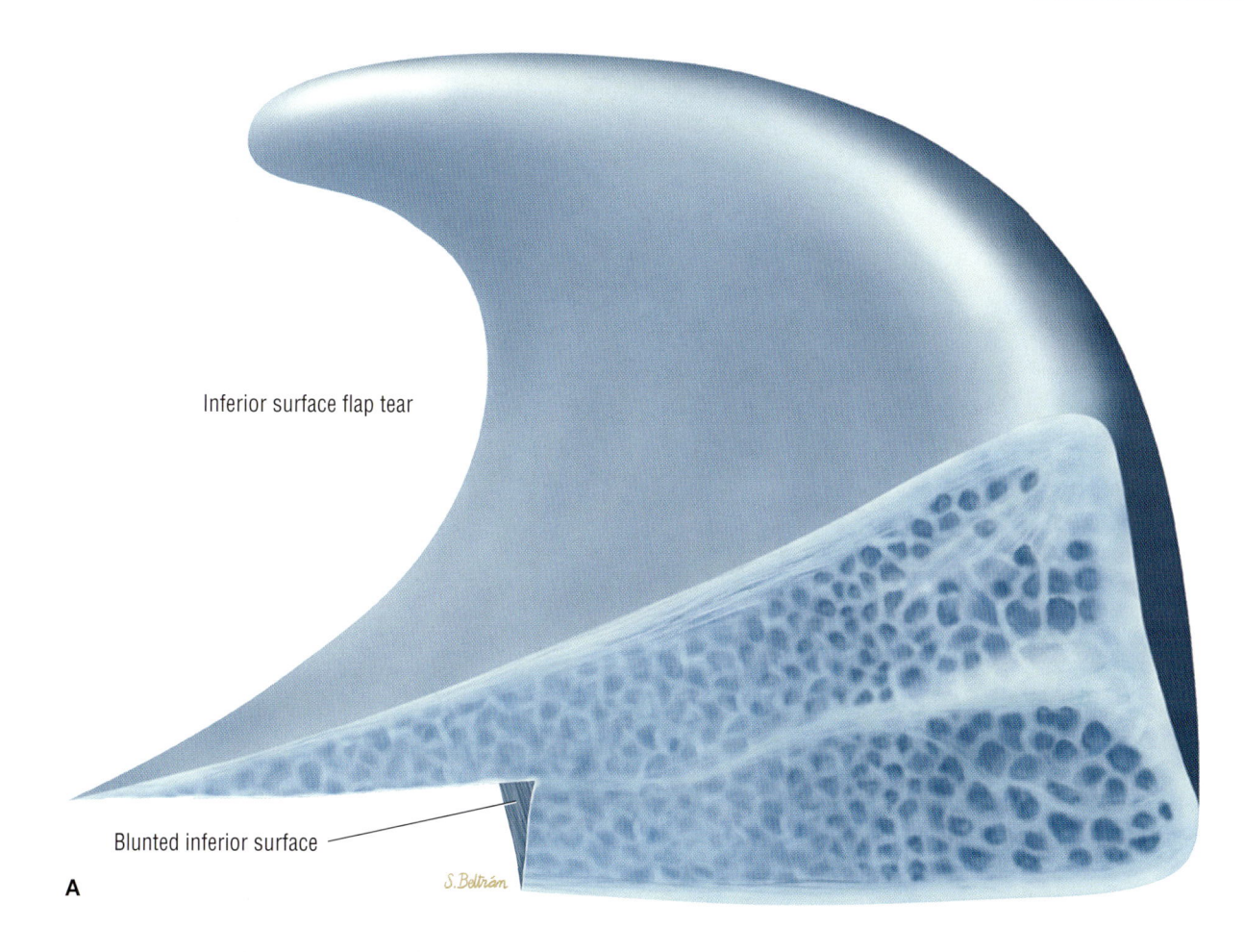

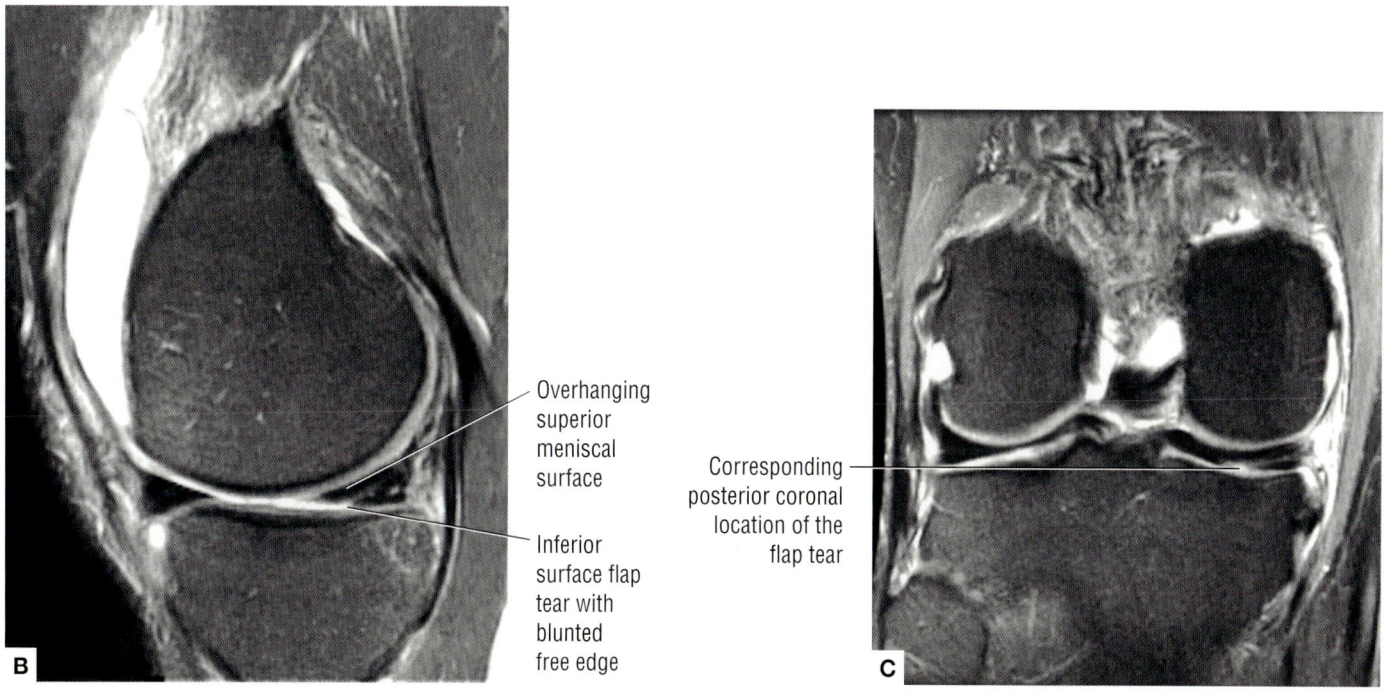

FIGURE 4.104 (**A**) Illustration of inferior surface flap tear subtype. (**B**) Corresponding sagittal FS PD FSE image. (**C**) Foreshortened and blunted inferior leaf is illustrated on a corresponding posterior coronal image. The flap tear pattern is specific on sagittal images, and the posterior coronal image location is confirmatory.

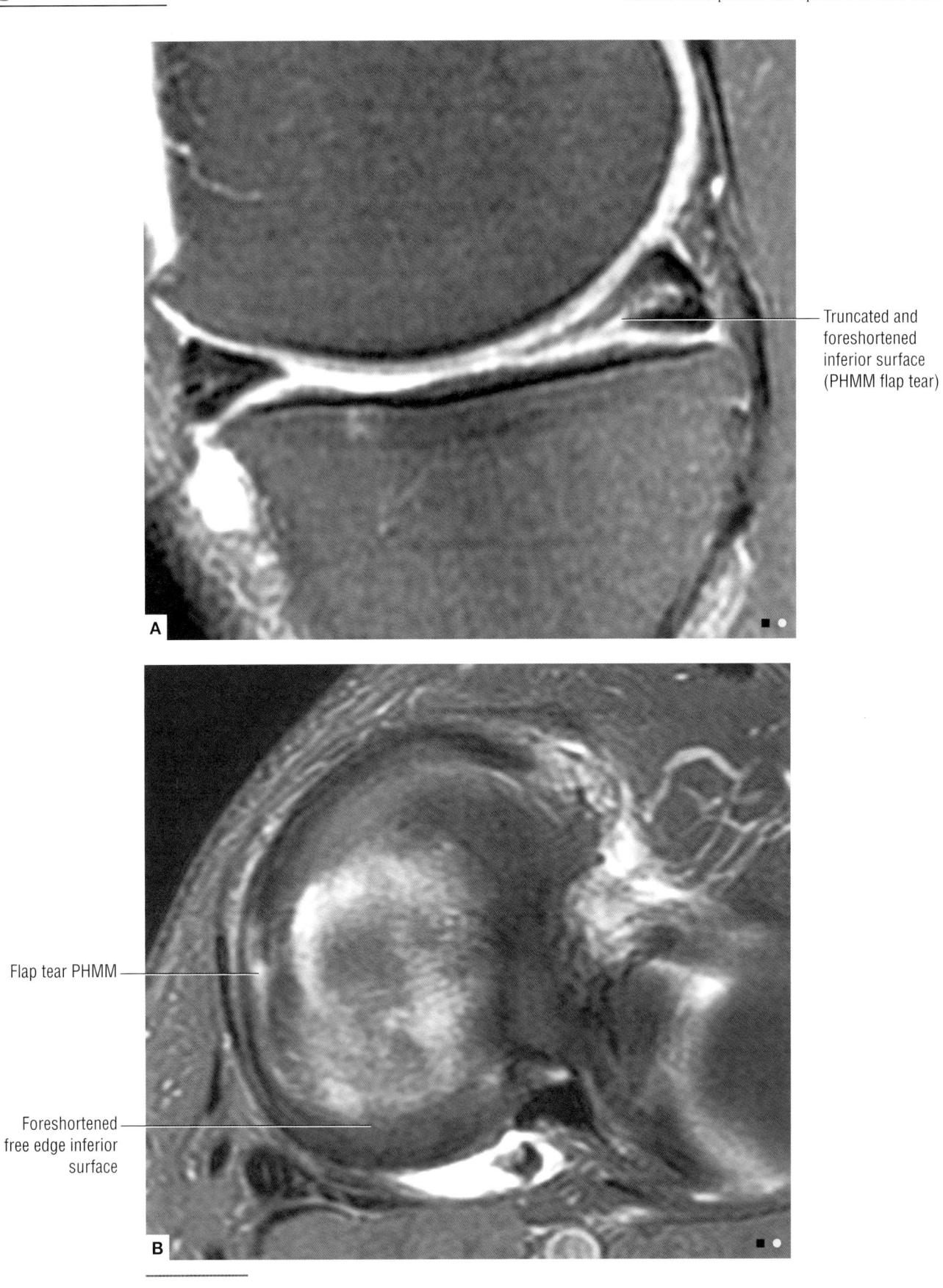

FIGURE 4.105 Flap tear with inferior surface extension. The relative absence of inferior surface meniscal tissue is associated with flap morphology provided there has not been a partial meniscectomy. The medial meniscus tear plane is horizontal oblique in sagittal section. The surface tear pattern is directly visualized as a flap tear with extension to the free edge. FS PD FSE sagittal (**A**) and axial (**B**) images.

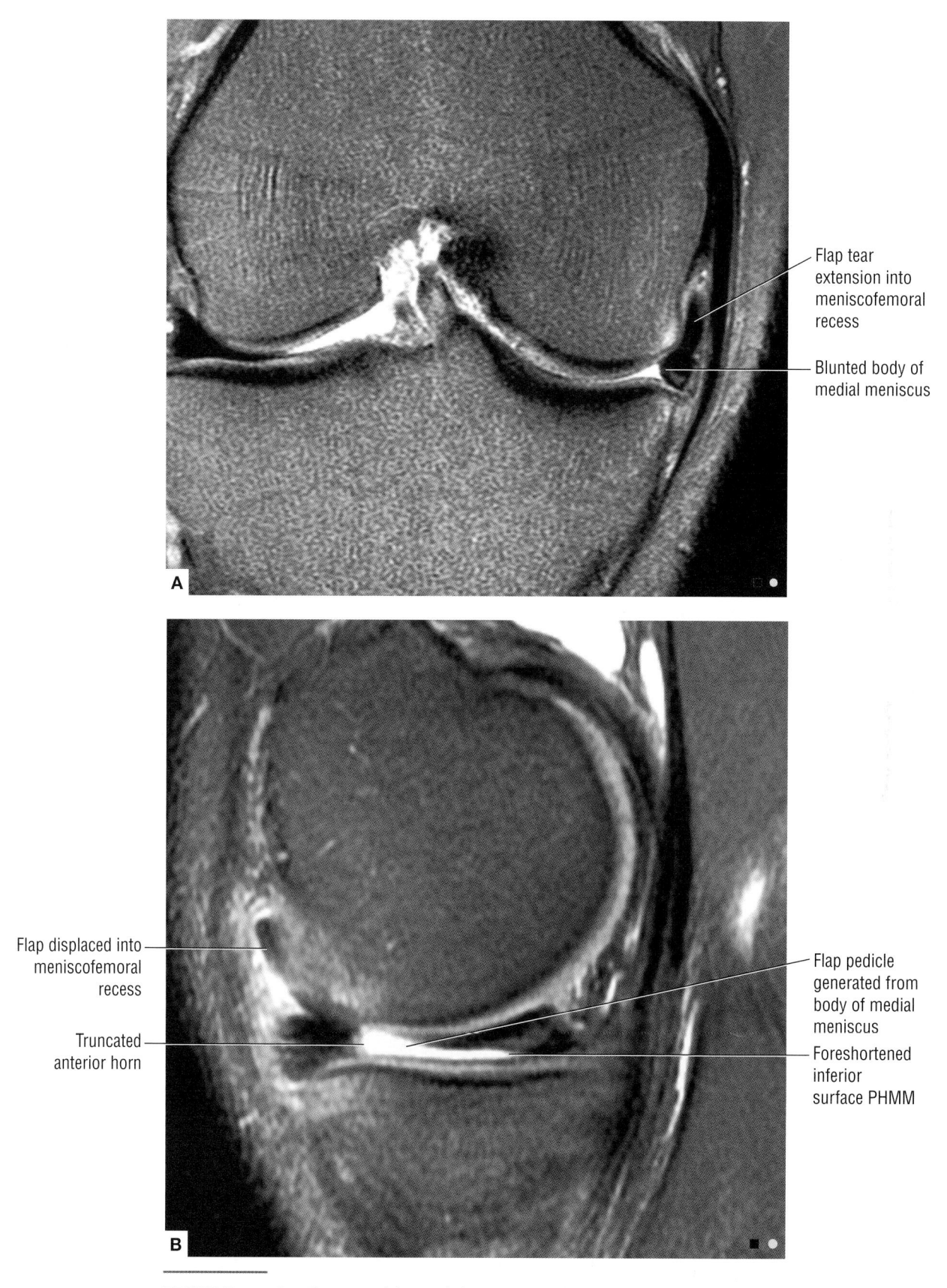

FIGURE 4.106 Flap tear of the medial meniscus with extension into meniscofemoral recess. (**A**) FS PD FSE coronal image. (**B**) FS PD FSE sagittal image.

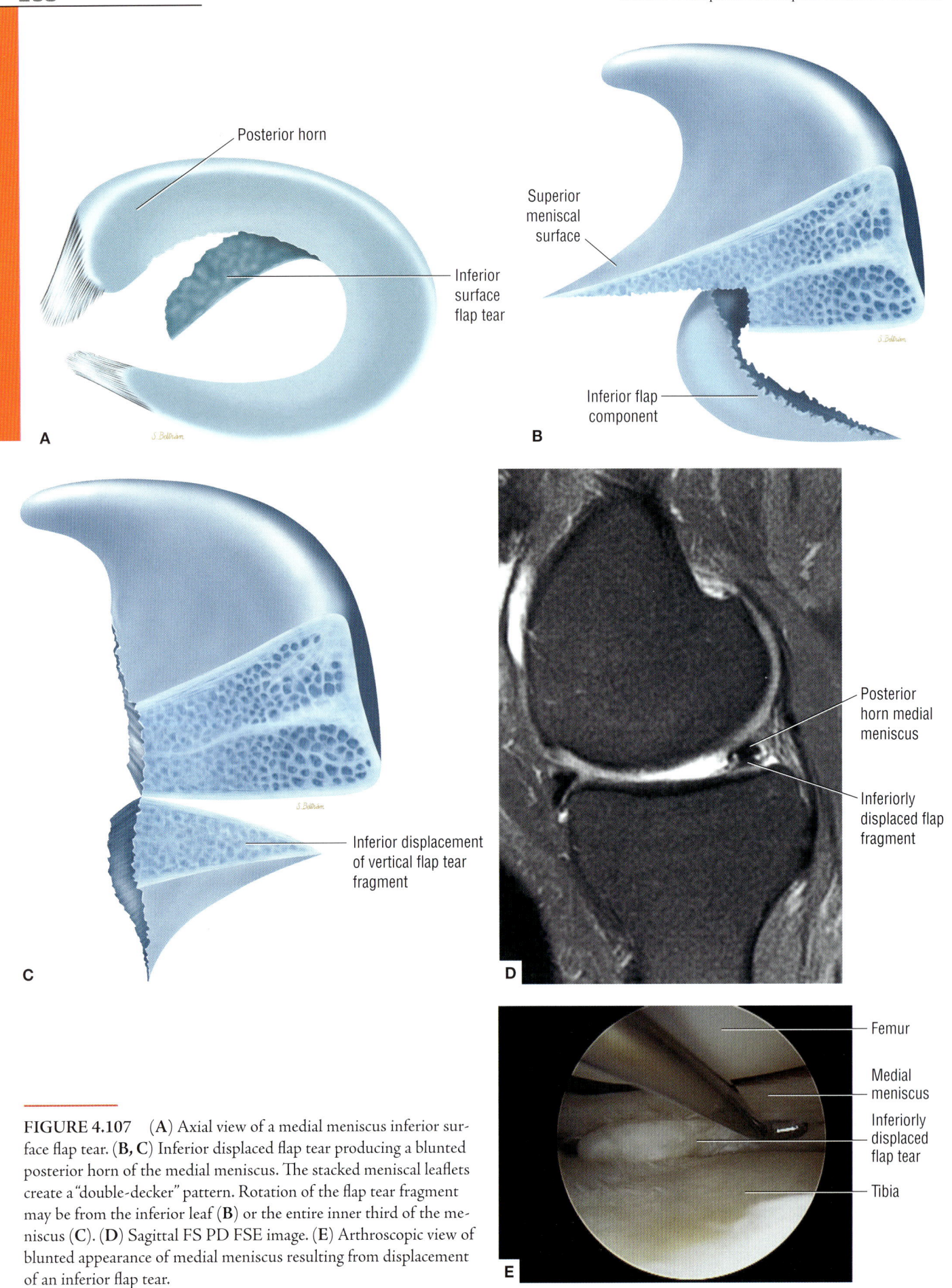

FIGURE 4.107 (**A**) Axial view of a medial meniscus inferior surface flap tear. (**B, C**) Inferior displaced flap tear producing a blunted posterior horn of the medial meniscus. The stacked meniscal leaflets create a "double-decker" pattern. Rotation of the flap tear fragment may be from the inferior leaf (**B**) or the entire inner third of the meniscus (**C**). (**D**) Sagittal FS PD FSE image. (**E**) Arthroscopic view of blunted appearance of medial meniscus resulting from displacement of an inferior flap tear.

The Meniscus   269

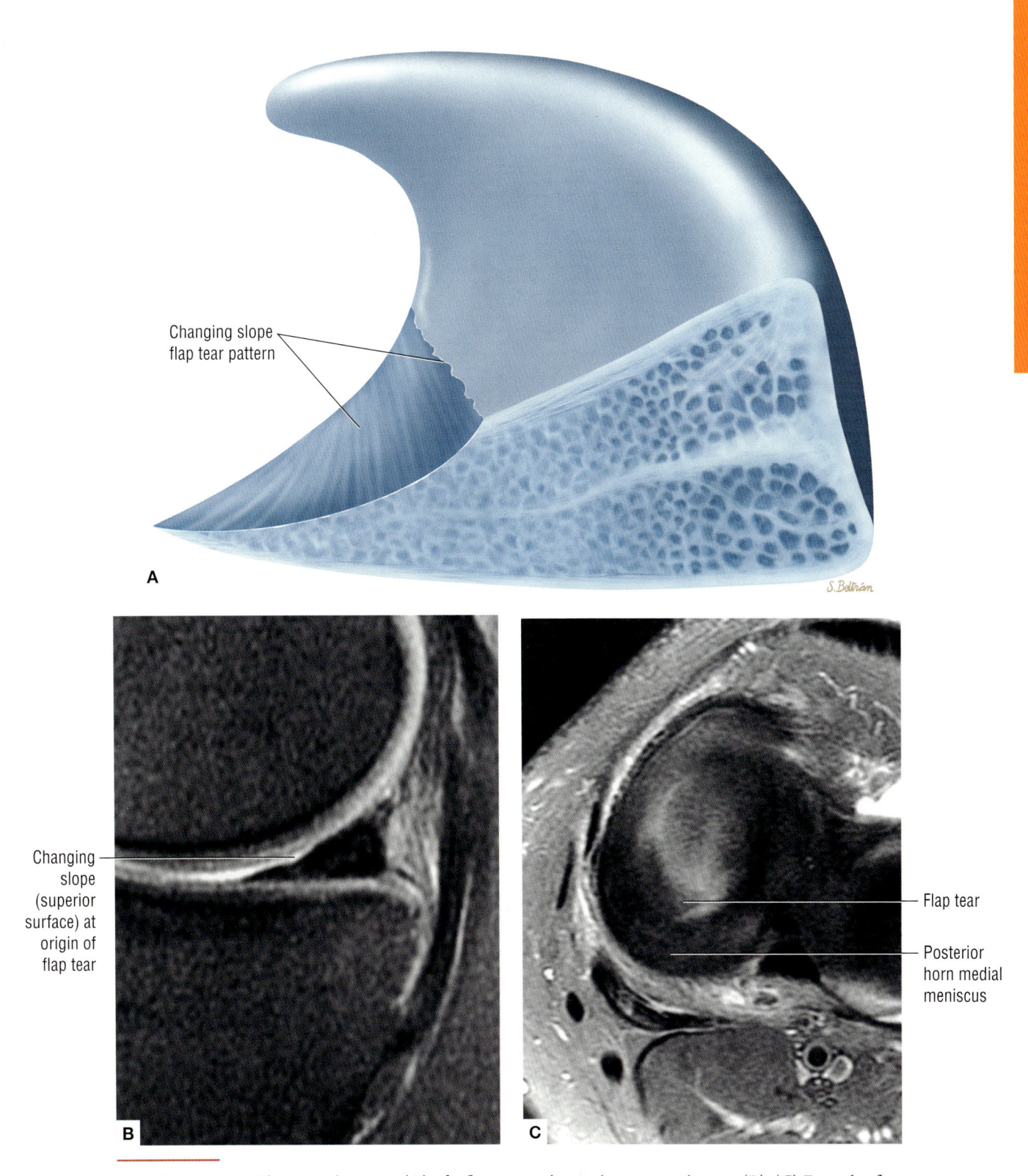

FIGURE 4.108 Changing slope sign (**A**) of a flap tear with correlative sagittal image (**B**). (**C**) Free edge flap component is seen on this corresponding axial image. The nondisplaced component of a flap tear may demonstrate a changing slope contour of its superior surface.

Displaced flap tear posterior notch

Body-posterior horn junction

Subchondral edema medial femoral condyle

Change in slope of superior surface

Inferior surface flap tear donor site

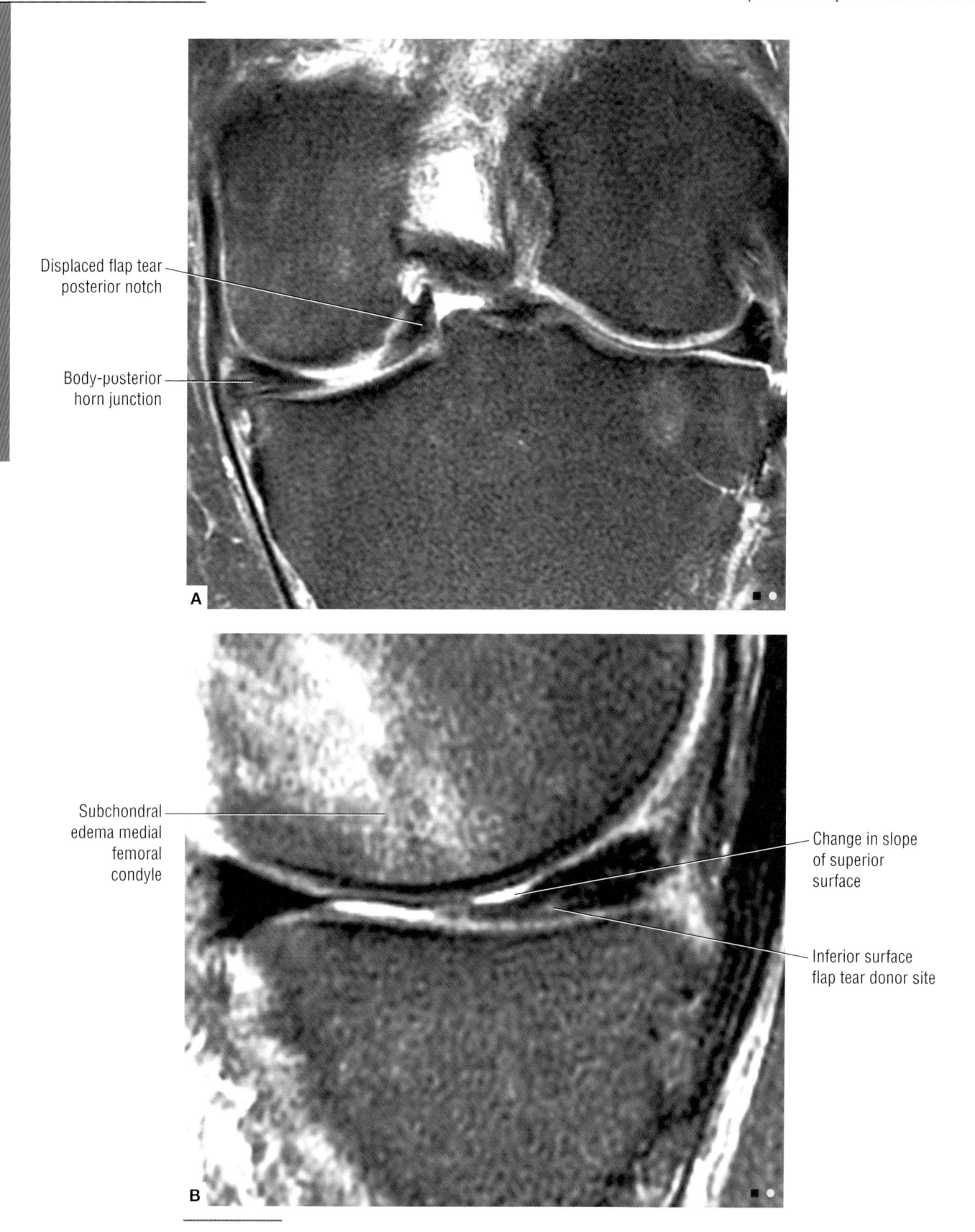

FIGURE 4.109 Central notch displacement of a medial meniscus flap tear on a posterior coronal image (**A**). This is not a bucket-handle tear since there was not anterior extension of the tear. Flap tears may demonstrate a changing slope of the meniscal surface (**B**). FS PD FSE coronal (**A**) and sagittal (**B**) images.

The Meniscus 271

FIGURE 4.110 Separation of a displaced medial meniscus flap fragment with inferior displacement into coronary recess on color coronal section.

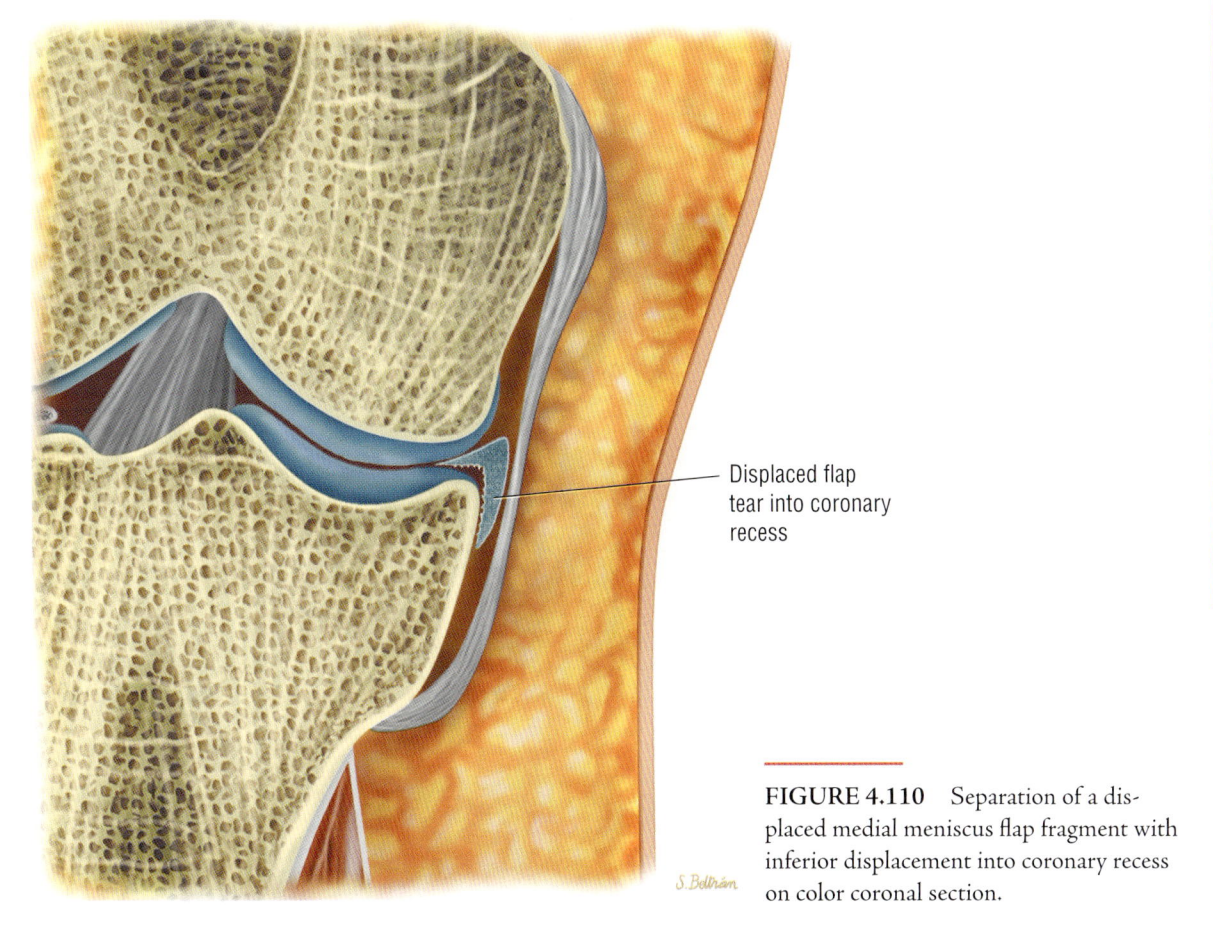

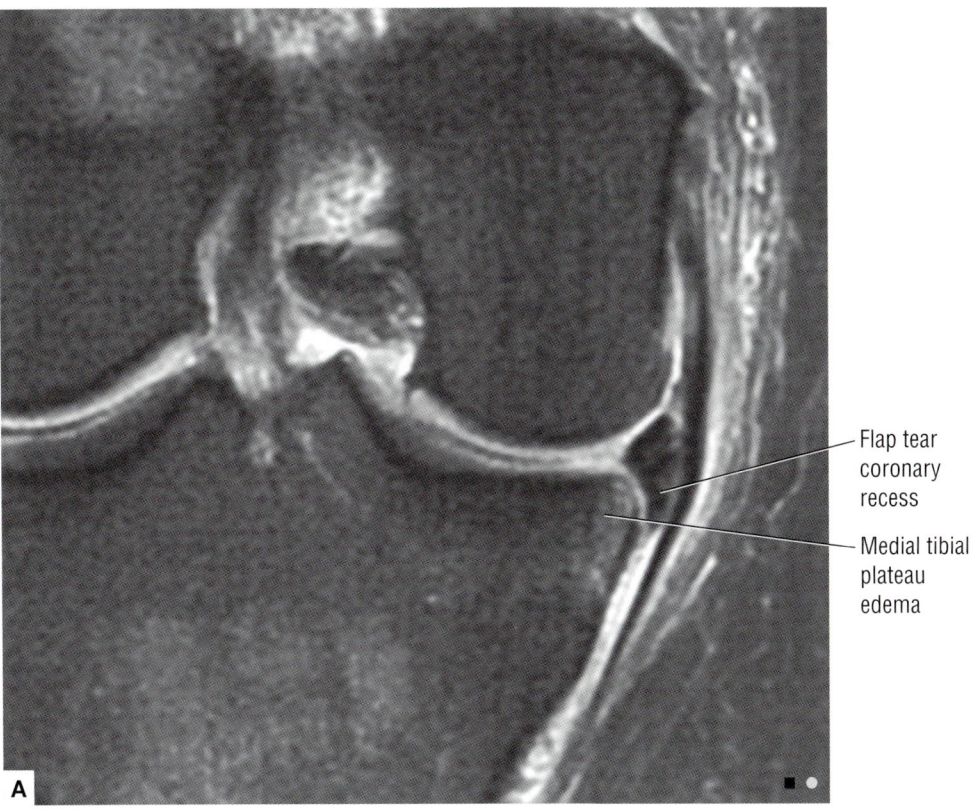

FIGURE 4.111 Meniscotibial displaced flap fragment originating from the body/posterior horn of the medial meniscus. The flap displaces or pivots from the central third of the body segment to the anterior aspect of the coronary recess. FS PD FSE coronal (**A**) (*Continued*)

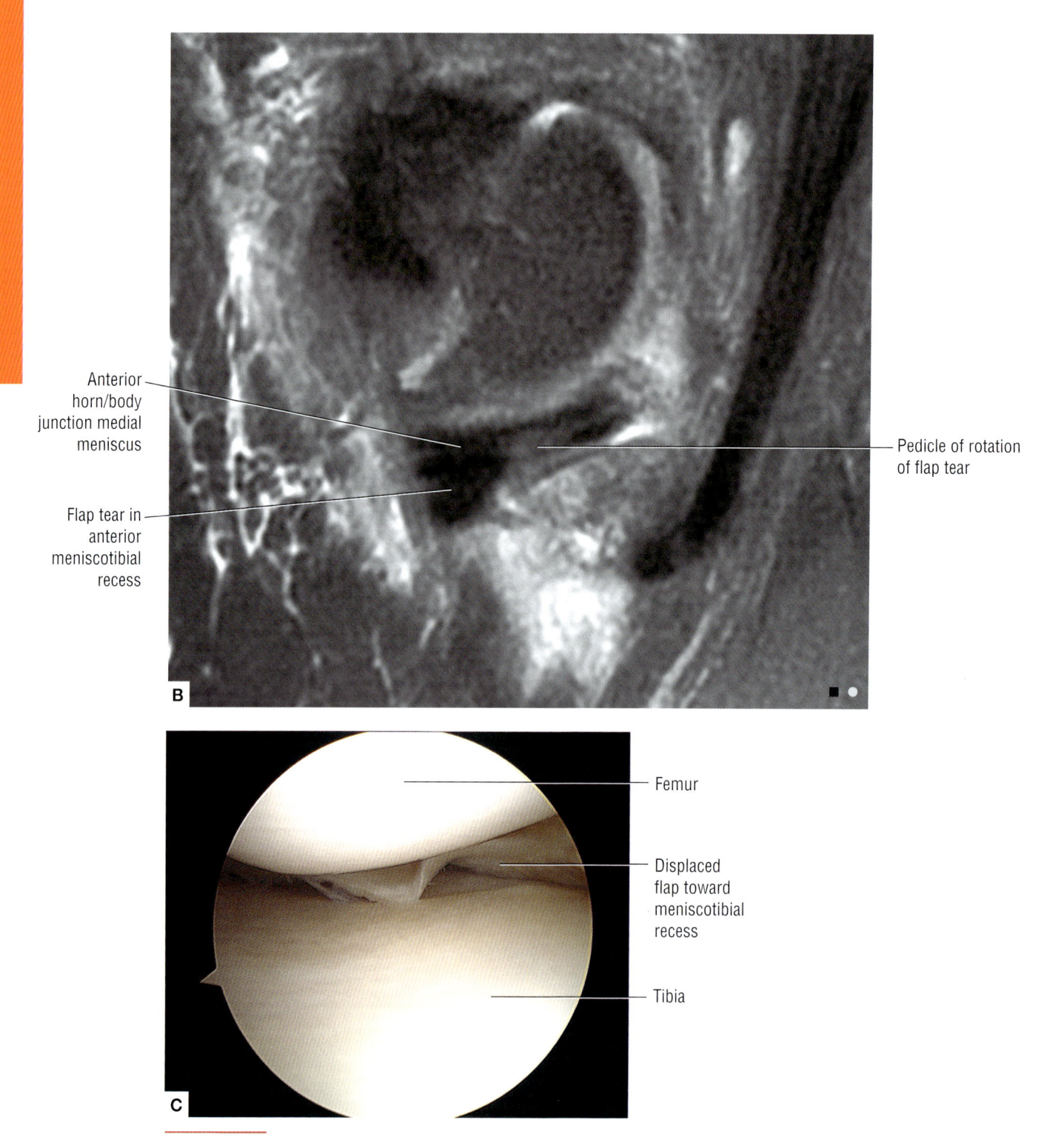

FIGURE 4.111 (*Continued*) and sagittal (**B**) images. (**C**) Arthroscopic view of a hidden flap tear showing a rolled appearance in the posterior horn as the flap fragment displaces into the meniscotibial recess.

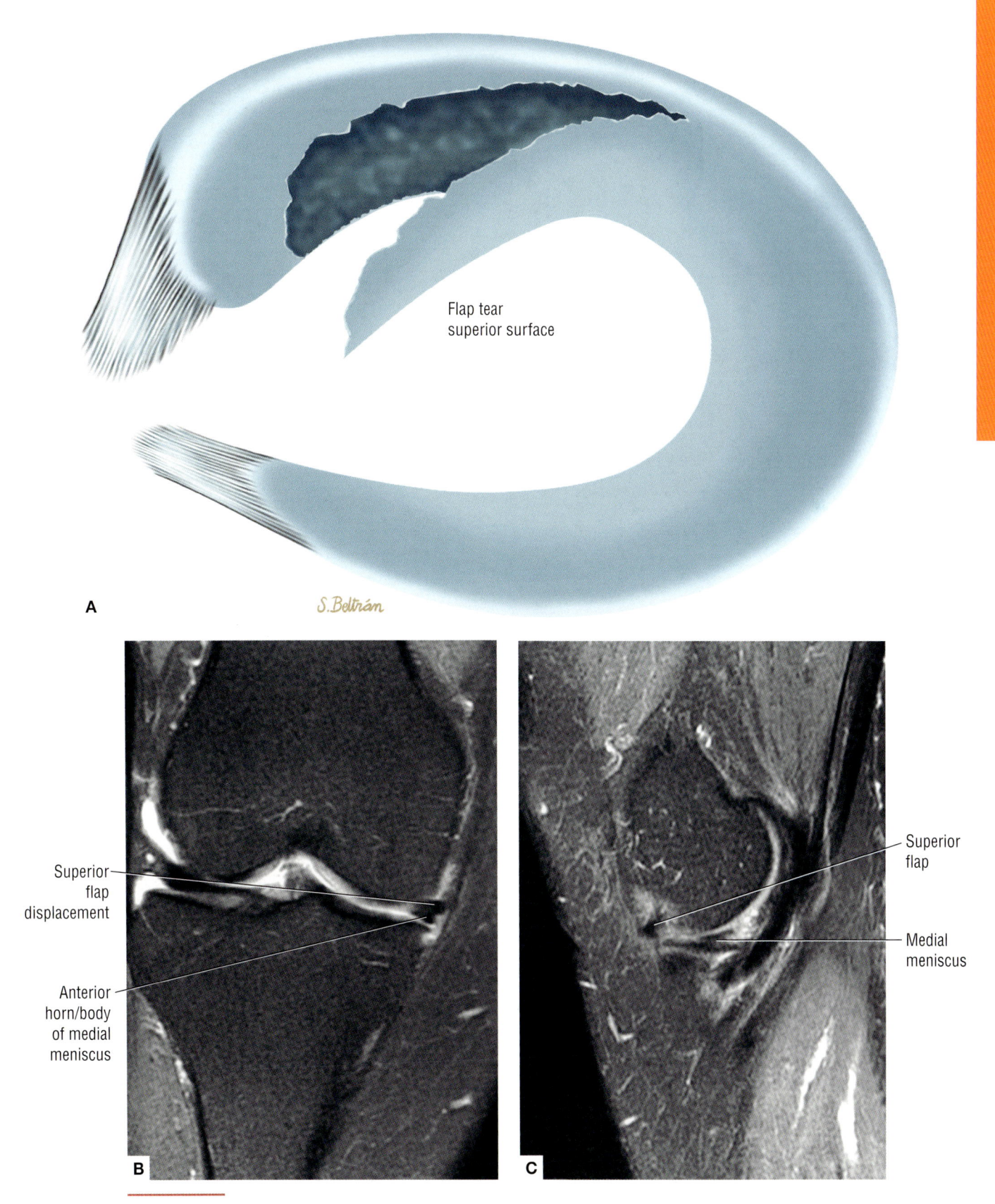

FIGURE 4.112 Superior flap rotation (**A**) producing the "double-decker" morphology of the medial meniscus in the coronal plane (**B**). Anterior displacement of the superior flap is best identified on the corresponding FS PD FSE sagittal image (**C**).

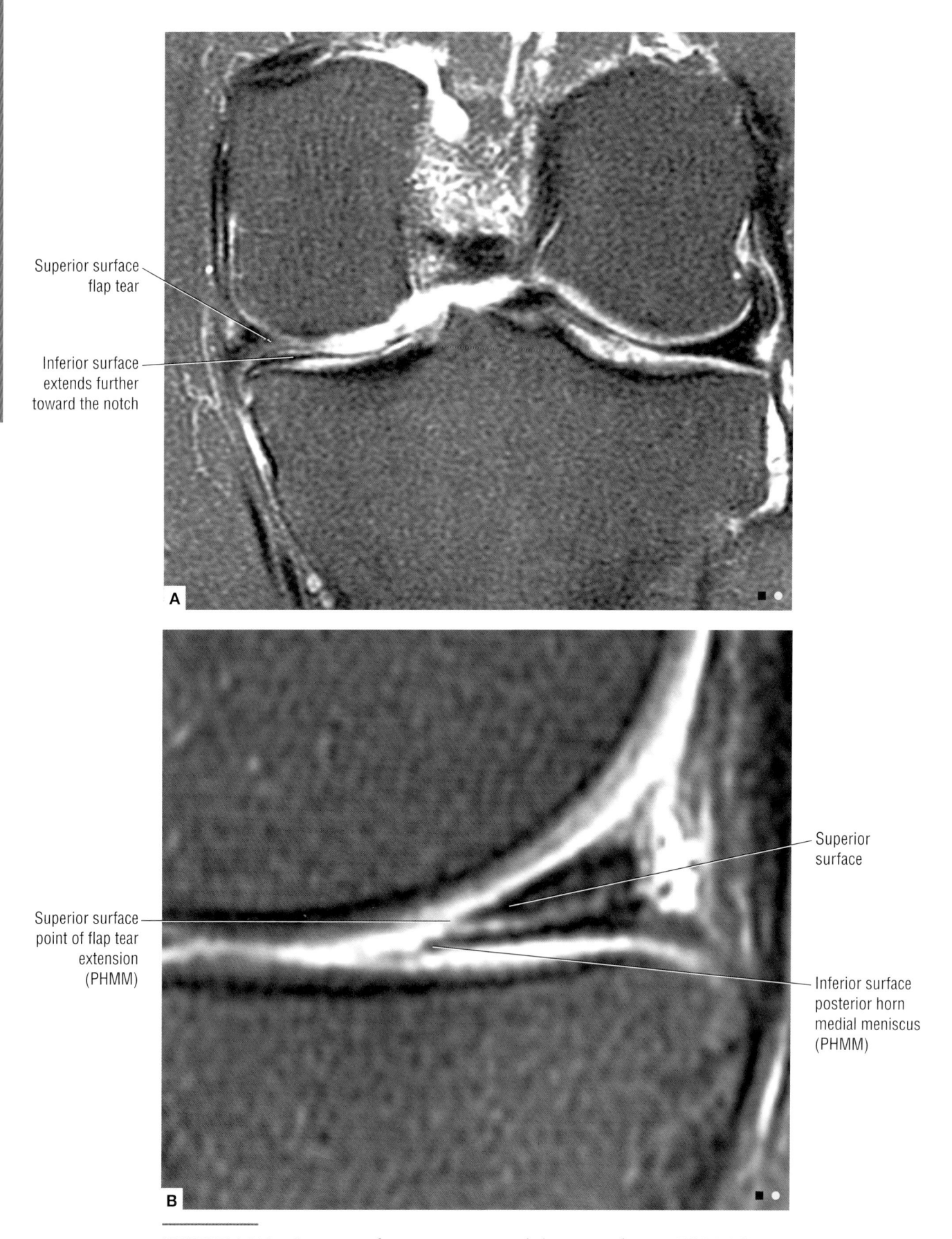

FIGURE 4.113 Superior surface extension in a medial meniscus flap tear. FS PD FSE coronal (**A**) and sagittal (**B**) images.

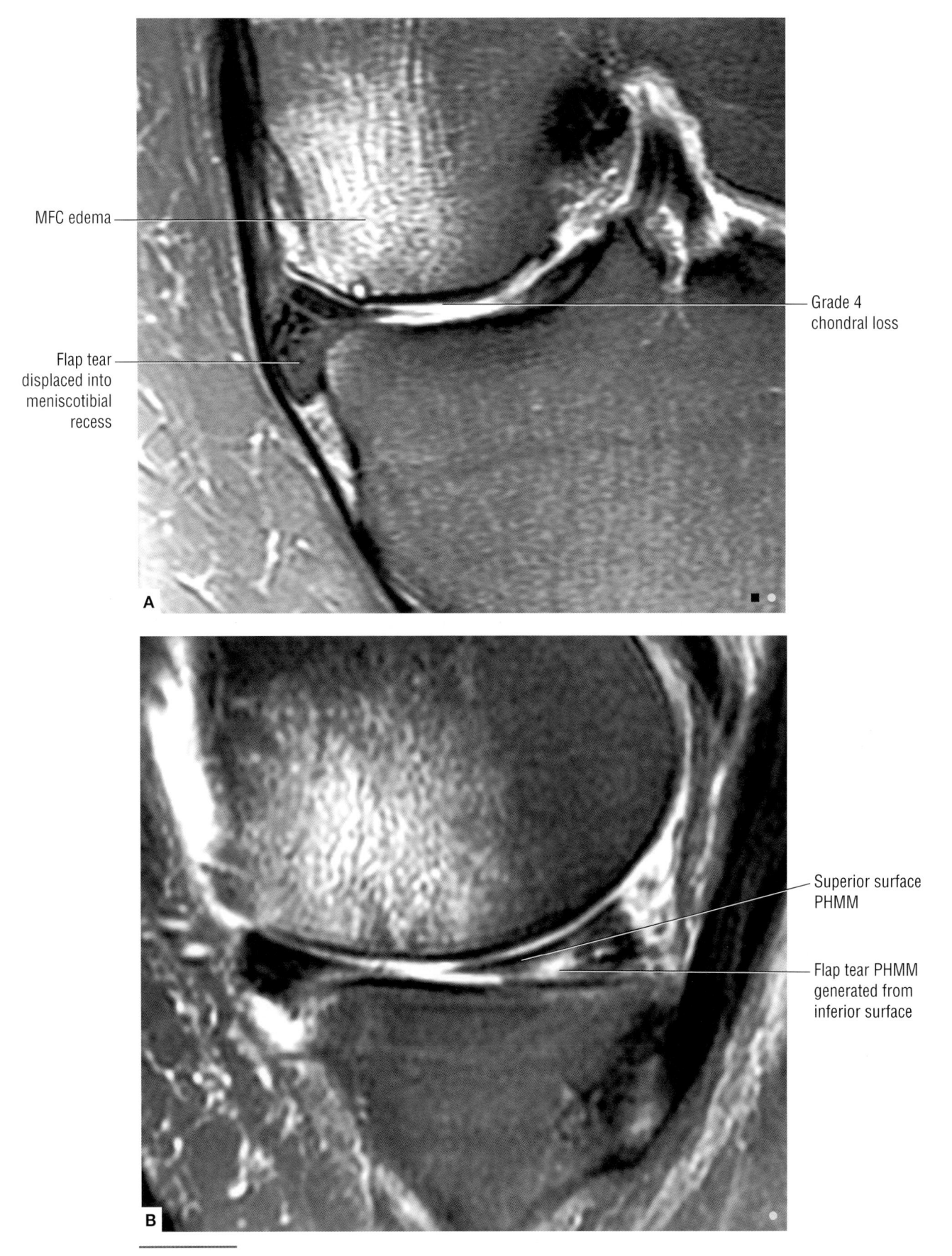

FIGURE 4.114 Coronary recess or meniscotibial displacement of a flap tear involving the body/posterior horn medial meniscus. FS PD FSE coronal (**A**) and sagittal (**B**) images.

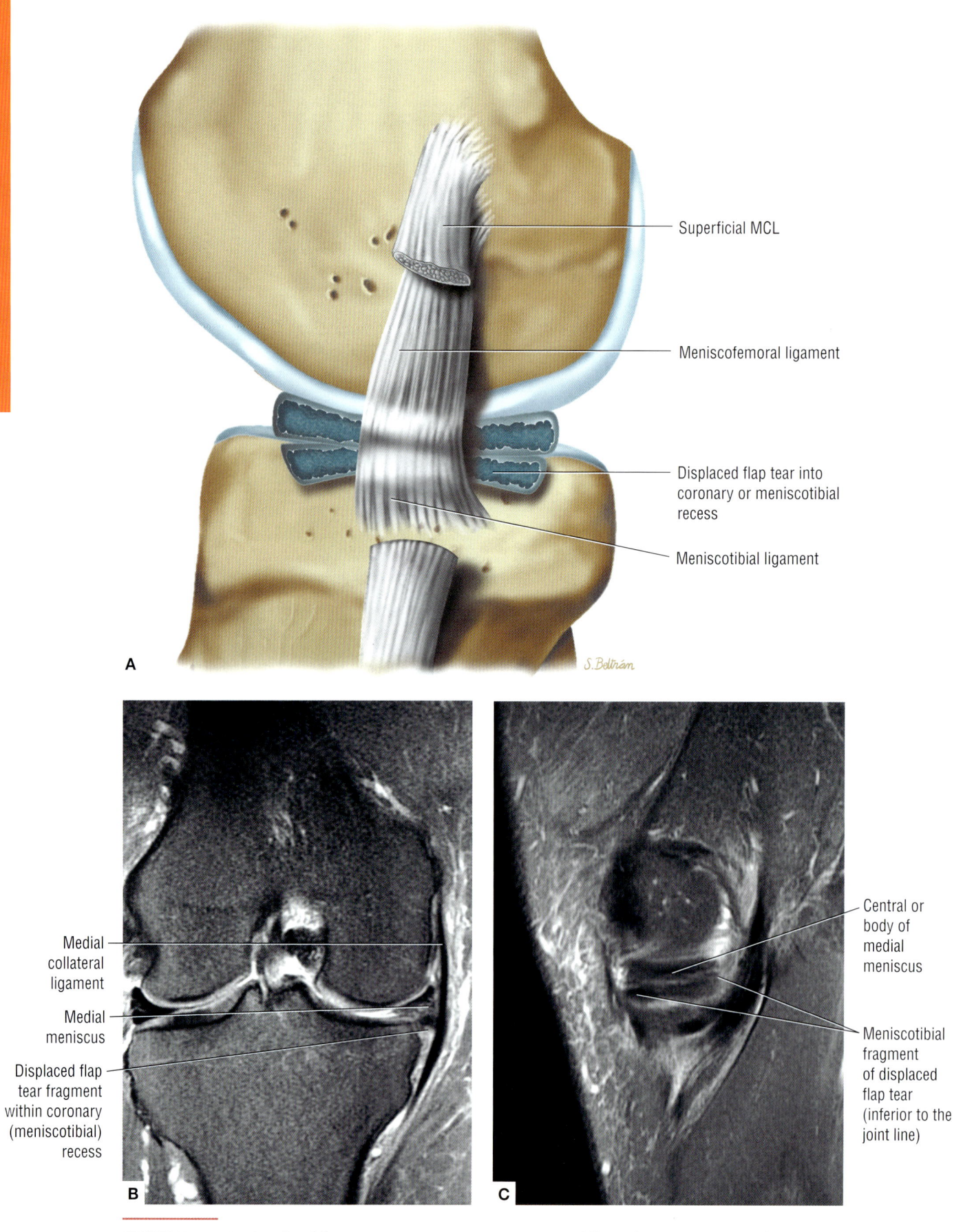

FIGURE 4.115 Displaced flap tear into coronary recess on sagittal (lateral) color illustration (**A**), FS PD FSE coronal image (**B**), and sagittal image (**C**).

The Meniscus

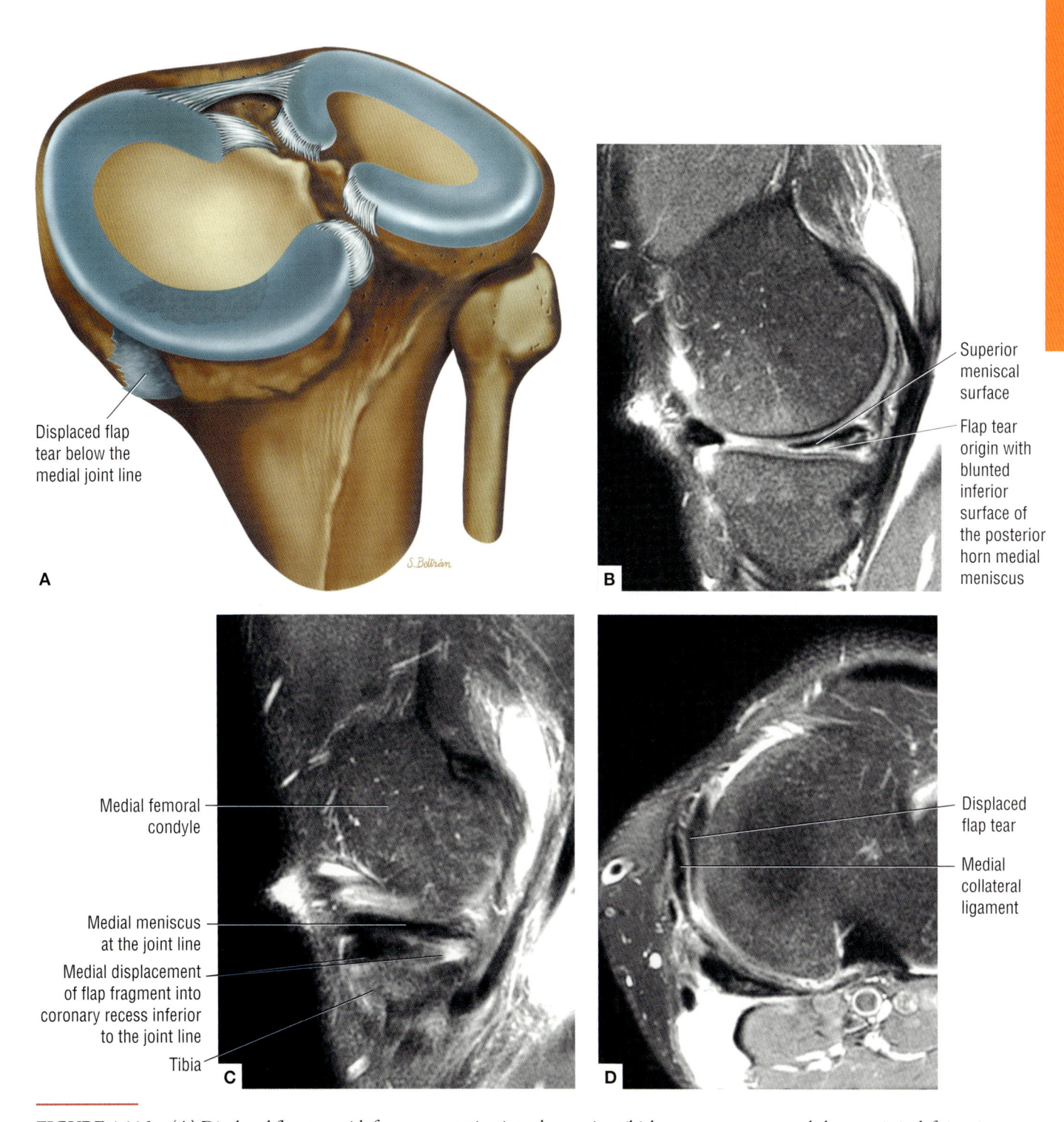

FIGURE 4.116 (**A**) Displaced flap tear with fragment rotation into the meniscotibial or coronary recess and characteristic deficient inner margin or inferior leaf on color illustration. (**B**) The superior medial perspective is shown on this sagittal image. Meniscal extrusion with inferior displacement of the flap can be seen on corresponding sagittal (**C**) and axial (**D**) images.

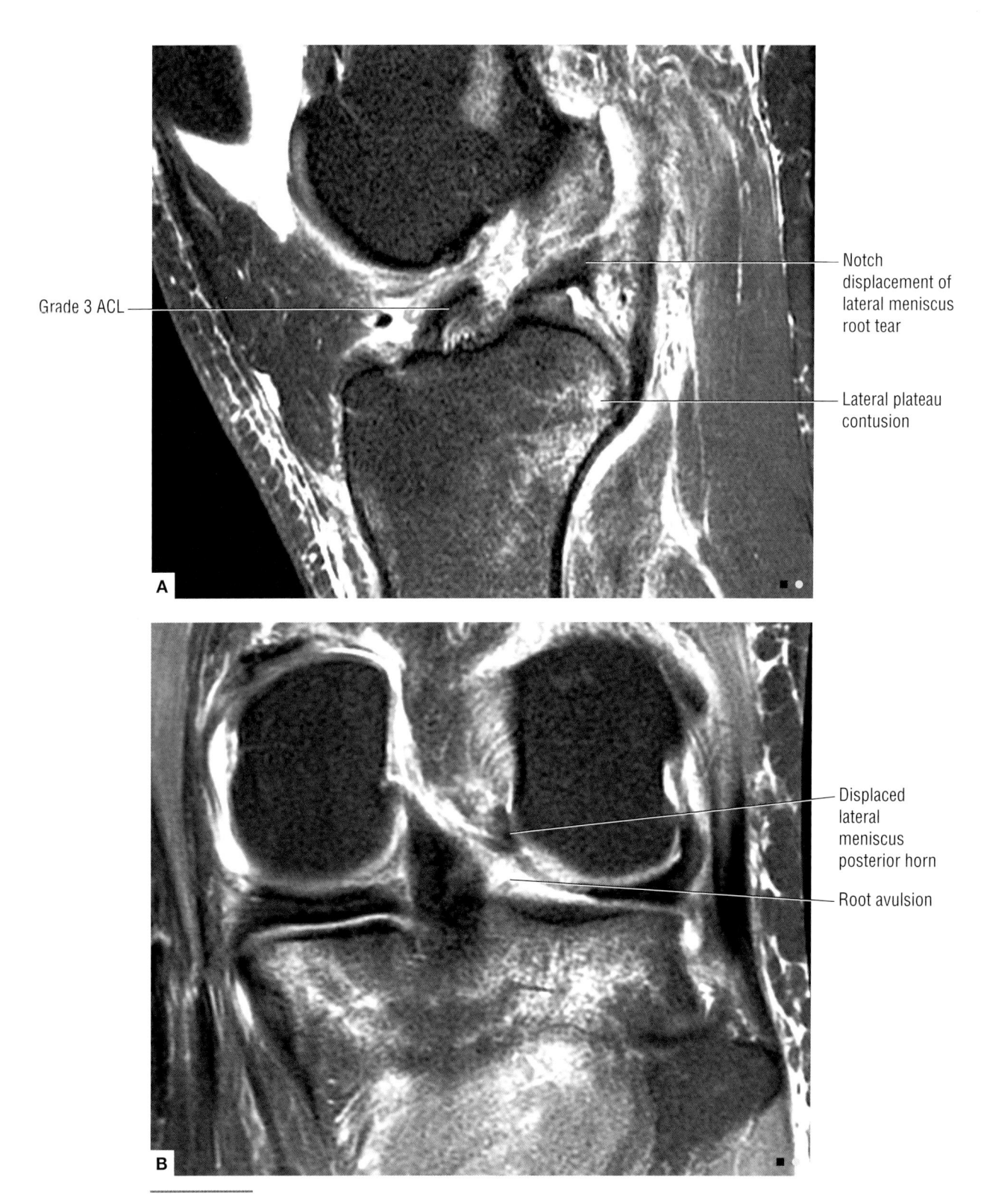

FIGURE 4.117 Displaced lateral meniscus root tear associated with a grade 3 ACL tear. FS PD FSE sagittal (**A**) and coronal (**B**) images.

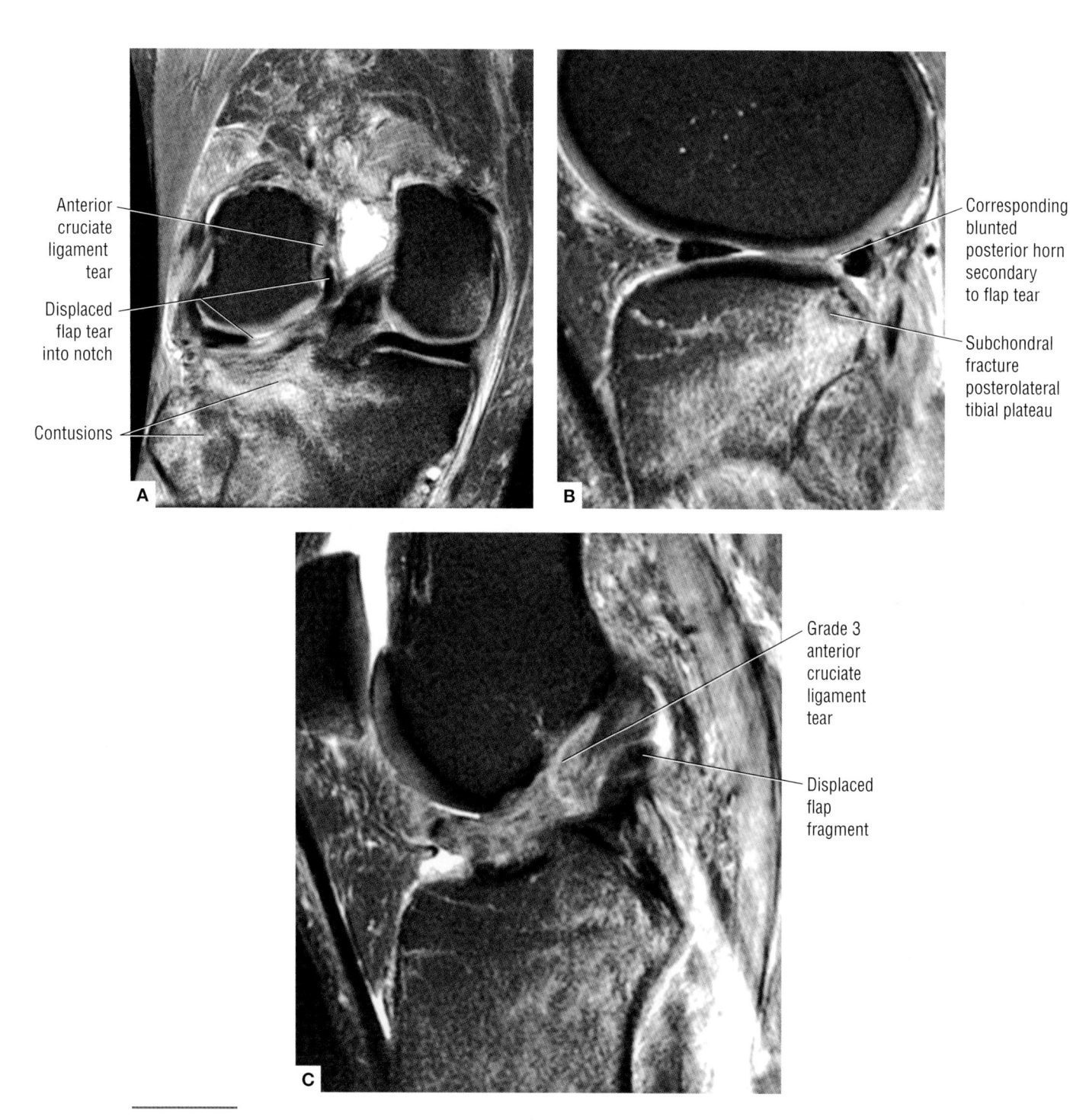

FIGURE 4.118 Displaced flap tear associated with ACL disruption. The posterior horn fragment is displaced into the posterior intercondylar notch posterior to the ACL. ACL-associated flap tears result from combined radial and longitudinal tear components. There is extension of the tear adjacent to the lateral meniscus root. (**A**) Coronal FS PD FSE image. (**B, C**) Sagittal FS PD FSE images.

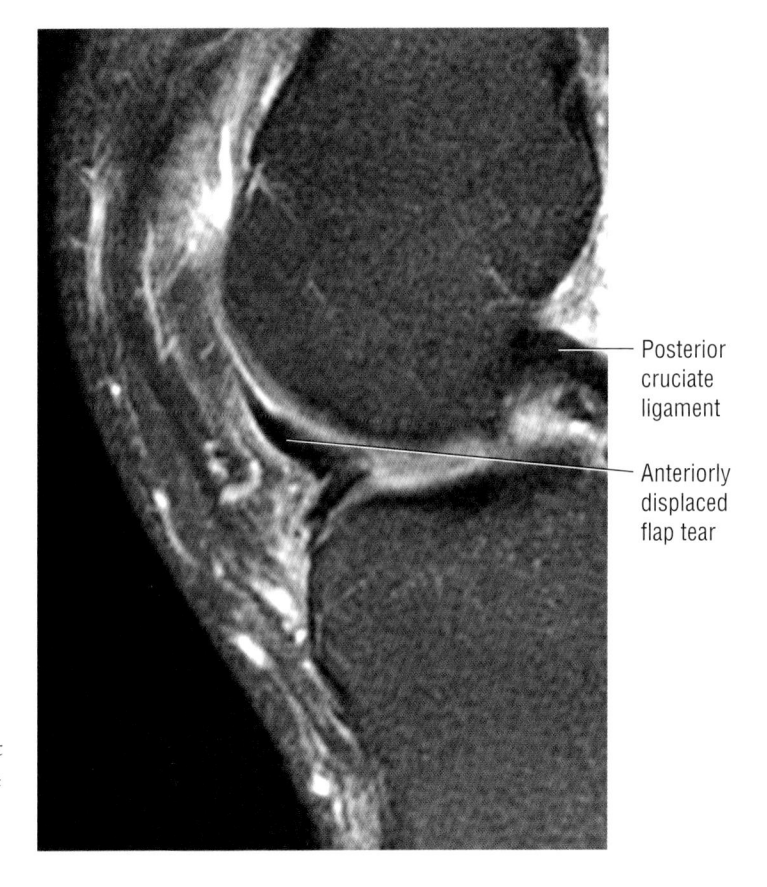

FIGURE 4.119 Flap tear variant with vertical superior folding of the anterior fragment (sagittal FS PD FSE image).

- Posterior cruciate ligament
- Anteriorly displaced flap tear

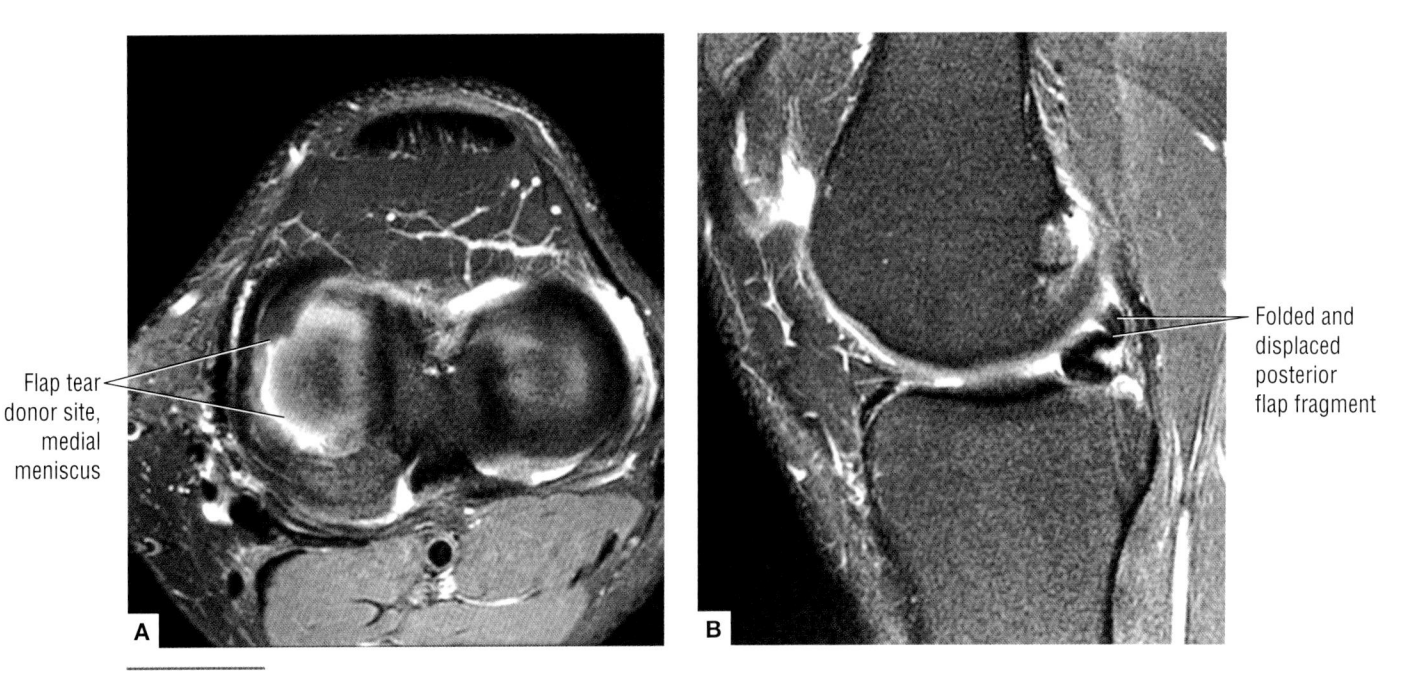

FIGURE 4.120 Flap tear variant involving the body and posterior horn producing vertical superior folding of the rotated flap fragments (the reverse S sign of a complex flap tear). (**A**) Axial FS PD FSE image. (**B**) Sagittal FS PD FSE image.

- Flap tear donor site, medial meniscus
- Folded and displaced posterior flap fragment

The Meniscus 281

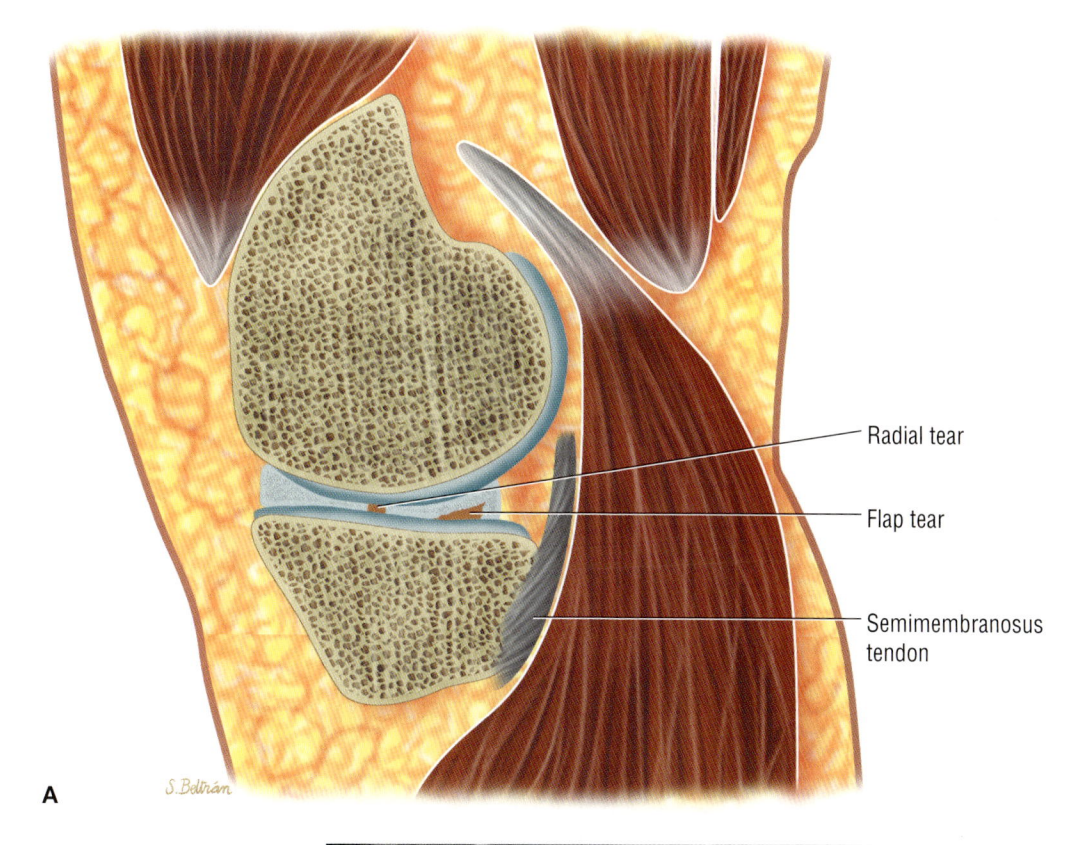

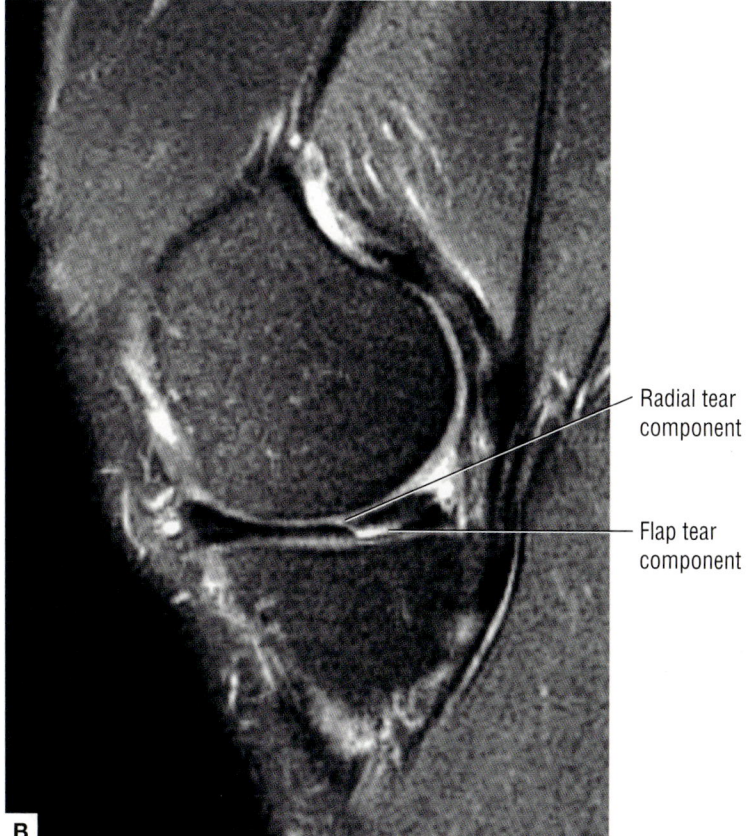

Labels (A): Radial tear; Flap tear; Semimembranosus tendon

Labels (B): Radial tear component; Flap tear component

FIGURE 4.121 Continuity of a radial tear and flap tear pattern in the medial meniscus. The tear initiates as a radial tear, then changes direction with a longitudinal component to create the flap pattern. The relative deficiency of the inner margin of the inferior leaf with blunting of the remaining inferior leaf is characteristic of a flap tear. (**A**) Sagittal color illustration. (**B**) FS PD FSE sagittal image.

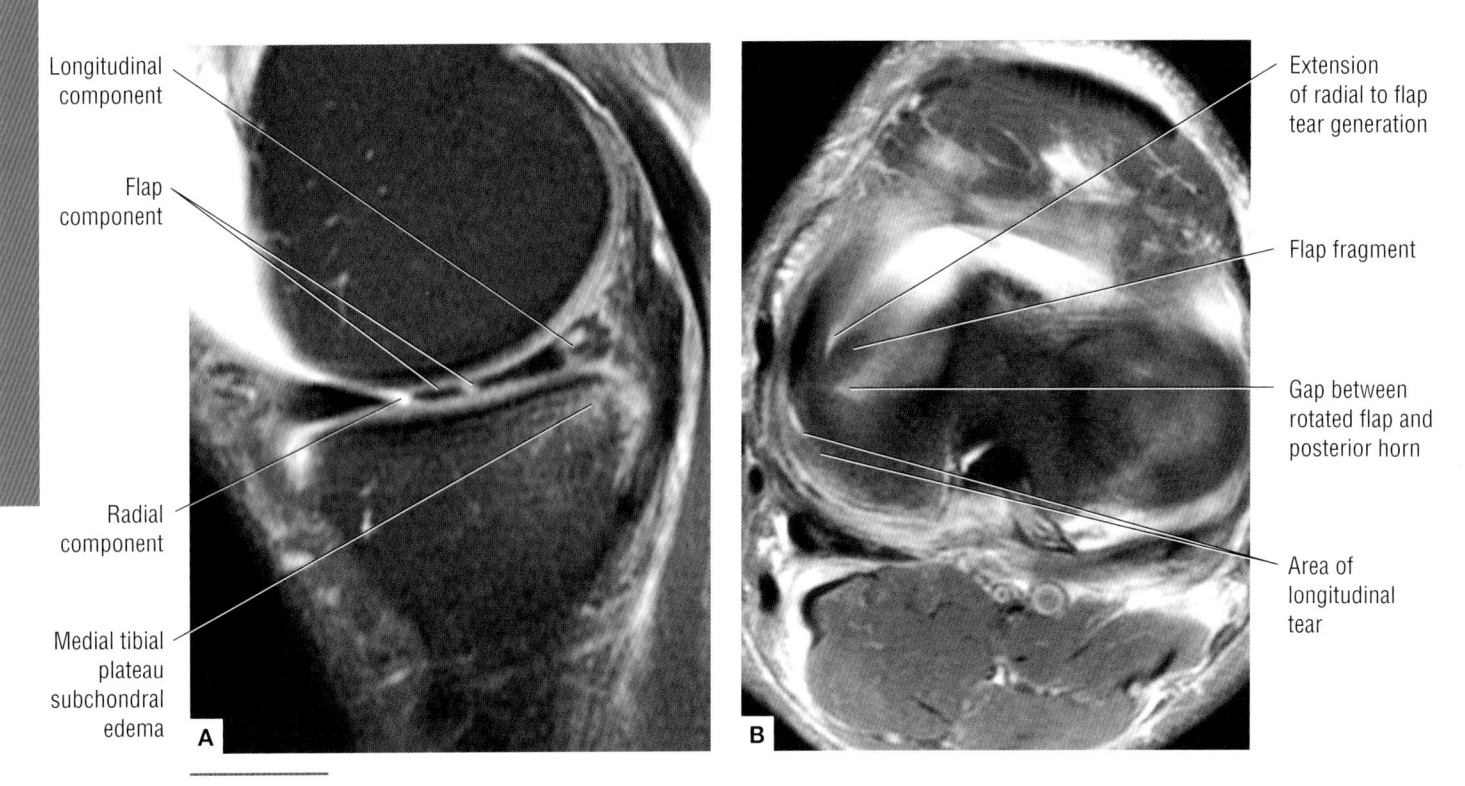

FIGURE 4.122 (**A**) FS PD FSE sagittal image illustrating a complex tear with radial tear, longitudinal tear, and flap tear components. (**B**) Corresponding FS PD FSE axial image identifies both the flap and radial components.

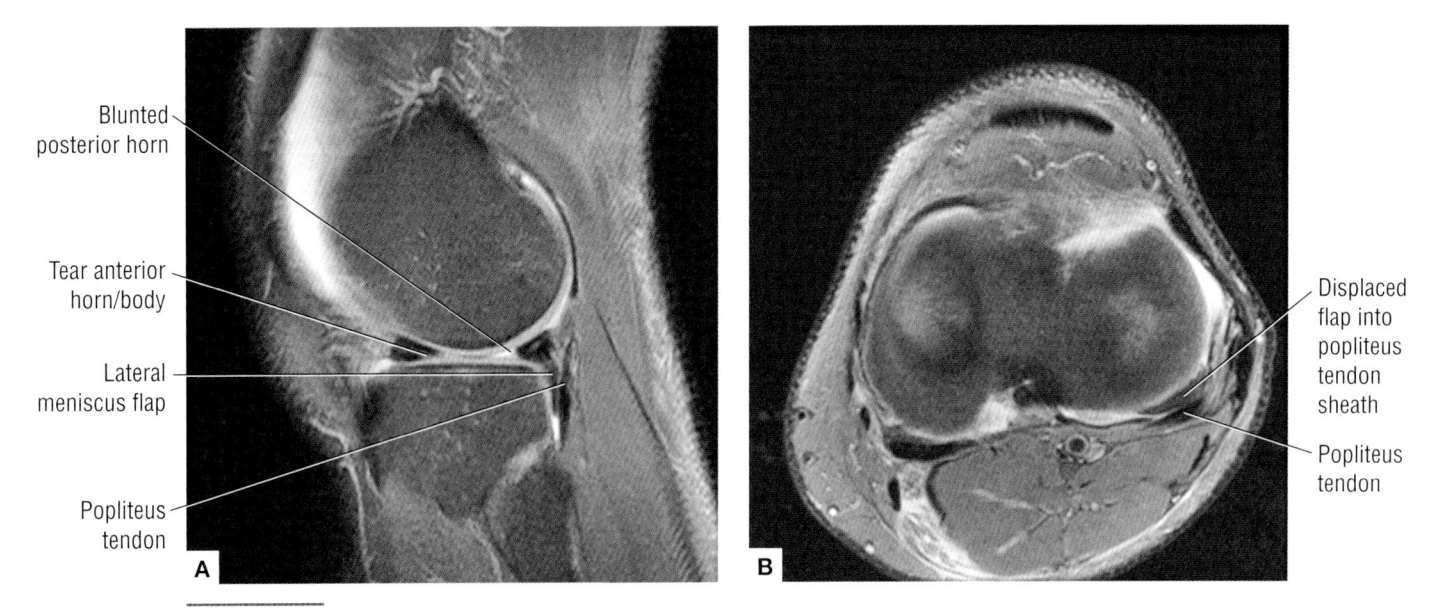

FIGURE 4.123 Displaced lateral meniscus flap tear in the popliteus tendon sheath. Tear can be seen inferior to the lateral joint line and anterior to the popliteus tendon. (**A**) Sagittal FS PD FSE image. (**B**) Axial FS PD FSE image.

The Meniscus 283

FIGURE 4.124 Medial tibial plateau marrow edema associated with medial meniscus flap tear. Compressive loading of the medial compartment associated with meniscal dysfunction leads to increased load transference to both the articular cartilage and subchondral bone.

- Medial collateral ligament
- Medial meniscus
- Flap tear in coronary recess
- Subchondral edema of medial tibial plateau

- Proximal posterior cruciate ligament
- Posterior meniscal flap anterior to meniscal root

- Flap tear on posterior coronal image

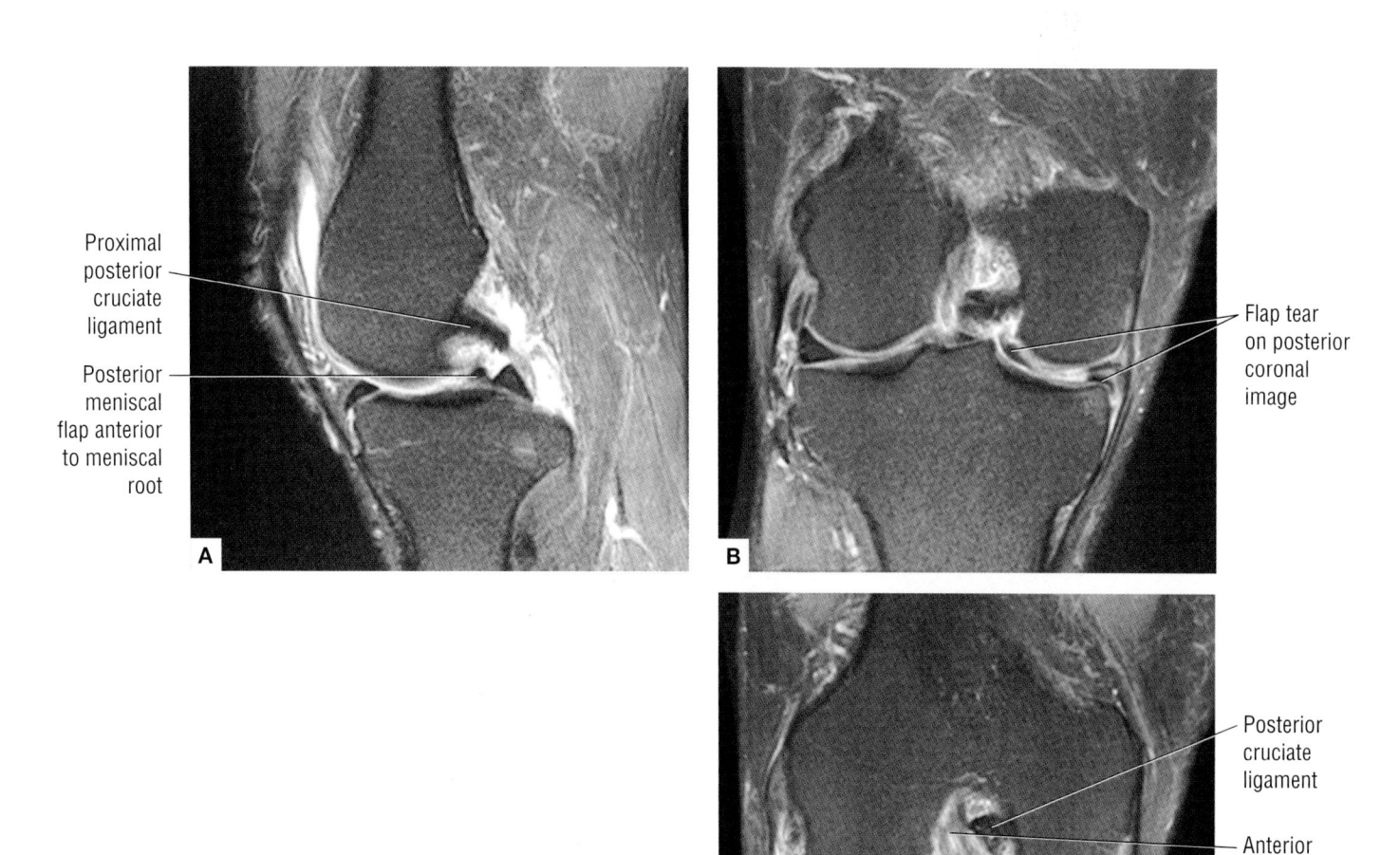

FIGURE 4.125 Flap tear mimicking a bucket-handle tear. (**A**) Posterior double delta sign on sagittal image. (**B**) Corresponding posterior coronal image showing intercondylar notch displacement. (**C**) Anterior coronal images, however, do not show anterior extension of the displaced meniscal flap fragment. Diagnosis of a true bucket-handle tear requires identification of displaced meniscal tissue on both posterior and anterior coronal images.

- Posterior cruciate ligament
- Anterior cruciate ligament
- Blunted free edge
- Coronary recess flap displacement

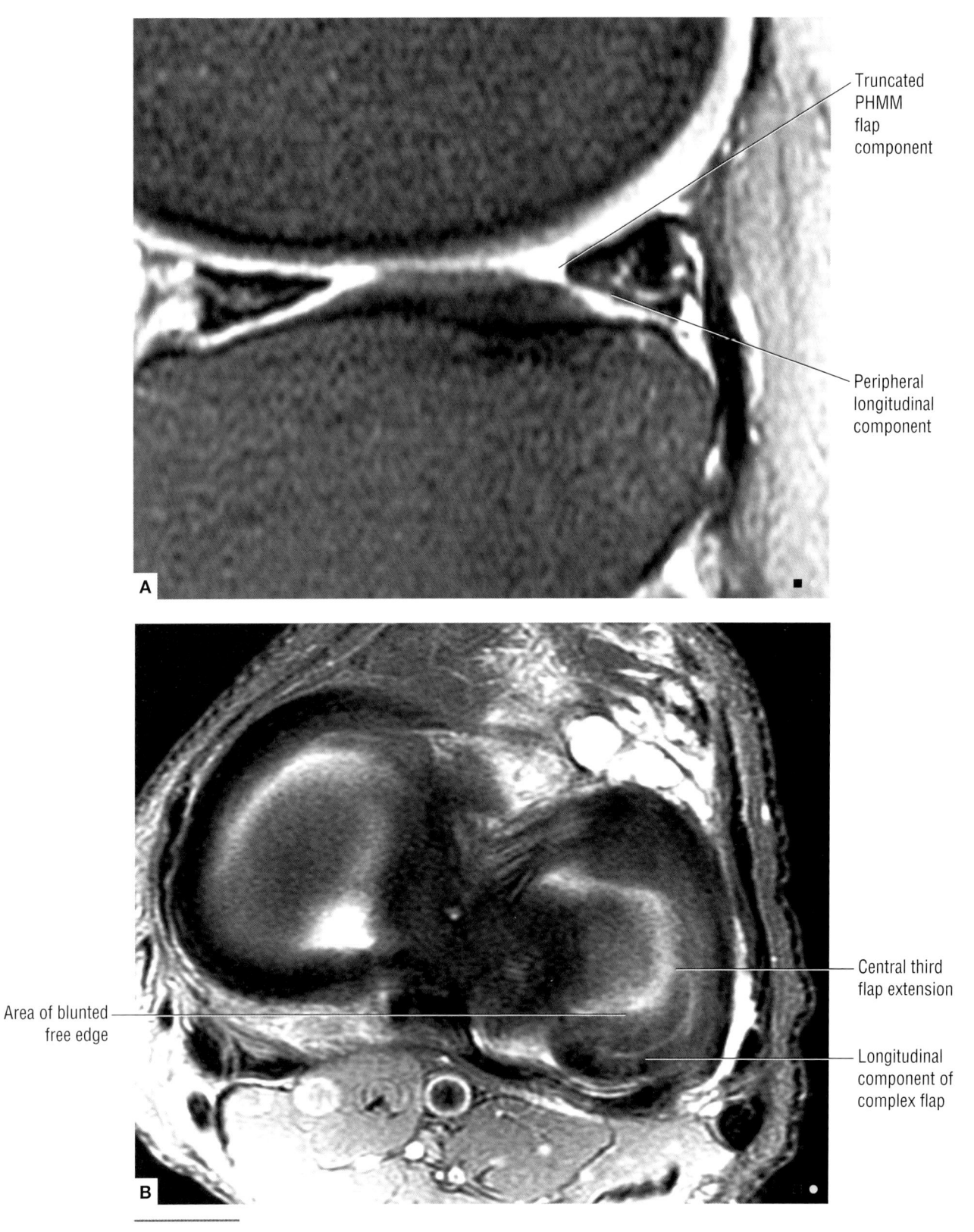

FIGURE 4.126 Complex meniscal tear with truncated free edge flap component and longitudinal component on sagittal (**A**) and axial (**B**) FS PD FSE images.

The Meniscus

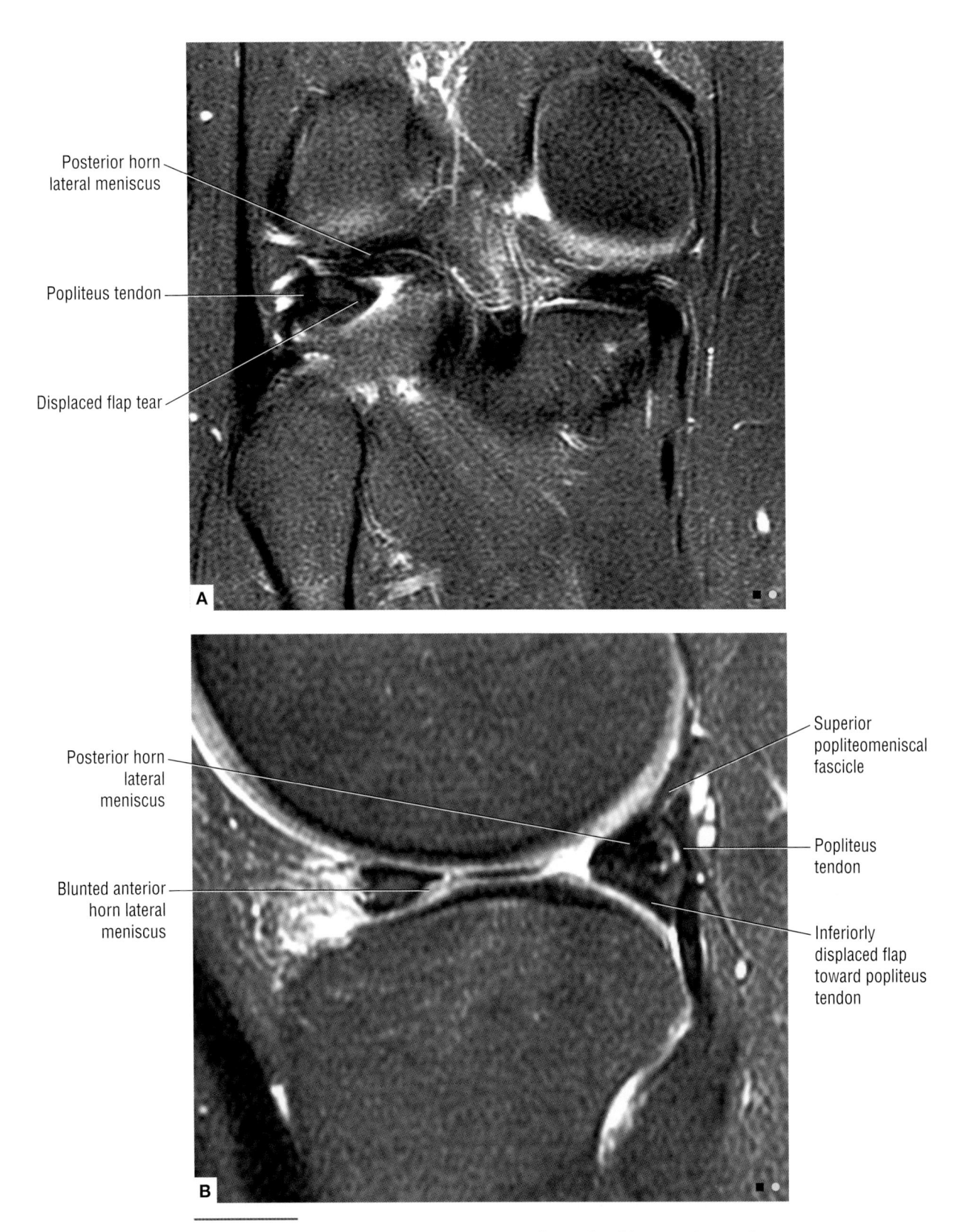

FIGURE 4.127 Flap tear displacement into the popliteal hiatus. FS PD FSE coronal (**A**) and sagittal (**B**) images.

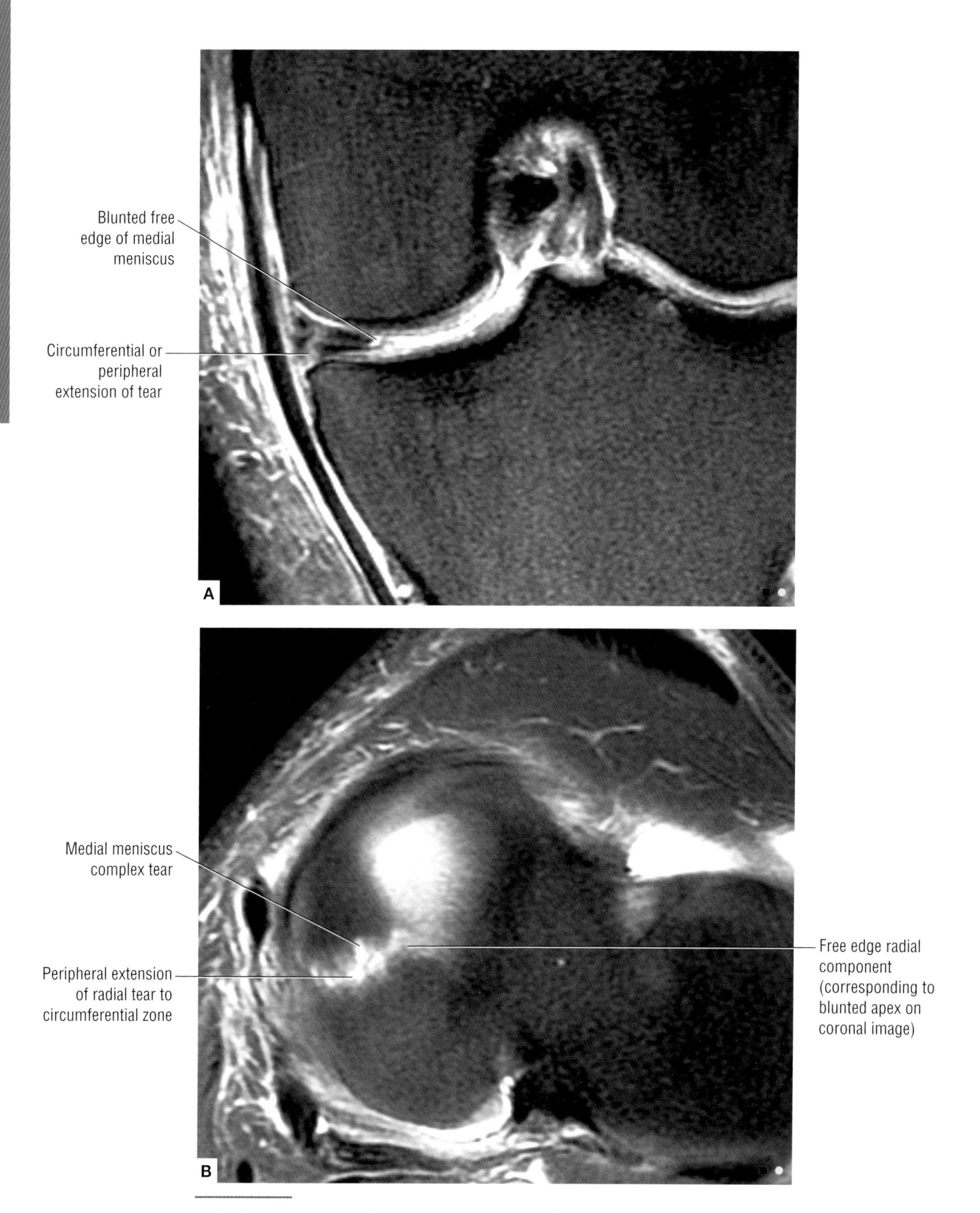

FIGURE 4.128 Complex tear as a peripheral third extension of a medial meniscus radial tear. The margins of the tear are irregular. FS PD FSE coronal (**A**) and axial (**B**) images.

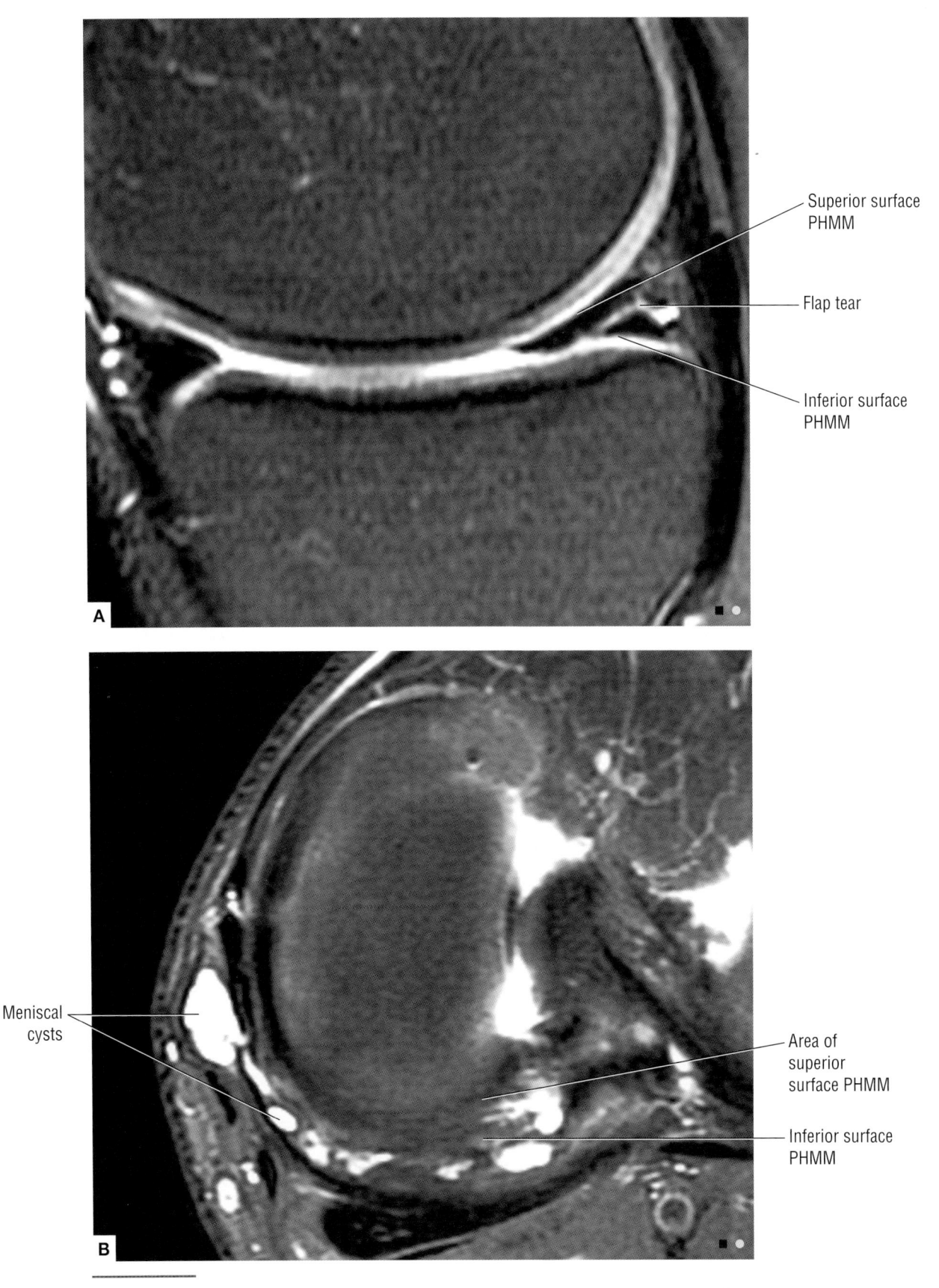

FIGURE 4.129 Meniscal cyst development along the course of a flap tear involving the body and posterior horn of the medial meniscus. FS PD FSE sagittal (**A**) and axial (**B**) images.

MR Accuracy in Detection of Meniscal Tears

- Sensitivity of MR imaging of meniscal tears is between 80% and 100% compared with arthroscopy.[302,456]

- With fast three-dimensional (3D) MR imaging, there is a 95% concurrence between MR imaging and arthroscopy in the detection of meniscal tears and a 100% correlation for meniscal degeneration.

- Correlation of peripheral meniscal signal intensity on sagittal MR images with coronal plane images of the corresponding menisci may reduce the incidence of false-positive MR findings (especially in the posterior horn of the medial meniscus).

- MR is particularly useful in cases of multiple or complex knee lesions.
    - The accuracy of the clinical knee examination drops from 72% for a single lesion to 30% for multiple lesions.[404]

- The possibility of an associated meniscal tear in the presence of a clinically deficient ACL knee or an existing MCL tear is a clinical indication for MR referral.

- The sensitivity of MR in the detection of chondral lesions using FS FSE techniques improves clinical diagnostic accuracy for treatment and patient care.

- MR findings of grade 2 signal intensity in the posterior horn of the medial meniscus correlate with histologic studies showing that the posterior horn of the medial meniscus receives the greatest femoral tibial forces during biomechanical loading and is the most frequent site of grade 2 signal intensity.

- Depiction of grade 2 signal intensity in asymptomatic patients cannot be used to prospectively predict progression to fibrocartilaginous weakening.

- It is essential that clinical examination findings be addressed with MR studies, based on the prevalence of meniscal tears in asymptomatic persons.

- Variations in the accuracy rates of MR compared with those of arthroscopy may be the result of:
    - Differences in the learning curves of radiologists in interpreting MR signal intensities
    - Differences in the experience of several arthroscopists participating in the correlative studies
    - False interpretation of areas of fibrillation or fraying as meniscal tears
    - Inability of arthroscopy to detect intrasubstance degenerative cleavage tears
    - Obstructed arthroscopic visualization of the posterior horn of the medial meniscus by the medial femoral condyle
    - Difficulty in accurately imaging the periphery of the meniscus at the meniscocapsular junction
    - Variability in examinations using different MR imaging equipment and surface coils at a variety of field strengths

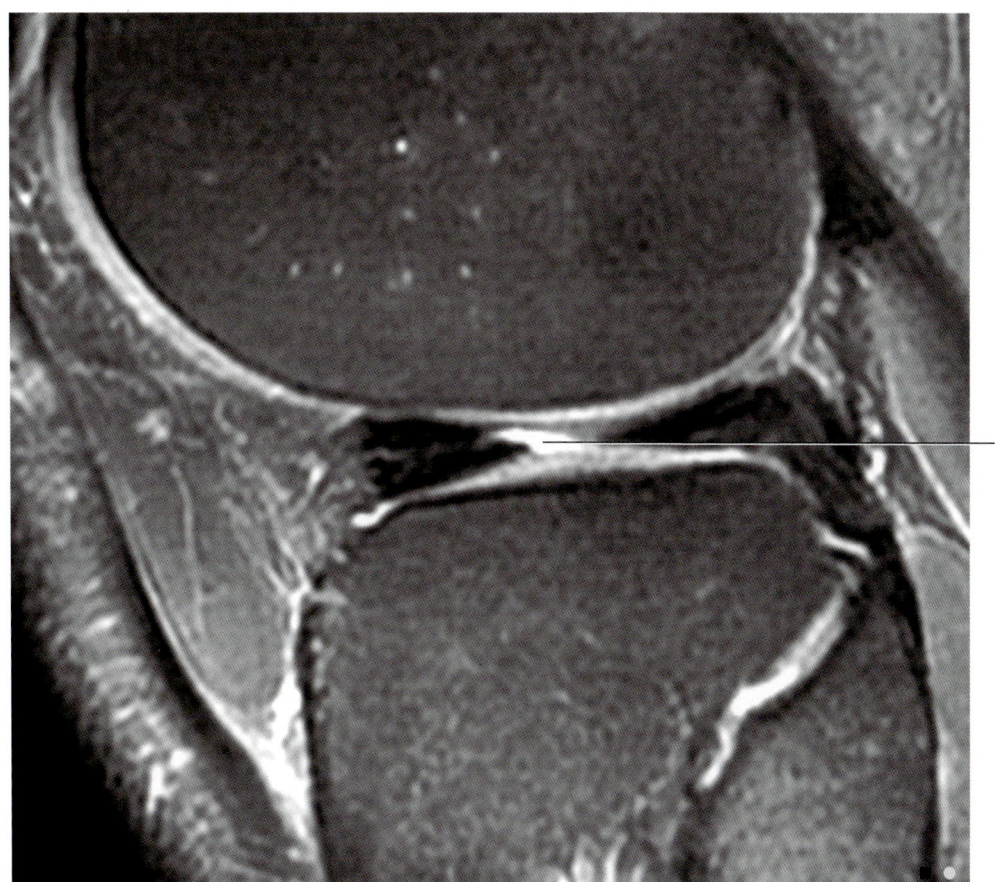

FIGURE 4.130 Flap tear with extension to free edge of meniscus. Sagittal FS PD FSE image.

Discoid Meniscus

Key Concepts

- **Discoid Meniscus**
    - Incomplete discoid menisci can be differentiated from complete discoid types by the degree of discoid morphology.
        - No anterior or posterior horn equivalents are identified in the complete discoid meniscus (type A).
    - Prominent or cavitary grade 2 signal intensity in a discoid meniscus may be associated with positive clinical signs and symptoms related to the lateral compartment.
    - The popping or snapping knee syndrome is associated with the Wrisberg variant (absence of the posterior coronary ligament).

Discoid Meniscus

- Dysplastic meniscus that has lost its normal or semilunar shape and has a broad disc-like configuration[7,20,108,515]
- Lateral discoid menisci are more common than medial discoid menisci.
    - The degree of enlargement varies from mild hypertrophy to a bulky slab of fibrocartilage.
- Incidence of discoid menisci is reported to be 1.4% to 15.5%.[7]
- Watanabe's classification groups discoid menisci into:
    - Incomplete or complete
        - Refer to the degree or extent to which the meniscus demonstrates discoid morphology with an intact posterolateral meniscotibial ligament
        - Incomplete with a superior surface concavity on sagittal MR images; may see separate anterior and posterior horns centrally toward notch
        - Complete without concavity to superior surface of meniscus on sagittal images; covers the tibial plateau without central anterior and posterior horn development. The meniscus does not taper toward the central notch.

- Wrisberg-ligament type (Wrisberg variant)[20,88]
    - Meniscal morphology is normal, and the deformity is defined either by the absence of the posterior capsular attachment (the posterior meniscotibial coronary ligament) or by the coverage area of the lateral tibial plateau.
    - The deficiency or lack of posterior capsular attachment is thought to result in incomplete mediolateral motion, trauma, and secondary hypertrophy of the hypermobile meniscus.[149]
    - There is no medial meniscus counterpart to the Wrisberg-ligament type discoid lateral meniscus.
- Discoid menisci:
    - Congenital deformities
    - Frequently bilateral
    - Usually asymptomatic
        - McMurray's test may be negative on clinical examination.
        - Symptomatic when a meniscal tear develops (incomplete and complete types)
    - Present as fibrocartilaginous masses with an oval or circular shape
    - Thickness of the fibrocartilage varies from 5 to 13mm.[7]
    - Are susceptible to tears and cysts
- Young patients often present with symptoms of torn cartilage.
    - Clinical symptoms of a discoid lateral meniscus may not develop until adolescence.
        - Often asymptomatic until adult life
        - Physical findings of intraarticular pathology include quadriceps atrophy, lack of full extension, and joint line tenderness.
    - Pain, clicking or snapping, and locking are common clinical findings in children.[22]
    - Wrisberg ligament variant associated with snapping knee
        - Snapping knee syndrome associated with meniscal subluxation through flexion and extension
- A complete discoid meniscus extends to the intercondylar notch.
- An anterior megahorn discoid meniscus occurs when the posterior horn is normal but the anterior horn and body form a solid mass of fibrocartilage.

- The Wrisberg-ligament type of discoid meniscus may present earlier with lateral joint pain with or without an audible or palpable "clunk."

- Differential diagnosis of a discoid meniscus:
    - Any condition that presents as a "snapping knee" on physical examination (a snapping sound during knee flexion and extension)
    - Conditions include:
        - Patellofemoral joint subluxation or dislocation
        - Meniscal cysts
        - Congenital subluxation of the tibiofemoral joint
        - Subluxation or dislocation, or both, of the proximal tibiofibular joint
        - Snapping of the tendons about the knee on an osteophyte or roughened surface
        - A displaced flap tear or bucket-handle tear

- Treatment of the unstable inner segment of a discoid meniscus requires saucerization or resection (partial meniscectomy) to a stable rim.
    - Create a contoured, 6mm stable meniscal rim.

- The Wrisberg-ligament type of discoid lateral meniscus is prone to medial displacement into the intercondylar notch and is best treated with a total meniscectomy.[69,193]
    - May displace medially, laterally, or anteriorly and is unstable.

- Some patients with symptomatic discoid menisci undergo saucerization and partial resection in the presence of intrasubstance degeneration without a surface tear.[20]
    - On MR examination, these menisci demonstrate prominent or thick horizontal grade 2 signal intensity oriented along the middle collagen bundle or shear plane of the meniscus.

- Menisci with grade 2 signal intensity are not usually treated at arthroscopy except for cases of discoid menisci.[20,118]

- Osteochondritis dissecans of the lateral femoral condyle if present is associated with a poorer prognosis.

- Imaging findings in the evaluation of discoid menisci include:
    - Plain-film radiographs may show:
        - Widening of the involved compartment
        - Hypoplastic lateral femoral condyle
        - High fibular head
        - Chondromalacia
        - Cupping of the lateral tibial plateau
        - Squared-off lateral femoral condyle[419]
    - Arthrography demonstrates an elongated and enlarged meniscus that extends toward the intercondylar notch.
    - On sagittal MR images, using a 4-mm slice thickness, a discoid meniscus exhibits a continuous or bowtie appearance on three or more consecutive images.[22,419]
        - Demonstration of the anterior and posterior horns is limited to one or two sagittal sections adjacent to the intercondylar notch.
        - Central tapering, which is visualized on sagittal images in the normal meniscus, is lost in discoid fibrocartilage.
        - Thick grade 2 signal intensity present on sagittal images correlates with mucinous degeneration within a more cavitary area of degeneration.
    - The increased inferior-to-superior dimensions of the meniscus can be appreciated on both coronal and sagittal images.
        - A discoid meniscus may be as much as 2mm higher than the opposite meniscus.[441]
        - Coronal images show the extension of the discoid meniscus apex toward or into the intercondylar notch.
    - Less common presentation of both medial and lateral discoid meniscus as rare variant

- Complete discoid meniscus:
  - Meniscal fibrocartilage without distinct anterior and posterior horns
    - Usually interposed between the femoral condyle and the tibial plateau on every sagittal image through the involved compartment

- Incomplete discoid meniscus:
  - More common than complete discoid meniscus
  - The meniscus does not extend into the intercondylar notch on coronal images.

- If the radial diameter (shown on coronal images) through the body or central third of the meniscus measures 13mm from the capsular margin to the free edge, a discoid meniscus is probable.[88]
  - Normally, the central coronal image displays the smallest radial cross-section of the meniscal body.

- In the presence of an effusion, the enlarged meniscus is outlined with high-signal-intensity fluid on FS PD FSE, T2*-, or STIR-weighted images.

- Axial images demonstrate the circumferential morphology of both incomplete and complete discoid menisci.
  - Axial images prescribed from the sagittal plane parallel to the lateral joint line will optimize visualization of the discoid morphology on a single image.
  - Grade 2 signal intensity and discoid menisci may correlate with intrameniscal cavitations or cysts.
  - Many orthopaedic surgeons recommend meniscectomy for a symptomatic discoid meniscus, even without grade 3 signal intensity.
  - Discoid menisci usually demonstrate a prominent and thickened grade 2 signal intensity that may correlate with an intrasubstance cleavage tear.

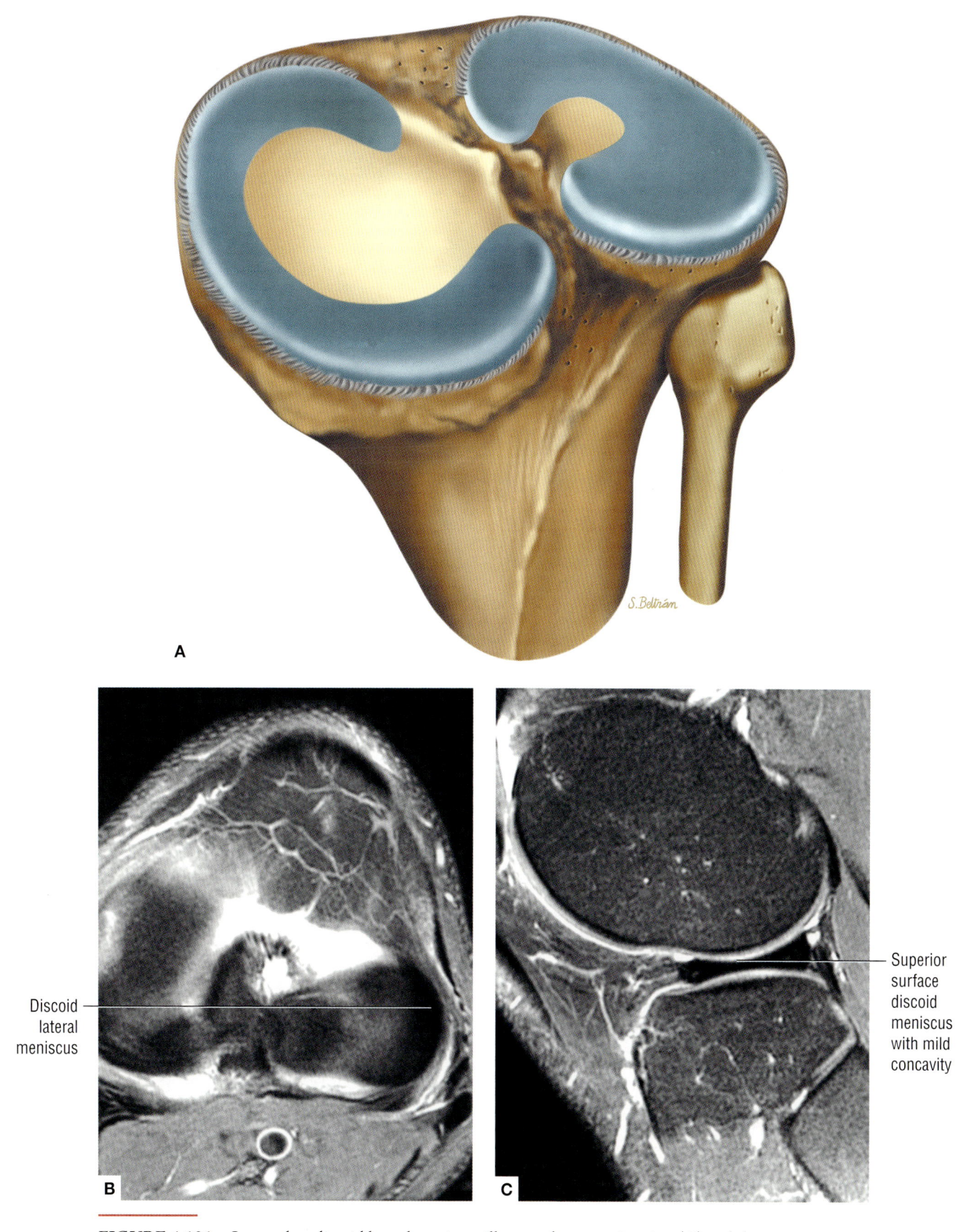

FIGURE 4.131 Incomplete discoid lateral meniscus illustrated on superior view (**A**) and shown on corresponding axial (**B**) and sagittal (**C**) FS PD FSE images. Note there is slight surface concavity in the body of the partial discoid fibrocartilage on the sagittal image (**C**).

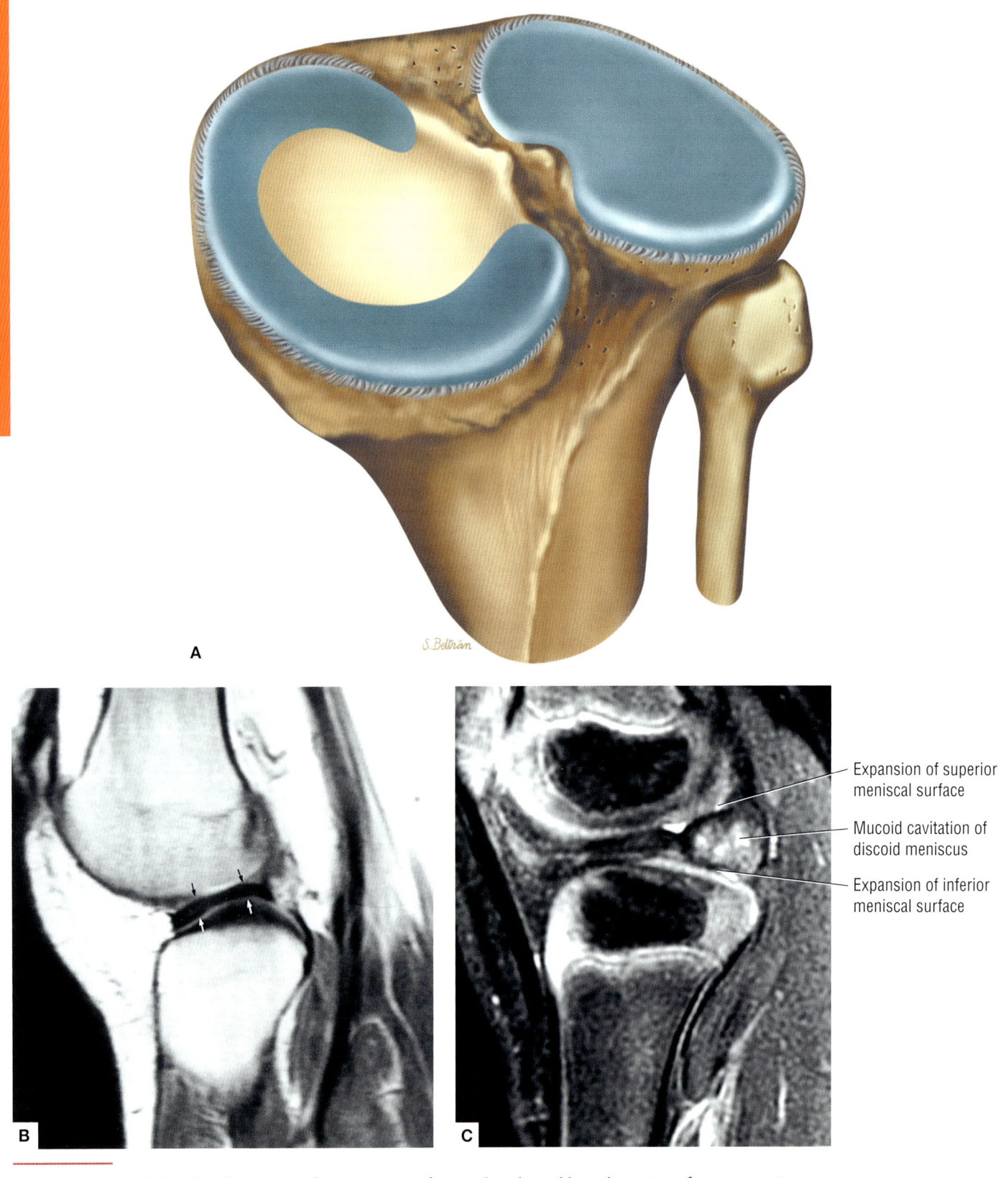

- Expansion of superior meniscal surface
- Mucoid cavitation of discoid meniscus
- Expansion of inferior meniscal surface

FIGURE 4.132 (**A**) Color illustration of superior view of a complete discoid lateral meniscus from a posterior perspective. (**B**) The thick slab of lateral meniscal fibrocartilage is seen as a continuous low-signal-intensity band on corresponding sagittal image (*arrows*). The superior surface of the complete discoid meniscus has no concavity. (**C**) Symptomatic discoid lateral meniscus in a three-year-old with mucoid expansion of the posterior aspect of the lateral meniscus.

The Meniscus

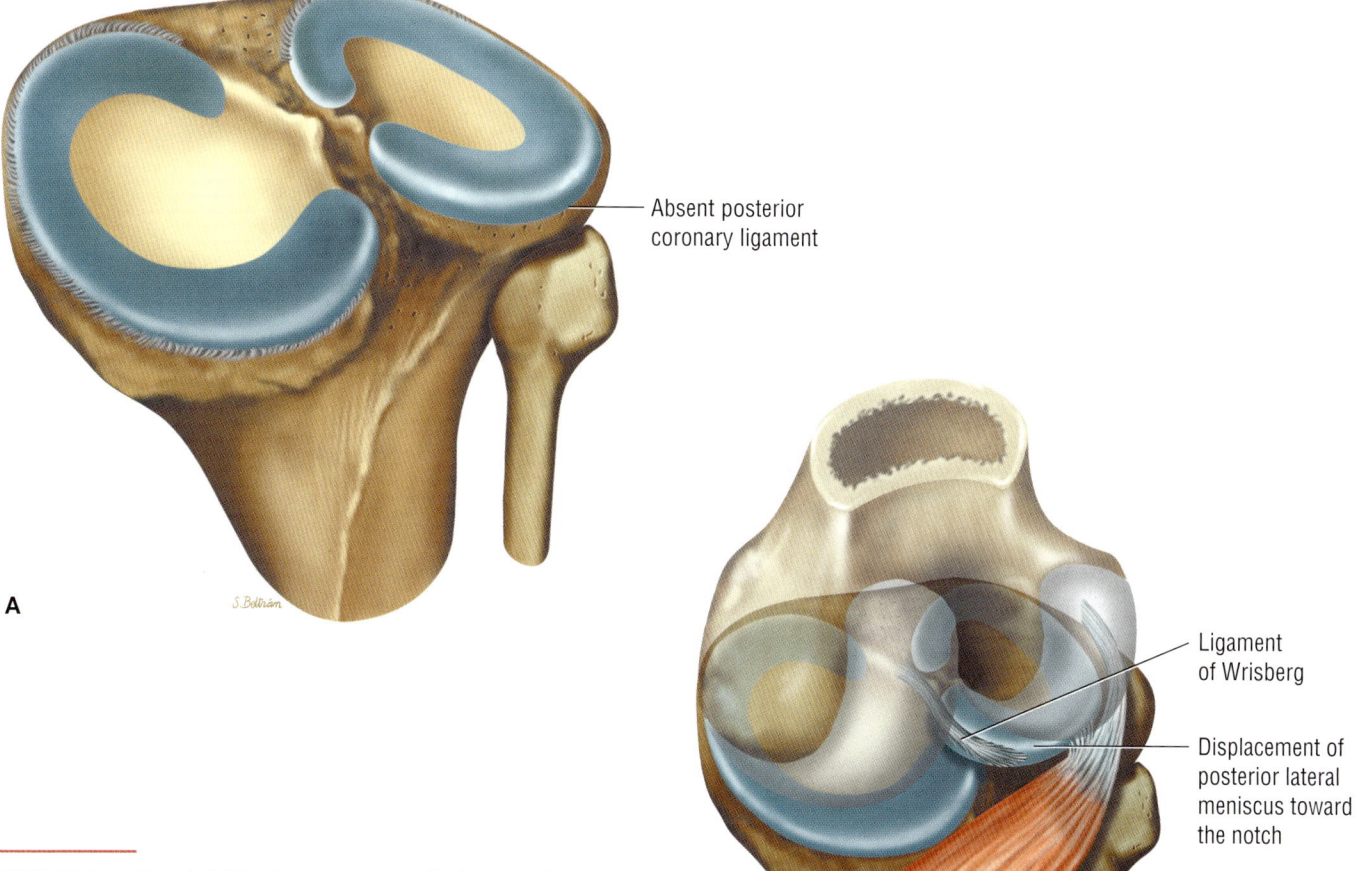

FIGURE 4.133 (**A**) Wrisberg variant with absence of the posterior coronary ligament on posterior superior view. (**B**) Without meniscotibial restraint, there is potential for entrapment of the posterior aspect of the fibrocartilage. In extension, the attached Wrisberg ligament pulls and displaces the posterior aspect of the meniscus into the intercondylar notch.

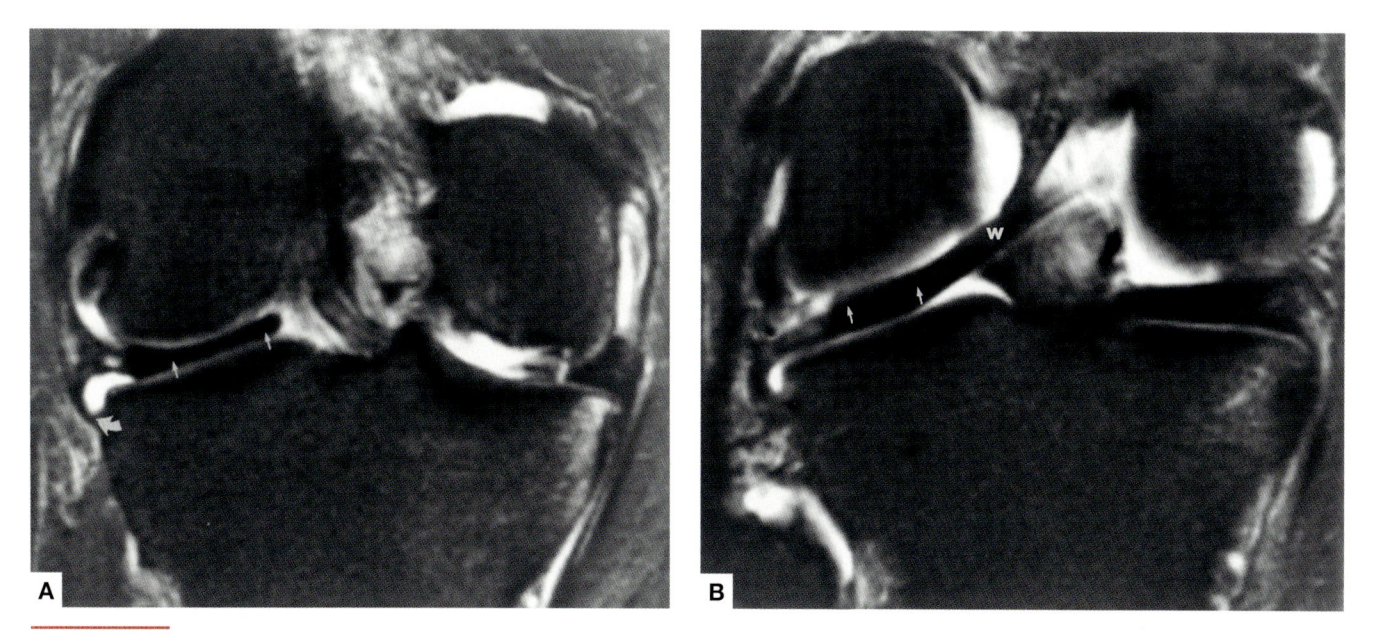

FIGURE 4.134 A complete discoid meniscus (*small arrows*) interposed between the lateral femoral condyle and tibial plateau extending to the intercondylar notch on FS PD-weighted FSE coronal images. An intact meniscotibial ligament (**A**, *curved arrow*) and Wrisberg's ligament (**B**, W) are shown.

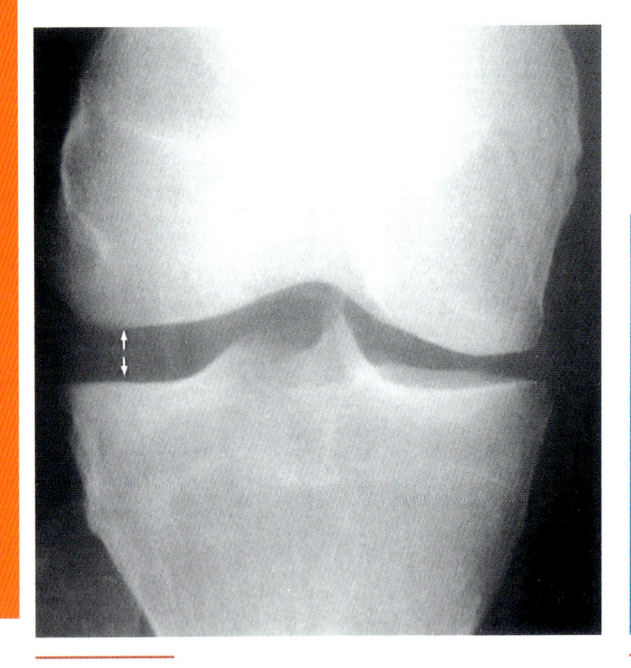

FIGURE 4.135 Convention radiographs show lateral joint space widening in complete discoid menisci.

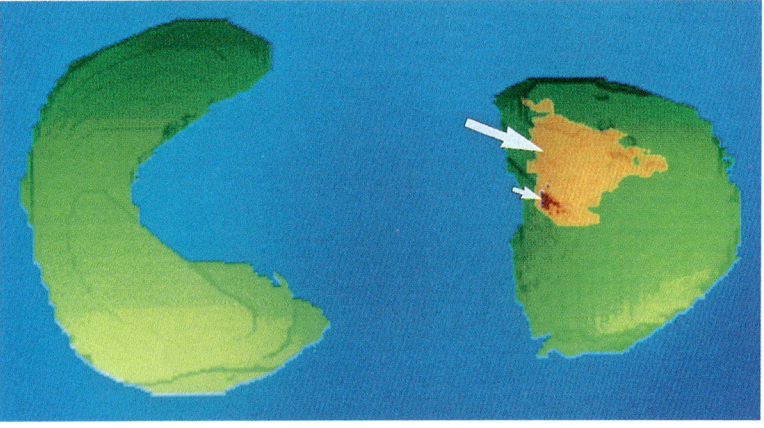

FIGURE 4.136 A 3D MR rendering shows intrasubstance degeneration (*orange and large arrow*) and a superior surface tear (*red and small arrow*).

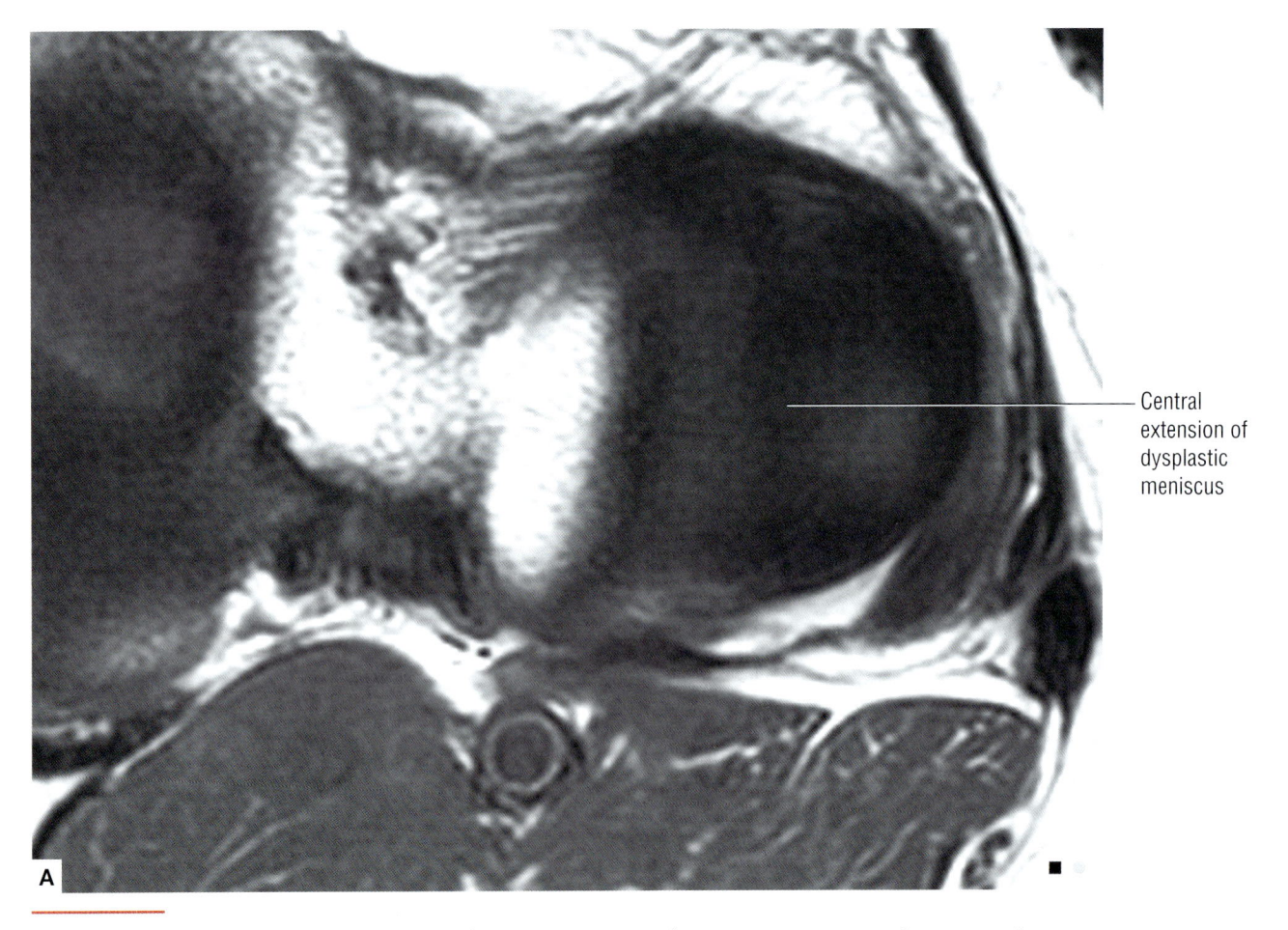

Central extension of dysplastic meniscus

FIGURE 4.137 Discoid-like (partial discoid) lateral meniscus with a concave superior surface covers a large area of the tibial plateau. PD axial (**A**).

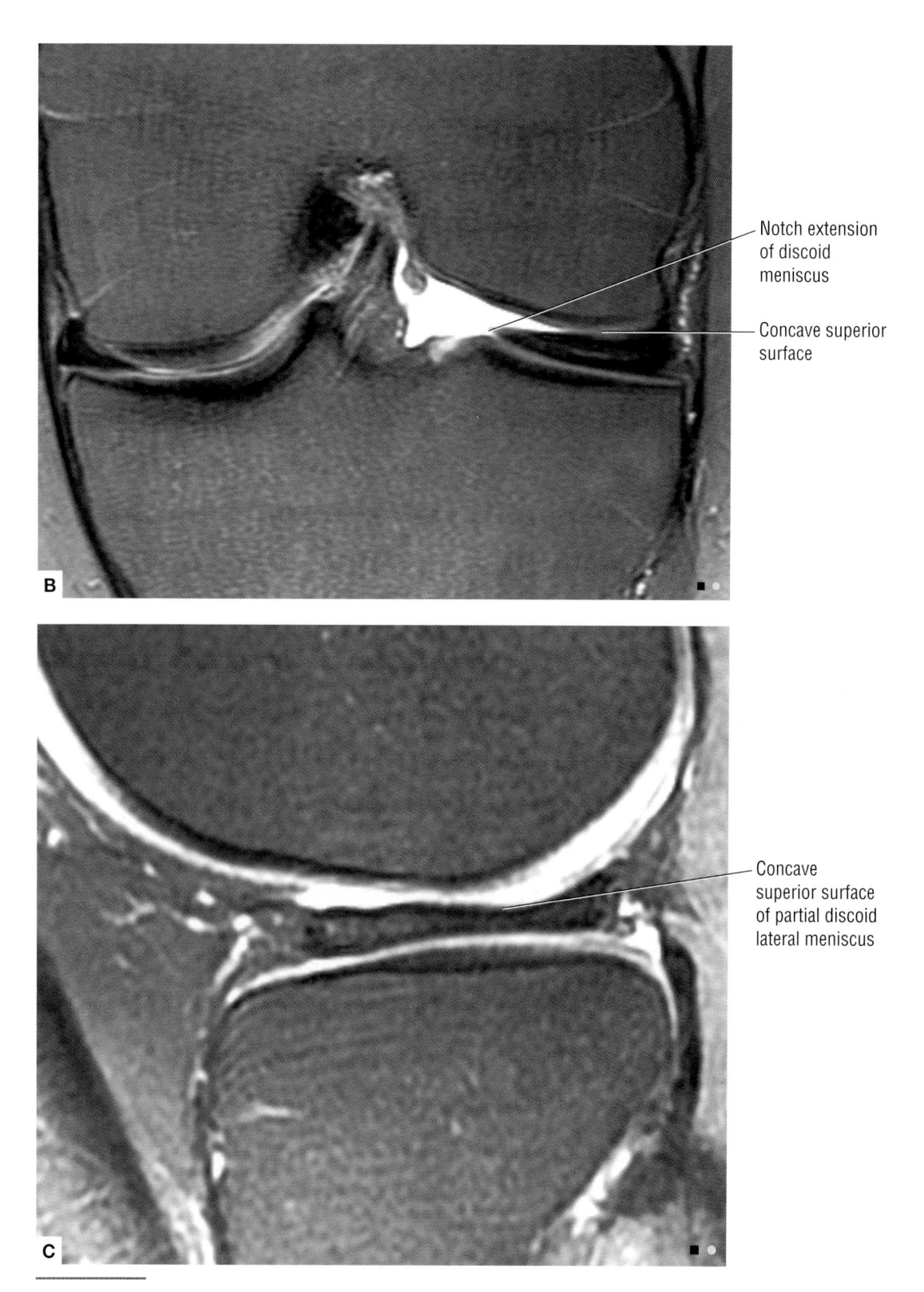

FIGURE 4.137 *(Continued)* FS PD FSE coronal (**B**), and sagittal (**C**) images.

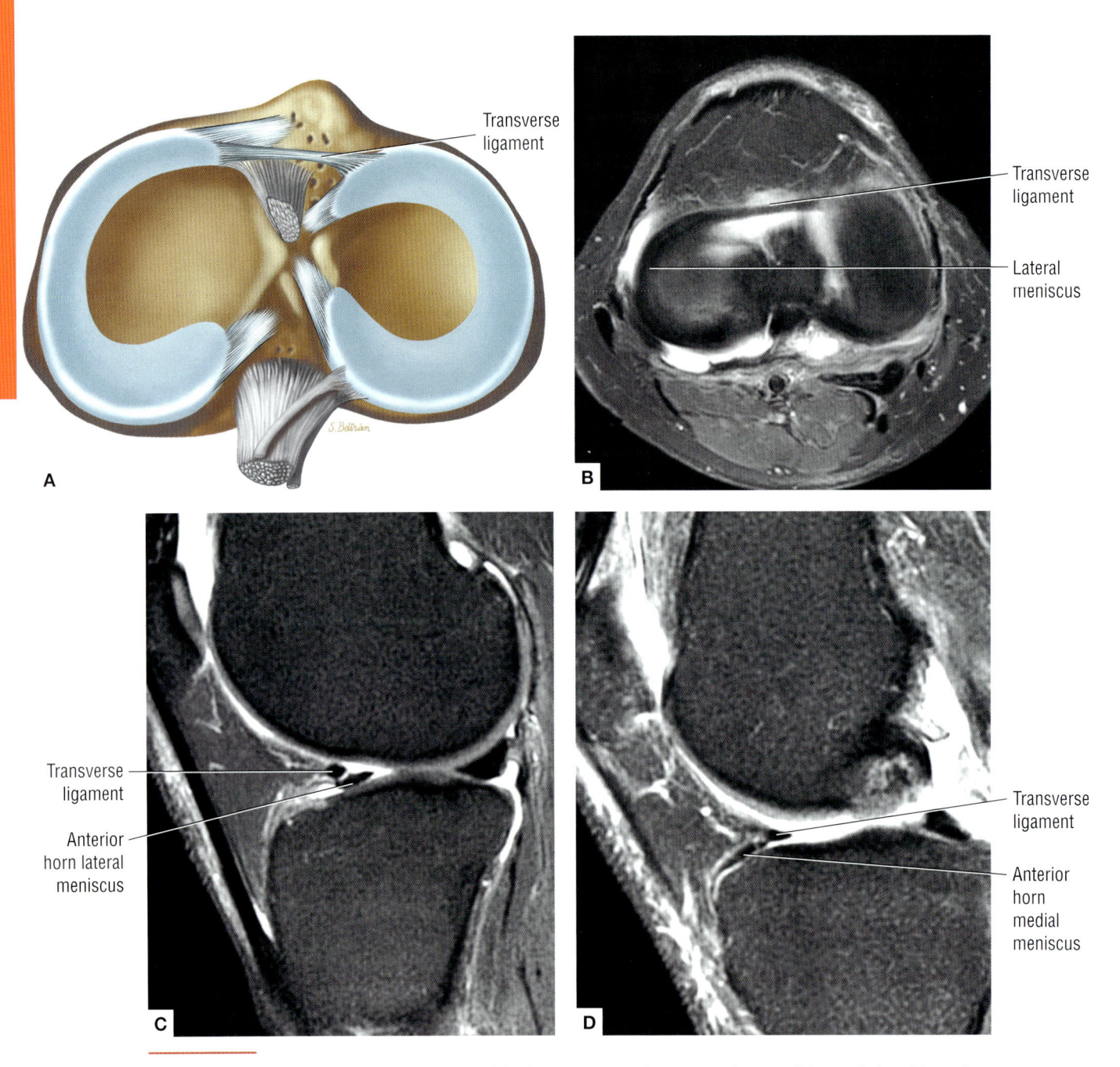

FIGURE 4.138 The transverse ligament of the knee connects the anterior horns of the medial and lateral menisci. (**A**) Axial superior view color illustration showing the transverse ligament coursing anterior to the anterior horn of the lateral meniscus. In the medial compartment, anterior horn fibrocartilage extends anterior to the transverse ligament attachment. Axial (**B**) and sagittal (**C, D**) FS PD FSE images. The transverse ligament (**B**) is located anterior to the anterior horn of the lateral meniscus (**C**) and posterior to the anterior horn of the medial meniscus (**D**). The anterior horn of the medial meniscus extends anterior to the more superiorly located transverse ligament. The transverse ligament is also located directly posterior to the free edge of Hoffa's fat pad.

Pitfalls in Interpretation of Meniscal Tear Findings

- Meniscal Tears
    - Attenuation of grade 3 signal intensity extension to an articular surface is associated with a closed meniscal tear.
    - External rotation of the knee may accentuate the course of the meniscofemoral ligaments.
        - The ligament of Wrisberg is often mistaken for a peripheral tear of the posterior horn of the lateral meniscus.
    - Meniscal flounce does not indicate the existence of or increased association with a meniscal tear.
- Grade 2 vs. Grade 3 Signal Intensity
    - Sometimes it is difficult to distinguish articular surface extension of signal intensity.
        - Evaluation of the morphology of the meniscus as well as the degree and thickness of increased signal intensity may facilitate a more accurate interpretation.
    - Weakening or decreased signal intensity of a grade 3 lesion as it approaches an articular surface is indicative of an intrasubstance closed tear.
        - May require surgical probing at arthroscopy for detection
    - In the presence of a joint effusion, grade 3 signal:
        - Becomes more conspicuous with conventional T2 weighting
        - Corresponds to a disrupted meniscal surface
            - Facilitates the influx of free water molecules (i.e., T2 prolongation)
        - Chronic grade 3 signal may not allow the influx of synovial fluid and persist as intermediate signal intensity.

- Correlation with corresponding coronal images may be helpful:
    - In patients with peripheral signal intensity
    - When grade 2 and grade 3 signal intensities cannot be differentiated
    - Extension to the superior or inferior surface of the meniscus or meniscal apex can be more easily determined.[377]
- Artifact
    - Peripheral signal artifact (also called *annefact* or *star artifact*):
        - Can appear as either a bright spot or as a ribbon of bright signal smeared through the image
        - Occurs when signals are generated outside the field of view (FOV) and the receiver coil is able to detect them
        - Best visualized when a body coil is used to transmit radiofrequency and a phased-array coil is used to receive the signal
        - On long-axis images, sagittal or coronal, the artifact typically occurs if the phase encoding is selected along the superior-to-inferior (S-I) direction and the receiver coils extend beyond the imaging FOV.
            - Bright signal originates outside the FOV and is aliased back into the image.
        - Artifact may overlap the meniscus in the sagittal plane when using FSE sequences.
        - Steps to reduce the likelihood of producing artifact include:
            - Use S-I frequency when possible.
            - Ensure that the imaging FOV matches the receiver coil coverage, or use a smaller radiofrequency coil with reduced S-I coverage when possible.
                - If using a CTL spine coil, select only that needed for the FOV.

The Meniscus

- Offset the FOV along the S-I or left-right direction to change the position of the artifact.
    - Sometimes the best method to achieve usable images without changing phase and frequency coils
    - Only a few centimeters of offset may be sufficient to shift the artifact so that it no longer overlaps the critical area of the meniscus at the level of the joint line.

- **Truncation artifact**
    - *Less common pitfall*
    - May mimic a meniscal tear when a 128 × 128 matrix with a 128-pixel phase-encoded axis is oriented in the S-I direction[325]
    - Minimized when a 192 or 256 × 256 matrix is used
    - Most conspicuous two pixels from the high-contrast interface between the meniscus and the articular cartilage
    - A pseudo-tear may be seen when the high-signal-intensity artifact is projected over the low-signal-intensity meniscus.[323]

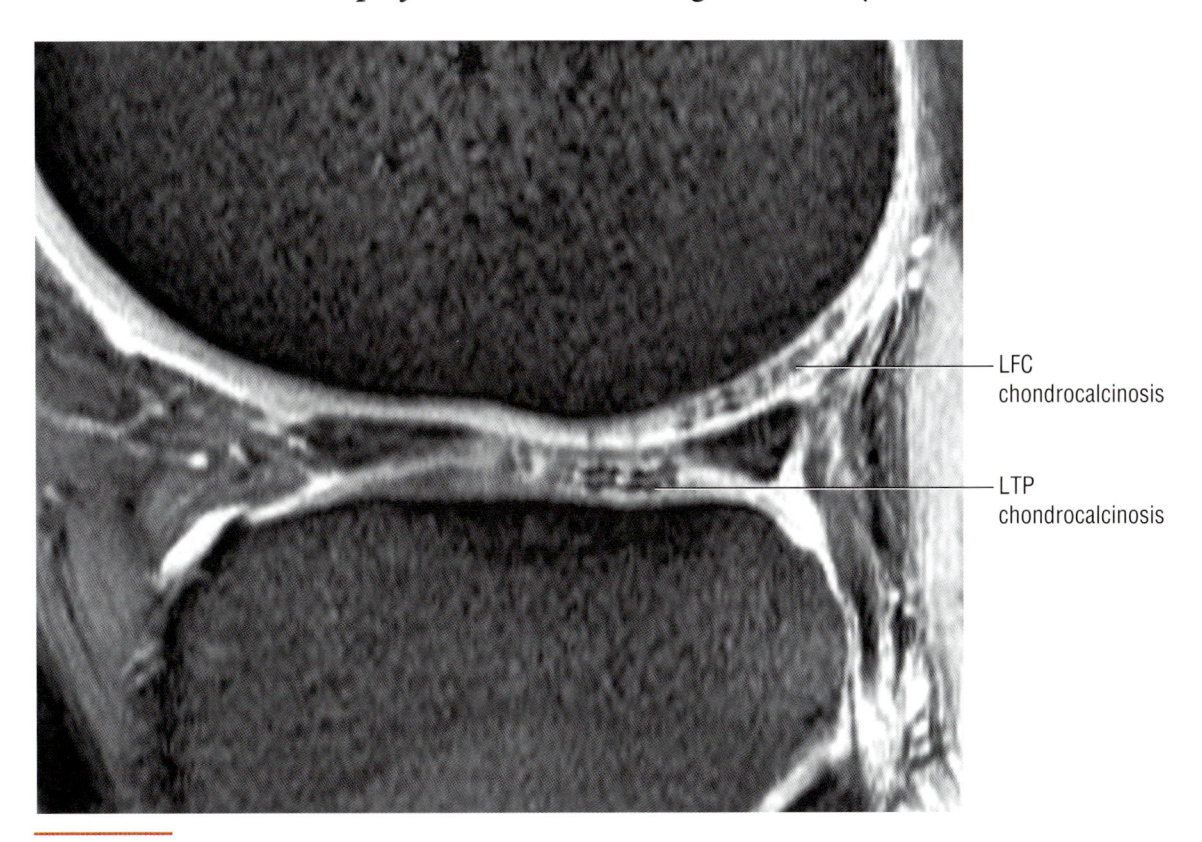

FIGURE 4.139 Chondrocalcinosis as hypointense foci within the chondral surfaces: lateral femoral condyle (LFC) and lateral tibial plateau (LTP). Sagittal GRE image.

- **Transverse Ligament**
  - The transverse ligament of the knee:
    - Connects the anterior horns of the medial and lateral meniscus
    - Can simulate an oblique tear adjacent to the anterior horn of the lateral meniscus
    - Originates anterolateral to the central rhomboid attachment of the lateral meniscus
      - The central rhomboid attachment may normally demonstrate linear increased signal intensity.
    - Varies in diameter
    - Absent in 40% of gross specimens
  - On sagittal or axial images, the transverse ligament courses between the tibial attachment of the ACL and Hoffa's infrapatellar fat pad to its insertion on the anterior superior aspect of the anterior horn of the medial meniscus.
  - In the presence of a joint effusion, increased signal intensity may be present in the interface between the transverse ligament and the anterior horn of the lateral meniscus on FS PD FSE images.
  - In up to 30% of MR examinations, the fat that surrounds the low-signal-intensity ligament mimics grade 3 signal intensity.
  - In 15% of MR examinations, the transverse ligament can be followed in its entire medial-to-lateral extent.[323]
  - Infrequently, the medial extent of the transverse ligament may simulate a tear adjacent to the anterior horn of the medial meniscus.
    - Unrelated to the transverse ligament, the anterior root of the medial meniscus may insert along the far anterior tibial margin and be mistaken for anterior meniscal extrusion.[462]
  - Axial images demonstrate the course of the transverse ligament as a low-signal-intensity band traversing Hoffa's infrapatellar fat pad.

The Meniscus

- On serial sagittal images, the round transverse ligament may be traced from the anterior horn of the lateral meniscus to the anterior horn of the medial meniscus.

- The central attachment of the anterior horn of the medial meniscus is located anterior to the transverse ligament when viewed in the sagittal plane.

    - A connection between the ACL and the anterior horn of the medial meniscus may exist through the meniscocruciate ligament (not usually apparent on MR).[462]

- The transverse ligament is always identified anterior to the anterior horn of the lateral meniscus.

- In external rotation, the transverse ligament may assume a more linear morphology in the attachment to the anterior horn of the lateral meniscus.

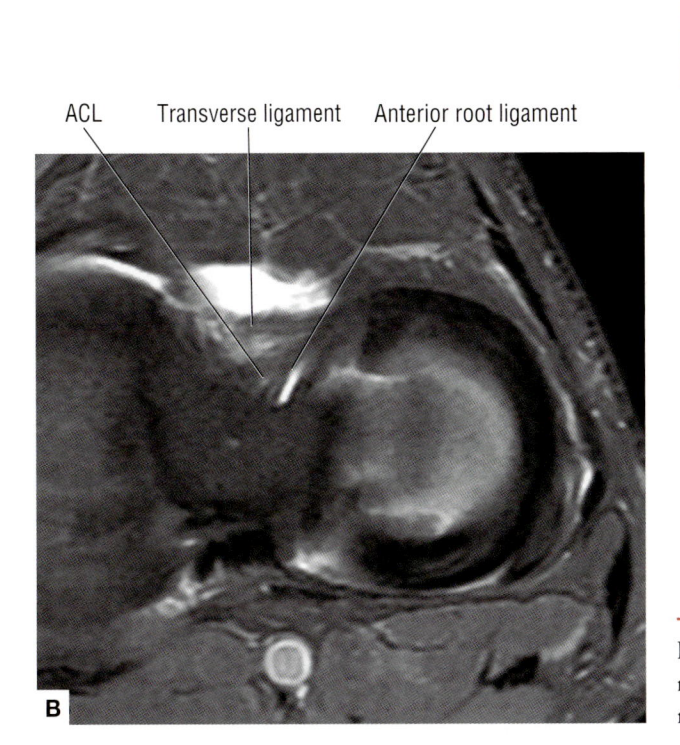

FIGURE 4.140 Proximity and contiguous fibers between the anterior root ligament of the lateral meniscus (LM) and the anterior cruciate ligament (ACL). Axial illustration (A) and axial FS PD FSE image (B).

- **Anterior Horn of the Lateral Meniscus**
  - Isolated tears of the anterior horn of the lateral meniscus:
    - Can be easily differentiated from transverse ligament pseudo-tears
    - Relatively uncommon compared to other meniscal tear locations
  - The central anterior ligamentous rhomboid attachment of the anterior horn of the lateral meniscus may be mistaken for a meniscal tear.
    - Attachment is normally directed obliquely upward on sagittal images and frequently contains increased internal signal intensity.
      - In this location, the increased signal intensity is sometimes referred to as "speckled."
      - The striated appearance of the medial aspect of the anterior horn is related to the contiguous fibers between the anterior root ligament of the lateral meniscus and the ACL.[462]
      - Although not as apparent on MR imaging, a similar connection may exist between the ACL and the anterior horn of the medial meniscus.
  - It may be visualized on one or two sagittal images adjacent to the intercondylar notch and occurs near the origin of the transverse ligament.
  - Excessive external rotation of the knee results in pseudo-foreshortening of the anterior horn of the lateral meniscus relative to the posterior horn and is associated with apparent anterior-to-posterior elongation of the femoral condyle.
    - Always review the location of sagittal image prescriptions on corresponding axial images to appreciate the effects of knee rotation on MR findings.

- **Fibrillation**
  - Fraying of the concave free edge of the meniscus facing the intercondylar notch
    - Seen as increased signal intensity restricted to the apex of the meniscus in the presence of normal meniscal morphology
  - If abnormal morphology (truncation or foreshortening of the meniscus) is present, a meniscal tear (radial or flap tear) is likely.
    - A flap tear, for example, may exist adjacent to the free edge of the meniscus as an interridge tear.
  - FS PD-weighted FSE images:
    - Useful in defining the meniscal outline or morphology
    - Less sensitive to the detection of intrameniscal signal intensity
  - Sometimes difficult to differentiate between the MR characteristics of fraying and tearing of the meniscus[230]
  - A macerated meniscus imbibes synovial fluid throughout its substance and demonstrates a diffuse increase in signal intensity (multiple grade 3 tears).
  - Posttraumatic diffuse increased intrameniscal signal intensity without a discrete meniscal tear may be seen in a more acute setting.
    - Loosely referred to as *meniscal contusion* or *posttraumatic meniscal edema*[79]
      - The terms meniscal edema or contusion are not commonly used (more accurate to describe the hyperintensity).
    - Amorphous meniscal signal should not be confused with meniscocapsular or medial meniscal posteroinferior corner tears that occur in association with ACL disruption.

Popliteus Tendon

- In the posterior horn of the lateral meniscus, the popliteus tendon sheath may be mistaken for grade 3 signal intensity and can be falsely interpreted as a tear.

- The popliteus tendon sheath is intermediate in signal intensity on T1- and FS PD- or T2-weighted images and courses in an oblique, anterosuperior-to-posteroinferior direction, anterior to the low-signal-intensity popliteus tendon.

- In the presence of a joint effusion, fluid in the popliteus sheath demonstrates bright signal intensity on T2- or T2*-weighted images.

- In addition, the superior and inferior fascicles of the posterior horn of the lateral meniscus are best displayed on T2-weighted images (including FS PD-weighted FSE or T2*-weighted sequences) in the presence of a joint effusion.

- A fascicle tear should not be confused with the normal superior and inferior meniscocapsular defects, which allow passage of the popliteus tendon through the popliteus hiatus.

- In the sagittal plane, the most lateral image through the popliteus tendon displays the anatomy of the inferior fascicle, with normal deficiency of the superior fascicle.

- More medially, both the superior and inferior fascicles are visualized.

- The most medial image through the popliteus tendon and sheath displays the superior fascicle with normal deficiency of the inferior fascicle.

- The course of the popliteus muscle and tendon can be followed on serial axial, sagittal, and posterior coronal images.

- The thickness of the popliteus tendon sheath is variable and may be identified as a thin line or a thick band.

- A true peripheral lateral meniscal tear usually presents with a different obliquity than that described for the popliteus tendon sheath.

- A vertical tear of the posterior horn of the lateral meniscus, however, may parallel the popliteus tendon sheath. In such cases, the popliteus tendon should be used as a landmark for the location of the peripheral edge of the meniscus.

- After lateral meniscectomy, the low-signal-intensity popliteus tendon may be mistaken for a retained posterior horn remnant. Continuity with the popliteus tendon helps to avoid this misdiagnosis.

Partial Volume Averaging

- The concave peripheral meniscal edge may produce the appearance of grade 2 signal intensity on peripheral sagittal images through the body of the meniscus.[186]

- This appearance is more commonly seen in the medial meniscus and is caused by partial volume averaging of fat and neurovascular structures lying in the concavity of the meniscus.

- This artifact has been reported in up to 29% of medial and 6% of lateral menisci.[323]

- Corresponding thin-section radial or coronal images, however, display an intact meniscal structure and may display the concave margin of the meniscus.

Meniscofemoral Ligaments

- Laterally, the meniscofemoral ligament consists of the *ligament of Humphrey*, which extends anterior to the PCL, and a posterior branch of the *ligament of Wrisberg*, seen posterior to the PCL.

- The meniscofemoral ligament most commonly has direct attachment to the lateral meniscus and is obliquely oriented to its insertion on the medial femoral condyle.

- The posterior branch of the meniscofemoral ligament, the ligament of Wrisberg, is the larger of the two branches and may appear to be half the cross-sectional diameter of the PCL.[323]

- The anterior meniscofemoral ligament has been reported to be present in 34% of anatomic dissections and the posterior meniscofemoral ligament in 60%.

- MR visualization has been reported in 33% of cases for either ligament, and in 3% of MR examinations, both structures are identified.

- One branch of the meniscofemoral ligament usually predominates.[462]

    - Separate from the anterior meniscofemoral ligament of Humphrey, there may exist a rare anterior meniscofemoral ligament connecting the anterior horn of the medial meniscus to the roof of the intercondylar notch (best seen in the sagittal plane). This anterior meniscofemoral ligament may be mistaken for an infrapatellar plica.

- The ligament of Humphrey can be best seen on sagittal images, whereas the ligament of Wrisberg is best shown on posterior coronal images.

- The ligament of Humphrey can, however, be identified on coronal images.

- Meniscal insertion of the meniscofemoral ligament may mimic the appearance of a vertical tear in the posterior horn of the lateral meniscus.[493]

- This pseudo-tear, the result of fat and or fluid interposed between the meniscus attachment and the meniscofemoral ligament, can be seen extending obliquely from the superior meniscal surface and is directed posteriorly and inferiorly toward the inferior meniscal surface.

- With external rotation of the knee, the interface between the meniscofemoral ligament and the posterior horn of the lateral meniscus becomes more prominent.

    - In this location, the ligament of Wrisberg is more likely than the ligament of Humphrey to be mistaken for meniscal pathology.

- Oblique meniscomeniscal ligaments, which pass between the ACL and PCL, also may be mistaken for a displaced flap tear or bucket-handle tear.[414]

- The oblique meniscomeniscal ligament passes from the anterior horn of one meniscus to the posterior horn of the opposite meniscus.

Pseudo–Bucket-Handle Tear

- On posterior coronal images that traverse both the body and the posterior horn of the lateral meniscus, separate portions of the posterior horn may be mistaken for a lateral bucket-handle tear.
    - This is more likely to occur with the knee positioned in external rotation.

- This appearance is not usually encountered on posterior coronal images through the medial meniscus.

- Correlation with sagittal images shows normal meniscal morphology without tearing.

Pseudohypertrophy of the Anterior Horn (Anterior Flipped Meniscus)

- Complex meniscal tears may present with a unique MR appearance.

- In the lateral meniscus, the posterior horn may be absent or truncated, or it may be displaced or flipped anteriorly, occupying the space adjacent to the anterior horn, creating pseudohypertrophy of the anterior horn fibrocartilage.

- This pattern is commonly seen in bucket-handle tears of the lateral meniscus.[529]

- The two meniscal horns are separated by an interface of fluid.

- The flipped posterior horn tissue is posterior to the anterior horn.
    - The anterior horn may be more deformed (blunted on its free edge).
    - The displaced posterior horn may be mistaken for the anterior horn.

- **Lax Meniscal Sign or Meniscal Flounce**
    - Sometimes a lax or redundant folding, buckling, or flounce in the meniscus contour is present without any associated fibrocartilage tear.
        - This finding is seen more commonly in the medial meniscus and is best visualized when there is an associated effusion and/or joint laxity.
    - A flounce contour without associated meniscal pathology may also be seen in the lateral meniscus.
    - The lax or "buckled meniscus" sometimes simulates a central or peripheral meniscal tear.
        - This phenomenon may disappear with joint manipulation or subsequent imaging.
    - A true meniscal flounce or fold represents a normal variant, provided there are no other associated indicators of meniscal pathology.
    - The presence of a meniscal flounce is not associated with an increased prevalence of meniscal tears.

- **Vacuum Phenomenon**
    - The magnetic susceptibility of normal amounts of intraarticular gas may produce a low-signal-intensity void or blooming artifact on GRE images.
    - This artifact may be mistaken for a meniscal tear or articular cartilage injury.

- **Pseudo–Loose Body**
    - Normal high-intensity fat intercondylar notch signal may be mistaken for a loose body on $T2^*$-weighted or FS coronal or sagittal images.
        - Unlikely to occur if T1-weighted images are correlated with corresponding GRE or FS images

- **MCL Bursa**
    - The bursa of the MCL is seen between the periphery of the body of the medial meniscus and the MCL.[393]
    - On T2-weighted images, fluid within the bursa may be falsely mistaken for a peripheral meniscocapsular tear.

- **Magic-Angle Phenomenon**
    - On short-TE images, the magic-angle phenomenon may be responsible for increased signal intensity in the upward-sloping portion, or medial segment, of the posterior horn of the normal lateral meniscus.[371]
        - This effect is a function of the anisotropic behavior of normal meniscal fibrocartilage.
            - Seen in meniscal sections oriented at approximately 55 degrees relative to the static magnetic field (B zero) along the long axis of the magnet bore

- **Capsular Attachment**
    - The region between the posterior horn of the medial meniscus and the capsular periphery may be mistaken for a peripheral vertical tear of the medial meniscus.
    - Fat and peripheral vessels in this region produce a signal that can be mistaken for a meniscocapsular separation. T2* GRE images are useful in appreciating the lack of low-spin-density meniscal signal in the normal capsular junctional zone between the capsule and the meniscus.
    - FS PD FSE images can be windowed to appreciate the difference between meniscal and capsular signal intensity.
    - The identification of a complete and well-defined fluid plane between the meniscus and the capsule, or the presence of a corner tear of the posterior horn of the medial meniscus adjacent to the capsule, may be seen in association with meniscocapsular injuries.
    - In this area, the normal capsular attachment of the meniscus is not as prominent as the well-defined condensation of the meniscofemoral and meniscotibial ligaments that occurs in the central third of the meniscocapsular interface.

- **Popliteal Artery**
    - The popliteal artery within the popliteal fossa neurovascular bundle is located posterior to the posterior horn of the lateral meniscus.
    - If phase and frequency direction are not swapped, pulsation artifacts produce an artificial signal in the area of the posterior horn of the lateral meniscus and obscure accurate visualization of the ACL in the sagittal plane.
    - Phase and frequency are also swapped in the axial plane to improve visualization of the patellofemoral articular cartilage.

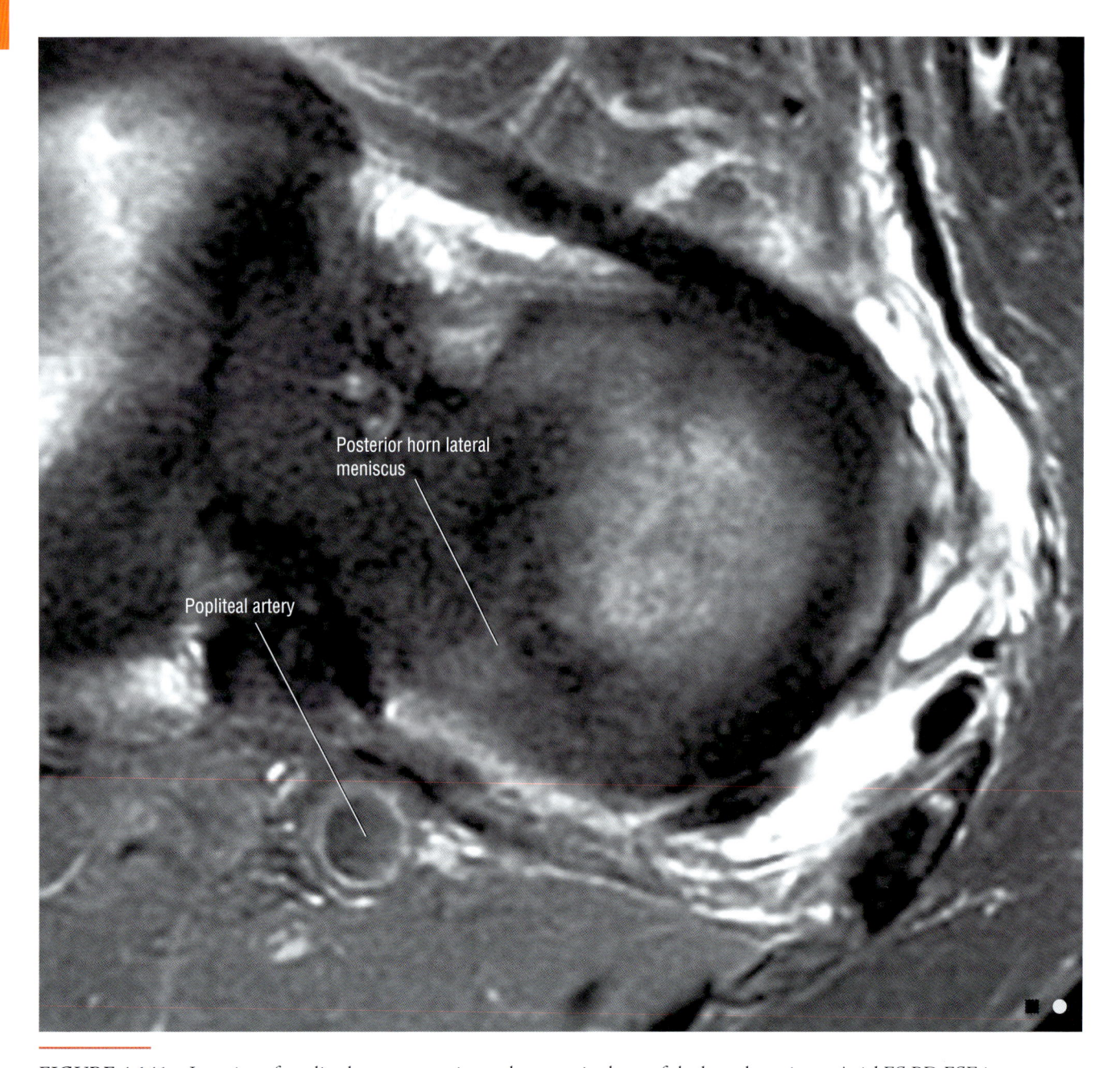

FIGURE 4.141 Location of popliteal artery posterior to the posterior horn of the lateral meniscus. Axial FS PD FSE image.

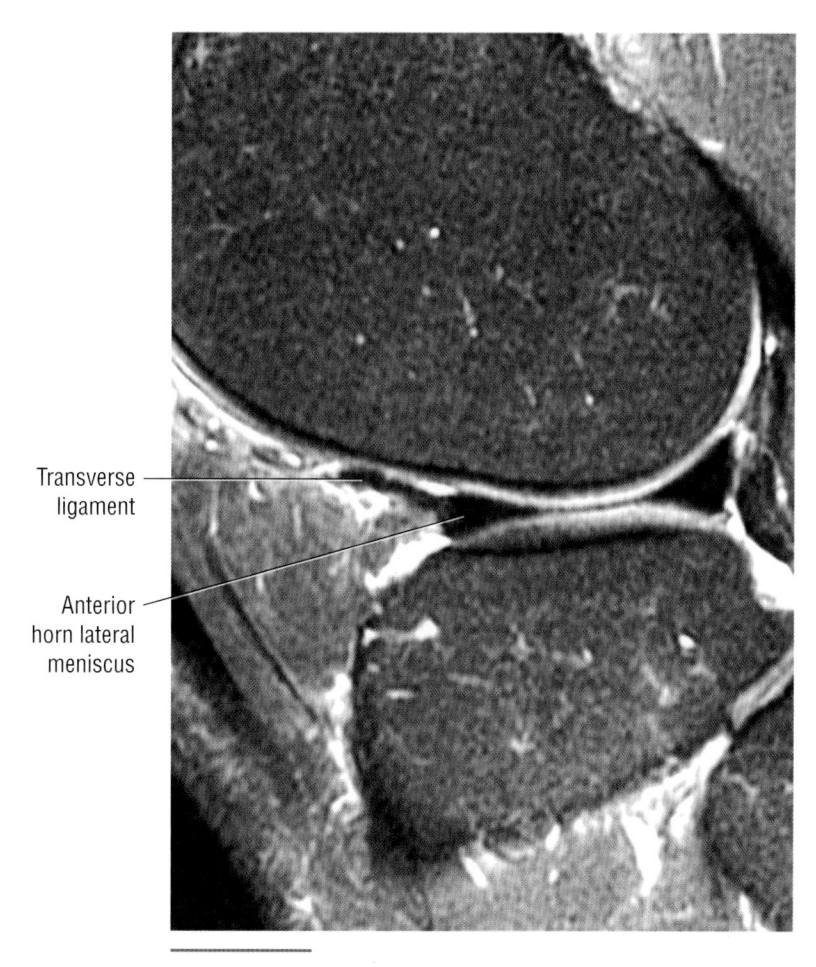

FIGURE 4.142 Sagittal FS PD FSE image shows a linear morphology of the transverse ligament.

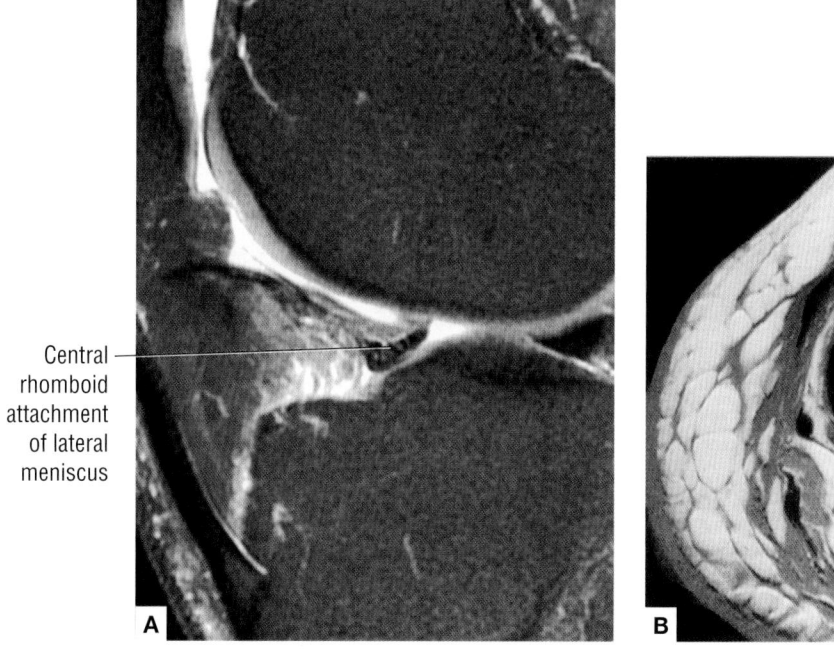

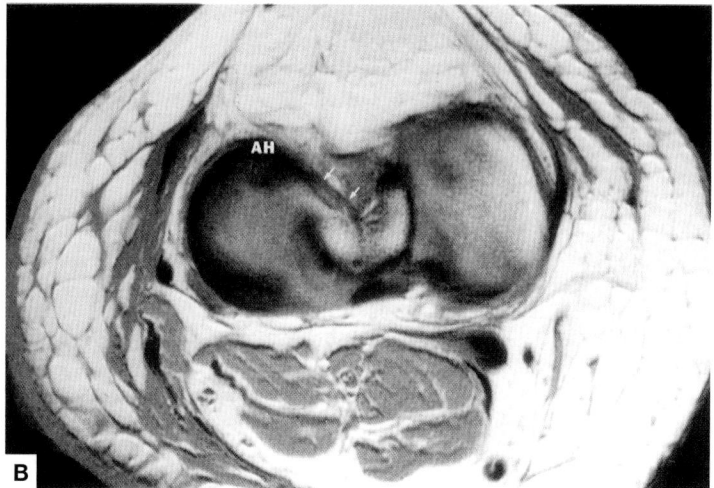

FIGURE 4.143 (**A**) Sagittal FS PD FSE image shows the speckled pattern of the normal central rhomboid attachment of the anterior horn of the lateral meniscus. (**B**) T1-weighted axial image of the central rhomboid attachment (*small arrows*) of the anterior horn (AH) of the lateral meniscus.

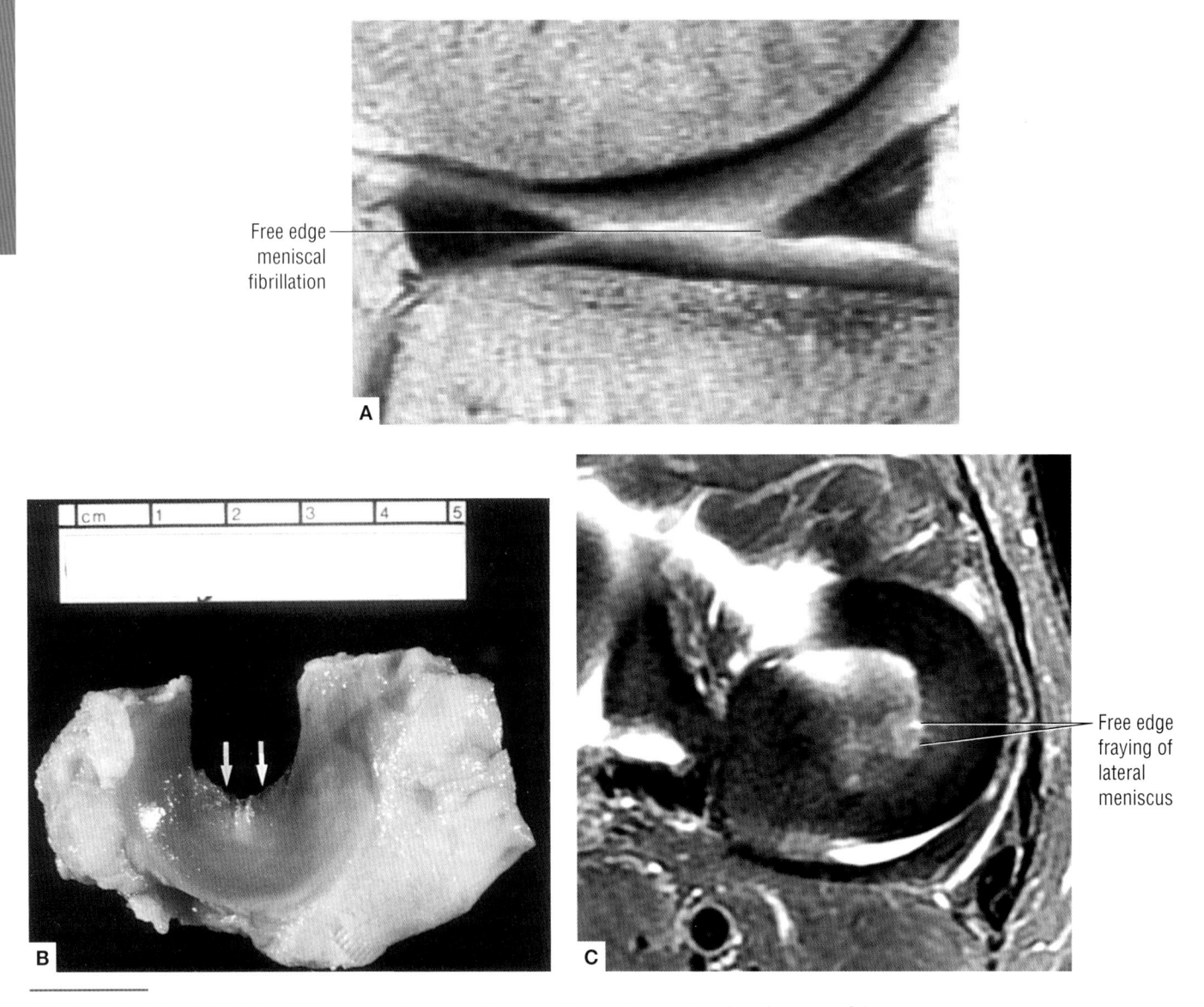

FIGURE 4.144 (**A**) Minimal blunting and intermediate signal intensity restricted to the apex of the meniscus representing degenerative fibrillation or fraying. These changes may be mistaken for a radial tear. (**B**) Gross specimen shows a meniscus with fibrillation along the concave free edge (*arrows*). (**C**) Free edge lateral meniscal fraying without defined meniscal tear.

The Meniscus

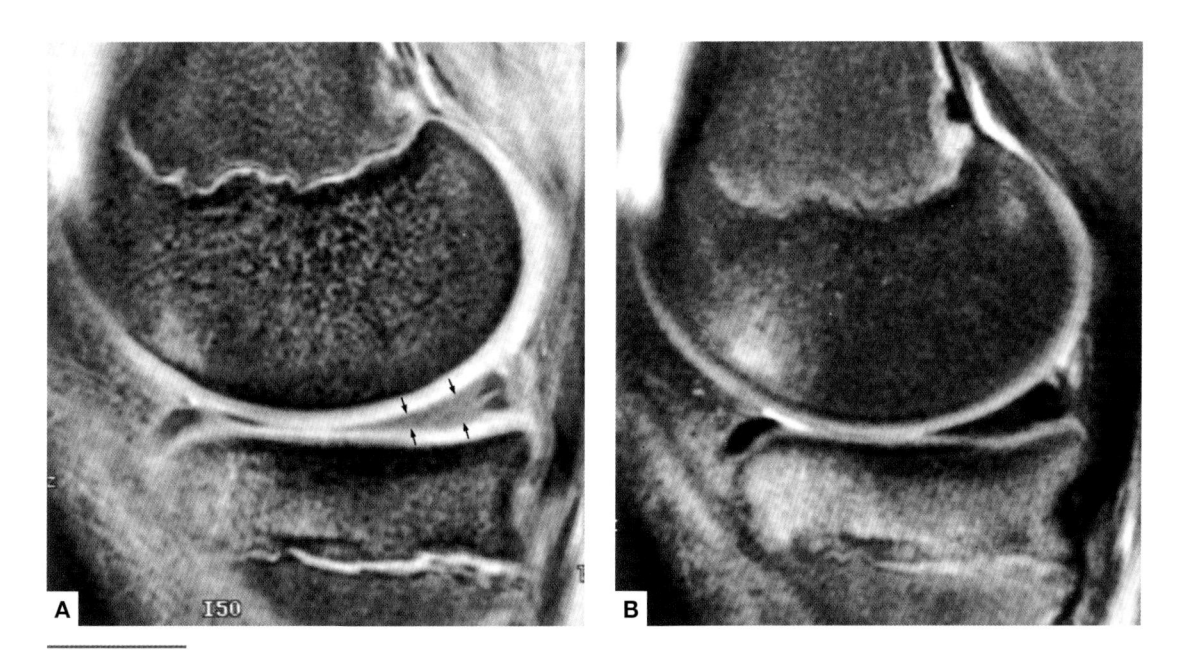

FIGURE 4.145 (**A**) Acute posttraumatic diffuse "meniscal edema" (*arrows*) is hyperintense on this T2*-weighted sagittal image. (**B**) On a corresponding FS PD-weighted FSE sagittal image, however, the posterior horn of the medial meniscus demonstrates normal morphology without tearing. Associated anterior medial compartment bone contusions can be seen on this sequence.

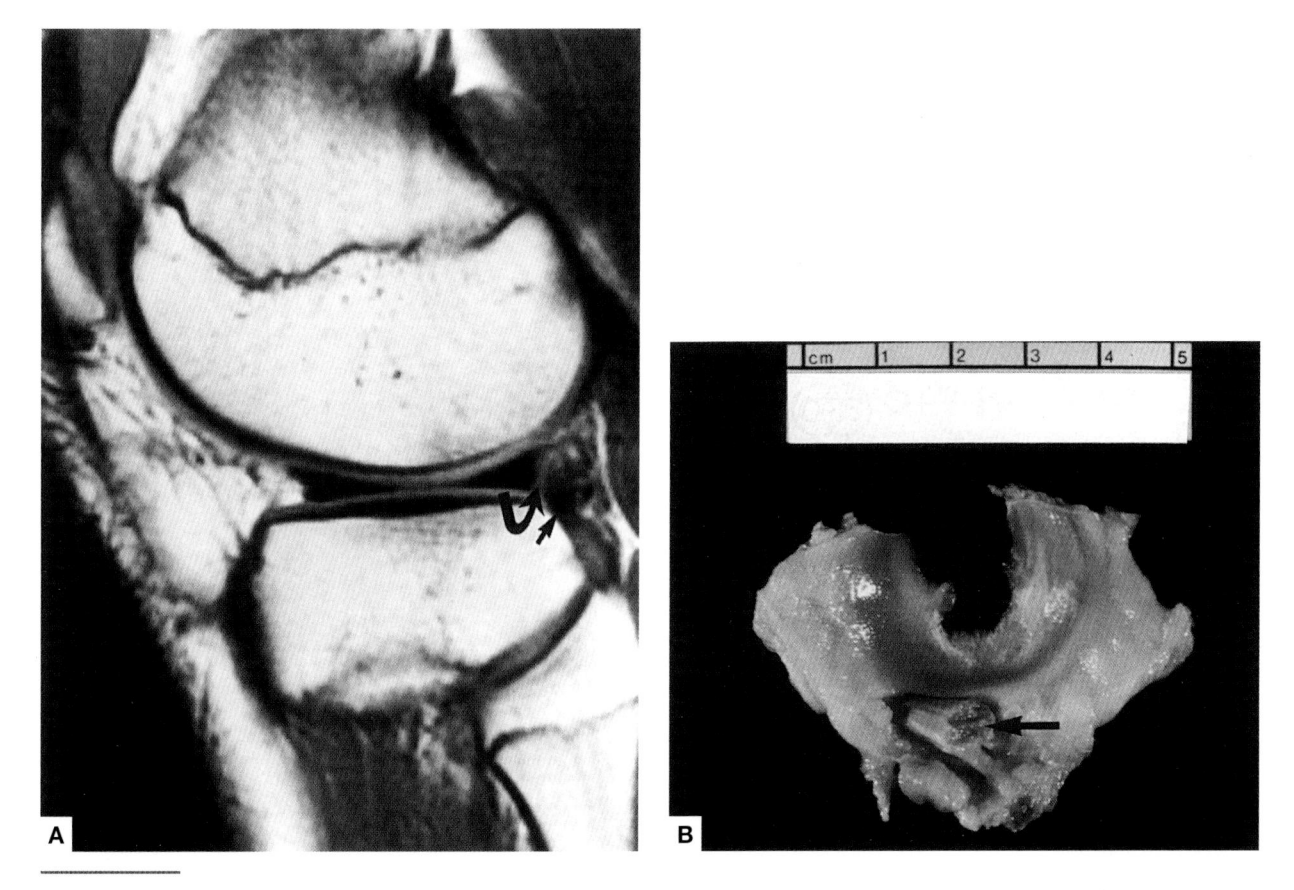

FIGURE 4.146 Popliteus tendon and sheath. (**A**) T1-weighted sagittal image demonstrating the intermediate-signal-intensity popliteus tendon sheath (*curved arrow*) and the low-signal-intensity popliteus tendon (*straight arrow*). (**B**) The corresponding gross specimen shows the course of the popliteus tendon (*arrow*) along the posterior horn of the lateral meniscus.

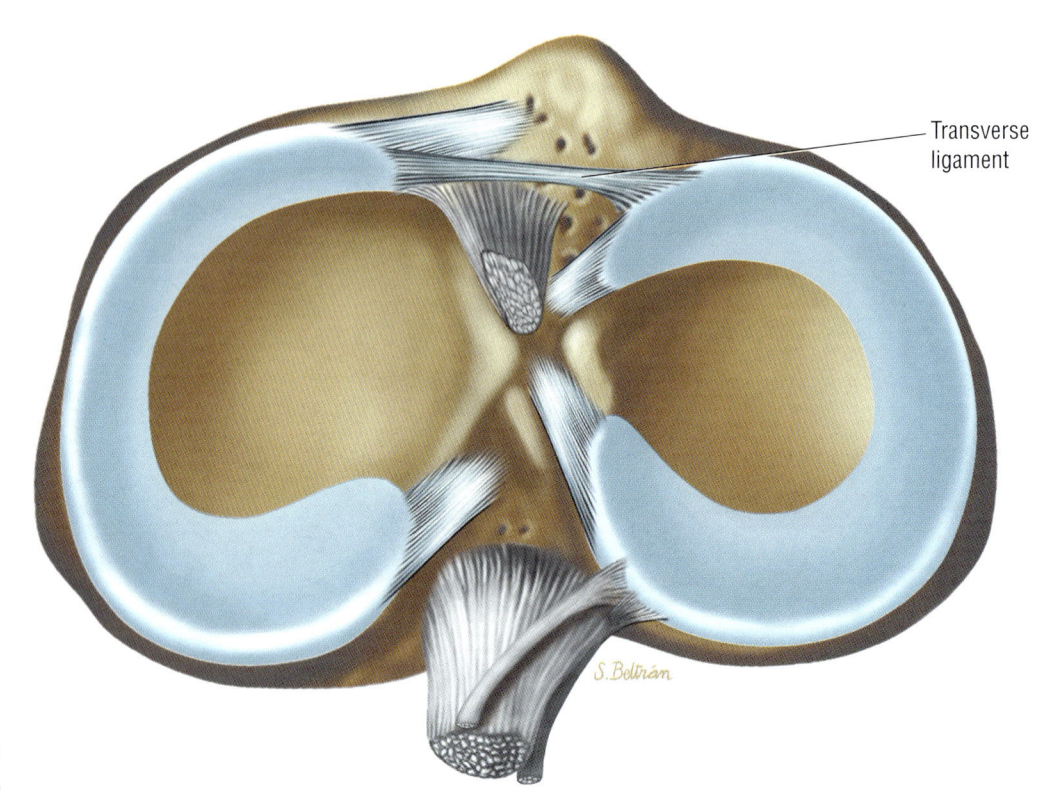

FIGURE 4.147 The transverse ligament of the knee connects the anterior horns of the medial and lateral menisci. Axial superior view color illustration showing the transverse ligament coursing anterior to the anterior horn of the lateral meniscus. In the medial compartment, anterior horn fibrocartilage extends anterior to the transverse ligament attachment.

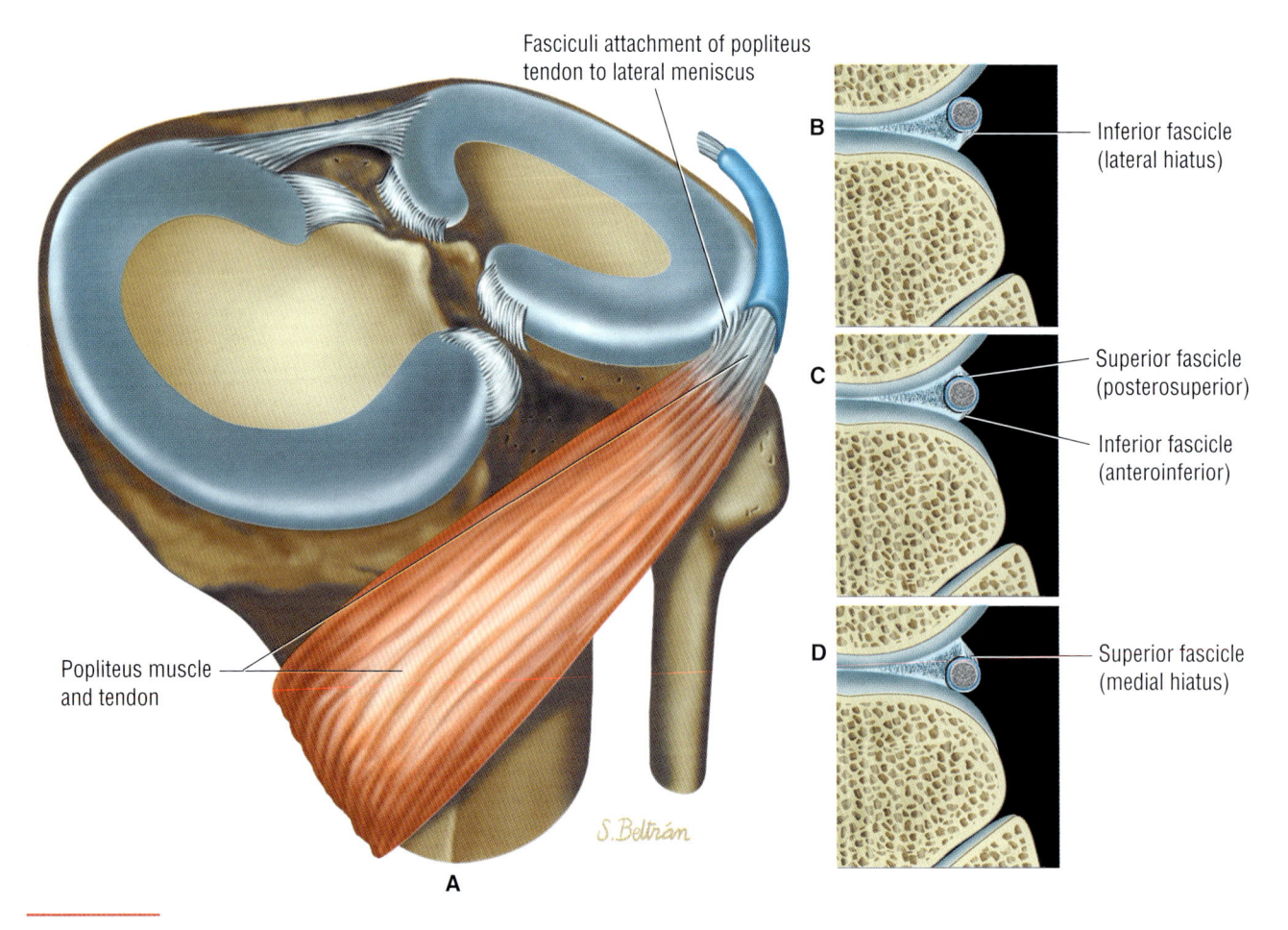

FIGURE 4.148 (**A**) The popliteus tendon is extraarticular but intracapsular and susceptible in posterolateral corner injuries. It is covered by a synovial membrane on its medial aspect. The popliteal hiatus is bound anteroinferiorly by the superior fascicle. These fascicles are also referred to as popliteomeniscal ligaments. Normal deficiencies of the fascicle allow passage of the popliteus tendon from the lateral (**B**) to the medial (**D**) aspect of the hiatus. Both superior and inferior fascicles are shown at the mid-portion of the hiatus (**C**).

The Meniscus

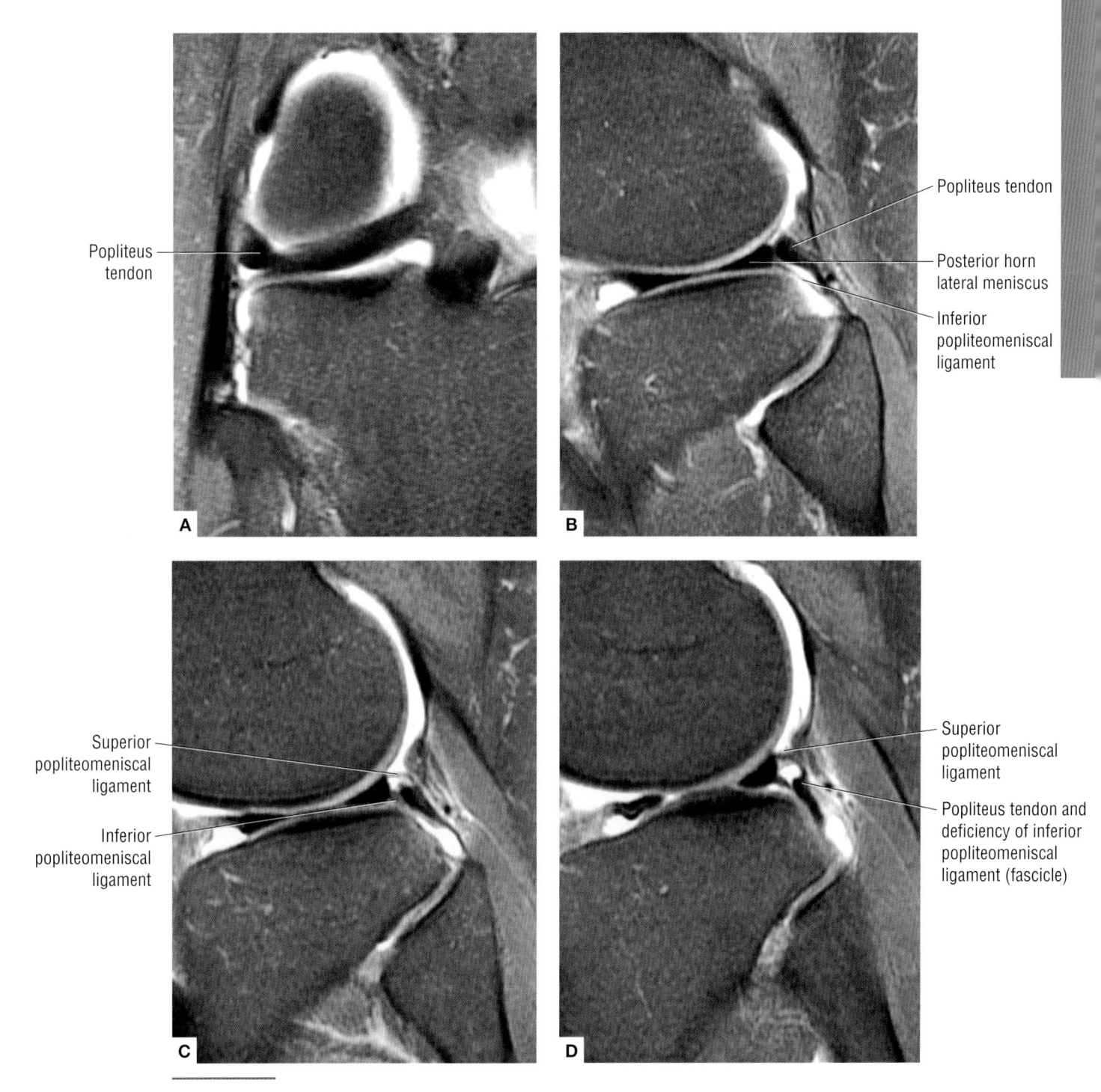

FIGURE 4.149 Coronal (**A**) and sagittal (**B**) images at the level of the superior popliteomeniscal ligament or fascicle deficiency on a lateral peripheral image. (**C**) Both inferior and superior fascicles are visualized between the lateral and medial sagittal sections through the hiatus. (**D**) A more medial section through the hiatus showing the normal inferior popliteomeniscal ligament (fascicle) deficiency.

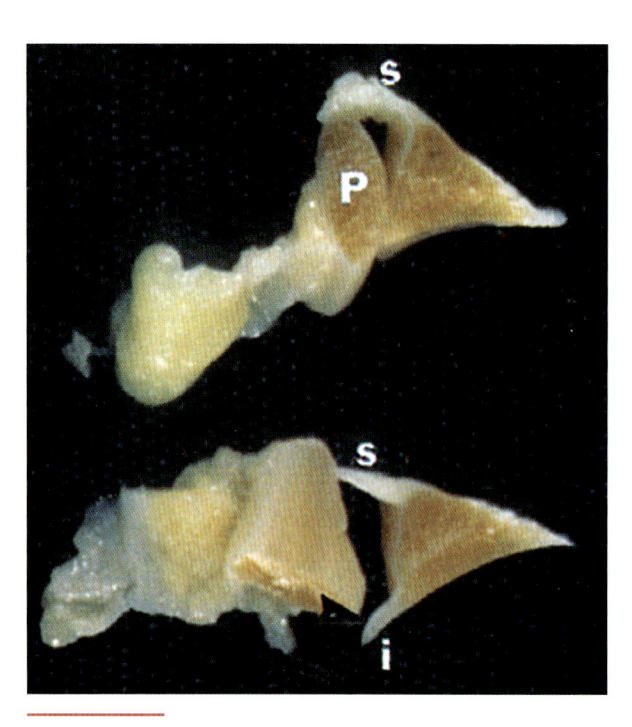

FIGURE 4.150 Examination of a gross anatomic specimen allows identification of the superior (s) and inferior (i) fascicles. The popliteus tendon (P) passes normally through defects in the inferior and superior fascicles.

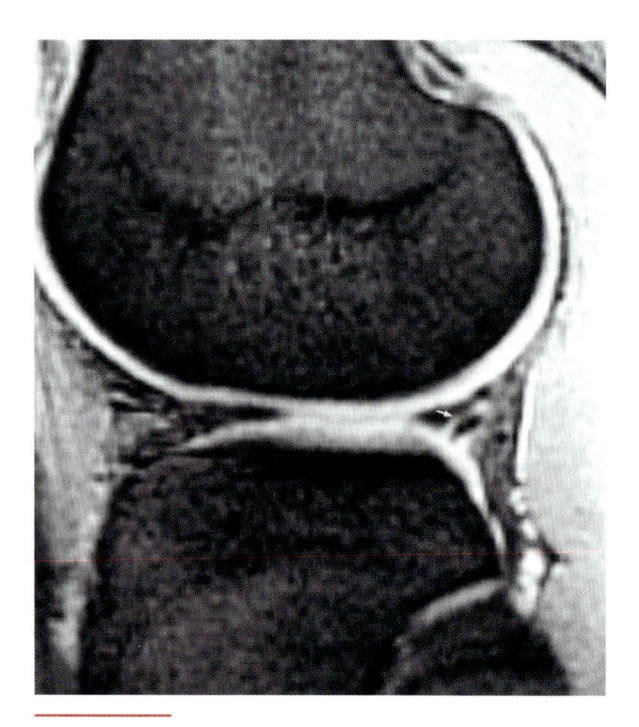

FIGURE 4.151 A tear (*arrow*) of the posterior inferior corner of the lateral meniscus on a T2*-weighted sagittal image. The oblique direction of the tear is opposite to the expected course of the popliteus tendon. The superior meniscal fascicle is intact and is shown in continuity with the posterior horn of the lateral meniscus.

The Meniscus

Meniscofemoral and Intermeniscal Ligaments

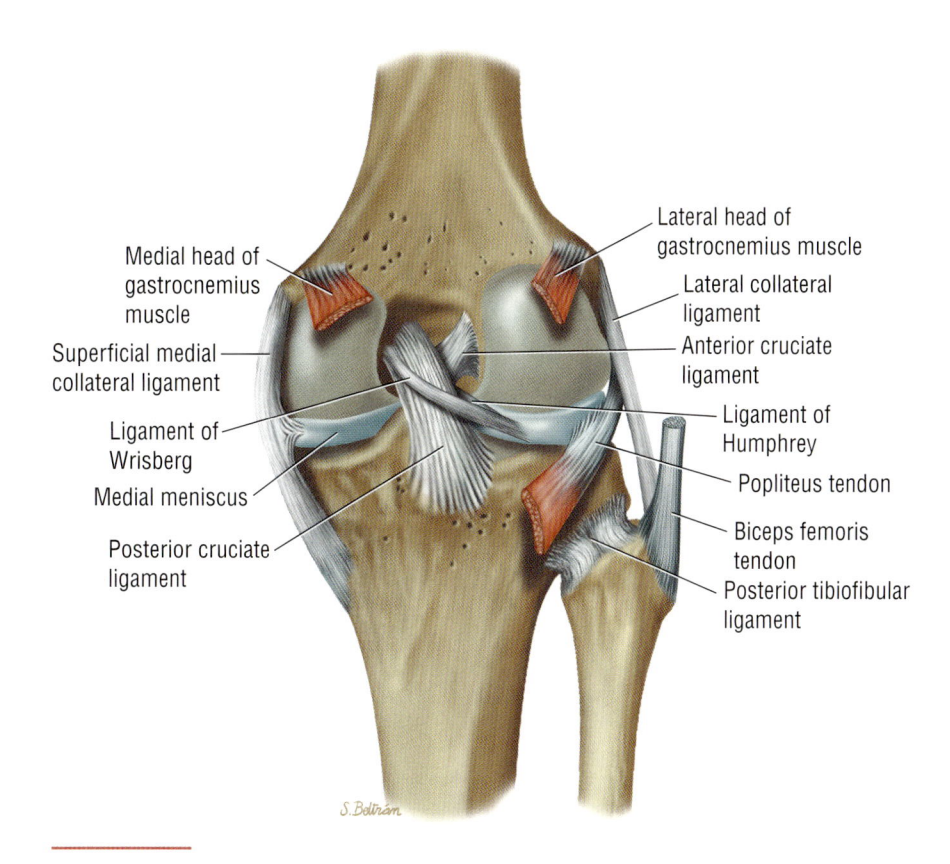

FIGURE 4.152 The ligaments of Humphrey and Wrisberg attach the lateral meniscal posterior horn to the medial femoral condyle. Partial insertion of the popliteus tendon into the posterolateral aspect of the lateral meniscus occurs through the superior and inferior fasciculus forming the popliteal hiatus.

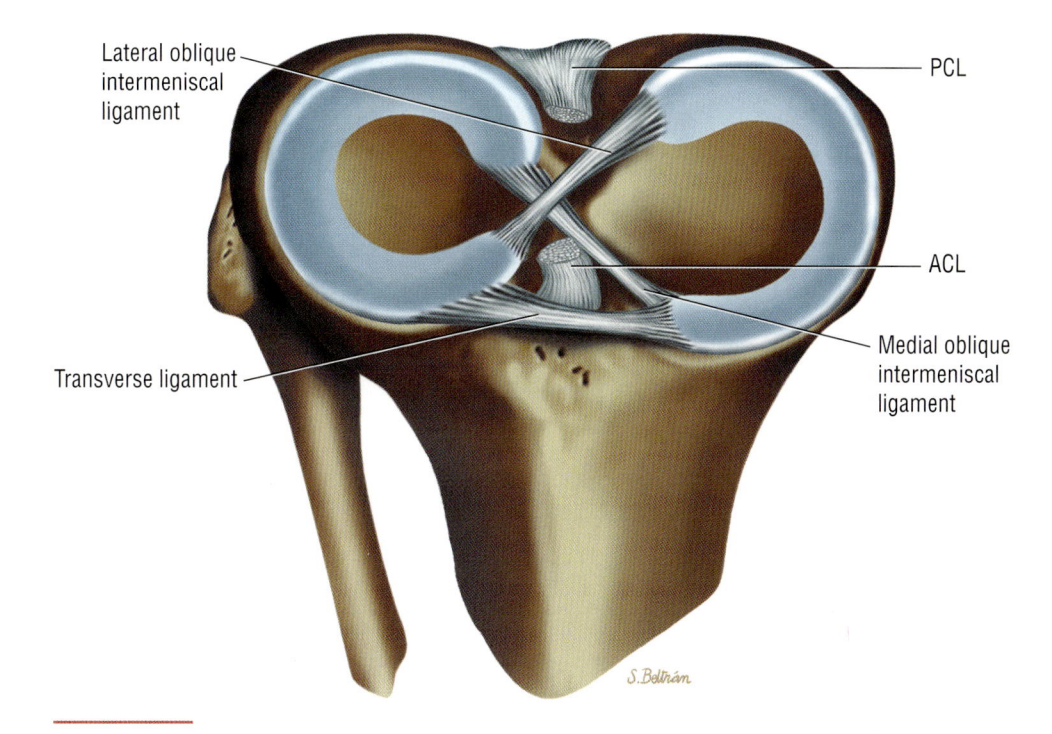

FIGURE 4.153 The course of the oblique intermeniscal ligaments can be seen from the anterior horn of the medial meniscus to the posterior horn of the lateral meniscus. Superior view of both oblique meniscal ligaments.

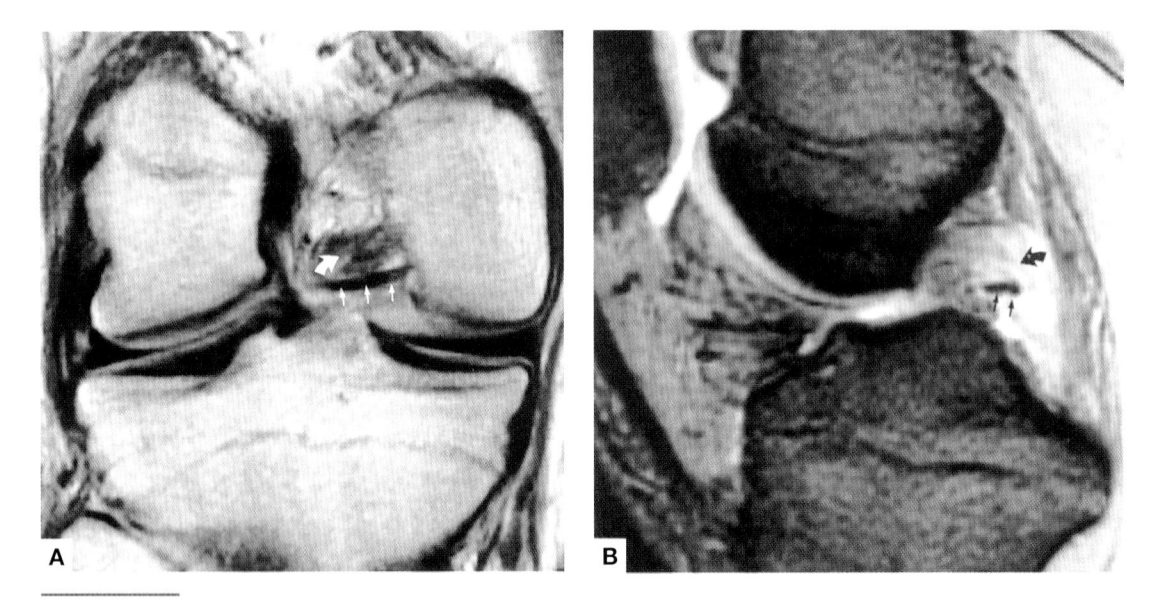

FIGURE 4.154 (A) Intermediate-weighted coronal and (B) T2*-weighted sagittal images show the anatomy of the ligament of Humphrey (*straight arrows*). A complete tear of the PCL (*curved arrow*) is also present.

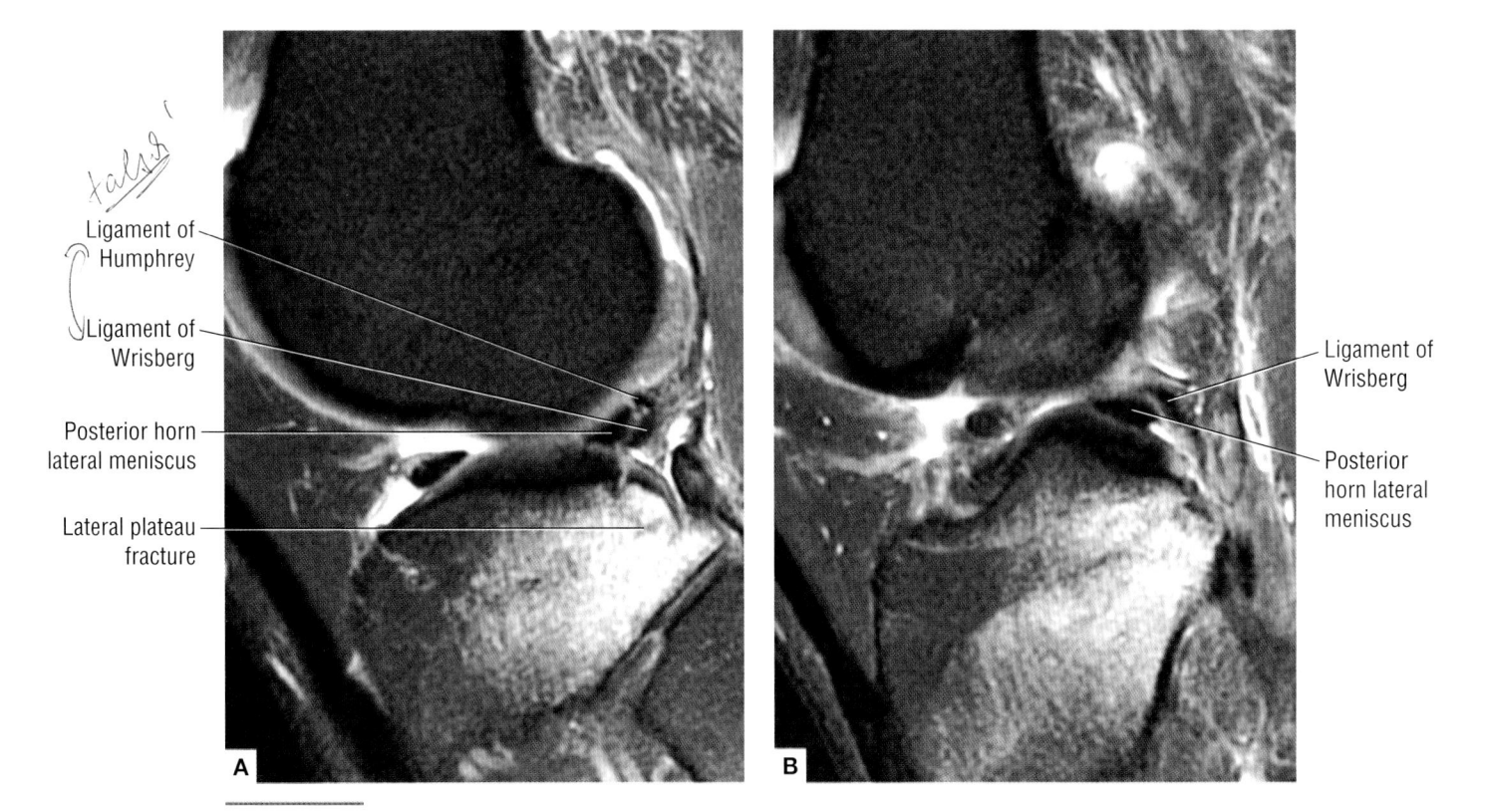

FIGURE 4.155 Sagittal FS PD FSE images of the normal meniscofemoral ligaments without a meniscal tear. (A) The ligaments of Humphrey and Wrisberg can be seen posterior to the posterior horn of the lateral meniscus. (B) On next medial sequential image through the lateral compartment, the ligament of Wrisberg courses superiorly to pass posterior to the PCL within the intercondylar notch. The hyperintense interface between the lateral meniscus and meniscofemoral ligament is normal, even though a fracture of the posterior lateral tibial plateau can be seen on this image.

The Meniscus 323

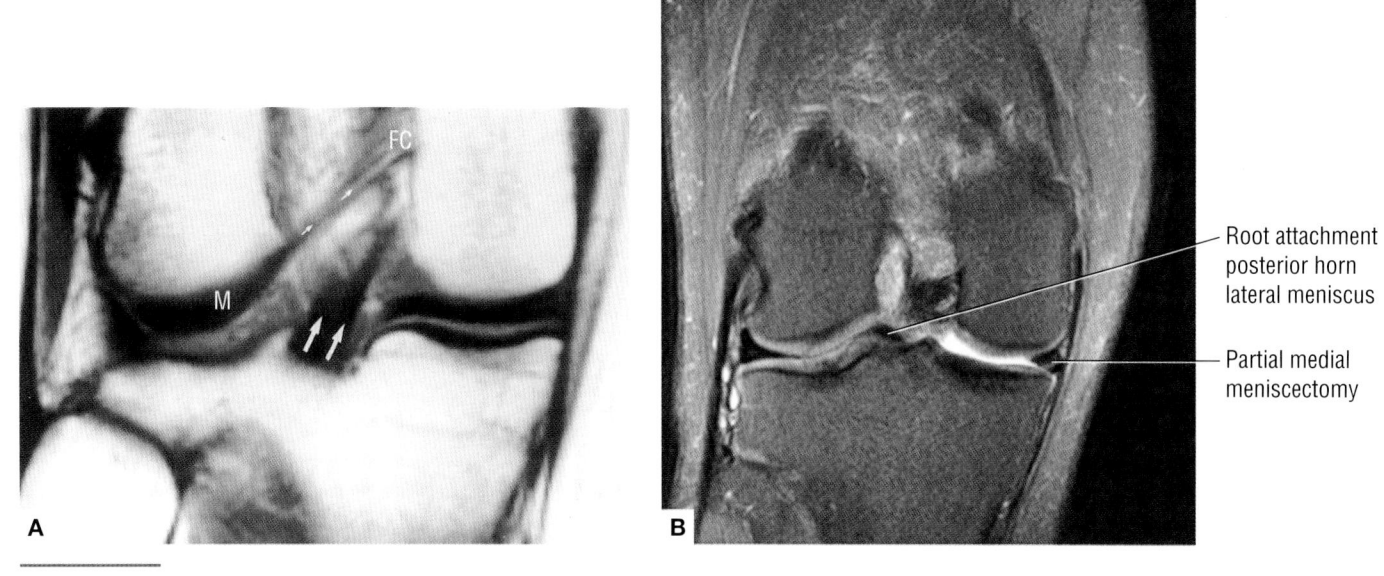

FIGURE 4.156 (**A**) The ligament of Wrisberg (*small arrows*) and the PCL (*large arrows*) are seen on a T1-weighted posterior coronal image. The attachments of the ligament of Wrisberg to the posterior horn of the lateral meniscus (M) and the posteromedial femoral condylae (FC) are evident. (**B**) The posterior root attachment of the lateral meniscus is often mistaken for a displaced meniscal fragment, including a bucket-handle tear. Incidental post–partial meniscectomy changes are also seen in the medial meniscus, which is foreshortened and has residual grade 3 signal intensity (coronal FS PD FSE image).

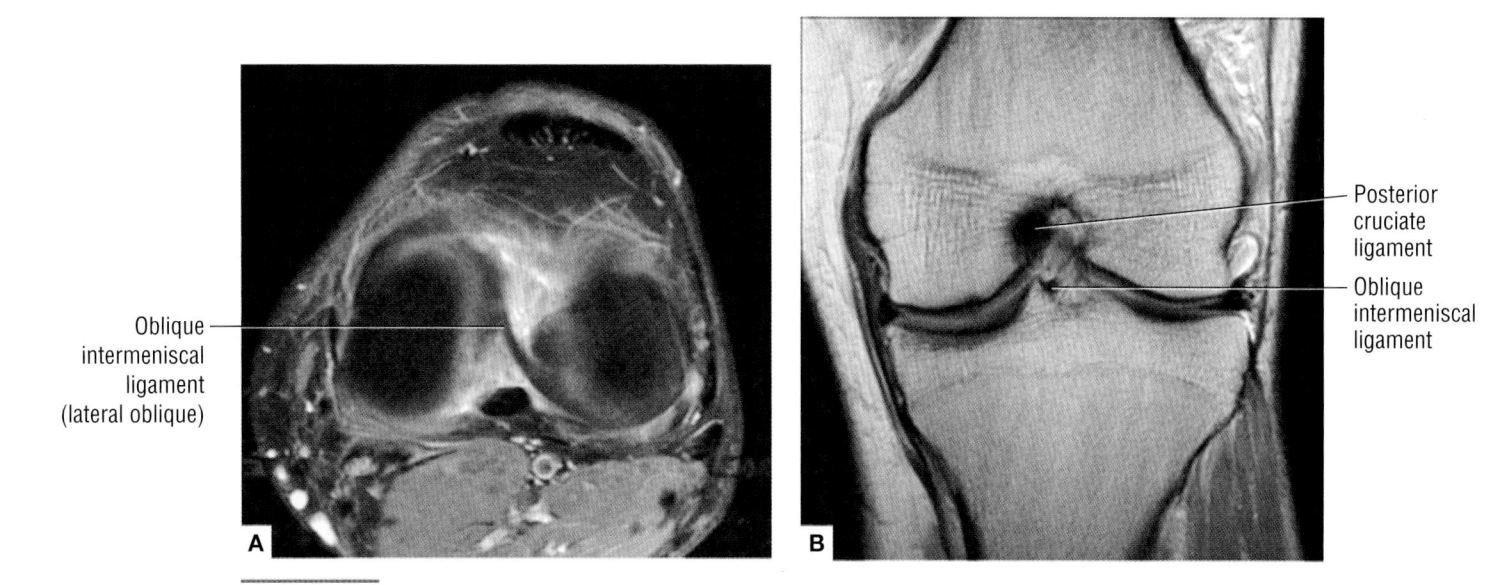

FIGURE 4.157 The course of the oblique intermeniscal ligaments can be seen from the anterior horn of the medial meniscus to the posterior horn of the lateral meniscus. (**A**) Axial FS PD FSE image. (**B**) Anterior coronal PD FSE image.

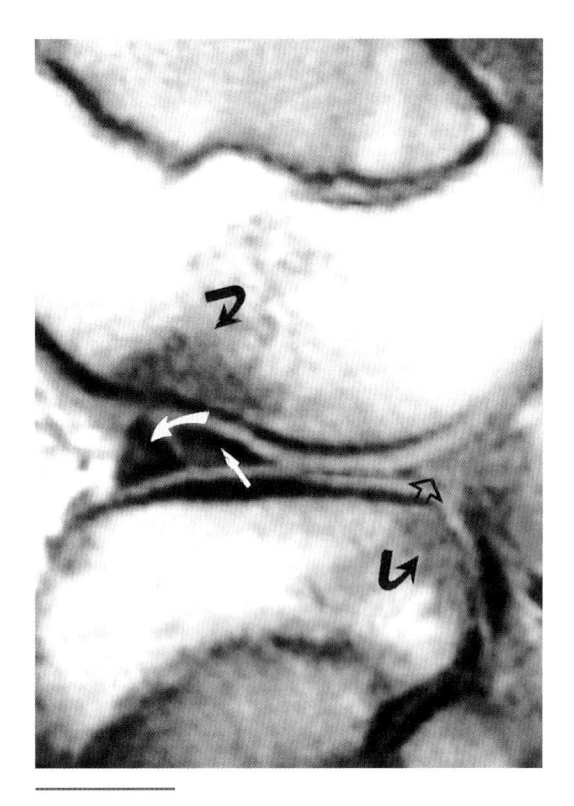

FIGURE 4.158 The posterior horn of the lateral meniscus (*open arrow*) is displaced toward (*straight arrow*) the anterior horn of the lateral meniscus (*curved arrows*). Trabecular bone contusions are of low signal intensity relative to the adjacent bright fatty marrow epiphysis on a T1-weighted sagittal image.

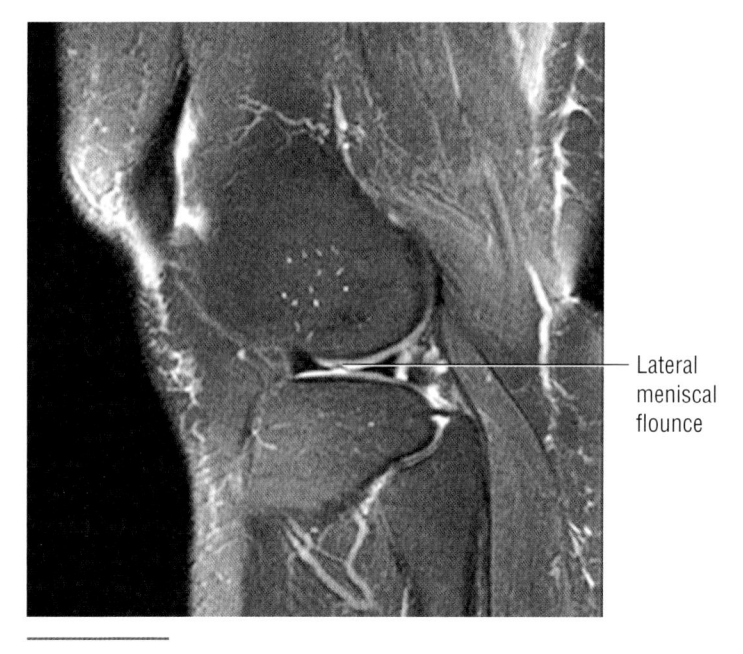

FIGURE 4.159 Less common lateral meniscal flounce on FS PD FSE sagittal image.

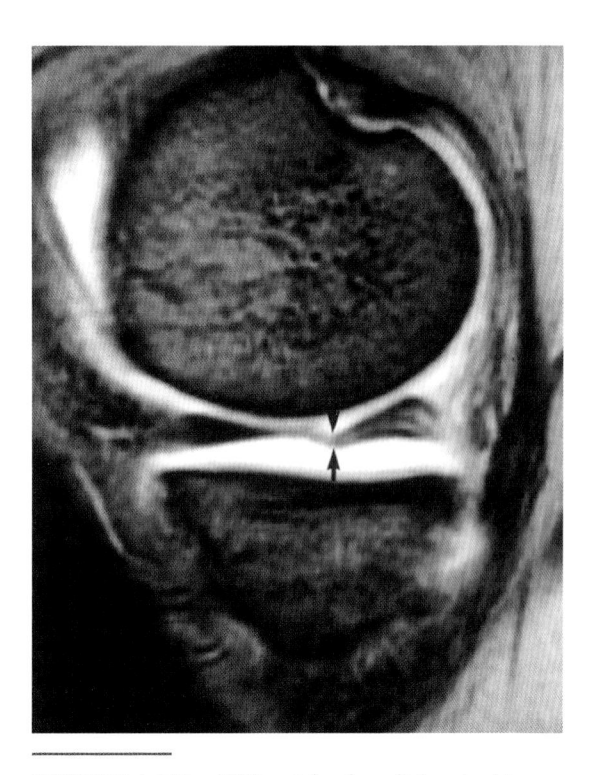

FIGURE 4.160 T2*-weighted medial sagittal image demonstrates that a wavy folded contour may be a normal variant of the intact meniscus.

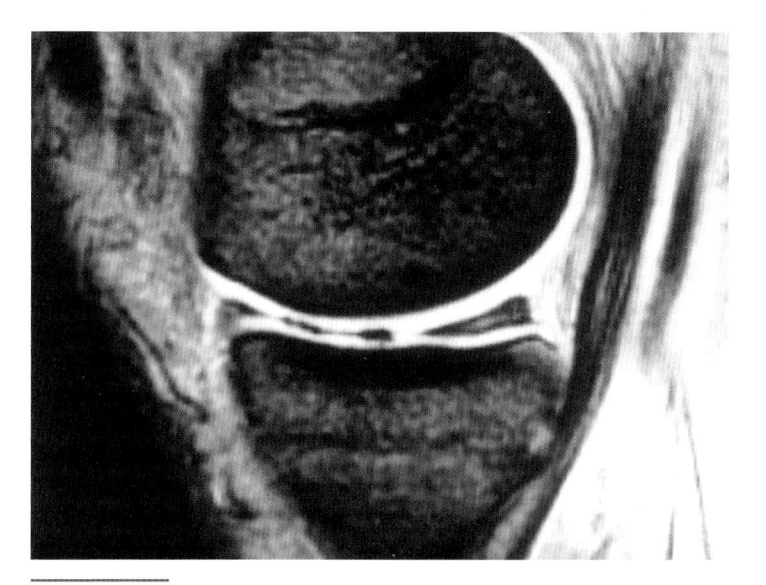

FIGURE 4.161 The vacuum phenomenon. Normal intraarticular gas is identified as a signal void between the femoral and tibial articular cartilage. This T2*-weighted sagittal image demonstrates blooming of the signal void from magnetic susceptibility of the intraarticular gas.

The Meniscus

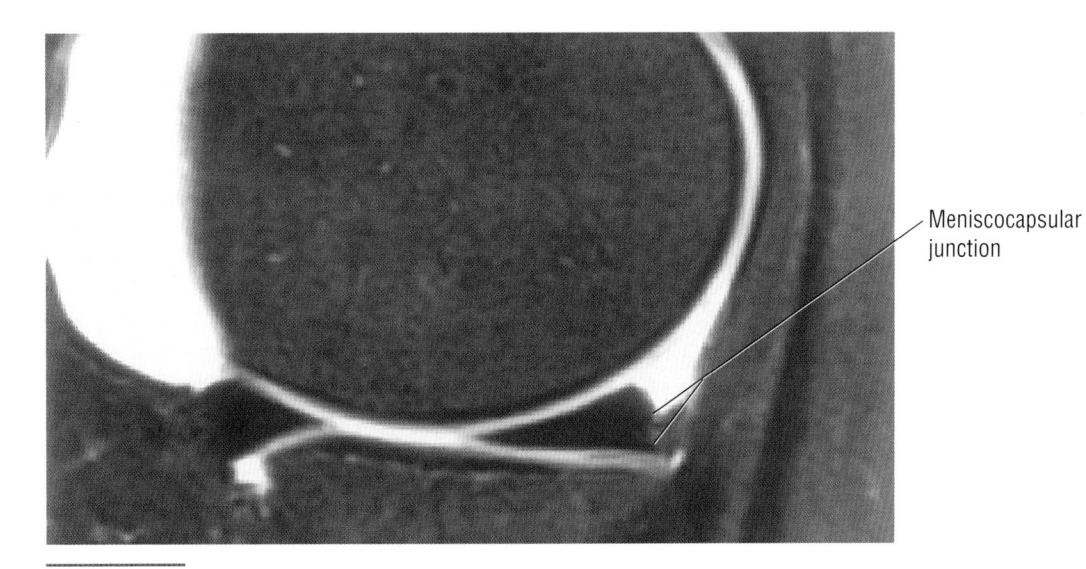

FIGURE 4.162 FS PD FSE sagittal image displaying the normal medial meniscocapsular attachment with an intact meniscus–capsular interface junction at the periphery of the posterior horn of the meniscus.

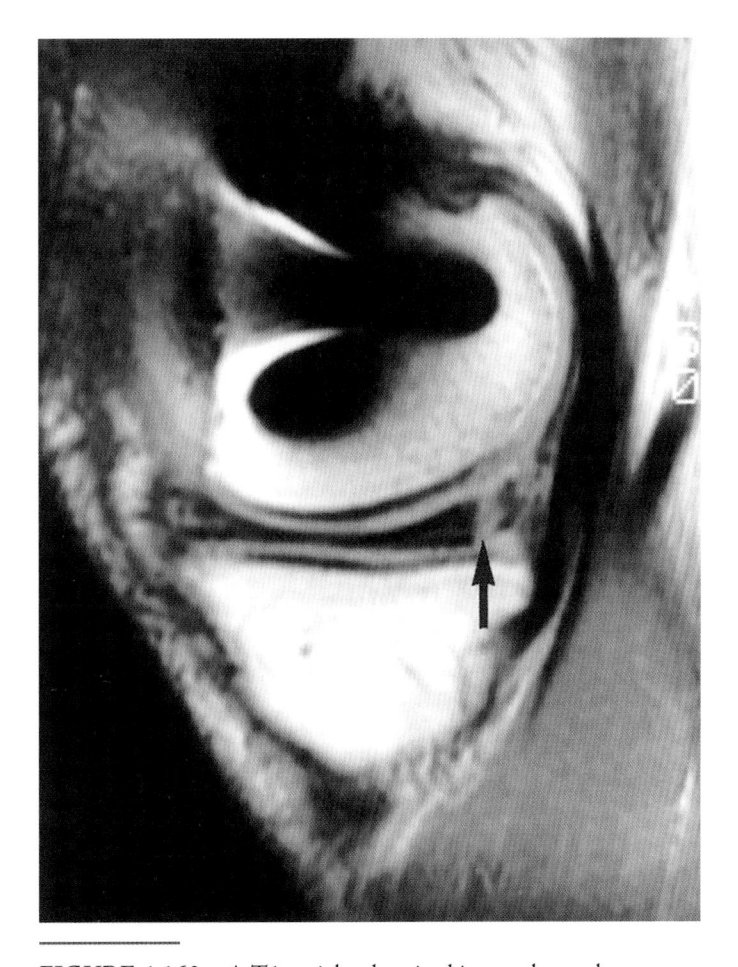

FIGURE 4.163 A T1-weighted sagittal image shows that peripheral grade 3 signal intensity (*arrow*) in a postmeniscal transplant represents suture attachment with healing, not a vertical tear.

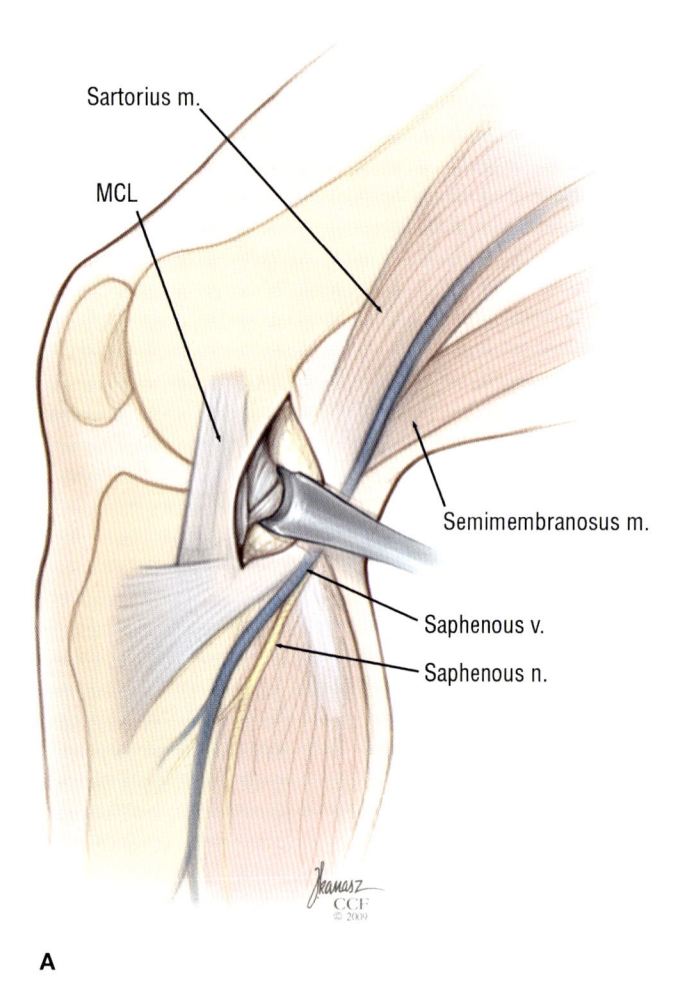

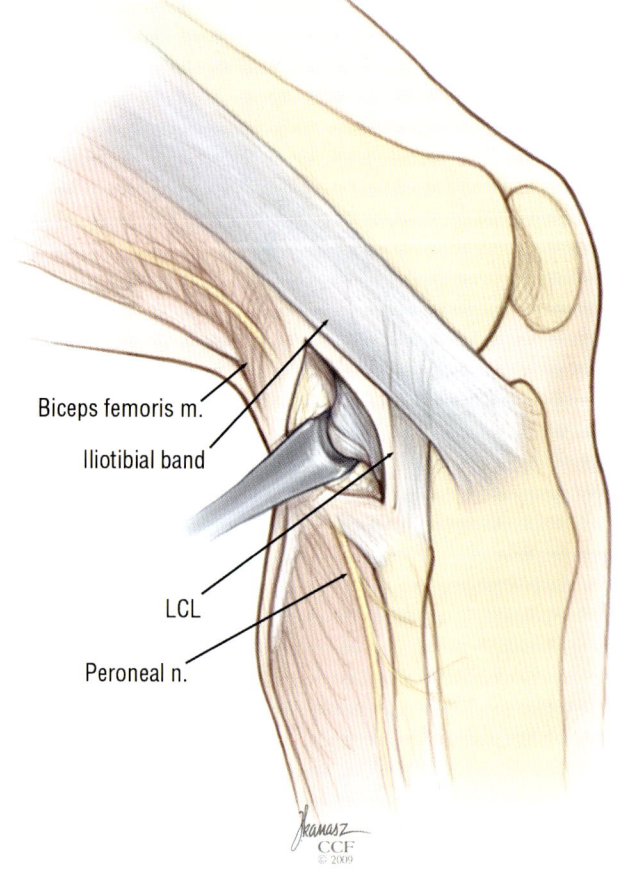

FIGURE 4.164 (**A, B**) Medial and lateral exposures of the peripheral joint capsule as used for surgical access for meniscal repair. (Reprinted from Fu FH. *Master Techniques in Orthopaedic Surgery: Sports Medicine.* Philadelphia, PA: Lippincott Williams & Wilkins; 2010, with permission.)

Meniscal Replacement

- Allograft transplants
    - Extensive meniscal defects
- Partial meniscus implants
    - Fill partial meniscectomy defects
        - Defects greater than two thirds of the meniscal width and less than 5cm
        - Intact anterior and posterior horns and root attachment
        - Stable peripheral rim at popliteus hiatus
- Total meniscus implants
- Allograft technique
    - Harvested from human donors usually with attached bone as anchors
    - Fixation of the allograft to the joint capsule
    - More commonly combined with another procedure
        - ACL reconstruction
        - Articular cartilage repair
        - High tibial osteotomy
- Implant technique
    - Synthetic scaffold implant can be custom fit to the size of the meniscus defect.
    - Synthetic scaffolds are porous, acellular, and bioresorbable.

Treatment of Meniscal Tears

- Treatment options for meniscal injury include:
    - Open meniscal repair, usually appropriate for peripheral tears that occur within 1 to 2mm of the meniscosynovial junction and involve the posterior third of the medial or lateral meniscus[90]

- Nonoperative treatment, sometimes indicated for partial thickness split tears that involve less than 50% of the meniscal width and for full-thickness tears less than 5mm in size with vertical or oblique tear patterns
- Meniscectomy, used to treat complex tears, degenerative tears, and large radial and flap tears[61]
- Meniscal replacement
- Meniscal transplantation, used to delay the development of degenerative disease after meniscectomy

- The inside-out technique of meniscal repair is the gold standard and is indicated for tears of the body and posterior horn.[379]

- Meniscal repairs are frequently performed in conjunction with ACL reconstructions because of the association of meniscal tears with ACL-deficient knees.

- Results of meniscal repairs performed in conjunction with ACL reconstructions are better than those of isolated meniscal repairs.

- The vascularity of the posterior horn of the lateral meniscus permits repair of complex tears, and injection of a fibrin clot can be used as an adjunct in some cases.[64,185]

- Tears in the vascular or red-red zone tend to form a clot and heal compared to meniscal tears in the avascular central region or white-white zone, which do not.

- Meniscal tears in the red-white zone are common in location and require enhanced techniques to promote healing.
  - Technical suturing for a stable repair
  - Stimulation of the repair site by hematoma, fibrin clot or glue, cell growth factors, creating traumatic vascular channels, and adjacent synovial bleeding[40,147]

- Reparable meniscal tears, including peripheral vertical longitudinal and meniscocapsular injuries, have the following characteristics:
    - Tear is traumatic
    - Tear is located within the peripheral third (the vascular zone) of the meniscus
    - Relative preservation of the body segment of the meniscus
- Peripheral meniscal tears are often associated with hemarthrosis and frequently occur in sports injuries.
- The medial meniscus is more often affected in football and basketball injuries, whereas the lateral meniscus is more often torn in injuries sustained during wrestling or soccer.
- Tears involving the avascular zone may not be suitable for repair.
- As mentioned, vascular zone tears and unstable peripheral longitudinal vertical tears greater than 1cm in length, including displaced bucket-handle tears, are candidates for meniscal repair.[61]
- Also, meniscal repair may be appropriate for tears in avascular portions of the meniscus that are in communication with peripheral synovium and perimeniscal capsular plexus.
- Techniques such as abrasion of the perimeniscal synovium, meniscal rasping, and implantation of exogenous fibrin clots have increased and expanded the criteria for meniscal repair.
- Most tear types with rim widths of up to 5mm are considered candidates for meniscal repair, contingent on their ability to be stabilized and coapted.
- Because of the importance of the lateral meniscus in load transmission and the potential for severe degenerative disease in patients undergoing total lateral meniscectomy, meniscal repair techniques are usually attempted for most lateral meniscal tears.[480]
- Lateral meniscal tears are also more common in association with acute ACL injuries.

- Tears stable to arthroscopic probing (<3mm of translation on arthroscopic palpation) and short radial tears less than 5mm in length may not require resection.[61]

- There have been reports of patients in whom certain lateral meniscal tears (posterior horn avulsion tears, vertical tears posterior to the popliteus tendon, and stable vertical longitudinal and radial tears) were identified during ACL reconstruction and who had remained asymptomatic without treatment of their meniscal lesions.[140]

- Arthroscopic repair of the meniscal root back to its native insertion site (modification to meniscal transplantation technique)[462]
    - Lateral meniscal root tears commonly occur with ACL tears.
    - Medial meniscal root tears occur with other ligament injuries in sports trauma in younger patients (<40 years old) and in association with minor trauma in the age group over 40 years old.[379]

- The decision to perform a partial meniscectomy depends on the morphology of the tear and its extension to the free edge of the meniscus.[402]

- Horizontal tears should not be treated with primary meniscal repair.

- For longitudinal, vertical, or bucket-handle tears, when meniscal repair is not indicated, a partial meniscectomy is performed in which the displaced portion of the meniscus is reduced with a probe before resection of the meniscus until stable tissue is exposed.

- A horizontal component is often present at the meniscal rim.

- Radial tears greater than 5mm may be symptomatic and partially resected at arthroscopy.

- Although usually associated with horizontal tears, meniscal cysts may be associated with deep radial tears.

- Partial meniscectomy with removal of a flap is performed in oblique tears.

- The stability of the remaining portion of the meniscus can be tested with a probe at arthroscopy and varies as a function of the horizontal and vertical component to the tear.

- In horizontal cleavage tears, if one leaf is unstable, it is resected, leaving the stable leaf.

- A 3-mm flap may be left. In addition, avascular tears and tears associated with unstable ACL-deficient knees in patients older than 40 years are frequently treated by partial meniscectomy.[61]

- Meniscal Transplantation
    - Meniscal transplantation, developed by Garrett et al.,[157] is used to delay the development of degenerative disease after meniscectomy.
    - In this procedure, age- and size-matched allograft menisci are sutured to the resected meniscal rim.
    - The anterior and posterior meniscal horn and meniscotibial attachments are preserved so that they can function as firm anchors for the generation of hoop stresses.
    - Accurate restoration of the meniscal horns is achieved with the use of bony plugs or blocks.
    - This procedure is primarily used in young patients who have undergone total meniscectomy and who are likely to develop degenerative arthrosis by middle age.
    - Ideal patients for meniscus transplantation meet the following criteria:
        - Documented near-complete meniscectomy
        - Ligamentous stability
        - Early (grades I to II) chondral degeneration
        - Intact osseous alignment and congruence of articular cartilage[320]
    - Degenerative arthrosis develops more rapidly after lateral meniscectomy than after medial meniscectomy, and patients with significant joint space narrowing and chondral loss are not candidates for meniscal replacement.
    - Meniscal transplantation also contributes to stability in ACL-deficient knees with absent medial menisci and fibrocartilage.
    - It may also contribute to preservation of joint function as part of a three-stage reconstruction that includes the repair of the meniscus, the ACL, and any associated osteochondral lesion.

- MR is used preoperatively to evaluate the meniscal remnant, to determine proper sizing, and to identify associated chondral erosions.

- Postoperatively, MR is used to evaluate the integrity of the transplant and allograft and to follow peripheral healing at the suture site.

- During the process of peripheral revascularization after meniscal transplantation, persistent grade 3 signal intensity may be seen.

- New novel technique developed for meniscal transplantation using a three-tunnel technique for either the medial or lateral meniscus.

Medial meniscus allograft secured to the tibia and meniscal rim

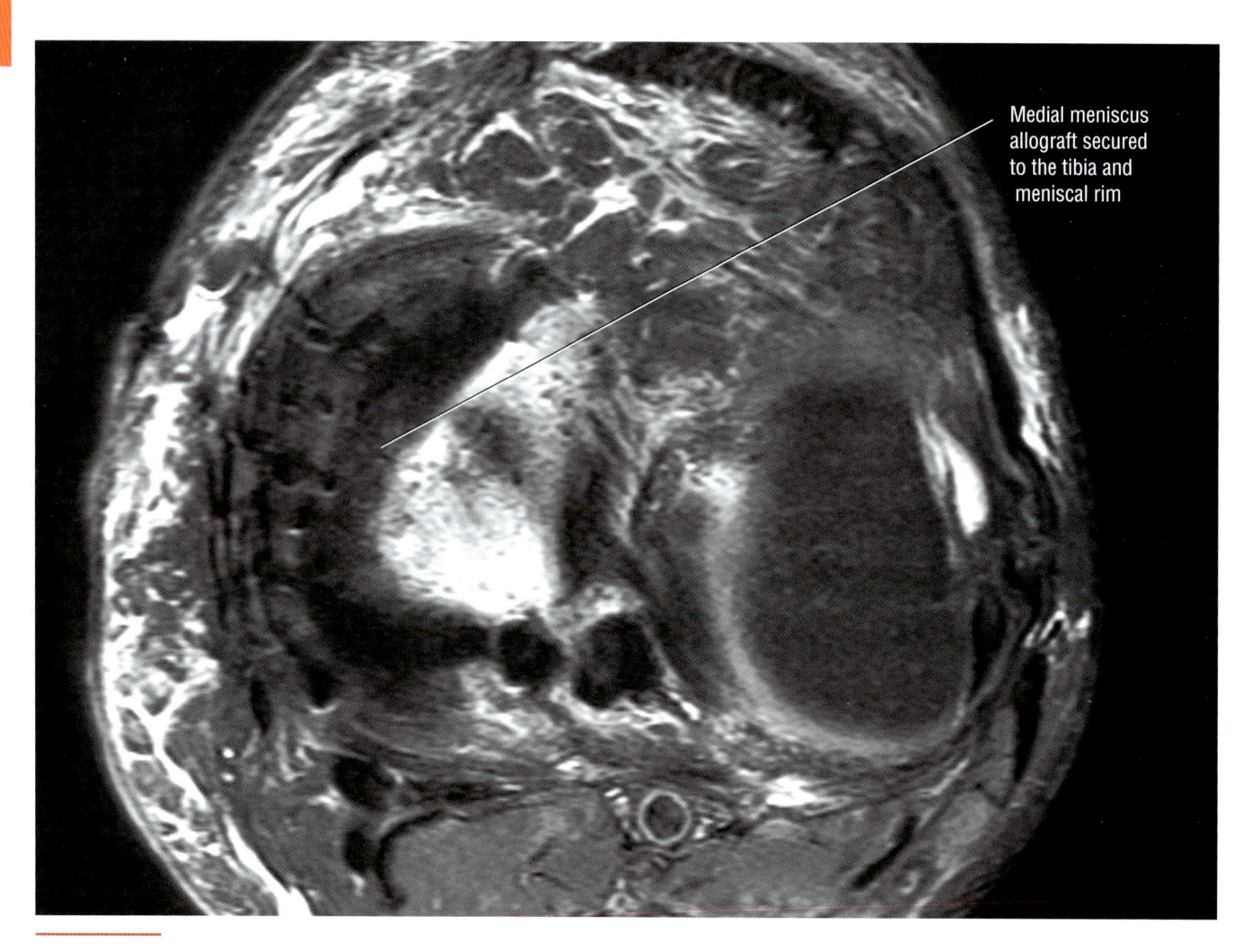

FIGURE 4.165 Medial meniscus transplantation using technique of three-tunnel fixation of the meniscus to the tibia and suturing the meniscus to the remnant native meniscus. Axial FS PD FSE image of the medial meniscus allograft.

Postoperative Appearance of the Meniscus

Key Concepts

- Postoperative Meniscus
    - Grade 3 signal intensity should not be mistaken for residual tear or retear in a stable meniscal remnant after partial meniscectomy.
    - Selective blunting of the inferior surface (leaf) is associated with partial meniscectomy of tears extending to the inferior articular surface of the meniscus.
    - Stable meniscal fibrovascular scars are intermediate in signal intensity on FS PD FSE images.
        - Direct linear extension of hyperintense fluid or intraarticular contrast, however, represents retear of the meniscal repair or extension of the tear into an unstable meniscal remnant.
    - MR arthrography is primarily used to evaluate post–primary repair menisci and in cases of more extensive partial meniscectomies.
- The postoperative evaluation of partial meniscectomies and primary repair offers unique challenges for MR imaging.
- Correlation of MR findings with preoperative MR studies or details of the arthroscopic surgery is useful in increasing the accuracy of MR diagnosis of a retear or persistent tear or a normal healing response to the meniscal fibrocartilage.
- It may be difficult to identify tears in the meniscal remnants after a partial meniscectomy.
- The free edge of the inferior leaf may be preferentially resected in tears demonstrating inferior surface extension.

MR Appearance After Meniscectomy

- Even in the absence of a retear, the meniscal remnant may demonstrate a residual grade 3 signal intensity, also referred to as *intrameniscal signal conversion*.

- FS PD FSE or T2* GRE (although the latter is subject to increased susceptibility artifact, as discussed below) images can be used to identify fluid directly extending into the cleavage plane of a tear in a meniscal remnant.

- This finding is more specific than the presence of grade 3 signal intensity on short-TE or T1-weighted images.

- A meniscal cyst may be associated with an unstable or symptomatic meniscal remnant or postrepair meniscus.

- A sharp, blunt, surgical truncation of the apex of the meniscus with foreshortening is often seen with partial meniscectomy.

- The meniscal tissue, however, may be contoured so that the remnant does not show obvious blunting.

- Residual signal intensity may also occur if one or both leaves of a cleavage component of a tear are removed. MR accurately demonstrates the degree of partial meniscectomy from less than 25% to 75% or greater.

- FS PD-weighted FSE images display the morphology of the postoperative meniscus with decreased magnetic susceptibility artifact in comparison with GRE techniques.

    - It is important to recognize the limitation of FSE technique in accurately identifying intrameniscal signal intensity, and it should be used in conjunction with either FS PD conventional spin-echo or GRE images.

- Postoperative meniscal fragments adjacent to the site of a meniscectomy may also be identified with MR imaging, especially using techniques of FSE with FS or conventional T2 spin-echo images.

- After meniscectomy, increased contact stress and elastic modulus between the femur and the tibia place the articular cartilage at risk of injury, and the meniscal remnants are less effective in diffusing loads to a greater area of the knee joint.

- No meniscal tissue is seen after a total meniscectomy; the joint space left after removal of fibrocartilage may be filled with fluid.

- Additional MR findings after partial or complete meniscectomy may include progressive joint space narrowing with articular cartilage loss and subchondral low signal intensity in the involved compartment before the appearance of radiographic sclerosis.

- The lateral compartment is especially at risk for arthrosis after partial or complete meniscectomy.

- Subchondral changes may display hypointensity on T1 or PD FSE images and hyperintensity on corresponding STIR or FS PD FSE images during stages of reactive hyperemia.

- Flattening or posterior ridging of the femoral condyles and tibial marginal spurring and sclerosis (indicative of previous meniscectomy) are chronic findings.[6]

- Smith et al.[446] have divided the MR characteristics of partial meniscectomy into three groups.

    - Group 1 menisci demonstrate near-normal length and no osteoarthritis.

    - Group 2 menisci are significantly shortened but do not show osteoarthritis.

        - In group 2 menisci, contour irregularities simulated meniscal fragmentation in 40% of segments studied; therefore, no rigid criteria for diagnosis of tearing in meniscal segments with partial meniscectomy contour irregularities were established in this study.

    - Group 3 menisci may be any length, but they demonstrate the development of osteoarthritis.

- Regenerated meniscal tissue (i.e., rim) is composed of fibrous tissue, is smaller than normal, and demonstrates low to intermediate signal intensity on T1-, PD-, T2-, or T2*-weighted images.

- Accurate correlation of the original tear pattern with the extent of the meniscectomy increases the usefulness of the finding of grade 3 signal intensity as an indicator of retear.

- An increased prevalence of radial tears has been observed in postoperative partial meniscectomy remnants and is attributed to the altered hoop mechanism of the meniscus secondary to meniscal resection.[520]

- The accuracy of MR diagnosis of recurrent tears in the postoperative meniscus may be improved with MR arthrography.[520]

- MR arthrography is useful in patients with meniscal resections of greater than 25%, provided that native joint fluid does not already extend into the meniscus.

- MR arthrography is not necessary in patients with minimal meniscal resection (<25%).[301,309,385]

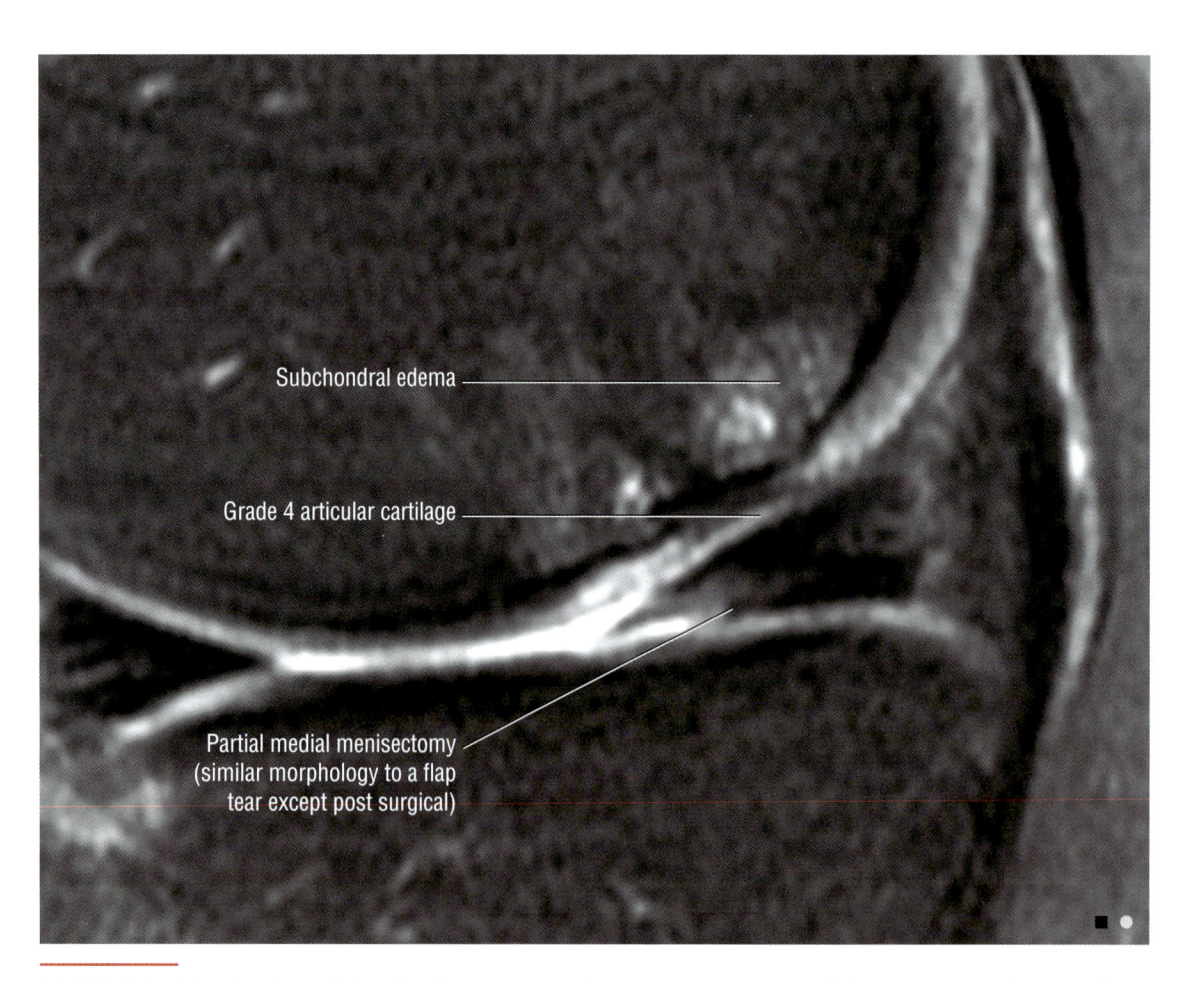

FIGURE 4.166 Accelerated chondral degeneration subsequent to a partial medial meniscectomy. Sagittal FS PD FSE image.

MR Appearance After Meniscal Repair

- Primary meniscal repairs may show grade 1, grade 2, or persistent grade 3 signal intensity on postoperative MR.[15,106,244]

- Second-look arthroscopy has shown that healed meniscal repair may demonstrate grade 3 signal intensity, making postoperative characterization of primary repairs difficult.[106]

- Criteria for retear of a primal meniscal repair are similar to those for a partial meniscectomy remnant.

- Signs of retear include:
    - Hyperintensity at the repair site on FS PD- or T2-weighted images
    - Displaced meniscal fragments
    - Increased signal intensity at a new location or site relative to the repair[281]

- Intraarticular gadolinium may be helpful in identifying imbibed synovial fluid extending into menisci that are retorn after primary repair according to the same principle underlying the use of long-TE or T2-weighted images to identify the direct extension of fluid into the cleavage plane of a tear to help increase diagnostic accuracy.

- Both IV and intraarticular gadolinium have been used to improve characterization of recurrent tears and meniscal surfaces.[14,119]

- Correlation of MR findings with second-look arthroscopic examination of post–primary repair menisci has shown that there may be conversion of grade 3 signal intensity into lower grades of signal intensity, primarily in areas of fibrovascular healing, which corresponds with the conversion of granulation or scar tissue to normal fibrocartilage.

- This process occurs over a period of months. Arnoczky et al.[15] evaluated MR signals in healing menisci in dogs.
    - They found that in full thickness radial tears, the normal fibrovascular scar tissue or repair tissue generated increased signal intensity on MR that persisted at 26 weeks, even though this fibrovascular repair tissue had converted from scar into fibrocartilage.

- This study supports the observation that normal fibrovascular repair tissue as well as conversion of fibrovascular repair tissue to fibrocartilage may demonstrate persistent grade 3 signal intensity in healing menisci.

- The findings by Deutsch et al.[106] of persistent signal intensity up to 27 months postoperatively demonstrate that the conversion process from fibrovascular tissue to fibrocartilage is protracted and may even be chronic.

- Intact meniscal fibrovascular scars are intermediate in signal on FS PD FSE images and maintain intermediate signal without allowing extension of intraarticular gadolinium-based contrast on corresponding MR arthrography.

- Types of repair techniques
  - Tears in the red-red zone (within 3mm of the meniscal periphery) represent the optimal location for repair with access to a well-developed blood supply.
  - Inside-out (with vertical mattress sutures)
    - Gold standard
    - Concomitant ACL reconstruction improves.
    - Achieves stabilization of large, longitudinal or bucket-handle tears
  - Outside-in
    - Anterior and middle segments
  - All-inside
    - Vertical longitudinal tears posterior horn
    - All applied to radial, horizontal, and root tears

- Key criteria on MR whether using arthrography or fluid-sensitive sequences is to identify the presence of free fluid in the plane of the repair.
  - If fluid extends greater than 50% of tear site, then repair of meniscus is considered not healed.

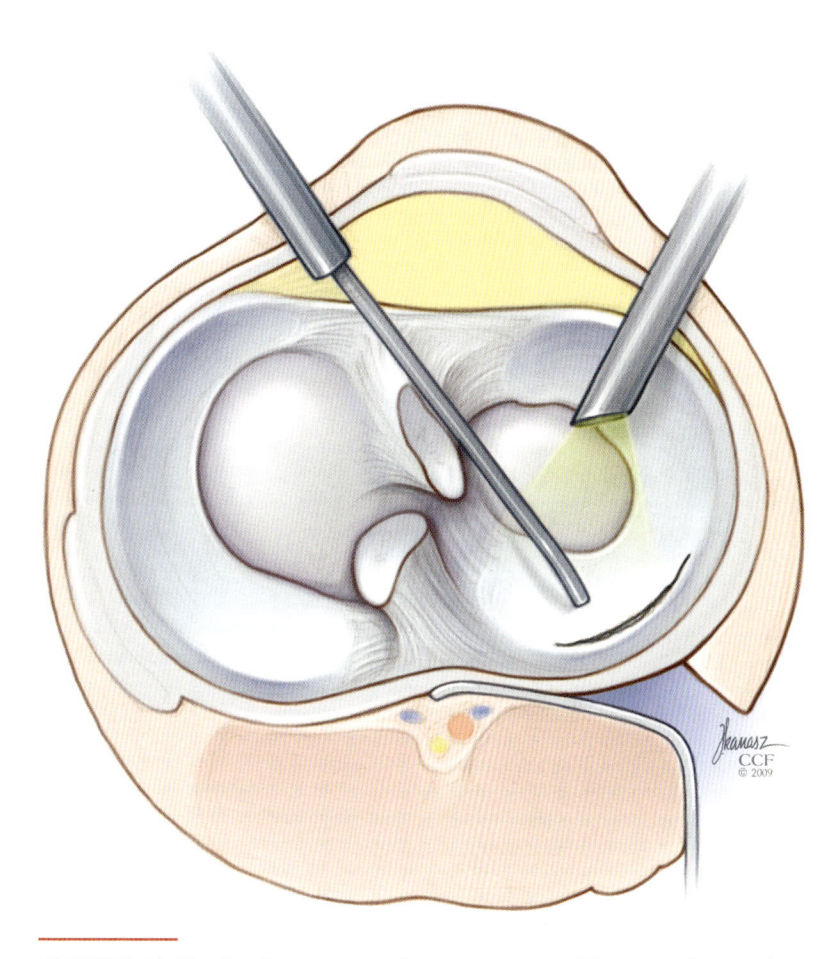

FIGURE 4.167 Inside-out meniscal repair technique. The circumferential location of a meniscal tear is important in the type of repair selected. Tears of the posterior horn and body are effectively treated with an inside-out technique, whereas anterior horn tears are often addressed with an outside-in approach. (Reprinted from Fu FH. *Master Techniques in Orthopaedic Surgery: Sports Medicine.* Philadelphia, PA: Lippincott Williams & Wilkins; 2010, with permission.)

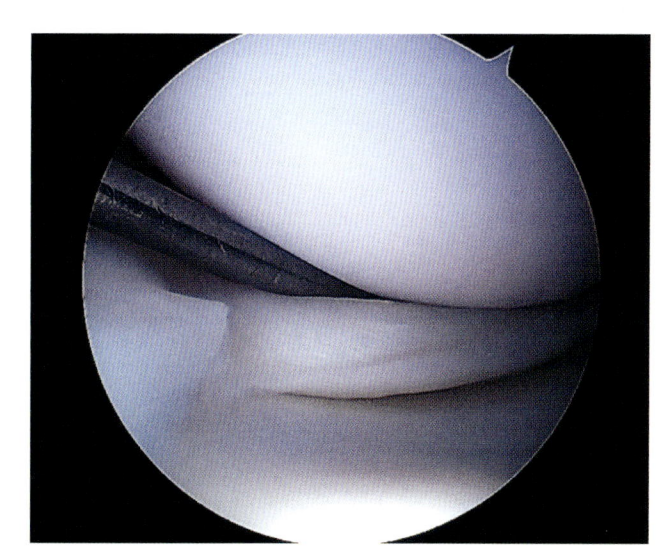

FIGURE 4.168 Example of an unstable peripheral longitudinal medial meniscus tear amenable to repair. This tear originates near the attachment of the medial collateral ligament and extends vertically through the meniscus from its femoral to its tibial surface. Repair is effective because the tear margins can be brought into close apposition and maintained with peripheral transcapsular sutures. (Reprinted from Fu FH. *Master Techniques in Orthopaedic Surgery: Sports Medicine.* Philadelphia, PA: Lippincott Williams & Wilkins; 2010, with permission.)

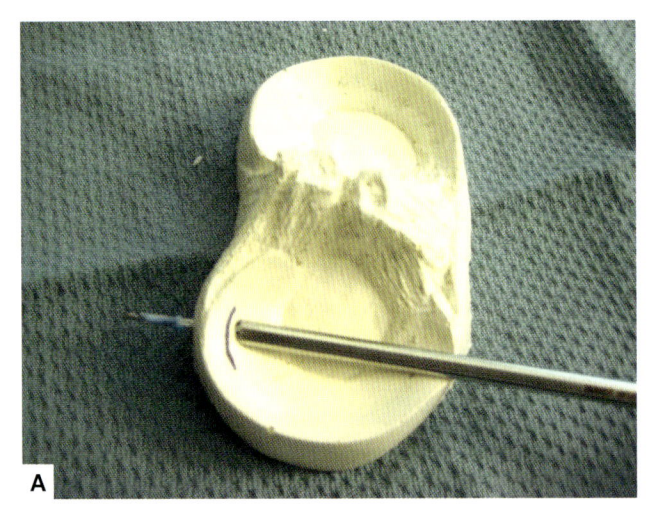

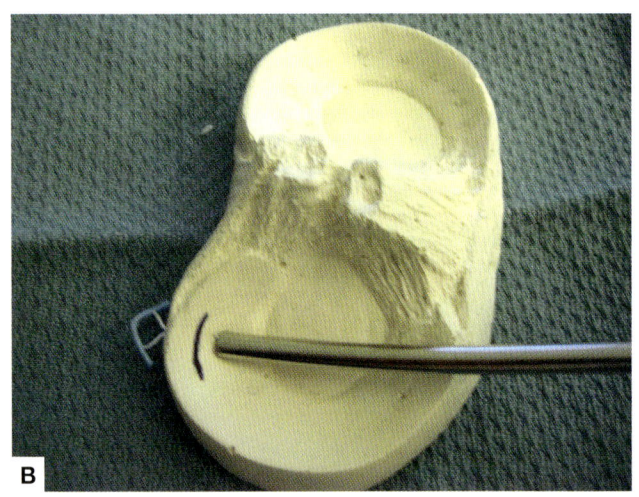

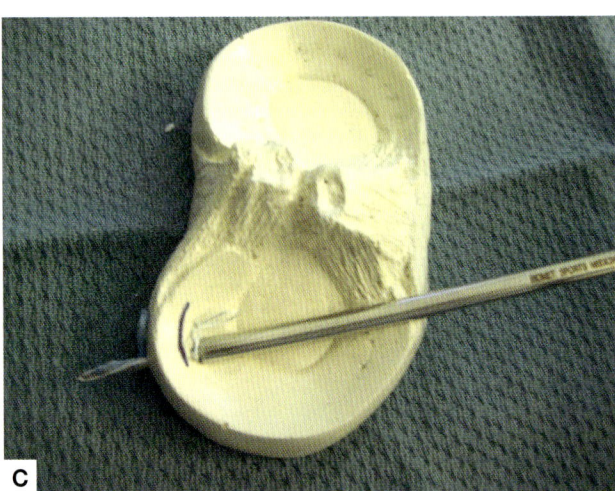

FIGURE 4.169 All-inside repair techniques are applied for more posterior meniscal tears and tears of the meniscal body sement. (**A**) While maintaining gentle but firm pressure on the meniscus, the first all-suture anchor is passed by advancing the green trigger to its forward mechanical stop. (**B**) Once the green lever has reached its forward mechanical stop, the green trigger is pulled back to its endpoint. (**C**) The cannula is repositioned 5 to 10mm away from the first anchor and toward the side corresponding with the red trigger of the inserter and the second anchor is fired. (Reprinted from Fu FH. *Master Techniques in Orthopaedic Surgery: Sports Medicine*. Philadelphia, PA: Lippincott Williams & Wilkins; 2010, with permission.)

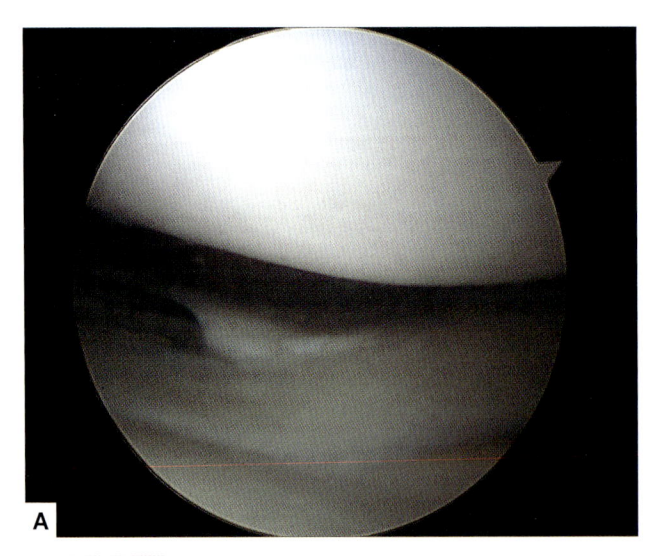

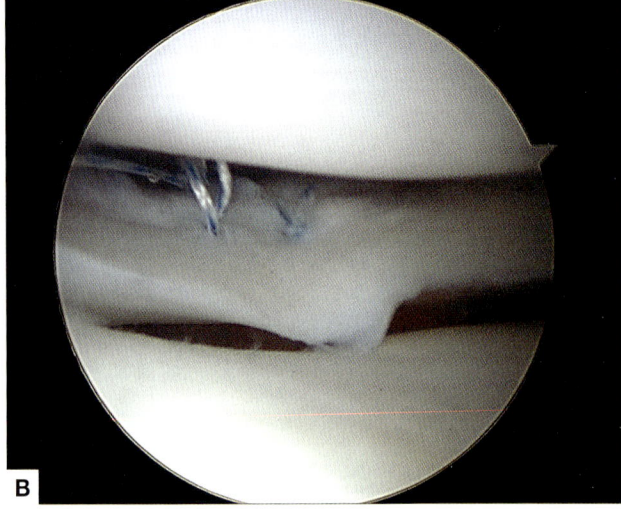

FIGURE 4.170 (**A**) Arthroscopic view of a longitudinal tear of the lateral meniscus in a left knee from the lateral portal. (**B**) Arthroscopic view of an all-inside meniscus repair of the lateral meniscus using two FAST-FIX devices. (Reprinted from Fu FH. *Master Techniques in Orthopaedic Surgery: Sports Medicine*. Philadelphia, PA: Lippincott Williams & Wilkins; 2010, with permission.)

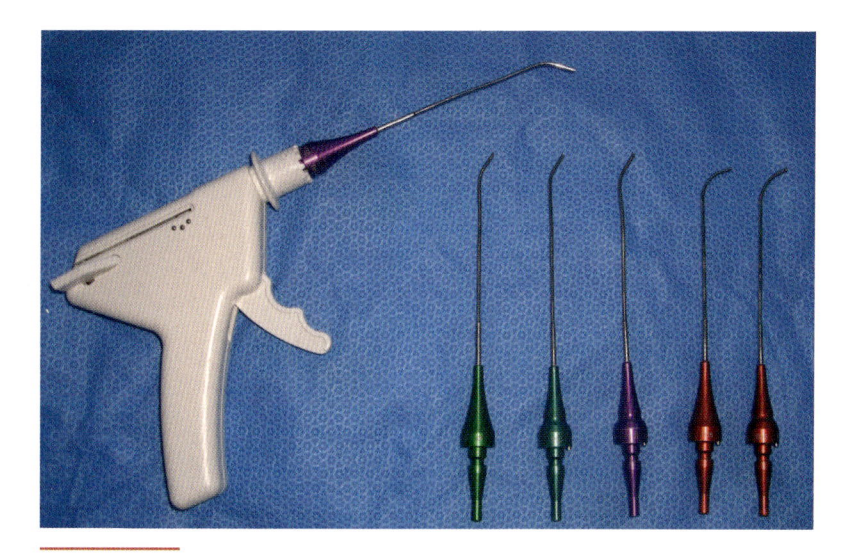

FIGURE 4.171 Sharpshooter as a suture passage device (for mattress suture placement) and zone-specific cannula attachments (ConMed Linvatec, Largo, Florida). The ratchet trigger allows single hand advancement of the suture through the joint capsule. (Reprinted from Fu FH. *Master Techniques in Orthopaedic Surgery: Sports Medicine*. Philadelphia, PA: Lippincott Williams & Wilkins; 2010, with permission.)

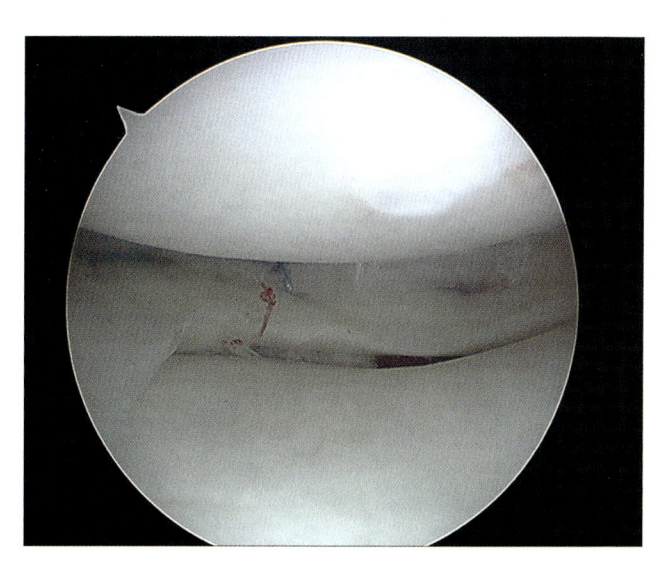

FIGURE 4.172 Composite lateral meniscus tear with alternating horizontal and vertical mattress sutures. The goal is use the minimum of fixation to create an approximated and stable meniscal repair. (Reprinted from Fu FH. *Master Techniques in Orthopaedic Surgery: Sports Medicine*. Philadelphia, PA: Lippincott Williams & Wilkins; 2010, with permission.)

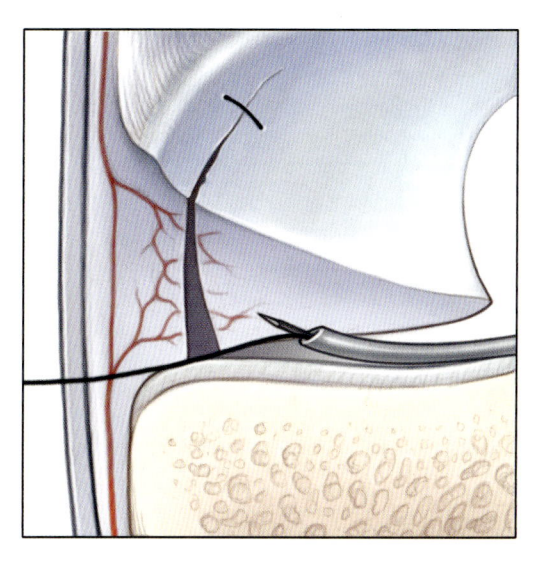

FIGURE 4.173 Vertical suture placement. Note how the meniscal tear is engaged with the suture central to the longitudinal tear. (Reprinted from Fu FH. *Master Techniques in Orthopaedic Surgery: Sports Medicine*. Philadelphia, PA: Lippincott Williams & Wilkins; 2010, with permission.)

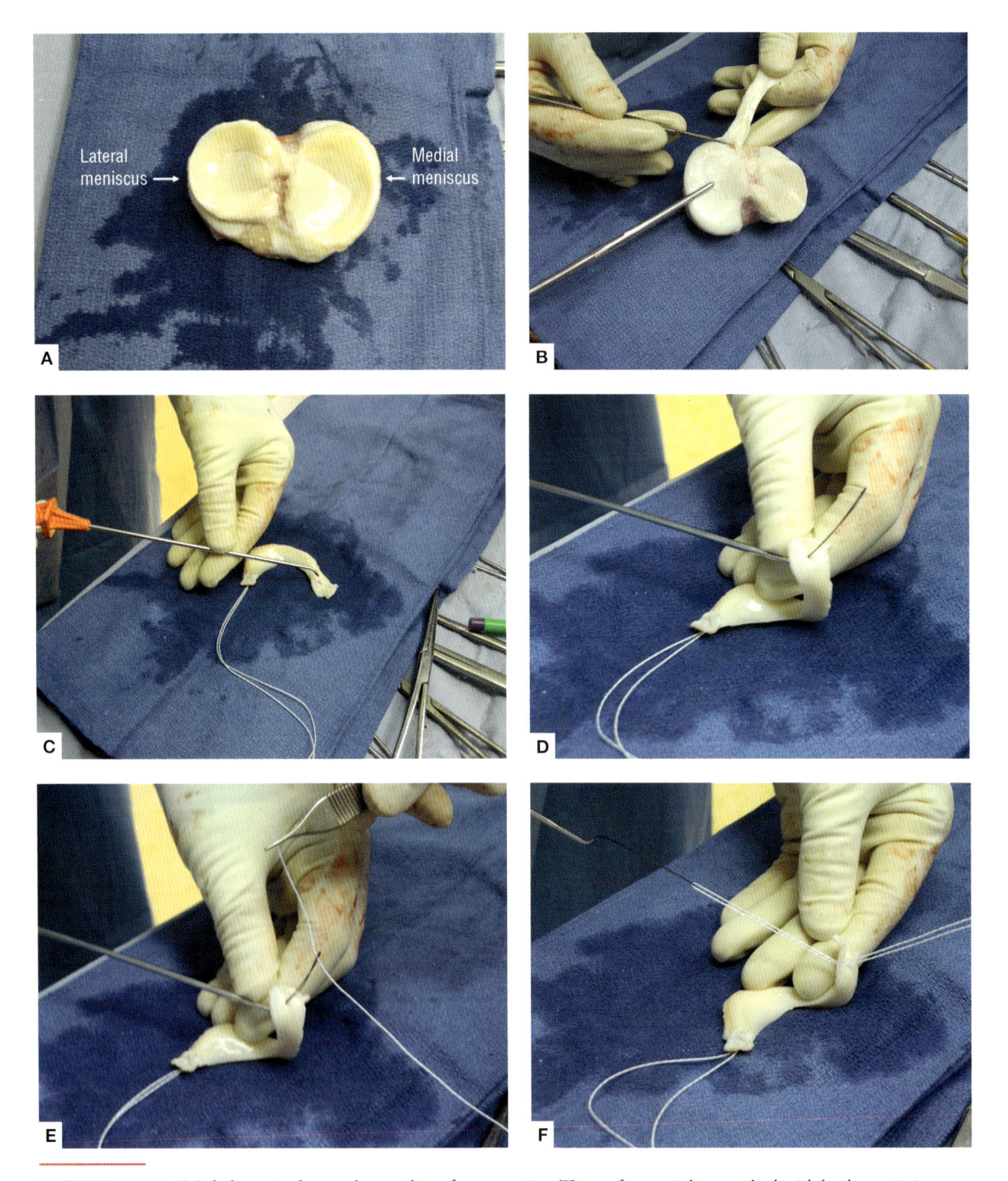

FIGURE 4.174 Medial meniscal transplant with graft preparation. The graft material is supplied with both menisci attached to the proximal tibia. The anterior and posterior root insertions are released through subperiosteal dissection. (**A**) Proximal tibial allograft with menisci intact. Medial and lateral menisci are labeled. (**B**) The posterior horn of the medial meniscus has been released and the anterior horn is released with a no. 15 blade scalpel at the anterior meniscus insertion. (**C**) The anterior meniscal horn is marked and an Acupass suture shuttle (Smith and Nephew, Andover, Massachusetts) is lined up for insertion. (**D**) The suture shuttle is inserted and advanced. (**E**) The suture shuttle is loaded with 2 Ultrabraid (Smith and Nephew). (**F**) The suture is advanced through the meniscal allograft.

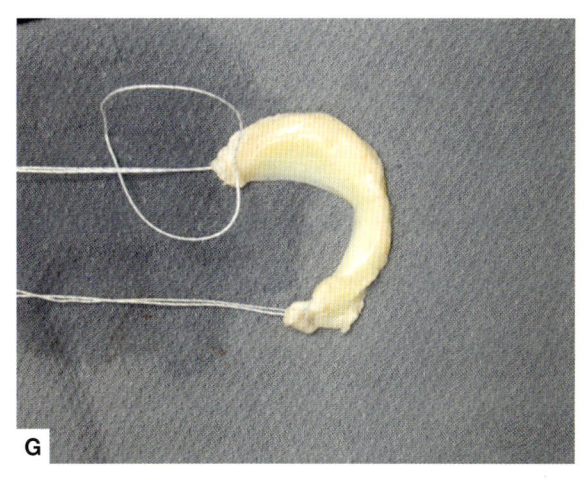

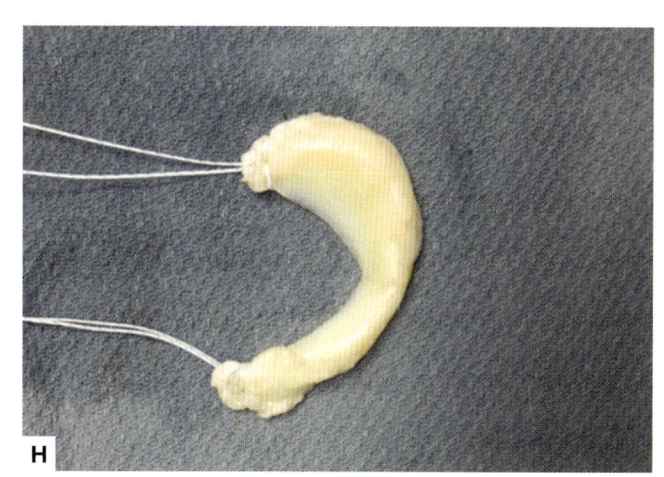

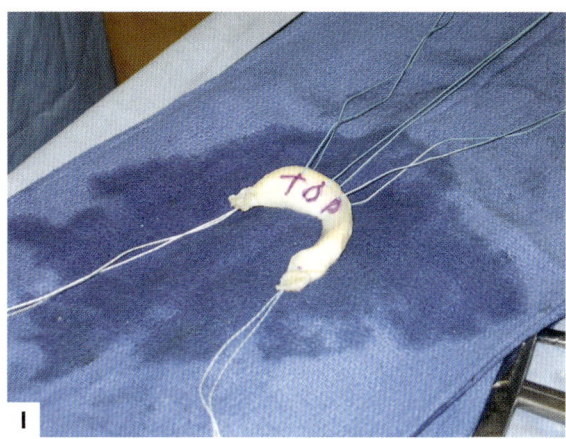

FIGURE 4.174 *(Continued)* (**G**) The suture ends are brought through the suture loop. (**H**) The loop is tensioned around the meniscal root. (**I**) The allograft is labeled for orientation, and additional 0 Cotton Polydek is placed in the periphery 1cm apart. The graft is now ready for placement. (Reprinted from Fu FH. *Master Techniques in Orthopaedic Surgery: Sports Medicine.* Philadelphia, PA: Lippincott Williams & Wilkins; 2010, with permission.)

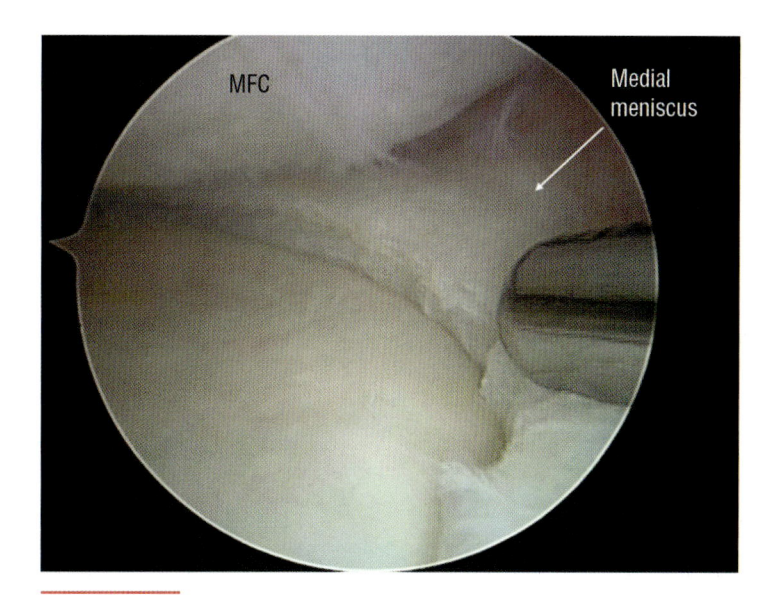

FIGURE 4.175 Preparation of medial compartment. The medial compartment is prepared by arthroscopic debridement of the remaining medial meniscus to a smooth outer rim. The peripheral one third should be preserved for the vascular and nerve contributions. MFC, medial femoral condyle. (Reprinted from Fu FH. *Master Techniques in Orthopaedic Surgery: Sports Medicine.* Philadelphia, PA: Lippincott Williams & Wilkins; 2010, with permission.)

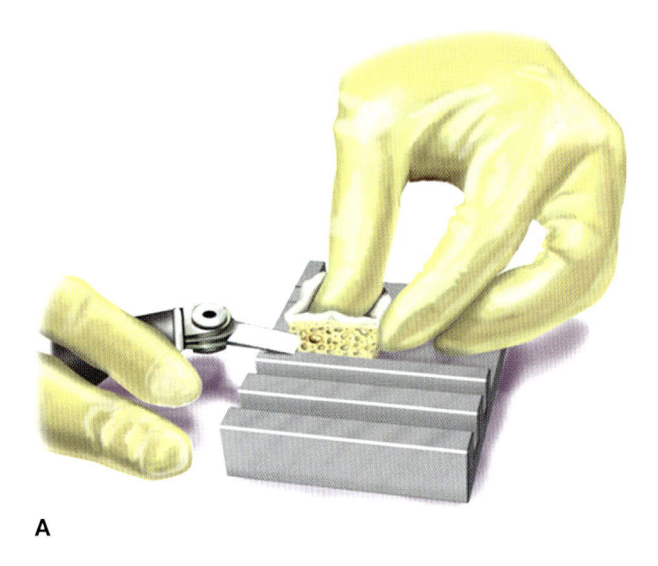

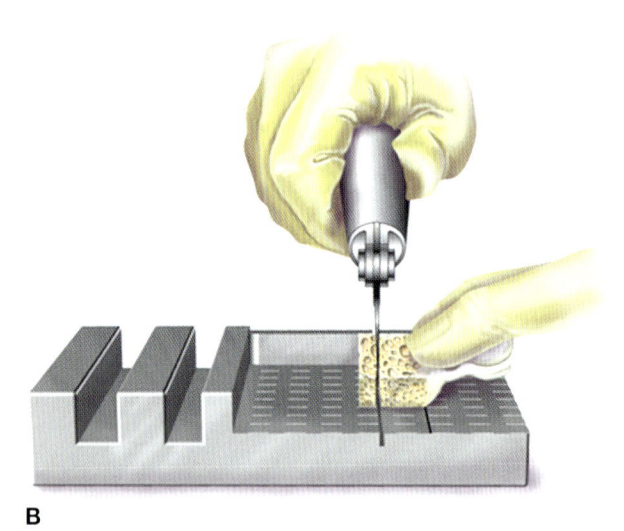

FIGURE 4.176 Lateral meniscus transplant technique with allograft bridge technique. (**A, B**) A diagram showing the allograft bone block being cut to appropriate size. (Courtesy of Stryker Endoscopy, San Jose, California.) (Reprinted from Fu FH. *Master Techniques in Orthopaedic Surgery: Sports Medicine*. Philadelphia, PA: Lippincott Williams & Wilkins; 2010, with permission.)

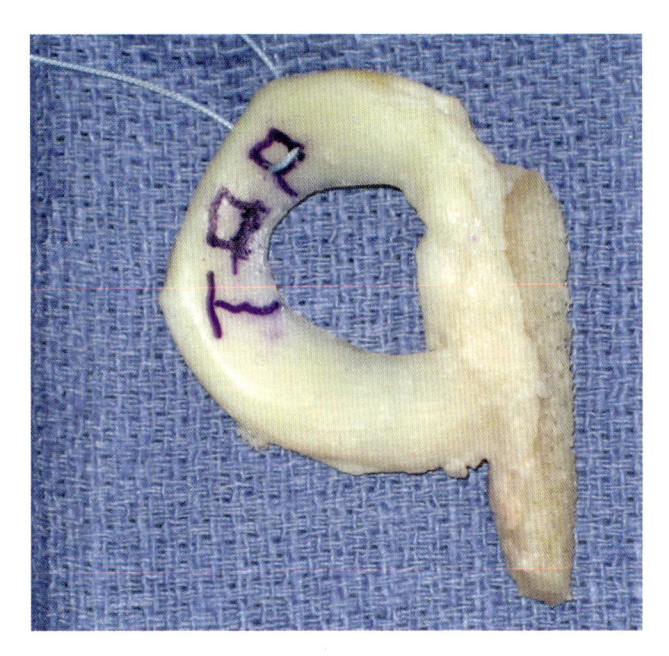

FIGURE 4.177 Lateral meniscal allograft with bone bridge cut to size and traction suture placed at the junction of the posterior and middle thirds. (Reprinted from Fu FH. *Master Techniques in Orthopaedic Surgery: Sports Medicine*. Philadelphia, PA: Lippincott Williams & Wilkins; 2010, with permission.)

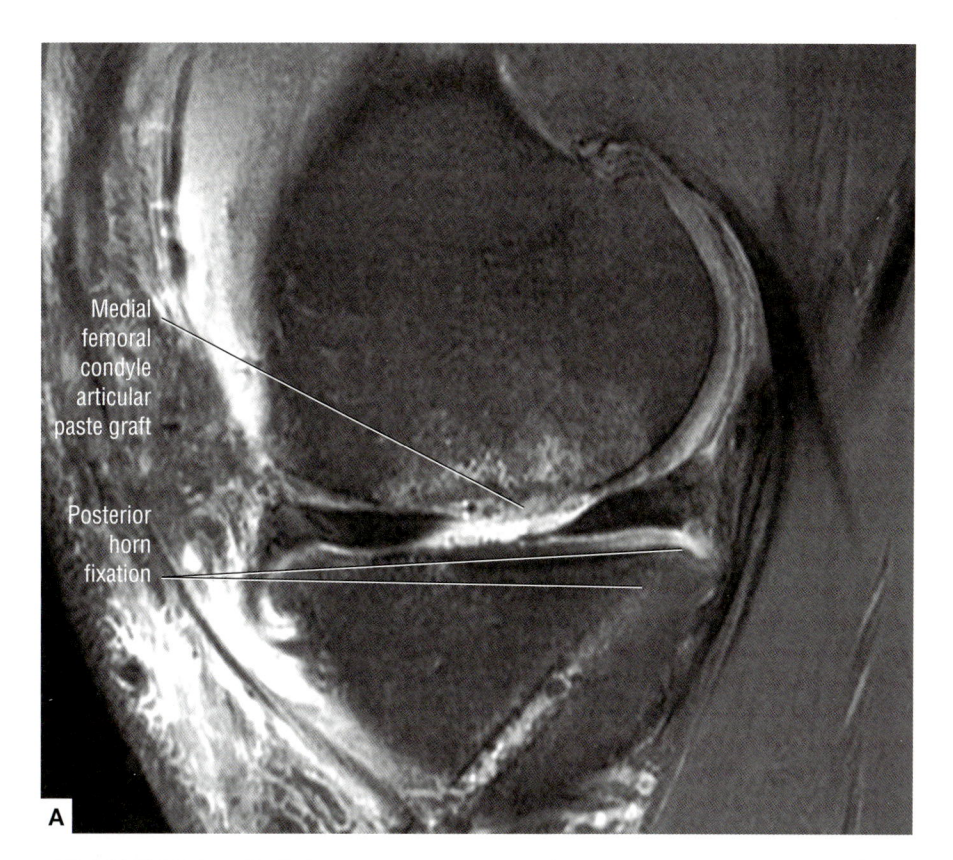

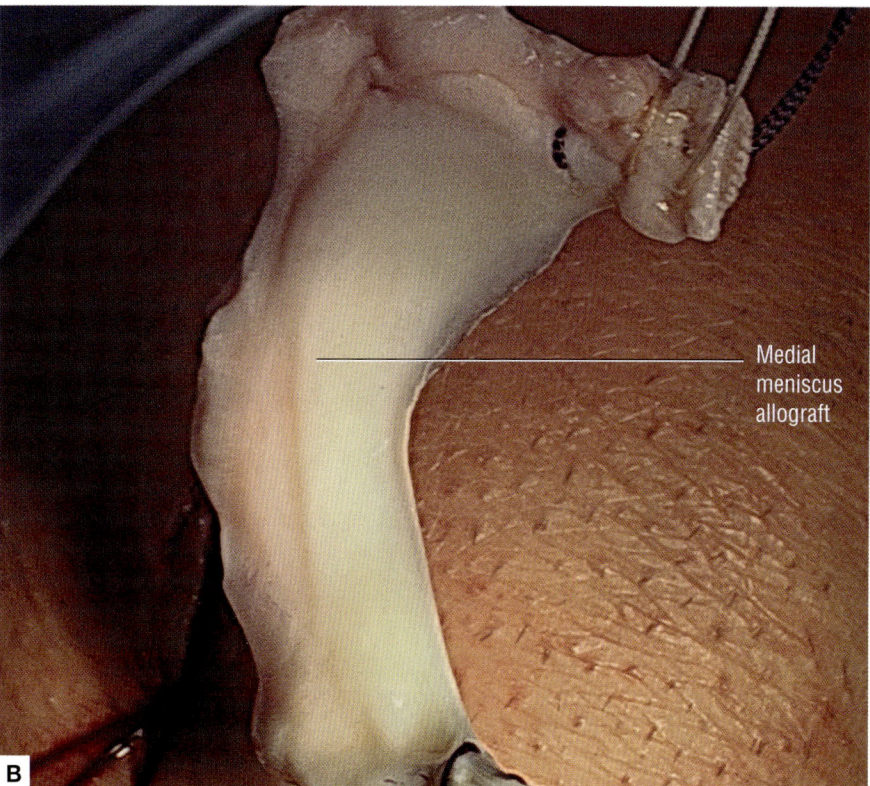

FIGURE 4.178 Case of medial meniscus transplantation using the novel technique of securing the allograft to the tibia at three sites using the three-tunnel fixation technique. Tunnel for fixation of the posterior horn of the meniscal allograft shown on sagittal FS PD FSE image (**A**). Medial meniscal allograft prepared with mattress sutures on the posterior horn (**B**).[471] The meniscal rim is preserved to prevent subluxation of the meniscus into the gutter. The allograft is sewn into the remnant rim. Articular cartilage paste graft is shown in area of medial femoral condyle 6 weeks postoperative. (*Continued*)

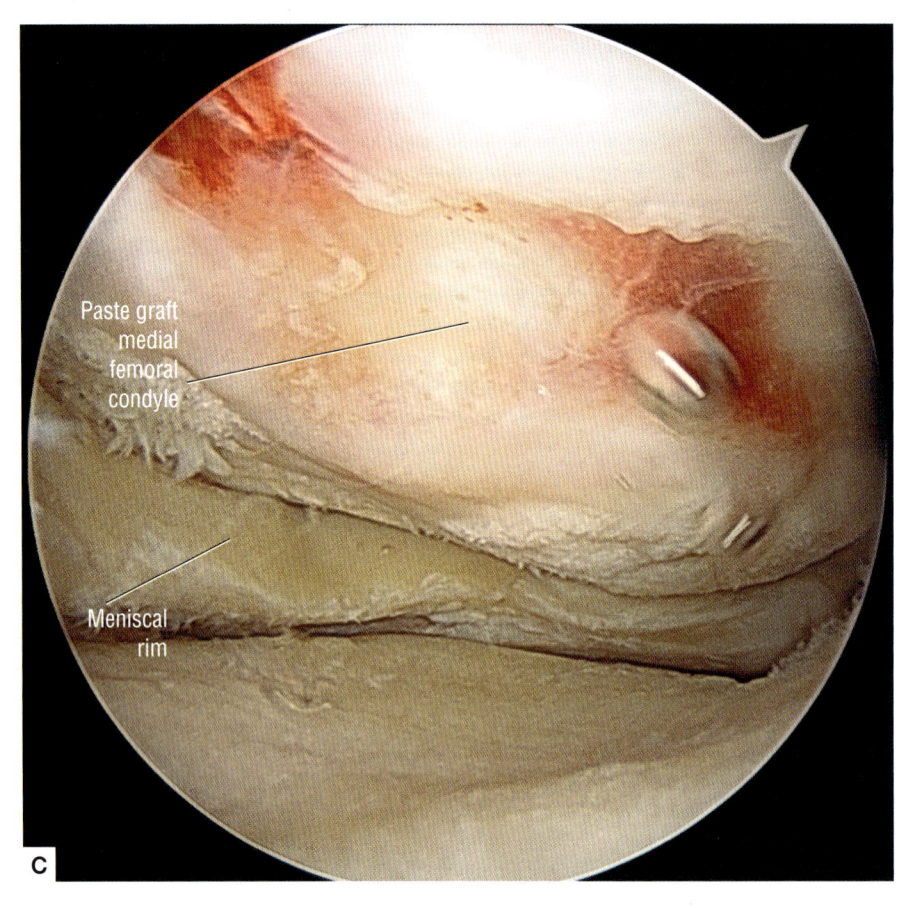

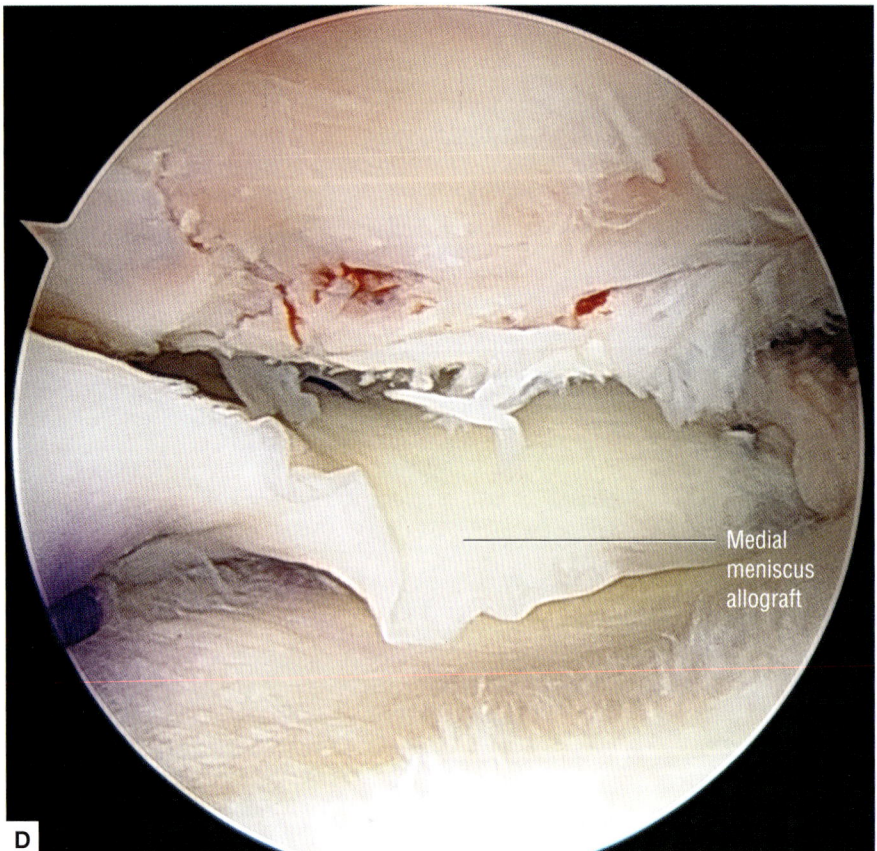

FIGURE 4.178 *(Continued)* **(C, D)** Arthroscopic view before and after allograft placement. (Courtesy of The Stone Clinic, San Francisco, California.)

The Meniscus

Three-Tunnel Technique Meniscus Allograft Plus Stem Cells For Meniscal Transplant

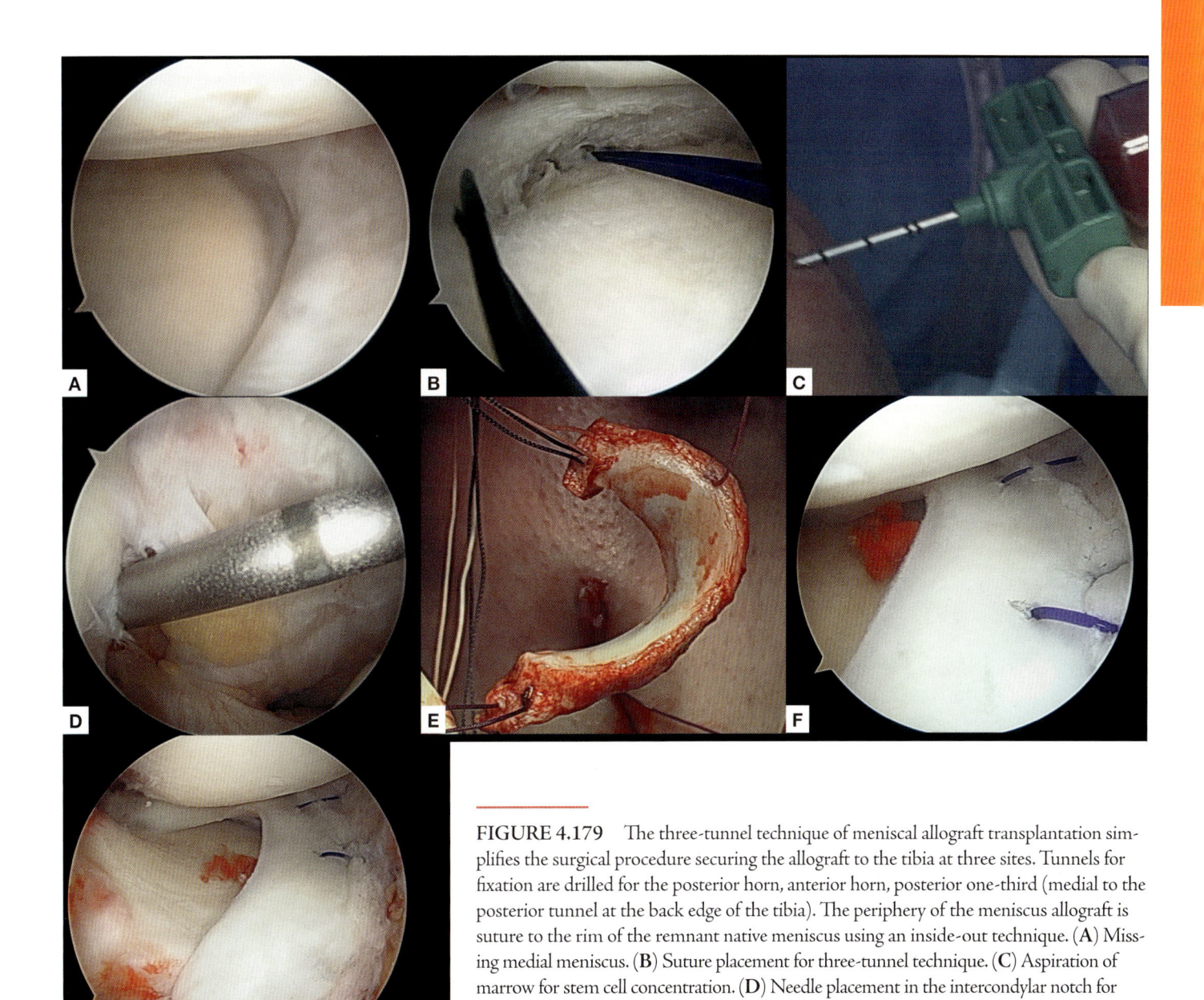

FIGURE 4.179 The three-tunnel technique of meniscal allograft transplantation simplifies the surgical procedure securing the allograft to the tibia at three sites. Tunnels for fixation are drilled for the posterior horn, anterior horn, posterior one-third (medial to the posterior tunnel at the back edge of the tibia). The periphery of the meniscus allograft is suture to the rim of the remnant native meniscus using an inside-out technique. (**A**) Missing medial meniscus. (**B**) Suture placement for three-tunnel technique. (**C**) Aspiration of marrow for stem cell concentration. (**D**) Needle placement in the intercondylar notch for aspiration of marrow and stem cells. (**E**) Meniscus allograft loaded by vacuum pressure with concentrated stem cells. (**F**) Placement of medial meniscus allograft. (**G**) Placement of medial meniscus allograft. (Courtesy of The Stone Clinic, San Francisco, California.)

Segmental Meniscus Reconstruction Using Allograft

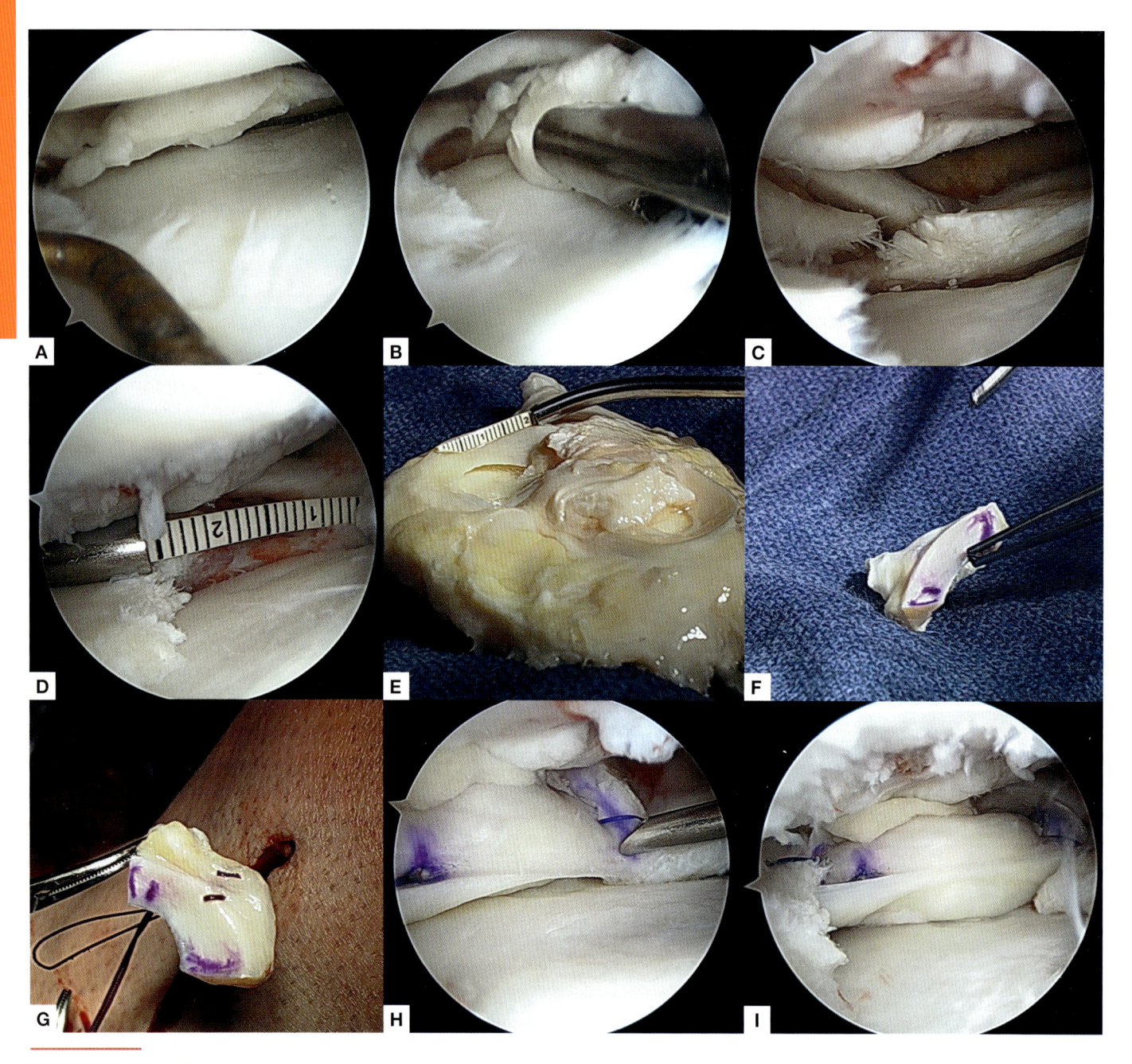

FIGURE 4.180 Technique for rebuilding portions of damaged or missing meniscal fibrocartilage. (**A**) Torn segment of lateral meniscus at popliteus hiatus. (**B**) Segmental defect of lateral meniscus. (**C**) Segmental defect of lateral meniscus. (**D**) Measurement of meniscus defect. (**E**) Measurement of donor meniscus for allograft segment preparation. (**F**) Allograft meniscus segment preparation. (**G**) Allograft meniscus prepared for placement. (**H**) Placement of allograft meniscus segment. (**I**) Placement of allograft meniscus segment. (Courtesy of The Stone Clinic, San Francisco, California.)

The Meniscus

Partial Menisectomy

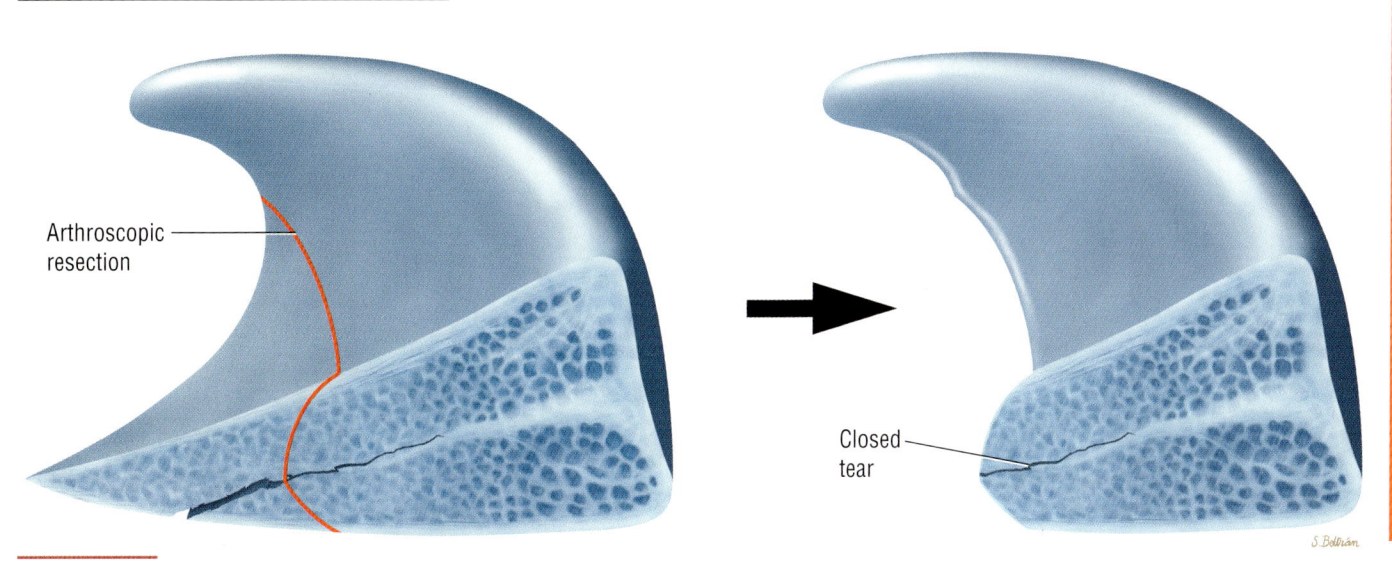

FIGURE 4.181 Boundary of partial meniscectomy to a stable meniscal rim. Residual degeneration or a closed tear is left to preserve the surrounding meniscal tissue.

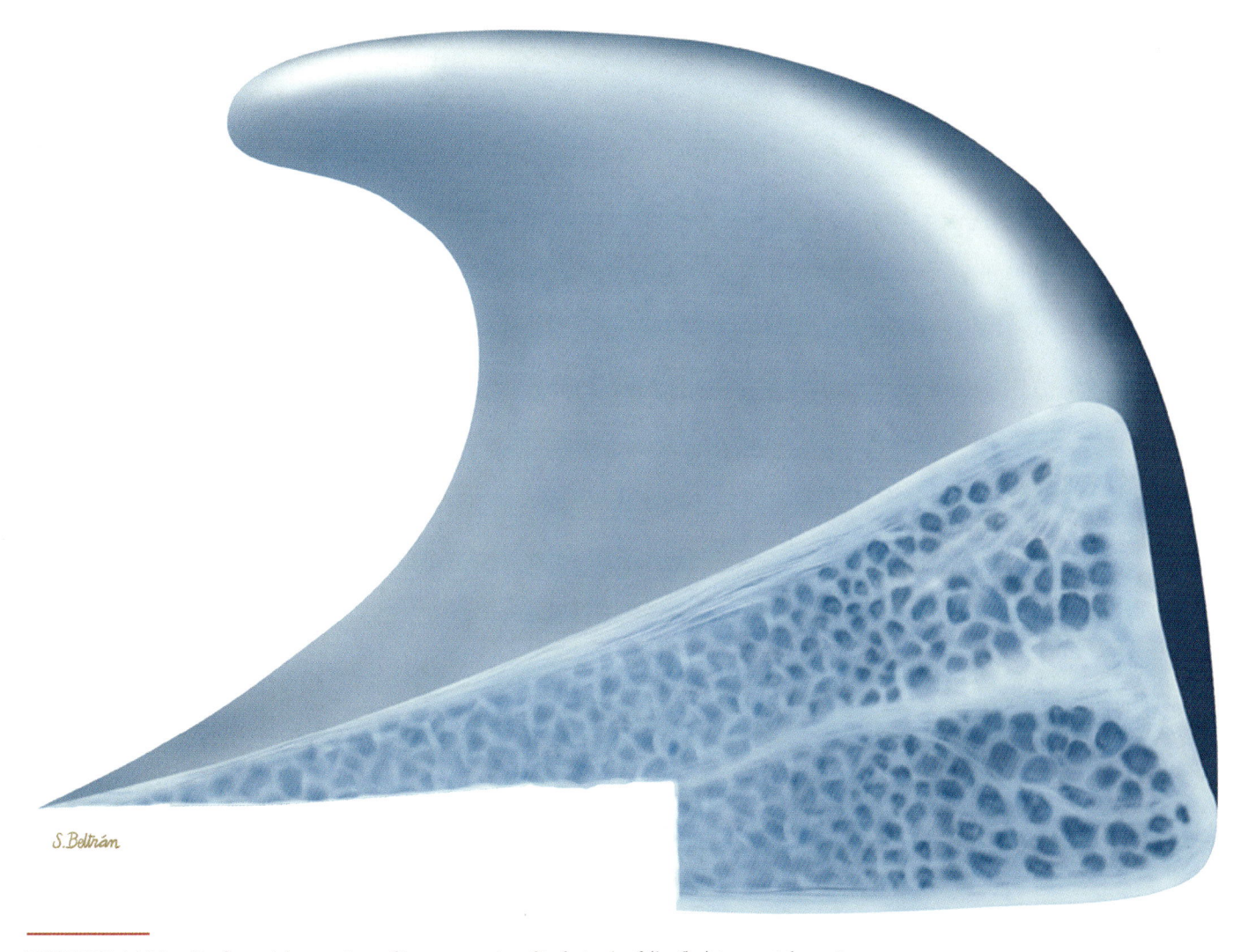

FIGURE 4.182 Preferential resection of inner margin of inferior leaf (leaflet) in partial meniscectomy.

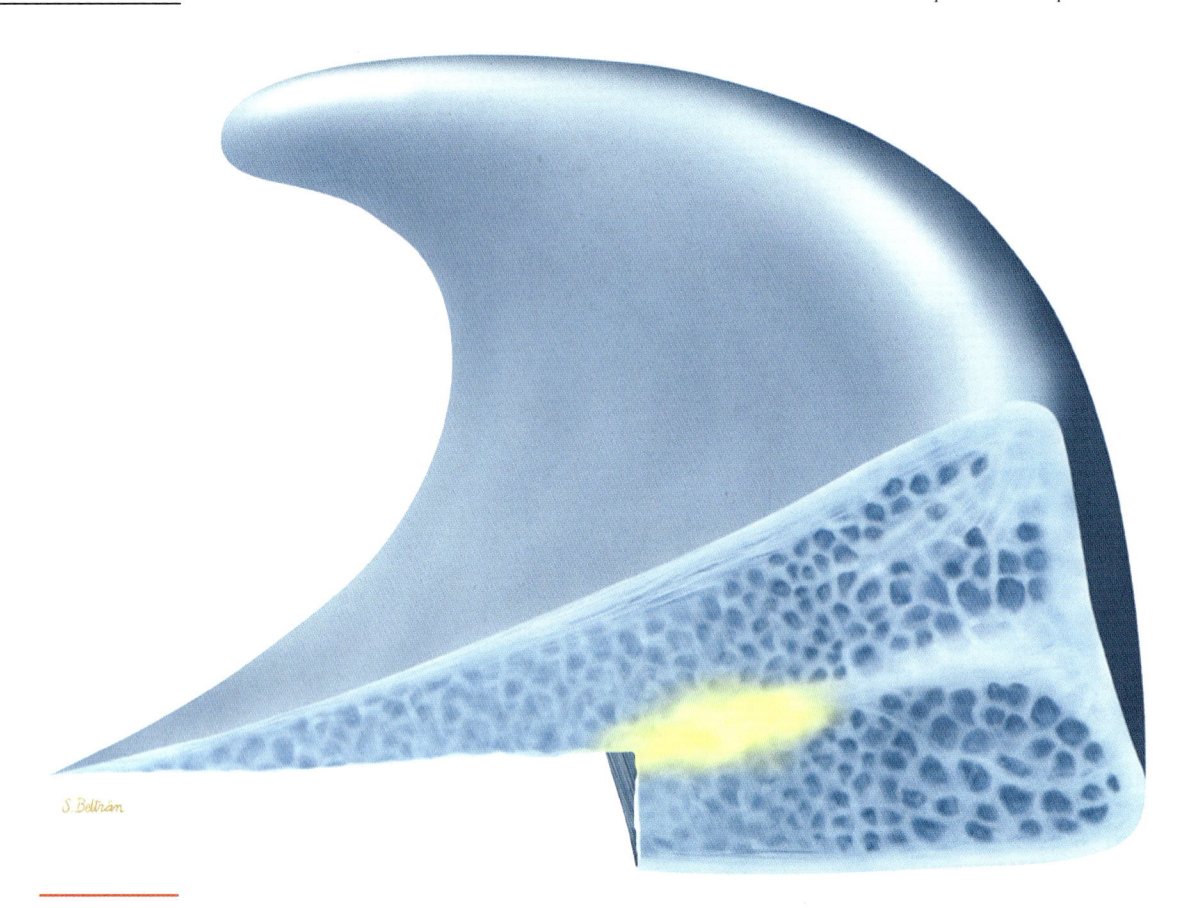

FIGURE 4.183 Partial meniscectomy. Residual meniscal degeneration (*yellow*).

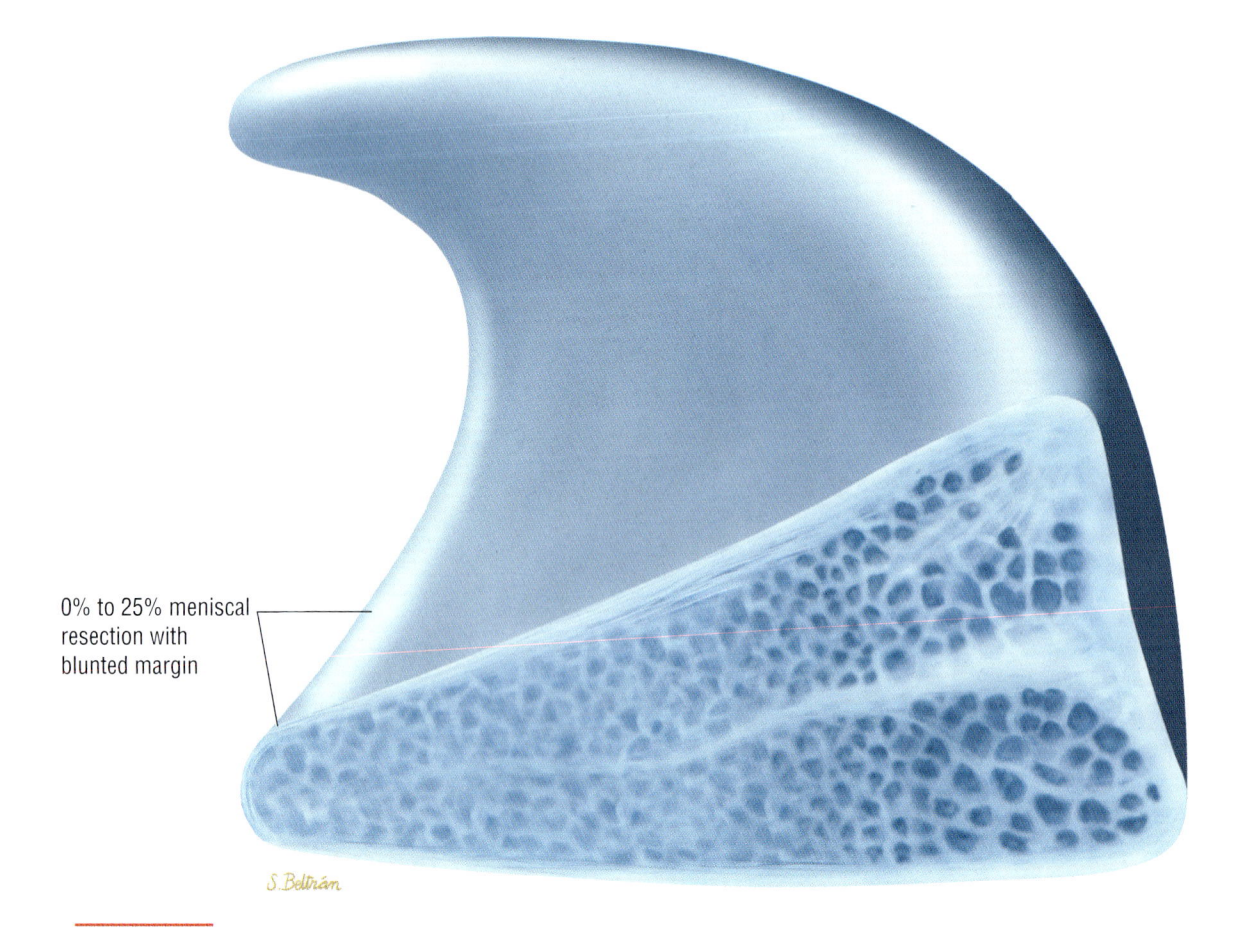

0% to 25% meniscal resection with blunted margin

FIGURE 4.184 Mild free edge blunting after a minimal or micro-partial meniscectomy.

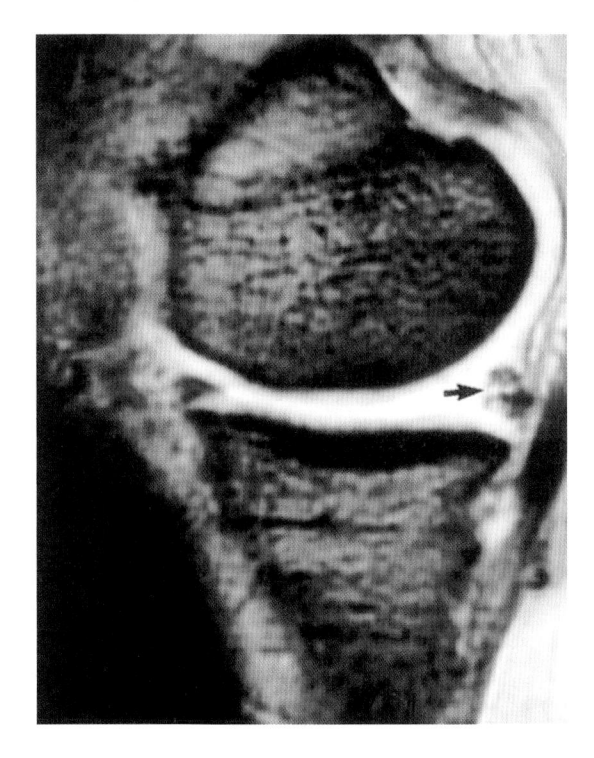

FIGURE 4.185 T2*-weighted image shows normal residual grade 3 signal intensity (*arrow*) in a partial remnant from a posterior horn medial meniscectomy. This intensity does not represent a retear in this stable meniscal rim.

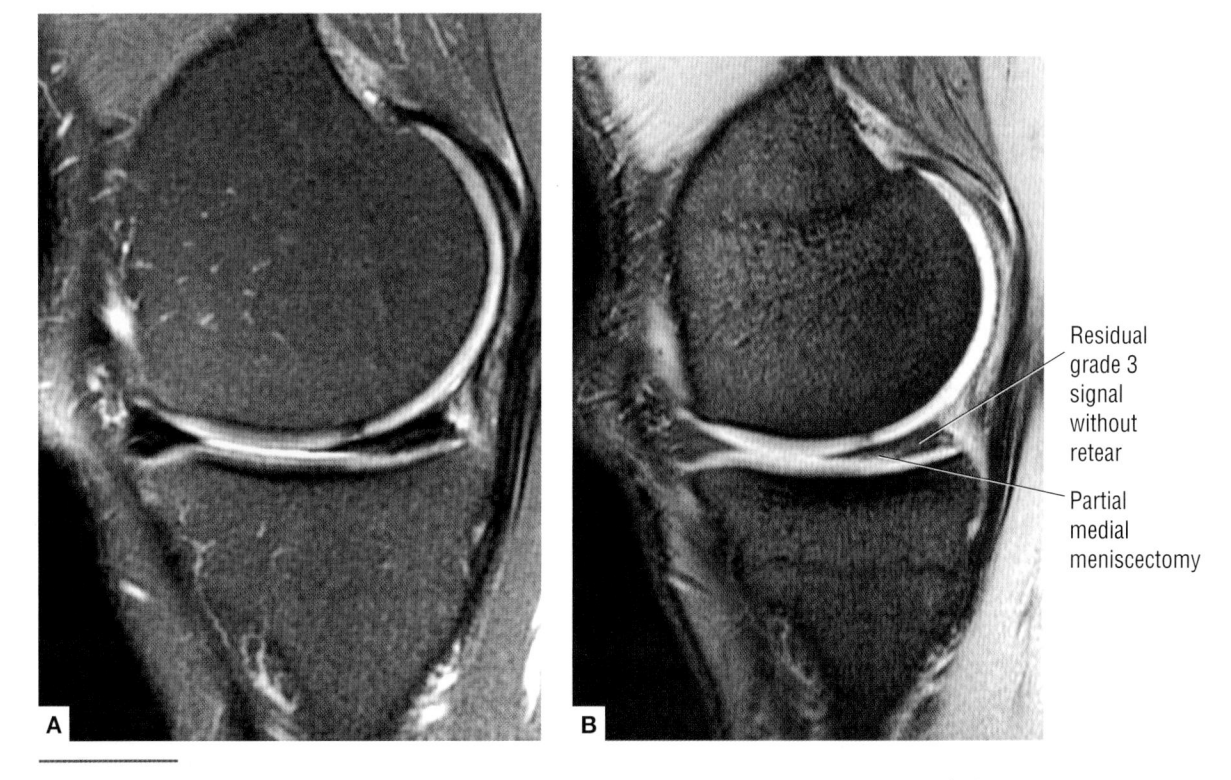

FIGURE 4.186 Partial medial meniscectomy posterior horn fibrocartilage on FS PD FSE (**A**) and T2* GRE (**B**) sagittal images. Residual grade 3 signal is best visualized with GRE T2* contrast.

Partial medial meniscectomy

Retear of posterior horn remnant medial meniscus

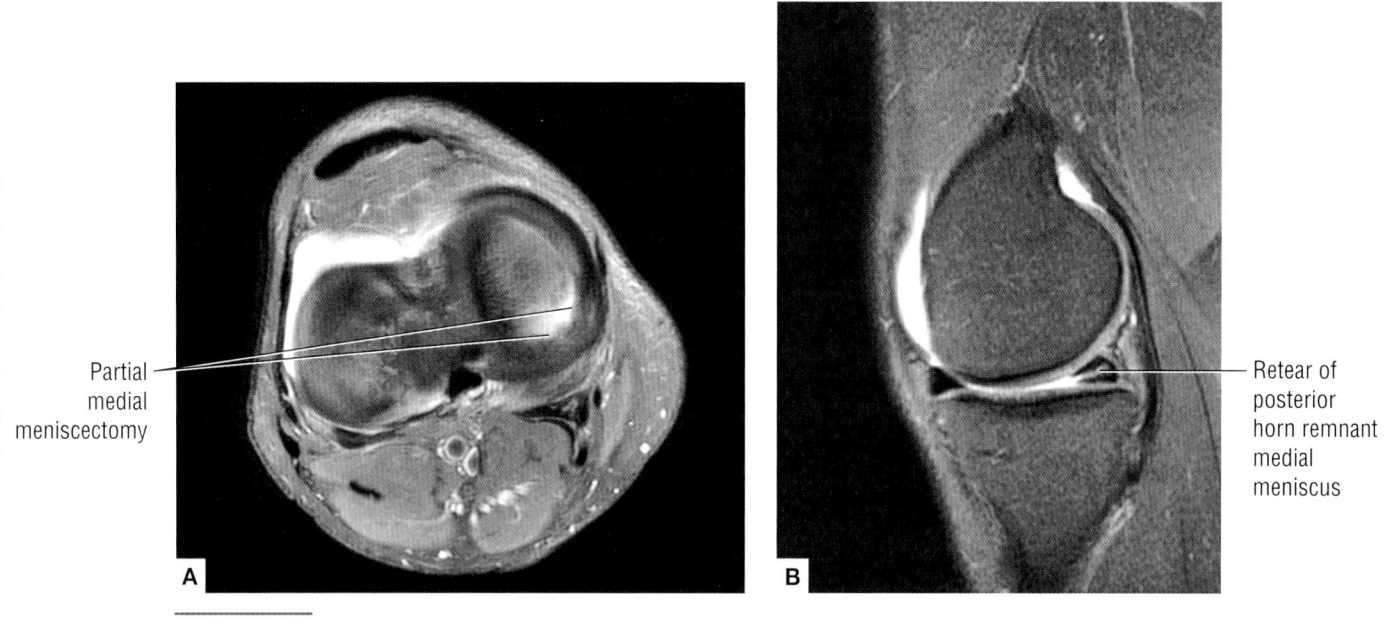

FIGURE 4.187 (**A**) Axial image showing post–partial medial meniscectomy. (**B**) Corresponding FS PD FSE sagittal image showing retear of the meniscal remnant.

Partial medial meniscectomy

Residual grade 3 signal intensity

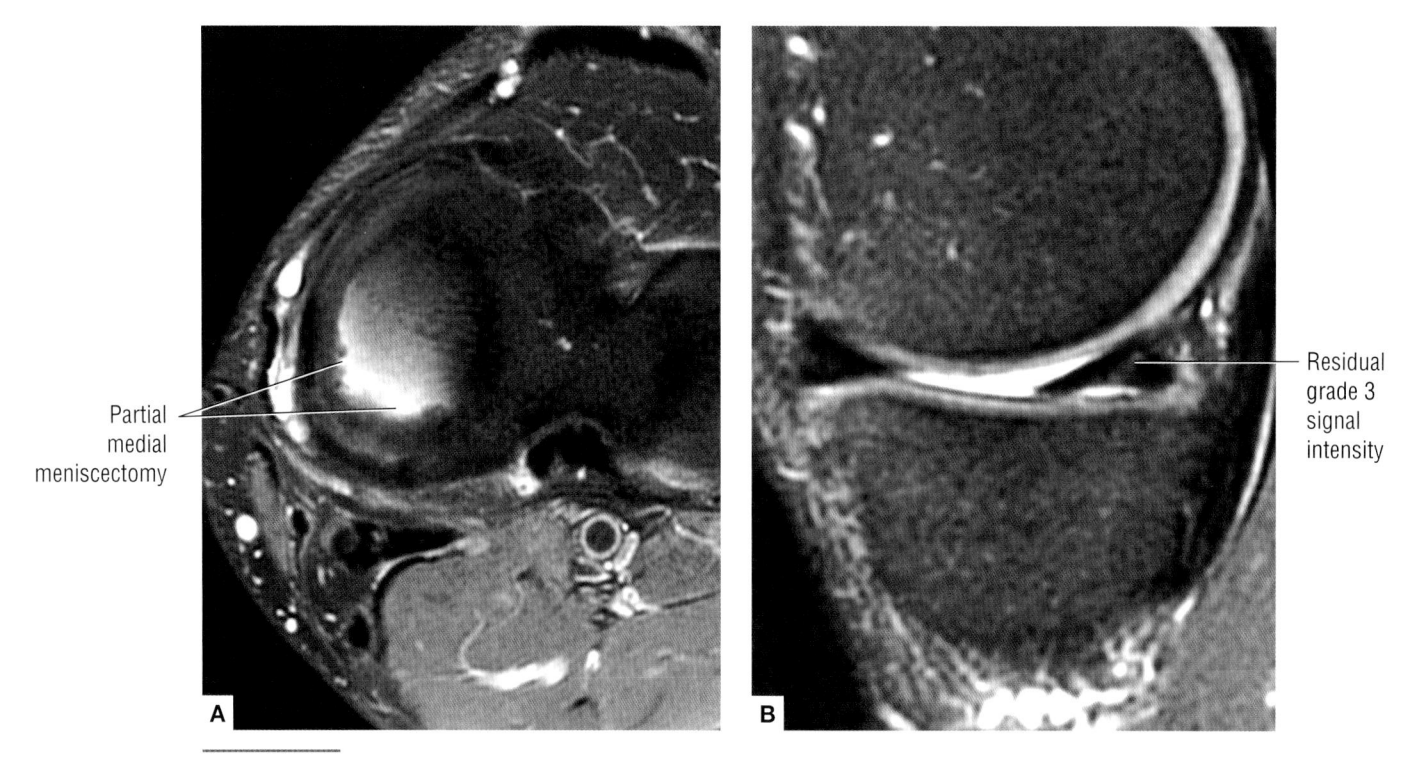

FIGURE 4.188 Contoured free edge (**A**) and inferior leaflet (**B**) after partial medial meniscectomy. Residual intrasubstance meniscal signal is present without retear. (**A**) Axial FS PD FSE image. (**B**) Sagittal FS PD FSE image.

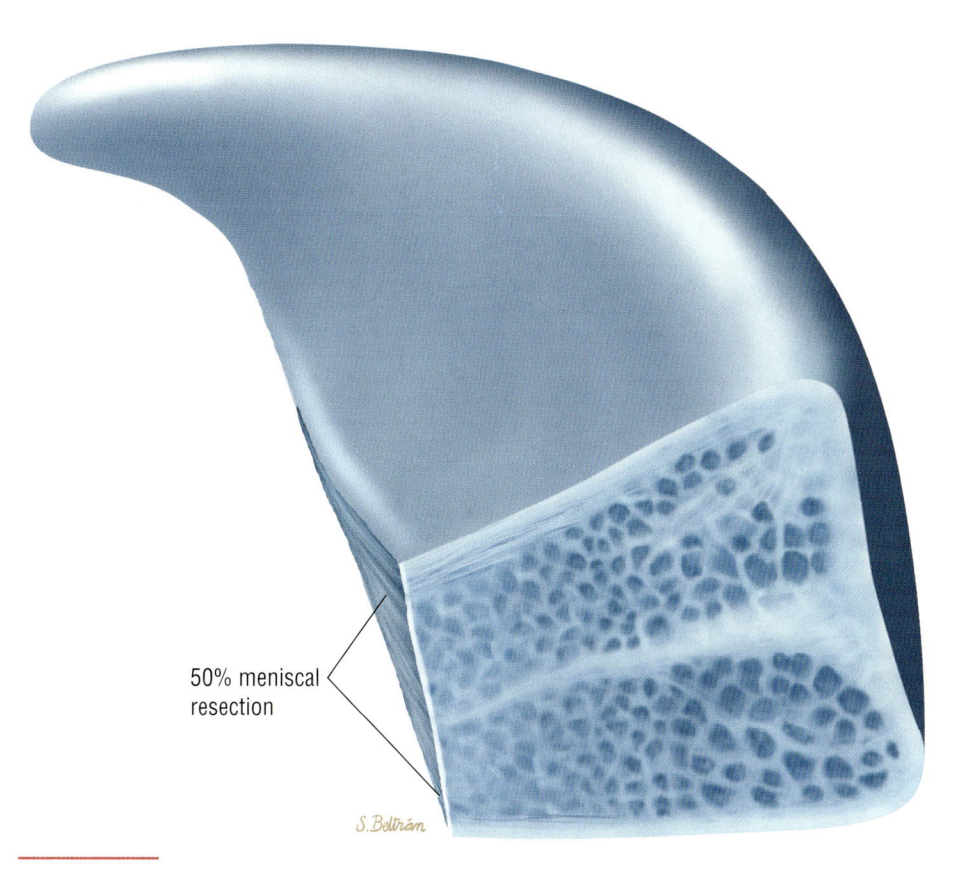

FIGURE 4.189 Fifty percent meniscal resection with blunted free edge.

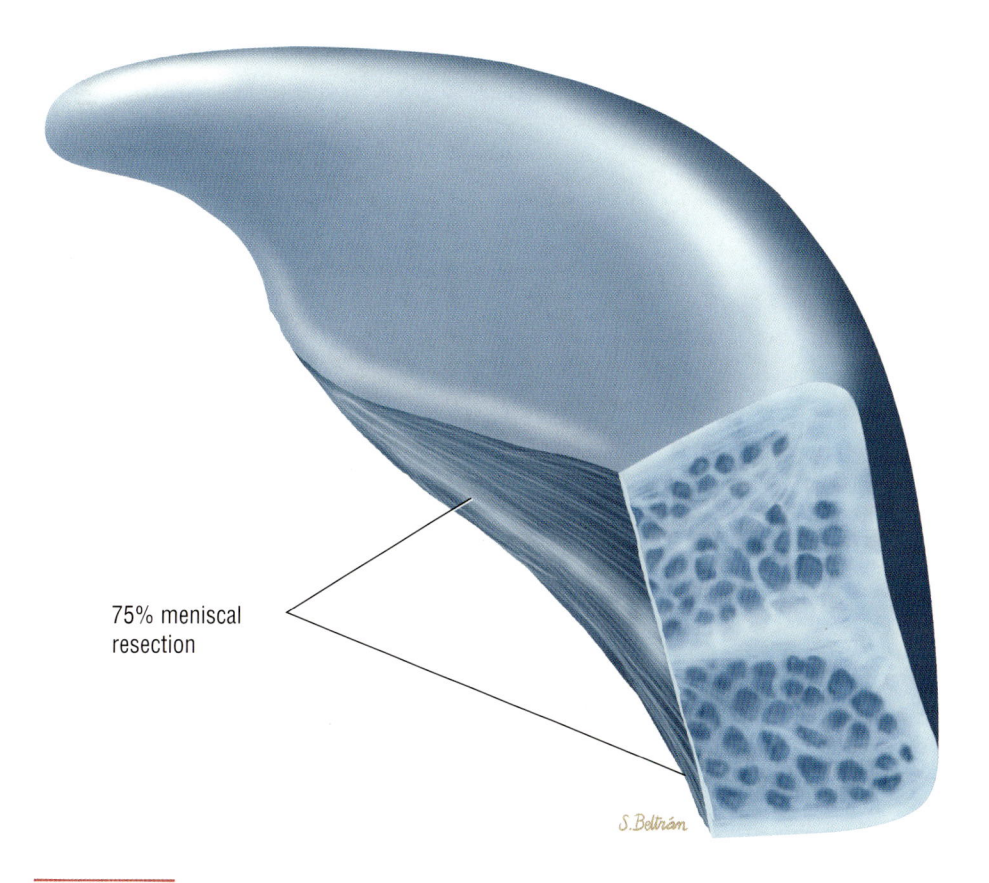

FIGURE 4.190 Cross-sectional sagittal illustration of a 75% resection of posterior horn lateral meniscus with a thick rim of meniscal remnant.

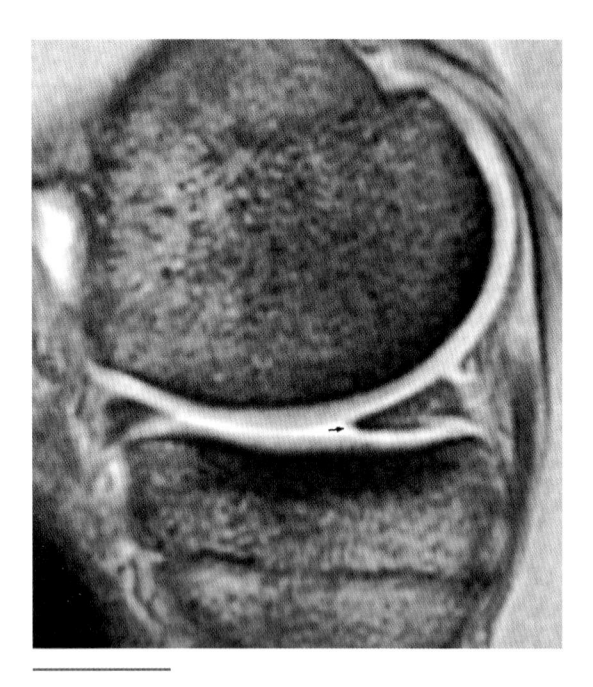

FIGURE 4.191 Mild free edge blunting after a minimal or micro-partial meniscectomy. FS PD FSE sagittal image.

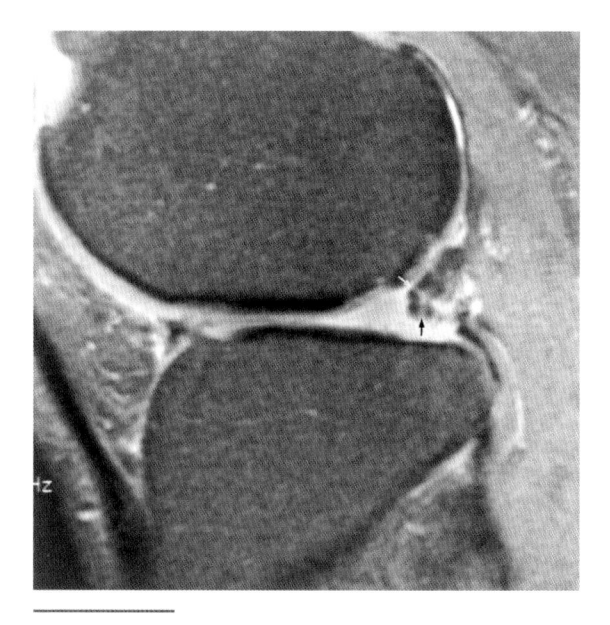

FIGURE 4.192 Fifty percent meniscal resection with blunted free edge. FS PD FSE sagittal image demonstrates persistence of grade 3 signal intensity (*arrows*) in the posterior horn remnant of the lateral meniscus.

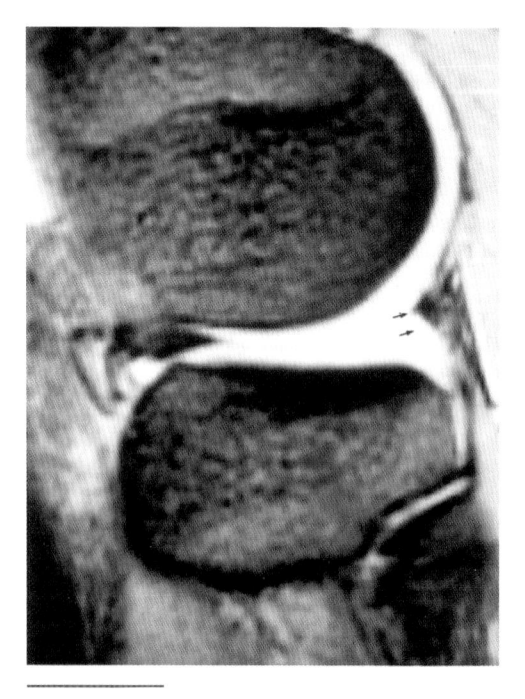

FIGURE 4.193 Seventy-five percent resection of posterior horn lateral meniscus with a thick rim of meniscal remnant. T2* GRE sagittal image.

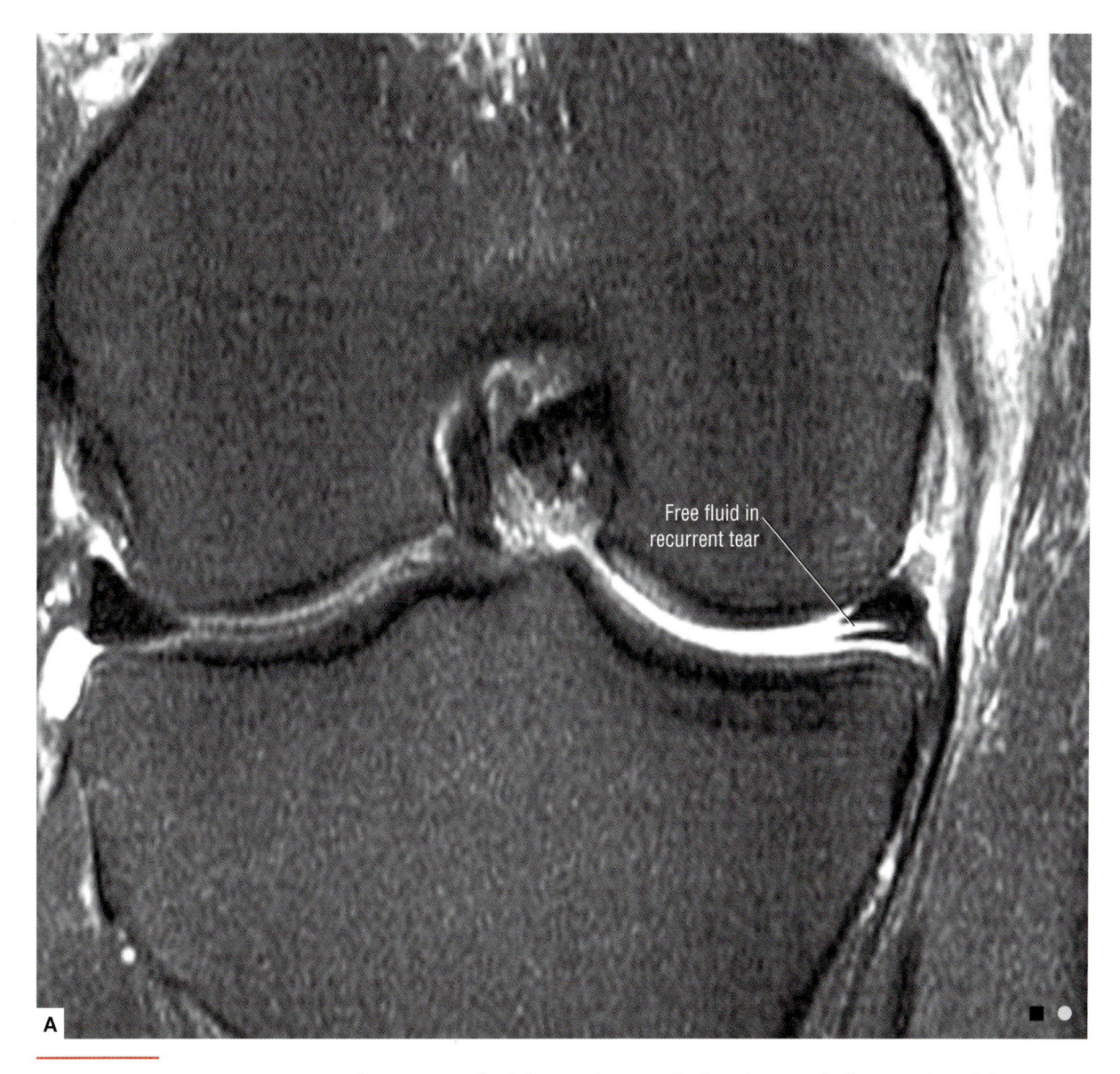

FIGURE 4.194 Recurrent tear as hyperintense fluid distinct from residual grade 3 signal after partial medial meniscectomy. (**A**) FS PD FSE coronal, (**B**) FS PD FSE sagittal, and (**C**) FS PD FSE sagittal images. (*Continued*)

- Direct signs of recurrent tear:
    - Present → Extension of fluid into area of grade 3 signal
    - Fragmentation of meniscal remnant
    - New meniscal tear pattern

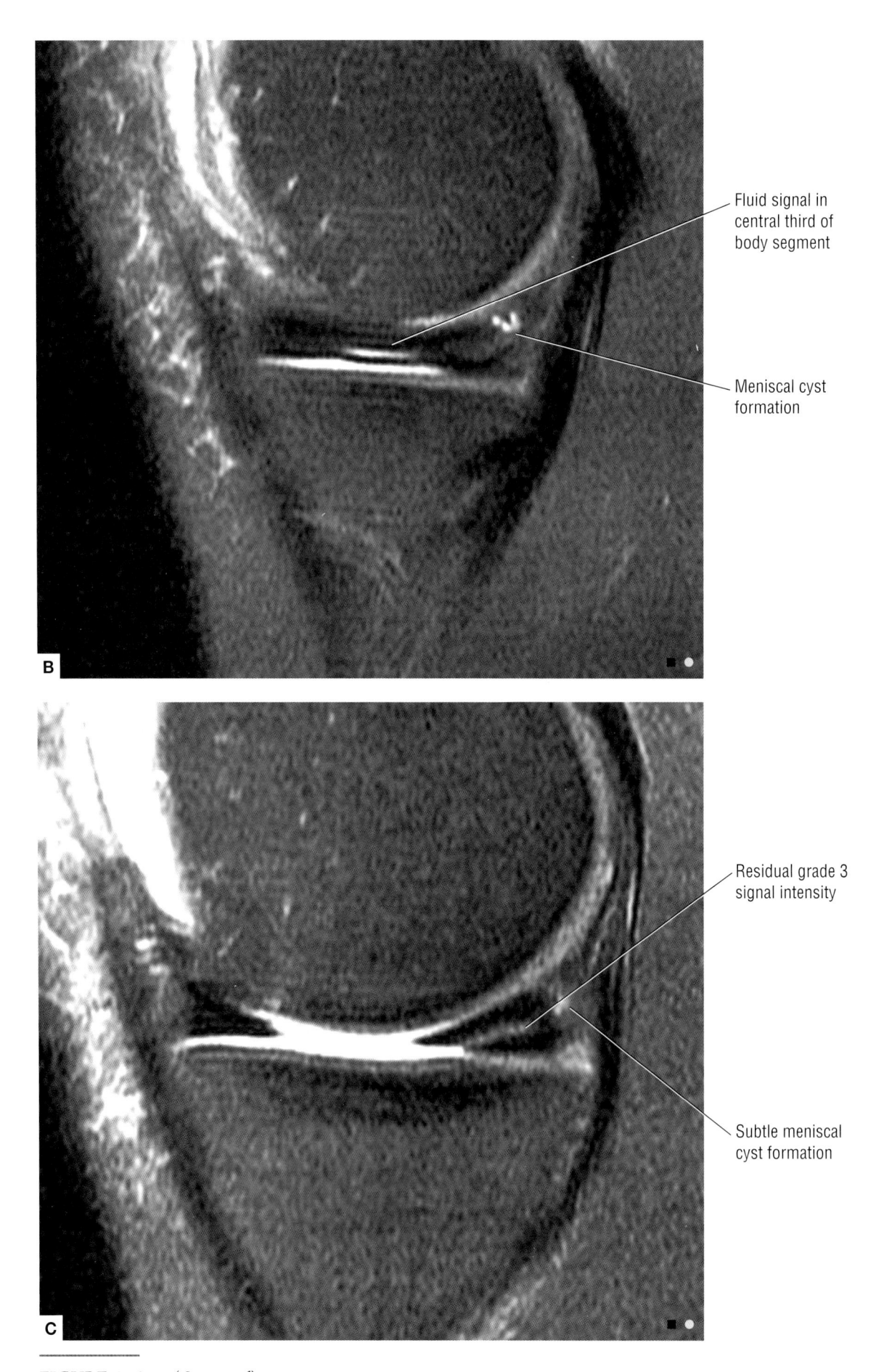

FIGURE 4.194 (Continued)

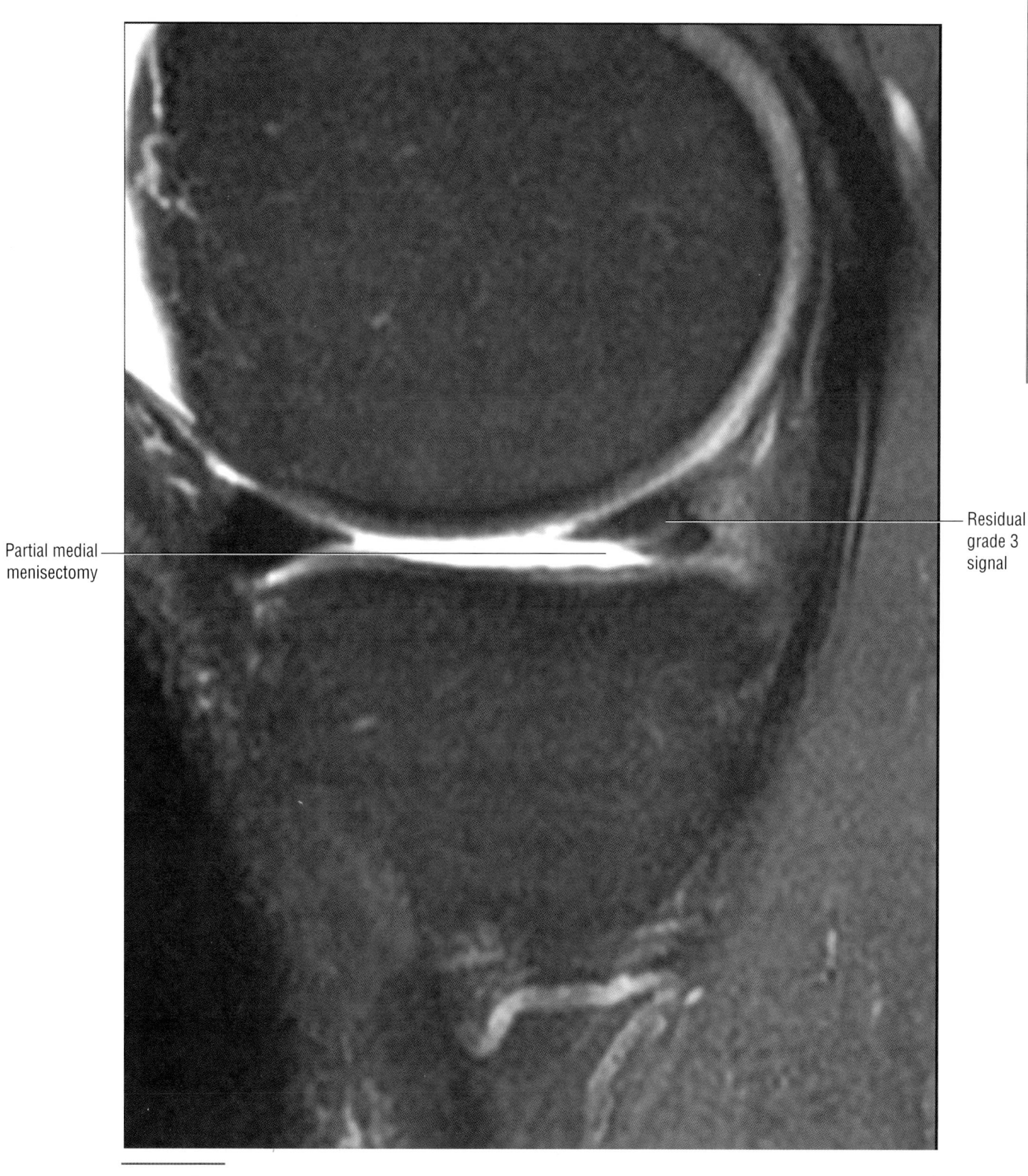

FIGURE 4.195 Normal appearance of posterior horn remnant. Residual grade 3 signal is intermediate with the influx of hyperintense joint fluid and without the formation of a meniscal cyst. FS PD FSE sagittal image.

Retear posterior horn remnant medial meniscus

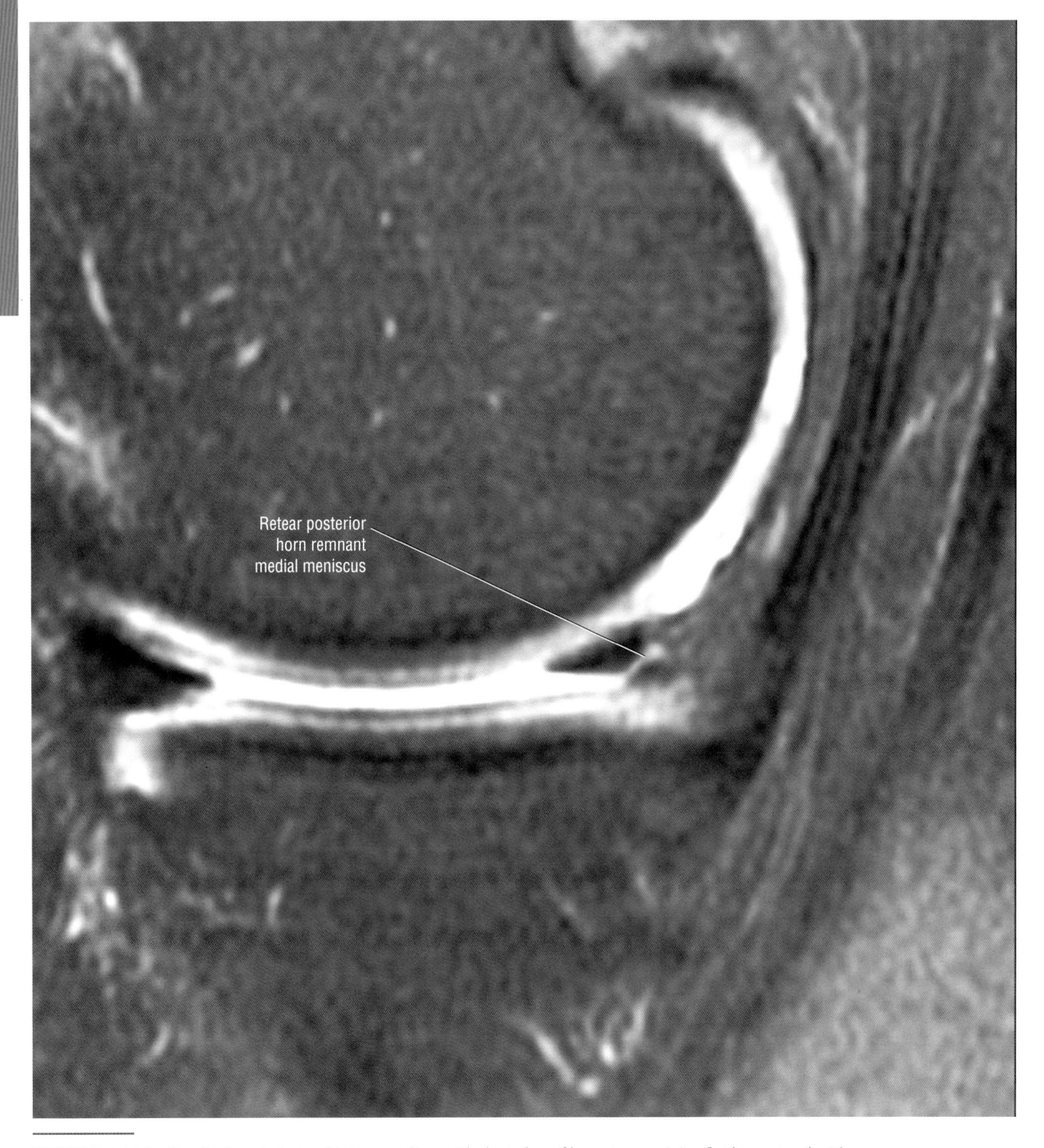

FIGURE 4.196 Residual grade 3 signal is intermediate with the influx of hyperintense joint fluid associated with a recurrent tear. FS PD FSE sagittal image.

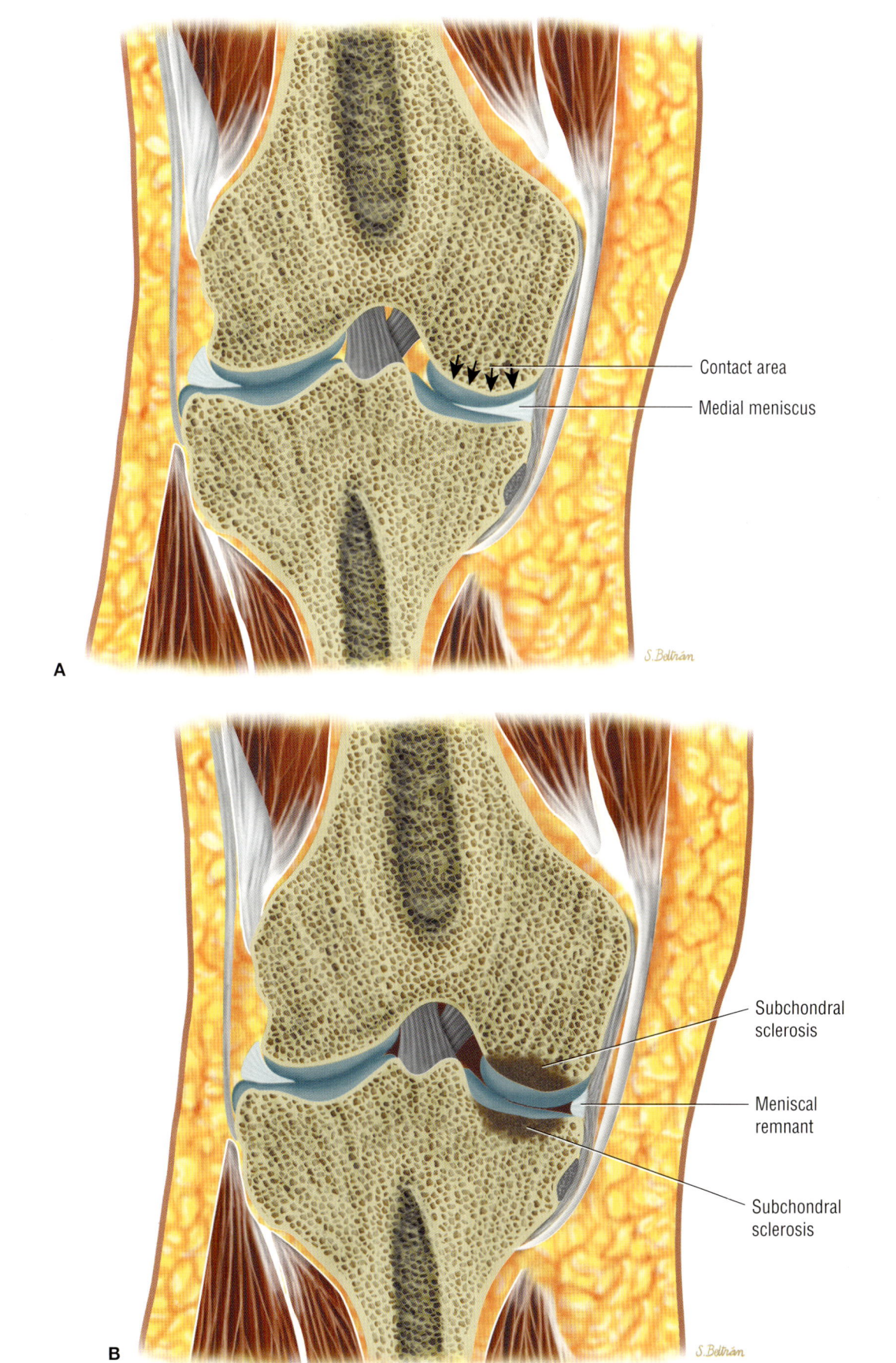

FIGURE 4.197 (**A**) A large contact area between the medial femoral condyle and the tibial plateau allows normal load transference to the intact meniscus. (**B**) Loss of the condylar meniscus contact area results in focally concentrated stress and medial compartment arthrosis after a partial meniscectomy.

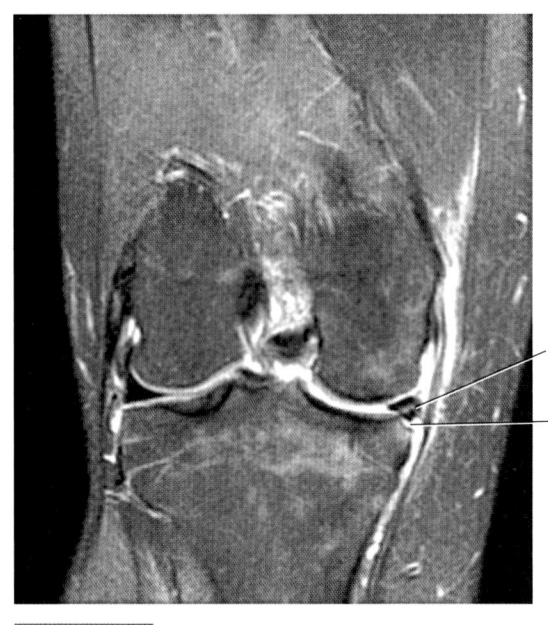

FIGURE 4.198 Coronal FS PD FSE image shows extrusion of a meniscus remnant and erosion of the medial tibial plateau.

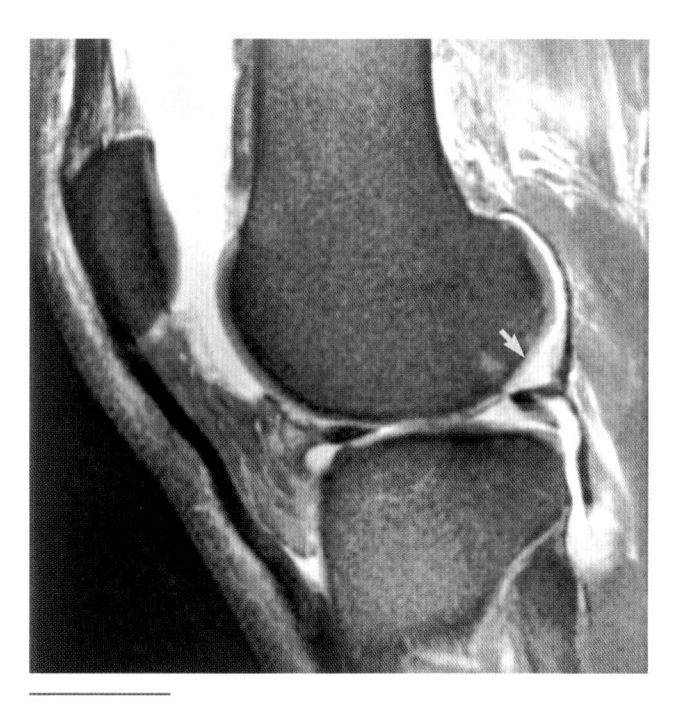

FIGURE 4.199 Loss of lateral femoral condyle articular cartilage (*arrow*) opposite the lateral meniscus posterior horn remnant shown on a FS T2-weighted FSE sagittal image.

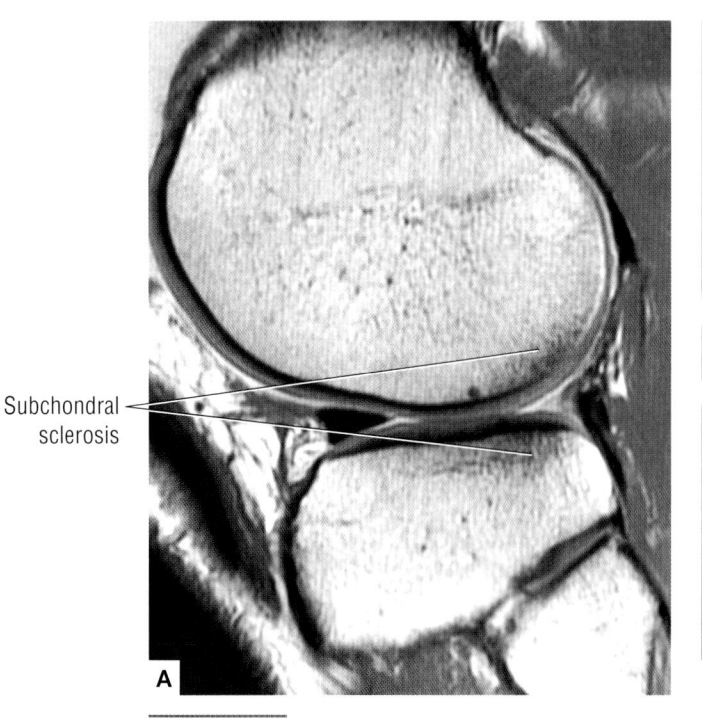

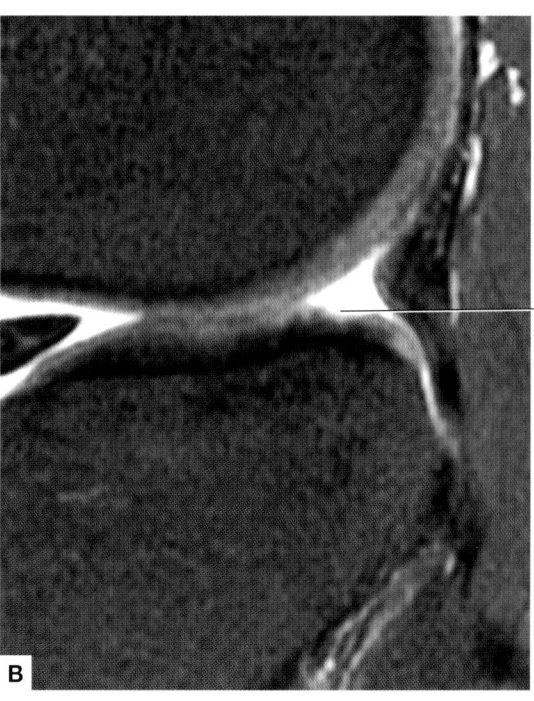

FIGURE 4.200 Partial lateral meniscectomy. (**A**) Sagittal PD FSE image showing early superficial surface subchondral sclerosis of the posterior lateral compartment. (**B**) Sagittal FS PD FSE image depicting chondral erosion subsequent to partial lateral meniscectomy.

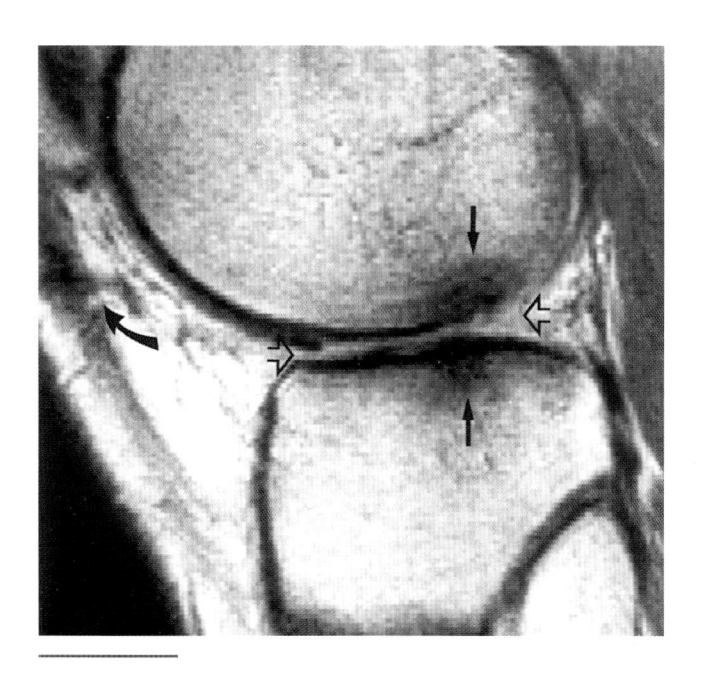

FIGURE 4.201 Lateral compartment arthrosis with advanced degenerative changes after lateral meniscectomy (*open arrows*). Hypointense subchondral sclerosis is demonstrated (*closed arrows*). Arthroscopy tract is seen anteriorly.

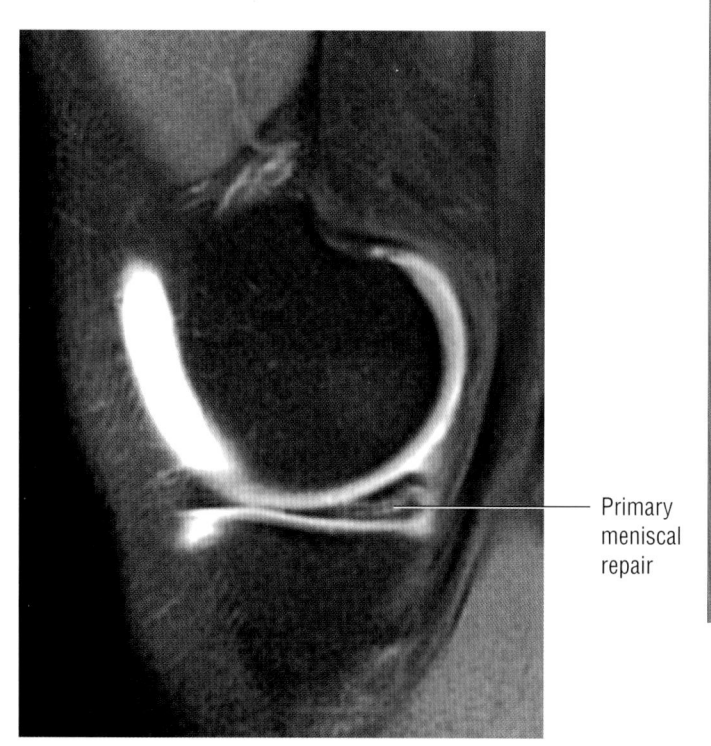

FIGURE 4.202 Primary meniscal repair with intrasubstance signal intensity not extending to an articular surface (sagittal FS T1 MR arthrogram image).

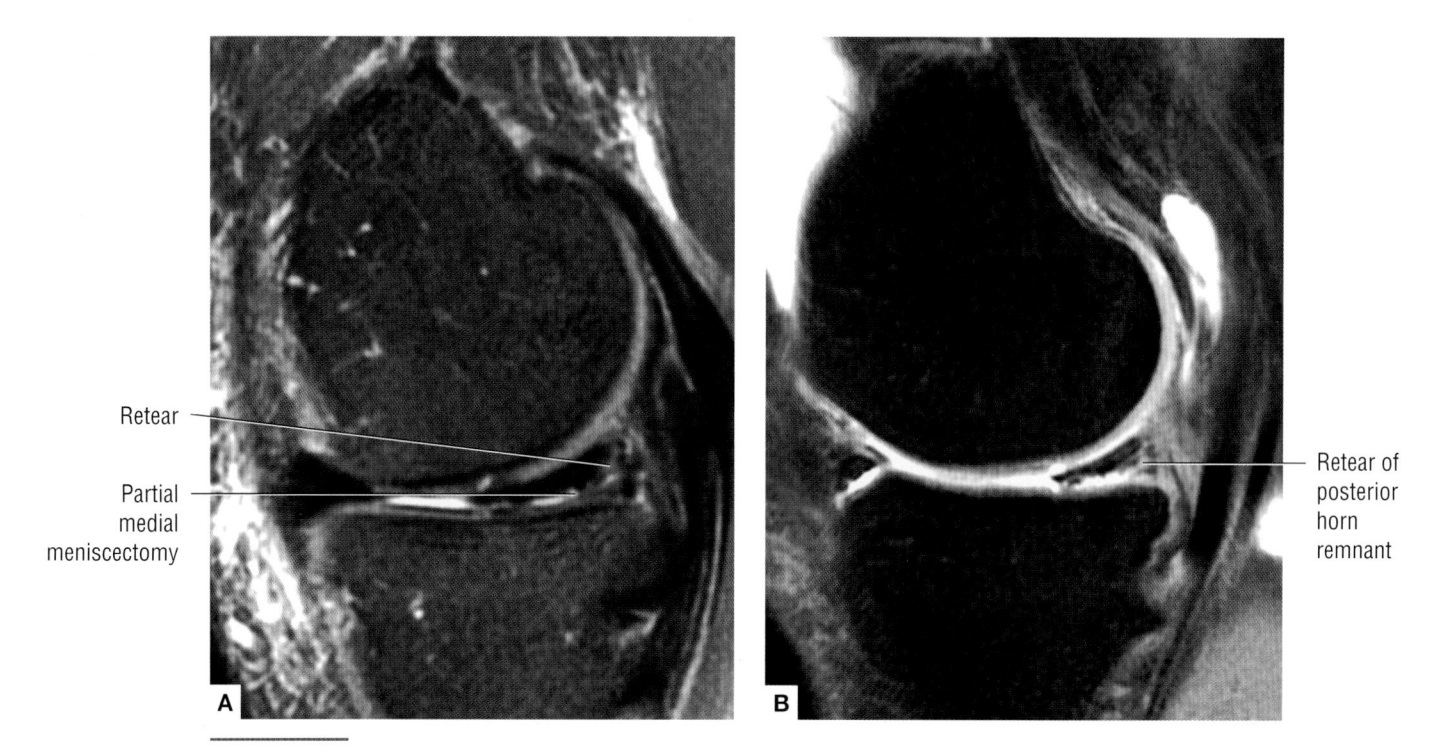

FIGURE 4.203 MR arthrogram. Retear of posterior horn remnant showing increased conspicuity of contrast between FS PD FSE (**A**) and FS T1-weighted (**B**) sagittal images. The meniscal extension of intraarticular contrast is best visualized on the FS T1-weighted image.

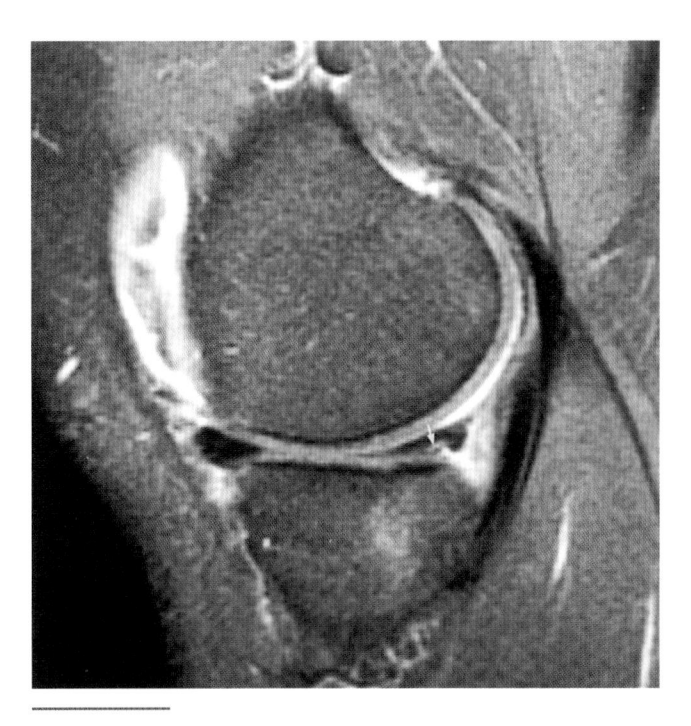

FIGURE 4.204 IV gadolinium enhancement facilitates identification of grade 3 signal intensity (*arrow*) extending to the irregular inferior surface of the postoperative meniscus on a FS T1-weighted image.

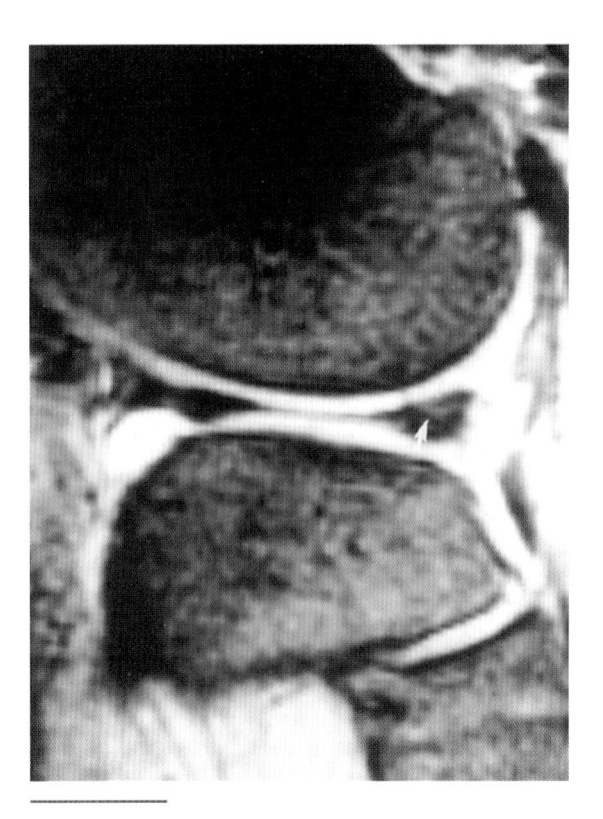

FIGURE 4.205 A T2*-weighted sagittal image made after primary repair of the lateral meniscus shows minimal residual signal intensity in the posterior horn.

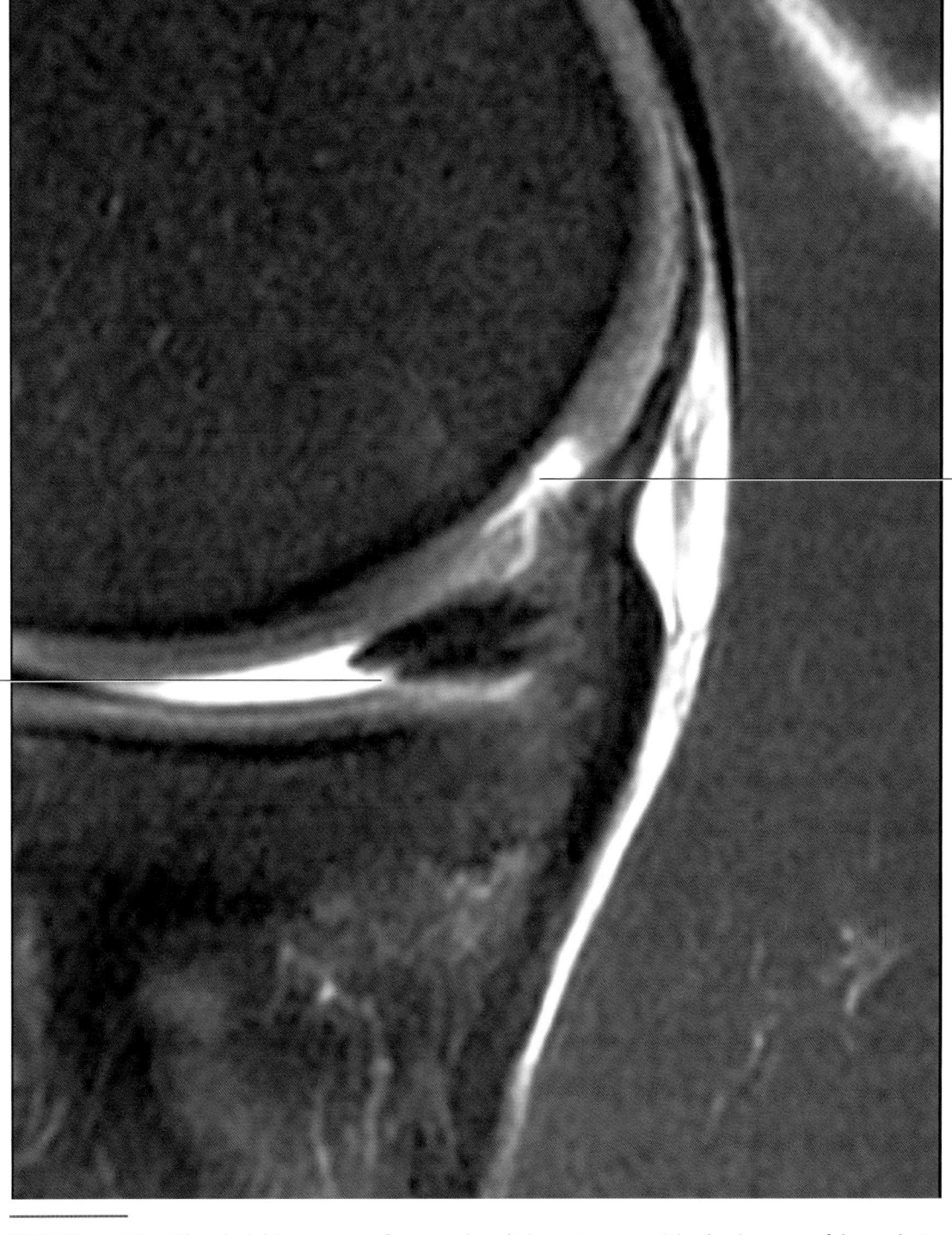

FIGURE 4.206 Chondral delamination after partial medial meniscectomy. The development of the grade 4 chondral lesion was accelerated by the repetitive axial loading from basketball activity.

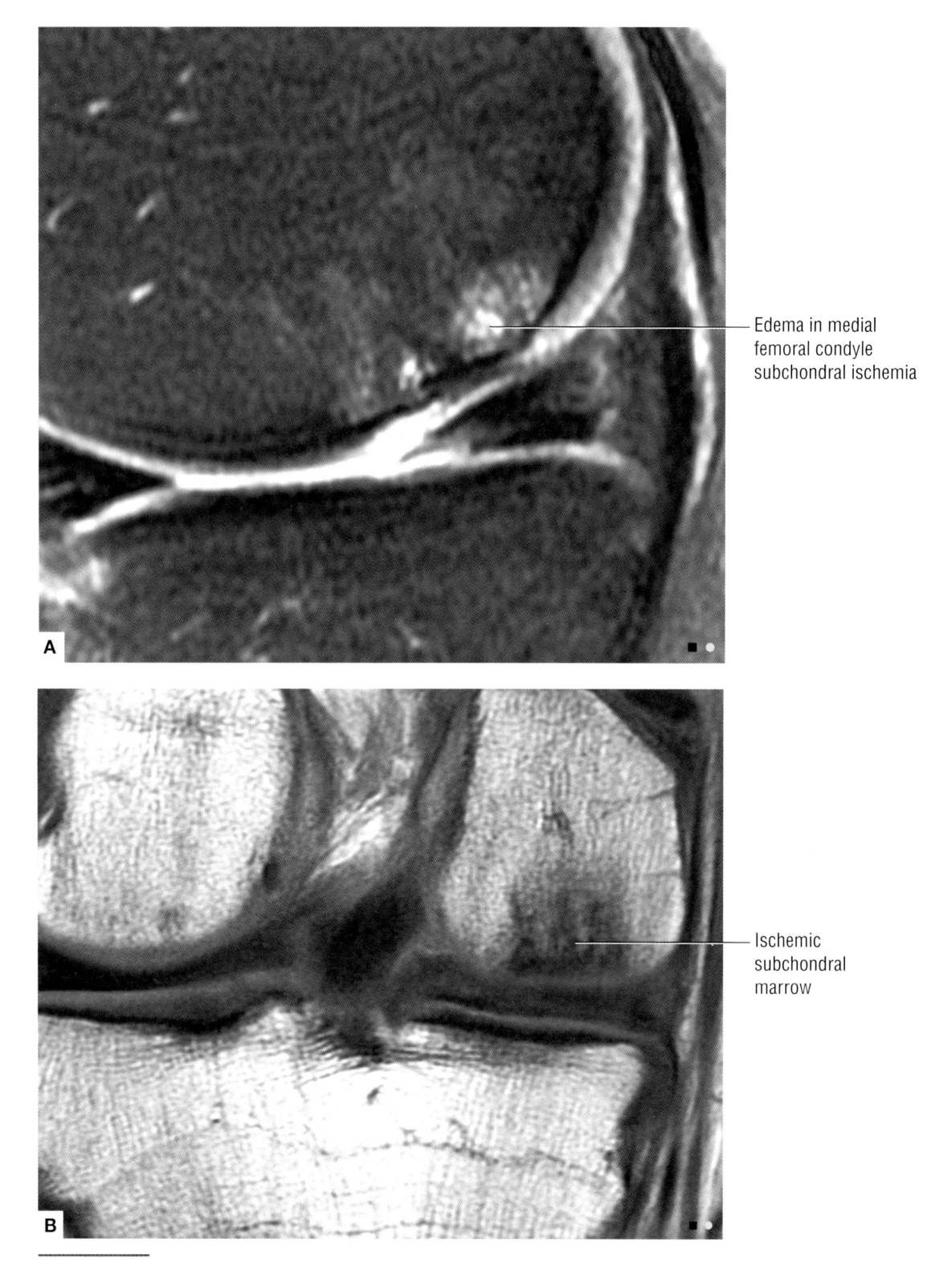

FIGURE 4.207 Ischemic change of the medial femoral condyle with grade 4 chondral degeneration subsequent to a partial medial meniscectomy. FS PD FSE sagittal (**A**) and coronal (**B**) images.

Miscellaneous Meniscal Pathology

Key Concepts

- **Meniscocapsular Separations**
    - The meniscocapsular ligaments consist of meniscofemoral and meniscotibial ligaments and are defined in layer 3 of the knee joint capsule.
    - Tears of the proximal MCL are associated with meniscofemoral ligament injuries.
    - Fluid interposed between the meniscus and capsular periphery posterolateral to the superficial MCL and deep MCL represents a form of meniscocapsular tearing and may be associated with a posterior medial meniscal corner tear in acute ACL injuries.
    - Meniscal avulsions involving the meniscotibial attachment occur in both the medial and lateral meniscus.

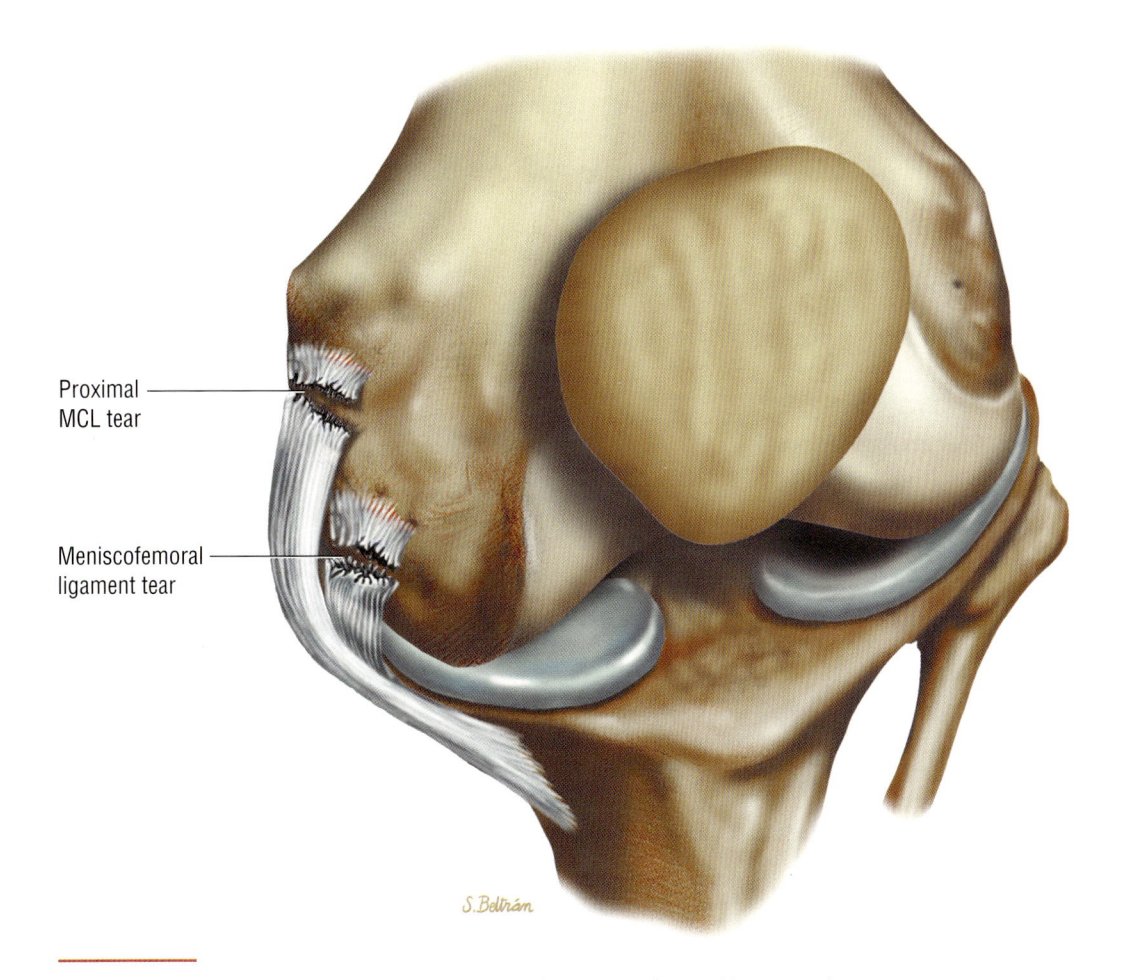

FIGURE 4.208 Coronal illustration showing the meniscofemoral ligament disruption in association with a proximally located MCL tear.

Meniscocapsular Separations

- Meniscocapsular separations or tears usually involve the less mobile medial meniscus.[323]

- The thick medial third of the joint capsule or medial capsular ligament is divided into meniscofemoral and meniscotibial components.[95,472]
    - Anteriorly, these fibers are separated from the superficial fibers of the MCL by an interposed bursa and can best be seen on routine FS PD FSE radial images through the medial compartment of the knee.

- The posterior horn of the medial meniscus, fixed to the tibia by meniscotibial or coronary ligaments, is especially susceptible to tearing at its capsular attachment.

- Even in the absence of grade 3 signal intensity through the meniscus, a separation at the meniscocapsular junction associated with pain may have clinical significance.

- Small or nondisplaced meniscocapsular tears may heal without surgical intervention because these tears occur through the vascularized periphery of the meniscus, adjacent to the perimeniscal capillary plexus.[324]

- Minor repair of these lesions also has a high success rate because of their peripheral location.

- On sagittal MR images, the tibial plateau articular cartilage should be covered by the posterior horn of the medial meniscus without an exposed articular cartilage surface.

- Displacement of the posterior horn of the medial meniscus by 5mm or more, uncovered tibial articular cartilage, and fluid interposed between the peripheral edge of the meniscus and capsule are suggestive of peripheral detachment.[324]

- Uncovering of the tibial articular cartilage, however, is not a specific sign for meniscocapsular injury, and quantitative measurements of meniscal displacement may be unreliable.

- In addition, the meniscus may have fluid within the superior and inferior capsular recesses without violation of the meniscocapsular junction.

- In true meniscocapsular separations, especially in association with ACL tears, sagittal images demonstrate fluid completely interposed between the peripheral portion of the posterior horn of the medial meniscus and the joint capsule.

- Coronal and sagittal images best display the anatomy of the deep capsular layer and its relation to the meniscus for identification of disruptions of the meniscofemoral and meniscotibial ligaments.

- MCL tears may also be seen in association with meniscocapsular separation.

- Complete peripheral detachment of the posterior horn is seen as a free-floating meniscus, especially if it is associated with a MCL tear.

- The interface between the posterior horn of the medial meniscus and posteromedial capsular tissue should be identified and defined on all sagittal images.

- Fluid extending completely across this interface (superior to inferior) or across the meniscotibial capsular attachment is an abnormal finding.

- In the posteromedial aspect of the knee, the capsule fuses with the gastrocnemius tendon superiorly and also attaches to the cortex of the posterior femoral condyle.

- A subgastrocnemius bursa is formed between the capsule and the gastrocnemius tendon.[96]

- In acute ACL tears, posterior inferior corner tears of the medial meniscus are frequently seen in association with posteromedial medial tibial osseous contusion or fractures.

- Peripheral tears are caused by contrecoup forces resulting from direct contact between the medial femoral condyle and medial tibial plateau subsequent to impaction between the sulcus terminals of the lateral femoral condyle and the posterolateral tibial plateau.

    - This area of meniscocapsular interface is more posterior and lateral (toward the notch) than the portion of layer 3 referred to as the deep MCL.

- Meniscal avulsion from the tibial plateau is associated with disruption of the meniscotibial attachment of the deep capsular layer.

- "Floating meniscus" describes the resultant appearance of fluid surrounding the detached meniscus in the setting of acute trauma with discontinuity of the meniscotibial capsular ligament.[31]
    - The meniscofemoral ligament is usually intact in this setting.
    - The prominent layer of fluid is localized between the meniscus and the tibial plateau.
- A "floating meniscus" may involve either the medial or lateral meniscus.
- A distal MCL tear may preferentially disrupt the meniscotibial ligament.

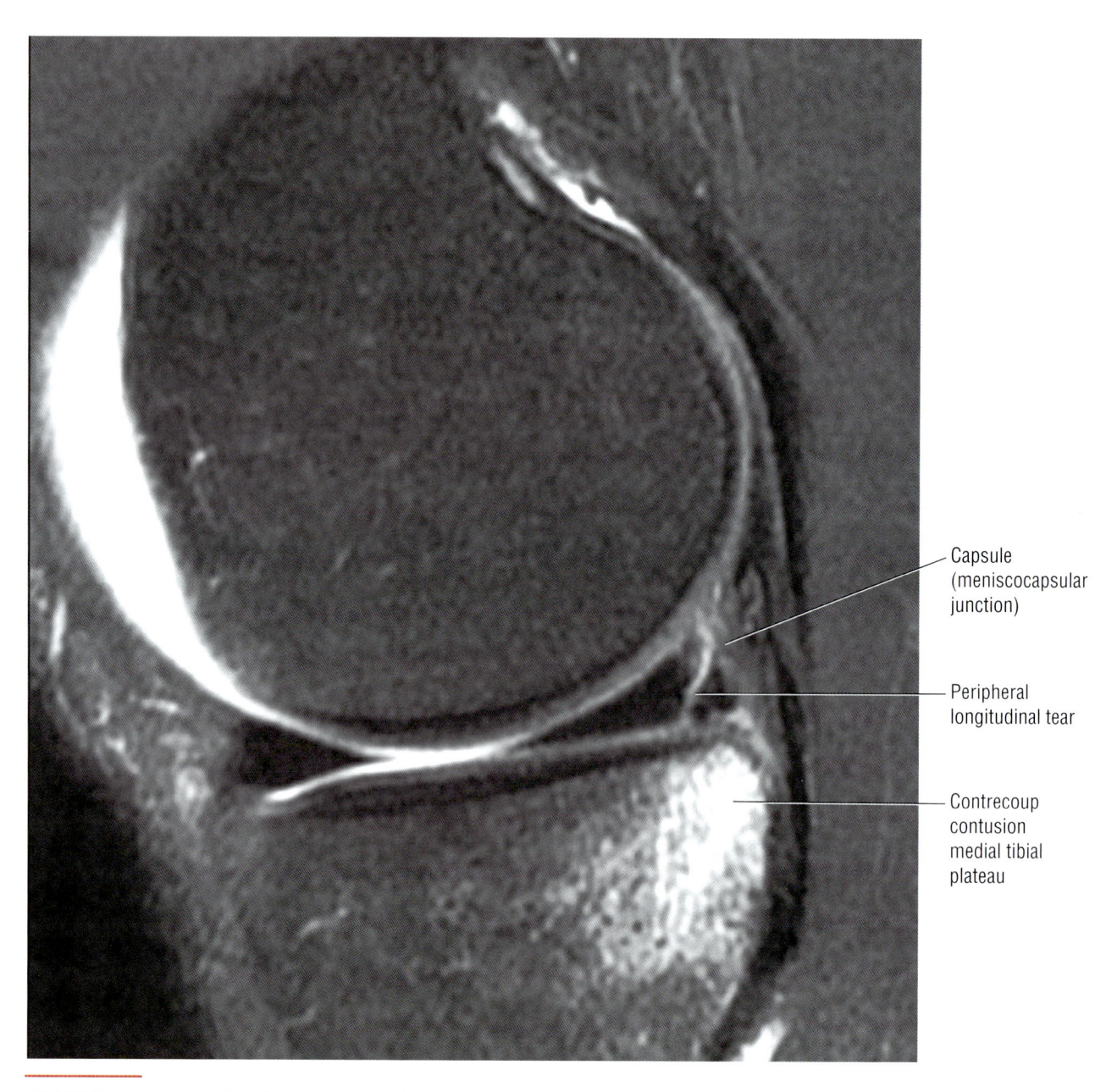

FIGURE 4.209 Peripheral vertical longitudinal tear adjacent to meniscocapsular junction in association with an acute ACL tear. Sagittal FS PD FSE image.

The Meniscus

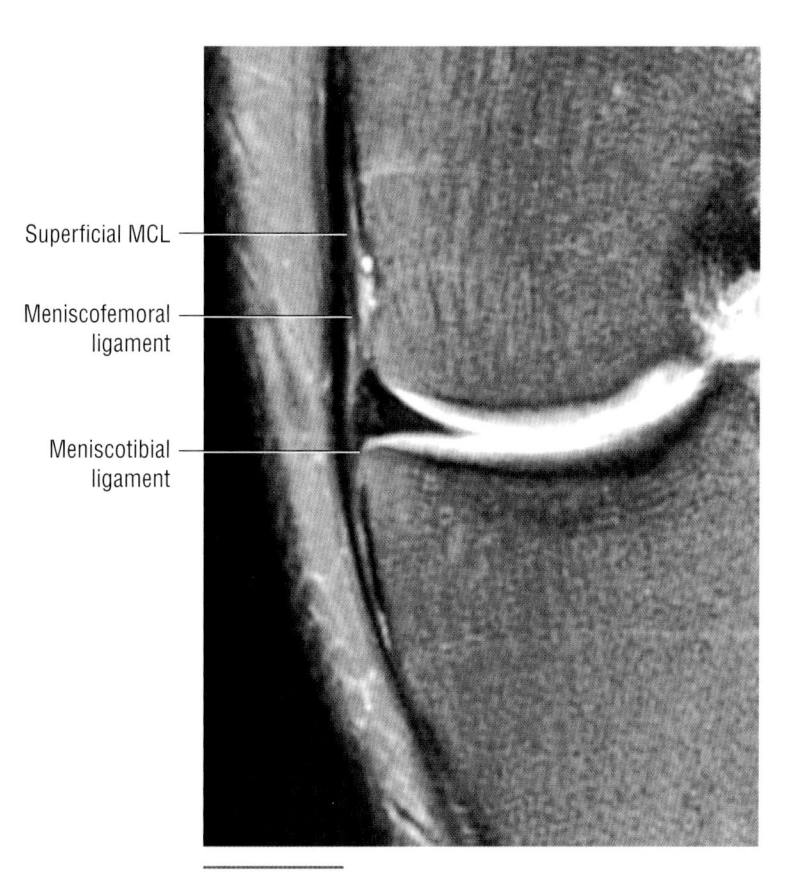

FIGURE 4.210 Coronal FS PD FSE image showing the medial meniscofemoral and meniscotibial ligaments proximal and distal, respectively, to the lateral joint line.

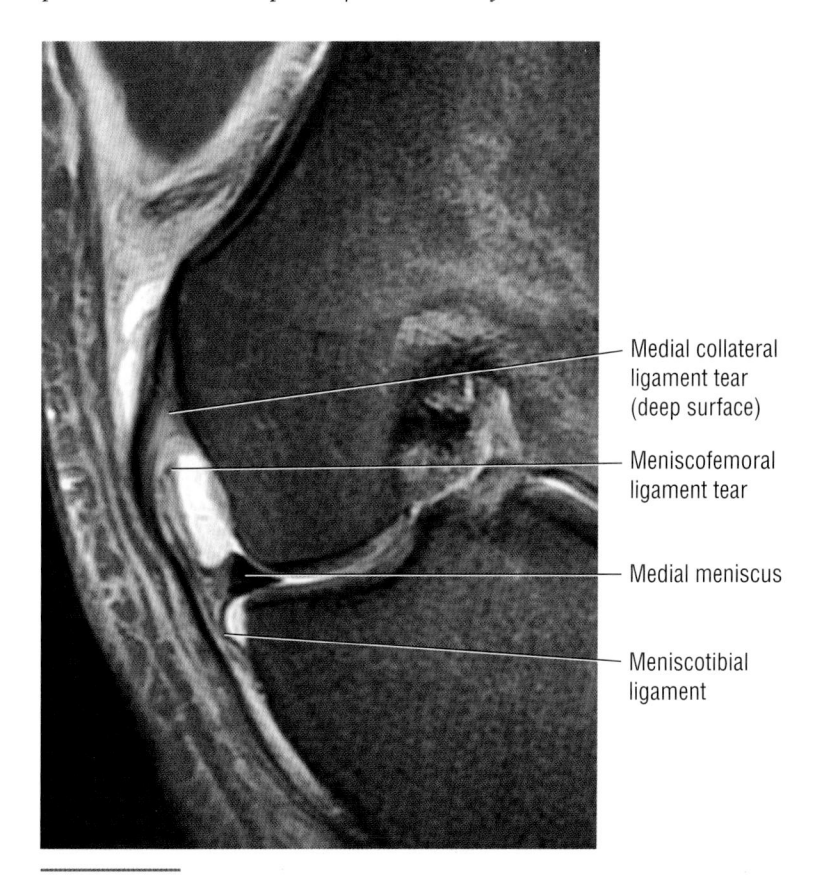

FIGURE 4.211 FS PD FSE coronal image showing meniscofemoral ligament disruption in association with a proximally located MCL sprain.

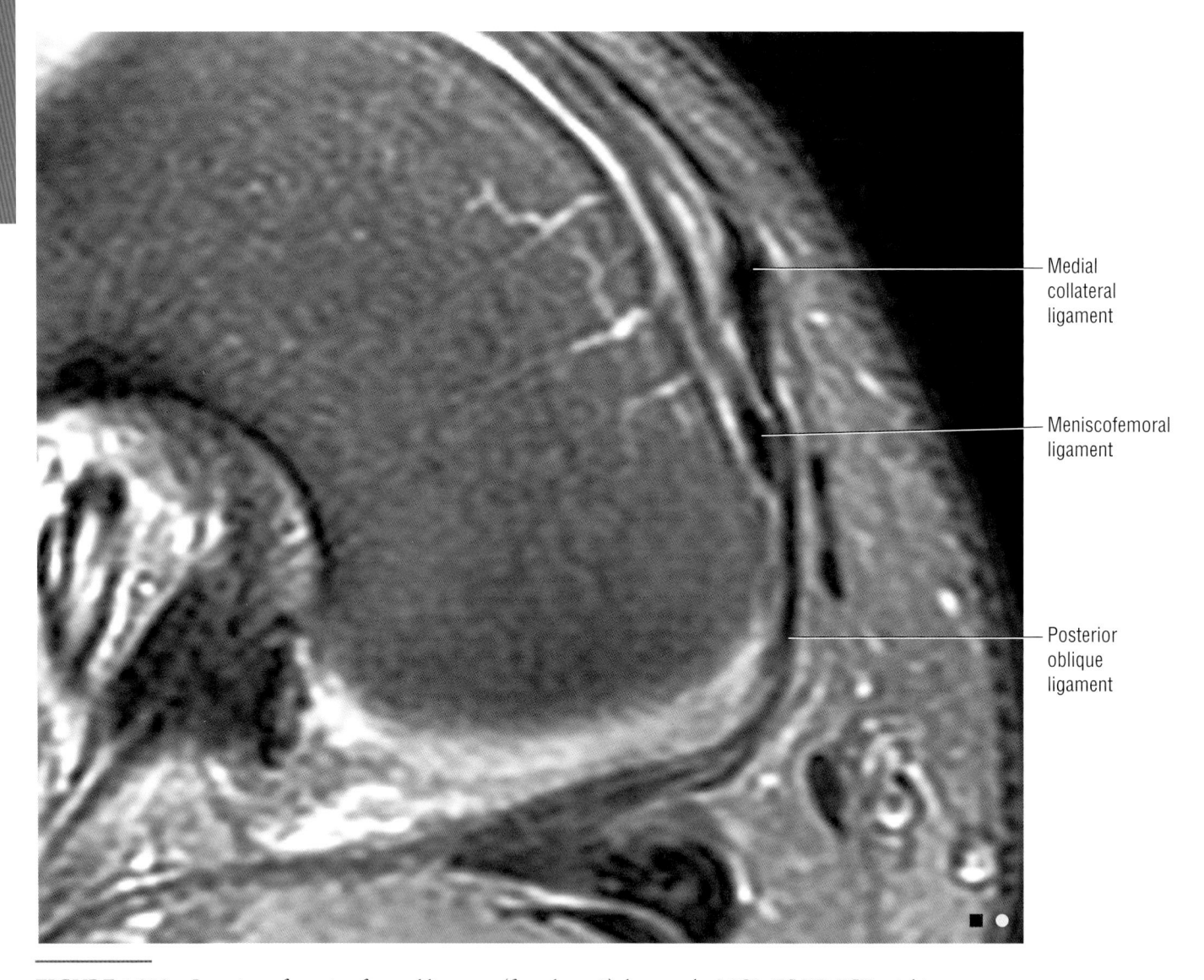

FIGURE 4.212 Location of meniscofemoral ligament (from layer 3) deep to the MCL. FS PD FSE axial image.

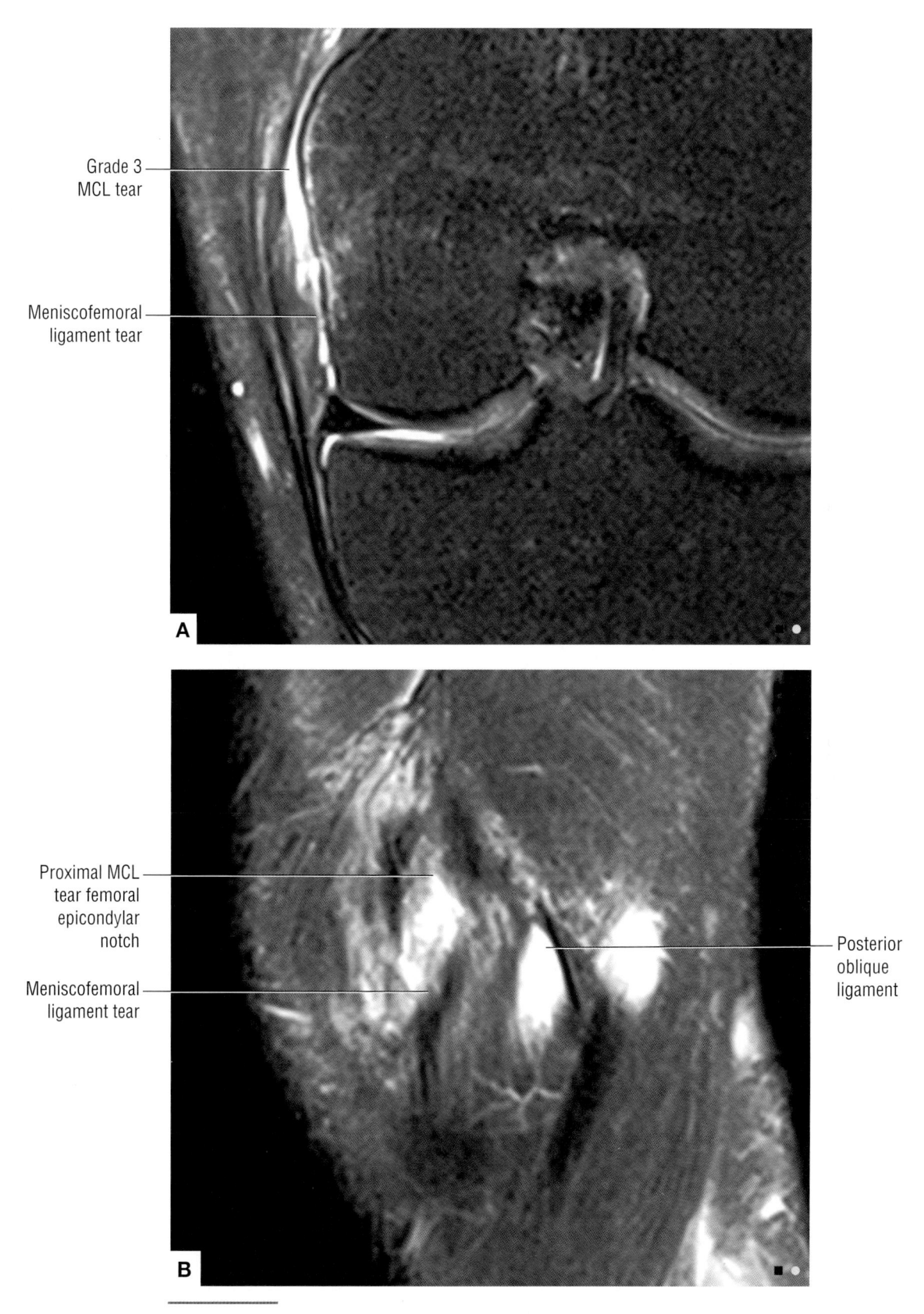

FIGURE 4.213 Disruption of the meniscofemoral ligament associated with a grade 3 proximal MCL tear. FS PD FSE coronal (**A**) and sagittal (**B**) images.

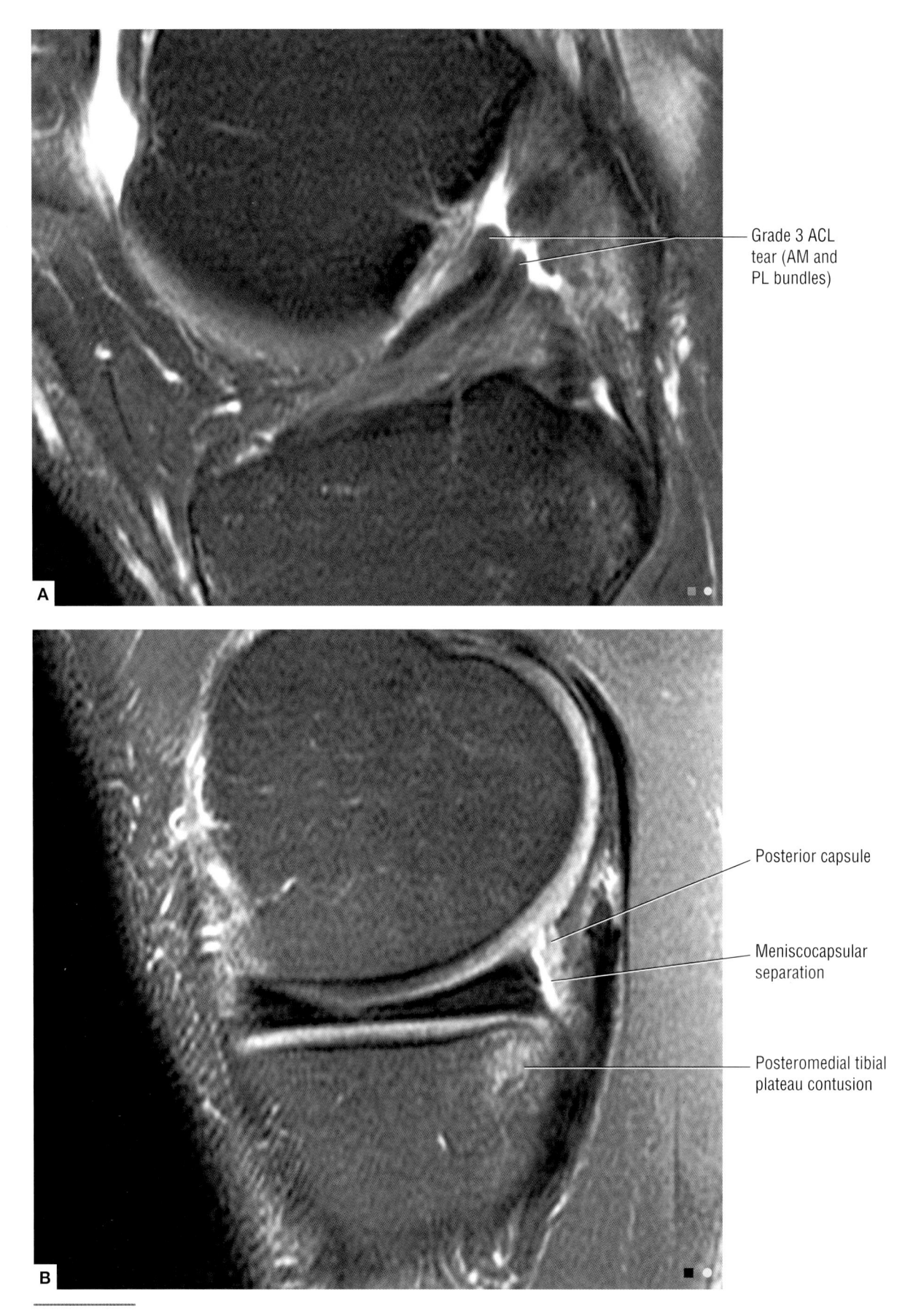

FIGURE 4.214 Grade 3 ACL tear with associated meniscocapsular tear and contrecoup medial tibial plateau contusion. (**A, B**) FS PD FSE sagittal images.

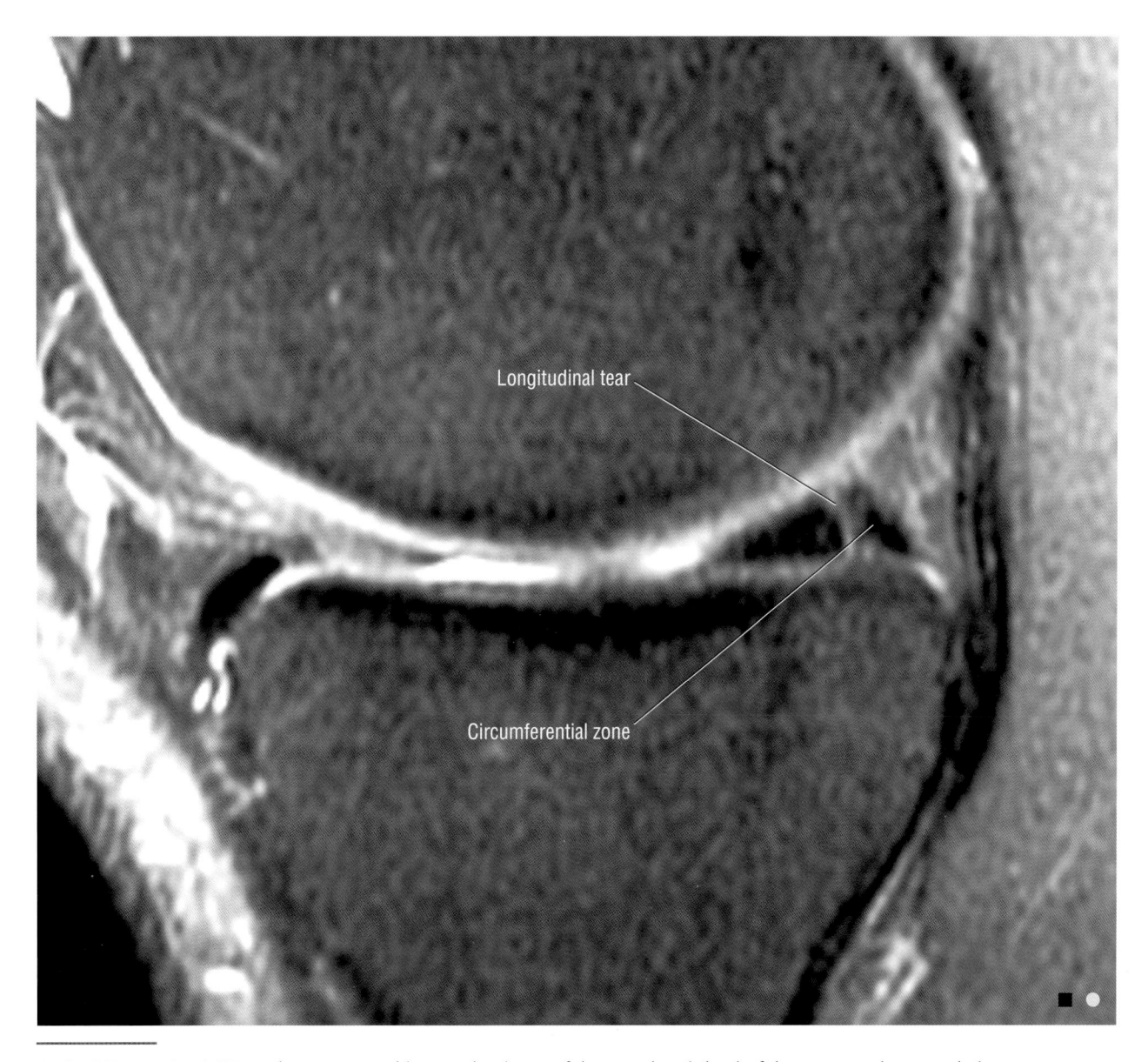

FIGURE 4.215 ACL grade 3 associated longitudinal tear of the peripheral third of the posterior horn medial meniscus. FS PD FSE sagittal image.

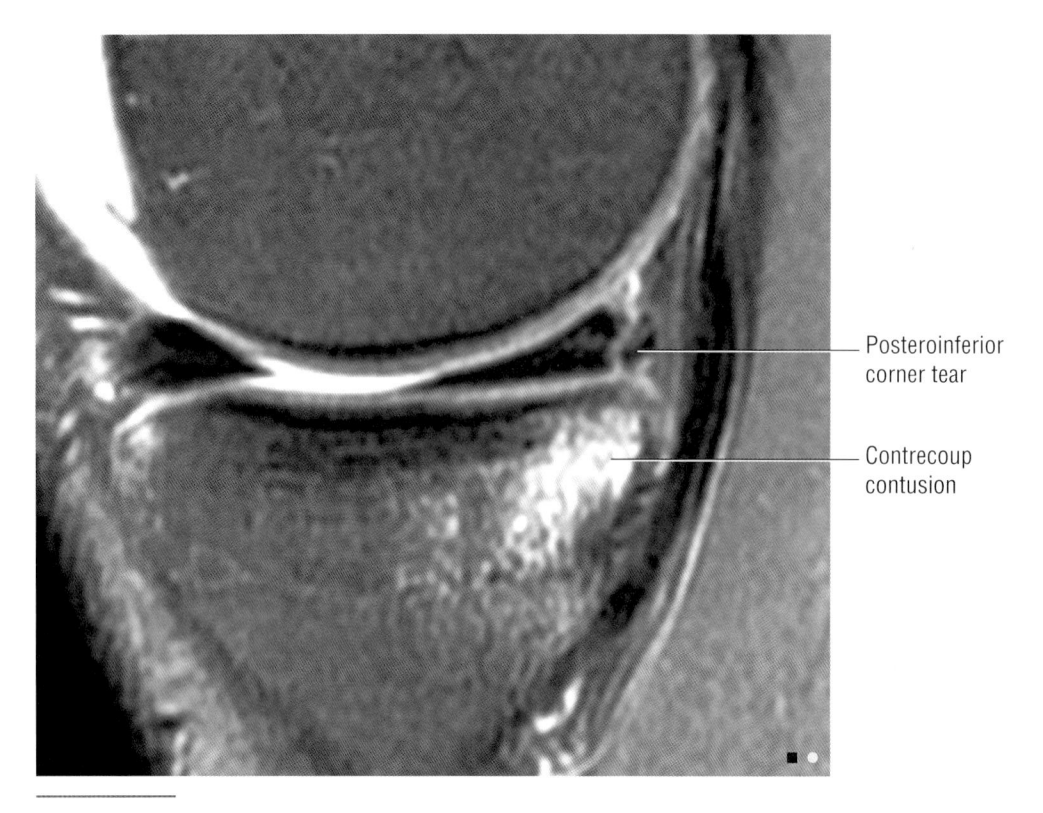

FIGURE 4.216 Posteroinferior corner tear of the posterior horn medial meniscus associated with a grade 3 ACL contrecoup injury. FS PD FSE sagittal image.

- Posteroinferior corner tear
- Contrecoup contusion

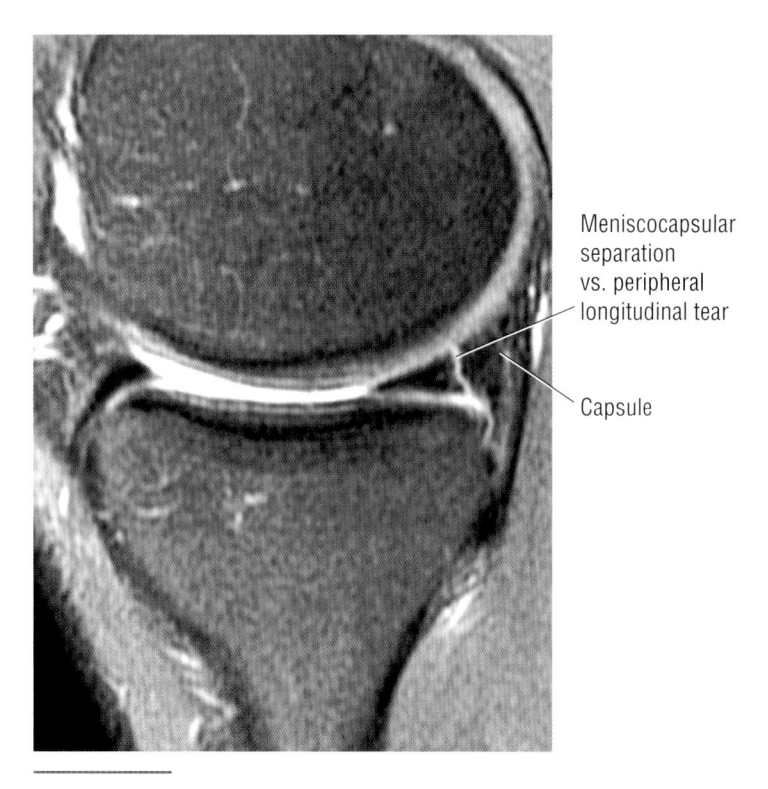

FIGURE 4.217 Sagittal PD FSE image with complete meniscocapsular separation at the interface of the posterior horn of the medial meniscus and the peripheral capsular tissue. Hypointense thick capsular tissue could not be mistaken for meniscal fibrocartilage in this case.

- Meniscocapsular separation vs. peripheral longitudinal tear
- Capsule

The Meniscus

Posteroinferior corner meniscal avulsion

Posteroinferior corner avulsion

Meniscotibial displacement

Lateral tibial plateau fracture

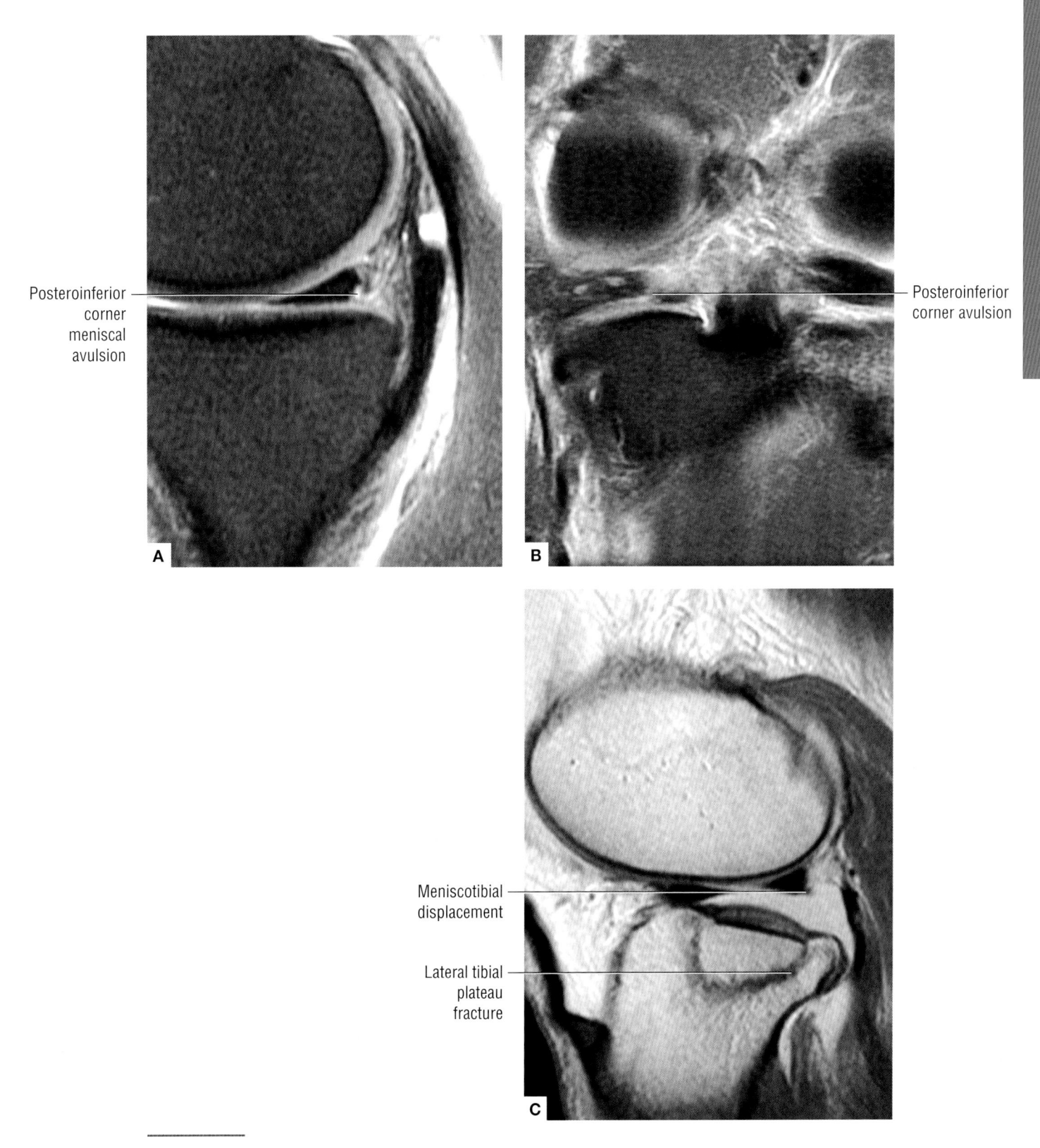

FIGURE 4.218 Posteroinferior medial meniscus corner avulsion at the meniscotibial ligament attachment site on FS PD FSE sagittal (**A**) and coronal (**B**) images. (**C**) Separate case with a "floating lateral meniscus" associated with a lateral tibial plateau fracture and disruption of the meniscotibial attachment.

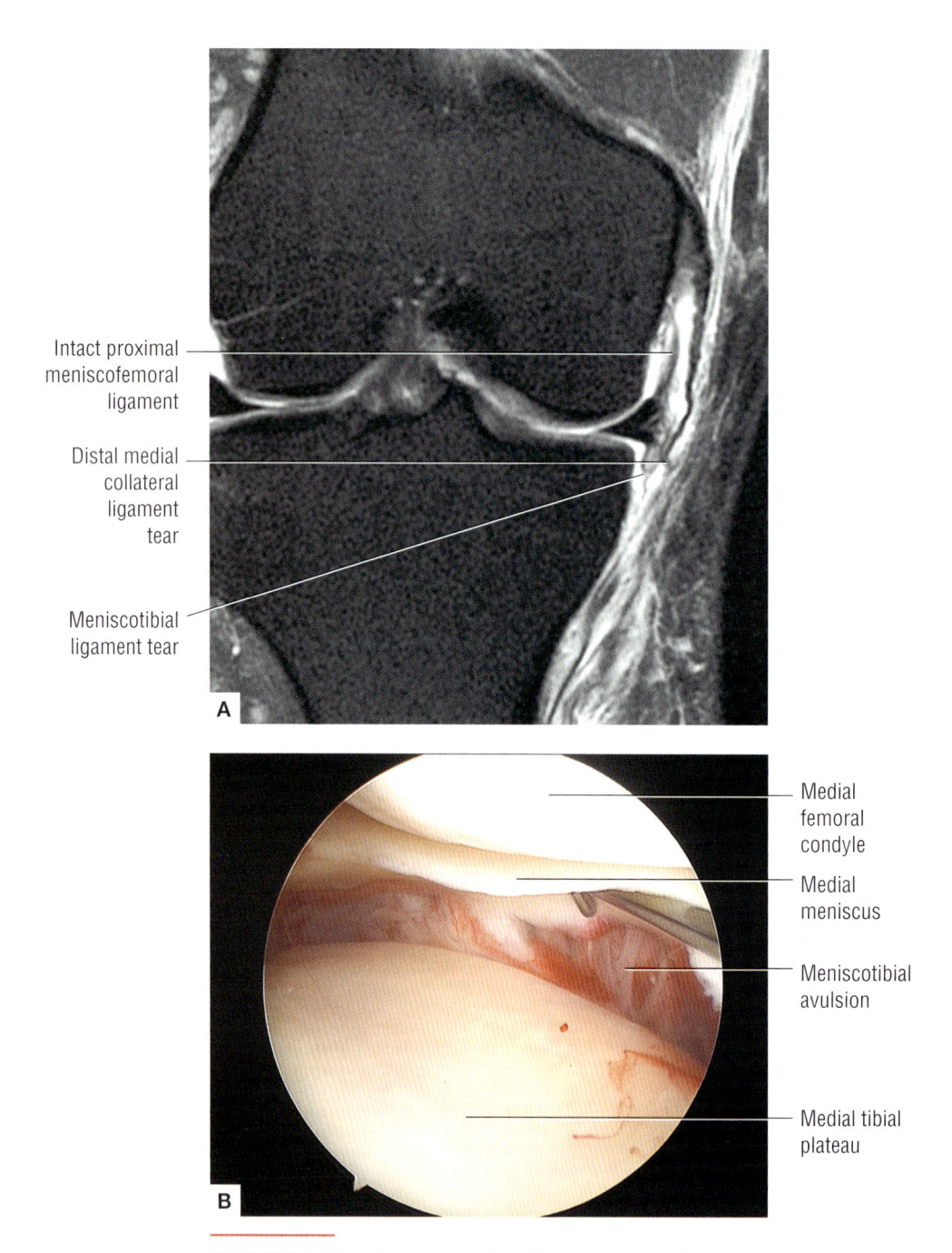

FIGURE 4.219 **(A)** A coronal FS PD FSE image demonstrating distal MCL avulsion associated with avulsion of the meniscotibial ligament. **(B)** Corresponding arthroscopic view shows a meniscotibial tear of the deep capsular layer of the MCL located between the elevated medial meniscus and medial tibial plateau.

Meniscal Cysts

- Meniscal Cysts
    - Meniscal cysts are related to either microscopic or macroscopic tears in meniscal fibrocartilage.
    - Horizontal cleavage tears or complex meniscal tears with a horizontal component are associated with the development of meniscal cysts.
    - Loculations, septations, and dissection of the cyst from the site of origin are common findings.
- Meniscal cysts (also referred to as ganglion cysts, a nonspecific and less descriptive term) have been reported in 1% of meniscectomies.[88,393]
- Meniscal cysts are classified into three types:
    - Intrameniscal cysts
        - Uncommon and represent intrameniscal fluid collections in continuity with meniscal tears.
    - Synovial cysts
        - Rare and are not associated with meniscal tears.
        - Represent cystic outpouching of the joint capsule.[88]
    - Parameniscal cysts
        - More common and most frequently present as loculated or simple fluid collections located at the periphery of the meniscus, often with a horizontal cleavage tear pattern on cross-section.
        - Usually present at the level of the joint line, either as a focal mass or a swelling.
        - May develop in response to trauma or degeneration and are associated with meniscectomy.[51,154]
- One theory holds that injuries or trauma generate tangential or compressive forces that initiate necrosis in the central peripheral aspect of the meniscus, leading to mucoid degeneration and cyst development.

- Lateral parameniscal cysts are three to seven times more common than medial cysts, and they often present at the medial third of the peripheral margin of the meniscus.

- The difference in the prevalence of lateral and medial meniscal cysts may be exaggerated because of underreporting of medial cysts.

- Diagnostic use of MR for meniscal lesions should provide more accurate statistics about these cysts.[58]

- Medial meniscal cysts may dissect through soft tissue (i.e., joint capsule and MCL) and often present in a different location than the meniscus tear origin.
    - Location common deep to the MCL or in the posteromedial corner, deep to the posterior oblique ligament

- The medial meniscus may appear intact in the presence of an associated external cyst if there is peripheral propagation of mucoid degeneration.

- Pericruciate meniscal cysts may arise from tears of the posterior horn of the medial meniscus.
    - May be mistaken for a posterior cruciate ganglion cyst[278]

- Small meniscal cysts also occur in asymptomatic knees.[485]

- Medial meniscal cysts can be visualized extending from the posterior horn and dissecting peripherally to present in a more anterior location.

- A thin stalk in continuity with the meniscus can usually be identified in these cases.

- A horizontal meniscal tear, a flap tear with a primarily horizontal component, or a complex tear frequently communicates with a meniscal cyst with decompression of synovial fluid.

- In 90% of cases, lateral meniscal cysts are also associated with:
    - Horizontal flap tear
    - Horizontal cleavage tear
    - Or a complex tear with horizontal and radial components

- Lateral meniscal cysts are usually located anterior to the LCL or between the LCL and popliteus tendon.

- Discoid lateral menisci are associated with fibrocartilaginous cavitary lesions (prominent grade 2 signal) and parameniscal cyst development.
- Large meniscal cysts usually present as painful, palpable masses near the joint line.
- A palpable mass that disappears with knee flexion is known as *Pisani's sign*.
- Lateral meniscal cysts tend to be larger than medial cysts because the soft tissue constraints are looser than on the medial side.
- Meniscal cysts are uniformly low in signal intensity on T1-weighted images and increase in signal intensity on FS PD-weighted FSE images, T2* GRE images, or STIR images.
- Cysts may contain bloody or gelatinous fluid with an increased protein content.
    - Variation exists in signal-intensity properties on T2-type sequences relative to the appearance and imaging characteristics of free synovial fluid.
- Loculations or septations may be seen in complex meniscal cysts.
    - Usually in those cysts removed in distance from their site of origin (meniscal tear)
- Erosion of the adjacent tibial condyle may occur with large, untreated lateral meniscal cysts.
- The differential diagnosis of parameniscal cysts includes:
    - Osteophytic spurring
    - Synovial cysts
    - Proximal tibiofibular cysts
    - Traumatic bursitis
    - Masses (including pigmented villonodular synovitis, hemangioma, lipoma, and synovial sarcoma)[412]
- Although aggressive malignant lesions such as synovial sarcomas may show hyperintensity on T2-weighted images, they tend to have a lower and more inhomogeneous signal intensity than that of synovial fluid.
- Sometimes synovial sarcomas mimic the appearance of a hemorrhagic or highly proteinaceous fluid collection.

- IV gadolinium contrast peripherally enhances a meniscal cyst in comparison to the more centralized enhancement of a soft tissue neoplasm.

- Treatment for meniscal cysts is arthroscopic resection and repair of the tear.

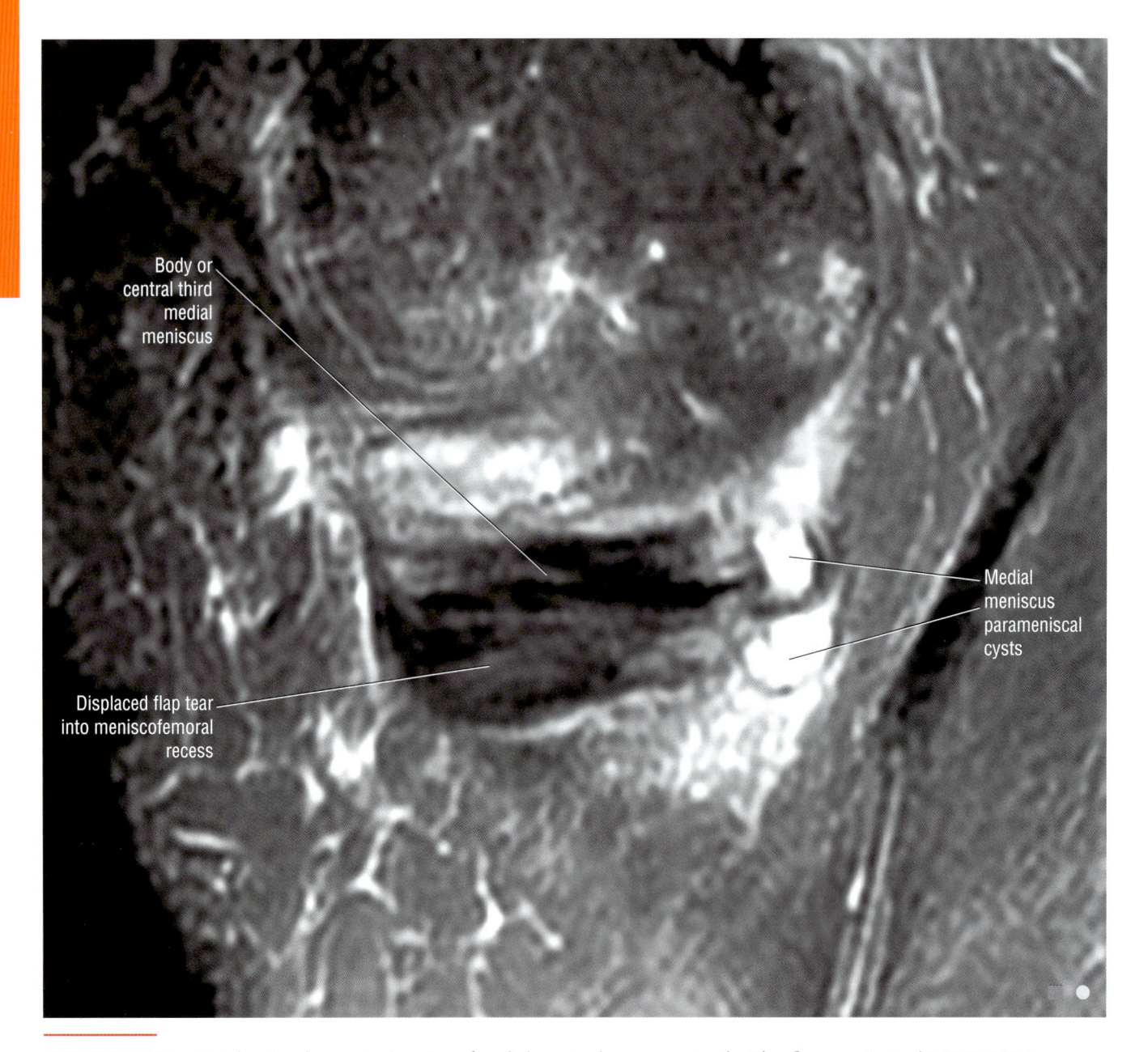

FIGURE 4.220 Peripheral and posterior location of medial meniscal cysts associated with a flap tear. Sagittal FS PD FSE image.

The Meniscus

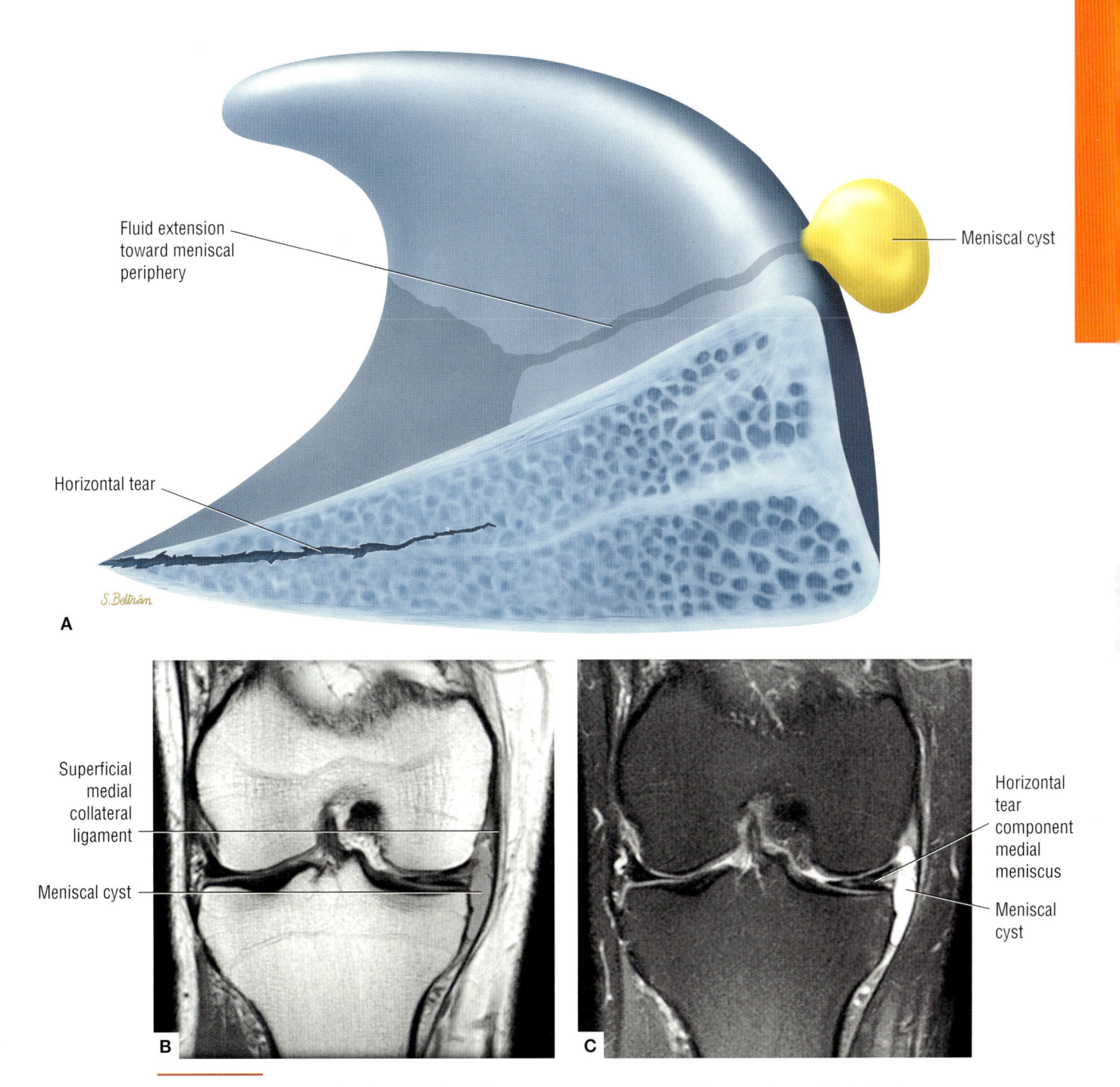

FIGURE 4.221 Peripheral meniscal cyst formation in continuity with horizontal tear. (**A**) Sagittal cross-section with parameniscal cyst in yellow. (**B**) Coronal PD FSE image. (**C**) Coronal FS PD FSE image.

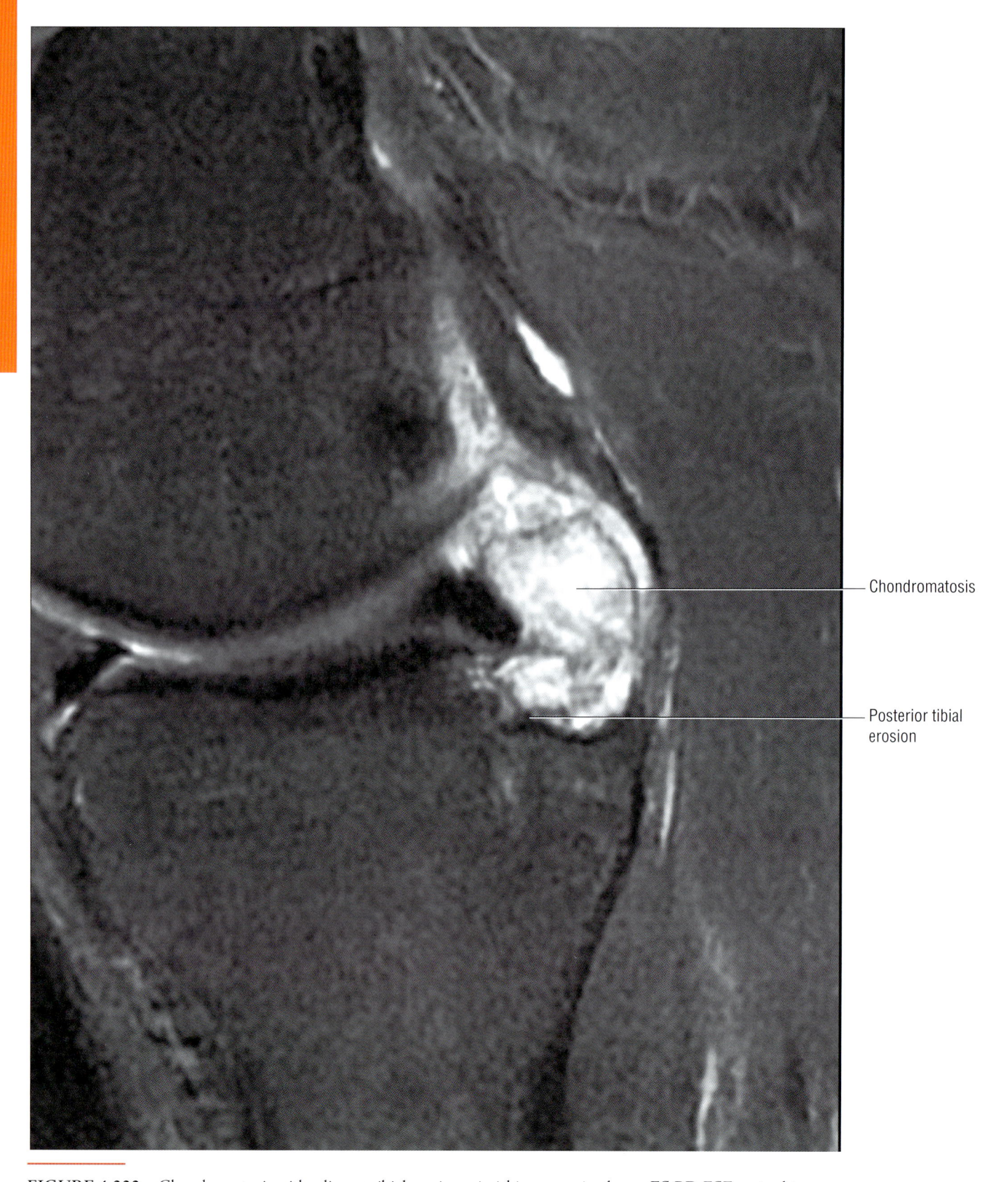

FIGURE 4.222 Chondromatosis with adjacent tibial erosion mimicking a meniscal cyst. FS PD FSE sagittal image.

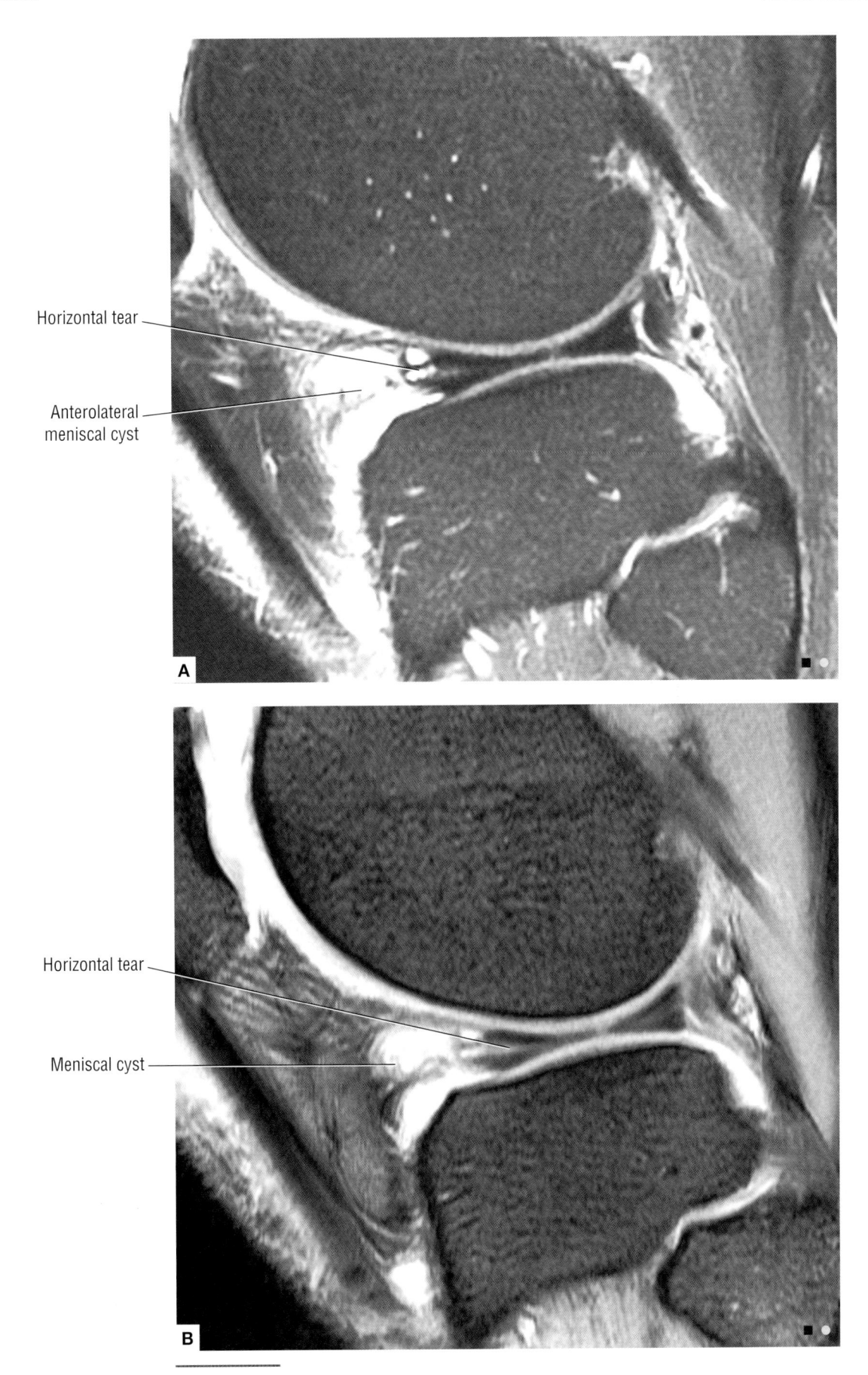

FIGURE 4.223 Anterolateral lateral meniscal cyst associated with a horizontal tear. Intrameniscal signal is more evident on gradient echo image. FS PD FSE (**A**) and gradient echo (**B**) sagittal images.

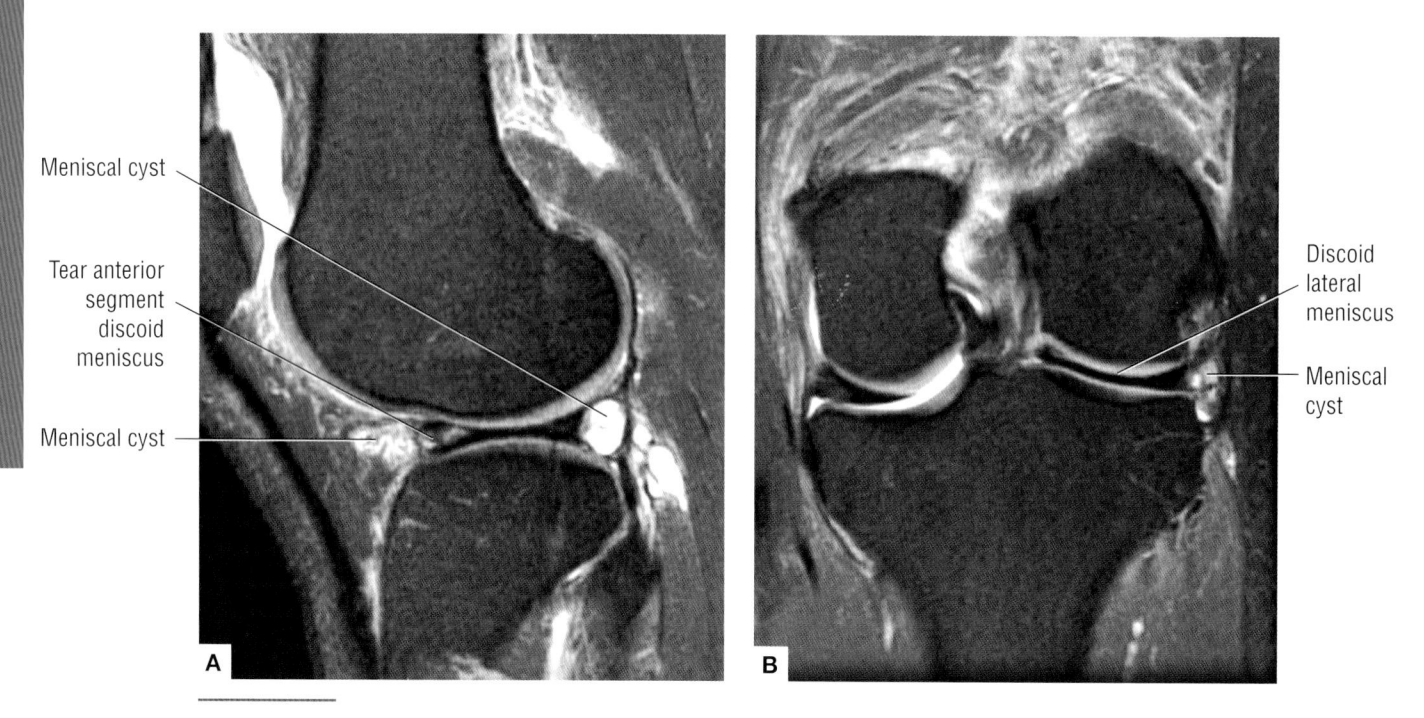

FIGURE 4.224 FS PD FSE sagittal (**A**) and coronal (**B**) images showing a discoid lateral meniscus forming fluid- and synovium-containing parameniscal cyst.

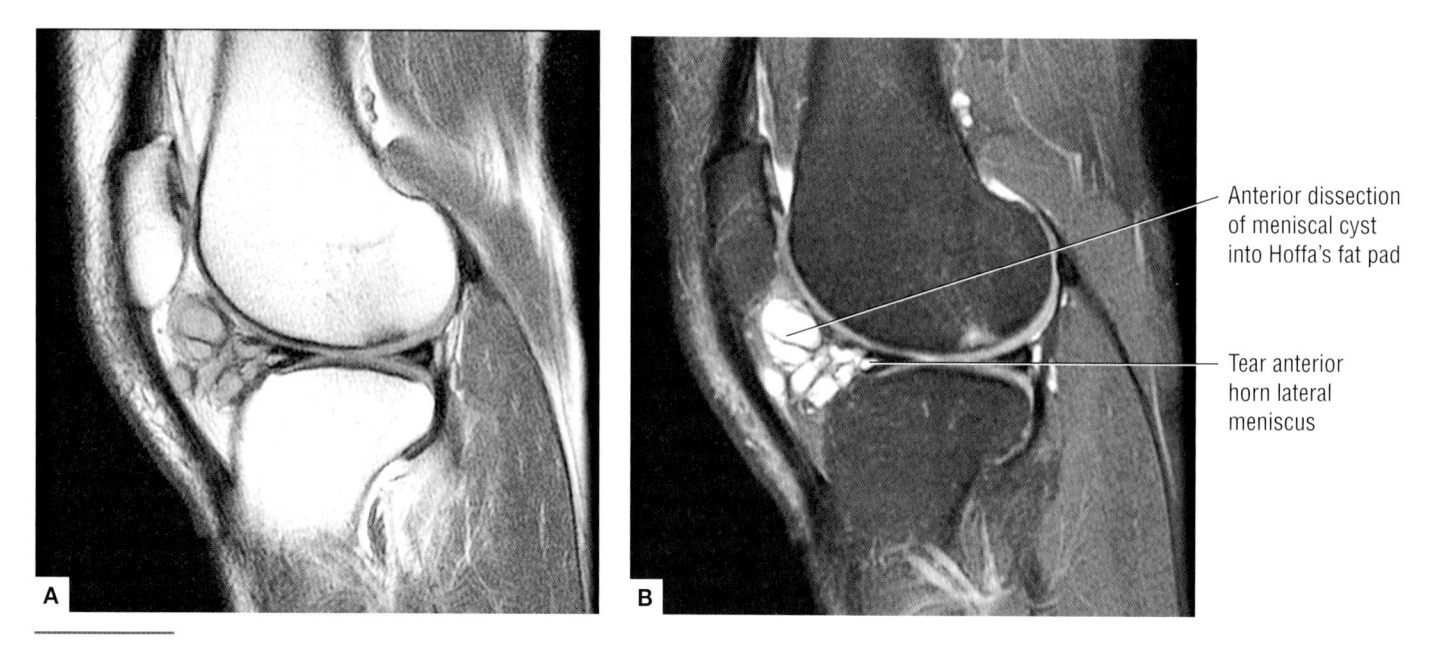

FIGURE 4.225 A large septated and multilobulated lateral parameniscal cyst dissecting freely into Hoffa's fat pad as seen on sagittal PD FSE (**A**), sagittal FS PD FSE (**B**).

The Meniscus 385

Lateral meniscal cyst posterior to Hoffa's fat pad

AHLM intrameniscal cyst

Anterior extension as a parameniscal cyst

Intrameniscal cyst

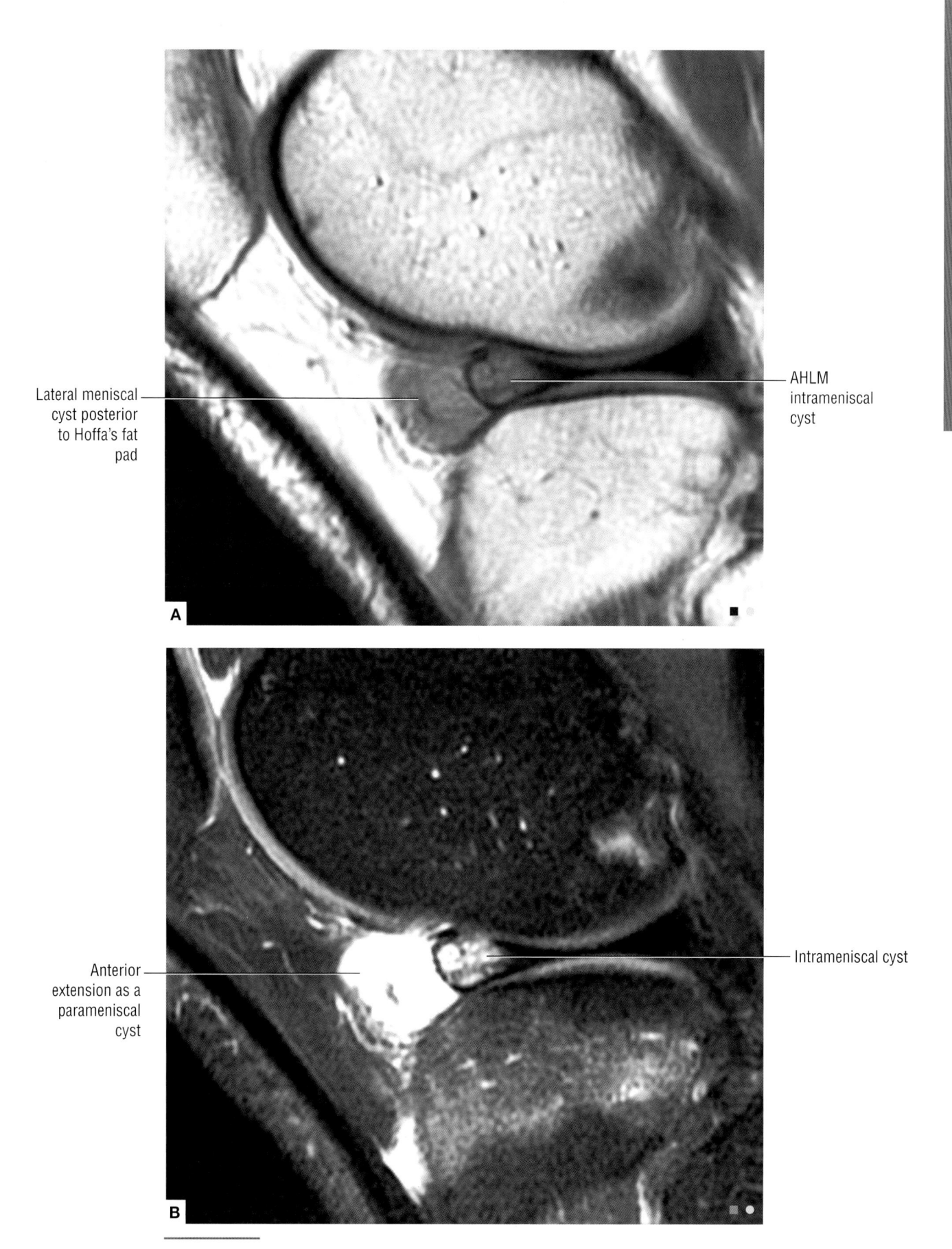

FIGURE 4.226 Intrameniscal and parameniscal cysts communicating with the anterior horn of the lateral meniscus. PD FSE (**A**) and FS PD FSE (**B**) sagittal images.

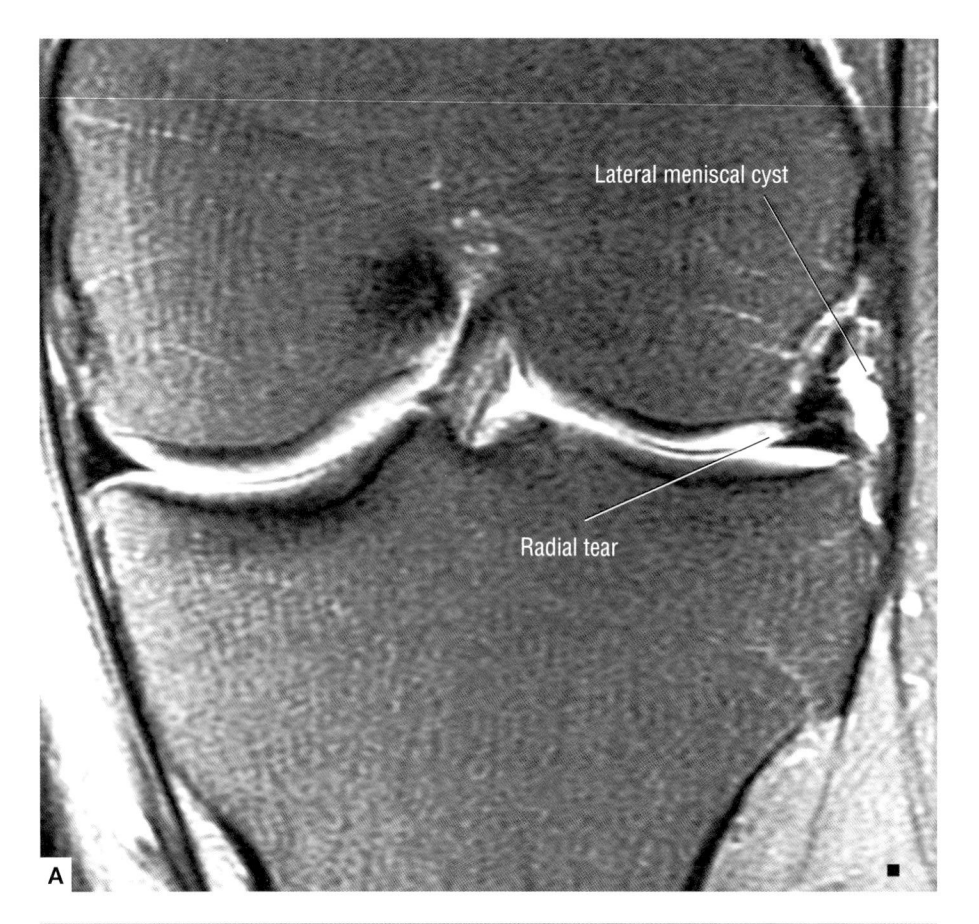

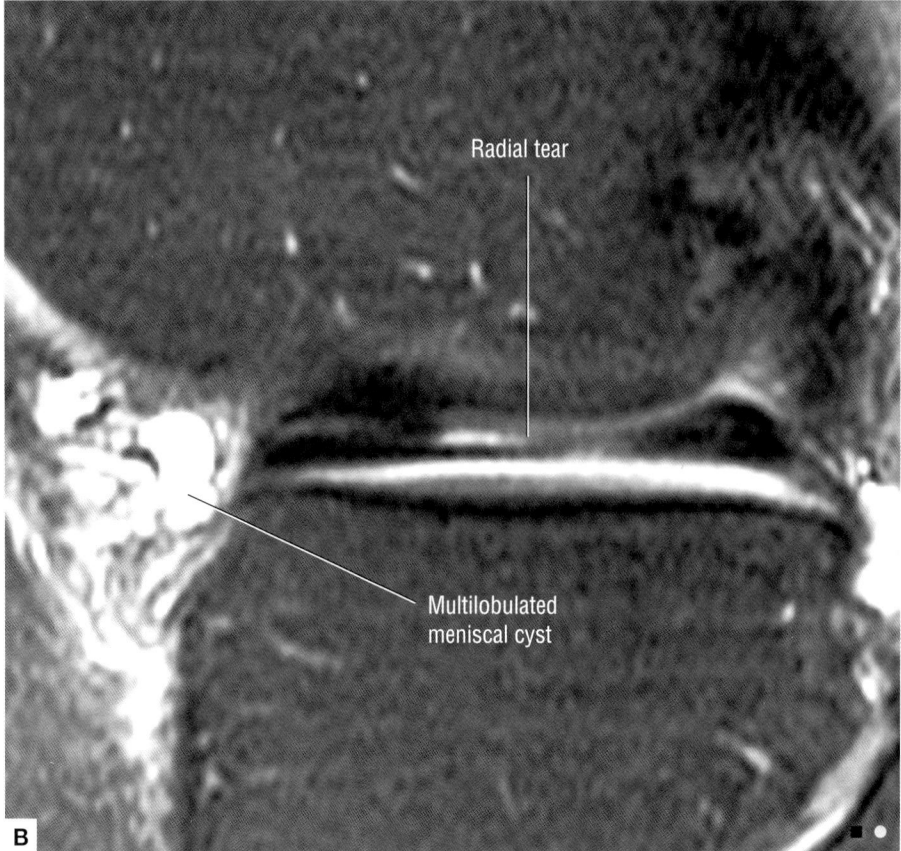

FIGURE 4.227 Lateral meniscal cyst (anterior lateral extension) with radial tear of the body of the lateral meniscus. FS PD FSE coronal (**A**) and sagittal (**B**) images.

The Meniscus 387

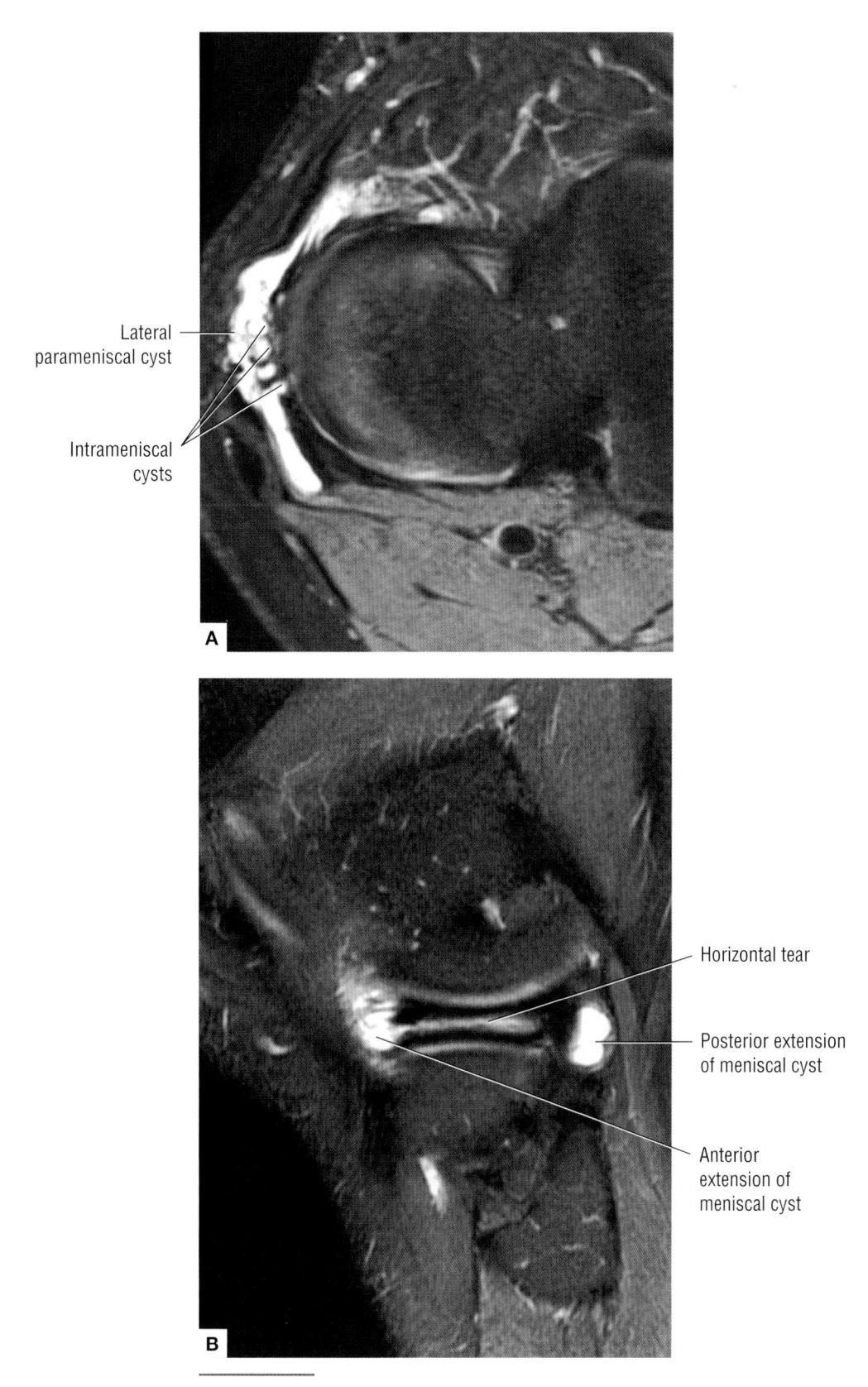

FIGURE 4.228 Lateral meniscus horizontal tear decompressing fluid into a series of intrameniscal cysts communicating with a larger peripheral parameniscal cyst. Anterior-to-posterior extension of the parameniscal cyst is shown on axial (**A**) and sagittal (**B**) FS PD FSE images.

Calcium Pyrophosphate Dihydrate Deposition Disease

- Calcium Pyrophosphate Dihydrate Deposition Disease
    - T2* GRE images are recommended for detection of punctate hypointense calcium pyrophosphate dihydrate crystal depositions.
    - High-contrast settings help identify meniscal tissue involvement.
    - Meniscal degeneration and tears may be underestimated secondary to localized susceptibility effects induced by crystal deposition, especially on T2* GRE images.

- In calcium pyrophosphate dihydrate deposition disease (CPDD), there is deposition of calcium pyrophosphate crystals in hyaline cartilage, synovial tissue, capsule, and/or meniscus. CPDD presents with the clinically separate yet related syndromes of:
    - Pseudogout, in which there is no urate, as is found in true gout
    - Tophaceous pseudogout, which produces pseudotumors
    - Familial CPDD, which is rare in the knee and presents at an earlier age
    - Pyrophosphate arthropathy, both osteoarthritic and neuropathic forms
    - Chondrocalcinosis, which is asymptomatic

- In chondrocalcinosis, meniscal calcifications are usually identified with conventional radiographic techniques.

- In patients with CPDD, MR studies using high-contrast settings for photography reveal focal, low-signal-intensity calcifications separate from adjacent low-signal-intensity meniscus.

- On T2*-weighted images, local susceptibility artifacts are seen around the foci of calcium pyrophosphate deposition, making them easier to identify.

- Crystals resulting from CPDD in either the meniscus or articular cartilage may dampen the signal intensity for meniscal degenerations and tears.
  - This may falsely produce grade 2 signal intensity in cases in which there is grade 3 signal intensity on corresponding T1- or PD-weighted images.
- Chondrocalcinosis, therefore, is more difficult to identify on non-GRE sequences.
- Increased signal intensity directly attributed to the effect of chondrocalcinosis may also decrease MR accuracy by producing false-positive tears on GRE sequences.[239]
- Dicalcium phosphate dihydrate, hydroxyapatite, and calcium oxalate are also responsible for cartilaginous calcifications.[69]
- A *meniscal ossicle* is larger and occurs as an isolated focus in asymptomatic patients without a history of antecedent trauma.[15]
- On MR, the marrow-containing corticated ossicle can be seen within the posterior horn of the medial meniscus.

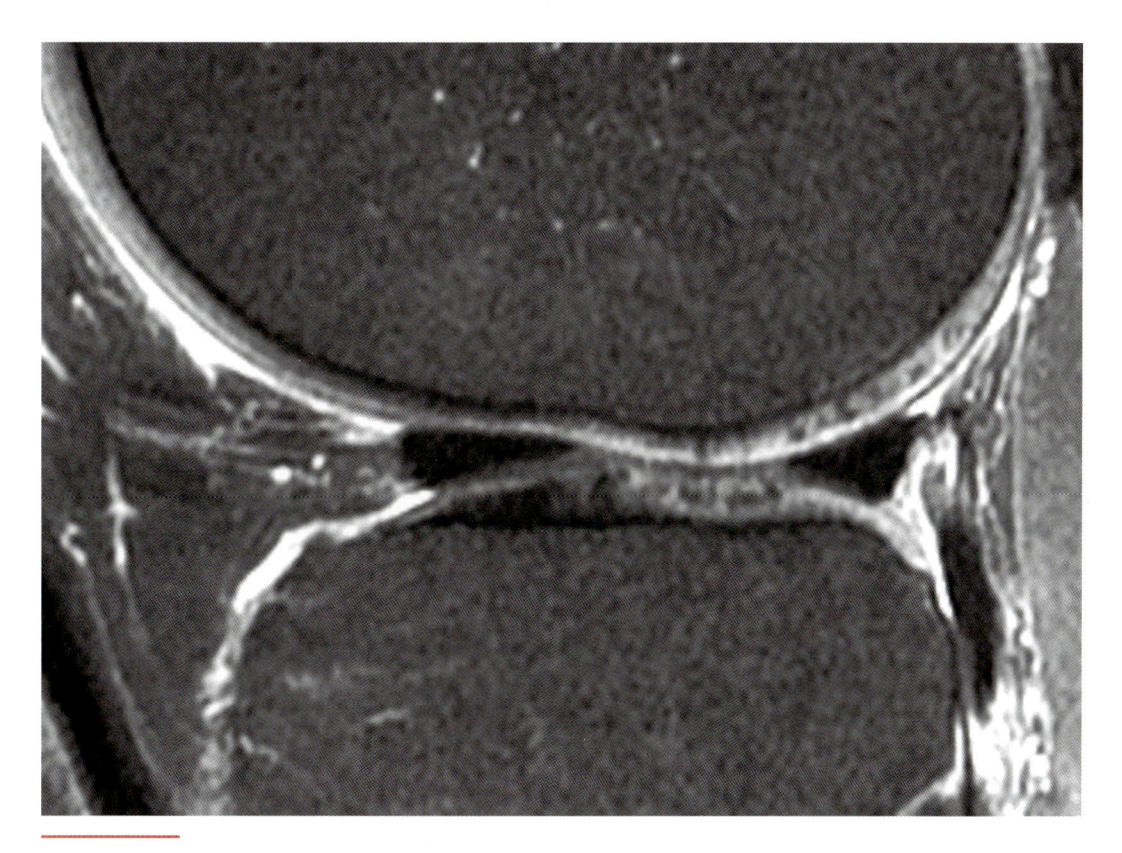

FIGURE 4.229 Chondrocalcinosis detected as punctate hypointense foci on sagittal FS PD FSE image.

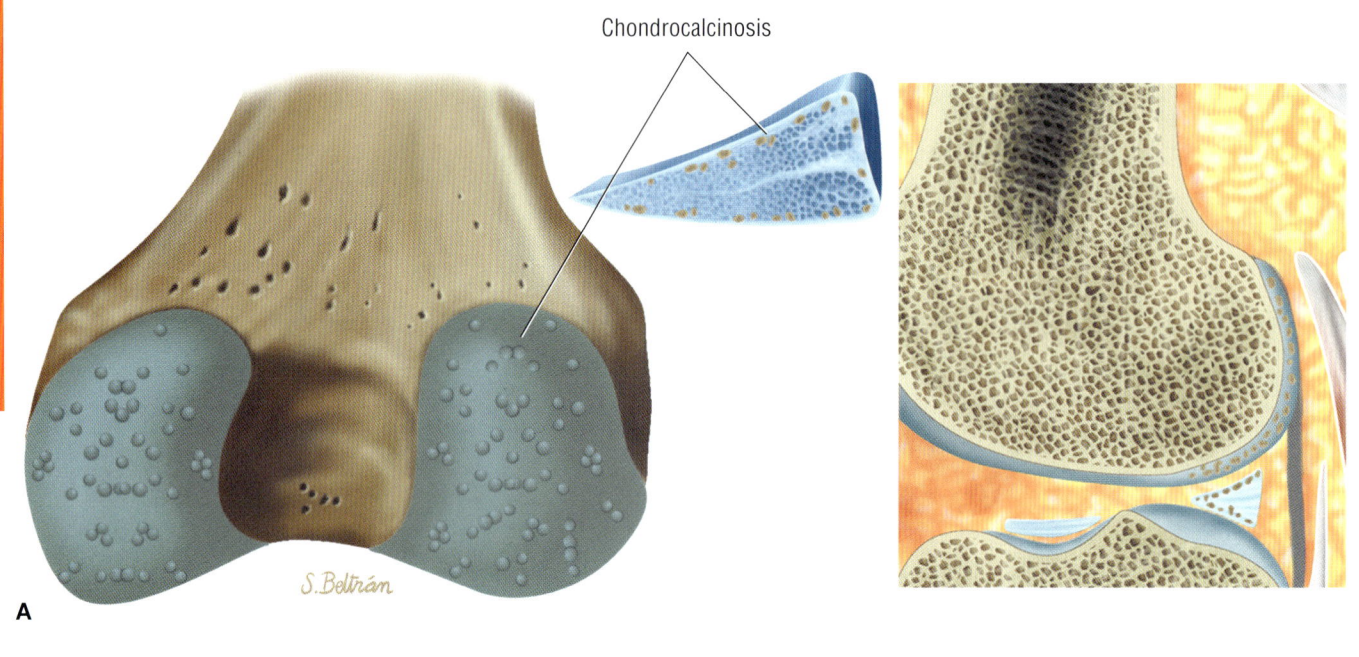

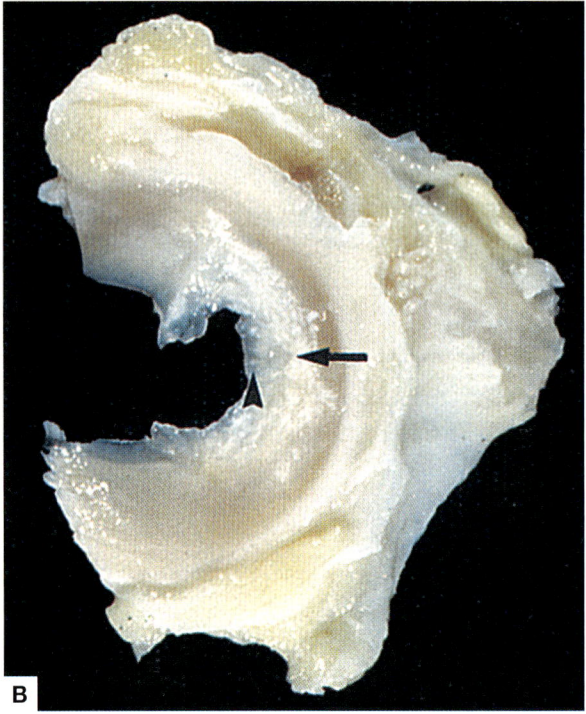

FIGURE 4.230 Chondrocalcinosis affecting both the articular cartilage and meniscus. (**A**) Posterior coronal and sagittal (lateral) cross-section illustration. (**B**) On a gross meniscal specimen, deposition resulting from chondrocalcinosis is seen in the lateral meniscus (*arrow*). Degenerative free edge of the meniscus is shown (*arrowhead*).

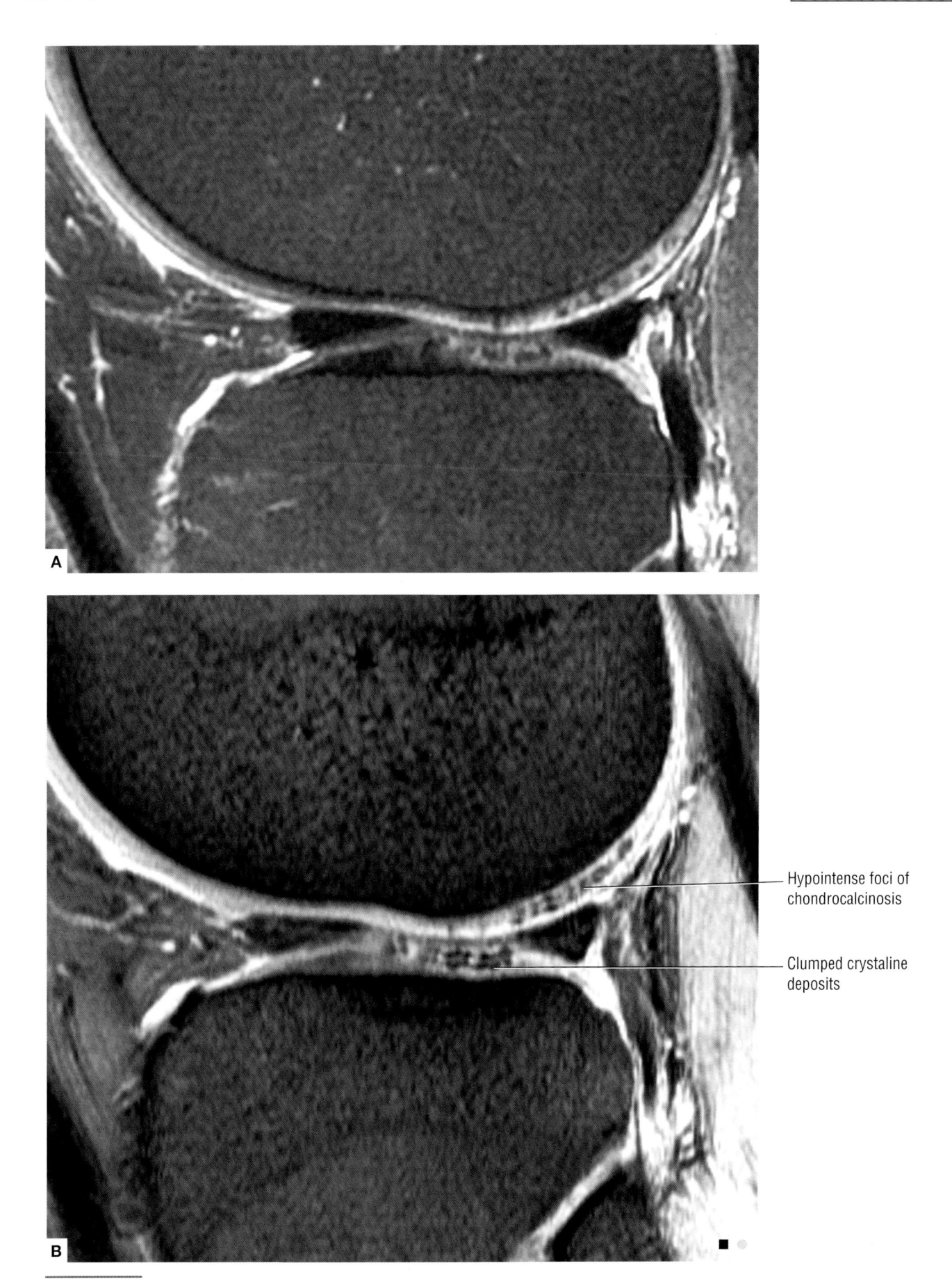

FIGURE 4.231 Improved conspicuity of hypointense foci of chondrocalcinosis comparing FS PD (**A**) and gradient echo (**B**) sagittal images.

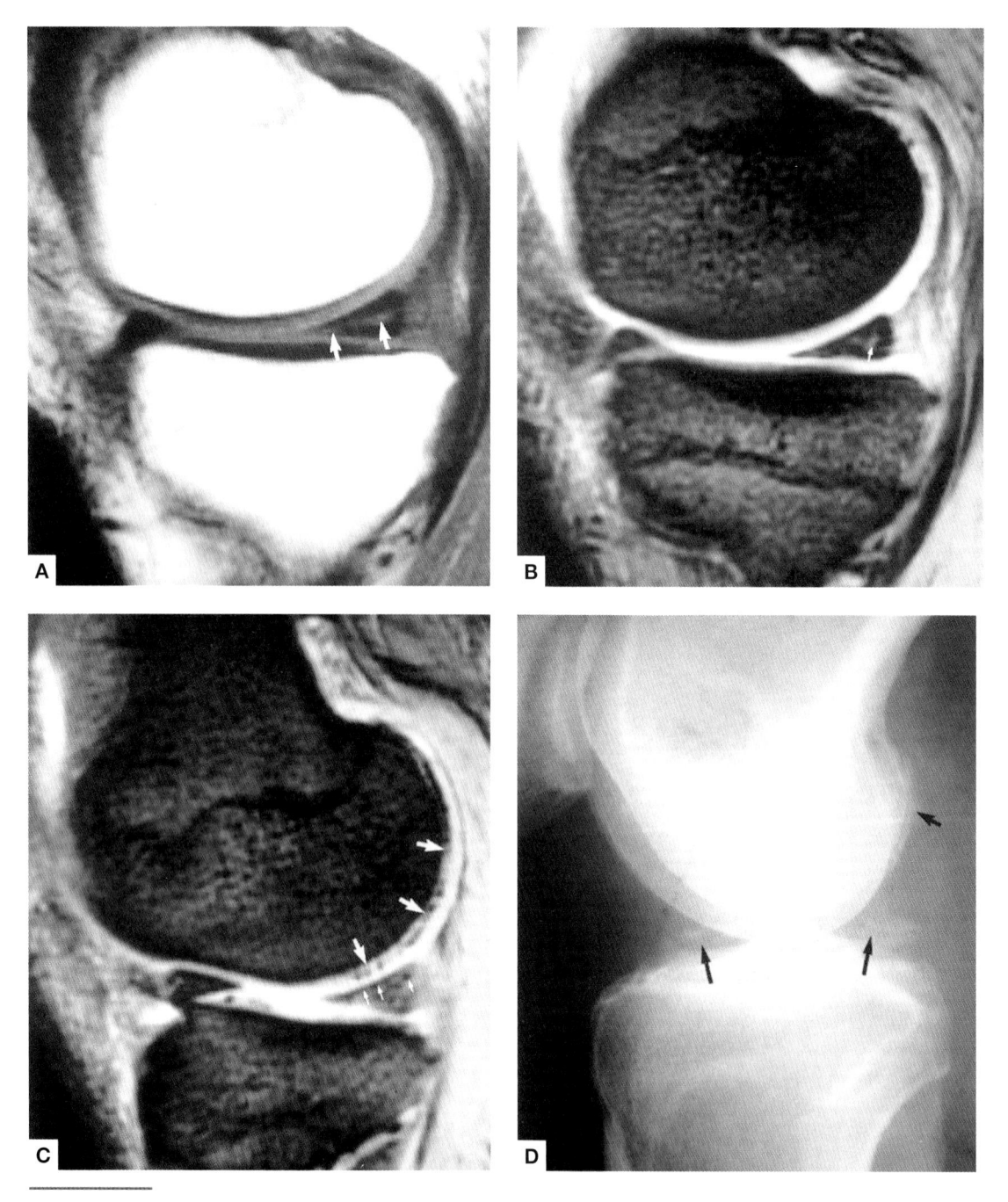

FIGURE 4.232 Chondrocalcinosis. **(A)** On a T1-weighted sagittal image, the posterior horn of the medial meniscus shows grade 3 signal intensity (*arrows*). **(B)** On the corresponding T2*-weighted sagittal image, chondrocalcinosis dampens the meniscal signal intensity (*arrow*) as a result of localized magnetic susceptibilities. **(C)** On a T2*-weighted sagittal image through the lateral compartment, multiple foci of deposition resulting from calcium pyrophosphate disease are evident within the articular cartilage (*large arrows*) and the meniscus (*small arrows*). **(D)** On the corresponding lateral radiograph, chondrocalcinosis is evident in a region of meniscal fibrocartilage (*large arrows*) and articular cartilage (*small arrow*).

The Meniscus 393

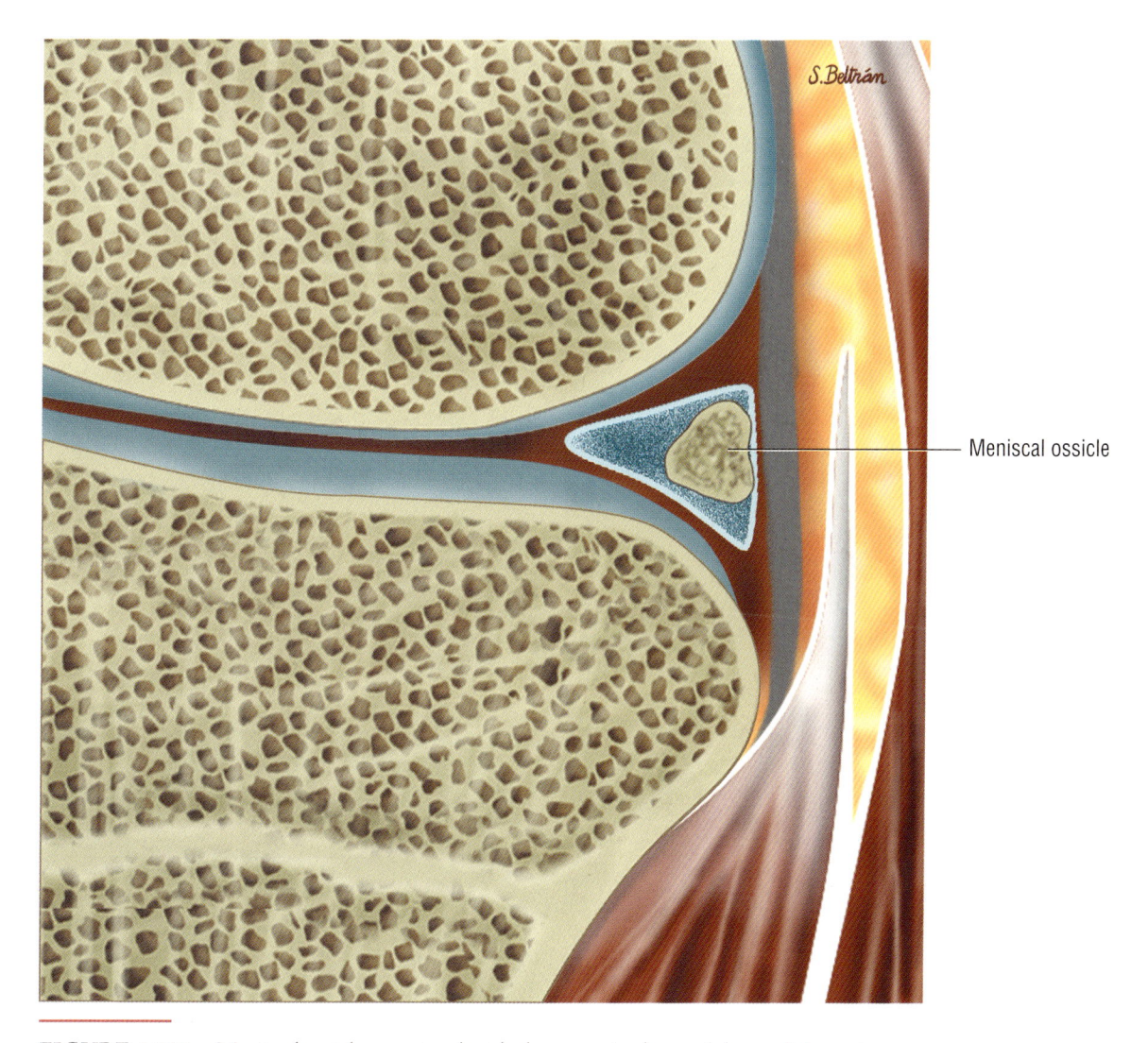

FIGURE 4.233 Meniscal ossicle associated with the posterior horn of the medial meniscus.

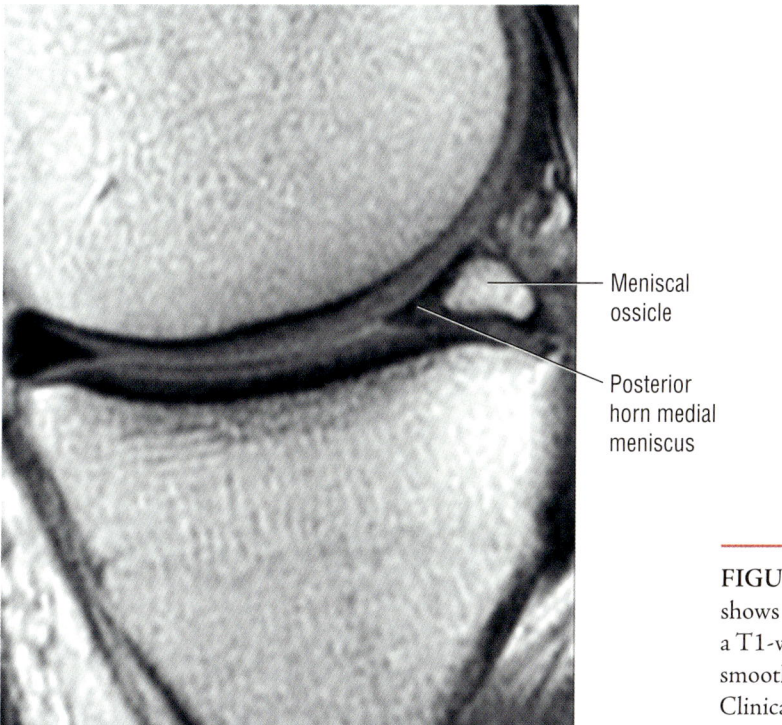

FIGURE 4.234 The meniscal ossicle shows bright marrow-fat signal intensity on a T1-weighted sagittal image. The ossicle has smooth margins and there is no donor site. Clinical presentation may present with intermittent pain without joint locking.

5 Cruciate Ligaments

Anterior Cruciate Ligament (ACL) (pages 397–414)

Mechanism of Injury (pages 415–435)

Magnetic Resonance Imaging (pages 436–438)

ACL Tears (pages 439–464)

ACL-Associated Posterolateral Corner and Osseous Injuries (pages 465–469)

Osseous Injuries (pages 470–486)

Treatment of ACL Injuries (pages 487–488)

ACL Reconstruction (pages 489–498)

MR Evaluation of ACL Reconstruction (pages 499–539)

Posterior Cruciate Ligament (PCL) (pages 540–577)

Cruciate Ligaments

Anterior Cruciate Ligament (ACL)

Key Concepts

- Two-bundle ligament with a small anteromedial and large posterolateral bundle
    - Nonisometric structure
- Primary restraint to anterior tibial displacement
    - Posterolateral bundle provides principal resistance to hyperextension forces.
    - Functional ACL fiber recruitment is more complicated than assignment to one of the two fiber bundles.
        - Both bundles nonisometric during flexion and extension

Functional Anatomy

- Intracapsular and extrasynovial
    - Enveloped by a fold of synovium originating from the posterior intercondylar area of the knee[225]
- ACL fiber attachment areas on the femur and tibia fan out at 3.5 times the size of the mid-substance of ACL.
- Proximal attachment to a fossa on the posteromedial aspect of the lateral femoral condyle[116,472]
    - 16 to 24mm in diameter at its origin[116]
        - Proximal-distal diameter 13.9mm = 9.5mm
        - Anterior-posterior diameter 9.3mm = 7.1mm[40]
    - Center of origin is 15mm from junction of posterior femoral shaft and proximal aspect of lateral femoral condyle (over-the-top position).
    - Over-the-top position is critical landmark in placement of femoral tunnel when reconstructing the ACL.

- In extension:
    - Anteromedial (AM) bundle located most anterior and proximal aspect of femoral insertion site
    - Posterolateral (PL) bundle originates at posterodistal area of femoral attachment.[40]
- 11mm wide and 31 to 38mm long[30]
    - Cross-sectional area increases from the femur to the tibia and changes with flexion and extension.
- Distal attachment to a fossa anterior and lateral to the anterior tibial spine, between the anterior attachments of the menisci
    - ACL reaches maximum diameter as it inserts on the tibia.
    - Tibial attachment anterior and lateral to medial intercondylar tubercle (eminence)
    - Tibial footprint[40]
        - AM bundle (AMB) inserts anteromedially.
        - PL bundle (PLB) inserts posterolaterally.
        - Tibial footprint has greater attachment area variation compared to the more consistent individual attachment areas of the femoral footprint.
    - Extends inferior and medial to the anterior tibial intercondylar area
    - Broader or larger than femoral attachment and passes deep to transverse ligament of the knee[116]
- Ligamentous branches of middle geniculate artery form vascular plexus that supplies both ACL and posterior cruciate ligament (PCL).
- Individual fascicles of ACL divided into AM and PL bundles[116,131,243]
    - AM and PL are distinct functional and anatomic fiber bundles.
    - Longer and stronger AM tightens with knee flexion.[525]
    - Smaller and shorter PL tightens with knee extension.[525]
    - In extension, as PLB becomes tight, the AMB becomes moderately loose.[40]
        - AMB and PLB are parallel to each other in extension.

Cruciate Ligaments

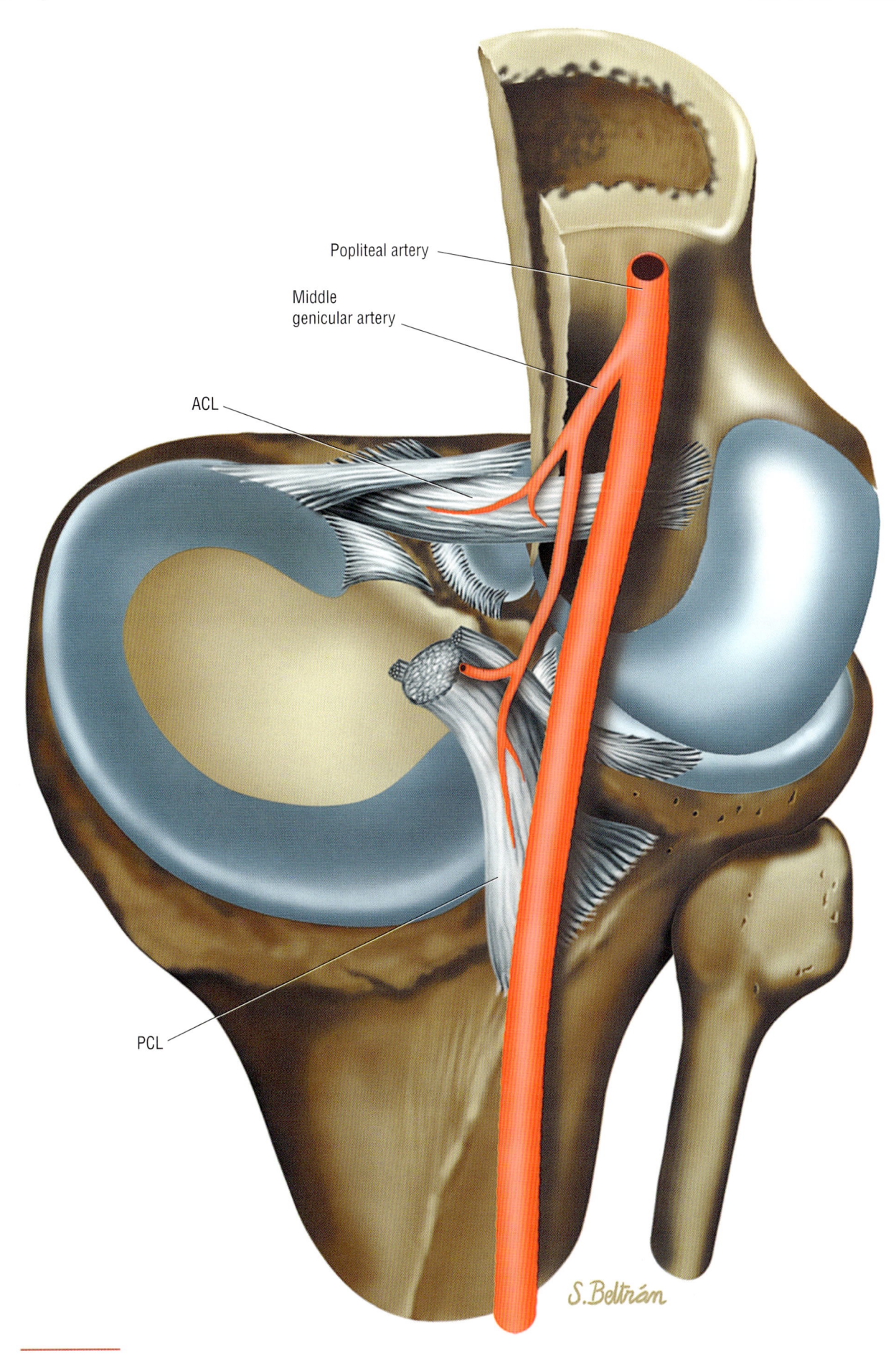

FIGURE 5.1 The vascular supply to the cruciate ligaments via the middle geniculate (genicular) arterial branch of the anterior popliteal artery. There is no blood supply derived from the ACL ligament to the bone insertion site.

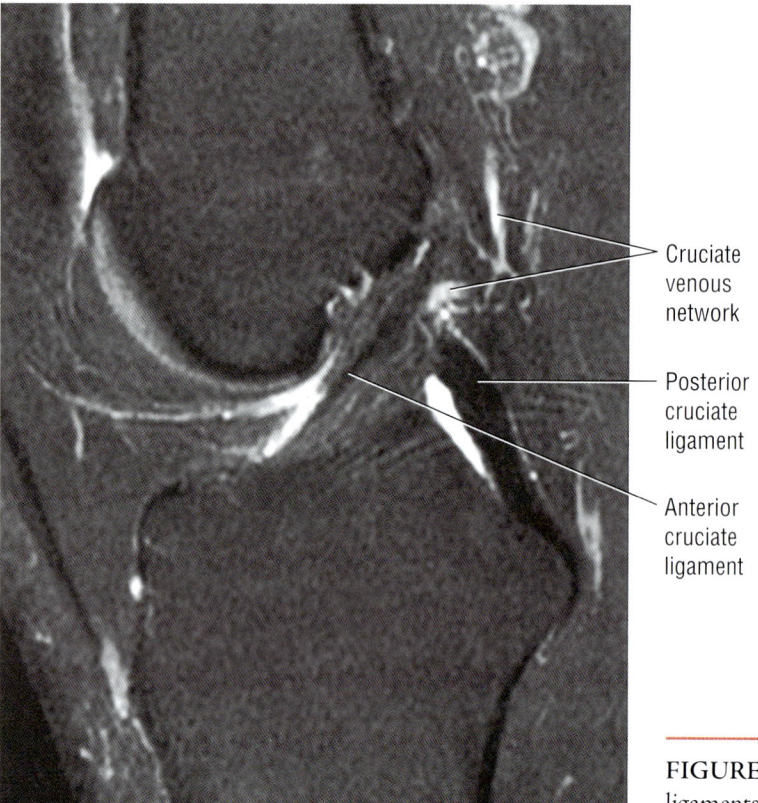

FIGURE 5.2 Return venous network for the cruciate ligaments corresponding to the ligamentous arterial anastomosis (sagittal FS PD FSE image).

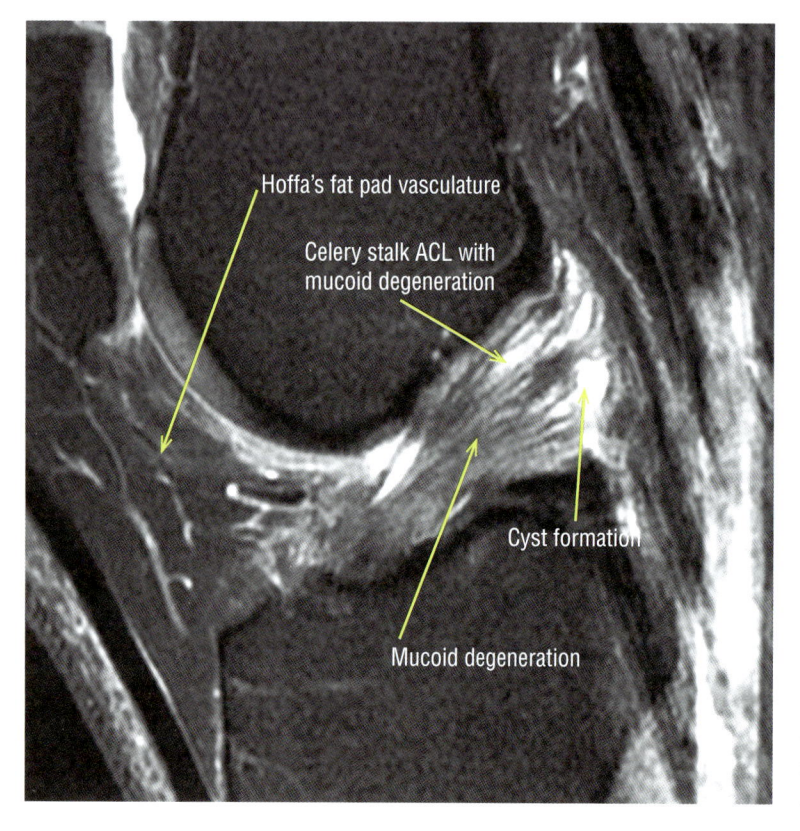

FIGURE 5.3 The middle genicular artery enters the posterior knee joint through the distal capsule through the dorsal capsule. The vascular density of the ACL decreases from proximal to distal ligament. Secondarily, small arteries from Hoffa's fat pad penetrate the ligamentum mucosum. The distal ACL receives blood supply from infrapatellar branches of the inferior genicular arteries. FS PD FSE sagittal image.

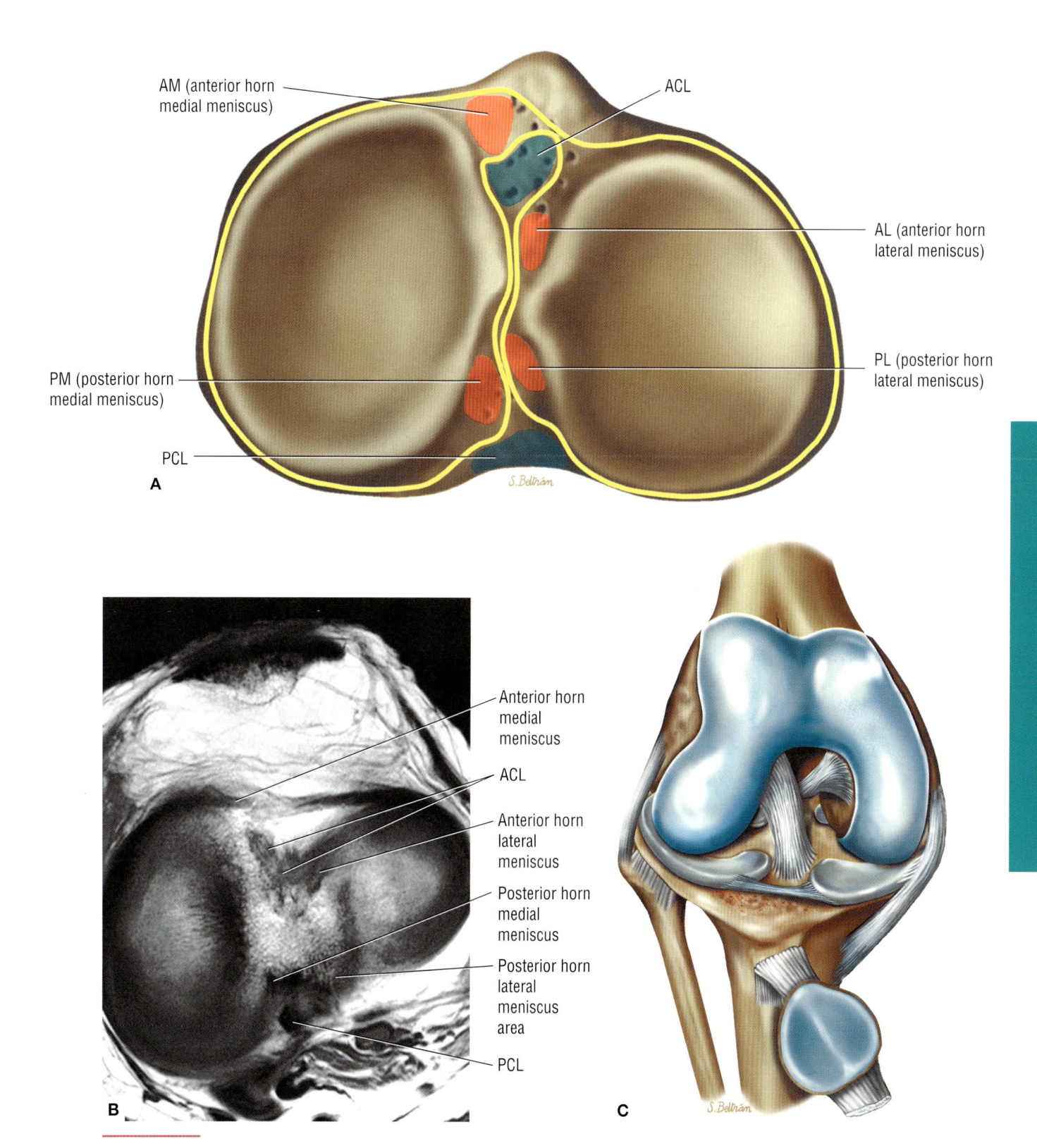

FIGURE 5.4 **(A)** Tibial insertion sites for the anterior cruciate ligament (ACL) and posterior cruciate ligament (PCL). Insertions are also indicated for the meniscal fibrocartilage. The ACL inserts between the anterior attachments of the menisci. The PCL attaches to the posterior intercondylar area and posterior tibial surface. **(B)** Corresponding axial MR image demonstrating hypointense cruciate ligament insertions. **(C)** Anterior tibial insertion sites of the ACL and menisci on anterior coronal perspective.

- In flexion, femoral attachment of ACL assumes more horizontal orientation, resulting in AM tightening and PLB loosening.[116]
    - AMB lengthens and becomes tight in flexion.
    - PLB slackens toward flexion.[40]
- In flexion, AM fibers twist or spiral over the PL fibers.[404]
    - Parallel fiber orientation is lost.
    - Femoral insertion becomes more horizontal.
    - AM wraps around the PLB.
    - With extreme flexion beyond 90 degrees, the PLB will then retighten toward full flexion.[40]
- Continuum of dynamics between AM and PL results in some portion of ACL being taut in both flexion and extension.[116]
    - Nonisometric two-bundle model

- ACL prevents anterior translation of the tibia and resists posterior translation of the femur.
- Both ACL and PCL regulate screw-home mechanism of the knee.[148]
- Highest loads in ACL occur with extension.
    - Anterior tibial loading near extension
    - Thus necessity of having a stronger PLB[40]

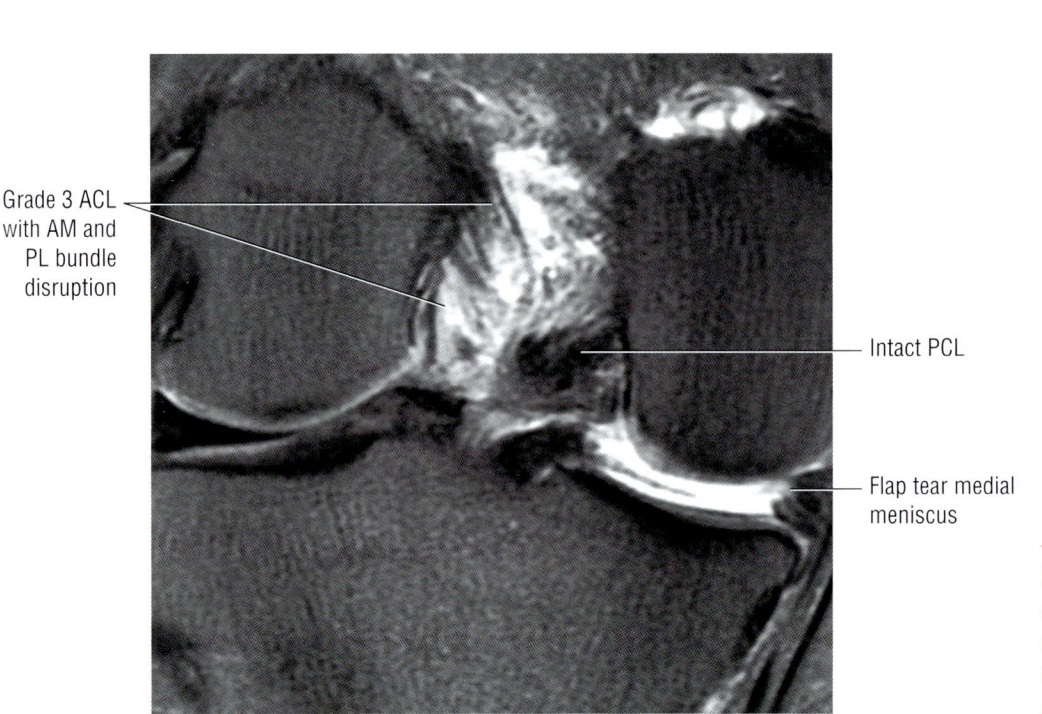

FIGURE 5.5 Intact PCL in a knee demonstrating disruption of ACL and medial meniscus. Coronal FS PD FSE image.

Grade 3 ACL with AM and PL bundle disruption

Intact PCL

Flap tear medial meniscus

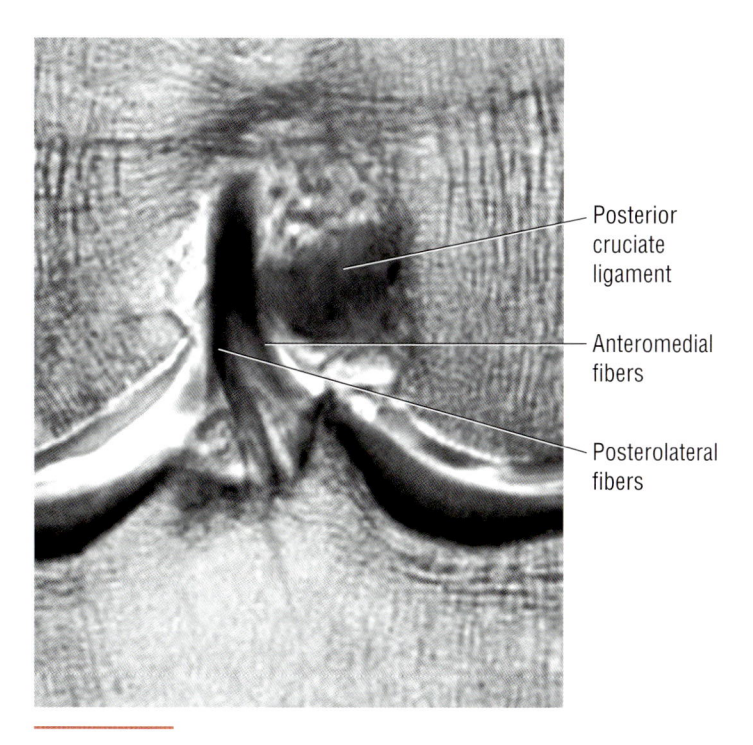

FIGURE 5.6 Coronal MR image demonstrating separate anteromedial and posterolateral fibers of the distal ACL in extension.

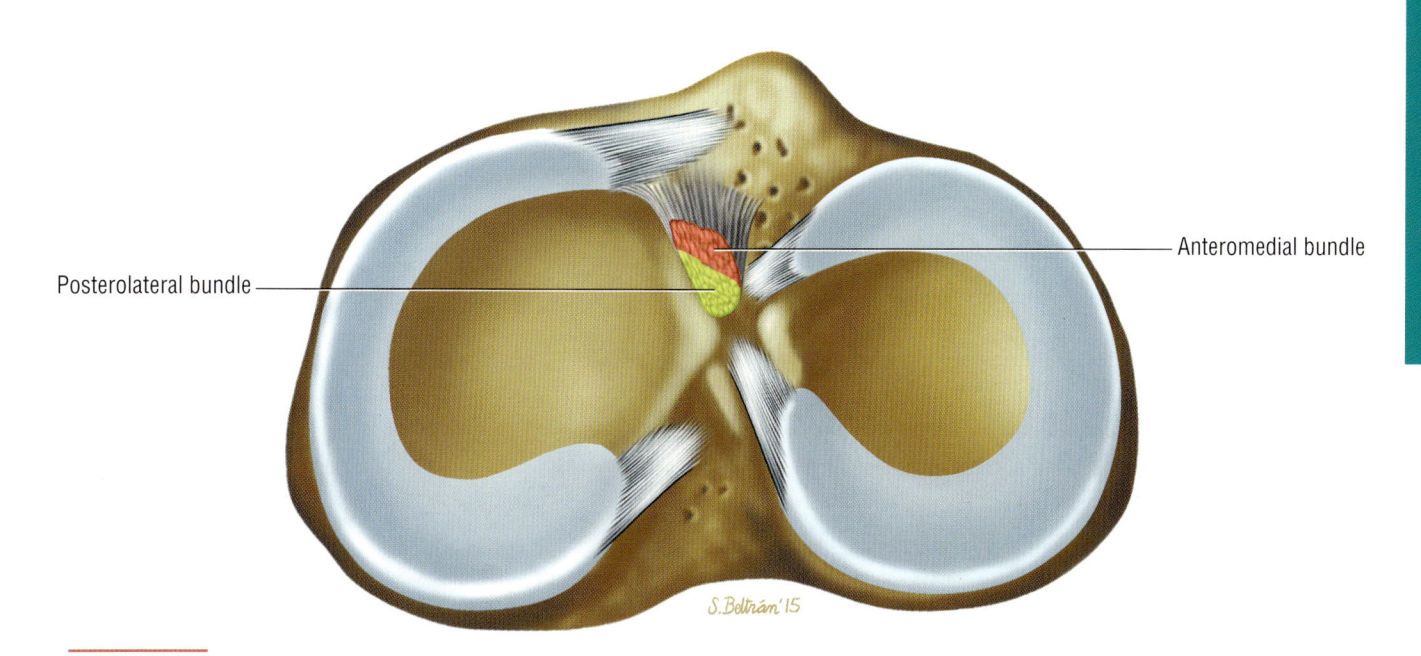

FIGURE 5.7 Tibial footprint of the anteromedial (AM) and posterolateral (PL) bundles of the ACL. The location of the AM and PL bundle attachment areas may show relative variation compared to the consistent femoral footprint of the proximal fibers.

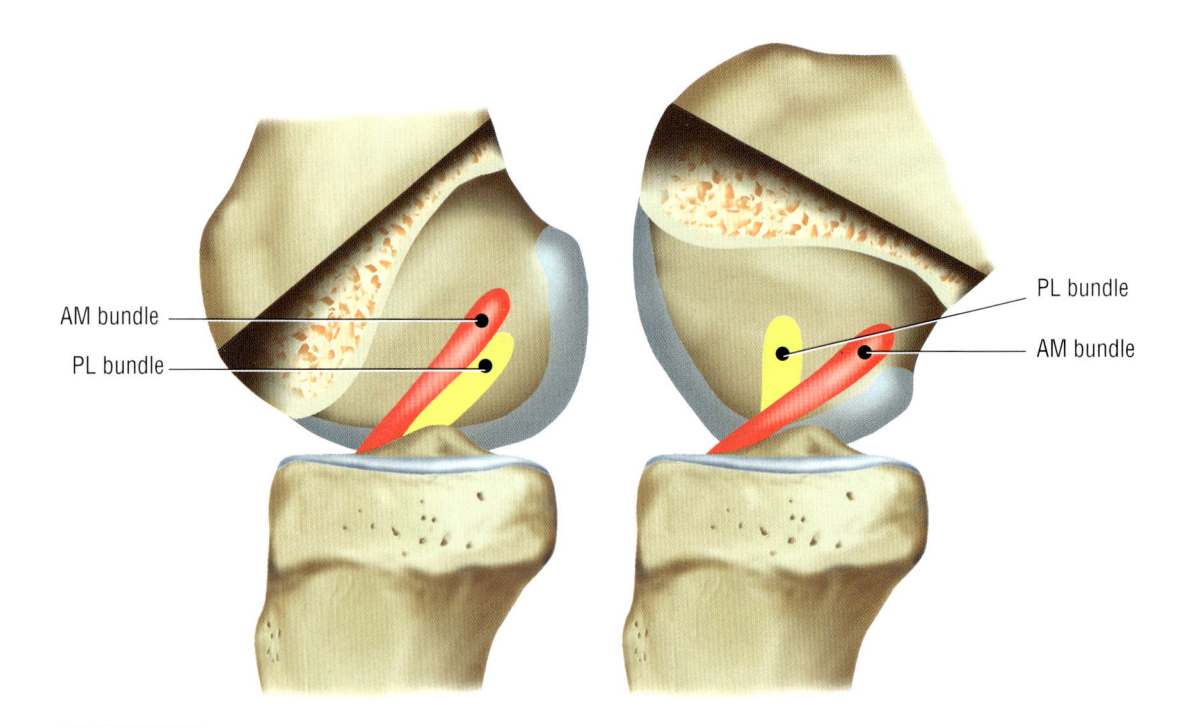

FIGURE 5.8 The anteromedial and posterolateral bundles are nonisometric in flexion-extension motion. The two bundles are parallel in knee extension with the PL bundle tight and the AM bundle moderately lax. The AM bundle becomes tight in flexion, and the PL bundle becomes more lax. With progressive flexion, the femoral insertion of the ACL becomes more horizontal, and the proximal AM bundle fibers are located posterior to the proximal PL bundle as the AM bundle wraps around the PL bundle.[40]

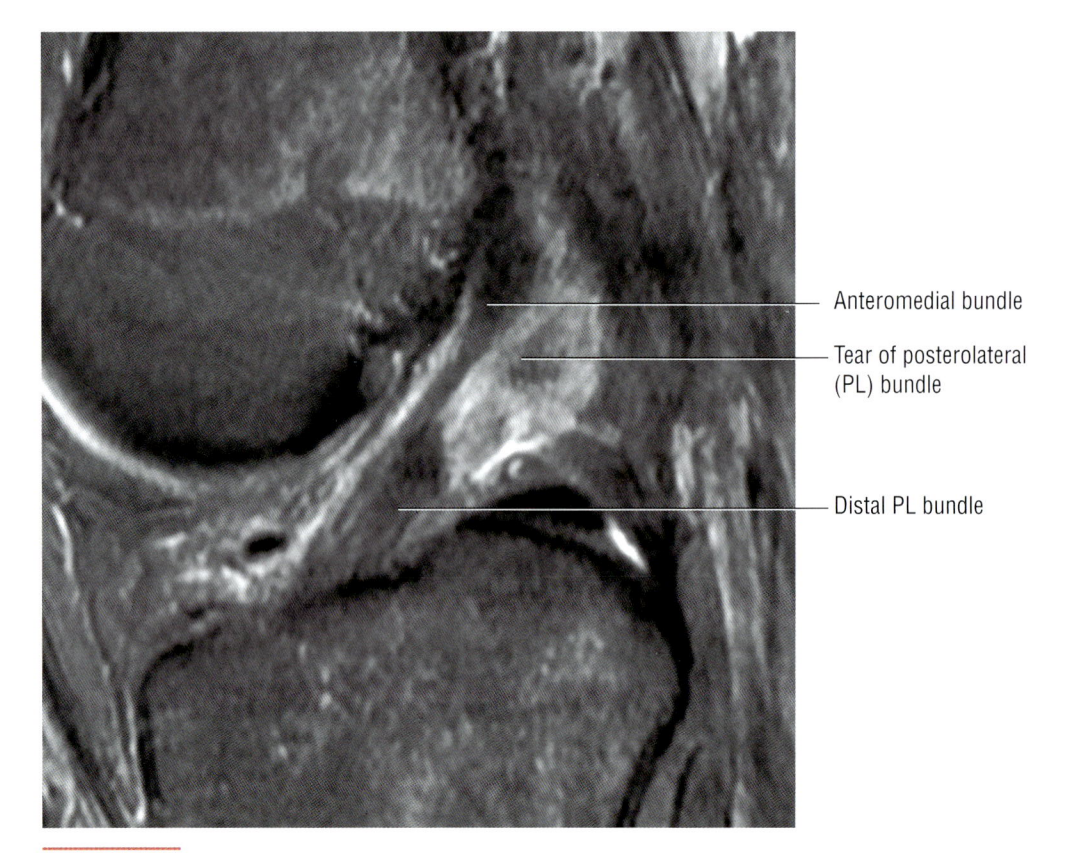

FIGURE 5.9 Selective posterolateral bundle tear with absent femoral attachment posterior to the proximal AM bundle. The knee is positioned in extension. FS PD FSE sagittal image.

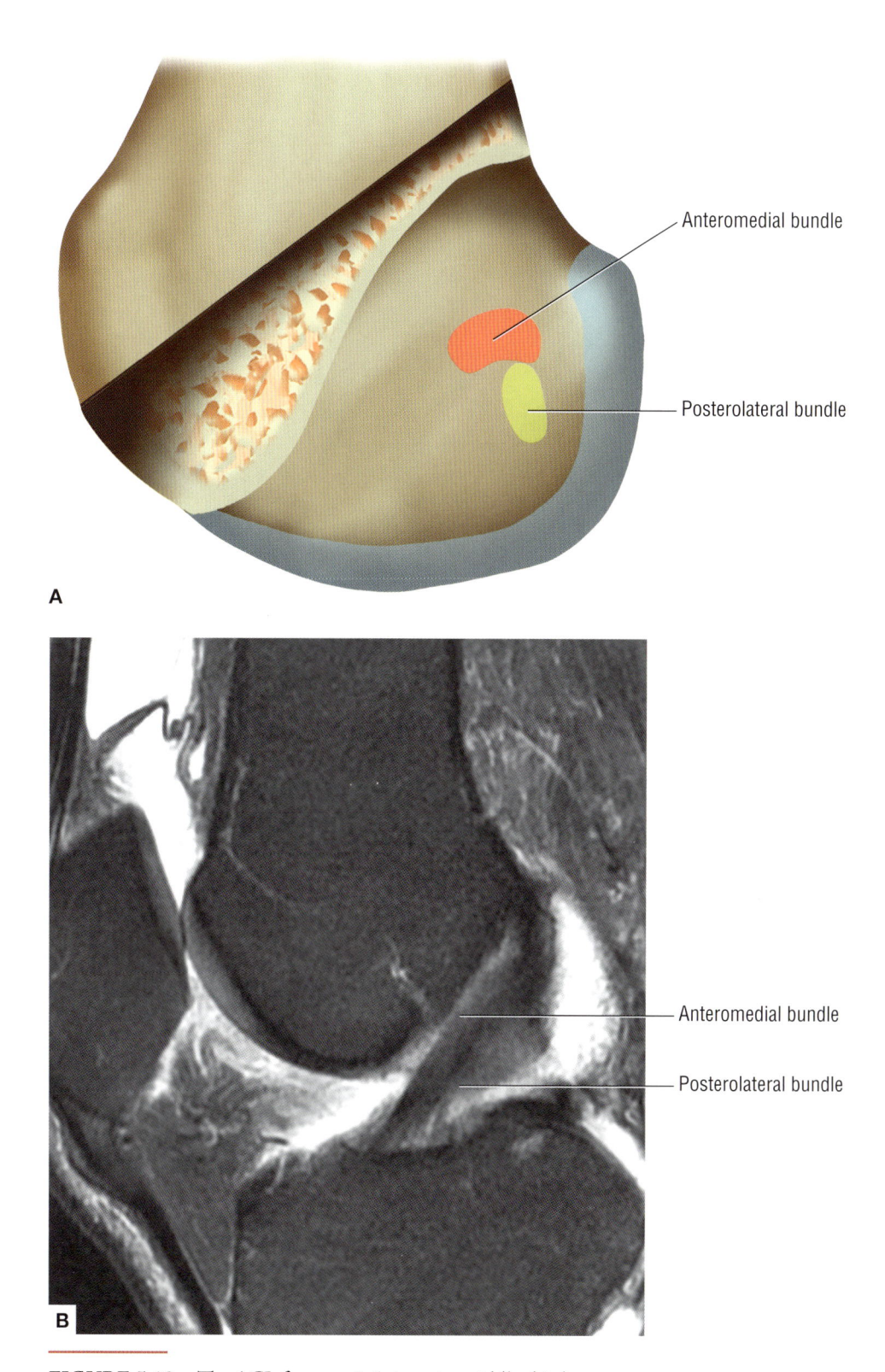

FIGURE 5.10 The ACL fans out 3.5 times its middle third or mid-substance size at both its femoral and tibial attachment sites. The femoral attachment occurs on the inner surface (medial aspect) of the posterolateral femoral condyle. In extension, the AM footprint fibers originate on the anterior and proximal aspect of the femoral insertion, while the PL bundle originates from the posterolateral aspect of the femoral ACL attachment. (**A**) ACL femoral attachment on sagittal section of the distal femur exposing the lateral femoral condyle. (**B**) FS PD FSE sagittal image.[40]

Intact AM bundle   PL bundle tear

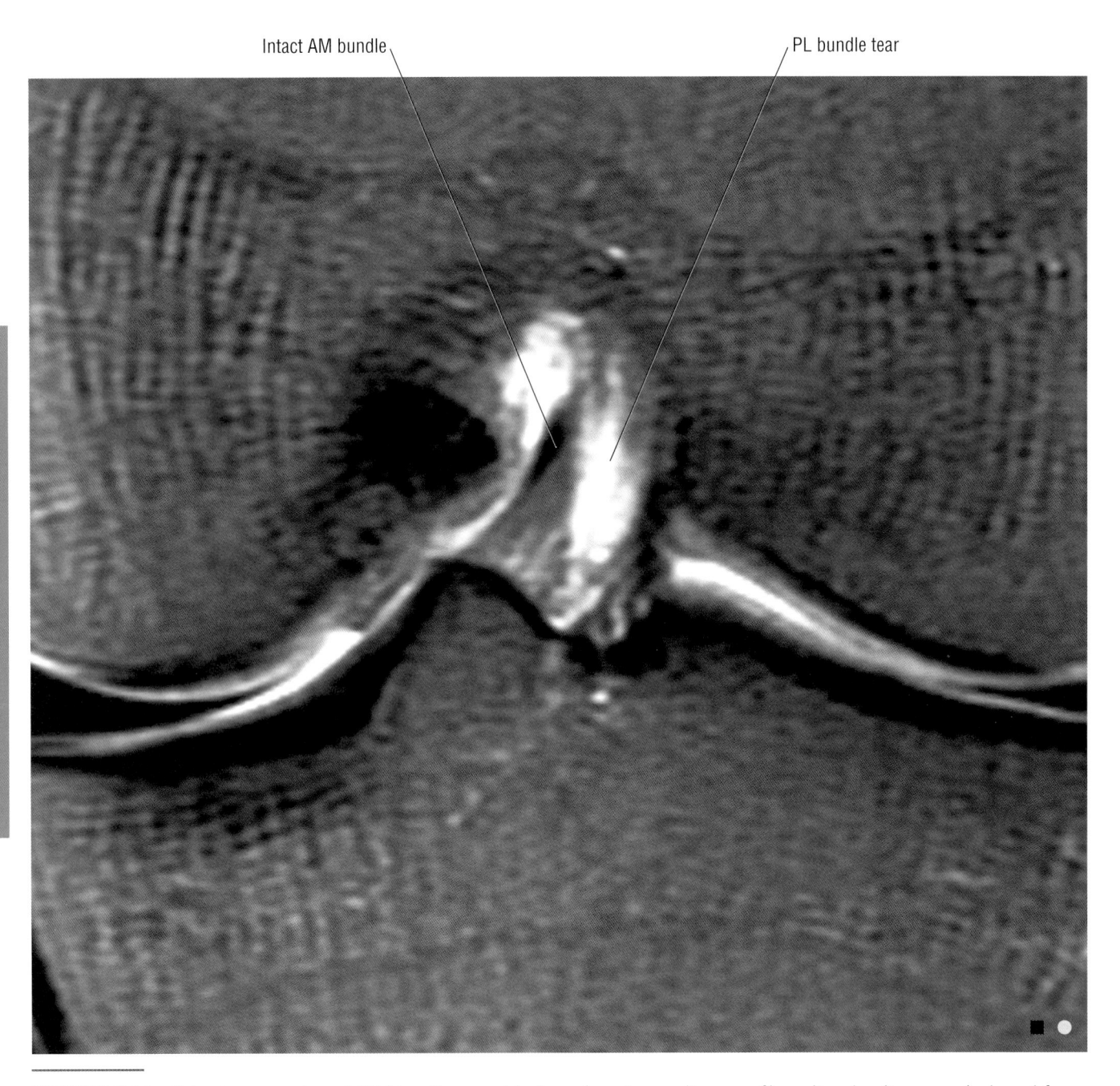

FIGURE 5.11 Selective posterolateral (PL) bundle tear with absent hypointense ligament fibers directly adjacent to the lateral femoral condyle. Anteromedial (AM) bundle is intact. FS PD FSE coronal image.

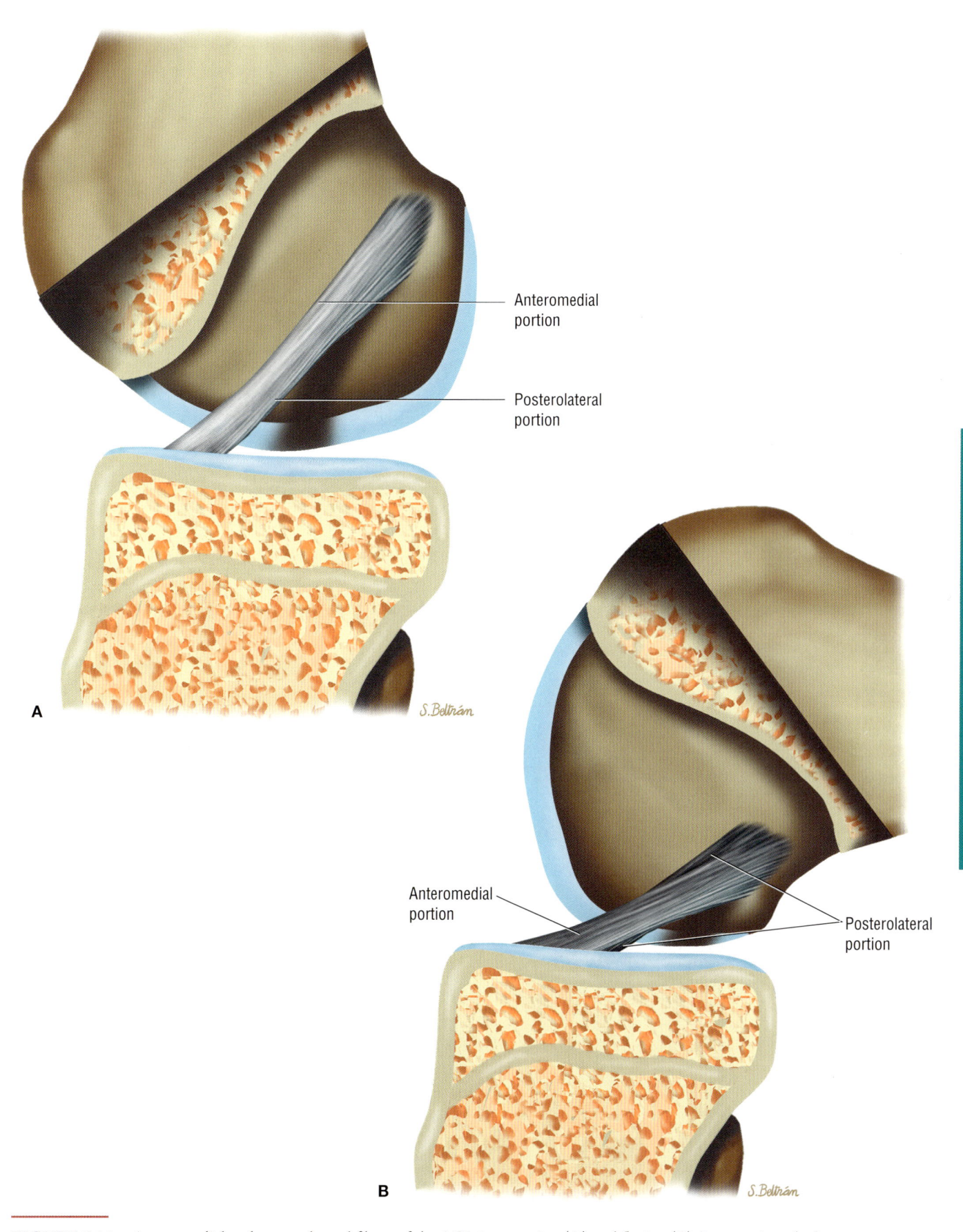

FIGURE 5.12 Anteromedial and posterolateral fibers of the ACL in extension (**A**) and flexion (**B**). In extension, the longer anteromedial fibers are identified anterior to the shorter posteriorly located posterolateral fibers. In flexion, the ACL ligament twists and the posterolateral fibers rotate beneath the anteromedial fibers. The ACL, therefore, is more cord-like in flexion, with the anterior superior portion comprising of posterolateral fibers.

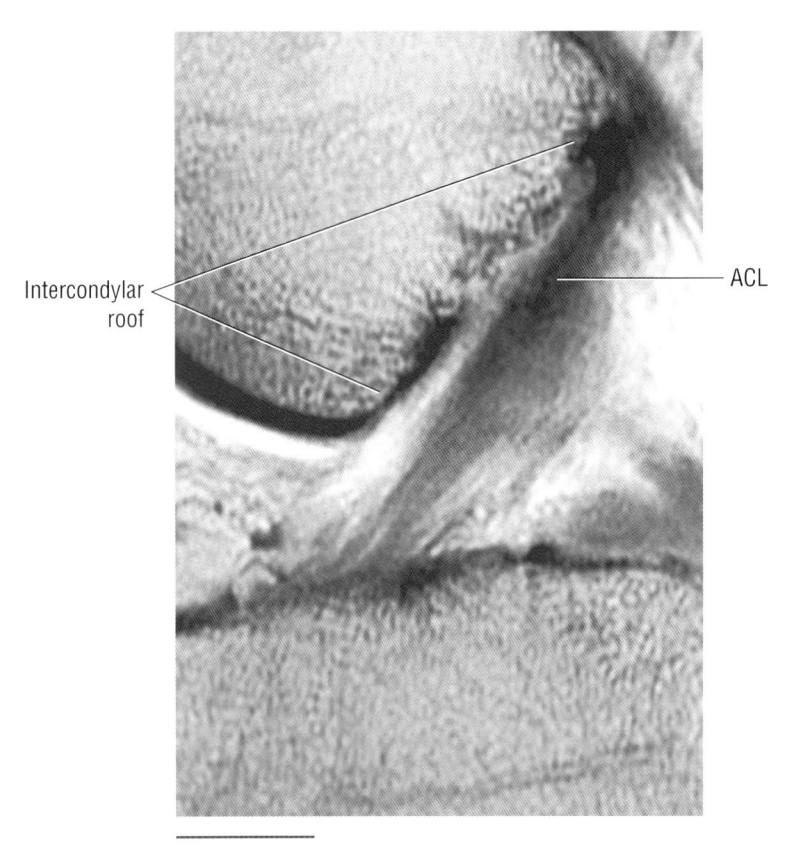

FIGURE 5.13 Sagittal plane through the intercondylar notch. The ACL is parallel to the intercondylar roof.

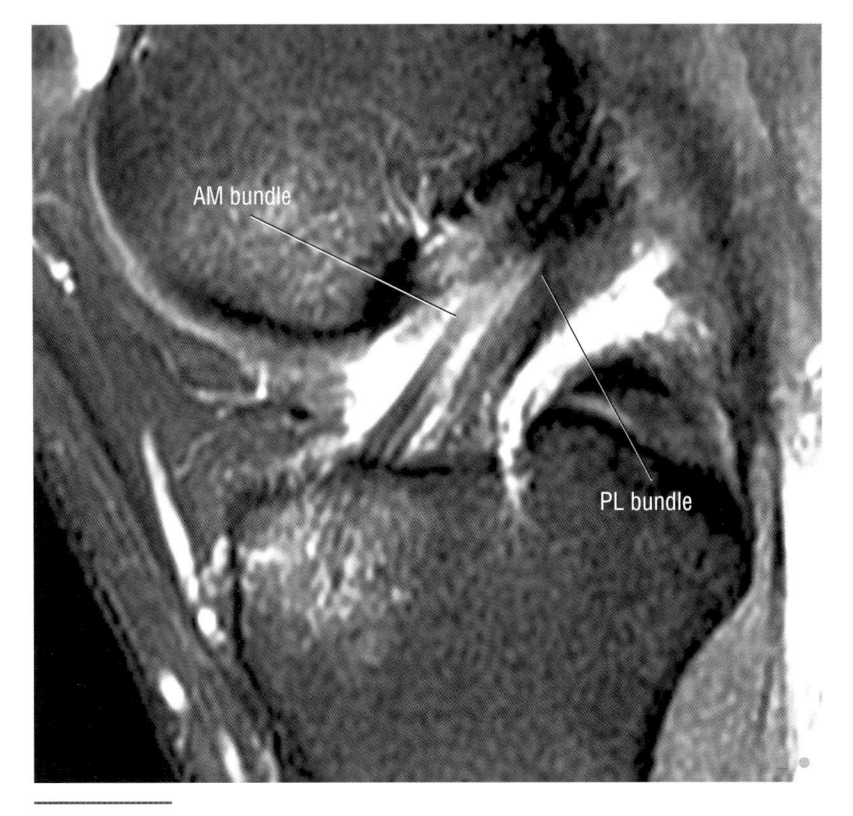

FIGURE 5.14 Double-bundle anatomy of the ACL with distinct AM and PL bundle femoral and tibial footprints. FS PD FSE sagittal image.

Cruciate Ligaments

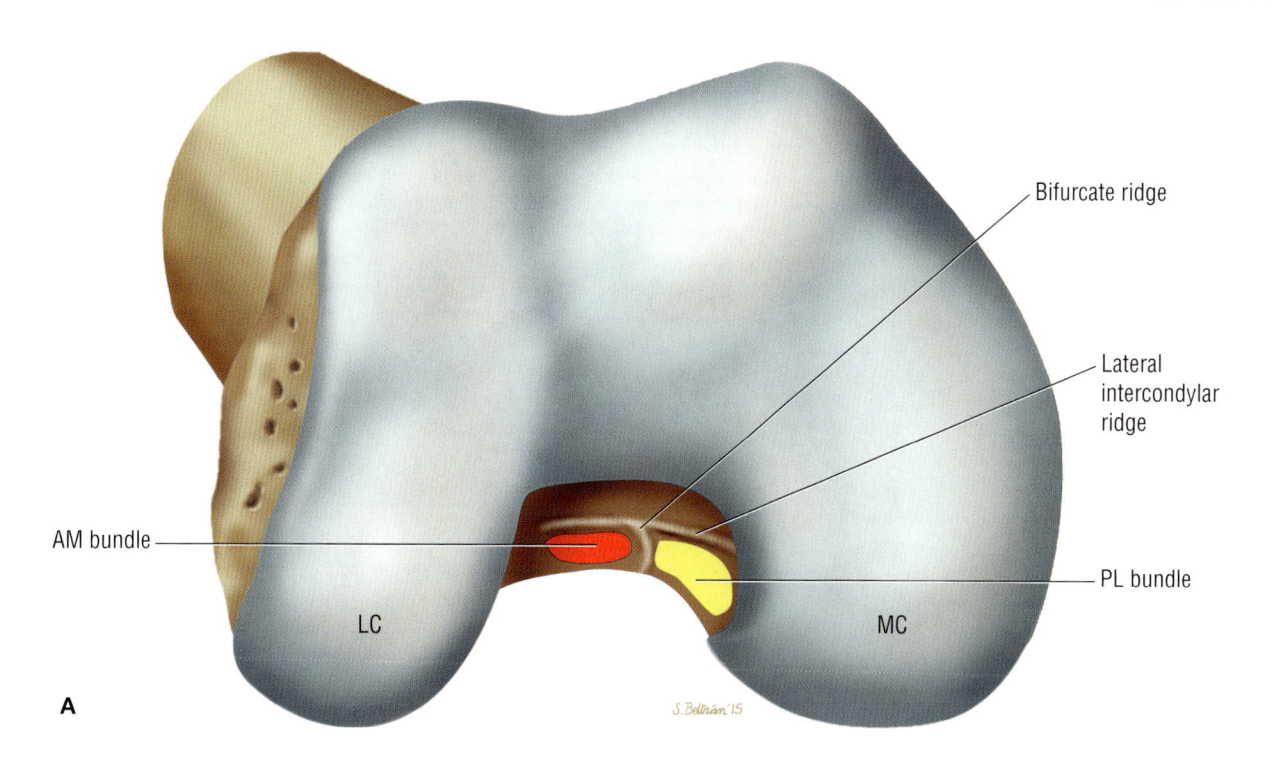

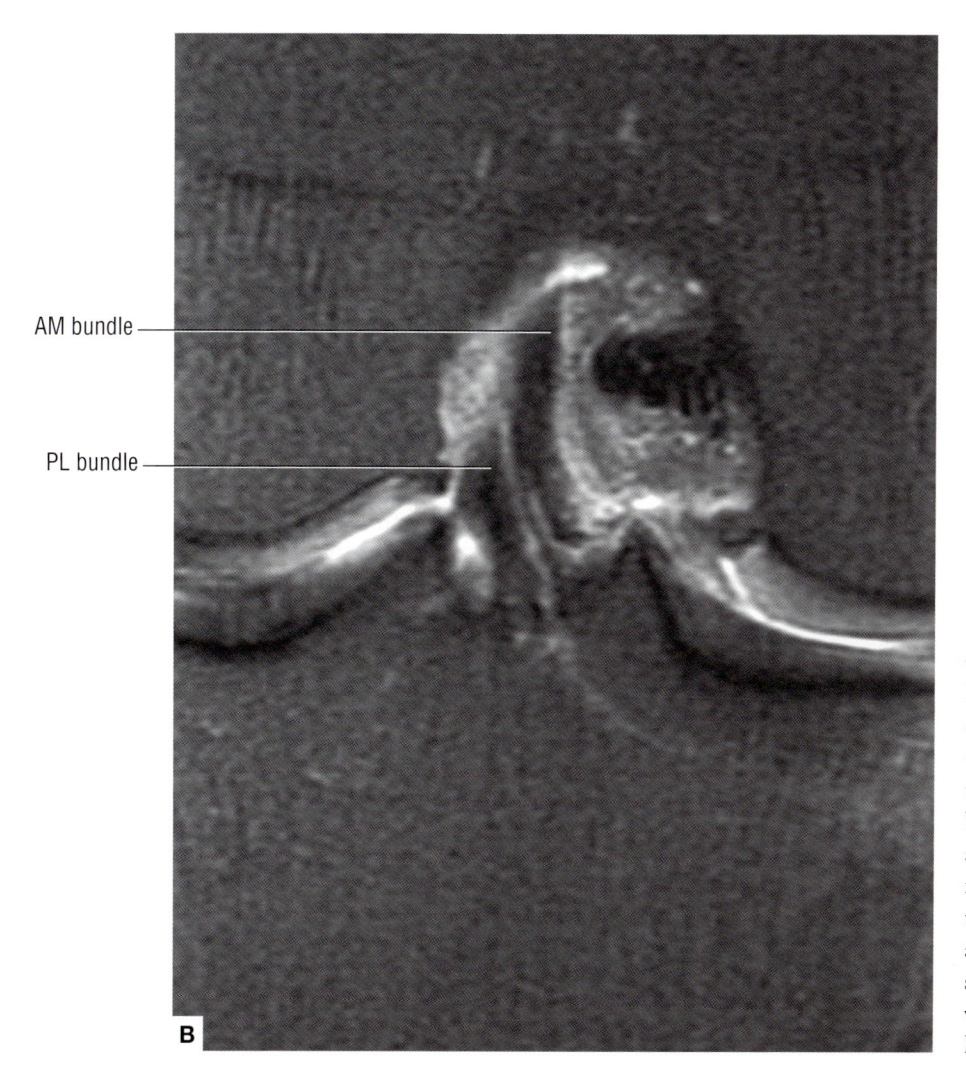

FIGURE 5.15 The lateral intercondylar ridge defines the anterior border (superior limit in 90-degree flexion of the knee) of the ACL footprint. The bifurcate or lateral bifurcate ridge separates the AM and PL bundle femoral insertion sites. As a surgical landmark, the AM and PL femoral footprints are below the equator of the lateral sidewall. (**A**) Femoral ACL landmarks viewing from the notch, (**B**) FS PD FSE coronal image.[147]

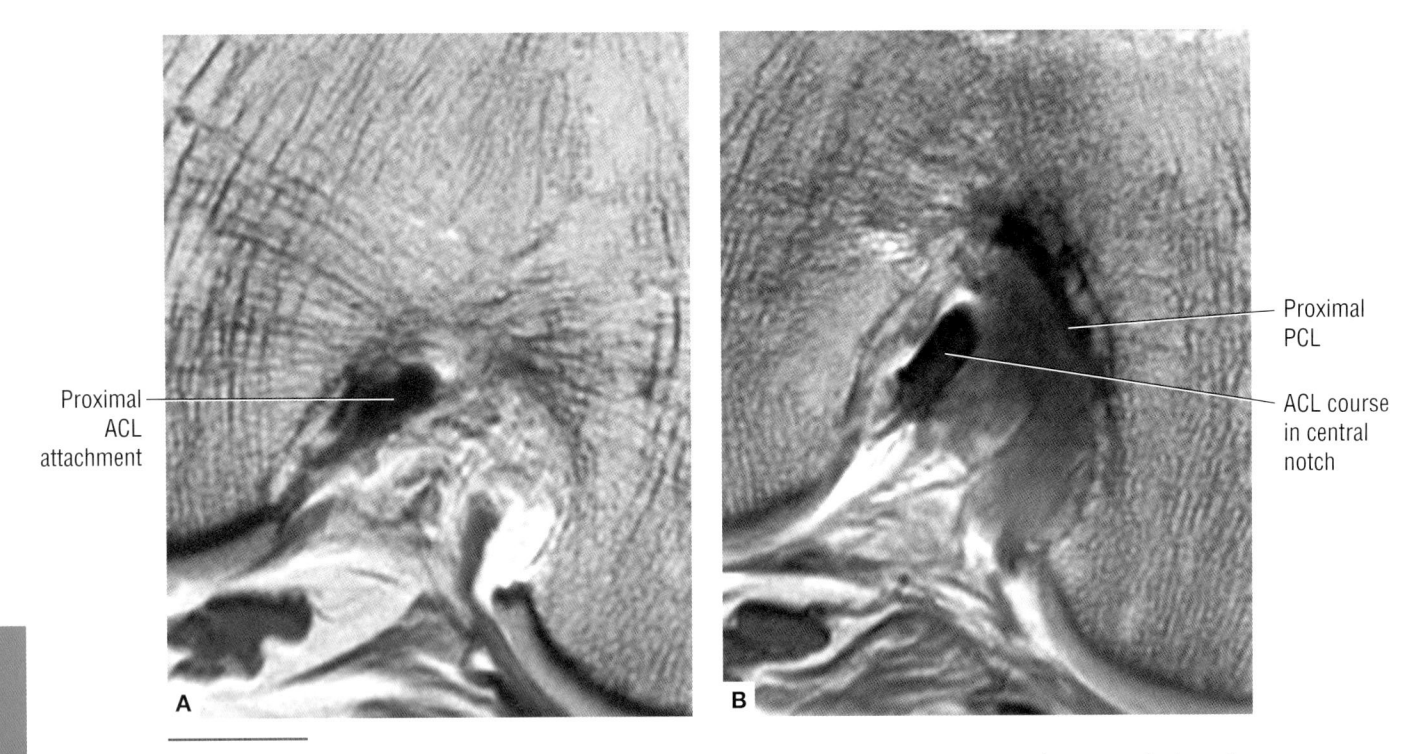

FIGURE 5.16 Axial intercondylar anatomy of the ACL and PCL. Proximal ACL attachment to the lateral femoral condylar side wall (**A**) and a more central notch axial section (**B**) are demonstrated.

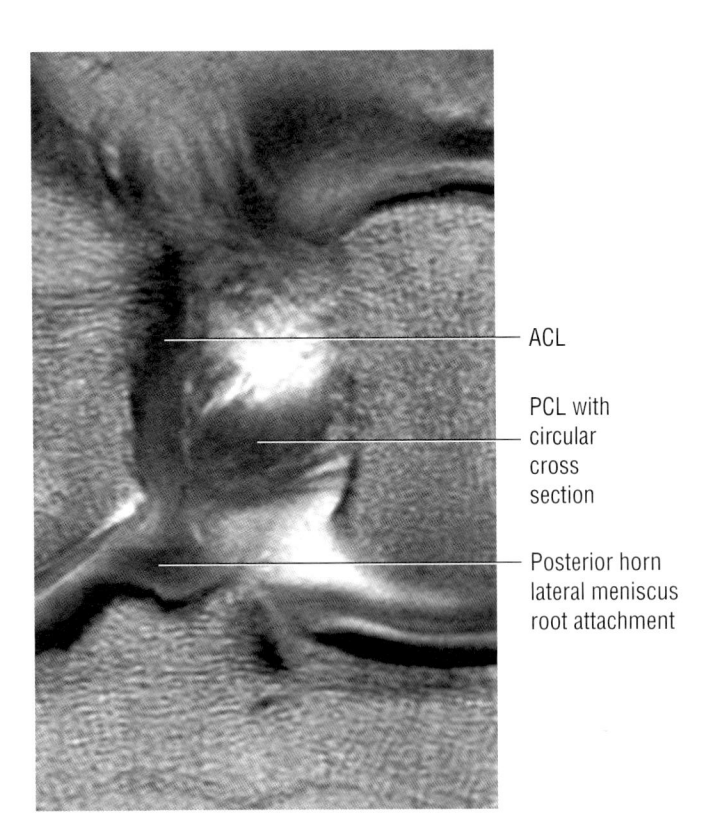

FIGURE 5.17 The anatomy of the ACL and PCL in the coronal plane. The ACL is band-like in morphology, whereas the PCL is circular in cross-section. The PCL has a course opposite to the ACL and attaches to the posterior intercondylar area and posterior tibial surface. The anterior root attachment of the lateral meniscus should not be mistaken for the ACL insertion.

Microanatomy and Component Structure

- Epiligament covers cruciate ligaments as a vascular layer.[40]
- Deep to epiligament
    - Parallel fibers with fascicles surrounded by a paratenon
    - Fascicles divided in subfascicles covered by an epitenon
        - Subfascicular units composed of collagen fibers
- Direct femoral and tibial osseous insertion
    - Transition from ligamentous tissue to bone
        - Zone of fibrocartilage
        - Zone of mineralized cartilage
- Myofibroblast
    - Contractile property
    - Crimp (regular fiber wave pattern)
    - Ligament healing
- Extracellular components
    - Extracellular volume mostly collagen fibers
    - Collagen
        - Type I is most abundant type and oriented in parallel fashion and responsible for tensile strength
        - Type II at femoral and tibial insertion sites associated with fibrocartilaginous regions (indication of applied pressure or shear)
        - Type III in loose connective tissue that separates type I collagen bundles and generated during graft ligamentization process
        - Type IV in basal lamina of intra- and periligamentous vessels
        - Type VI along complete length of ligament and more abundant in ACL. Serves as a gliding component between functional fibrillar units. Highest concentration near attachment sites where higher strains exist.
        - Glycosaminoglycans ground substances in association with proteoglycans. Contribute to viscoelastic properties and protection against repetitive loading.
        - Elastic components facilitate ligament length changes and are concentrated along mid-substance.[40]

Biomechanics

- ACL is primary constraint for anterior tibial translation.[40]
- Limits internal rotation as a secondary stabilizer
  - In conjunction with medial collateral ligament (MCL) and posteromedial structures
- Structural and viscoelastic characteristics (seen in both cruciate ligaments)
  - Elongation during loading
  - Ligament stiffness associated with fiber recruitment and ligament straightening
  - Yield load
    - Nonreversible structural damage in the ACL
    - Linear long-elongation relationship changes to nonlinear
    - Maximum or failure loads associated with destruction of ligamentous integrity and occur after yield load is exceeded
  - Viscoelastic behavior
    - Time-dependent changes in ligament loading and elongation
    - Stress relaxation related to constant stretch for a continuous time for a load to maintain elongation and reach a steady state
    - Creep describes ligament lengthening when exposed to a constant load over a period of time until steady state is obtained.[40]

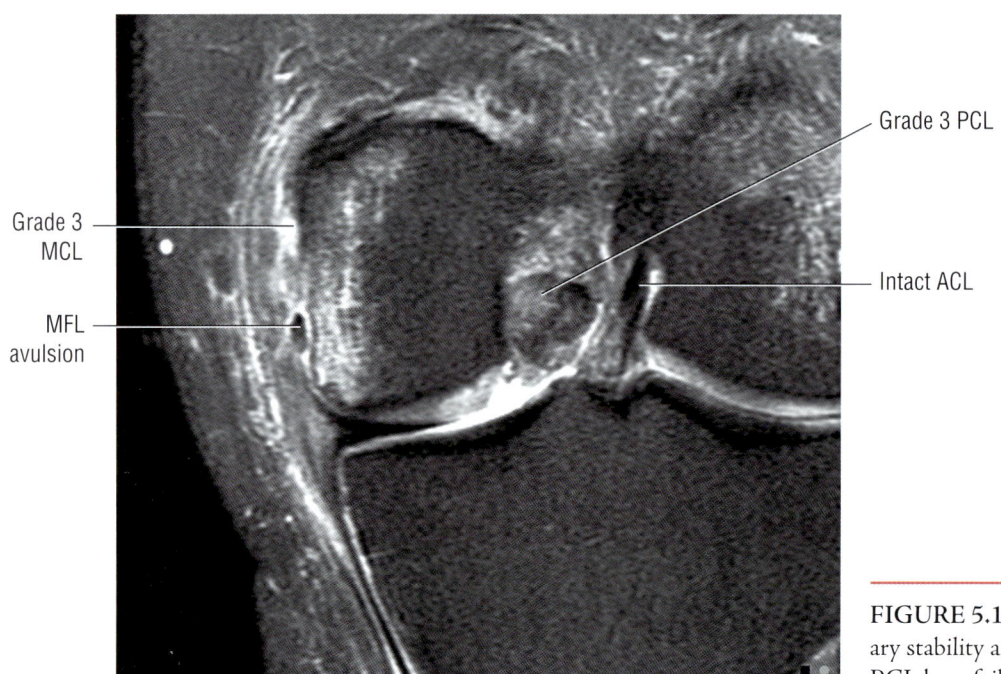

FIGURE 5.18 Intact ACL providing secondary stability after the superficial deep MCL and PCL have failed. Coronal FS PD FSE image.

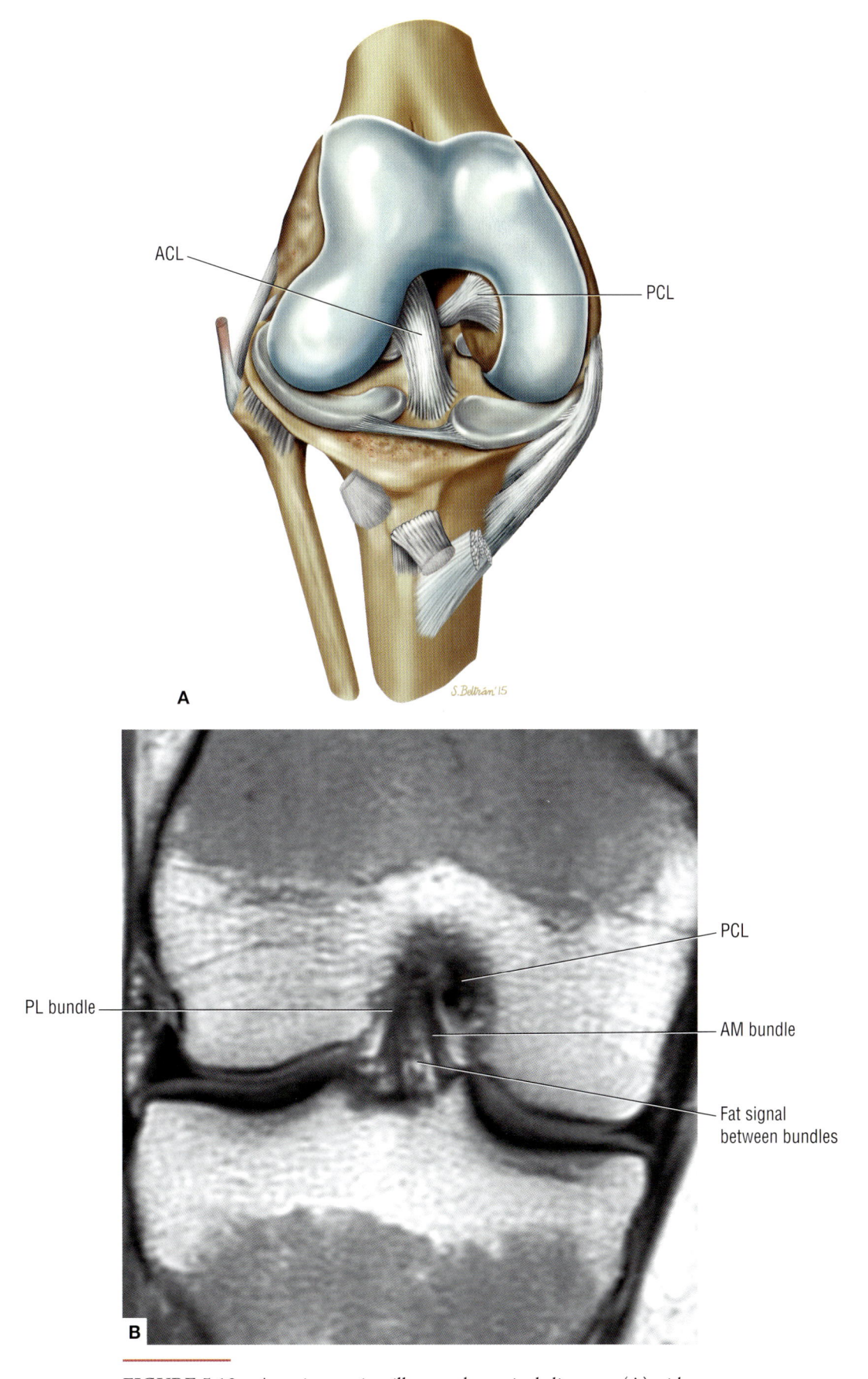

FIGURE 5.19 Anterior cruciate illustrated as a single ligament (**A**) with double-bundle morphology demonstrated on coronal PD image (**B**). The interdigitation of fat signal between ACL bundles is normal in the distal third of the ligament.

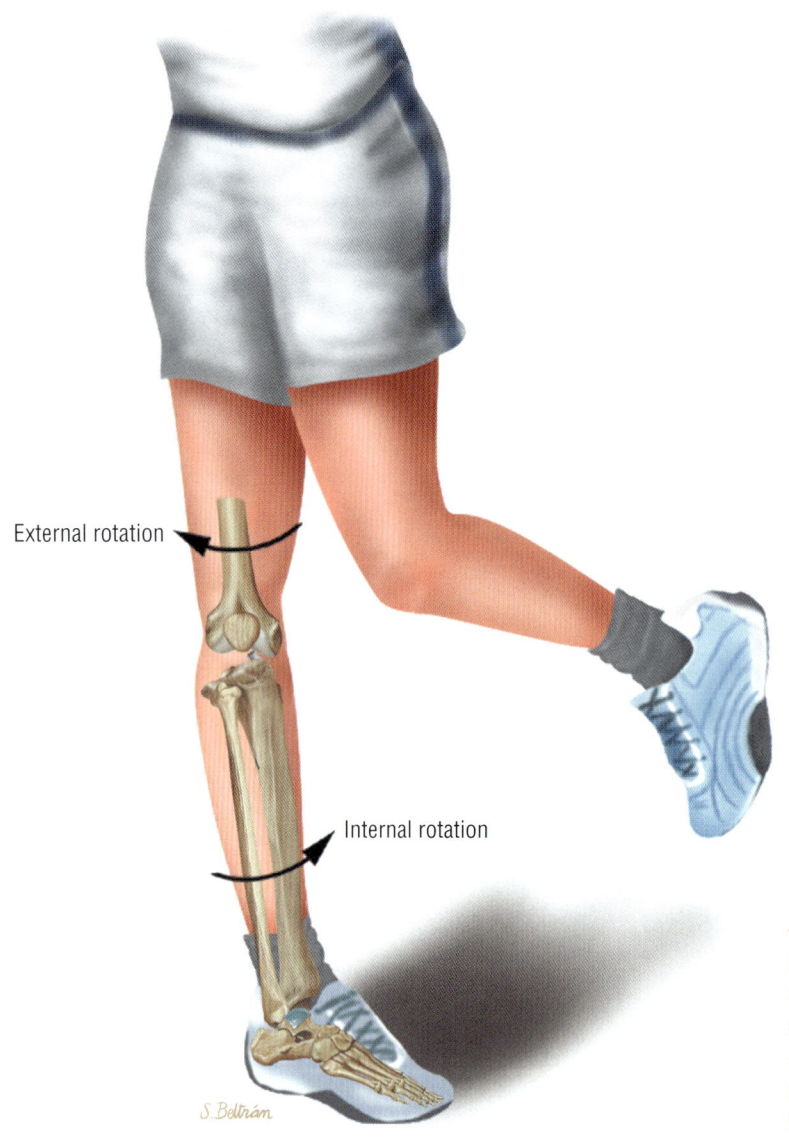

FIGURE 5.20 Grade 3 tear of the anterior cruciate ligament associated with a twisting injury of the hyperextended knee. This is the mechanism of landing after a basketball jump shot.

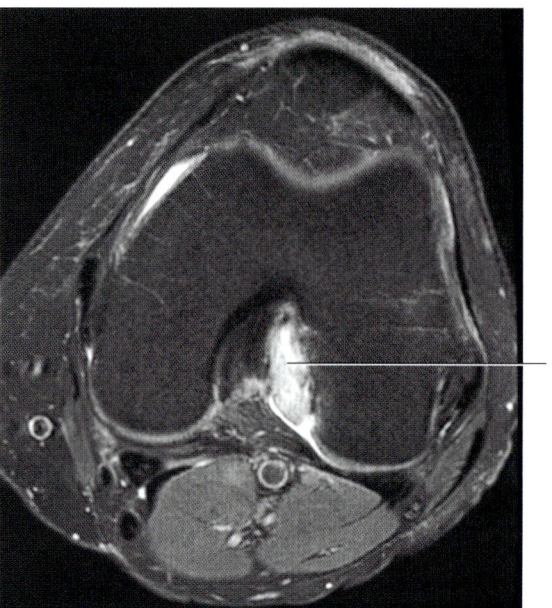

FIGURE 5.21 Disruption of proximal femoral attachment of the ACL. FS PD FSE axial image.

Mechanism of Injury

Key Concepts

- **ACL Injury**
  - **Pivot Shift Injury**
    - Noncontact injury in skiers or American football players
    - Valgus load, flexion and external rotation of tibia, or internal rotation of femur
    - ACL rupture and lateral compartment contusions
  - **Dashboard Injury**
    - Applied force to anterior proximal tibia with knee in flexion
    - Associated with anterior tibial and posterior patellar edema and rupture of the PCL and posterior joint capsule
  - **Hyperextension Injury**
    - Direct force applied to anterior tibia with planted foot
    - Direct injury secondary to car bumper impacting anterior tibia of a pedestrian
    - Indirect force as caused by forceful kicking motion
    - Kissing contusions of anterior femoral condyle and anterior tibial plateau (hyperextension with applied valgus force shifts bone contusions medially)
    - Associated soft tissue injuries include ACL, PCL, and/or meniscal injury.
    - Knee dislocation with at-risk structures including ACL, PCL, popliteal neurovascular structures, and posterolateral complex injuries
  - **Clip Injury**
    - Contact injury secondary to pure valgus stress to a partially flexed (10 to 30 degrees) knee
    - Seen in American football players
    - Osseous contusion of lateral femoral condyle from direct blow with medial femoral epicondylar edema related to MCL avulsion stress
    - Associated soft tissue structures at risk include proximal MCL and ACL due to increased knee flexion (O'Donoghue's triad includes medial meniscus).

ACL Mechanisms of Injury

- Three general mechanisms of ACL failure:
    - External rotation and abduction with hyperextension
    - Direct forward displacement of tibia
    - Internal rotation with knee in full extension[349,415]
- Noncontact mechanism occurs in 70% to 80% of cases of ACL tears.
- Loading on affected leg (one leg) then falling with a twisting valgus force while maintaining quadriceps contraction[40]
- With varus or valgus stress, ACL injury occurs after collateral ligament failure.
- Most common mechanism of contact-mediated ACL rupture injury is forced valgus in external rotation, causing disruption of MCL and medial supporting structures (valgus collapse of the knee).[30,135,223,243]
    - O'Donoghue's triad
        - ACL, MCL, and medial meniscus injuries
        - Associated with valgus stress in external rotation (clip injury)
        - Also associated with tears of posterior horn of the lateral meniscus (more serious injury)
- Second most common mechanism of injury (30% of patients) is hyperextension associated with meniscal tear
- Third most common pattern of injury is direct blow to flexed knee with ankle flexed (e.g., turf injuries)
    - PCL and posterior capsule also damaged in severe contact hyperextension injuries
    - May be associated with disruption of posterolateral complex, resulting in posterolateral instability
- Increasing frequency of noncontact or indirect mechanisms of injury
    - Isolated ACL injuries less common, but can occur with pivoting during deceleration (e.g., downhill skiing), causing forced internal rotation of femur
    - Classic knee injury in skiing is forward fall catching the inside edge of the ski (external rotation in valgus stress)

Cruciate Ligaments

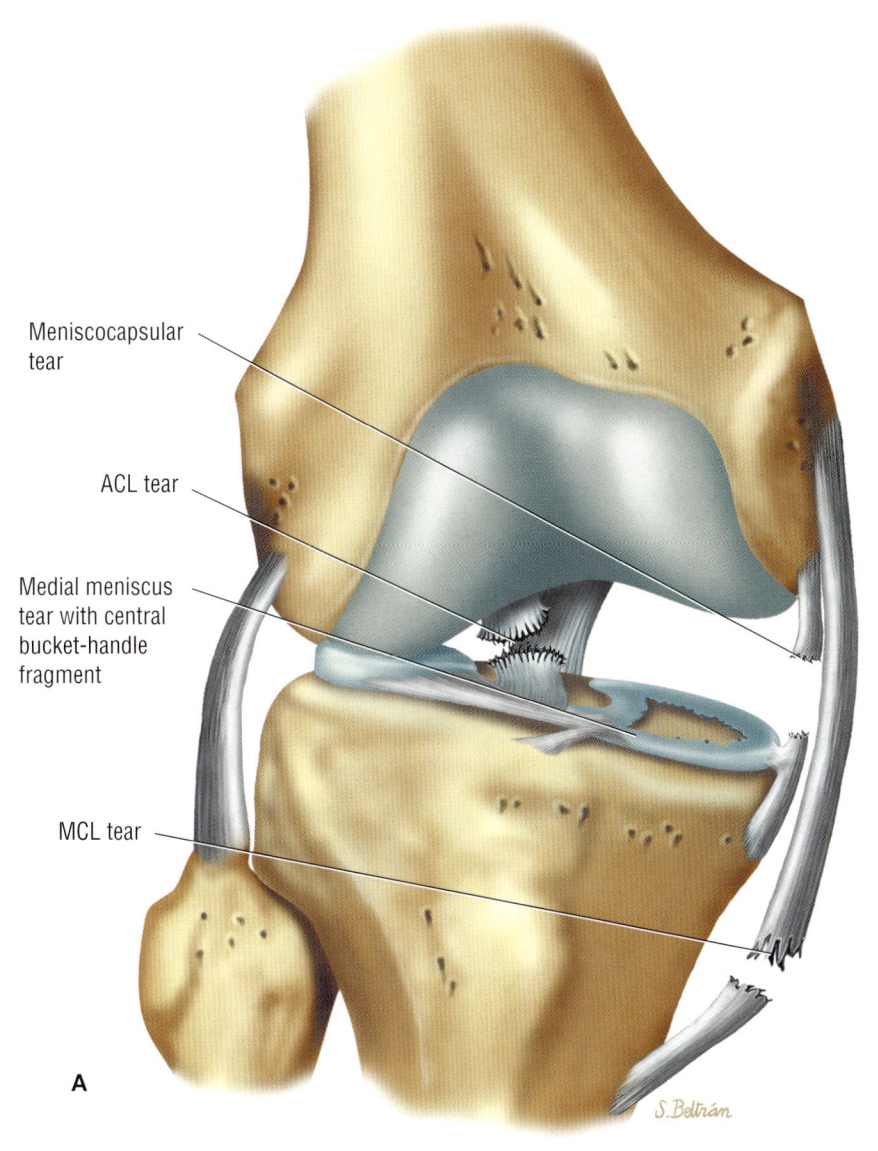

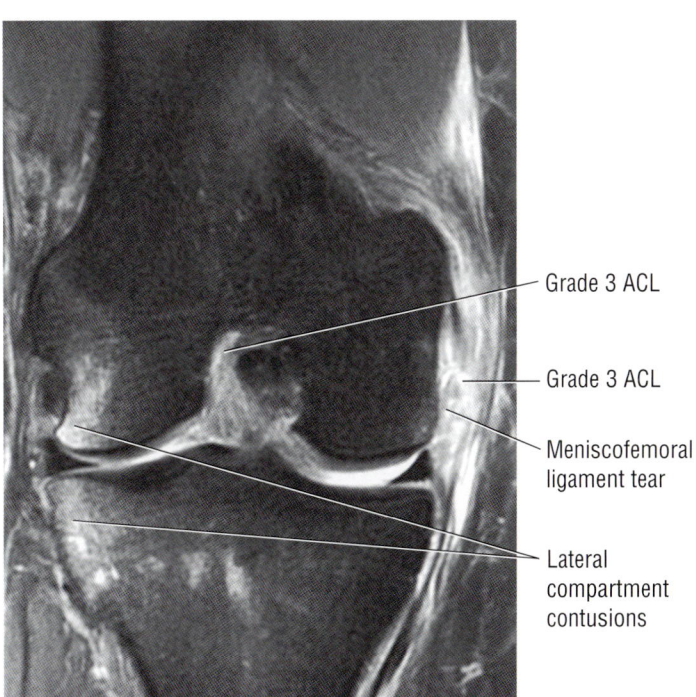

FIGURE 5.22 (A) O'Donoghue's triad is usually the result of a noncontact twisting injury with rupture of the MCL and ACL plus associated tearing of the medial meniscus. (B) Grade 3 MCL tear and lateral compartment contusions associated with an ACL tear on FS PD FSE coronal image.

418　Stoller's Orthopaedics and Sports Medicine: The Knee

- Intercondylar roof
- Proximal ACL rupture

A

- Effusion
- Proximal ACL disruption
- Lateral tibial plateau contusion

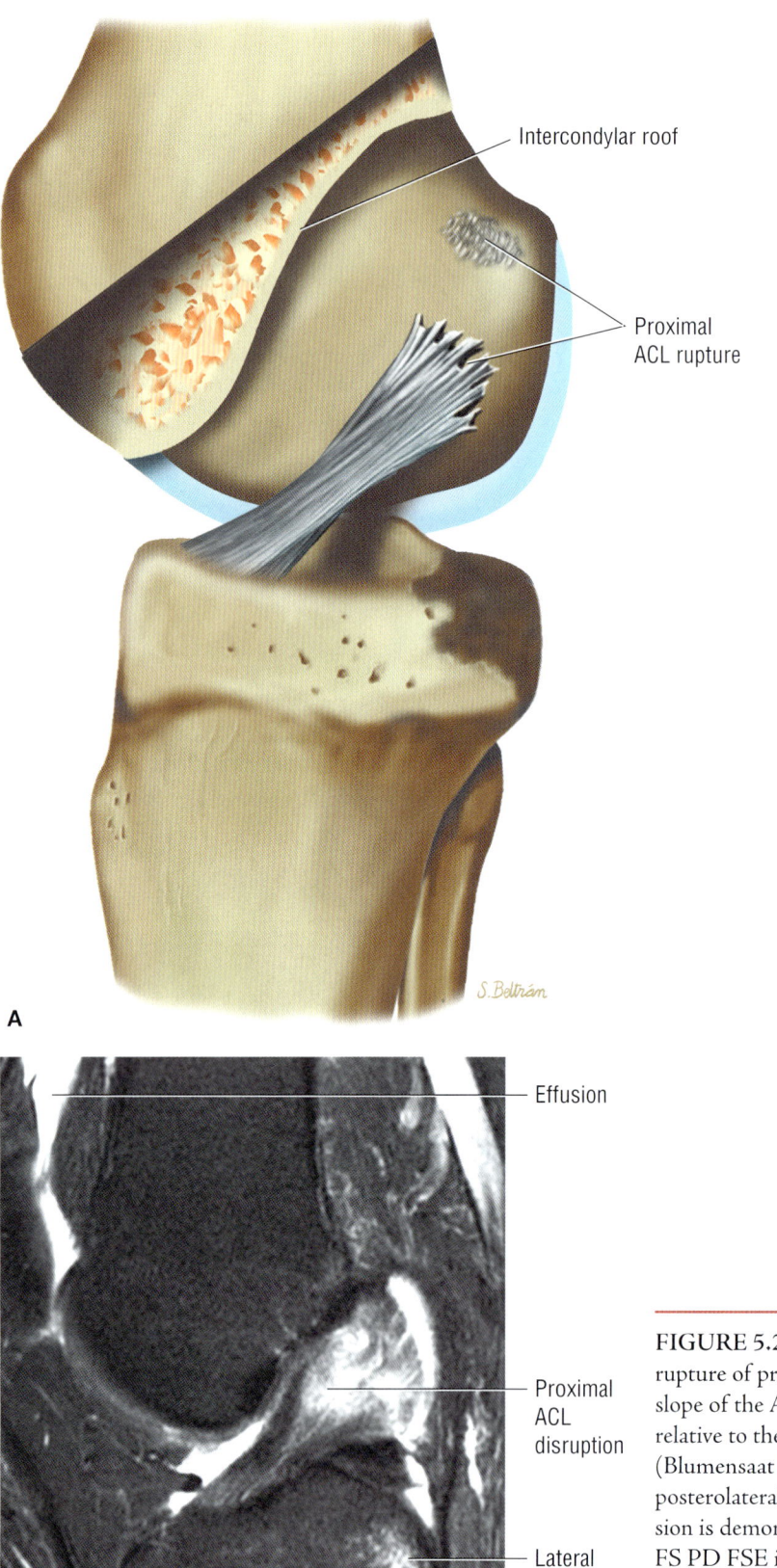

B

FIGURE 5.23 (**A**) Acute ACL rupture of proximal fibers. The slope of the ACL is decreased relative to the intercondylar roof (Blumensaat line). Characteristic posterolateral tibial plateau contusion is demonstrated. (**B**) Sagittal FS PD FSE image of a grade 3 ACL tear. Complete loss of proximal ligament continuity with the lateral femoral condyle side wall is shown in the sagittal plane. Acute findings of a joint effusion and posterior tibial plateau contusion are present.

Cruciate Ligaments

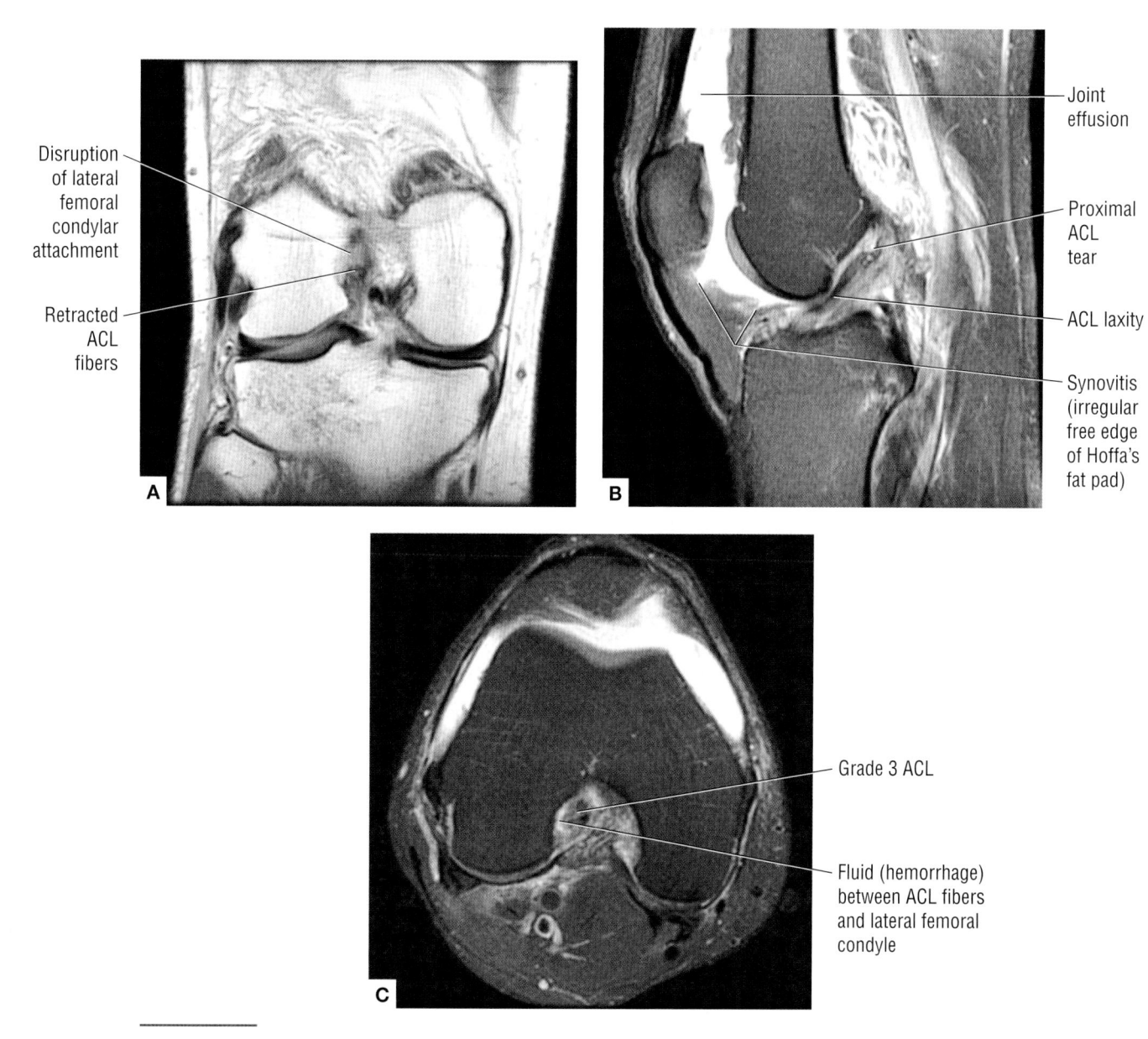

FIGURE 5.24 Acute ACL tear evaluated in three separate planes. (**A**) Coronal PD FSE image. (**B**) Sagittal FS PD FSE image. (**C**) Axial FS PD FSE image.

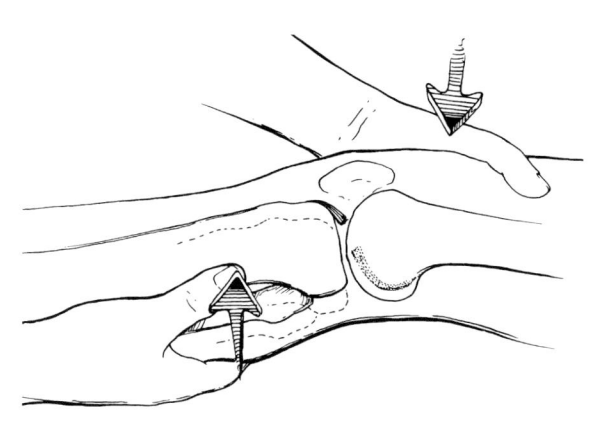

FIGURE 5.25 The Lachman test is performed in 20 to 30 degrees of knee flexion. Anterior laxity is tested assessing the degree of anterior tibial translation and endpoint using the contralateral knee laxity for comparison. (Reprinted from Fu FH. *Master Techniques in Orthopaedic Surgery: Sports Medicine.* Philadelphia, PA: Lippincott Williams & Wilkins; 2010, with permission.)

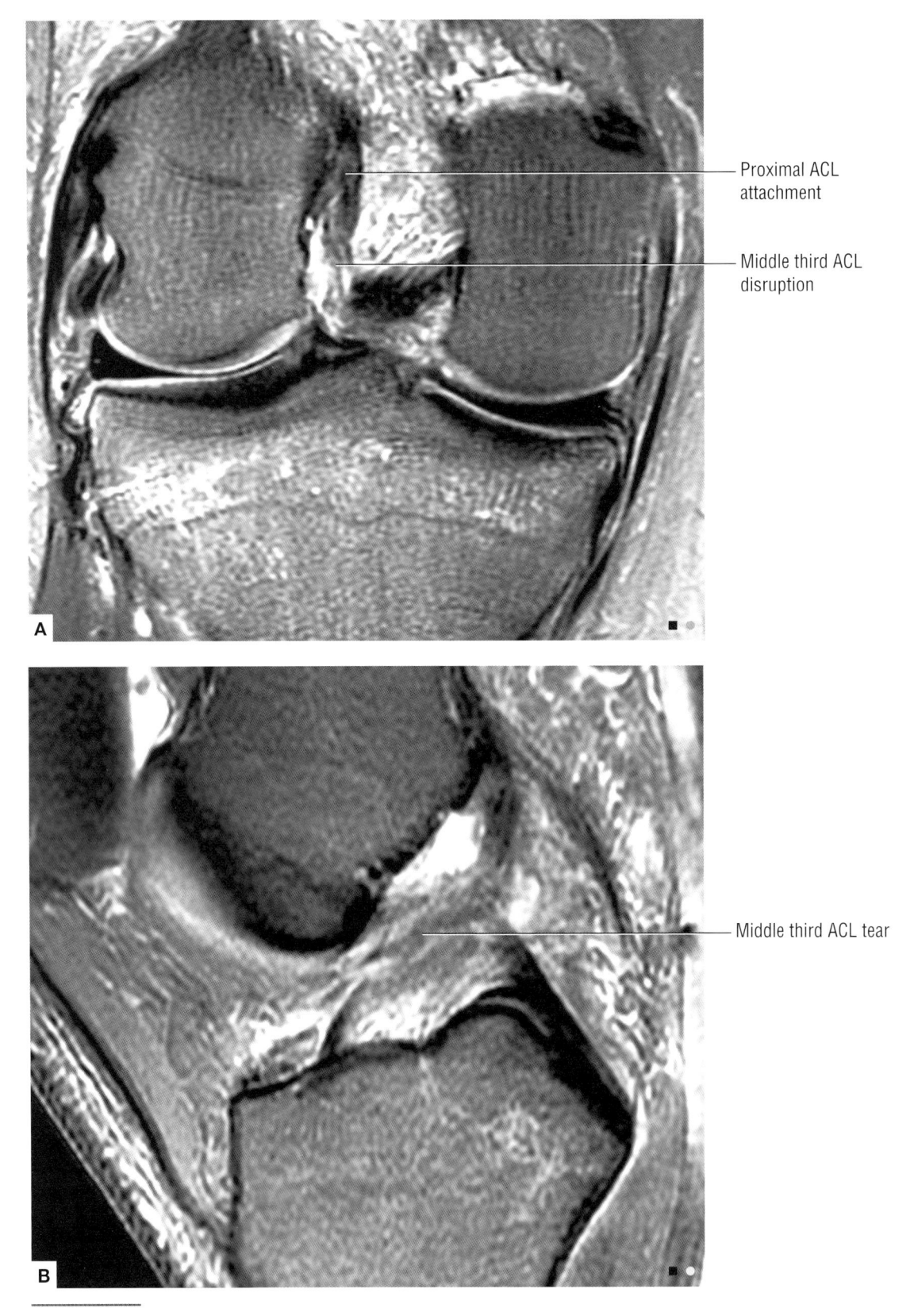

FIGURE 5.26 Middle third ACL tears should always be evaluated in at least two planes because intact femoral and tibial stumps may be mistaken for ligament fiber continuity. FS PD FSE coronal (**A**) and sagittal (**B**) images.

Cruciate Ligaments 421

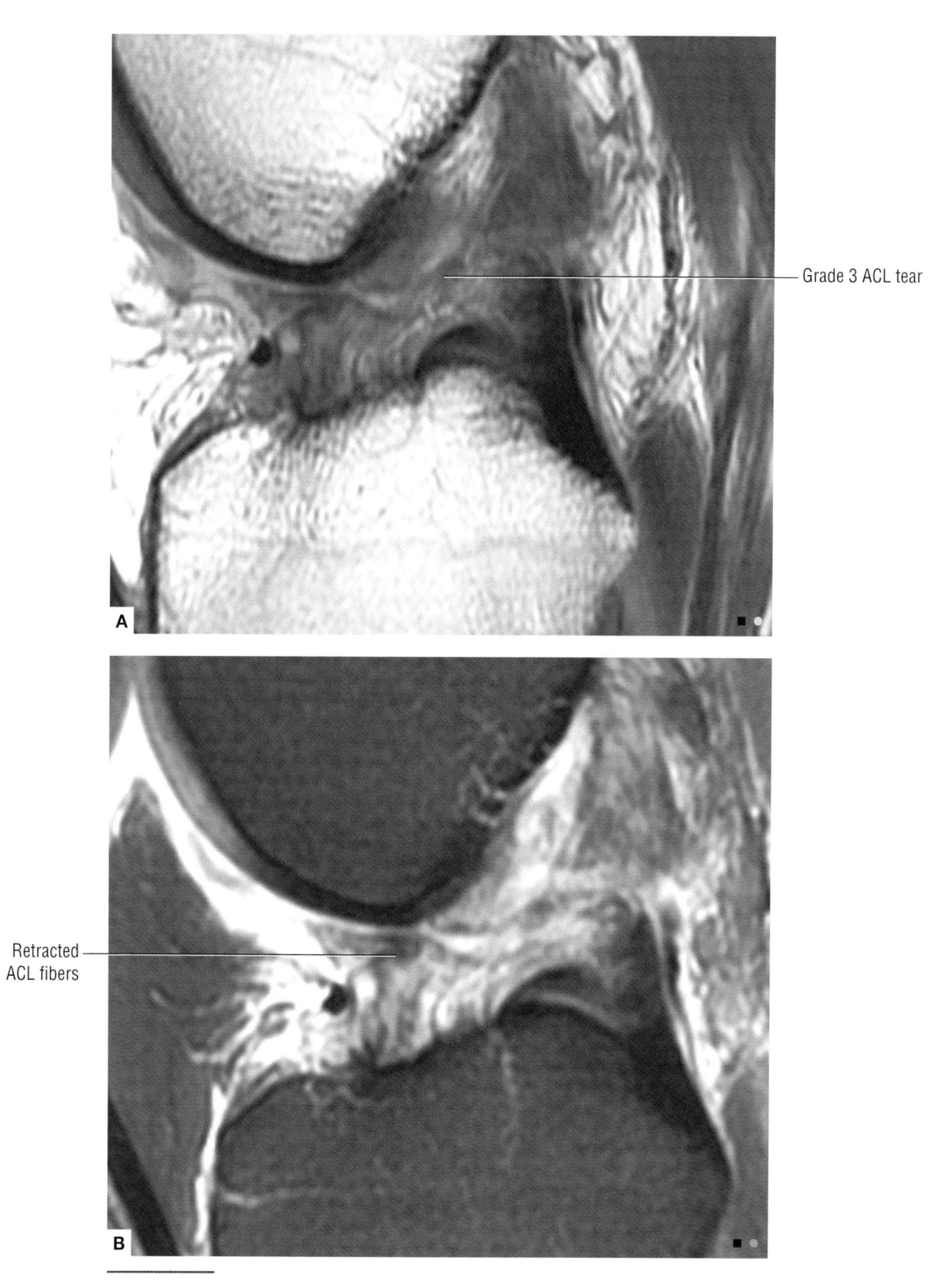

— Grade 3 ACL tear

Retracted ACL fibers

FIGURE 5.27 Grade 3 proximal ACL tear with complete loss of ligament architecture and fiber continuity. PD (**A**) and FS PD FSE (**B**) sagittal images.

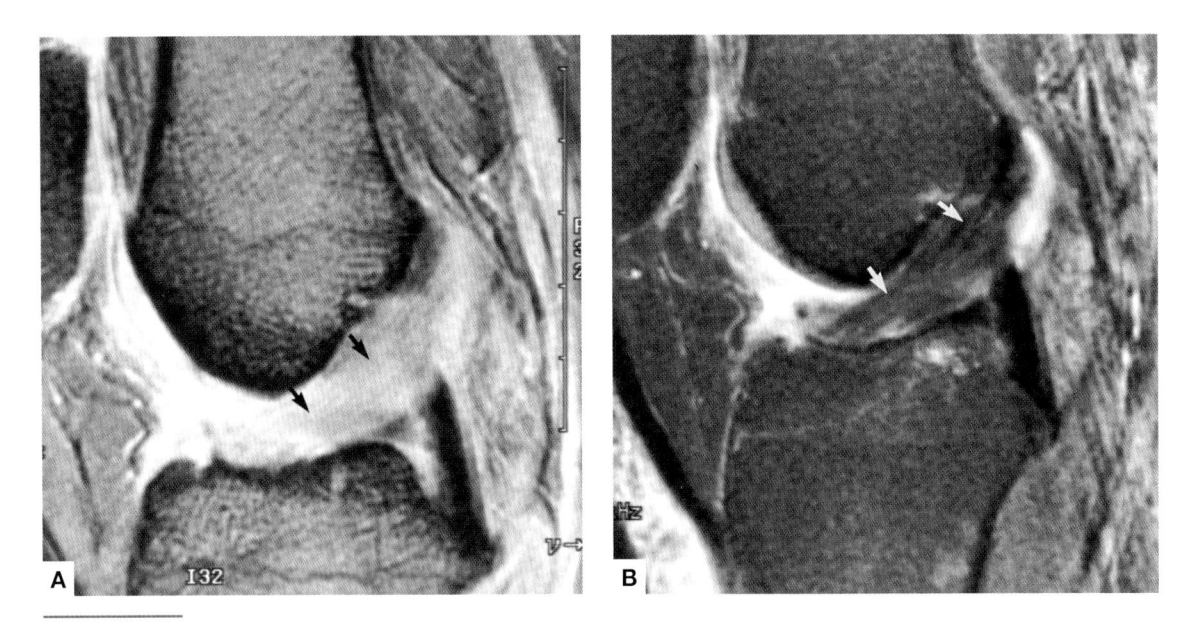

FIGURE 5.28 An interstitial tear. (**A**) An ACL interstitial tear pattern with diffuse hyperintensity (*arrows*) along the entire course of the ligament on a T2*-weighted sagittal image. (**B**) A thickened and posteriorly bowed ACL (*arrows*) is visualized with decreased signal intensity on a corresponding FS PD-weighted FSE sagittal image. The GRE image thus overestimates the degree of ligamentous tearing and should only be used in conjunction with a more specific FS PD or T2-weighted FSE sequence for this application.

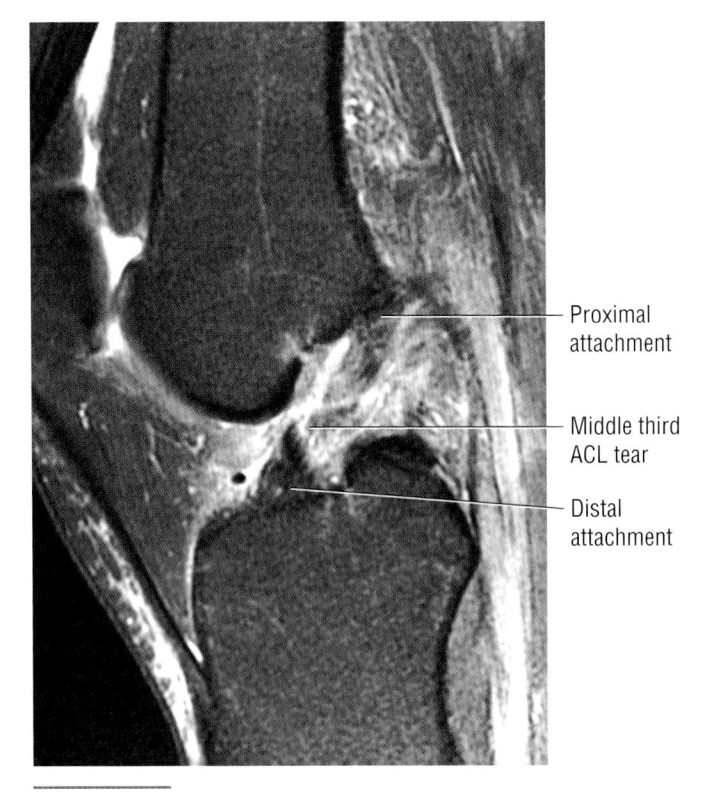

FIGURE 5.29 Disruption of the middle third of the ACL (FS PD FSE sagittal image).

- - May have associated posterolateral complex and lateral meniscus injuries
    - Forceful quadriceps contraction with passive anterior force (from forward movement of the ski boot) may result in isolated ACL injury.[30]
  - Can also occur in basketball and football players
    - Sudden deceleration to change direction can produce anterior drawer force on proximal tibia from forceful quadriceps contraction.
    - Noncontact isolated ACL tears also seen in hyperextension injuries in basketball players who rebound and in gymnasts who miss a dismount[223]
  - Increased prevalence of ACL tears in female high school and collegiate athletes, attributed to both extrinsic factors (e.g., increased muscular strength) and variety of intrinsic factors (e.g., increased joint laxity, limb alignment, and notch size)

Associated Intraarticular Pathology

- Meniscal tears
  - Associated with 41% to 68% of acute isolated ACL injuries[30,66,207]
  - Associated with 85% to 91% of chronic ACL-deficient knees[313]
  - Reported in up to 79% of pediatric patients
  - Better prognosis for successful meniscal repair when performed in conjunction with ACL reconstruction[63]
  - Higher incidence of lateral meniscal tears with acute ACL injuries, while medial meniscal tears more common with chronic ACL injuries[21,120]
- Articular cartilage lesions observed in 23% of acute and 54% of chronic injuries[207]
- Injury to meniscus and articular cartilage associated with episodic anterior tibial subluxation (especially medially)[30]
- Current mechanisms of injury more frequently represented by triad of injury to ACL, MCL, and lateral meniscus (in contrast to O'Donoghue's triad)[120]

Clinical Assessment of ACL Injury

- Classification of ACL tears
    - Grade 1: intraligamentous injury without change in ligament length
    - Grade 2: intraligamentous injury with increase in ligament length
    - Grade 3: complete ligamentous disruption
- Acute ACL tears associated with hemarthrosis (75%) and audible pop (34%) at the time of injury[30,69]
    - Hemarthrosis evident within first several hours in >70% of patients[223]
- ACL can resist loads as great as 2000N with maximum loading (primary stabilizer for anterior tibial displacement).[30,528]
- AMB of ACL must be disrupted for positive anterior drawer sign (knee in 90 degrees of flexion).
    - Anterior drawer sign also usually requires disruption of the medial capsule.[352]
- Lachman's test (anterior drawer test performed between 15 and 30 degrees of flexion) and pivot-shift test (performed with valgus stress and flexion) are positive in almost all patients with ACL disruption.
    - Tests for anterolateral rotary instability designed to elicit pivot-shift phenomenon (momentary anterior subluxation of tibia relative to femur at 25 degrees of knee flexion)
    - Pivot-shift test difficult to perform in acutely injured knee due to guarding[223]
- Classic anterior drawer sign may give false-negative result in isolated ACL tears.
    - Medial tibial plateau and meniscus abut convex surface of medial femoral condyle in flexion, limiting anterior tibial translation.
    - Isolated tears best identified with Lachman's test[487]
- In subacute tears, adhesions or attachments to PCL may result in decreased laxity.
- Partial ACL tears present in 24% to 39% of ACL injuries and frequently involve AMB
    - Commonly progress to complete tears within 1 year of initial injury[238]

Cruciate Ligaments

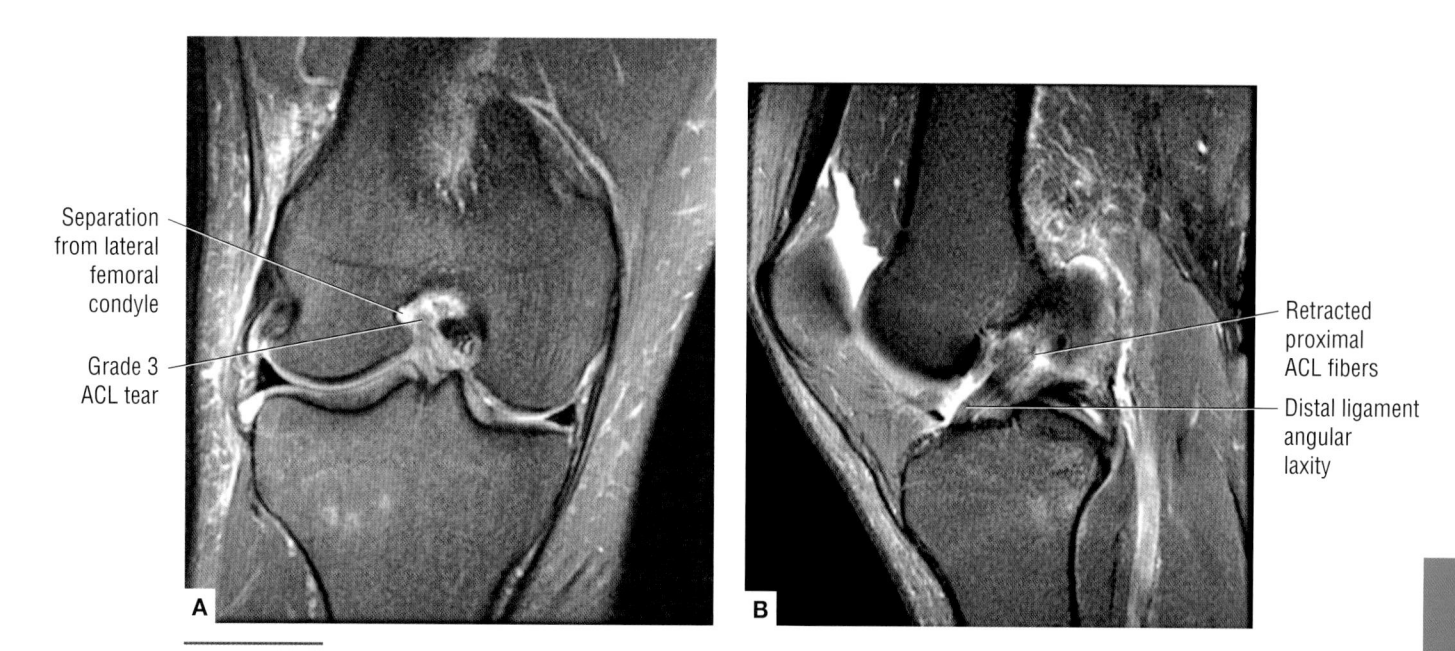

FIGURE 5.30 Coronal (**A**) and sagittal (**B**) FS PD FSE images show subacute ACL tear with angular deformity of the distal third fibers secondary to proximal grade 3 disruption.

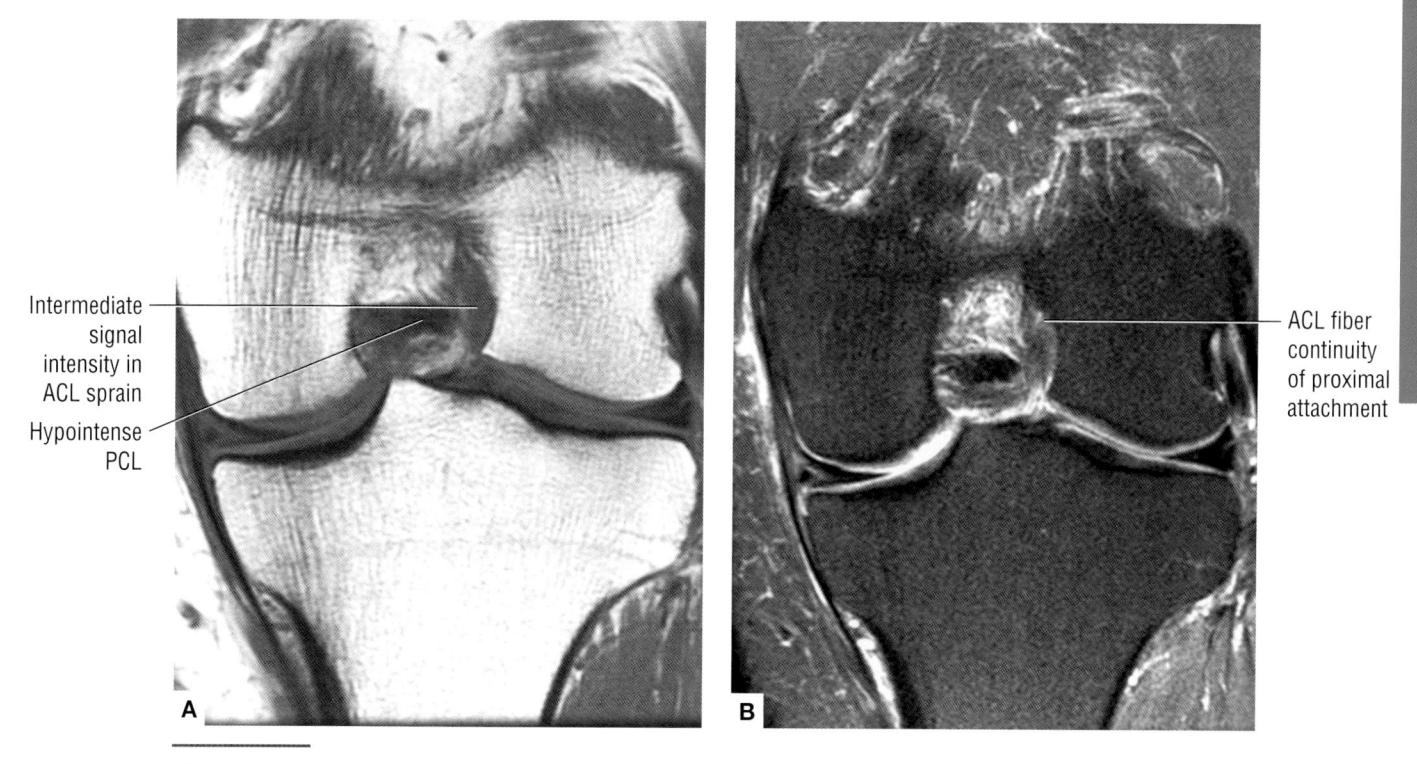

Labels (A): Separation from lateral femoral condyle; Grade 3 ACL tear
Labels (B): Retracted proximal ACL fibers; Distal ligament angular laxity

FIGURE 5.31 Grade 1 to 2 ACL sprain. (**A**) On PD FSE images, the ligament demonstrates intermediate signal intensity. (**B**) On corresponding FS PD FSE coronal images, the ligament demonstrates continuity. Loss of ligament hypointensity on a T1- or PD-weighted sequence is a sensitive sign of ligamentous strain or scarring. The FS PD sequence is specific for ligament continuity and can be used to differentiate a grade 2 from a grade 3 ACL sprain.

Labels (A): Intermediate signal intensity in ACL sprain; Hypointense PCL
Labels (B): ACL fiber continuity of proximal attachment

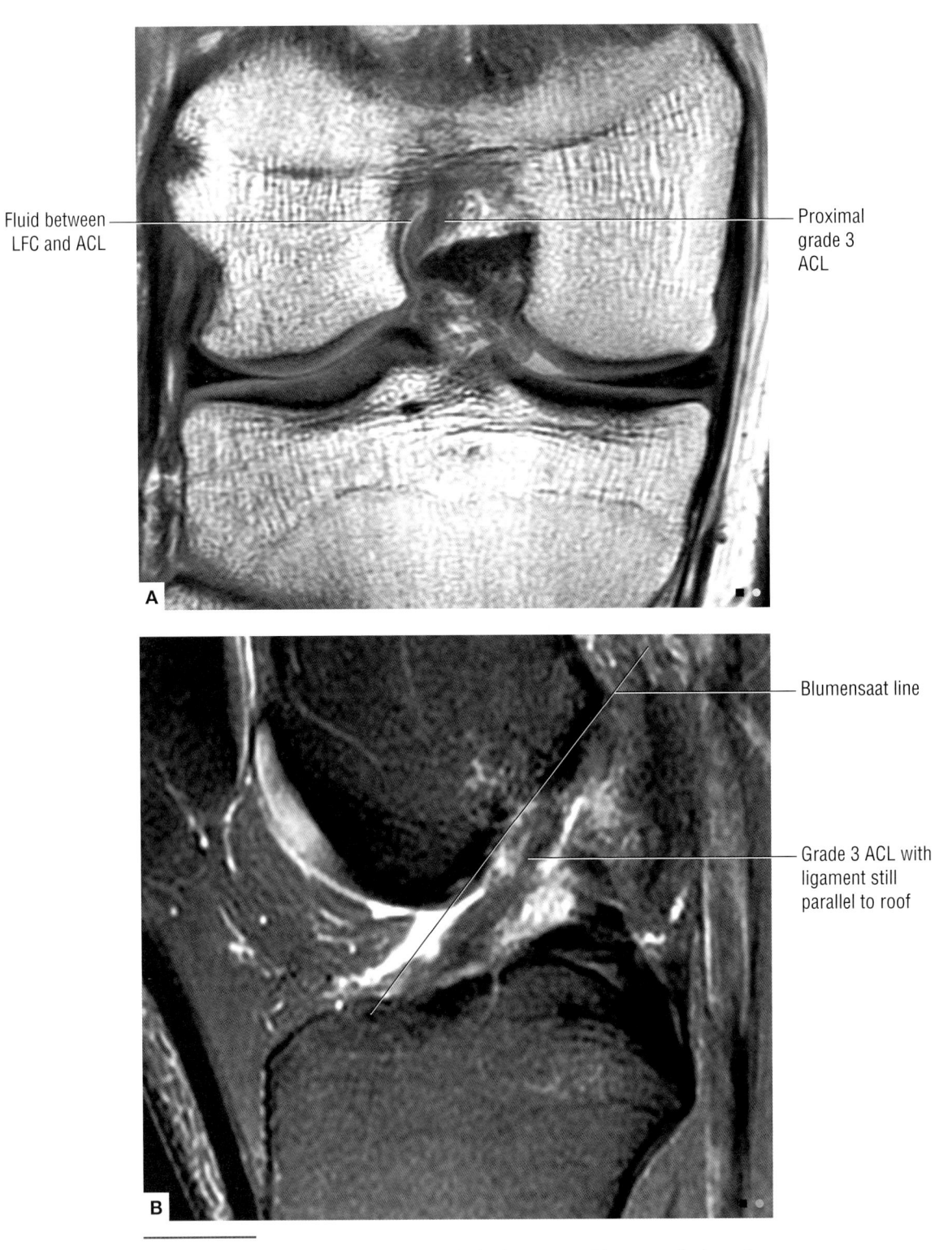

FIGURE 5.32 Grade 3 ACL tear with fluid interposed between the lateral femoral condyle (LFC) sidewall and proximal fibers. The ACL, although torn, remains relatively parallel to Blumensaat line and may be falsely interpreted as intact. Coronal PD (**A**) and sagittal FS PD FSE (**B**) images.

Cruciate Ligaments

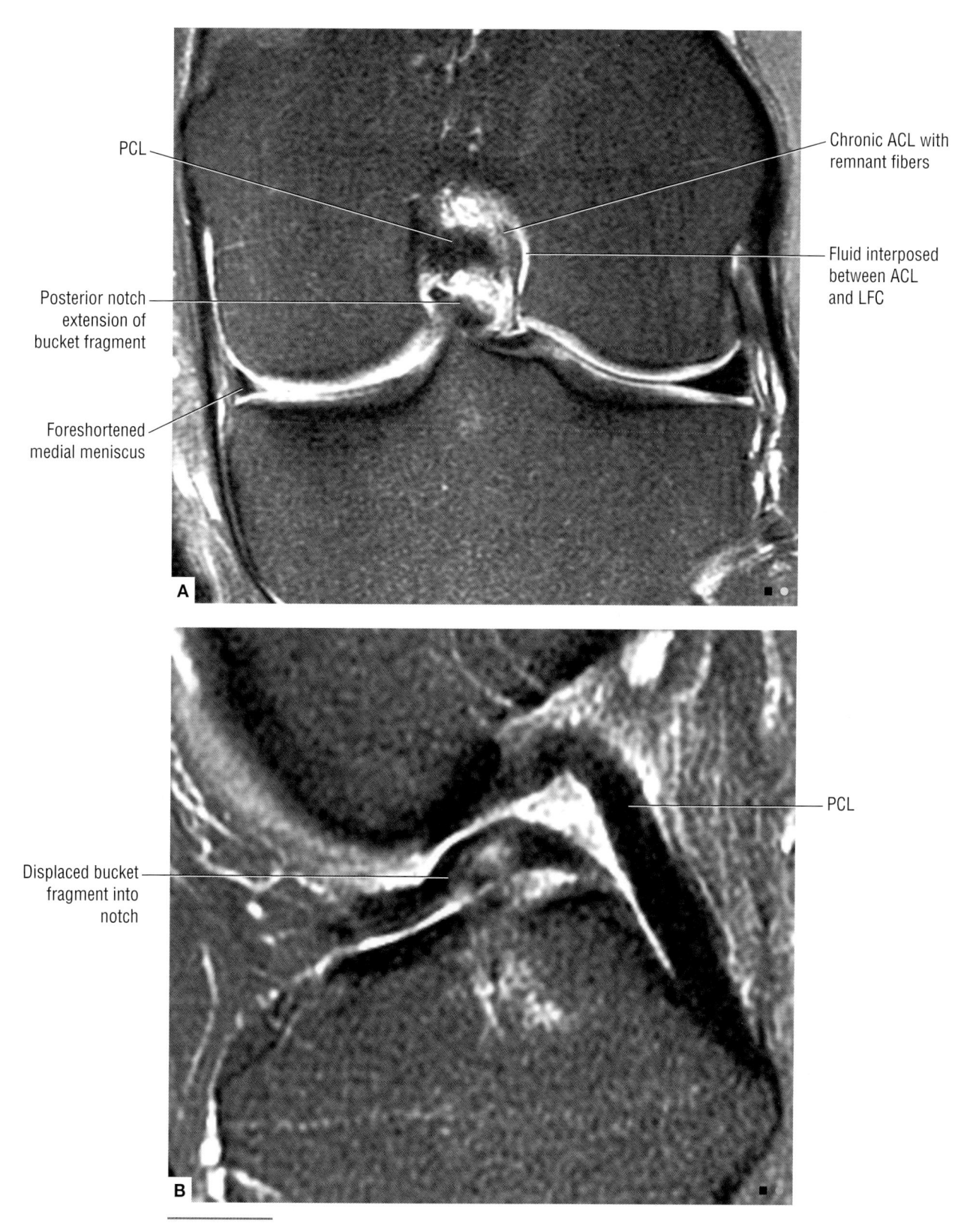

FIGURE 5.33 Association of medial meniscus bucket-handle tears with ACL-deficient knees. Coronal (**A**) and sagittal (**B**) FS PD FSE images.

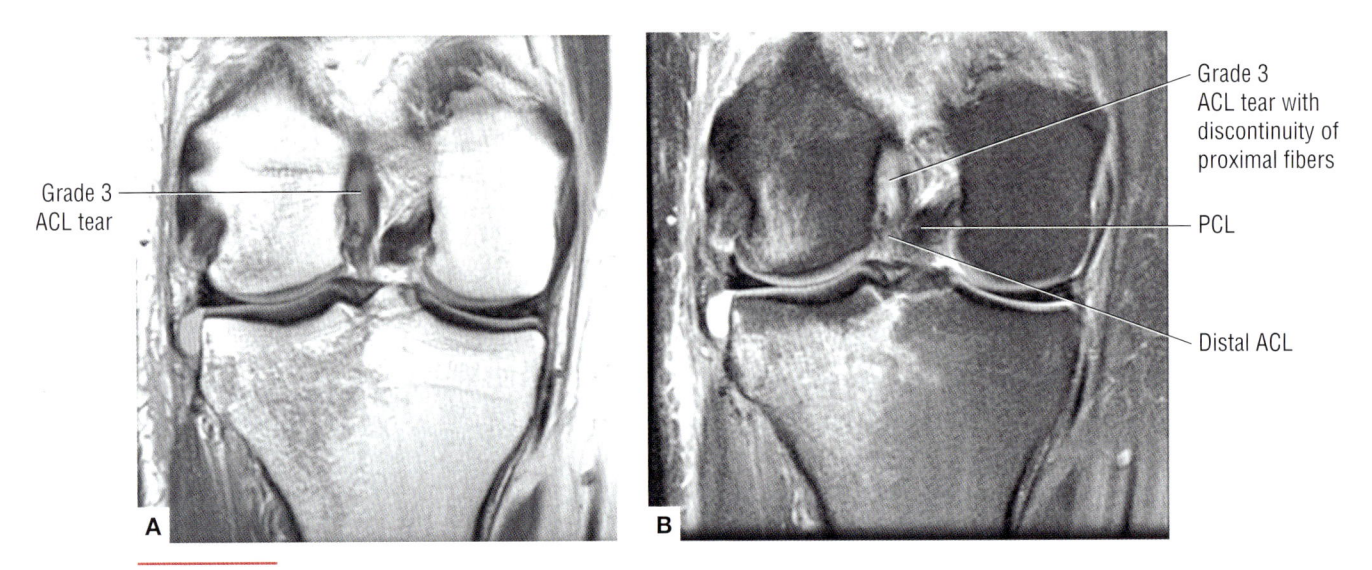

FIGURE 5.34 Grade 3 ACL tear with ligament discontinuity from the side wall of the lateral femoral condyle on coronal T1 (**A**) and coronal FS PD FSE (**B**) images.

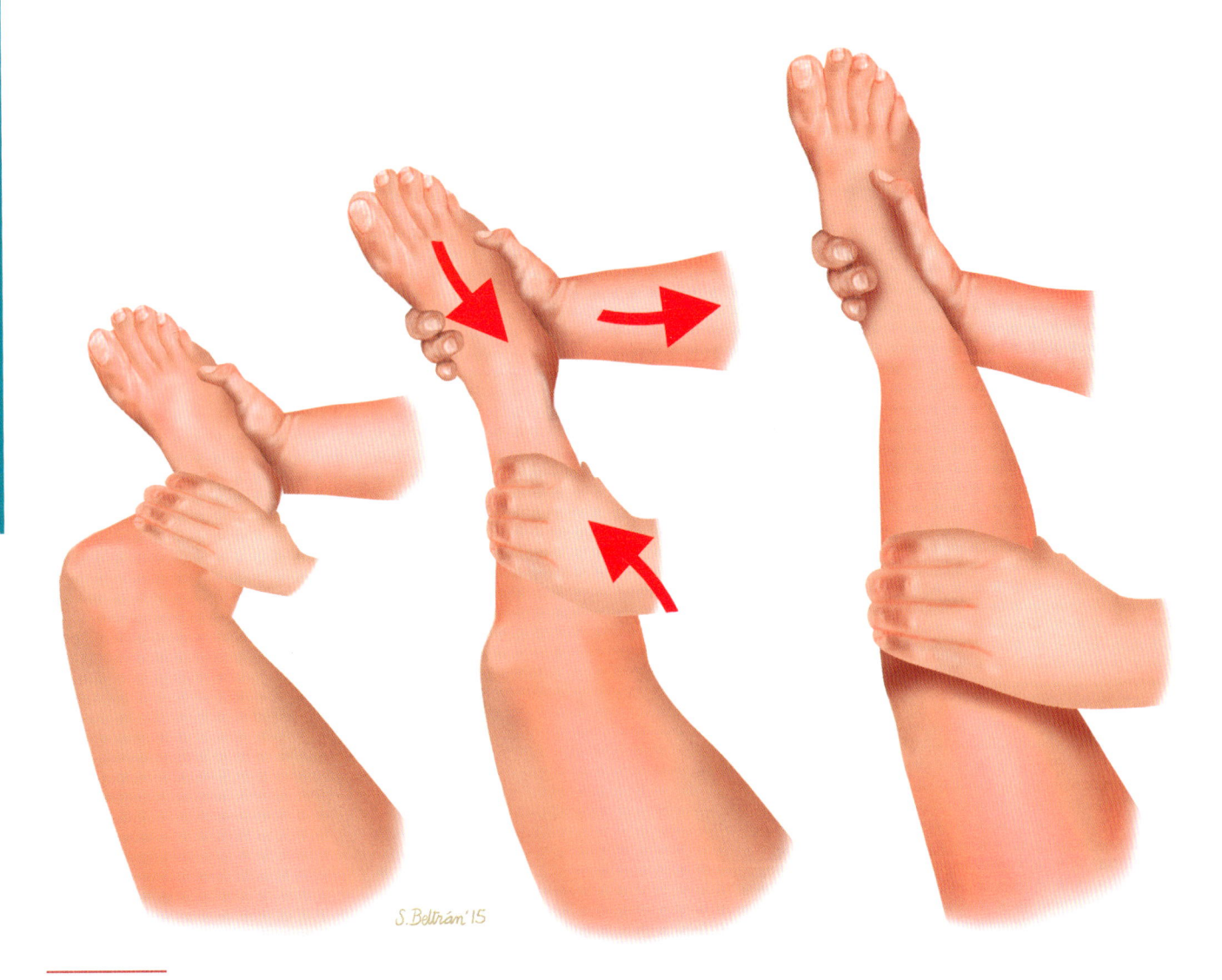

FIGURE 5.35 Pivot shift test to assess the rotational component of ACL competency. The pivot shift test is based on the lateral tibial plateau subluxing with flexion. The test requires an intact MCL with an applied valgus force, axial load, and internal rotation in extension and proceeding to flexion of the knee. In ACL deficiency, a reduction of the tibial subluxation occurs at approximately 30 degrees of flexion. The pivot shift test is best suited to be performed under anesthesia.

- KT-1000 and KT-2000 (Medmetric, San Diego, CA) arthrometers and knee laxity tester (Ortho System, Hayward, CA)
    - Instrument measurement systems that document tibial displacement by tracking tibial tubercle in relation to patella[223]
    - Knee subjected to 28- to 40-pound anterior load test → anterior tibial translation or subluxation 3mm greater in involved knee than uninvolved knee indicates ACL ligament disruption
- Limited intrinsic healing capacity of ACL possibly due to heterogeneity of collagen fibers or fibroblast function within synovial environment[148]
    - Poor capacity for healing may lead to chronic disability, including stretching of secondary knee restraints, articular cartilage destruction, and meniscal tearing.[238]

Diagnosis of ACL Injuries

- Majority by history and physical examination performed by experienced clinician
- Magnetic resonance (MR) arthrometer measurements usually used for confirmation
- MR used primarily to evaluate associated lesions (meniscal and chondral lesions in ACL-deficient knee)[21]
- Arthroscopy may be indicated when examination results are equivocal.
    - At arthroscopy, ACL may appear intact if proximal stump remains within intercondylar notch and adherent to PCL.[223]
    - Proper placement of knee to identify empty lateral wall and vertical strut signs (vertical orientation of retracted ligament fibers) can improve visualization of torn ACL.
- In an animal model study, positive MR findings for ACL pathology combined with normal arthroscopy did not necessarily represent a false-positive MR result; MR may reveal intrasubstance tears not detected on arthroscopy.[118]

Radiography and Arthrography

- Findings of acute ACL injuries on routine radiography
  - Soft tissue swelling and joint effusions
  - Irregularity in contour of Hoffa's fat pad on lateral projection (similar to irregular fat-pad sign on sagittal MR images in presence of synovitis)
    - Further evaluated by comparison of density of irregular free edge of the fat pad in contrast to adjacent fluid
  - Synovitis results from hemarthrosis, a synovial irritant.
    - Other causes of acute hemarthrosis must be considered (e.g., patellar dislocation and osteochondral fractures).
    - Fractures[393]
  - Avulsion of anterior tibial eminence
  - Lateral tibial rim (Segond) fracture
  - Posterior fracture of lateral tibial plateau
  - Osteochondral fracture of the lateral femoral condyle[148]
- Findings of acute ACL injuries on arthrography
  - ACL only indirectly assessed by observing air and contrast along reflected synovial surface
  - Absent or wavy anterior synovial surface on lateral projection
  - Normal ligamentum mucosum may be mistaken for intact ACL
  - Arthrographic findings can be subtle, and proper examination requires a high level of technical experience to produce acceptable accuracy rates.[393]

Cruciate Ligaments

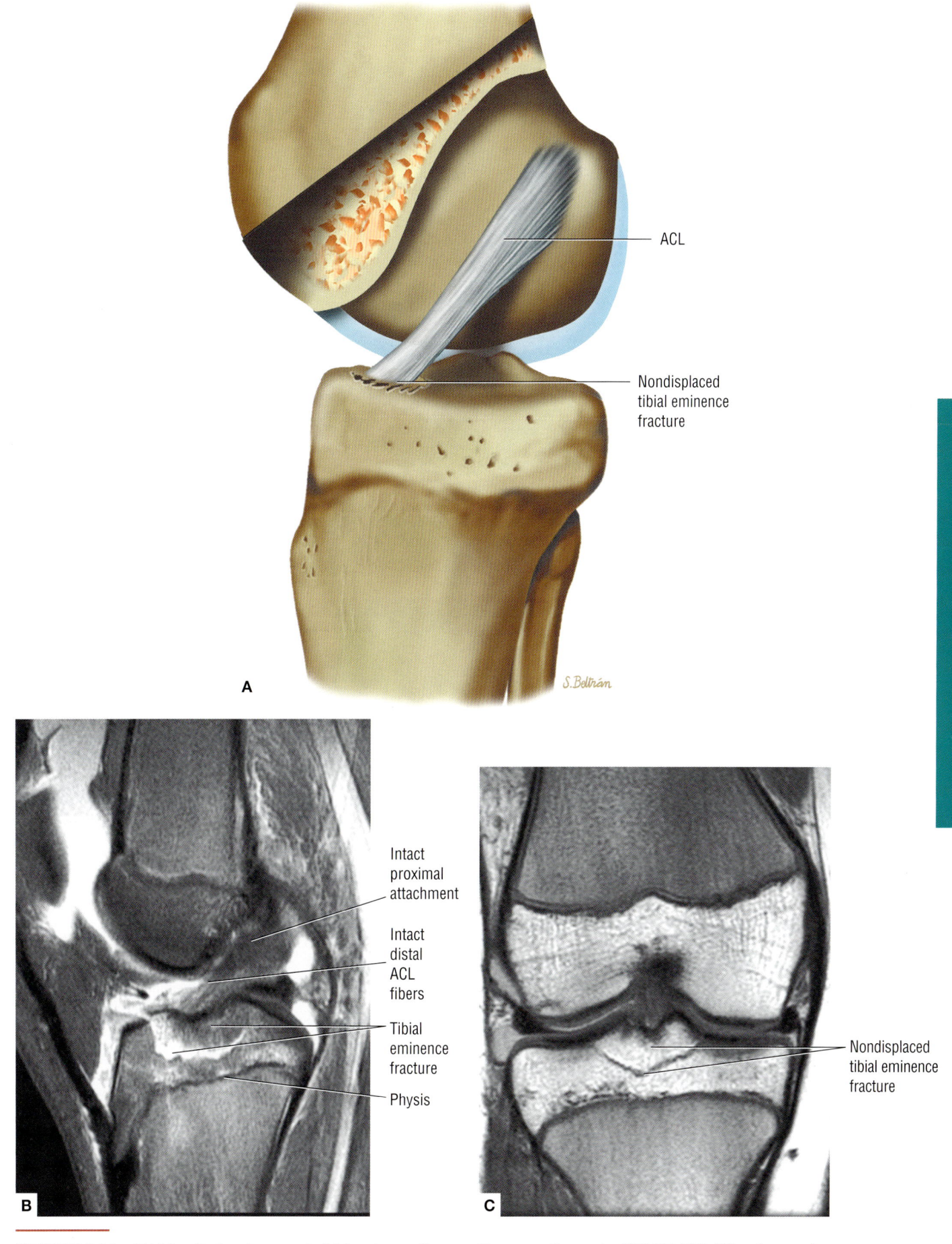

FIGURE 5.36 (**A**) Nondisplaced or type I tibial eminence fracture. Corresponding sagittal FS PD FSE (**B**) and coronal T1-weighted (**C**) images.

Avulsed ACL footprint

Eminence fracture

Intact ACL fibers

Displaced tibial eminence fracture at ACL insertion

Secondary trabecular fracture extension

Posterior capsule rupture

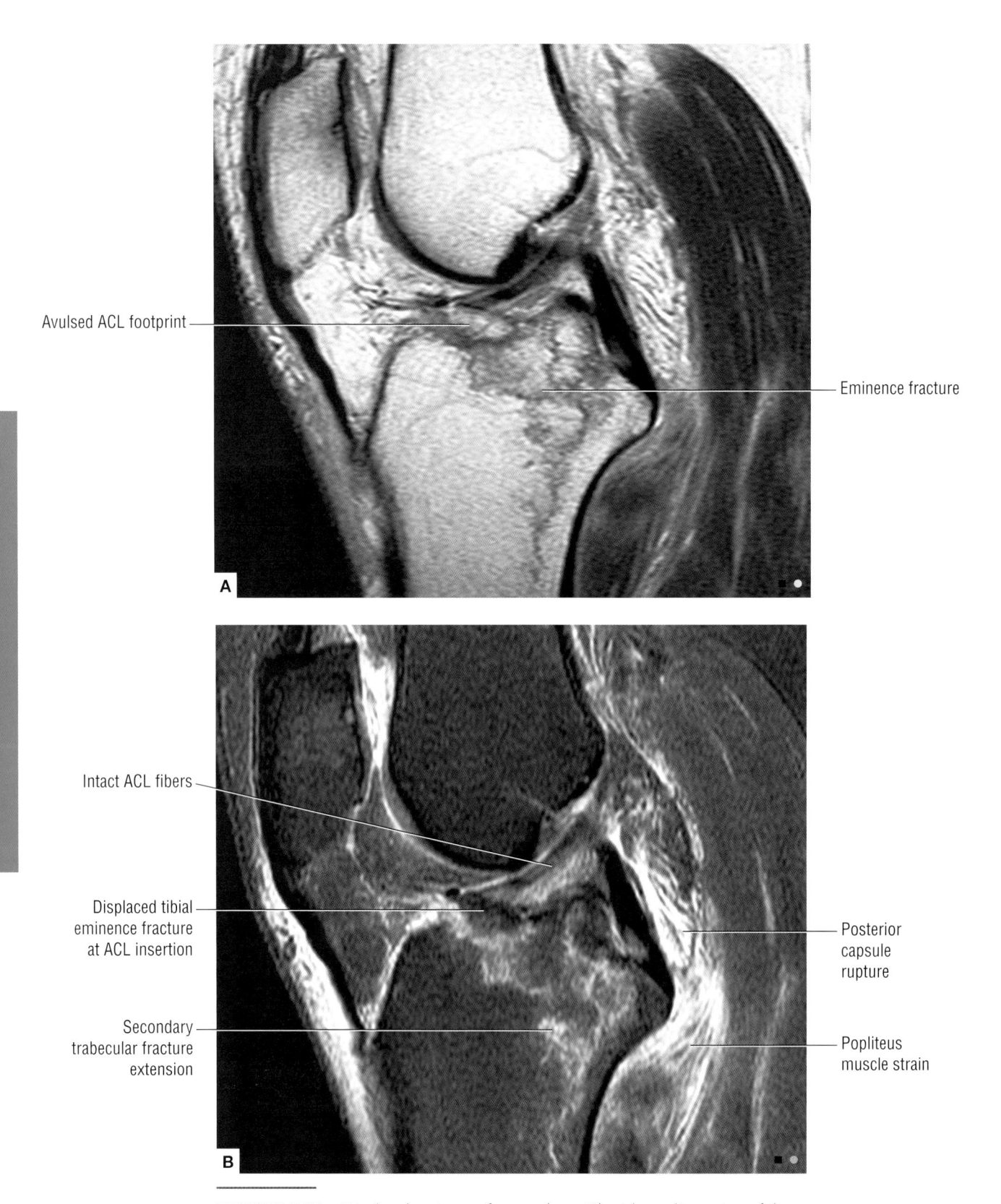

Popliteus muscle strain

FIGURE 5.37 Displaced eminence fracture (type II) without disruption of the ACL bundles from the tibial footprint. Sagittal PD (**A**) and FS PD FSE (**B**) images.

Cruciate Ligaments

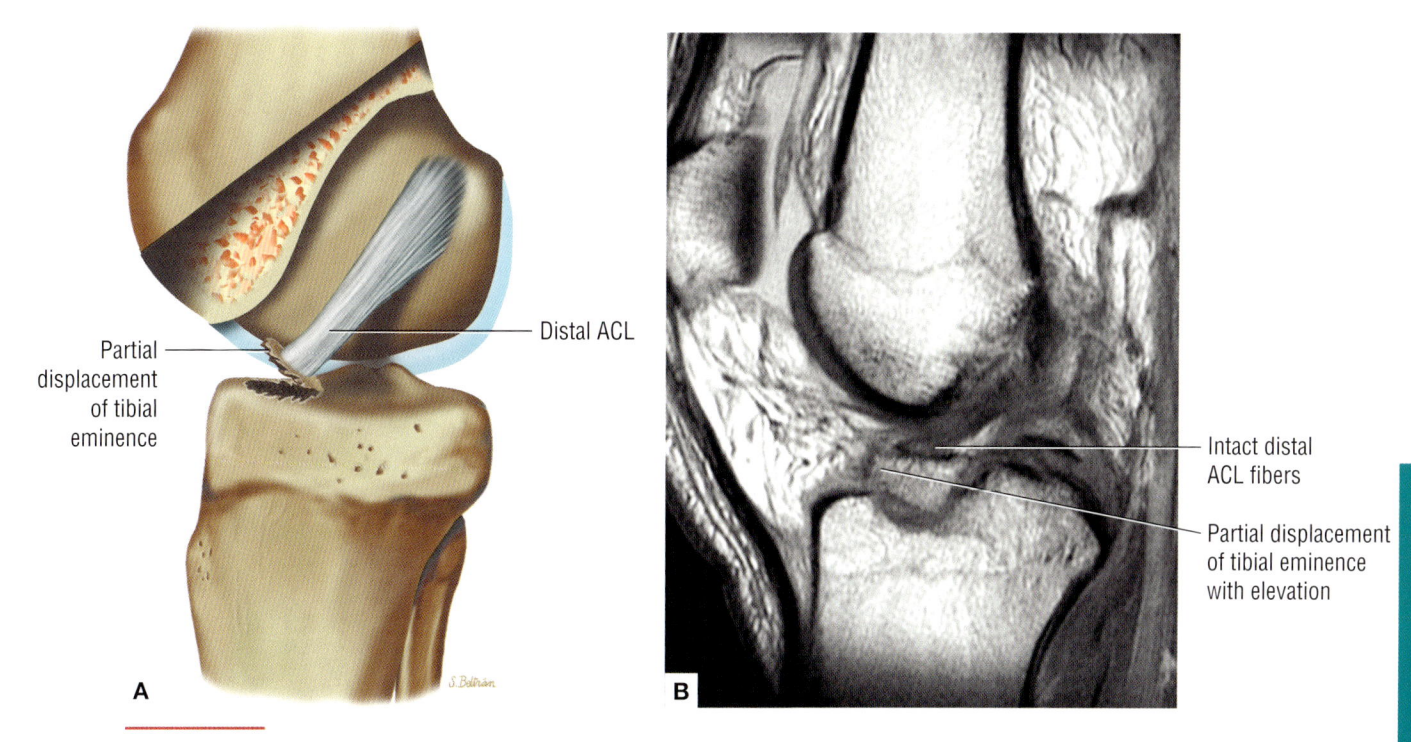

FIGURE 5.38 (**A**) Partially displaced or type II tibial eminence fracture with anterior osseous elevation. Corresponding sagittal PD FSE image (**B**).

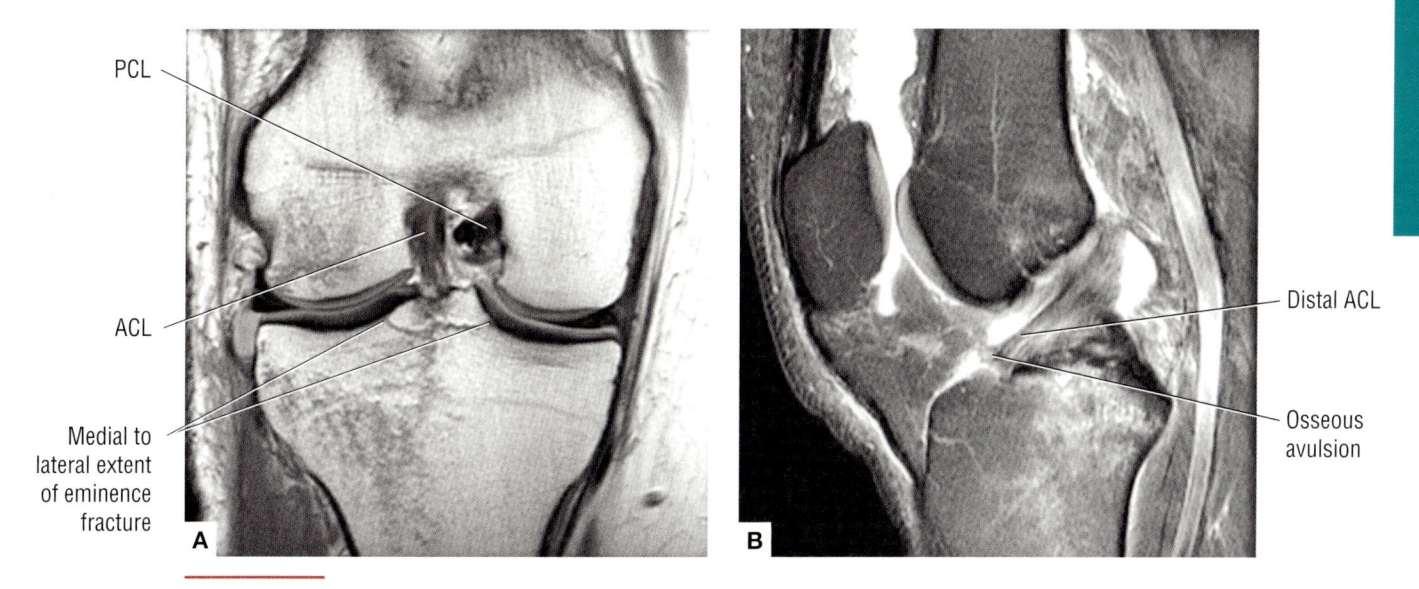

FIGURE 5.39 Type II tibial eminence fracture. Both coronal (**A**) and sagittal (**B**) images are used for accurate classification of the extent of the fracture. Medial-to-lateral extension across the eminence is best appreciated on the coronal image. (**A**) T1-weighted FSE coronal image. (**B**) FS PD FSE sagittal image.

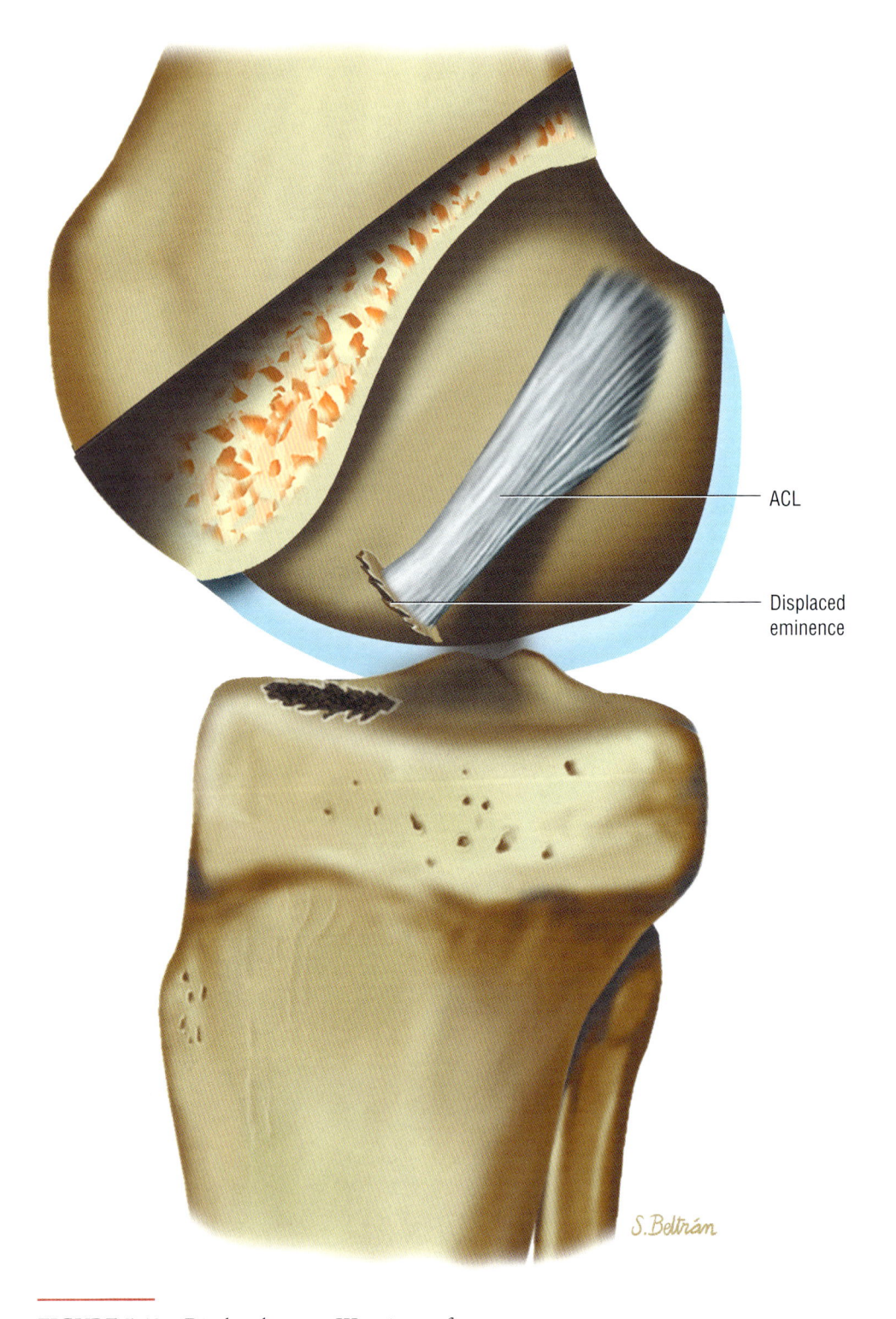

FIGURE 5.40 Displaced or type III eminence fracture.

Cruciate Ligaments

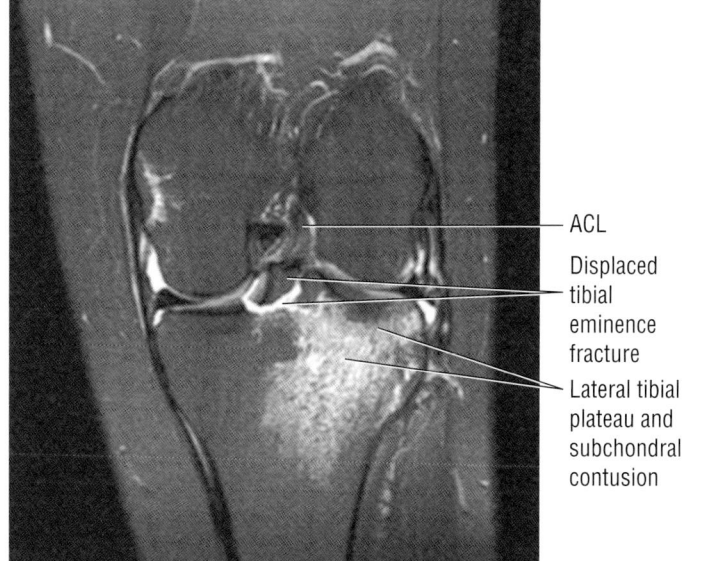

FIGURE 5.41 FS PD FSE coronal image demonstrating complete fragment elevation and rotation.

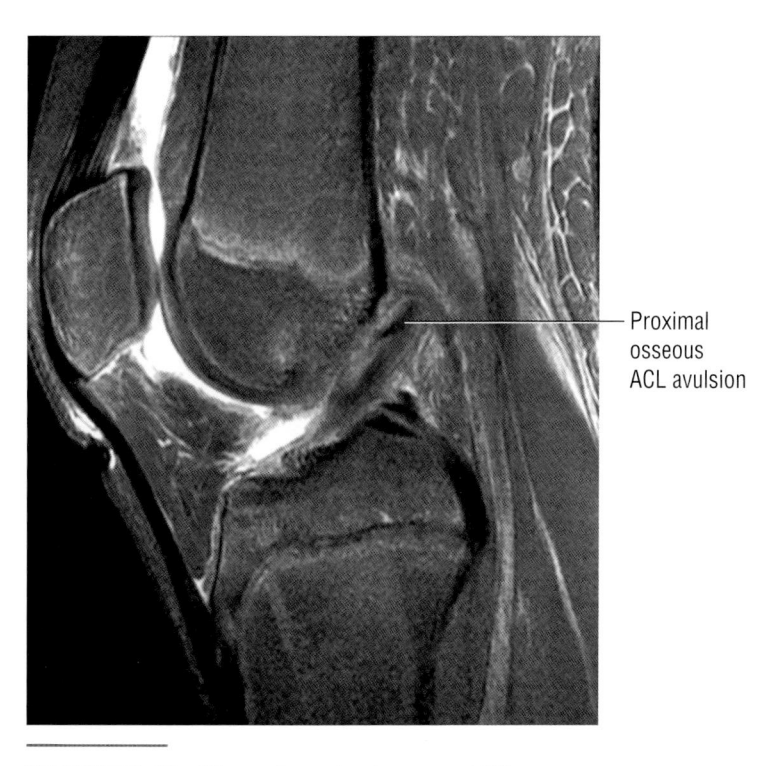

FIGURE 5.42 Unusual proximal osseous ACL avulsion (sagittal FS PD FSE image).

Magnetic Resonance Imaging

Key Concepts

- ACL Imaging
    - Sagittal images oriented parallel to lateral femoral condylar wall (optimizes ligament visualization in sagittal plane)
    - Axial image used as landmark to prescribe sagittal oblique plane
    - Elongation of anterior-to-posterior aspect of lateral femoral condyle is associated with excessive external rotation of the knee and may compromise accurate interpretation of the lateral meniscus.

MR Techniques for ACL Imaging

- For routine MR examinations, position the knee in 10 to 15 degrees of external rotation (to orient ACL with sagittal imaging plane)
    - Less critical as section thickness decreases (≤4mm)
- Entire sagittal sequence performed in oblique sagittal plane relatively parallel to orientation of ACL as determined on an axial image
    - Sagittal plane prescribed parallel to lateral femoral condylar wall at the level where the osseous condyles fuse together to bridge the intercondylar roof
- Excessive external rotation results in elongation of anterior-to-posterior dimensions of femoral condyles and limits accurate imaging of menisci.
- Excessive internal rotation may increase partial volume effect of proximal ACL attachment with lateral femoral condyle and may produce a pseudomass.
    - Pseudomass does not appear on corresponding coronal or axial images and does not demonstrate increased T2 signal intensity.[238]
- We routinely use axial, sagittal, and coronal plane images to evaluate the ACL.
    - Sagittal scans best demonstrate femoral and tibial attachments on one or two images and represent the primary plane for ACL analysis.
        - Typically 3- to 4-mm slice thickness
    - Axial and coronal scans particularly useful in demonstrating relation of proximal ACL attachment to medial aspect of the lateral femoral condyle
        - Partial volume effect minimized with thin sections

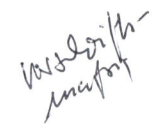

Cruciate Ligaments

- Properly obliqued sagittal images important in postoperative evaluation of ACL reconstruction
    - Coronal plane (rather than the axial plane) used as localizer for the course of the neoligament
- T1- and T2-weighted spin-echo or PD- and T2-weighted spin-echo images (to evaluate signal intensity changes in acute and subacute ACL injuries)
- T2*-weighted gradient echo (GRE) or FS PD-weighted FSE images (to demonstrate morphology and signal intensity changes within the ACL)
    - FS PD-weighted FSE excellent for demonstrating ACL contour, especially in ligament disruption, but may not demonstrate same degree of high signal intensity as shown on GRE
    - In postoperative imaging, PD-weighted FSE images have less magnetic susceptibility artifact than T2*-weighted scans.
    - PD FSE metal suppression sequences use higher bandwidth and echo train to minimize micrometallic artifact.
- All routine protocols include some form of T2 weighting (conventional or FSE) in all three planes to maximize sensitivity and specificity.
- T1-weighted images inadequate to appreciate edema and hemorrhage in disrupted ligament

Normal ACL Imaging Characteristics

- Band of low signal intensity on all three image planes with separate fiber striations visible near attachment points
- In full knee extension, ACL appears as 3- to 4-mm thick, single, low-signal band with straight or taut anterior margin.[238]
- Changing from extension to flexion is associated with decrease in signal intensity of cruciate ligaments.[448]
- Applied tension → decreased ACL signal intensity; release of tension → reciprocal increase in signal intensity
    - May explain higher signal intensity in ACL compared with PCL, because evaluations are performed in extension
- ACL may show more lax configuration with knee flexion, although biomechanically, the AMB tightens and the PLB loosens.

- On sagittal images, ACL parallels the orientation of the intercondylar roof.

- ACL may not be displayed in its entire course on a single sagittal image due to obliquity.
    - Can be minimized by proper oblique sagittal graphic prescription

- Individual low T1 fiber bundles may be separated by linear intermediate to bright T1 stripes believed to represent fat and synovium, usually at the tibial attachment.[238]

- AMB forms anterior border of the ACL.

- PLB represents the bulk of the ACL and may display intermediate T1 signal intensity.

- Axial plane helpful in spatially identifying partial tears corresponding to AMB and PLB

- Normal ACL fibers demonstrate low signal intensity on conventional T2, FS PD-weighted FSE, and T2*-weighted images.
    - Areas of eosinophilic degeneration in older persons may be visualized as regions of intermediate signal intensity.[189]

- Independent of partial volume effect, ACL may demonstrate greater signal intensity than the homogeneously low-signal-intensity PCL on T1-, conventional T2-, FSE PD-, and T2*-weighted images.

- Ligamentum mucosum, or infrapatellar plica, arises from the superior condylar notch, lies anterior to the ACL, and may be seen as distinct structure on MR.

- Coronal plane assessment of the ACL is more accurate than using the sagittal plane as the primary diagnostic plane of section (because the sagittal images usually obliquely section the ACL).
    - Identify hypointense signal in the proximal half of the AM and PL bundle in the coronal plane using either a T1 or PD (more commonly used) sequence. If intermediate signal in the ACL in this location is not normal, then use the corresponding fluid sensitive sequence to establish ligament continuity or lack of to the LFC and normal fiber striations.
    - Identify selective pathology of either the AM or PL bundle.

ACL Tears

Key Concepts

- Primary Signs
    - Abnormal ligament course (abnormal Blumensaat angle)
    - Abnormal ligament signal intensity (coronal images should be used in conjunction with sagittal images to compensate for segmental visualization in the sagittal plane)
    - Ligament discontinuity
- Secondary Signs
    - Lateral compartment osseous contusions (posterolateral tibial plateau is most specific)
    - Posteromedial tibial plateau contusion or fracture
    - Anterior tibial displacement (assessed in the lateral aspect of the lateral compartment)
    - Uncovered posterior horn lateral meniscus
    - Posterior cruciate line and angle
- Coronal T1 and PD FSE images identify increased signal intensity within ACL sprain or complete tear.
- Intact ligament remains hypointense and maintains ligamentous continuity on FS PD FSE coronal images on at least one image posterior to and including the plane of the MCL.
- Chronic ACL tears demonstrate resolution of osseous contusions, effusions, synovitis, and ligamentous hyperintensity (characteristic of acute injuries) unless seen in setting of an acute on chronic injury.
- Mucoid degeneration and ACL or intercondylar notch cysts may be symptomatic (restricted range of motion) without direct evidence of ACL sprain or partial tear.

ACL Tears

- Primary and accurate signs of ACL tear include discontinuity of the ACL and abnormal Blumensaat angle.[397,486]
    - Blumensaat line courses parallel to roof of the intercondylar notch (posterior surface of the femur).
    - Blumensaat angle is formed by the Blumensaat line and a line along the margin (including the distal portion) of the ACL.[276]
        - Negative (normal) Blumensaat angle: apex of angle directed superiorly
        - Positive (abnormal) Blumensaat angle: apex of angle directed inferiorly
- Other predictors of ACL tear
    - Discontinuity of ACL in one plane
    - Disruption of fascicles
    - Bone contusions on weight-bearing surface of the lateral femoral condyle and posterolateral tibial plateau (with or without posteromedial tibial plateau contusion)
    - Buckling of the PCL
    - Positive PCL sign or PCL angle
        - Positive PCL sign: failure of a line drawn along the posterior PCL on sagittal images to intersect the medullary cavity within 5cm of the distal femur
        - Positive PCL angle: decrease in normal obtuse shape of angle formed between lines drawn through the proximal and distal portions of the PCL (due to anterior tibial translation in ACL tears)
    - Positive posterior femoral line sign: failure of a line drawn at a 45-degree angle from the posterosuperior corner of the Blumensaat angle to intersect the flat portion of the proximal tibial surface or to intersect a point within 5cm of its posterior margin[312,397]
- Absence of secondary or indirect signs does not exclude ACL tear.[44]
    - Primary and secondary findings of ACL tears have shown high specificity in adult and pediatric populations.[486]
- Most accurate assessment for ACL tears requires combined use of axial, coronal, and sagittal images.[139]

Appearance of ACL in Acute Injury

- Loss of ligament continuity associated with wavy or lax contour (including posterior bowing or concavity of the anterior margin)
- More horizontal orientation of ACL on sagittal images
- Increased signal intensity of ACL on T2-weighted, FS PD FSE, or T2*-weighted images, although changes in signal intensity less pronounced with FSE or FS FSE techniques
    - Increased signal intensity on T2- or FS PD-weighted FSE images usually identified at femoral attachment on coronal images
    - Axial images excellent for showing fluid within proximal ligament fibers or between torn ACL and the lateral femoral condyle sidewall
    - Axial images especially helpful in evaluating injuries in skiers, in whom proximal ACL tears are more common compared with mid-substance distributions in nonskiers[238]
- Edematous soft tissue mass may be seen in region of torn fibers.[397]
- Widening of entire ligament associated with interstitial tear pattern
    - Interstitial disruption shows variable increases in T2 signal intensity.[238]
- Acute or focal angular deformity of ACL usually identified in association with discontinuous fibers
- Coronal plane particularly useful for differentiating grades of ACL injury, especially when sagittal images display ACL fibers only segmentally.
    - ACL is abnormal if fibers show intermediate signal intensity with or without loss of fiber striation on T1- or PD-weighted coronal images (assessed in same coronal plane as the MCL, where the femoral condyles fuse together and bridge the intercondylar roof).
    - Normal ACL should also be visualized on at least one coronal image posterior to this level.
    - Corresponding FS PD FSE coronal images must demonstrate ligament continuity to exclude a grade 3 ACL tear.
    - Coronal plane assessment increases MR specificity in distinguishing partial from complete ACL tears.

- Associated osseous injuries in acute ACL tears
    - Avulsions of the tibial intercondylar eminence occur in 5% of patients.
        - Tibial eminence fractures may be nondisplaced, partially displaced with anterior segment elevation, or completely displaced.
        - Careful evaluation of marrow signal on T1 or GRE images is important for minimally displaced or nondisplaced fractures.
        - Avulsion injuries might be missed on T2- or FS PD-weighted FSE images. Osseous avulsions from the femoral condyle are unusual.
    - Anterior subluxation or displacement of the tibia on lateral sagittal images is a secondary sign of anterolateral instability.[495]
        - Anterior drawer, or more properly Lachman's sign (because the knee is in extension), is dependent on degree of knee flexion, positioning, and design of extremity coil.
        - Limited by lack of comparison with the contralateral knee
        - Vertical line drawn at a tangent to the posterolateral femoral condyle should intersect the posterolateral tibial plateau if ACL is intact.
        - Anterior tibial subluxation of greater than 7mm has been reported in ACL tears (but is secondary sign only).[495]
        - Anterior subluxation in the medial compartment seen only with significant anterior translation of the tibia
        - Coronal visualization of the lateral collateral ligament (LCL) may be improved as the tibia translates anteriorly.
- Hemarthrosis associated with acute ACL tears
    - Characterized by synovitis with irregular free concave edge of Hoffa's infrapatellar fat pad
    - Occurs most often in complete acute ACL disruptions but may be present in partial tears
    - Ligament edema or hemorrhage may be associated with blurring of cruciate fascicles.
    - Fluid within the substance of the ACL or occupying the extrasynovial triangular space between the cruciate ligaments is abnormal.[277]

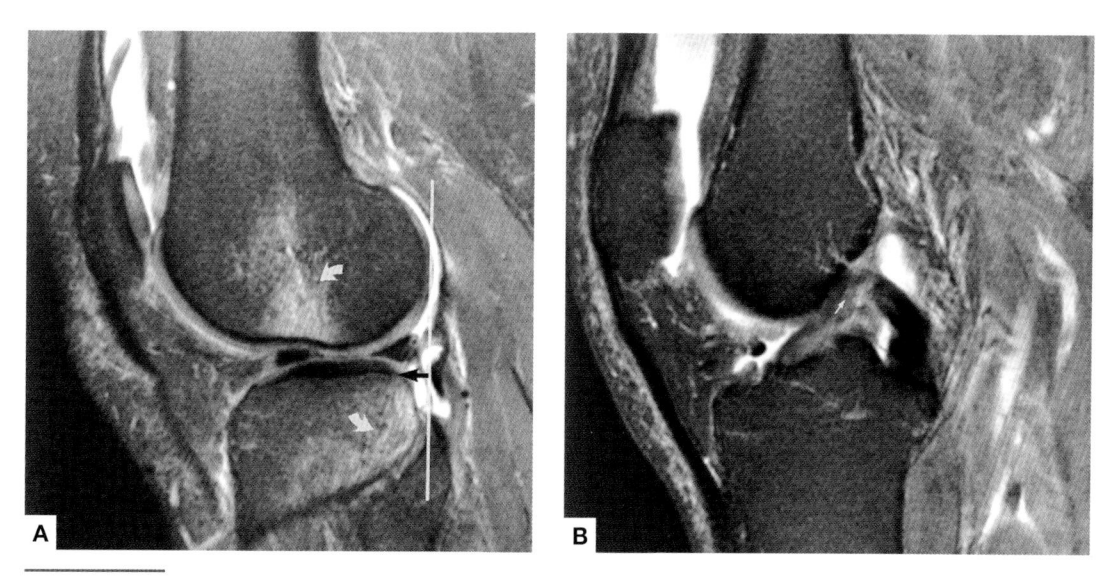

FIGURE 5.43 An acute ACL tear. (**A**) An MR anterior drawer sign (specifically, Lachman's sign) on an FS T2-weighted FSE sagittal image. Note anterior displacement of the lateral tibial plateau (*straight arrow*) relative to a plumb line (*long white line*) extrapolated from the posterior lateral femoral condyle. Hyperintense bone contusions (*curved arrows*) are shown in the lateral femoral condyle and posterior lateral tibial plateau. (**B**) An associated ACL tear (*arrow*) is shown on an FS PD-weighted FSE sagittal image.

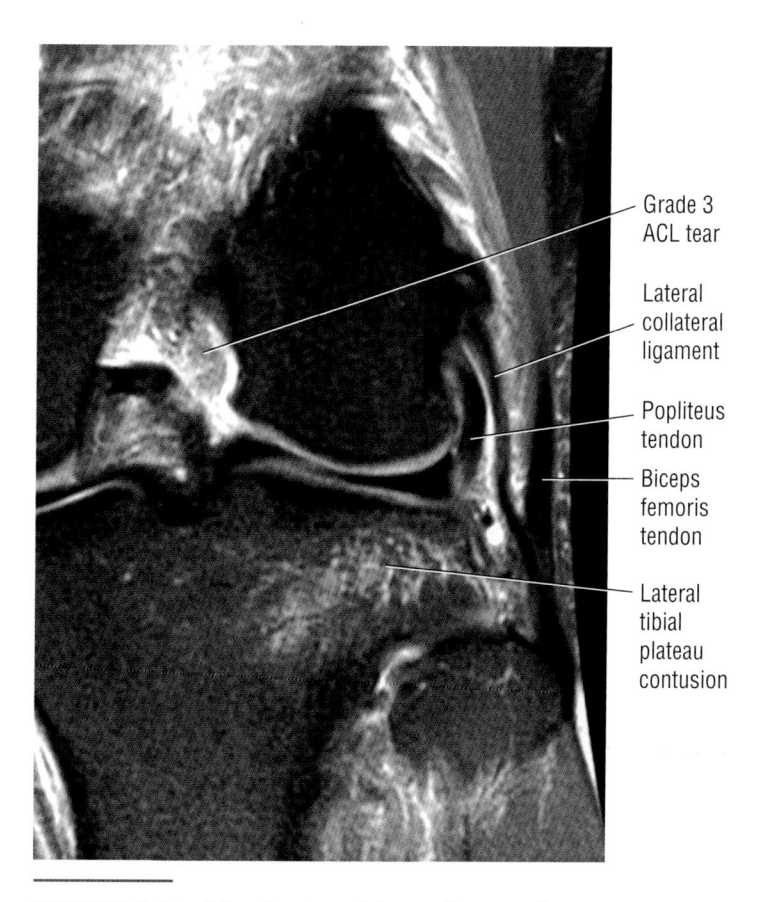

FIGURE 5.44 Visualization of the popliteus tendon, LCL, and biceps femoris on a single coronal image. Anterior translation of the tibia associated with an acute ACL disruption reorients the LCL into a more coronal course (coronal FS PD FSE).

- **Acute ACL stump entrapment**
    - May contribute to decrease or block to knee extension after rupture of the ACL[199]
    - Type 1: nodular mass at anterior aspect of the intercondylar notch
        - Involves proximal third of ACL and is associated with fibrosis at the free end of the stump, creating a bulbous configuration susceptible to anterior recess entrapment
    - Type 2: discrete and well-defined tongue-like extension of ACL stump associated with angulation
        - Completely displaced stump lies out of and anterior to the intercondylar notch in the anterior joint recess posterior to Hoffa's fat pad.
        - Caused by tears at the proximal femoral attachment, which can produce a long distal stump susceptible to anterior displacement and folding
    - Cyclops lesion, which may represent the end stage of a displaced ACL stump, presents with complete discontinuity of the ACL tibial attachment.
- **Partial ACL tears**
    - Discrete area or focus of increased signal intensity within the substance of the ACL
        - Bulk of ligament appears intact with a relatively normal axis, but there may be localized angulation of the ligament at the site of fiber disruption.[238]
    - ACL tears involving less than 25% of the substance associated with more favorable clinical outcome than tears involving 50% or more, which predispose to ACL deficiency and reinjury[356,492]
    - Accurate assessment more difficult than for complete tears
    - Difficult to grade progressive degrees of partial tears and accurately correlate with clinical grading of ACL pathology
        - Intraligamentous injury without a change in ligament length is considered a grade 1 ACL injury.
        - Partial ACL tear corresponds to grade 2 ligament injury as defined by the American Medical Association Ligament Injury Classification System (incomplete tears with a small increase in laxity).[80,286]

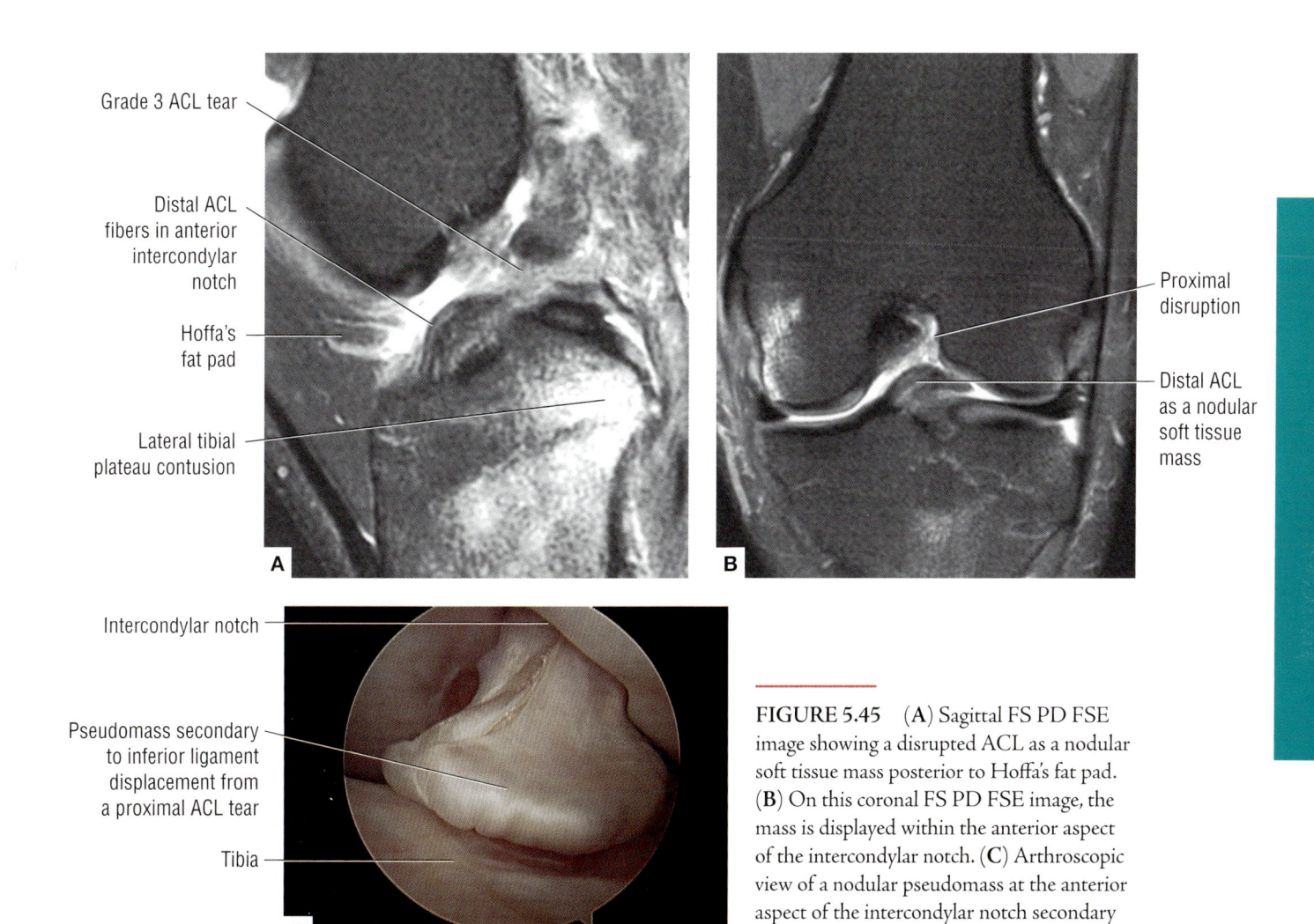

Cruciate Ligaments 445

FIGURE 5.45 (**A**) Sagittal FS PD FSE image showing a disrupted ACL as a nodular soft tissue mass posterior to Hoffa's fat pad. (**B**) On this coronal FS PD FSE image, the mass is displayed within the anterior aspect of the intercondylar notch. (**C**) Arthroscopic view of a nodular pseudomass at the anterior aspect of the intercondylar notch secondary to a more proximal ACL tear.

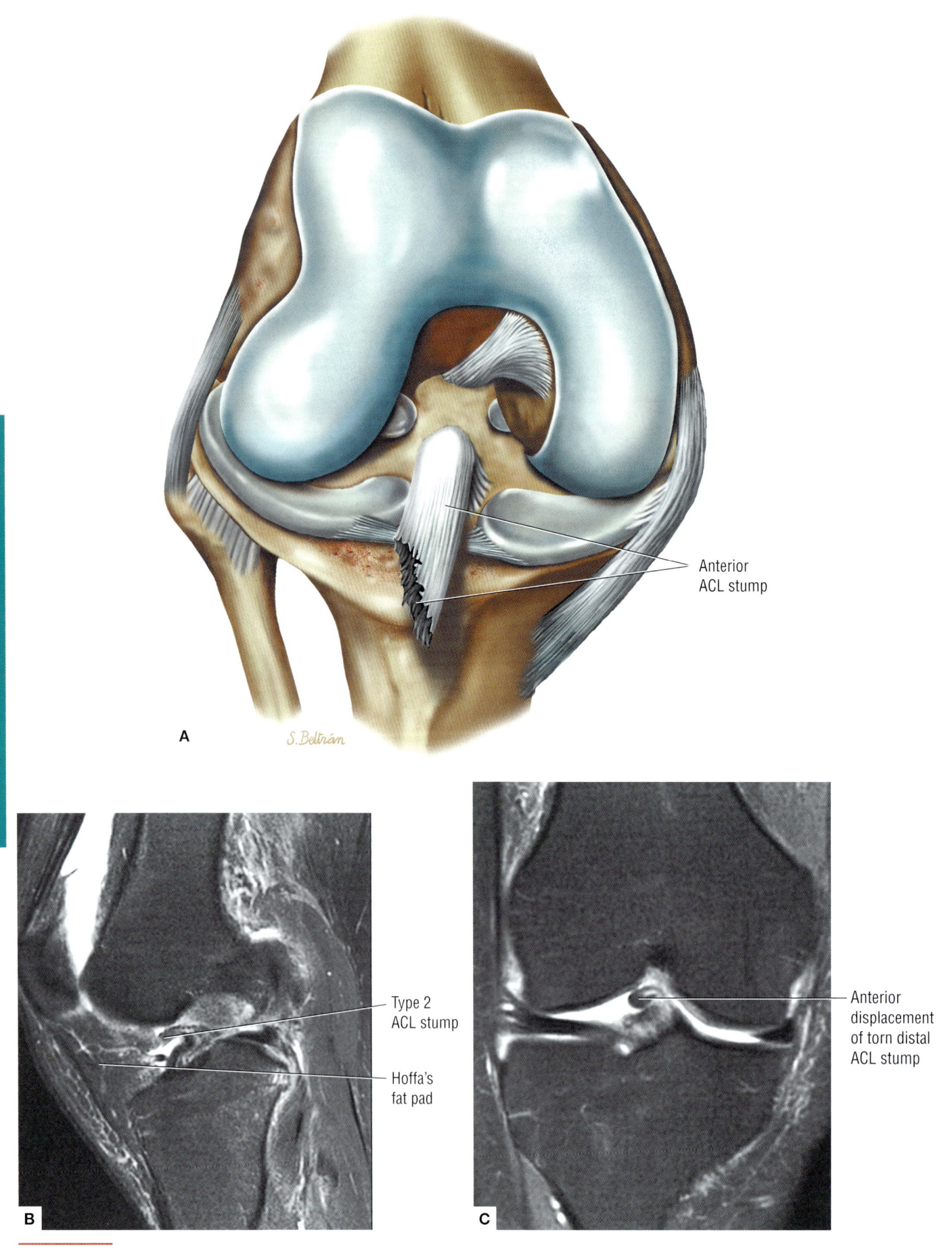

FIGURE 5.46 (**A**) Type 2 stump with a long distal segment of ligament displaced anteriorly. Ligament folding produces stump entrapment seen on corresponding FS PD FSE sagittal (**B**) and coronal (**C**) images.

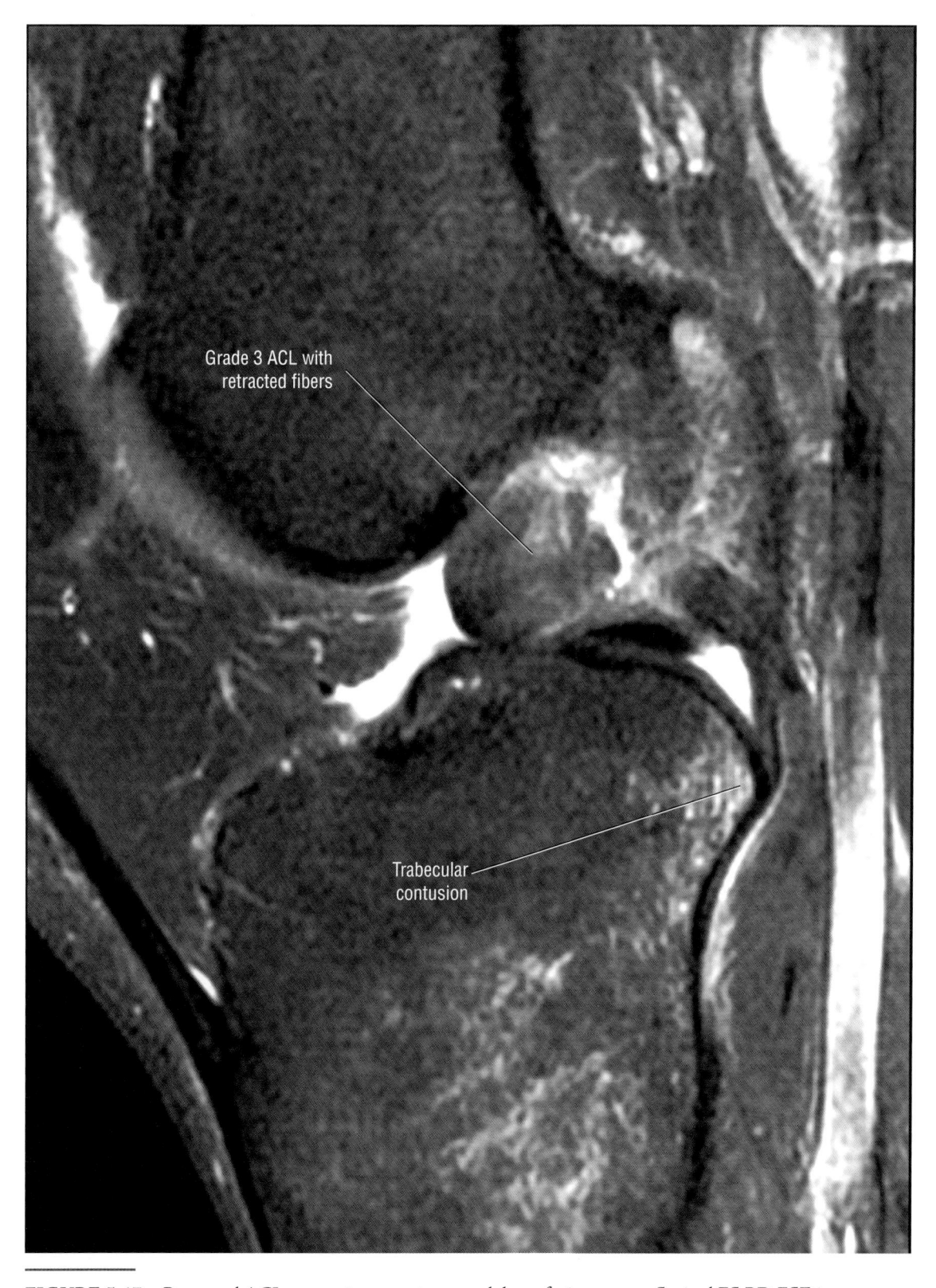

FIGURE 5.47 Retracted ACL presenting as an intercondylar soft tissue mass. Sagittal FS PD FSE image.

- Arthroscopy may not be as sensitive as MR to partial intrasubstance tears.[118]

- Specific designation of AMB versus PLB tears frequently not possible

- Difficulty in detecting partial ACL tears due to nonspecificity of intrasubstance abnormal signal intensity with concomitant morphology[492]

    - Abnormal signal intensity alone associated with either ligamentous sprain or disruption of collagen fibers,[189] which may remain arthroscopically occult

    - Sagittal FS PD-weighted FSE images and complementary coronal T1- or PD-weighting plus FS PD FSE T2-weighting are more accurate in correlating areas of increased signal intensity with partial tears than relying exclusively on abnormal signal on GRE images.

    - Some MR studies using GRE sequences show poor arthroscopic correlation for partial ACL tears.[492]

- AMB most commonly involved in incomplete or partial ACL tears[286]

    - More functional integration of ACL fibers, however, limits potential disruptive tension differences between the AMB and PLB.

    - Rupture of the AMB thought to be functionally equivalent to a complete ACL tear

    - Artificially created isolated tears of the AMB in cadaver knees could not be clinically detected by either physical examination or arthrometric testing[286]; thus, clinically diagnosed partial tears likely represent complete rupture of the ACL.

    - Progression from partial tear to symptomatic instability may represent a functionally incompetent ACL from the time of injury.[286]

    - Because differentiating partial from complete ACL tears is difficult clinically, the role of MR is particularly important.

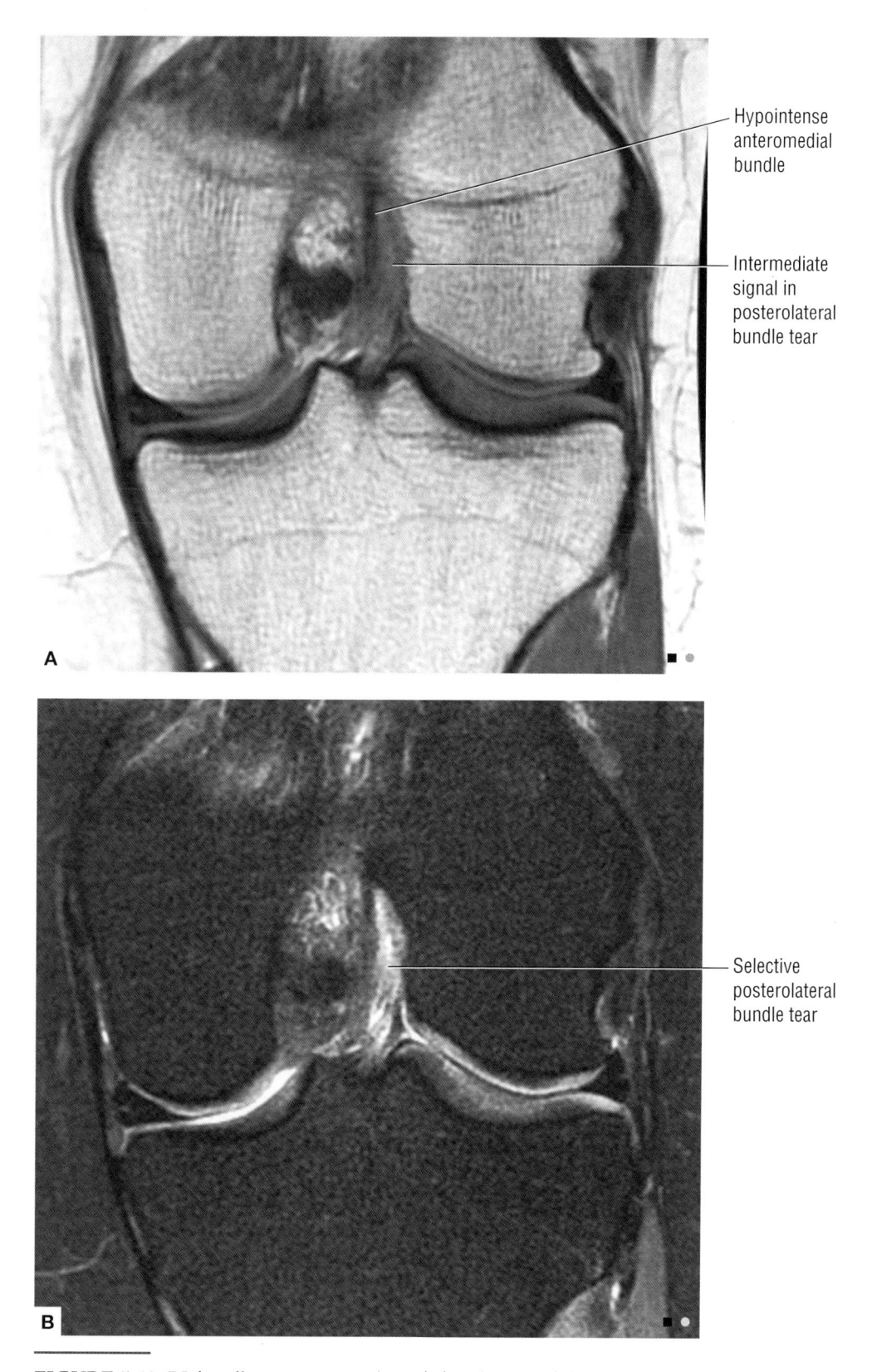

FIGURE 5.48 PL bundle tear on coronal PD (**A**) and FS PD (**B**) images. The intact AM bundle is hypointense relative to the torn PL bundle. (*Continued*)

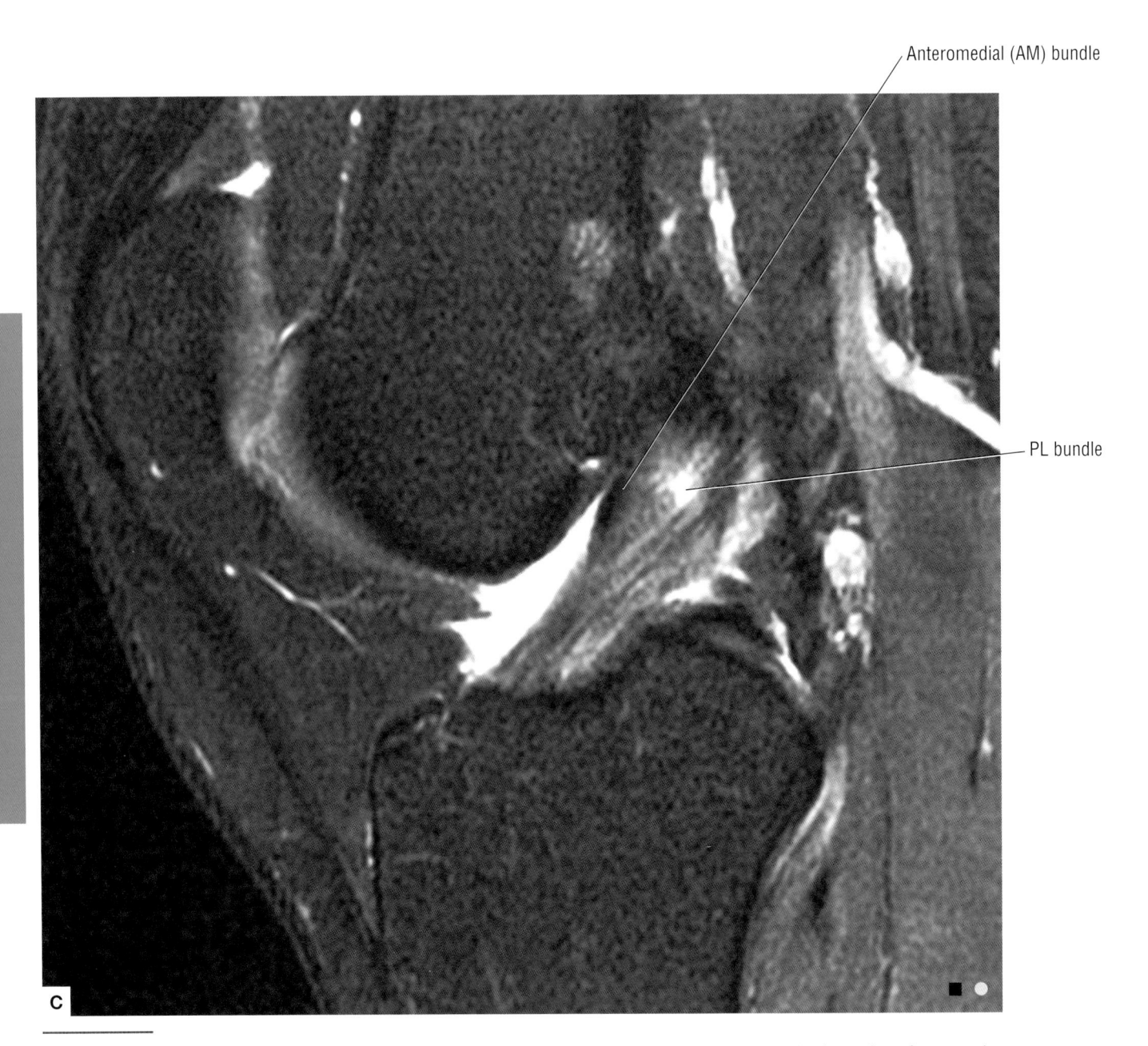

FIGURE 5.48 *(Continued)* (**C**) Corresponding sagittal FS PD FSE image with intact anterior leading edge of proximal AM bundle fibers and hyperintensity of posterior proximal fibers in area of PL disruption.

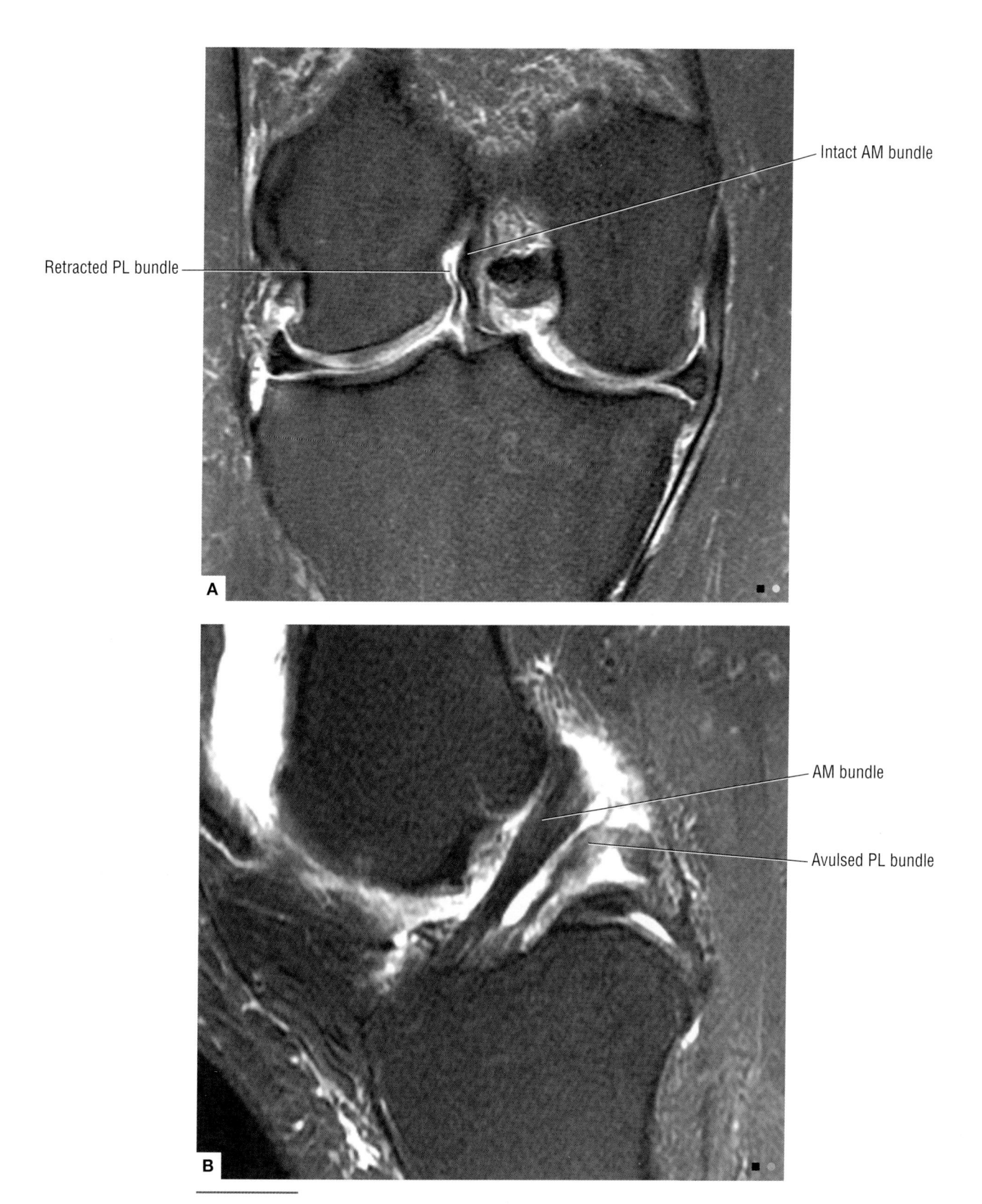

FIGURE 5.49 Avulsed and lax posterolateral bundle identified closest to the lateral femoral condyle on coronal image (**A**) and posterior to anteromedial bundle on sagittal image (**B**). Coronal (**A**) and sagittal (**B**) FS PD FSE images.

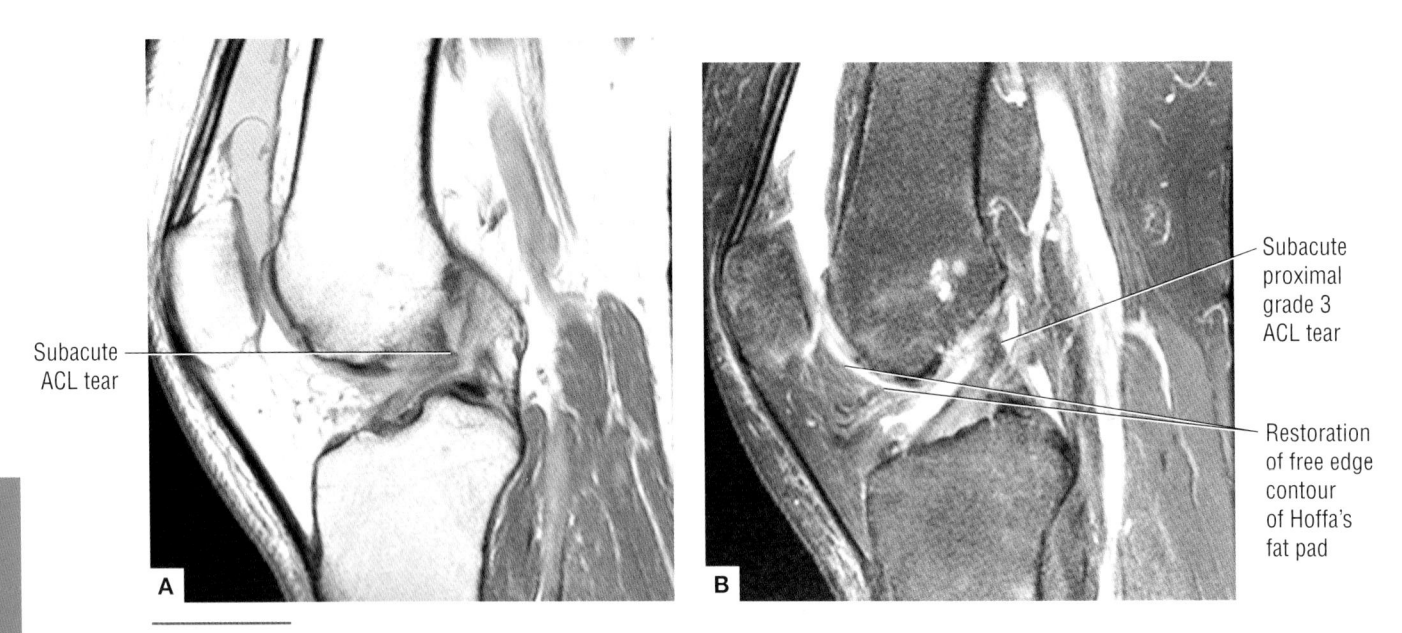

FIGURE 5.50 Subacute ACL tear showing proximal disruption on sagittal PD (**A**) and FS PD (**B**) FSE images. The ACL morphology is evident and the ligament is hypointense on FS PD FSE images (**B**). Since the initial injury, there has been a reduction in the increased interval signal intensity caused by synovitis and hyperextension contusions.

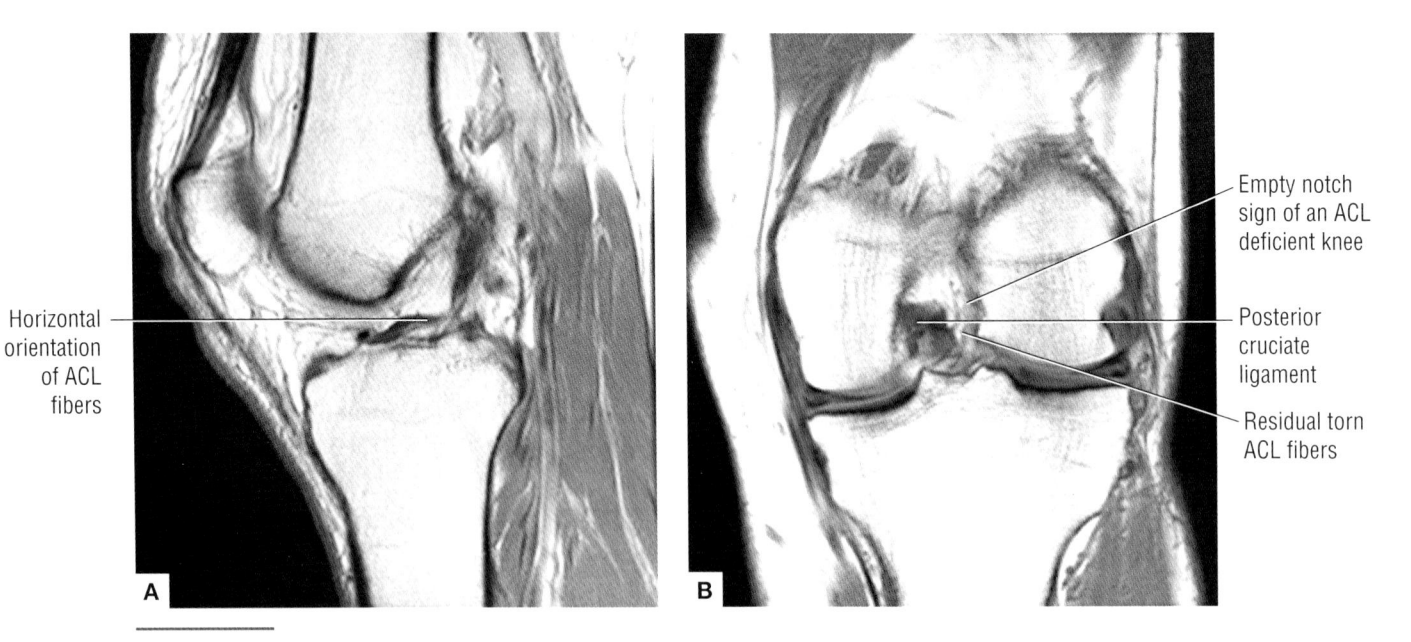

FIGURE 5.51 An empty notch sign. (**A**) A chronic ACL tear with a horizontally oriented ligament on a PD FSE sagittal image. (**B**) The ACL is essentially absent on the corresponding T1-weighted coronal image. Resolution of effusion synovitis and osseous contusions can also be seen.

- **Subacute ACL tears**
  - Morphology of torn ligament fibers may become less obscured as initial hemorrhage resolves.
  - Distal segment of ACL often assumes more horizontal location or orientation.
  - Fluid interposed in the ligamentous gap of the tear site usually more sharply defined
  - Associated bone contusions are usually persistent but may demonstrate decreased T2 signal intensity or extent of involvement.
  - Synovitis frequently detected but decreased compared to initial injury, as is the associated joint effusion
- **Chronic ACL tears**
  - Edema and synovitis usually not present
  - May show small chronic joint effusion
  - ACL may not be visualized on sagittal or coronal images.
    - Absence of ACL tissue in the lateral intercondylar notch → empty notch sign on coronal MR images (empty lateral wall)[397]
  - Chronically torn ACL often seen with horizontal axis or may display more vertical orientation and discontinuity/retraction of proximal attachment
  - Not uncommon for torn ACL to be adhered to PCL,[494] producing end point on anterior drawer test
  - ACL may appear attenuated.
  - Anterior translation of the tibia on the femur (MR anterior drawer sign) → static assessment of anterolateral instability
    - Uncovering of the undersurface of the posterior horn of the lateral meniscus (uncovered lateral meniscus sign)
    - Buckling of the foreshortened PCL[397]
  - Posterolateral capsular injuries without fluid extravasation or edema
  - Buckling or redundancy of the patellar tendon (although this can also be seen with knee hyperextension and quadriceps dysfunction)[393]
  - Indirect findings may be specific but not sensitive.
  - Supine imaging of patient with ACL-deficient knee causes tibia to fall in neutral alignment relative to the femur (because of gravity); with a PCL tear, the tibia subluxes posteriorly.

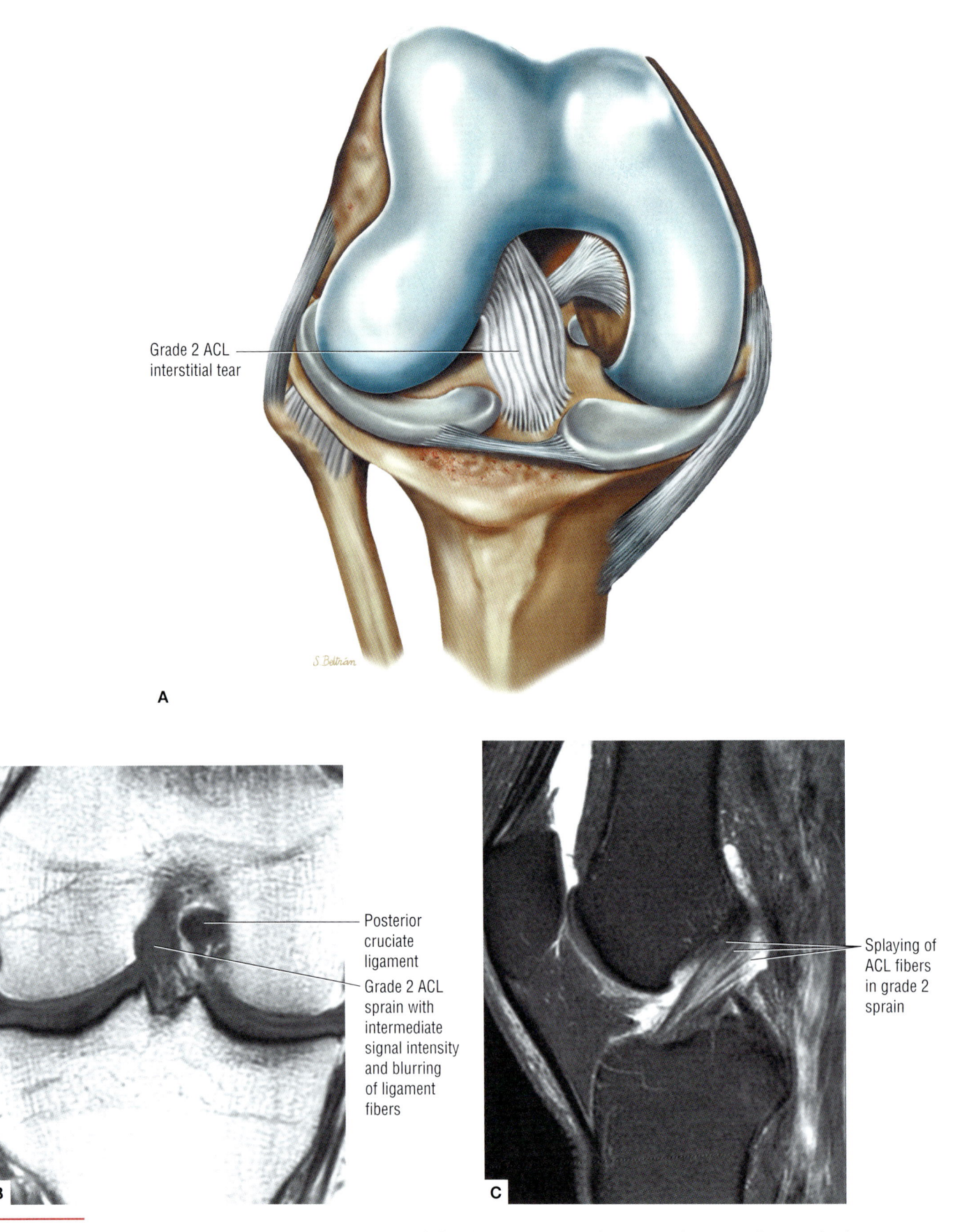

FIGURE 5.52 Grade 2 ACL sprain with ligamentous splaying (**A**) and edema is intermediate in signal on coronal T1-weighted images (**B**) and hyperintense on sagittal FS PD FSE images (**C**). The slope of the ACL remains parallel to the intercondylar roof.

Pitfalls in Interpretation of ACL Tear Findings: ACL Ganglia

- Intercondylar notch or ganglion cysts of the ACL (cruciate cysts) arise both on the surface and within the substance of the ACL.[103,232,287]
- Located in the middle and proximal portions of both ACL and PCL
- Thought to represent either mucinous degeneration of connective tissue or herniation of synovial tissue through capsular defect[287]
- Uniform increased signal intensity on FS PD FSE images, may be septated, no enhancement
- "Celery stalk" appearance with mucoid degeneration and fusiform enlargement
    - May be seen in isolation or with a well-defined ACL cyst
    - Mucinous or mucoid degeneration and ACL cysts may coexist and represent a spectrum of ACL response to degeneration and/or chronic trauma.
- May be symptomatic, causing either pain or intermittent swelling[232]
- May be associated with an ACL injury or other associated intraarticular joint pathology, or may present as incidental finding
- Often present with pain and clicking during terminal knee extension
- May produce pressure erosion of the adjacent lateral femoral condyle and present with pain during joint loading (e.g., running)
- Successfully treated with arthroscopic débridement[287]

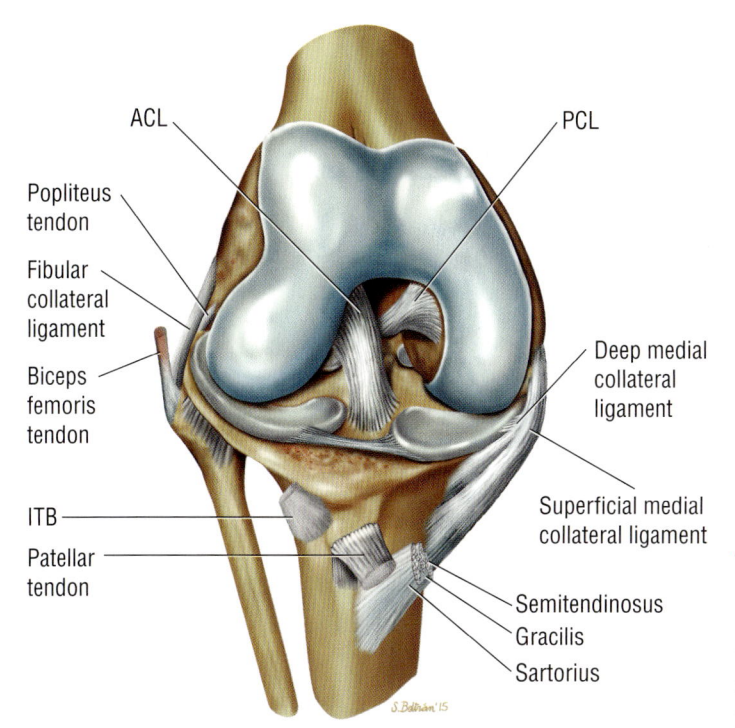

FIGURE 5.53 Normal notch anatomy. Notch cysts may be associated with mucoid changes in one of the cruciate ligaments. Intraosseous ganglion of the intercondylar roof can occur adjacent to an area of proximal ACL mucoid degeneration.

ACL Cyst and Mucoid Degeneration

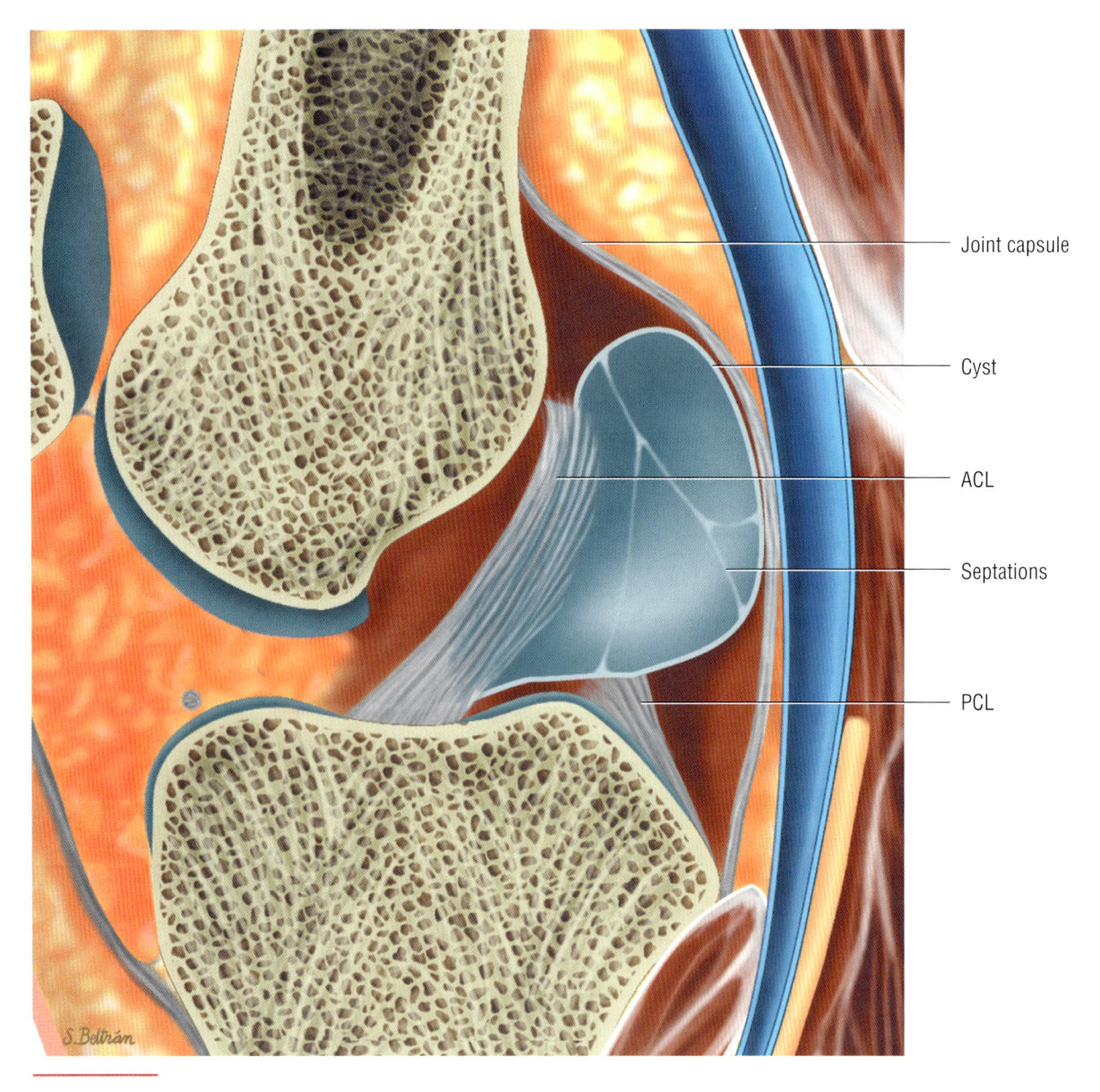

FIGURE 5.54 An ACL cyst in continuity with proximal ACL fibers.

Cruciate Ligaments

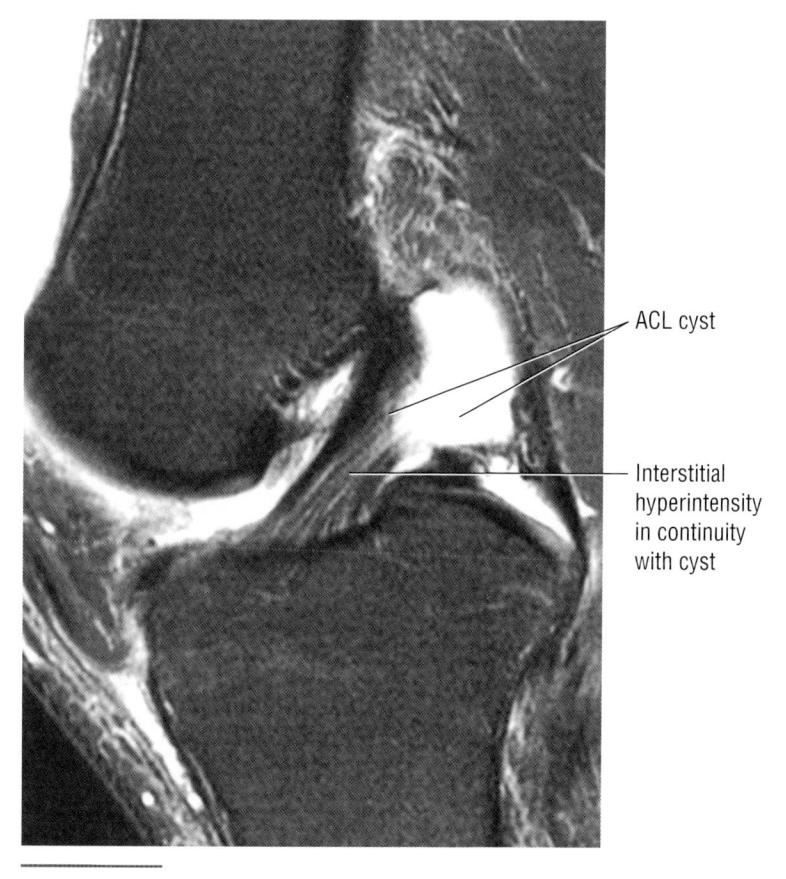

FIGURE 5.55 Sagittal FS PD FSE image demonstrates an intact ACL with associated proximal ganglion cyst.

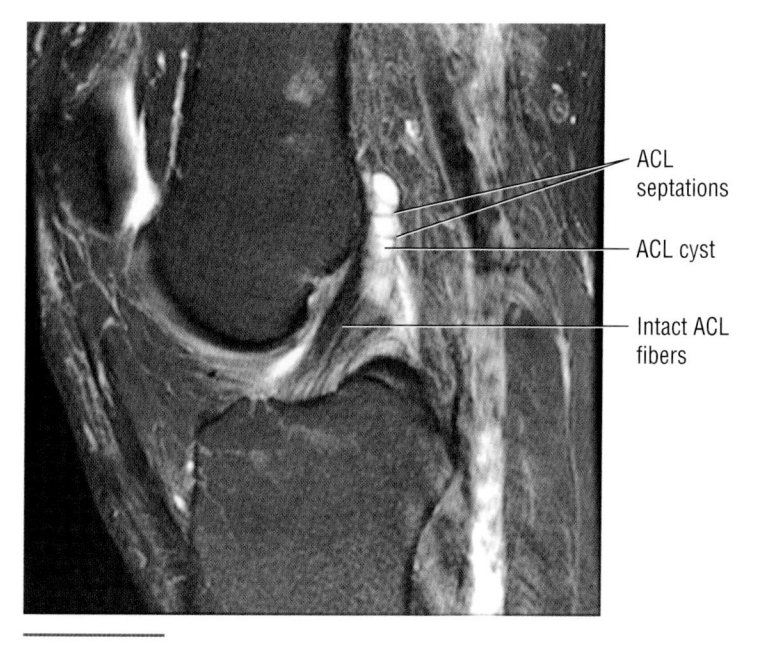

FIGURE 5.56 Septated ACL cyst extending proximally (sagittal FS PD FSE image).

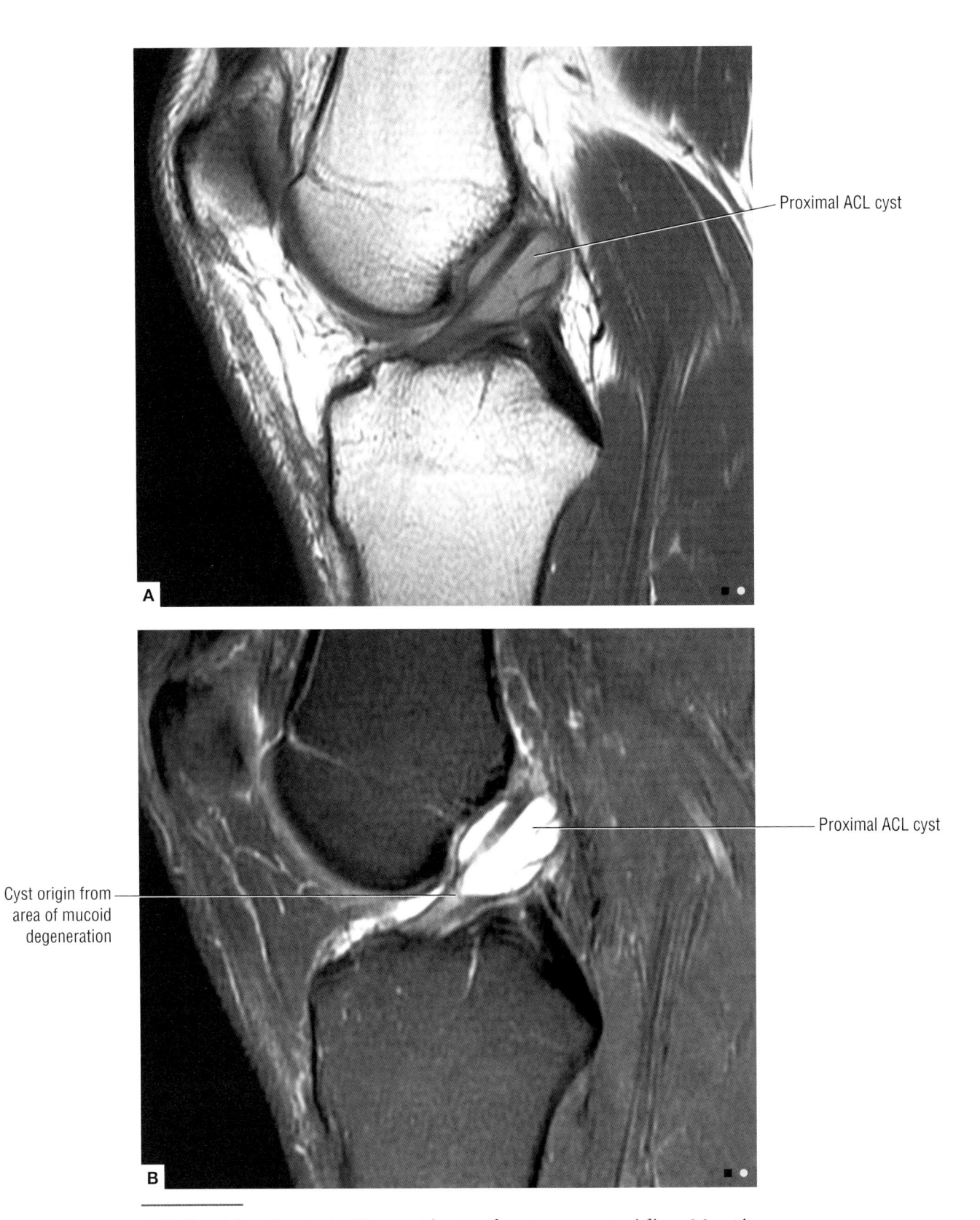

FIGURE 5.57 Proximal ACL cyst with origin from intact proximal fibers. Mucoid degeneration is present in distal fibers. Sagittal PD (**A**) and FS PD (**B**) images.

Cruciate Ligaments

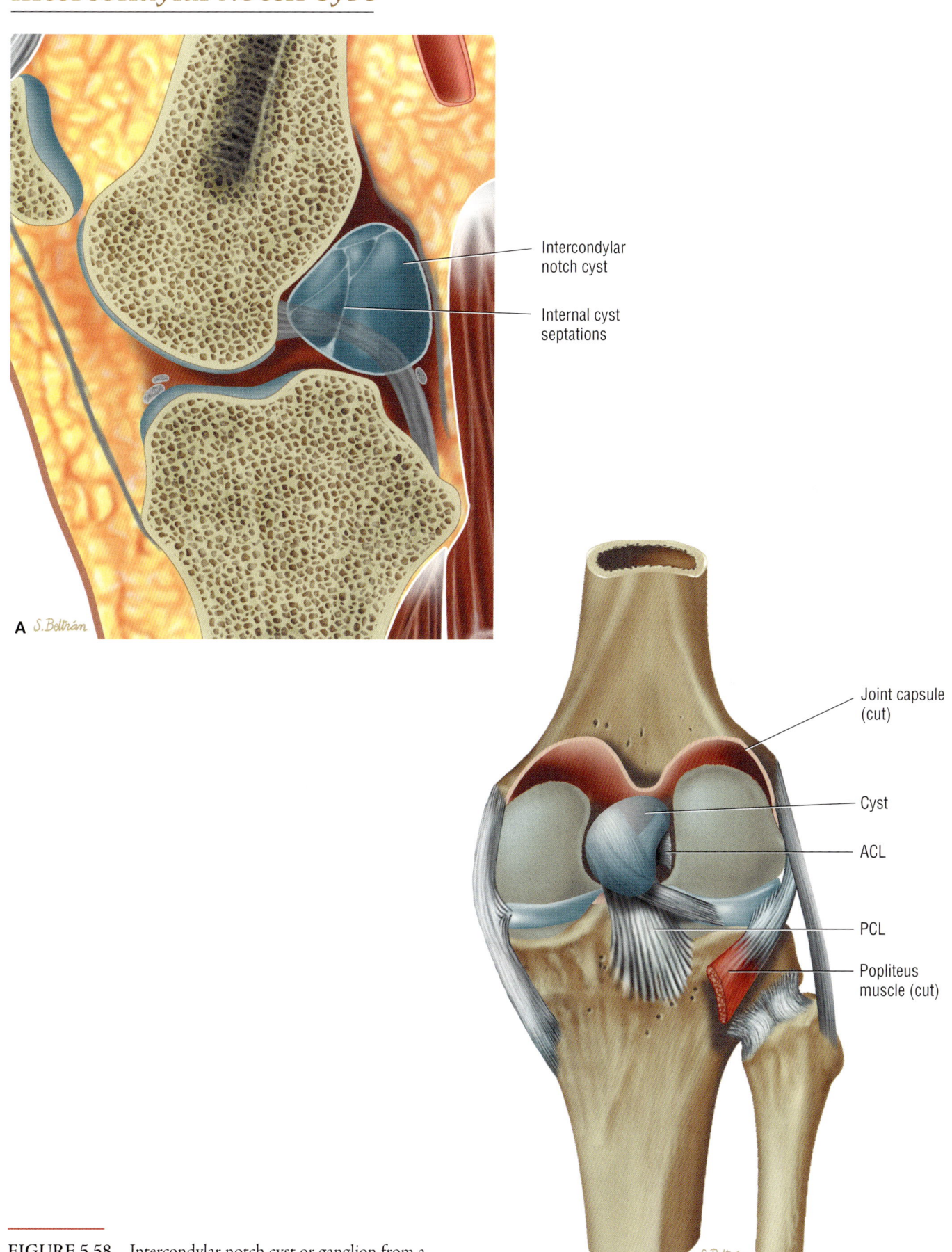

Intercondylar Notch Cyst

FIGURE 5.58 Intercondylar notch cyst or ganglion from a sagittal (**A**) and posterior coronal (**B**) perspective. (*Continued*)

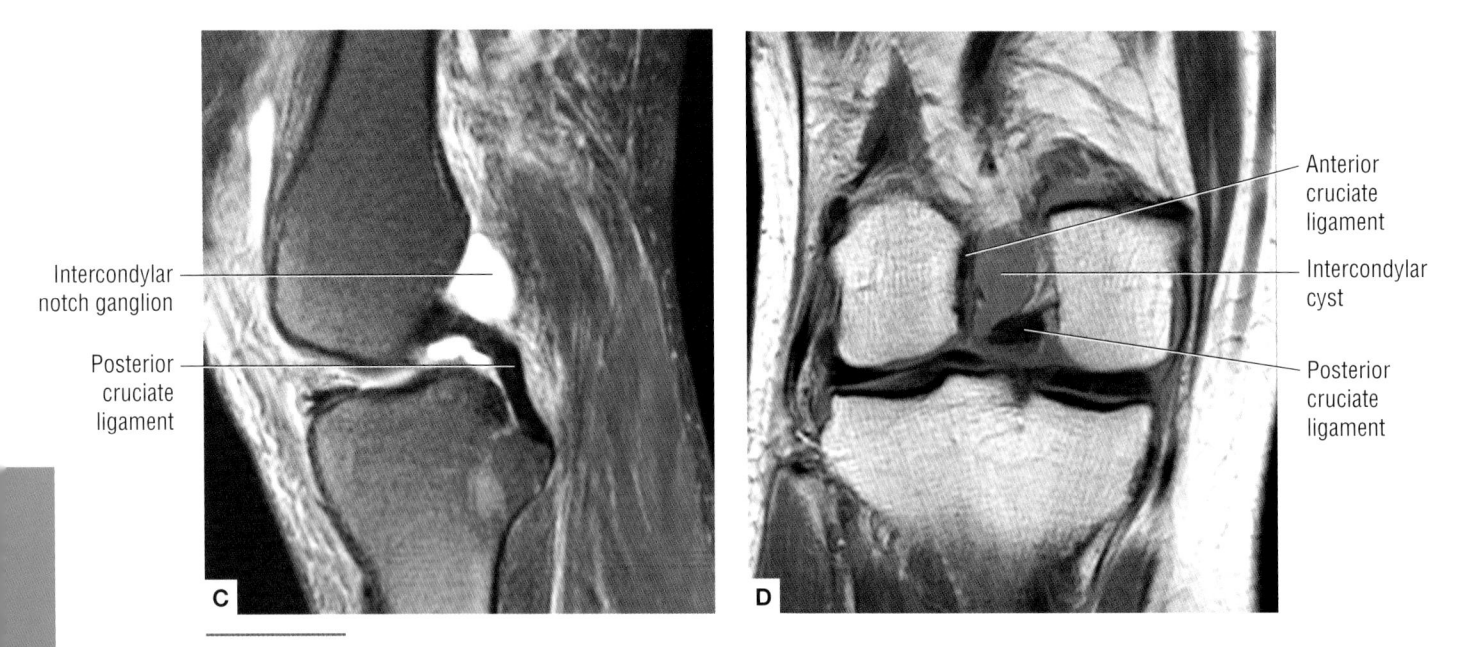

FIGURE 5.58 (*Continued*) The ganglion is hyperintense on a corresponding sagittal FS PD FSE image (**C**) and of intermediate signal on a PD FSE coronal image (**D**). The ganglion cyst is insinuated between the cruciate ligaments without a well-defined point of origin.

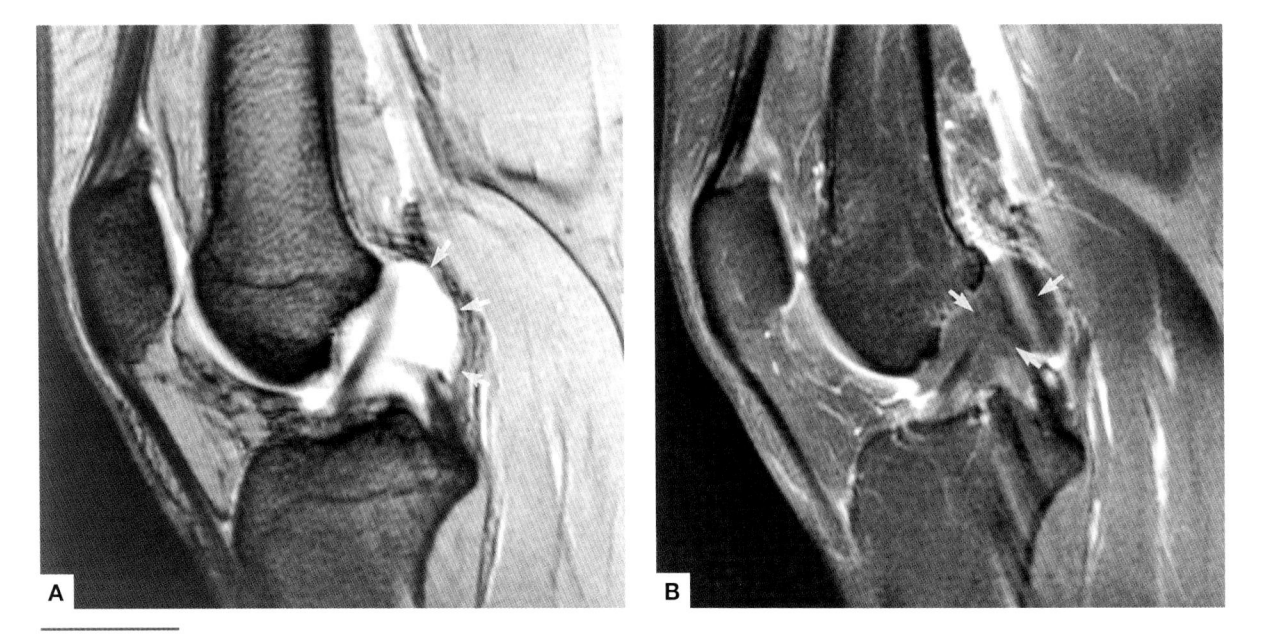

FIGURE 5.59 An intercondylar notch cyst (*arrows*) is hyperintense on a T2*-weighted sagittal image (**A**) and is not enhanced after intravenous administration of gadolinium–diethylene triamine pentaacetic acid on an FS T1-weighted sagittal image (**B**).

Cruciate Ligaments

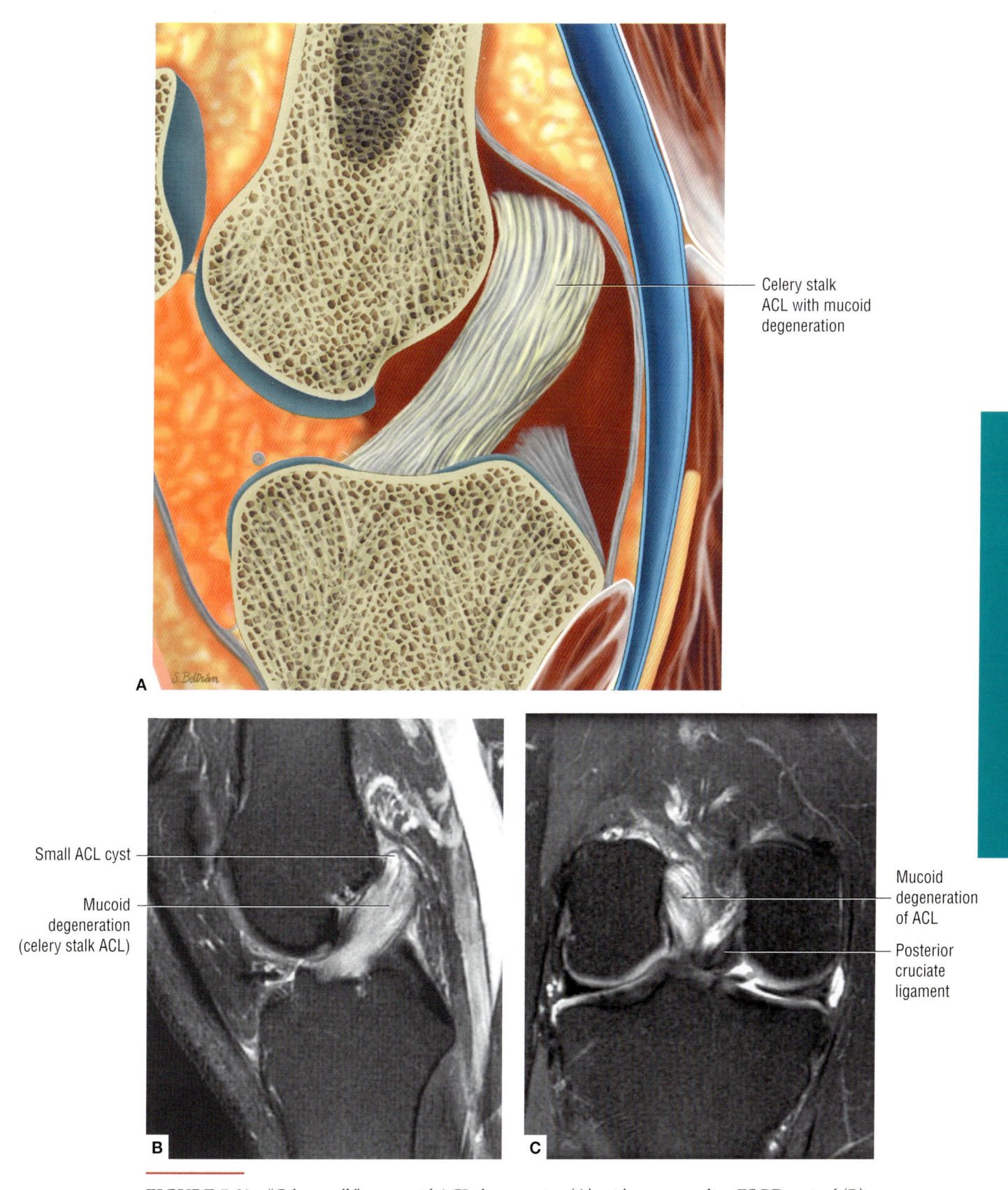

FIGURE 5.60 "Celery stalk" or mucoid ACL degeneration (**A**), with corresponding FS PD sagittal (**B**) and coronal (**C**) images. Note a small ACL cyst developing proximally in association with the mucinous changes.

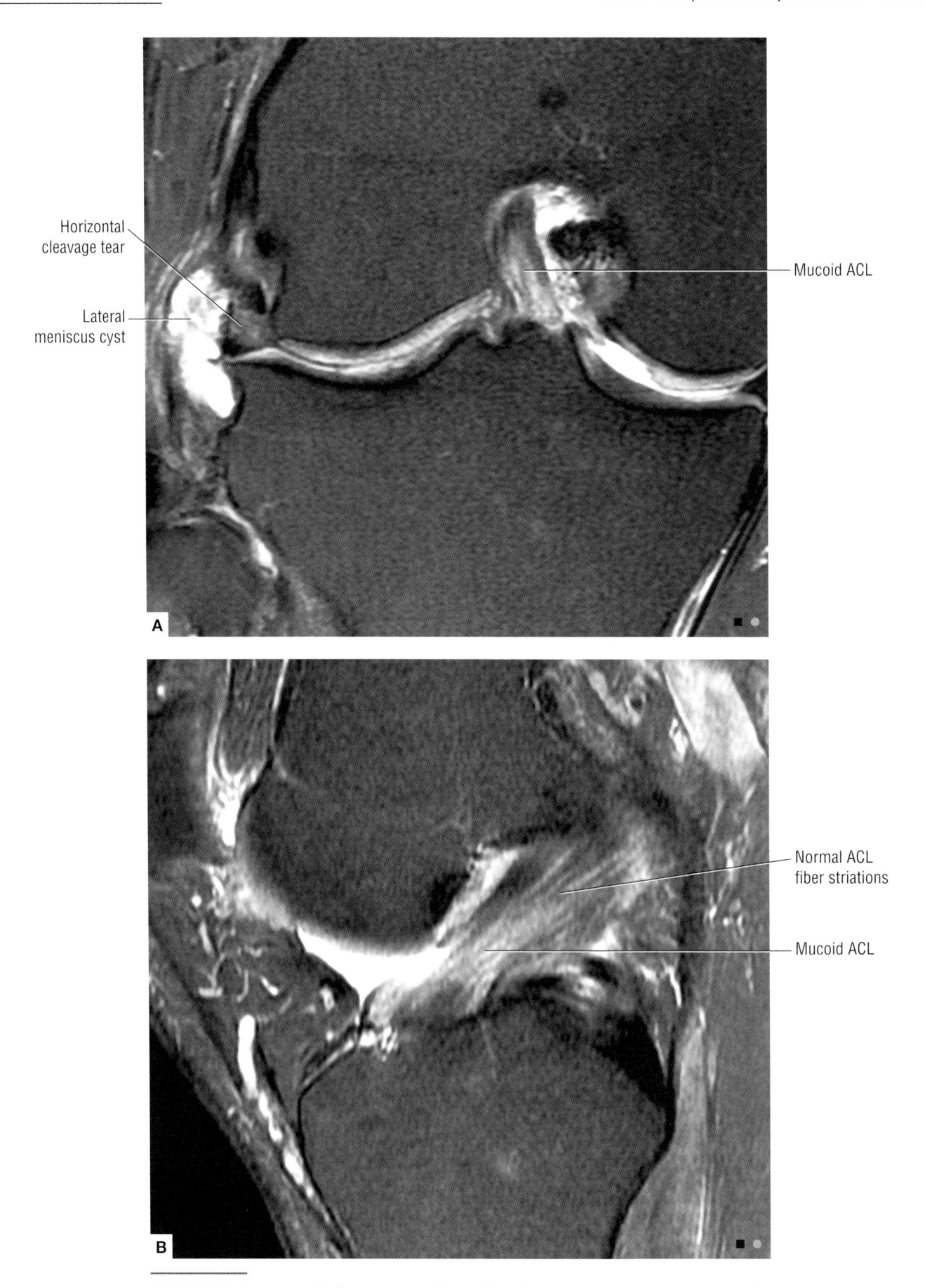

FIGURE 5.61 Mucoid degeneration of the ACL without any acute secondary signs of an ACL injury such as hyperintense lateral compartment contusions. If there is a component of associated anterior translation of the tibia, the mucoid changes may be associated with a remote ACL sprain. Coronal (**A**) and sagittal (**B**) FS PD FSE images.

Cruciate Ligaments

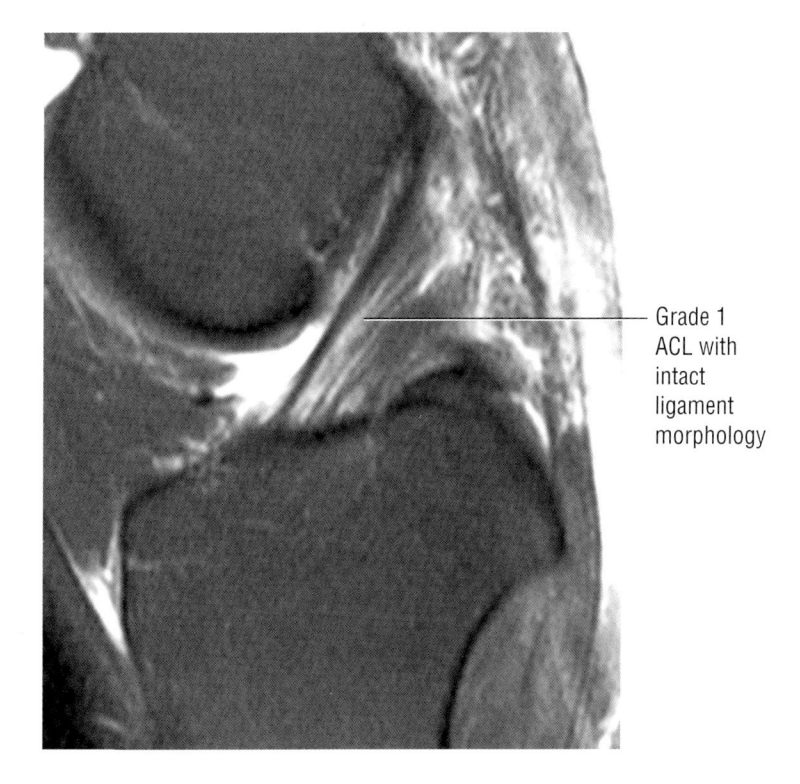

FIGURE 5.62 Grade 1 ACL sprain demonstrates hyperintense ligament edema without distortion of individual fibers or ligament laxity (sagittal FS PD FSE image).

Grade 1 ACL with intact ligament morphology

Partial loss of ACL parallel fiber orientation

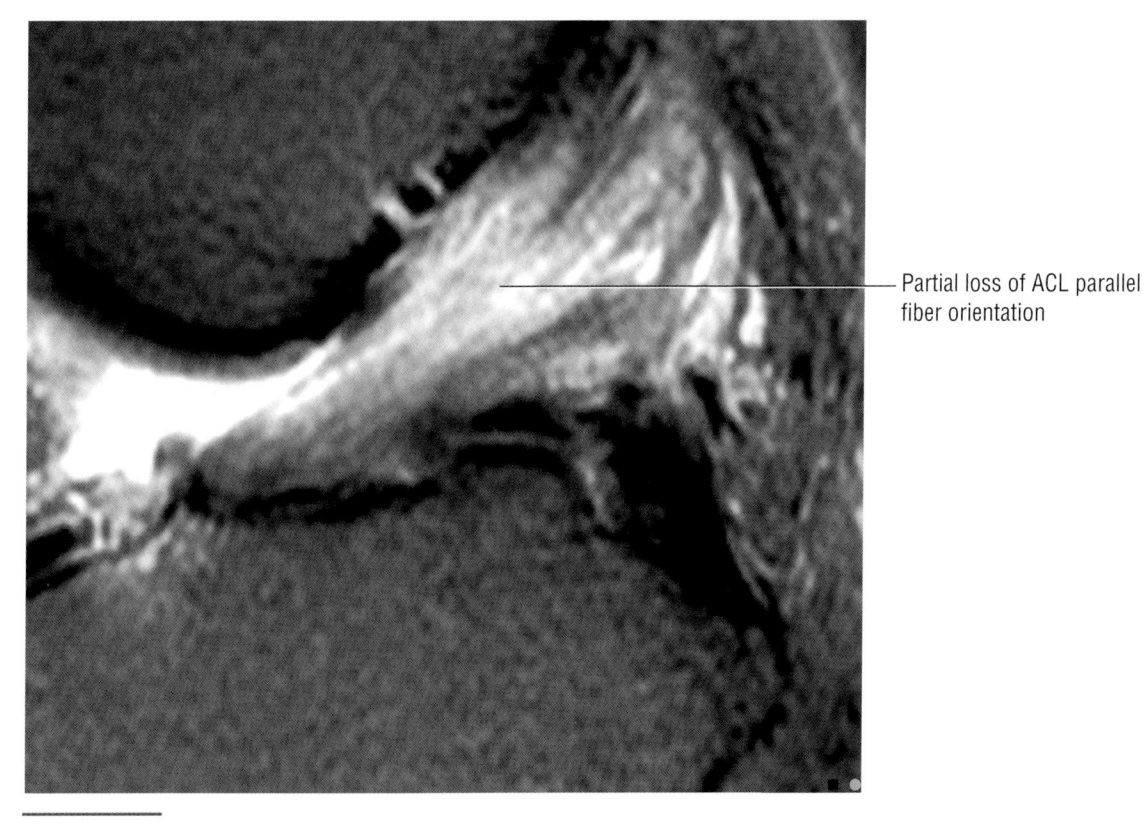

FIGURE 5.63 Subacute ACL sprain with partial loss of parallel fiber orientation relative to the intercondylar roof. Because a mucoid ACL could have a similar appearance, look for associated findings of anterior tibial translation or lateral compartment contusions. Grade 2 ACL sprains are usually associated with anterior tibial translation even if no lateral compartment contusions are detected. Sagittal FS PD FSE image.

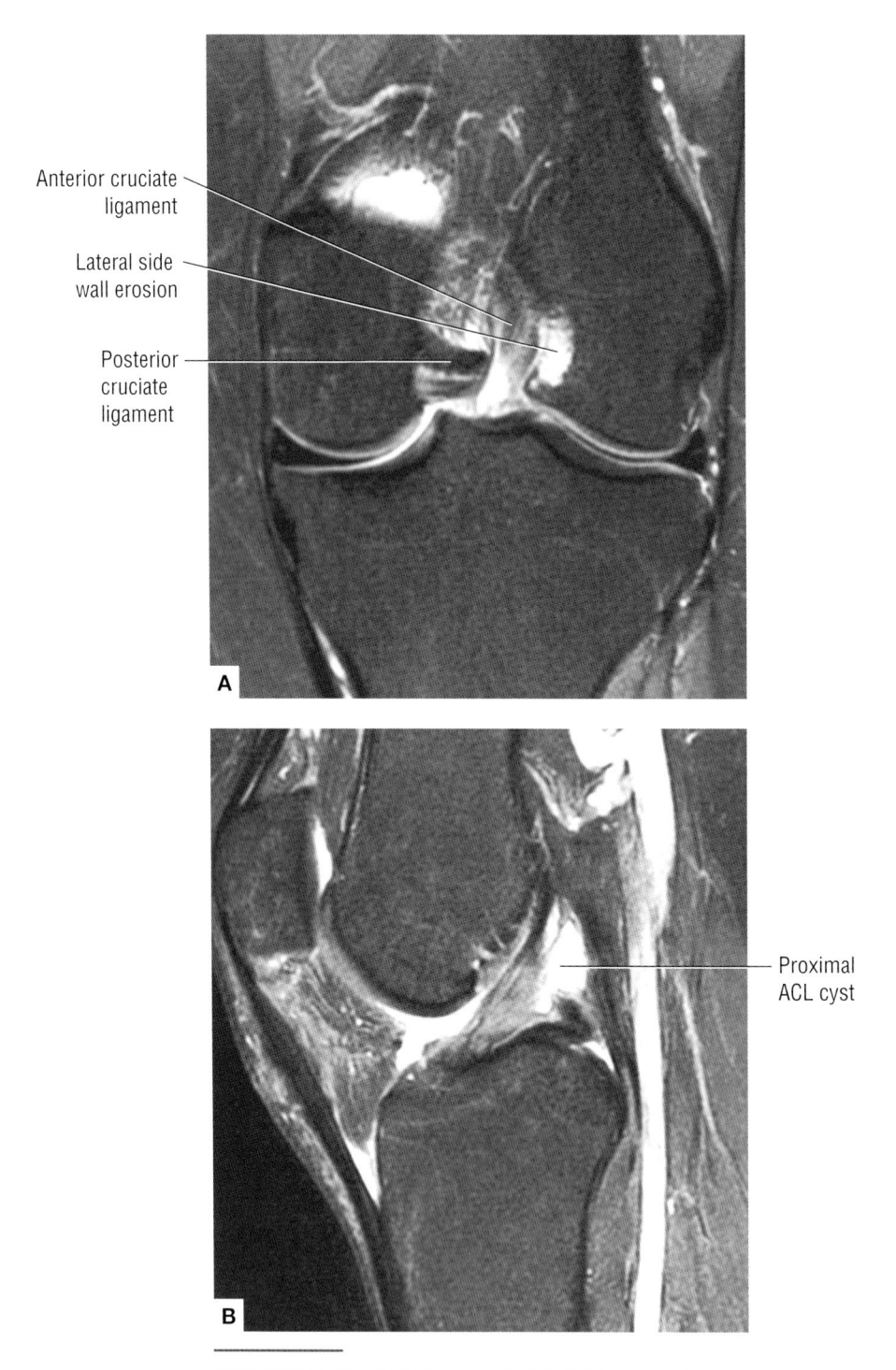

FIGURE 5.64 (**A**) Coronal FS PD FSE image of lateral side wall erosion. (**B**) Sagittal FS PD FSE image shows the cause to be an adjacent proximal ACL cyst in a long-distance runner.

ACL-Associated Posterolateral Corner and Osseous Injuries

Key Concepts

- Posterolateral corner (posterolateral or arcuate complex) includes:
  - Lateral collateral ligament
  - Popliteus muscle and tendon
  - Arcuate ligament
- Medial limb: courses over popliteus muscle and tendon, and joins oblique popliteal ligament
- Lateral limb: blends with capsule near condylar insertion of the lateral gastrocnemius muscle
  - Popliteofibular ligament
  - Popliteomeniscal fascicles
  - Fabellofibular ligament
  - Lateral head of gastrocnemius muscle
- Biceps femoris tendon and iliotibial band, although not usually listed as components of the posterolateral complex, contribute to stability of the lateral and posterolateral knee.

Posterolateral Corner Injuries

- Posterolateral corner = posterolateral or arcuate complex
- Posterolateral corner injuries associated with acute ACL (and PCL) tears[386]
- Uncommon to have isolated posterolateral corner injury[502]
- Functional failure of a reconstructed ACL can occur if reconstruction completed without repair of associated posterolateral corner injury.
- Anatomic structures of posterolateral corner include:
  - Lateral collateral ligament
  - Arcuate ligament (Y-shaped structure with medial and lateral limb)
  - Popliteus tendon
  - Popliteofibular ligament
  - Short lateral ligament
  - Fabellofibular ligament
  - Posterolateral part of capsule[341,504,512]

- Because terminology of these structures is inconsistent, it is best to refer to the anatomic organization of the posterolateral corner anatomy as three layers, as described by Seebacher et al.[423]
    - The popliteus complex and its attachments to the fibula and lateral meniscus represent key components of the posterolateral corner.
- Combined sectioning of ACL and posterolateral ligaments has shown maximal increases in primary anterior and posterior translation at 30 degrees of knee flexion.[502]
    - Increases also shown for primary varus, primary internal, and coupled external rotation
- Isolated posterolateral sectioning results in primary posterior translation, varus and external rotation, and coupled external rotation, maximal at 30 to 45 degrees of knee flexion.
- Hyperextension is most common mechanism in patients with combined ACL and posterolateral injury.[504] Common MR findings include:
    - Fluid posterior to popliteus tendon
        - Sign of trauma to attachment of arcuate complex
        - Fluid seen in expected location of medial limb of arcuate ligament (considered a separate but contiguous structure to the popliteus)[227]
    - Edema
    - Tearing of popliteus muscle and muscle–tendon junction
    - Direct visualization of arcuate ligament disruption (on FS PD FSE axial images)
- Acute repair or reconstruction of the posterolateral corner is performed at the time of ACL reconstruction.
- Extensive posterolateral injury may require primary repair, augmentation, or reconstruction of the popliteus muscle–tendon unit and the LCL.[355,504]

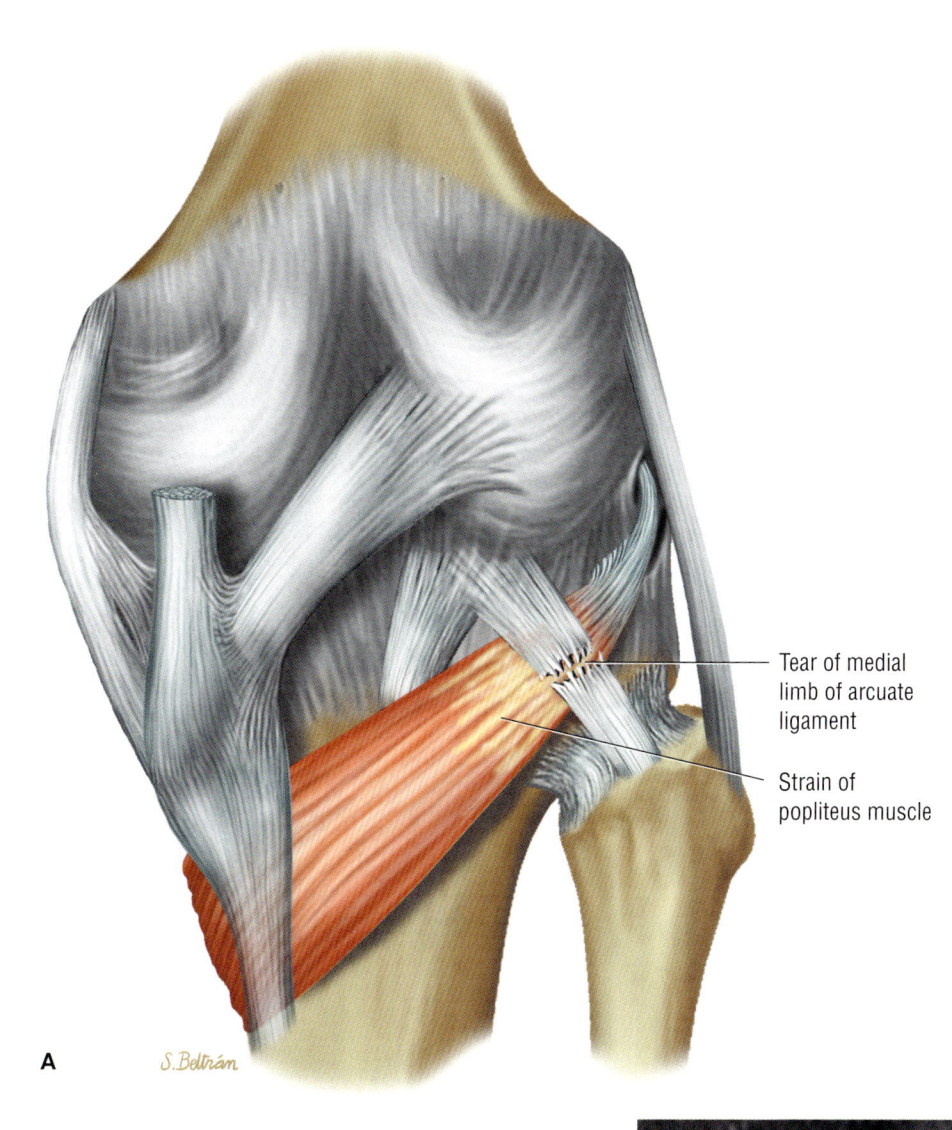

FIGURE 5.65 Posterolateral corner sprain. **(A)** Posterior coronal color illustration of a popliteus muscle strain and tear of the medial fibers of the arcuate complex. **(B)** Corresponding sagittal FS PD FSE image in an acute ACL tear demonstrating a posterolateral tibial plateau contusion, a fluid collection posterior to the popliteus tendon, and disruption of the medial limb of the arcuate ligament. Edema of the popliteal muscle tendon junction is a frequently associated finding.

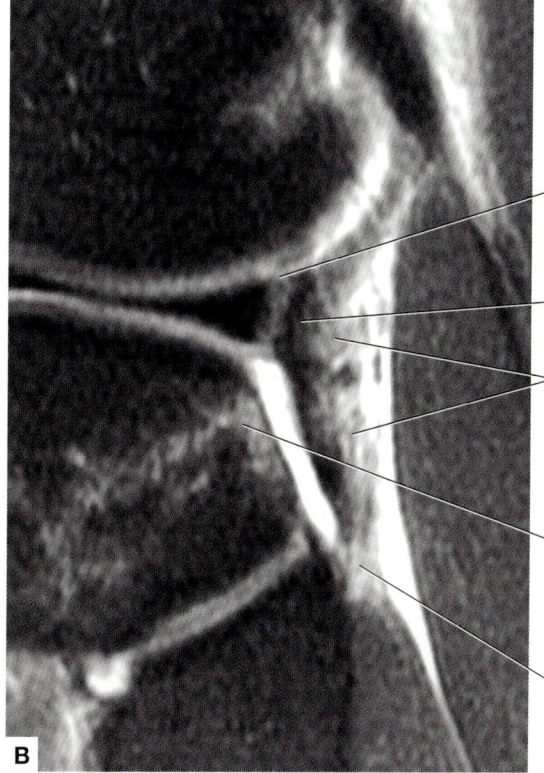

FIGURE 5.66 (**A**) Posterolateral capsular trauma in association with an acute ACL tear. (**B**) A popliteus muscle tear (*straight arrow*) with hyperintense hemorrhage on a FS PD-weighted FSE sagittal image. Note the anterior translation of the tibia relative to the femur. Osseous contusion (*curved arrow*) is indicated. (**C**) Hyperintensity of the popliteus muscle (*arrow*) on an axial FS PD-weighted FSE image.

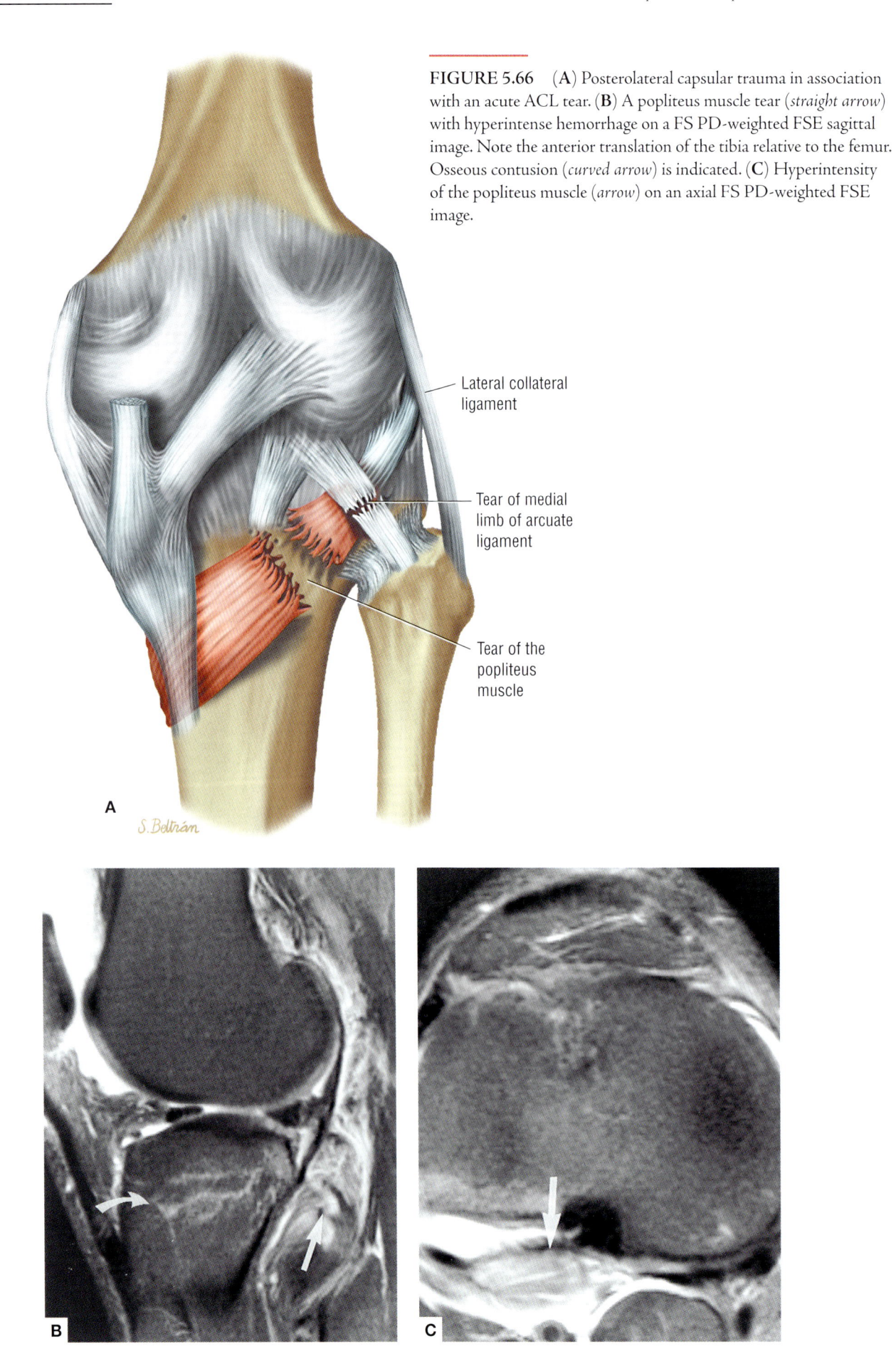

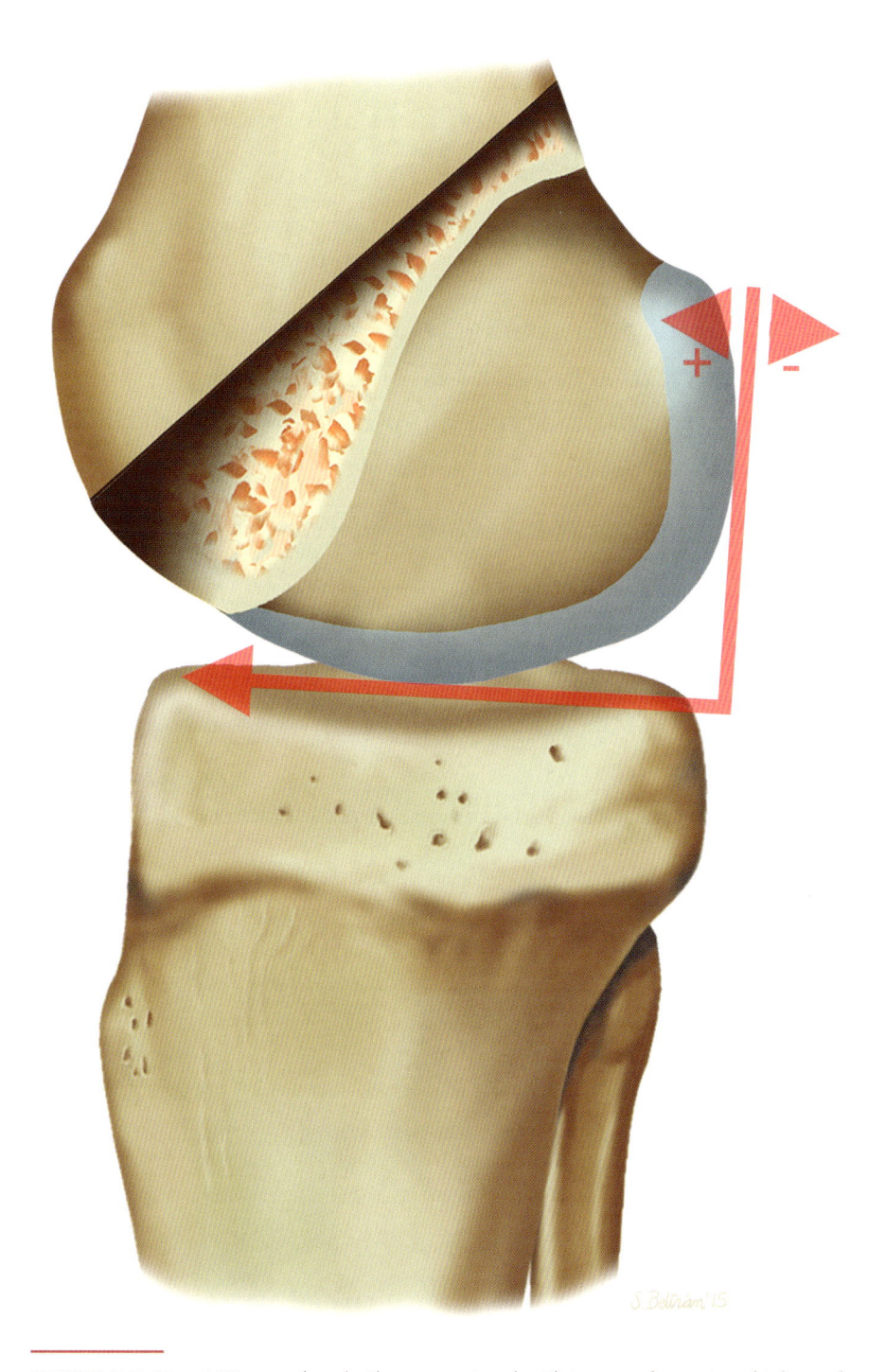

FIGURE 5.67 ACL tears (grade 3) are associated with increased anterior tibial translation relative to the femur as assessed at the level of the lateral femoral condyle (lateral compartment). Tibial translation is best assessed on sagittal MR images. Anterior tibial translation is seen in grade 2 and grade 3 injuries but may be seen in cases of ACL laxity without disruption. Significant anterior translation (greater than 7mm) is an indirect sign of ACL disruption.

Osseous Injuries

Key Concepts

- Posteromedial tibial plateau contusions or fractures represent contre-coup injuries.
    - Associated with lateral compartment osseous impaction and ACL rupture
    - Associated with posterior peripheral medial meniscus tears and meniscocapsular separations
- Segond fracture visualized on anterior coronal images at the location of the lateral compartment of the meniscotibial ligament
    - Associated with avulsion forces directed by the posterior fibers of the iliotibial tract
- Arcuate sign (associated with posterolateral corner injury) represents avulsion fracture of the fibular styloid process.
    - May involve popliteofibular ligament or arcuate and fabellofibular ligaments
- Avulsion fractures of the fibular head are associated with PCL tears.

Osseous Injuries

- Several types of osseous injuries associated with ACL tears[415]
- Lateral compartment osseous injuries
    - Most commonly bone contusions involving weight-bearing portion of the lateral femoral condyle and posterolateral tibial plateau
    - Posterior tibial contusions often coexist with nondisplaced trabecular fractures.
    - Careful evaluation of both coronal and sagittal images increases specificity for fracture identification.
    - Posterolateral tibial plateau (94%) and lateral femoral condyle (91%) subchondral bone impactions are relatively specific signs of acute ACL tear.[346]
        - Attributed to impact of lateral femoral condyle into posterior tibia during either initial rotary subluxation or recoil of the lateral femoral condyle

- Combination of valgus forces with anterior subluxation of the lateral tibial plateau produces impaction force on weight-bearing surface or midportion of the lateral femoral condyle, opposite or over the anterior horn of the lateral meniscus.[44,143,276,312,397,455,486]
  - FS PD-weighted FSE and short tau inversion recovery (STIR) images are most sensitive for demonstrating bone contusions.
- Resolve over time and are not as commonly seen 9 or more weeks after injury[393]
  - Decreased signal intensity and decrease in area of subchondral bone involvement seen during resolution phase of trabecular impactions
- Pattern of bone contusions may be seen in patients with chronic ACL tears.
  - Secondary to persistent or continued osseous impaction or trauma from initial injury
  - Secondary to reinjury from recurrent subluxation of the tibia due to ACL insufficiency[312]
- Lateral notch sign
  - Lateral femoral condylar notch or subchondral plate depression separate from the normal sulcus terminalis
  - Depression or condylar indentation greater than 1.5mm in depth at the condylopatellar sulcus
- Bone contusions show variable increases in signal intensity on conventional T2-weighted images compared with FS FSE or STIR techniques.
- Associated "kissing impaction" fracture of posterolateral tibial plateau usually present and should be identified, especially in hyperextension injuries[143]
- Bone contusions or impactions of the lateral tibial plateau may occur as an isolated finding (relatively specific for ACL injury) or in association with injury of the lateral femoral condyle.
- Flexion biomechanics may result in associated posteriorly located lateral femoral contusion.
- Segond fracture
  - Previously thought to represent bony ligamentous avulsion of the meniscotibial portion of the middle third of the lateral capsular ligament

- Currently attributed to avulsion injury of the posterior fibers of the iliotibial tract or anterior oblique band of the LCL[59]
- Associated with ACL rupture in 75% to 100% of cases[162,245,514]
- Small vertical avulsion of LCL insertion in the lateral aspect of the proximal tibia
- Elliptical fracture fragment may be seen at fracture site on coronal images.
- In acute or subacute injuries, fracture fragment demonstrates low signal intensity on T1- or PD-weighted images and high signal intensity on FS T2-weighted FSE or STIR images.
- In chronic injuries, fracture fragment shows normal fatty marrow signal with cortical offset.
- Associated with excessive internal rotation and varus stress, as commonly occurs in skiing, basketball, and baseball injuries
- Presents as anterolateral rotatory instability of the knee[245]
- Anterior oblique band of the LCL and posterior fibers of the iliotibial tract are critical lateral supporting structures involved in pathology of Segond fracture.

- Tibial spine avulsion
- Uncommon but specific finding for ACL injury[245]
- Frequently associated with distal ACL injuries because the distal fibers are relatively stronger than adjacent bone[245]
- Represent only 5% of ACL injuries in adults
- ACL injuries that are thought to be avulsion injuries are more likely to be intraligamentous or complete tears of the ACL.
- Posteromedial tibial plateau injury
- Contrecoup bone contusions (with or without involvement of the medial femoral condyle) that occur as the tibia reduces after ACL rupture[235]
- Posteromedial tibia and medial femoral condyle impact during knee reduction
- Occurs when there is compensatory varus alignment with internal rotation of the femur while the tibia is still anteriorly displaced

Cruciate Ligaments

- Smaller and less common than lateral femoral condyle and posterolateral tibial plateau injuries
- Impaction forces generally dissipate after initial lateral compartment impaction (unless there is excessive force as typically seen in sports-related trauma).
- Isolated medial compartment contusions have a different mechanism: major force is varus instead of valgus.
- Associated peripheral tears of the posterior horn of the medial meniscus and posteromedial meniscocapsular separations
  - Secondary to shearing force during subluxation of the tibia on the femur with simultaneous femoral rotation
  - Peripheral medial meniscal tears, including posterior inferior corner tears and/or meniscocapsular separations, may also result from direct posteromedial crush injury during contrecoup impaction.
- Arcuate sign
  - Avulsion fracture of the fibular head associated with injuries to the PCL and posterolateral ligaments[201,229]
  - Fractured elliptical fragment of fibular styloid process is attachment site of popliteofibular, arcuate, and fabellofibular ligaments.
  - LCL and biceps femoris tendon, in contrast, attach to lateral margin of the fibular head (avulsions of the LCL and biceps femoris are less common).

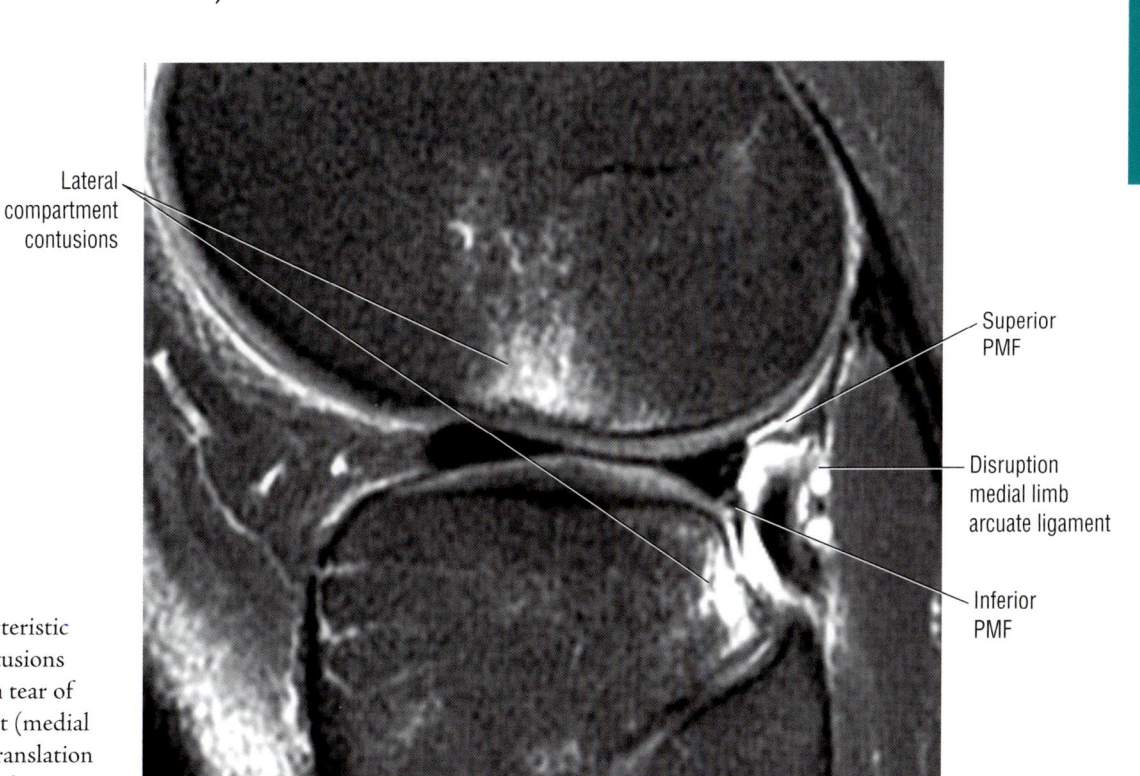

FIGURE 5.68 Characteristic lateral compartment contusions (trabecular fracture) with tear of the weak arcuate ligament (medial limb). There is anterior translation of the tibia relative to the femur. Sagittal FS PD FSE image.

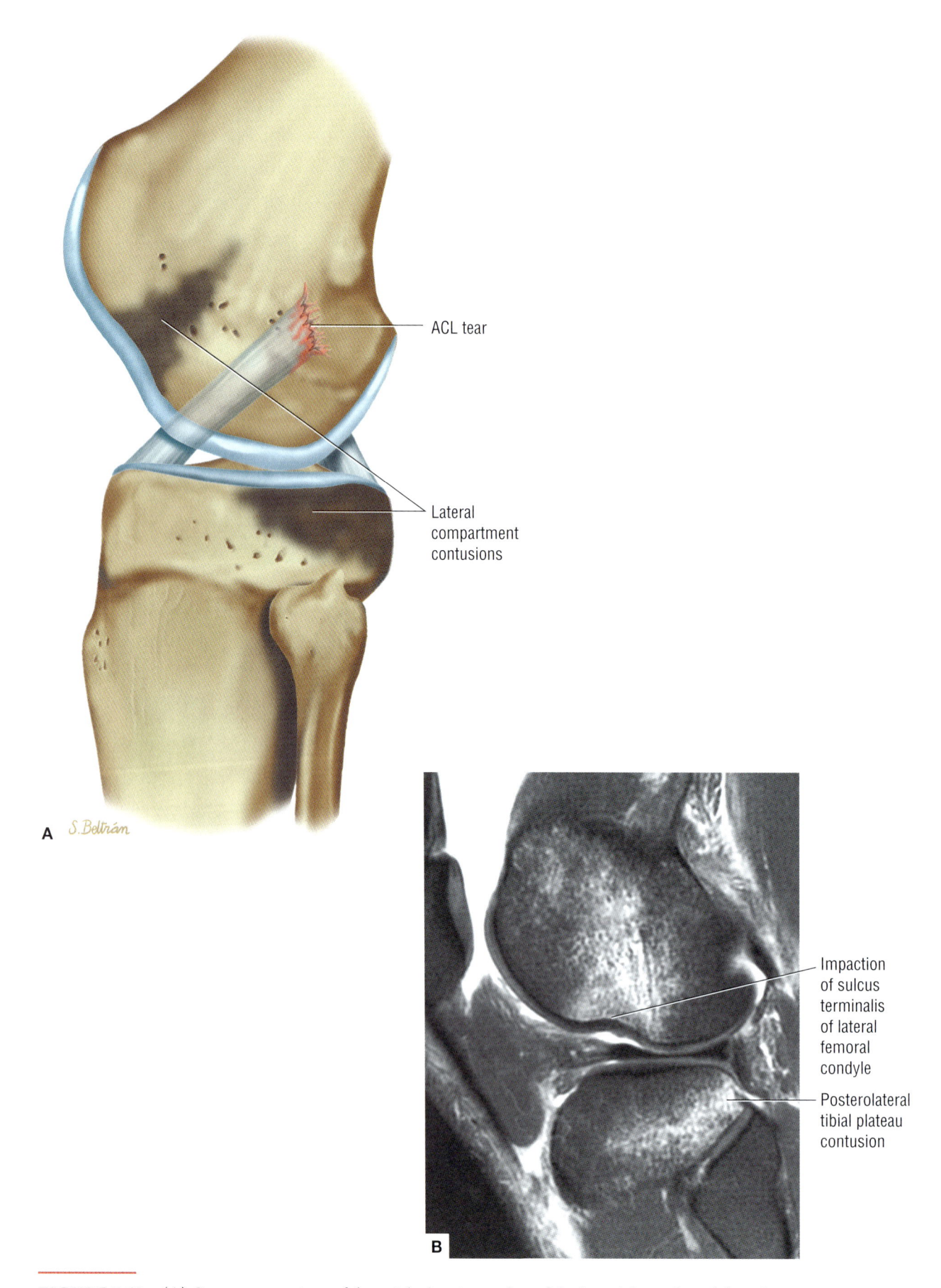

FIGURE 5.69 (**A**) Osseous contusions of the weight-bearing surface of the lateral femoral condyle and posterior lateral tibial plate are associated with an acute grade 3 ACL disruption. (**B**) Corresponding sagittal FS PD FSE image with lateral femoral condyle impaction and posterolateral tibial plateau contusion.

Cruciate Ligaments 475

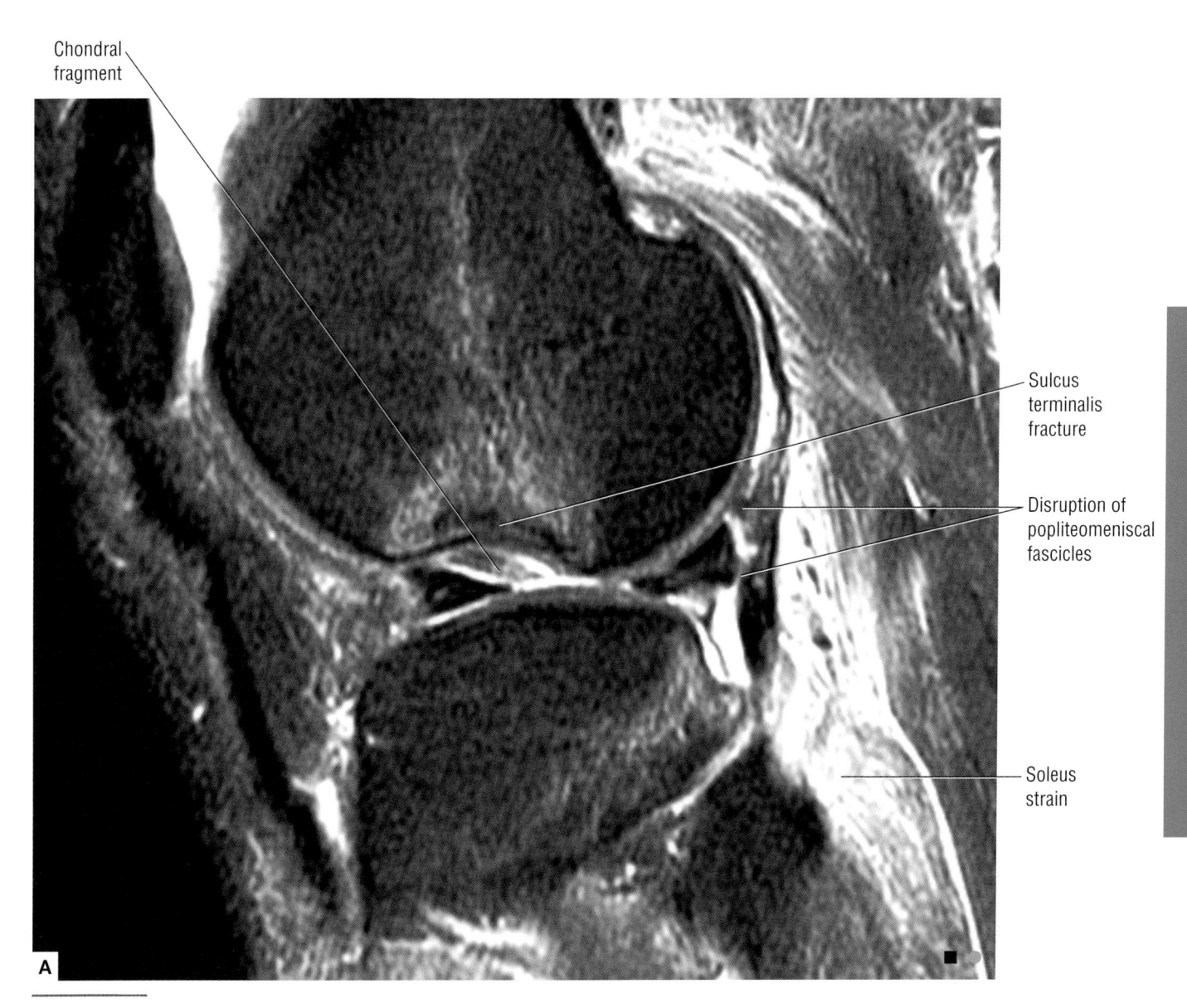

FIGURE 5.70 Posterolateral corner injury with grade 3 ACL (with sulcus fracture), grade 3 MCL, LCL sprain, popliteofibular ligament tear, tear of the popliteomeniscal ligaments, and root avulsion of the posterior horn lateral meniscus. Complex tear of the lateral meniscus and flap tear of the medial meniscus were associated findings. (**A**) Sagittal FS PD FSE. (*Continued*)

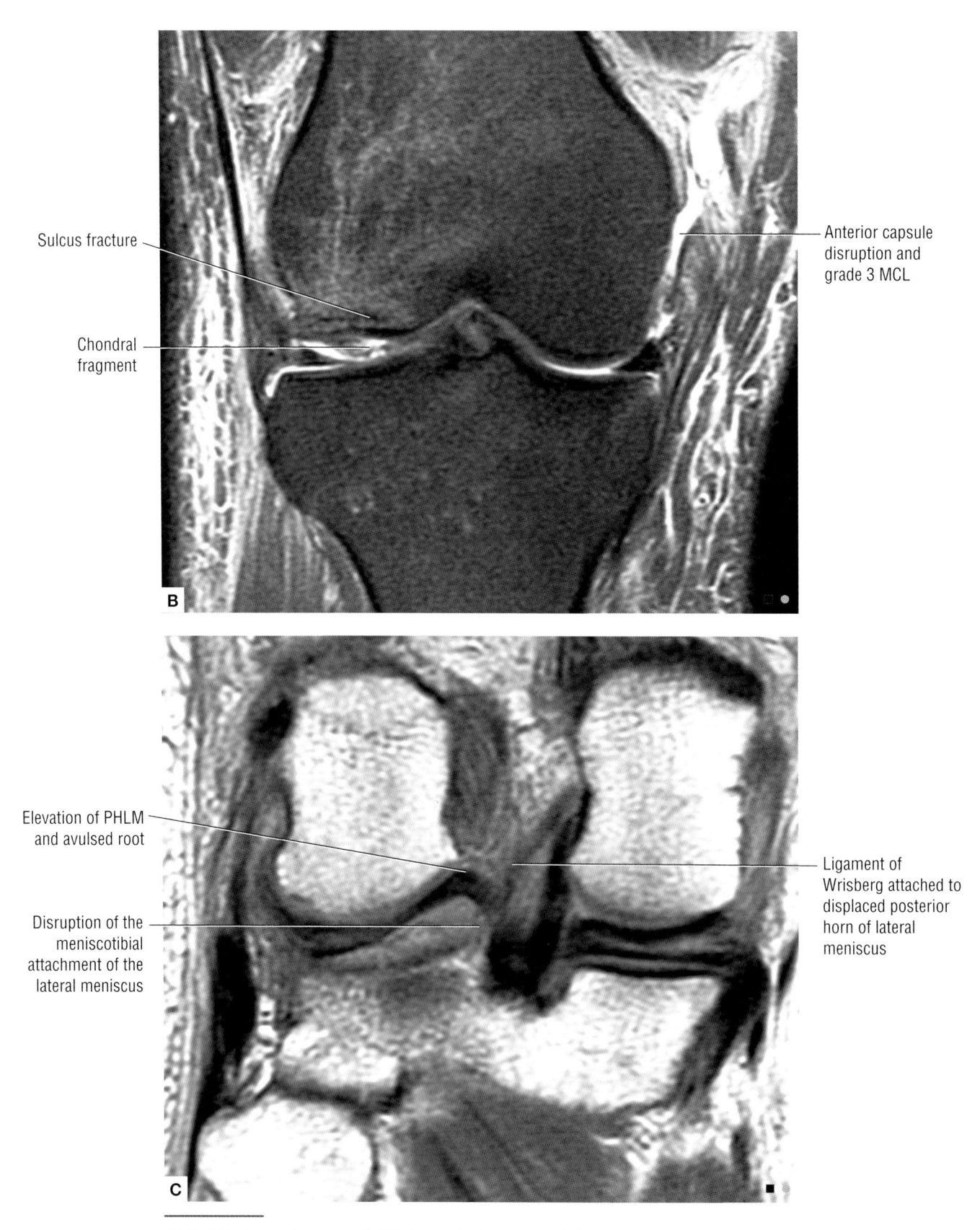

FIGURE 5.70 *(Continued)* (**B**) Coronal FS PD FSE. (**C**) Coronal PD FSE.

Cruciate Ligaments

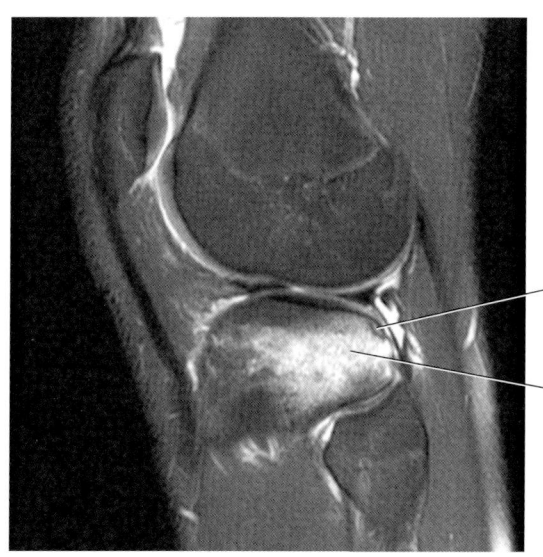

FIGURE 5.71 Nondisplaced posterolateral tibial plateau fracture secondary to ACL disruption on a sagittal FS PD image.

FIGURE 5.72 Lateral condylopatellar sulcus impaction with hyperintense subchondral marrow edema and depression of the subchondral plate. Bucket-handle lateral meniscal tear is shown (sagittal FS PD FSE image).

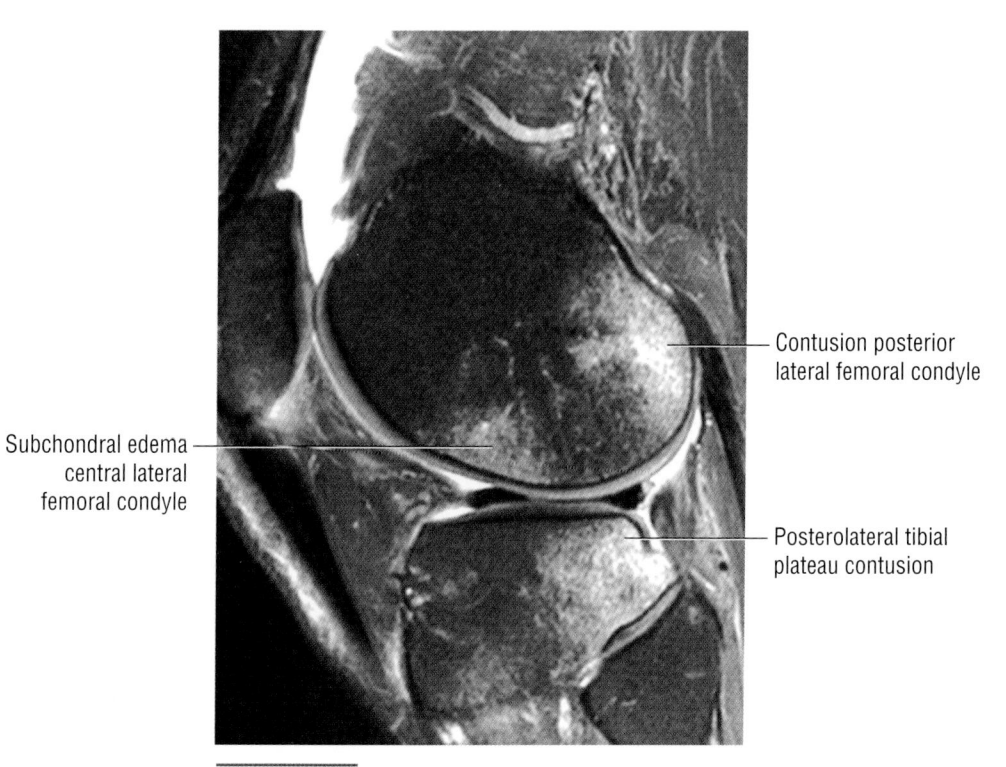

FIGURE 5.73 Osseous contusions of both the sulcus and posterior weight-bearing surfaces of the lateral femoral condyle. Note the osseous contusion of the posterior lateral tibial plateau and anterior translation of the tibia relative to the femur (sagittal FS PD FSE image).

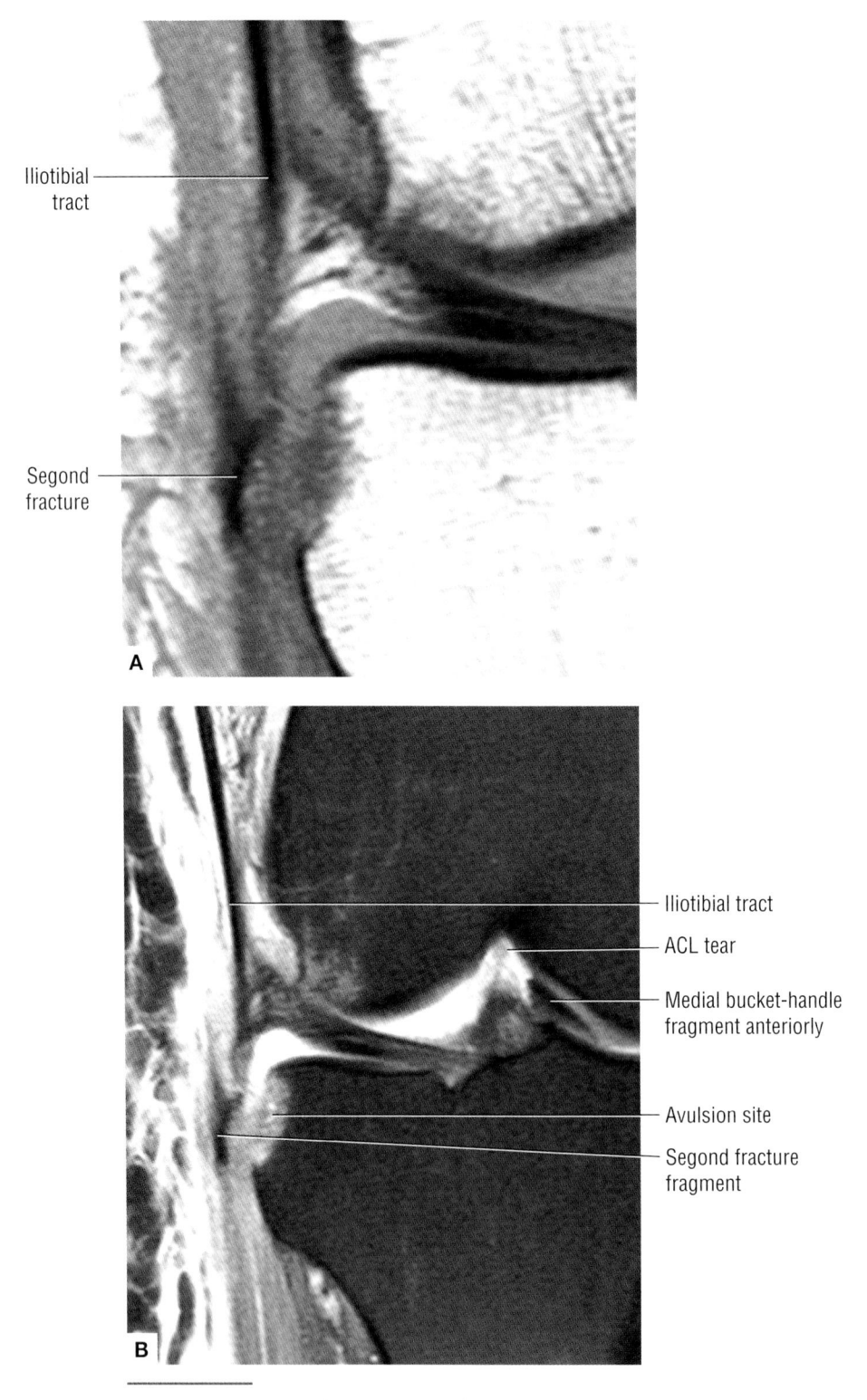

FIGURE 5.74 T1 (**A**) and FS PD (**B**) FSE coronal image of an acute Segond fracture associated with an ACL tear. The fracture is characteristically oriented along the long axis of the tibia, lateral and immediately inferior to the joint line (posterior and proximal to Gerdy's tubercle).

Cruciate Ligaments

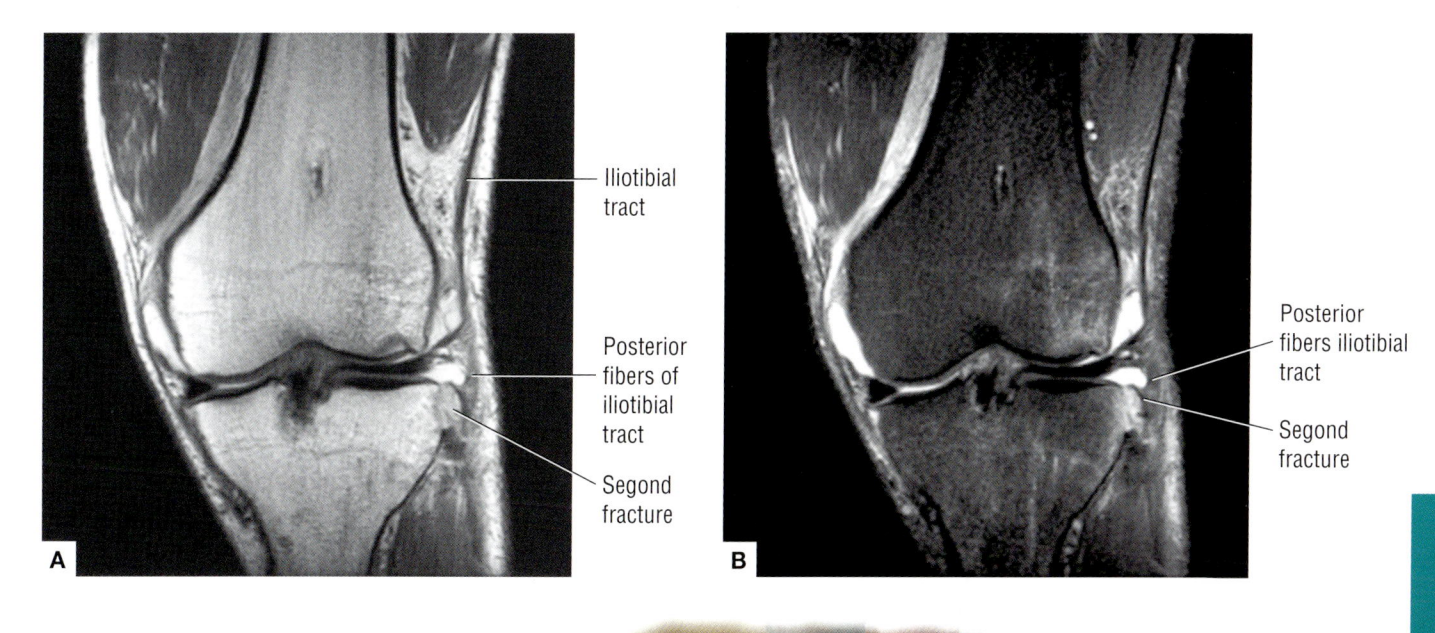

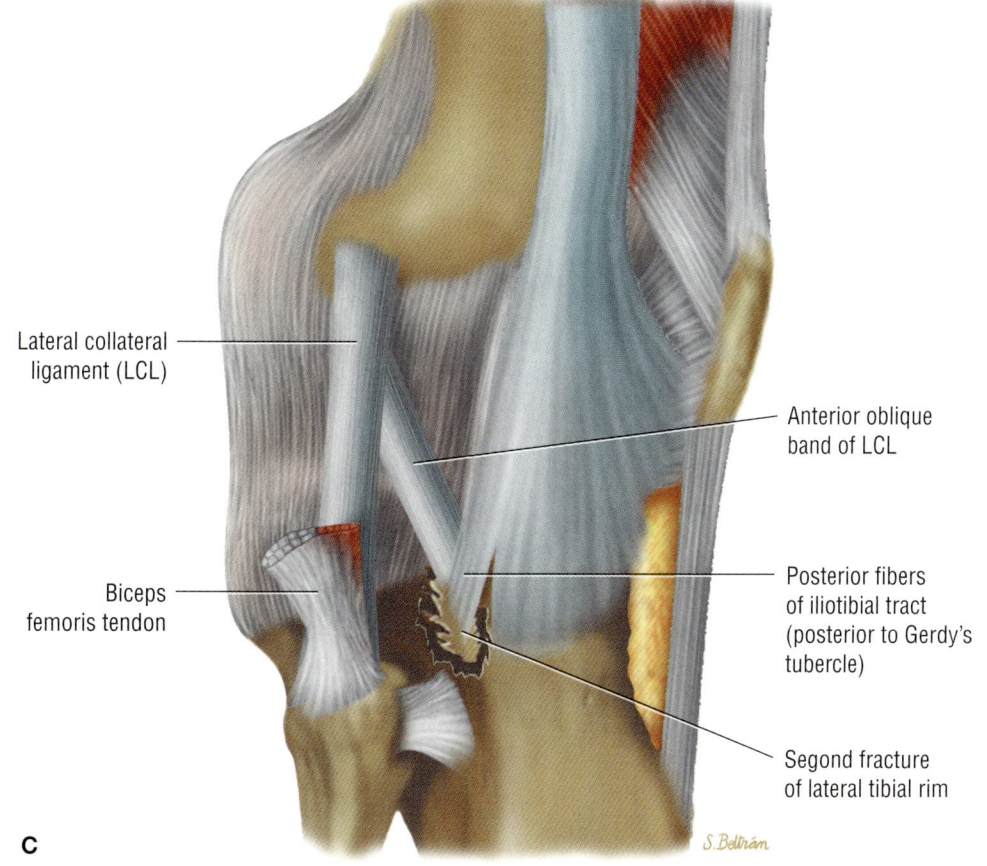

FIGURE 5.75 The posterior fibers of the iliotibial tract and anterior oblique band of the LCL are directly attached to the acute Segond fracture fragment as seen on coronal PD FSE (**A**) and FS PD FSE (**B**) images and a lateral view three-dimensional color illustration (**C**).

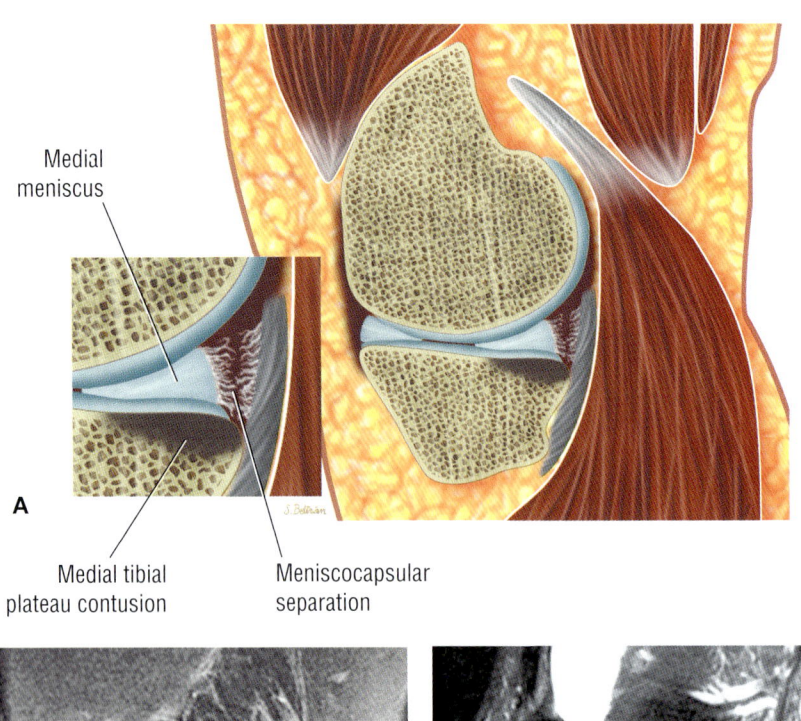

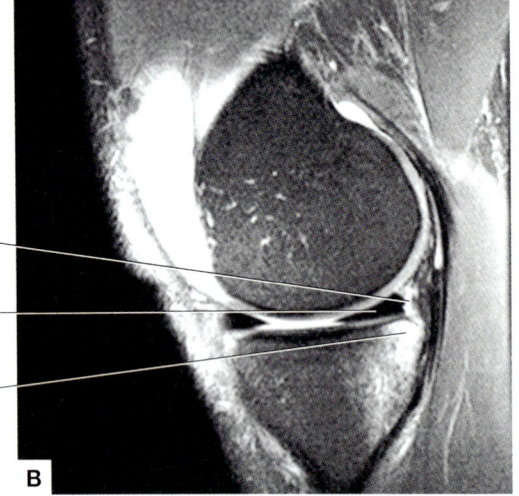

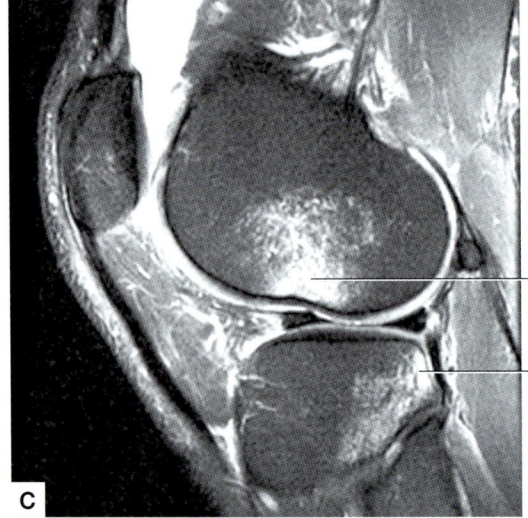

FIGURE 5.76 (**A**) Meniscocapsular separation with posterior medial tibial plateau contusion caused by an ACL rupture–related contrecoup injury. (**B**) Corresponding sagittal image displaying a hyperintense meniscocapsular separation and a medial tibial plateau contusion. Lateral compartment contusions (**C**) and the grade 3 ACL tear (**D**) are demonstrated. (**B–D**) Sagittal FS PD FSE images.

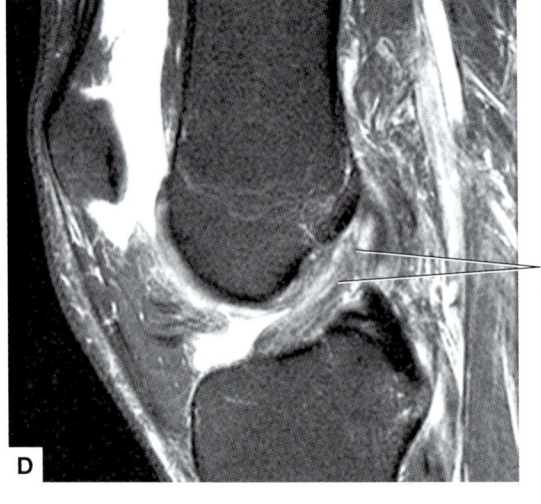

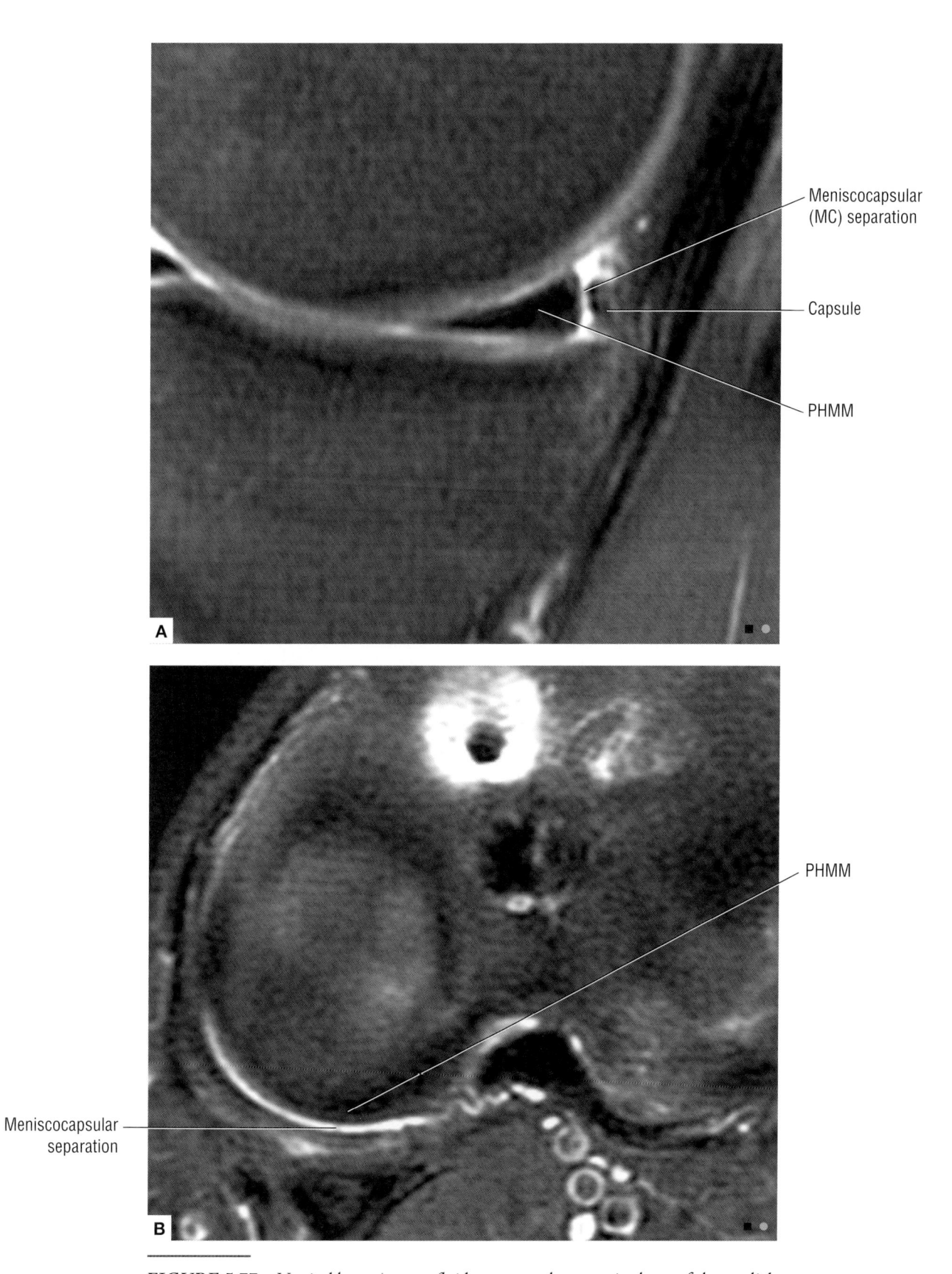

FIGURE 5.77 Vertical hyperintense fluid separates the posterior horn of the medial meniscus (posterior horn medial meniscus) from the peripheral posterior capsule. This finding (meniscocapsular separation) was the sequel of a grade 3 ACL tear and an associated contrecoup injury. An ACL reconstruction was performed. Sagittal (**A**) and axial (**B**) FS PD FSE images.

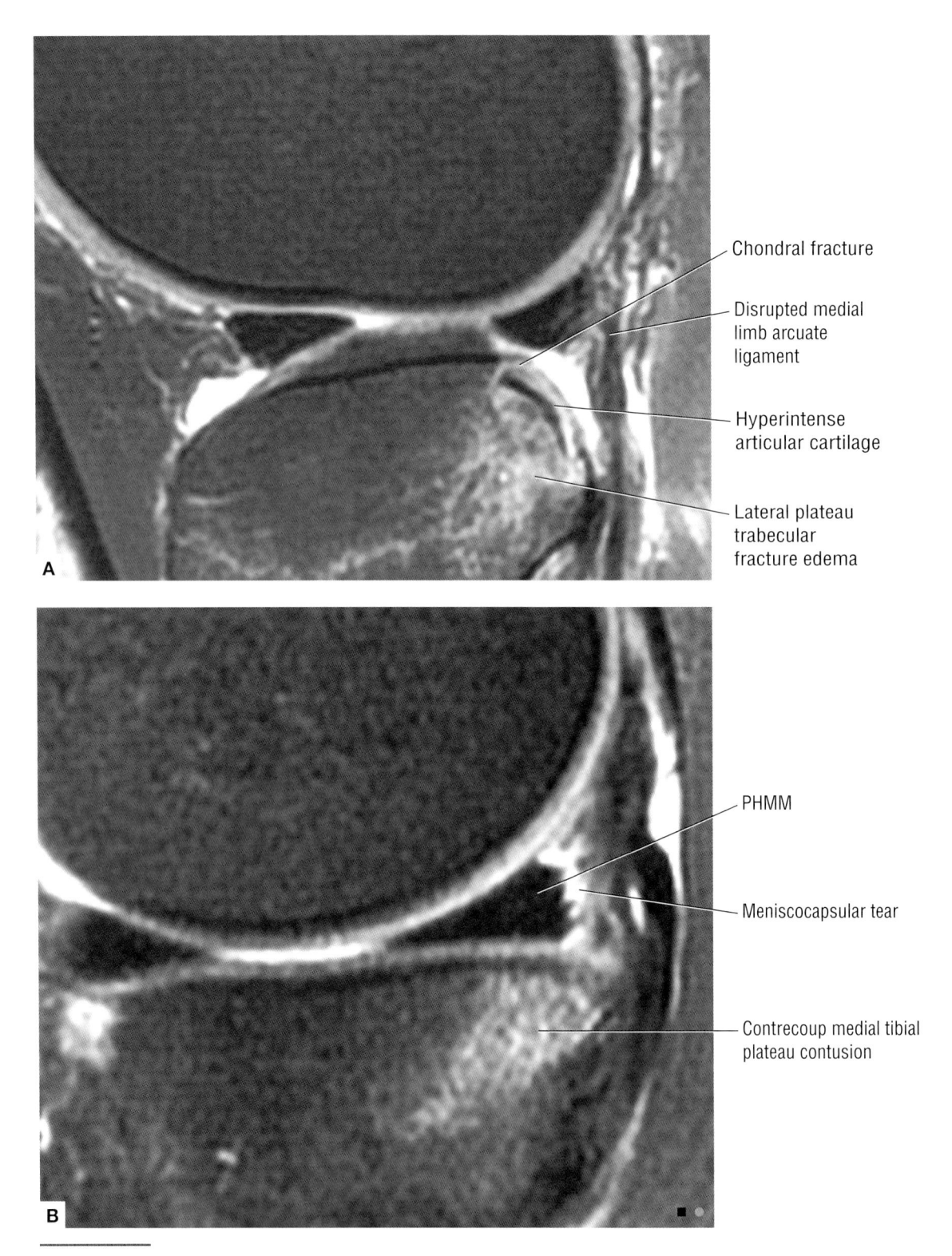

FIGURE 5.78 Grade 3 ACL-associated lateral tibial plateau fracture (**A**) and contrecoup medial tibial plateau trabecular contusion (**B**). Many ACL-related osseous contusions are in fact discrete subchondral fractures that demonstrate a linear component on T1/PD images. Hyperintensity within the involved articular cartilage surface overlying the contusion is associated with a traumatized cartilage matrix, which is a potential precursor lesion to posttraumatic arthritis. The medial tibial plateau contrecoup contusion or trabecular fracture is associated with meniscocapsular injuries or peripheral vertical tears of the posterior horn medial meniscus. Lateral (**A**) and medial (**B**) sagittal FS PD FSE images.

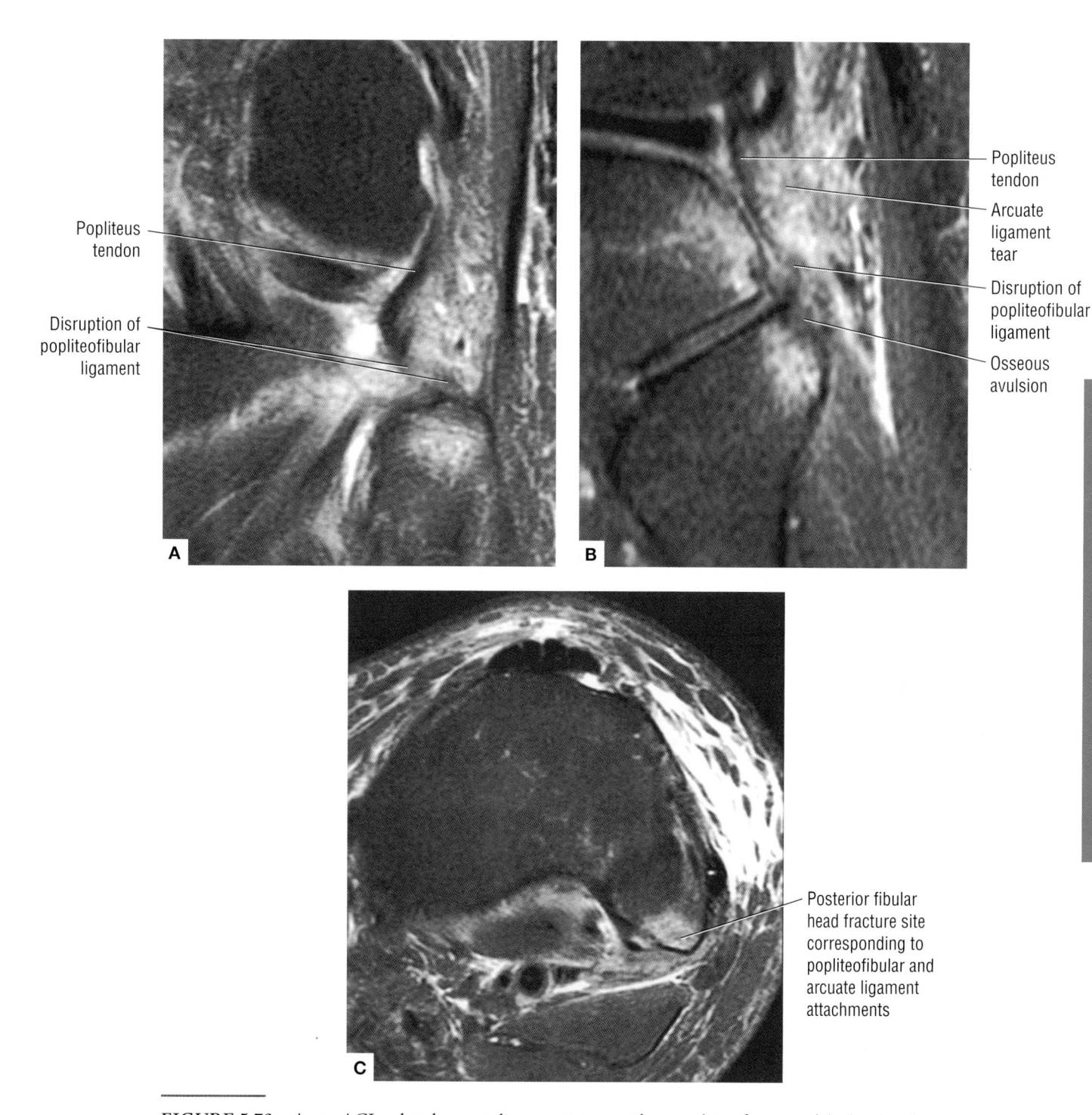

FIGURE 5.79 Acute ACL-related arcuate ligament injury with an avulsion fracture of the head at the attachment sites of the popliteofibular and arcuate ligaments. (**A**) Coronal FS PD FSE image showing the medial displacement of the popliteofibular ligament. (**B**) Sagittal FS PD FSE image showing arcuate ligament disruption. (**C**) Axial FS PD FSE image displaying the posterior involvement of the fibular head, corresponding to the attachments of the popliteofibular and arcuate ligaments.

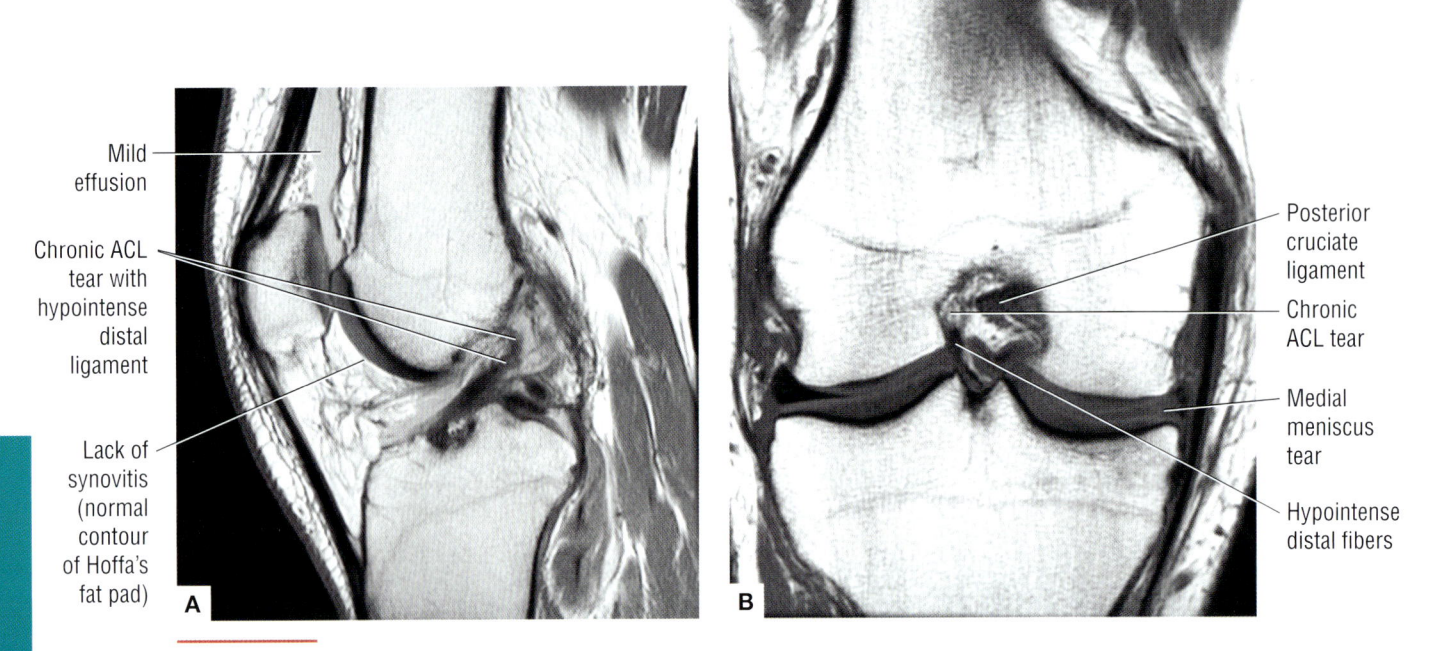

FIGURE 5.80 (**A**) Sagittal PD FSE image showing chronic ACL tear with mild residual effusion and synovitis. (**B**) Corresponding coronal PD FSE image with associated extensive tear of the medial meniscus.

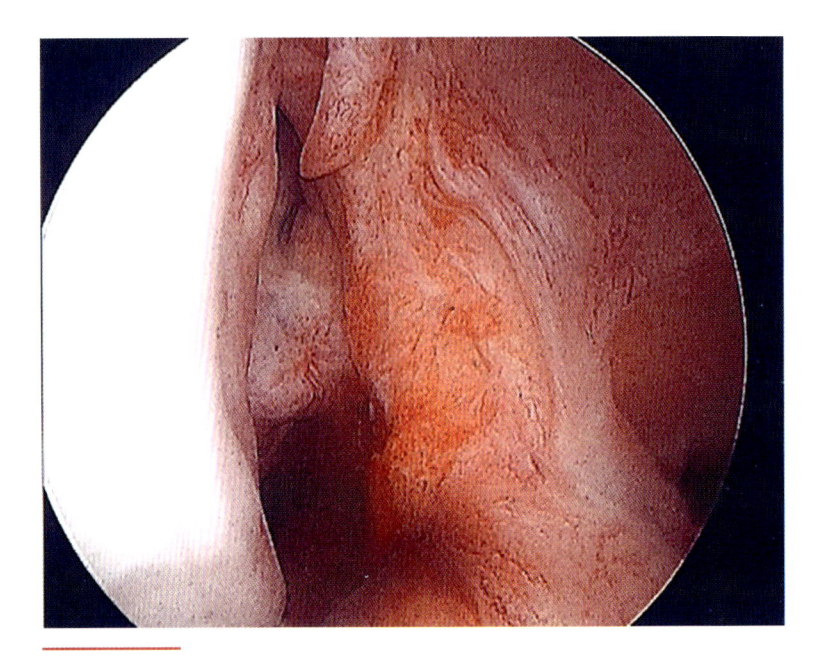

Labels (A): Mild effusion; Chronic ACL tear with hypointense distal ligament; Lack of synovitis (normal contour of Hoffa's fat pad).

Labels (B): Posterior cruciate ligament; Chronic ACL tear; Medial meniscus tear; Hypointense distal fibers.

FIGURE 5.81 Empty lateral wall seen on arthroscopy. (Reprinted from Fu FH. *Master Techniques in Orthopaedic Surgery: Sports Medicine*. Philadelphia, PA: Lippincott Williams & Wilkins; 2010, with permission.)

Cruciate Ligaments

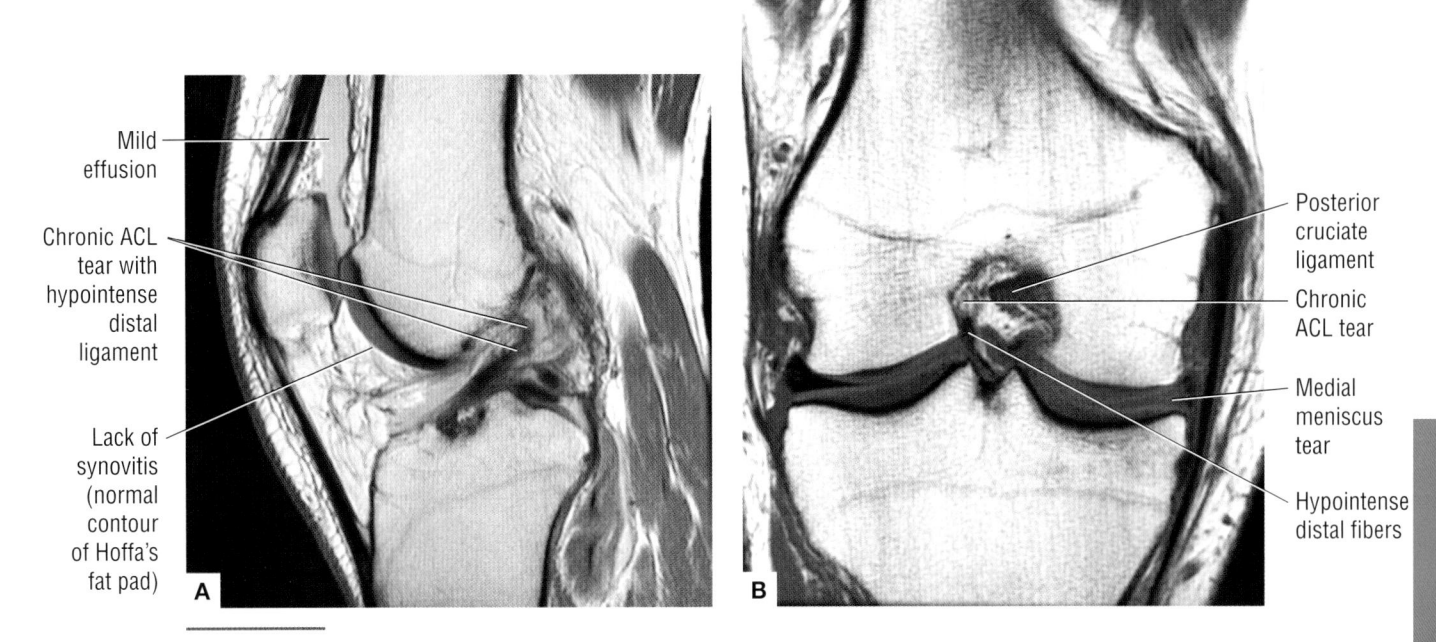

FIGURE 5.82 (**A**) Sagittal PD FSE image showing chronic ACL tear with mild residual effusion and synovitis. (**B**) Corresponding coronal PD FSE image with associated extensive tear of the medial meniscus.

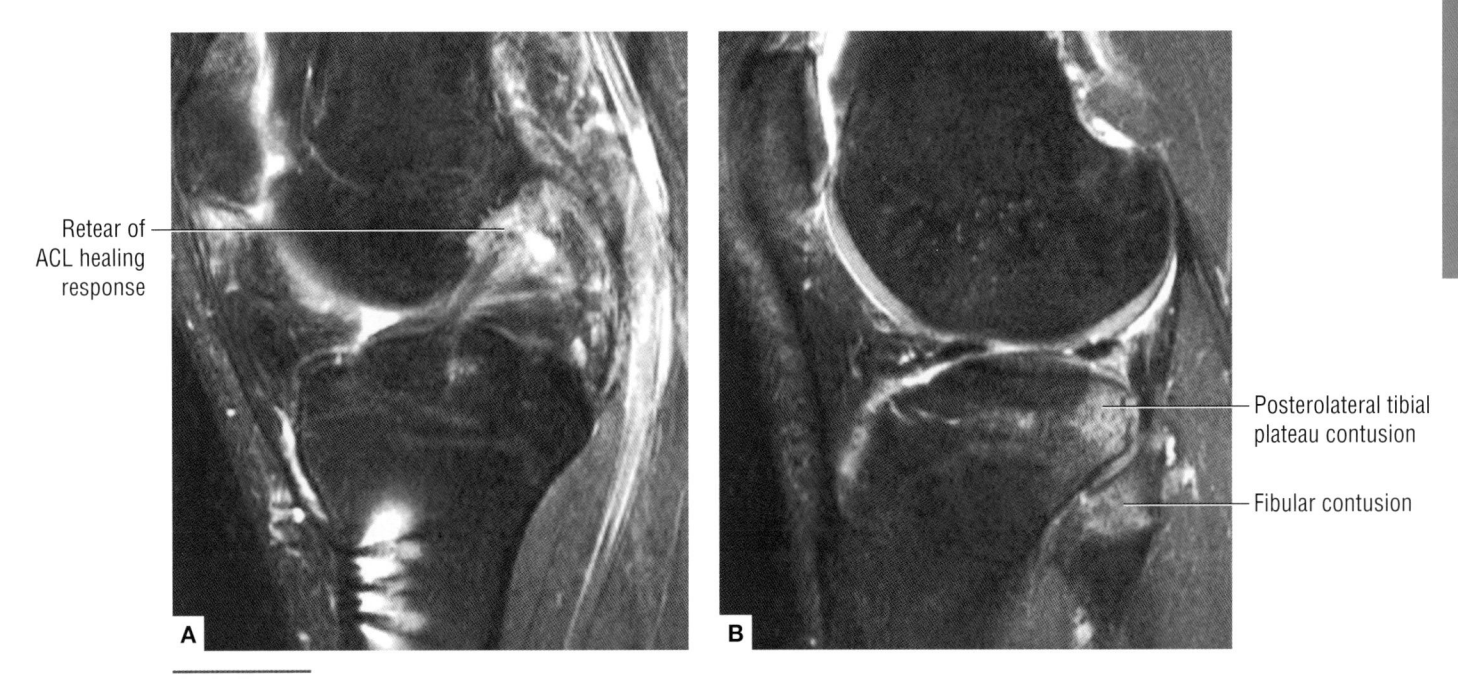

FIGURE 5.83 (**A**) Failed healing response treatment for a proximal ACL tear. Reinjury resulted in tearing of the scarred proximal fibers. (**B**) Acute lateral tibial plateau and fibular contusion indicate reinjury and instability. The posterior horn of the lateral meniscus was repaired at the time of the healing response procedure.

Accuracy of MR Imaging

- 95% accuracy of MR imaging in diagnosis of ACL pathology

- Accuracy, sensitivity, and specificity increase with inclusion of T2-weighted sequences.[327]

- 94% sensitivity of MR compared with 78% for anterior drawer test and 89% for Lachman's test[275]

- 100% specificity for ACL instability

- Use of nonorthogonal (sagittal oblique) plane compared to orthogonal plane increased accuracy from 61% to 66% and sensitivity from 70% to 100%; specificity remained at 100%.[500]

- 98% sensitivity when sagittal images are supplemented with coronal and axial images[139]

- Use of T1, PD, and FS PD FSE coronal images to document ACL injury and establish ligamentous continuity allows more accurate evaluation of partial ACL tears.

    - Lateral compartment bone contusions or other ancillary findings can be found in both partial and complete ACL injuries.

    - Partial tears may not warrant surgery at time of initial injury, although many eventually result in instability and ACL insufficiency.[312]

    - ACL deficiency also leads to intrasubstance meniscal degenerations and tears.

    - Menisci help stabilize anterior tibial translation in ACL-deficient knee.[69]

- Arthroscopy an imperfect or relative gold standard

    - Stretching or intrasubstance ACL injuries may go undetected despite positive MR findings.[118]

    - Initial experience has shown promising results in comparing arthrometric knee testing, MR, and second-look arthroscopic procedures for partial ACL tears.

Treatment of ACL Injuries

- Specific treatment for ACL injury depends on presence or absence of associated meniscal or second ligament injury.

- Associated meniscal tears, collateral ligament injuries, or patellofemoral instabilities are indications for ACL reconstructions.[237]

- Primary repair most successful when avulsion occurs at either femoral or tibial ACL attachment

- Avulsion from low T1 signal cortical bone without associated subchondral high T1 (marrow-containing) component may be more difficult to visualize.

- Visualization of cortical and trabecular bone may require use of GRE sequences.

- Mid-substance interstitial tears not good candidates for ACL repair

- ACL-deficient knee at risk for osteoarthritis, articular cartilage degeneration, and secondary meniscal tears
    - Secondary meniscal tears in as many as 20% of patients secondary to degenerative wear[238]
    - Potential for long-term disability and progressive deterioration
    - Treatment of ACL tears thus directed at reestablishing ACL function through repair or reconstruction

- Nonoperative/conservative treatment can be satisfactory in older, less active patients.[55]
    - Patients who are willing to accept some instability and risk for meniscal tear

- Factors influencing decisions related to conservative and surgical management of acute ACL injuries include:
    - Presence or absence of torn meniscus
    - Patient's age, occupation, and athletic participation
    - Degree of ligamentous laxity

- Recreational athletes treated with aggressive rehabilitation and functional bracing show fewer degenerative changes.[292]

- Satisfactory outcomes (83%) have been reported for nonoperative treatment of ACL rupture in middle-aged patients.[73]

- Healing response technique for treatment of proximal ACL tears in cases where slope of ACL was relatively parallel to intercondylar roof and proximal fibers in close proximity to lateral femoral condyle
    - Healing may be related to increased blood supply.
    - Functionally incompetent partial tears of proximal ACL can also be treated by modified healing response using microfractures to induce a blood clot.
- Patients with combined instabilities and desire to resume sports activity are better served by operative reconstruction.

ACL Repair

- Bony avulsion of distal ACL treated successfully with direct bone-to-bone fixation
- Primary repairs for mid-substance ACL tears frequently unsuccessful and not recommended
- Most patients have pain, stiffness, and instability at five-year follow-up of primary repairs.[131,353]
- Primary ACL repair and intraarticular augmentation produce better results than ACL repair alone (pivot-shift test, arthrometric testing, and activity levels).
- Results of ACL repair and synthetic augmentation (intraarticular polyester ligament augmentation device [LAD]) were poor.[353]

ACL Reconstruction

Key Concepts

- Incorrect placement of both tibial and femoral tunnels is the most common cause of ACL reconstruction failure.[40]
- Isometry
    - Historical focus related proper placement of femoral tunnel at intersection of posterior femoral cortex and posterior aspect of distal femoral physeal scar (on sagittal images).
    - Previous technique position of femoral tunnel at 11 o'clock and 1 o'clock positions in the right and left knees, respectively, produced grafts that were too vertical in both sagittal and coronal planes.
    - Previous teaching was to repair for constant length and tension of ACL graft throughout flexion and extension.
- Current goal of single-bundle ACL reconstruction is to produce proper obliquity in both sagittal and coronal planes to achieve proper biomechanics and not isometricity.[40]
- Anteriorly placed femoral tunnel associated with graft elongation and instability

ACL Isometry Revisited

- Isometry (maintaining ligament length) is a relative concept but not primary goal.
- Isometric behavior in its ideal definition implies linear separation of 1mm or less throughout the full range of flexion and extension.
- In fact, no femoral attachment site produces perfect isometry.
    - All grafts' femoral attachment sites associated with at least 2mm minimum change in graft length
- The previous recommended isometric location for femoral tunnel placement in the 11/1 o'clock position is now considered too vertical.
- Normal anatomic attachment placement is more important than trying to achieve exclusively optimized isometric points.
    - Proper anatomic attachment sites can also minimize change in graft length.
        - Minimize graft tension and prevent increased anterior translation[40,147]

ACL Reconstruction

- Goal of ACL reconstruction had been to establish sufficient isometric tension without regard to anatomic attachment sites.
    - Keep the distance between tibial and femoral attachment points from changing more than 2 to 3mm through zero to 90 degrees of flexion.[382]
    - This ACL isometry philosophy has since been modified.[40]
- Surgical reconstructions classified as extraarticular, intraarticular, or combined intra- and extraarticular[30,37]
- Extraarticular ACL reconstruction
    - Procedures (e.g., the MacIntosh, Ellison, and Andrews) include transfer of pes anserinus and various lateral techniques that use the iliotibial tract to provide restraint to anterior subluxation of the lateral tibial plateau.
    - Variable success
    - May be associated with persistent anterior tibial translation (e.g., pes anserinus transfer)
- Intraarticular ACL reconstruction
    - Bone–patellar tendon–bone construct achieves better results than extraarticular techniques.
    - Iliotibial band (ITB) may be transferred intraarticularly in lateral over-the-top reconstruction.
    - Other techniques use semitendinosus and gracilis tendons doubled or semitendinosus tendon quadrupled.
    - Autogenous, allograft, xenograft, and synthetic tissues can be used for ligament reconstruction for both acute and chronic ACL injuries.[18,30,144,539]
    - Allograft tissues: patellar and Achilles tendons
    - Synthetic allograft materials: carbon fiber, knitted Dacron (Invista, Wichita, KS), and braided polypropylene
    - Use of expanded polytetrafluoroethylene (Gore-Tex; W. L. Gore & Associates, Inc., Newark, DE) complicated by attenuation, rupture, and stretching of grafts
    - Bone–patellar tendon–bone graft using central (middle) third of patellar tendon remains most common and successful procedure for ACL reconstruction.

- 90% good outcome (defined as negative pivot-shift test and clinical stability)[238]
- Bone plugs taken from tibial tubercle and patella with central third of patellar tendon used as a free graft[238]
- Graft is 1.5 times as strong as the native ACL and can be placed arthroscopically.
- Bone plugs and interference screws allow stable fixation within tunnels.
- Advantages of bone-to-bone healing of the graft and easy arthroscopic accessibility to patellar tendon
- Complications include patellar fracture, tendon rupture or tendinitis, quadriceps weakness, and patellofemoral pain.
- Semitendinosus and gracilis tendons are transferred as free double-looped (folded) grafts since they are not as strong as the patellar tendon.
- Graft placed in 10-mm bone tunnel after proper sizing and contouring of bone plugs and graft
- Tibial tunnel usually located just posterior to midpoint of tibial ACL footprint to reduce impingement in extension and to decrease necessity for aggressive notchplasty
- Femoral tunnel recommendation of correct graft obliquity is the 2:30 to 9:30 position.[40]
- To limit impingement of graft on anterolateral aspect of condylar notch, especially in extension, notchplasty is usually performed.[237]
- Parallel osseous tunnels through lateral femur and anterior tibia created after isometric points selected
- Incorrect placement and positioning of graft can result in either slackening or overtension and stretching, resulting in increased laxity.[171]
- Isometry is relative because all of the graft fibers cannot maintain an isometric relation during flexion.
- Selection of femoral graft attachment is more dependent on fiber length.
- Anterior femoral tunnel may result in excessive strain during flexion.
- Posterior or distal femoral graft attachment may produce similar strain or elongation in extension.[393]
- Isometry is less affected by selection of the tibial attachment.

Graft Impingement

- Bone impingement on the graft can occur in either the roof and walls of the intercondylar fossa or at the intraarticular exits of the bone tunnels.[171]

- Impingement can result in stretching, abrasion, fibrocartilaginous remodeling, or tearing of the graft due to larger compressive stresses.

- Similarly, a congenitally narrow intercondylar notch may result in impingement of the native ACL.[187,269,454]

- Graft placed at anterior edge of ACL tibial attachment can result in impingement with intercondylar roof at full knee extension unless adequate superior notchplasty performed.
    - In full extension, normal ACL lies along roof of intercondylar fossa.
    - Anterior distal fibers of normal ACL curve around junction of intercondylar fossa and trochlear groove before insertion into tibia.
    - Distal fiber curvature not present in grafts → risk for impingement

- Extension loss or flexion contracture may be caused by either graft impingement or localized anterior arthrofibrosis.

- Side wall impingement with the intercondylar fossa is related to shape of the fossa, graft size, and presence of osteophytes.

- Impingement at intraarticular tunnel exits caused by knee flexion and bending of the graft, which may rub or abrade at the bone tunnel exit
    - Chamfering at the bone tunnel exit and drilling and alignment of the femoral tunnel through the tibial tunnel minimize this potential source of impingement.

Revascularization of ACL Graft

- Healing of native ACL is poor and significantly different from healing response of extraarticular ligaments.[42]

- In animal models, autogenous patellar tendon grafts show necrosis and lack of vascular or synovial attachment 2 weeks after intraarticular implantation.[42]

- "Ligamentization" describes histologic stages of incorporation of patellar tendon graft, which progresses through four stages of transformation:
    - Avascular necrosis (stage I)
    - Revascularization (stage II)
    - Cellular proliferation (stage III)
    - Remodeling (stage IV)

- After remodeling (stage IV), morphology and histology of ACL graft closely resemble native ACL, and there is evidence that further graft maturation occurs after the first year.

- Fibroblast healing thought to occur through the synovial membrane
    - Not intrinsic to patellar tendon graft
    - Revascularization from synovial fold and endosteal vessels in bone tunnels
    - Graft revascularization complete at 20 weeks, progressing from vascular synovial covering at 6 weeks and intrinsic vessel formation at 6 to 10 weeks

- Delayed vascularity of patellar tendon allografts compared to autografts
    - Autogenous patellar tendon grafts revascularized in early postoperative period and similar to original ACL at 1 year (by arthroscopy and light microscopy)[2]
    - But electron microscopic ultrastructural study suggests that grafts still immature at 1 year (presence of active fibroblasts with high cytoplasm-to-nucleus ratio)
    - May be necessary to reexamine aggressive rehabilitation programs that emphasize early return to full activity

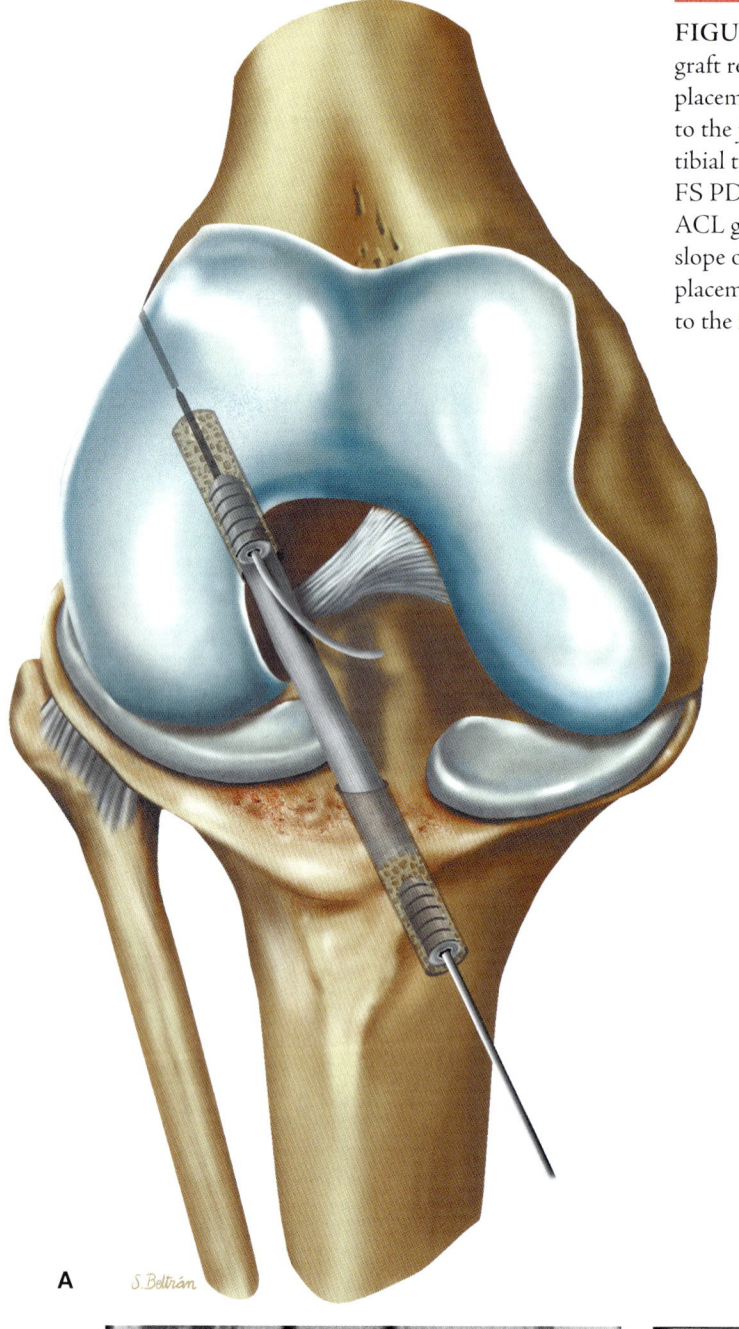

FIGURE 5.84 (**A**) Bone–patellar tendon–bone graft reconstruction components for ACL replacement. The tibial tunnel is at least 3cm distal to the joint line and about 1.5cm medial to the tibial tuberosity. Sagittal PD FSE (**B**) and sagittal FS PD FSE (**C**) images showing the hypointense ACL graft with tibial insertion posterior to the slope of the intercondylar roof. The femoral tunnel placement is correct, with the graft origin posterior to the femoral diaphyseal cortex.

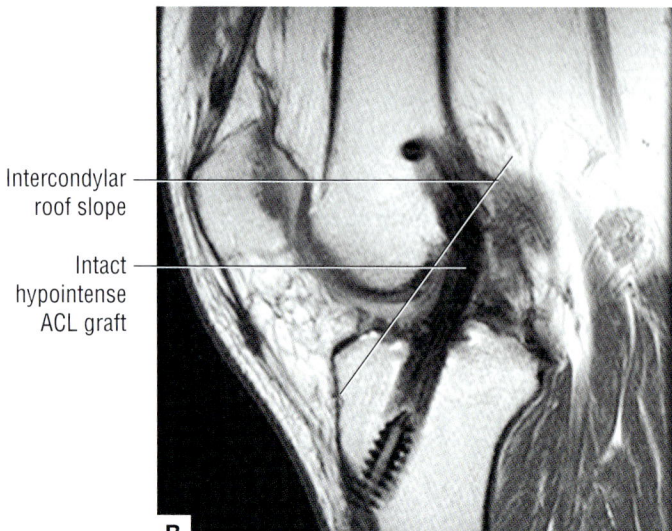

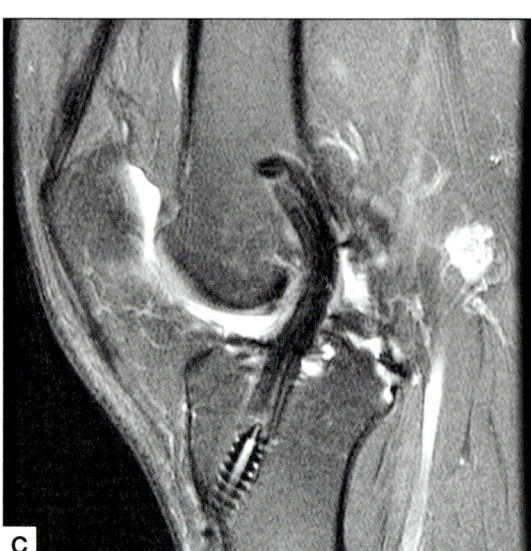

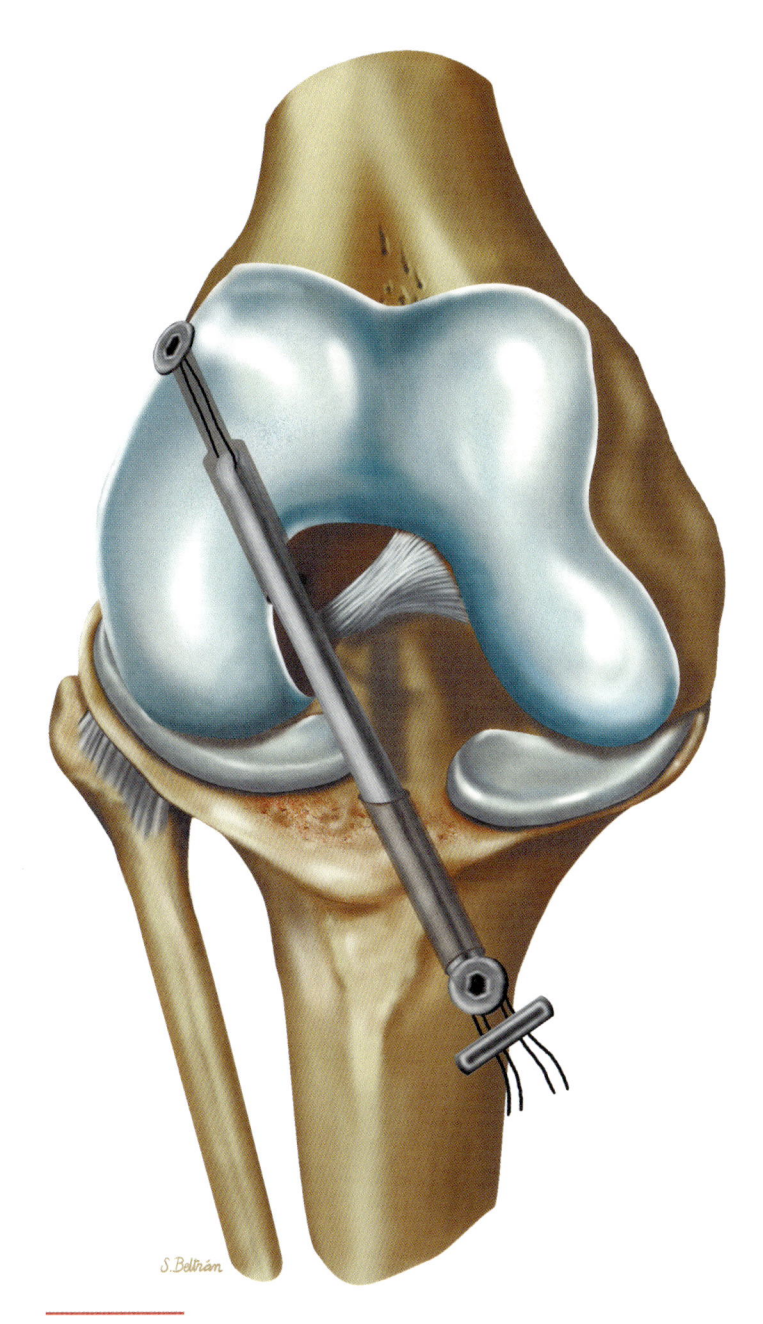

Cruciate Ligaments 495

FIGURE 5.85 Hamstring ACL graft.

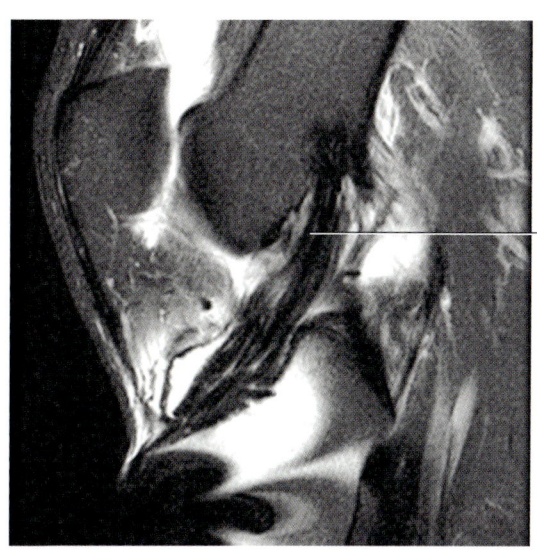

FIGURE 5.86 Intact hypointense hamstring graft. The gracilis and semitendinosus tendons are surgically harvested, then folded and endoscopically inserted as a single quadruple graft or as two separate doubled grafts during ACL reconstruction.

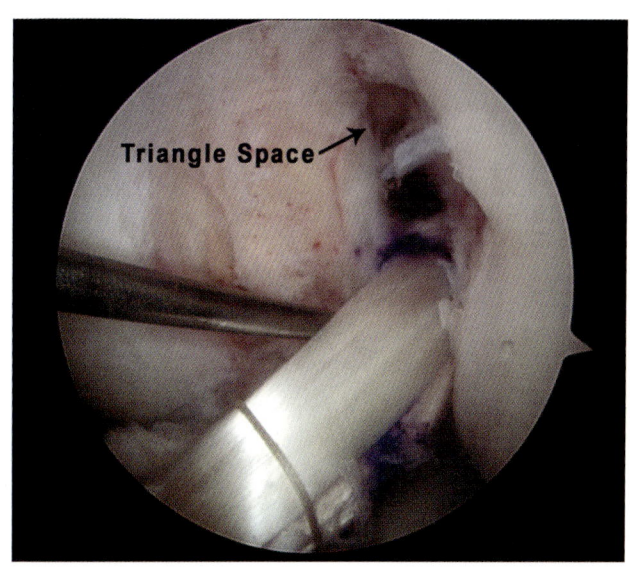

FIGURE 5.87 Final ACL construct with hamstring autograft single-bundle ACL reconstruction. Notice the space between the ACL graft and the native PCL. This "triangular" space is present in native knees. (Reprinted from Fu FH. *Master Techniques in Orthopaedic Surgery: Sports Medicine*. Philadelphia, PA: Lippincott Williams & Wilkins; 2010, with permission.)

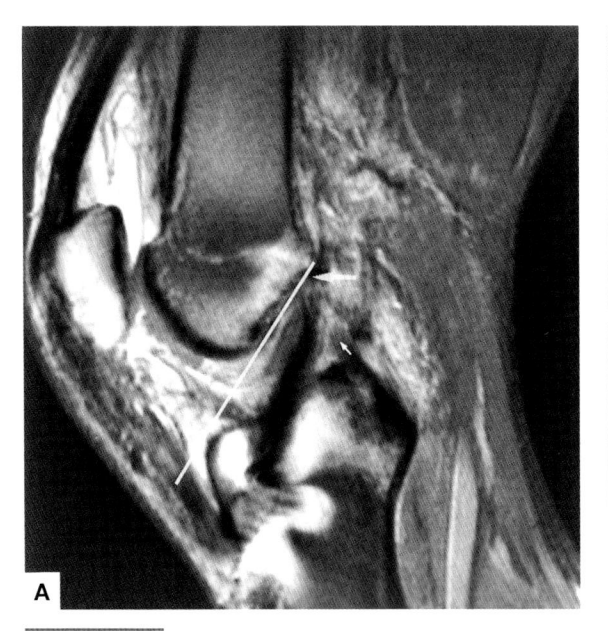

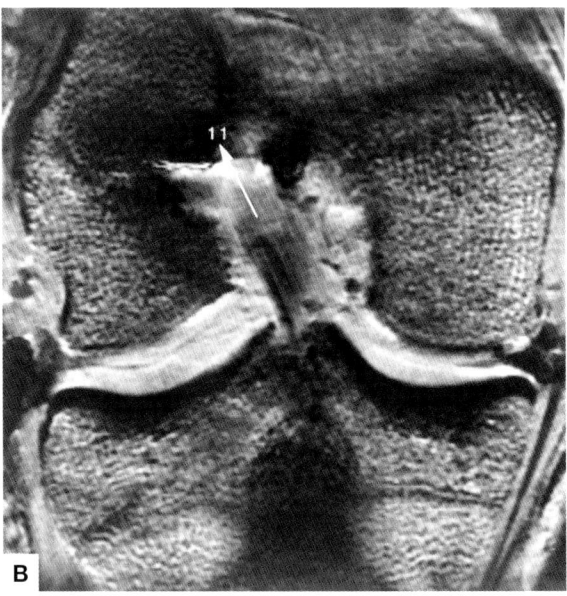

FIGURE 5.88 ACL autograft. (**A**) Unimpinged low-signal-intensity ACL graft with the tibial tunnel posterior to the slope (*long line*) of the intercondylar roof. The PCL is straight (*small arrow*) with the knee positioned in partial flexion. The isometric placement of the graft is indicated by the posterosuperior origin of the graft on the femur (*large arrow*) at the intersection of the posterior femoral cortex and the physeal scar (FS PD-weighted FSE sagittal image). (**B**) The 11-o'clock position (*11*) of the femoral tunnel on a spoiled gradient recalled coronal image. The high and very posterior graft placement in the classic (original) 11/1 o'clock position may result in symptomatic instability despite restricting anteroposterior laxity. Increased obliquity closer to the 9:30/2:30 position is now used to minimize graft tension and limit anterior translation with improved axial stability.

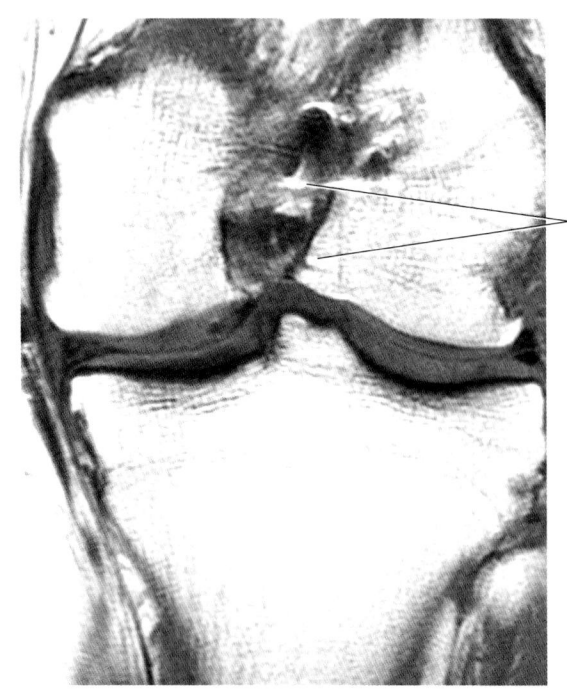

FIGURE 5.89 Failure of the ACL graft secondary to intercondylar notch stenosis. The space between the PCL, the lateral wall, and the intercondylar roof should be enlarged as appropriate during notch preparation (coronal T1-weighted FSE image).

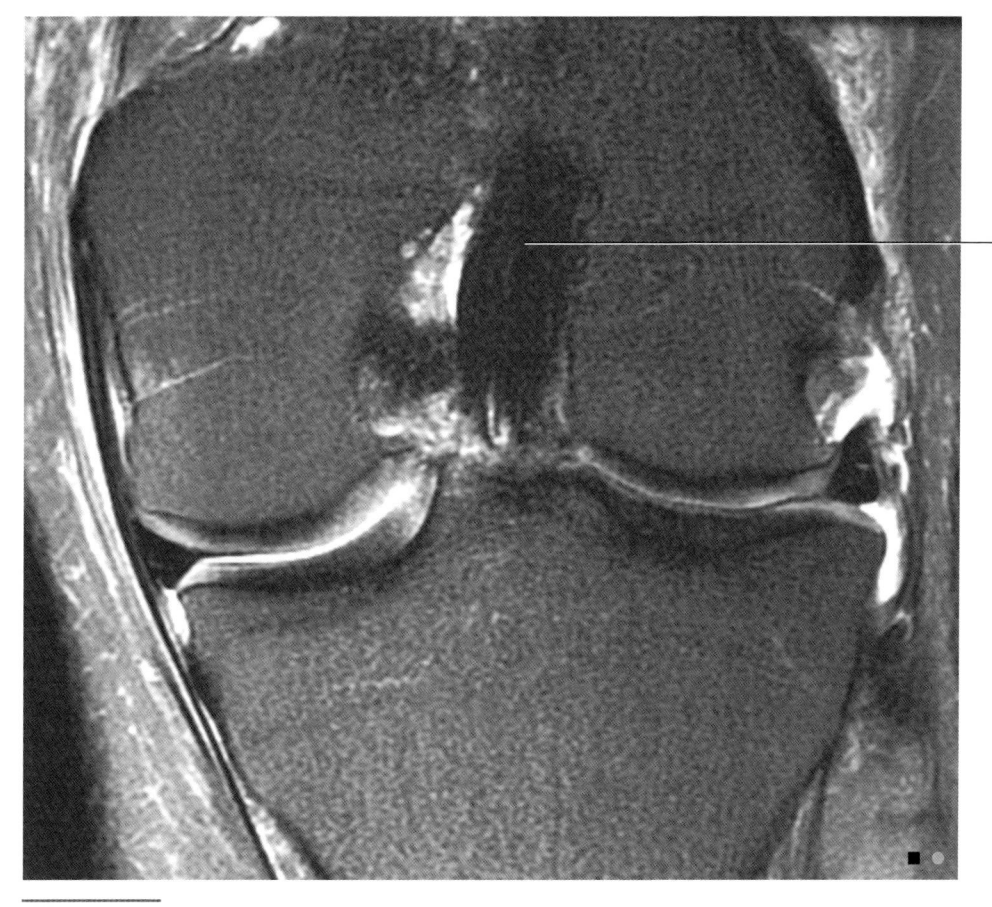

Cruciate Ligaments 497

FIGURE 5.90 Vertical ACL graft alignment in the coronal imaging plane. Grafts that are excessively vertical are less than effective in countering axial rotational stresses (as evident in a pivot shift test). Current practice is to place the ACL graft in the normal (more oblique in coronal and sagittal planes) anatomic attachments instead of selecting isometric points. Coronal FS PD FSE image.[40]

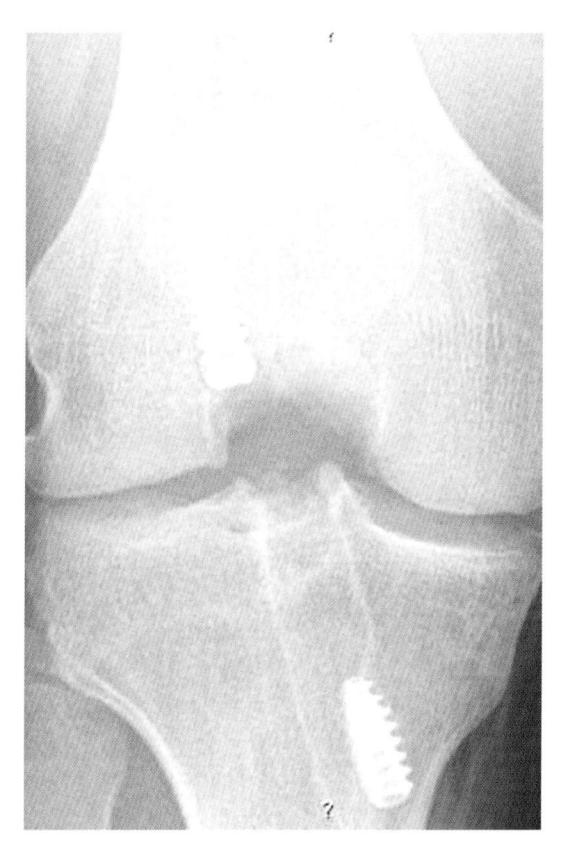

— Vertical orientation of ACL graft

FIGURE 5.91 Radiograph of a patient with a failed previous ACL reconstruction done via a transtibial technique. This image shows a vertical position of the prior graft. (Reprinted from Fu FH. *Master Techniques in Orthopaedic Surgery: Sports Medicine.* Philadelphia, PA: Lippincott Williams & Wilkins; 2010, with permission.)

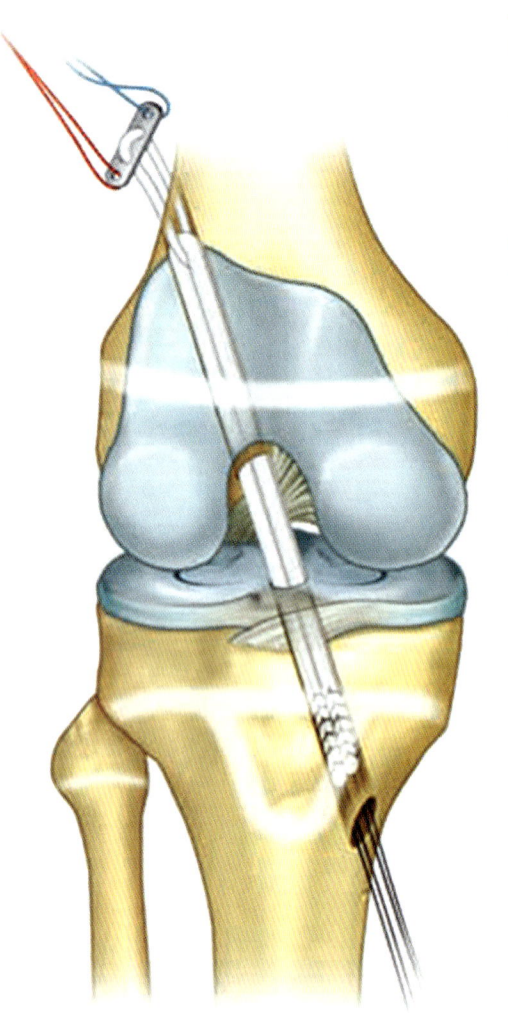

FIGURE 5.92 Example of a modified ACL reconstruction using a hamstring autograft in the skeletally immune patient. The graft is passed, and the Endo-Button is flipped on the femoral cortex. Since there is no potential femoral attachment site that allows for perfect isometry (2mm or less change in graft length), normal biomechanics and anatomy are more important principles. (Reprinted from Fu FH. *Master Techniques in Orthopaedic Surgery: Sports Medicine*. Philadelphia, PA: Lippincott Williams & Wilkins; 2010, with permission.)

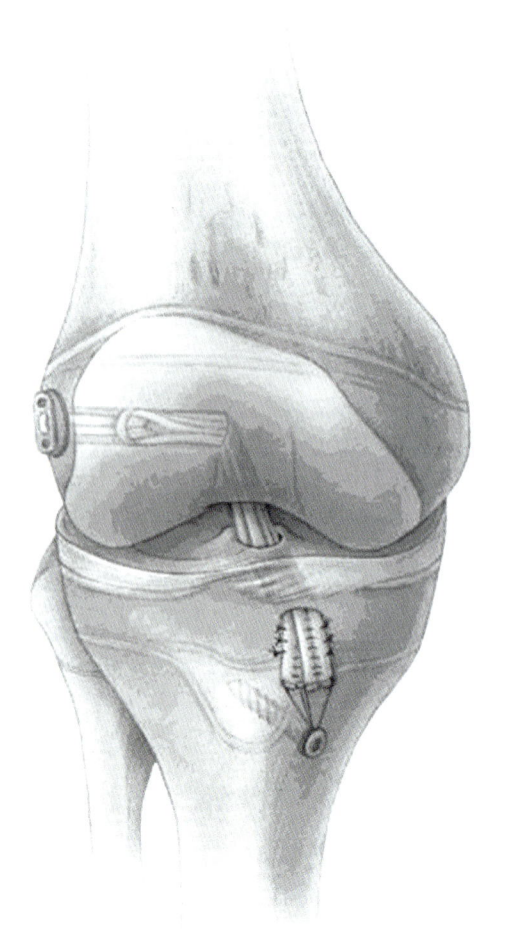

FIGURE 5.93 Physeal-sparing intraarticular ACL reconstruction with epiphyseal tunnels. (Reprinted from Fu FH. *Master Techniques in Orthopaedic Surgery: Sports Medicine*. Philadelphia, PA: Lippincott Williams & Wilkins; 2010, with permission.)

MR Evaluation of ACL Reconstruction

Key Concepts

- MR useful for assessing the following after ACL reconstruction:
    - Graft failure
    - Graft placement
    - Impingement
    - Arthrofibrosis (cyclops lesion)
    - ACL graft ganglia (related to graft tunnel)
    - Hardware placement
- Increased signal intensity may be seen in ACL grafts for 1 to 2 years after reconstruction with the bone–patellar tendon–bone construct.
- Uniform hypointensity of the graft demonstrated after 2 years

MR Evaluation of ACL Reconstruction

- Thin-section (≤3mm) sagittal or sagittal oblique MR images, parallel to ACL graft as prescribed on coronal images, recommended for accurate visualization of neoligament
- Conventional T2- or FS PD-weighted FSE images show less susceptibility artifact than GRE.
- Separate sagittal orthogonal plane may be required to prevent distortion and aid in interpreting meniscal pathology (depending on the magnitude of obliquity of sagittal oblique images).

Primary ACL Repair

- Nonaugmented primary repair of ACL not highly successful due to poor healing[42]
- Successfully sutured ACL ligament maintains low signal intensity except for focal areas of susceptibility artifact.
- Recent repairs may display edema and fluid within ACL.
- Orientation of primary repair should restore the parallel relation with the intercondylar roof that exists with a native ligament.

ACL Reconstruction

- Extraarticular reconstruction
- Thickening or micrometallic or ferromagnetic artifact of distal iliotibial band donor site on anterior coronal images[105]
- Intraarticular ACL reconstruction
- Evaluation of tunnel placement, graft impingement, and rupture[192]
- Criteria for MR evaluation of ACL graft tunnel positions extrapolated from standards developed with conventional radiographic studies
- Isometry primarily controlled by femoral tunnel placement, while graft roof impingement reflected in the location of the tibial tunnel; however, anatomic attachment sites are the primary goal while secondarily attempting to maintain isometry[192,197,212,333]
- Femoral tunnel cannot be more than a few millimeters anterior or inferior to anatomic origin of ACL on lateral wall of intercondylar notch without compromising isometry.
- In sagittal plane, intersection of low-signal-intensity posterior femoral cortical line with posterior intercondylar roof was used as the old intraarticular point of reference of femoral tunnel.[393]
  - A femoral tunnel aperture on Blumensaat line is now considered too high up in the notch (relative to the clock-face).
  - The optional position on the femoral side is distal to Blumensaat line that occurs on sidewall of notch.[40]
- Posterior superior edge of intercondylar roof closely corresponds to posterior edge of physeal scar on sagittal MR images.[105]
- Opening of femoral tunnel identified by either 2 o'clock/10 o'clock (right knee) or 2:30/9:30 (left knee) position on coronal images (closer to PLB attachment of native ACL)
- Femoral tunnel placed too far anteriorly contributes to tautness of graft in flexion and increased laxity in extension.
- Placement of graft in over-the-top position causes increased tension in extension.
- The 2:30/9:30 or even 3 o'clock/9 o'clock position may be associated with more relative anterior tibial translation on MR sagittal images but results in much improved rotational control.[40]

- The more anatomic position of the femoral tunnel (more oblique ACL graft) additionally helps keep the graft away from the PCL.
    - Decreases risk of impingement of the graft on the PCL
- Isometry on tibia is greater in sagittal plane and less sensitive to site of graft's tibial attachment (unlike small isometric zone for femoral tunnel).[505]
- Double-bundle technique
    - More effective at reproducing knee kinematics
- Causes for graft failure found on MR evaluation include:
    - Hardware malposition: interference screws and/or pins
    - Bone tunnel location
    - Bone plug dislodgement[309]
- T2 hyperintensity from vascular ingrowth may be seen in normal grafts for up to 2 years after placement.

Graft Impingement

- Potential sites of bone impingement
    - Intercondylar roof
- Side walls of intercondylar fossa
    - Intraarticular exits of osseous tunnels
- Roof impingement
- Lateral or excessive anterior placement of tibial tunnel (posterior placement of tibial tunnel or anterior placement of femoral tunnel produces instability)
- Placement of tibial tunnel parallel and posterior to Blumensaat line avoids roof impingement.
- Intermediate graft signal caused by vascularized periligamentous tissue, graft revascularization (seen up to 2 years after placement), or graft impingement
- Tibial tunnel positions that increase risk for impingement
- Centering tibial tunnel 5mm anterior and medial to the center of the ACL insertion and placing it within the ACL insertion puts graft at risk for impingement.[197]

Over-the-Top ACL Reconstruction

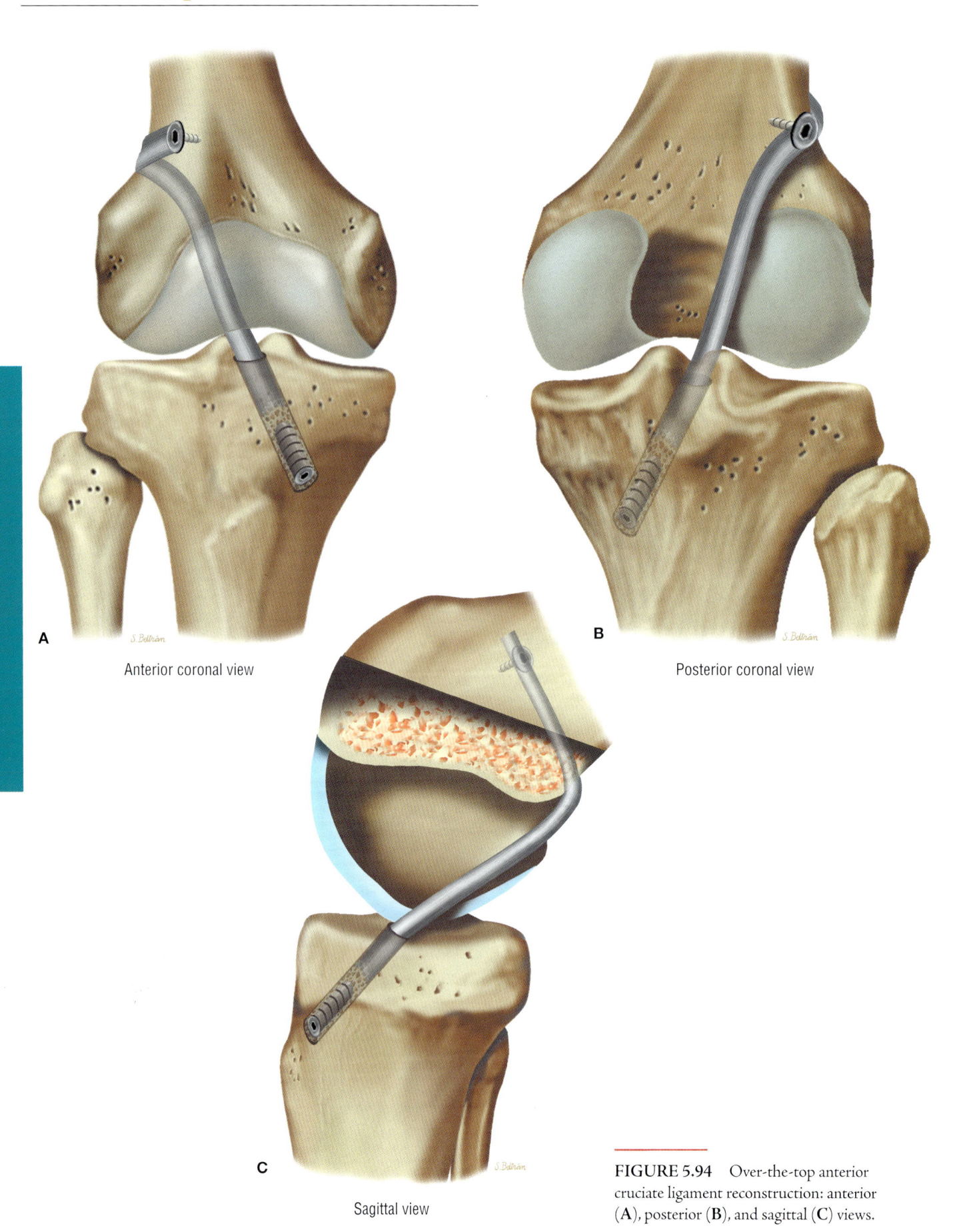

A Anterior coronal view

B Posterior coronal view

C Sagittal view

FIGURE 5.94 Over-the-top anterior cruciate ligament reconstruction: anterior (**A**), posterior (**B**), and sagittal (**C**) views.

Cruciate Ligaments

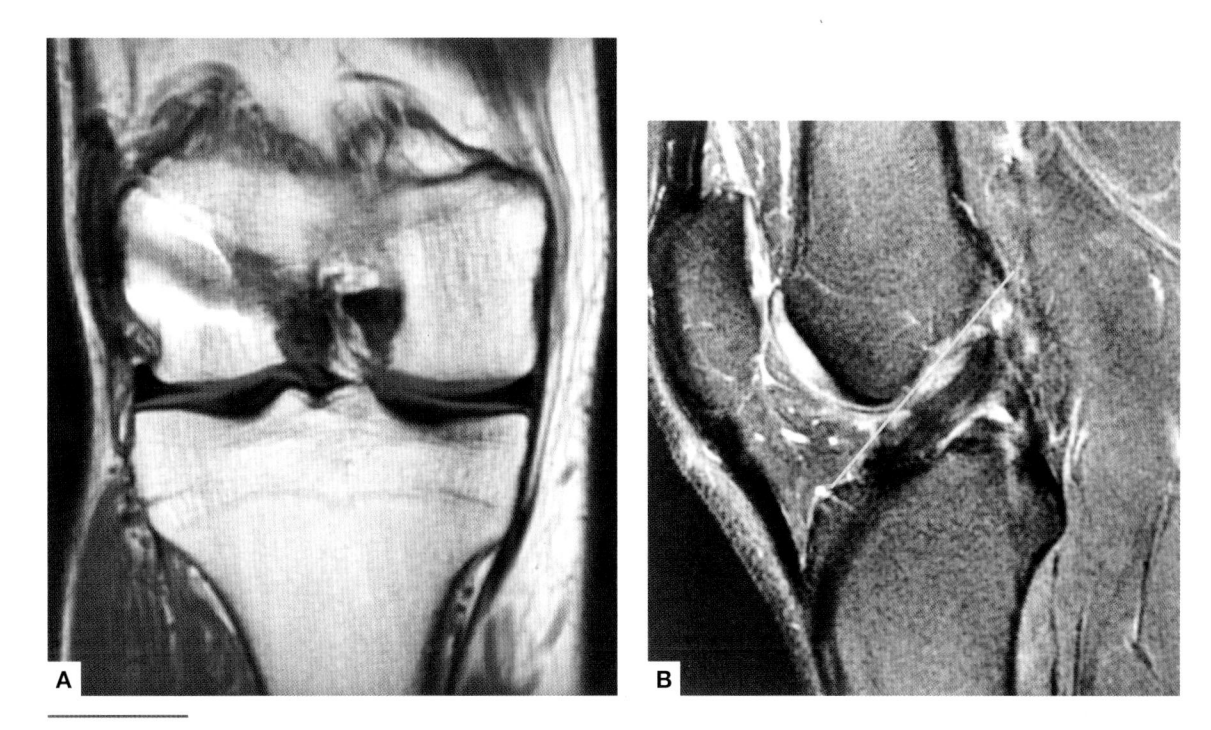

FIGURE 5.95 T1-weighted coronal (**A**) and FS PD-weighted FSE sagittal (**B**) images demonstrate a stable, low-signal-intensity ACL autograft without impingement. The tibial tunnel is placed posterior to the slope (*long white line*) of the intercondylar roof.

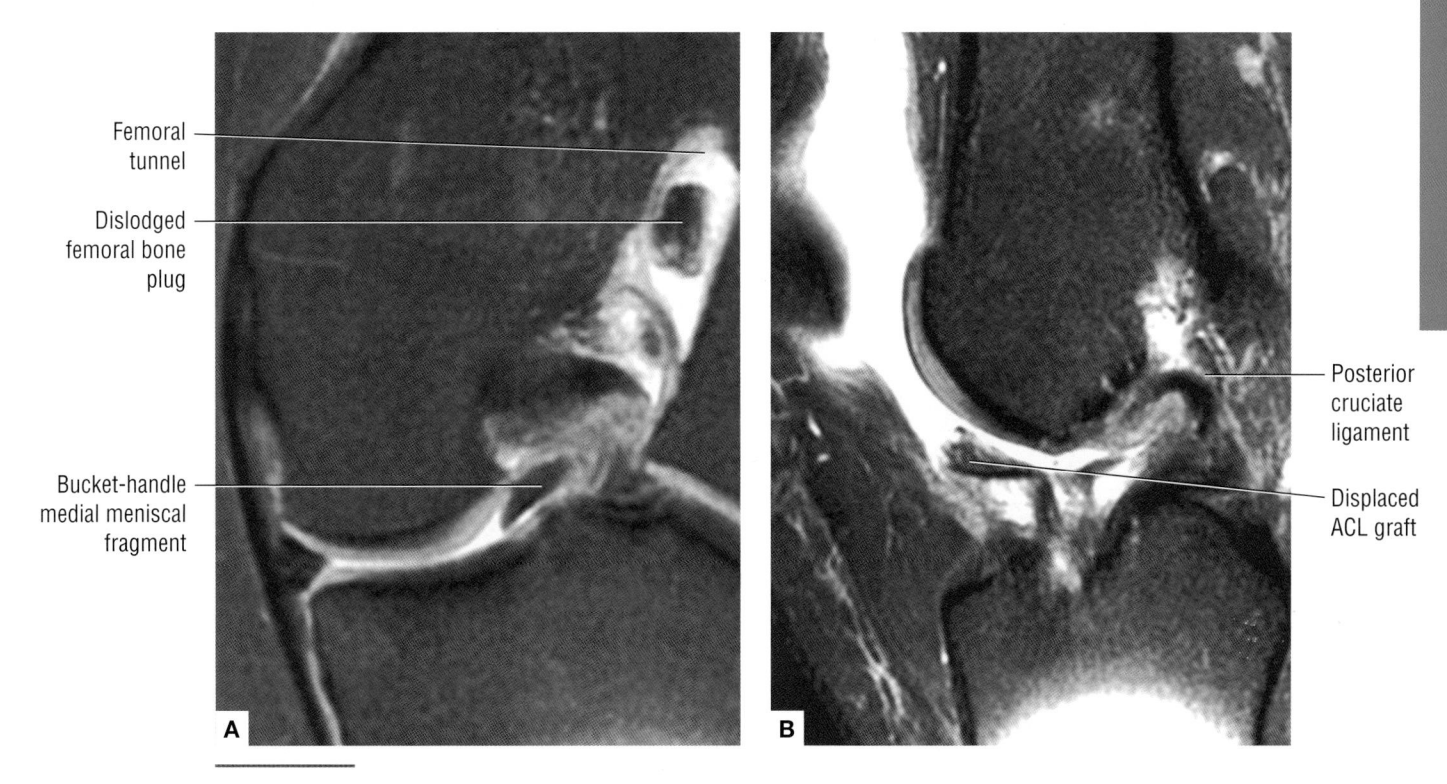

FIGURE 5.96 Dislodged femoral bone plug causing graft failure. The ACL graft has flipped anteriorly into the notch posterior to Hoffa's fat pad. A bucket-handle medial meniscus tear can be identified on coronal FS PD FSE image (**A**). (**B**) Sagittal FS PD FSE image.

Double Bundle ACL Reconstruction

ACL tear

Single-bundle graft

Double-bundle graft

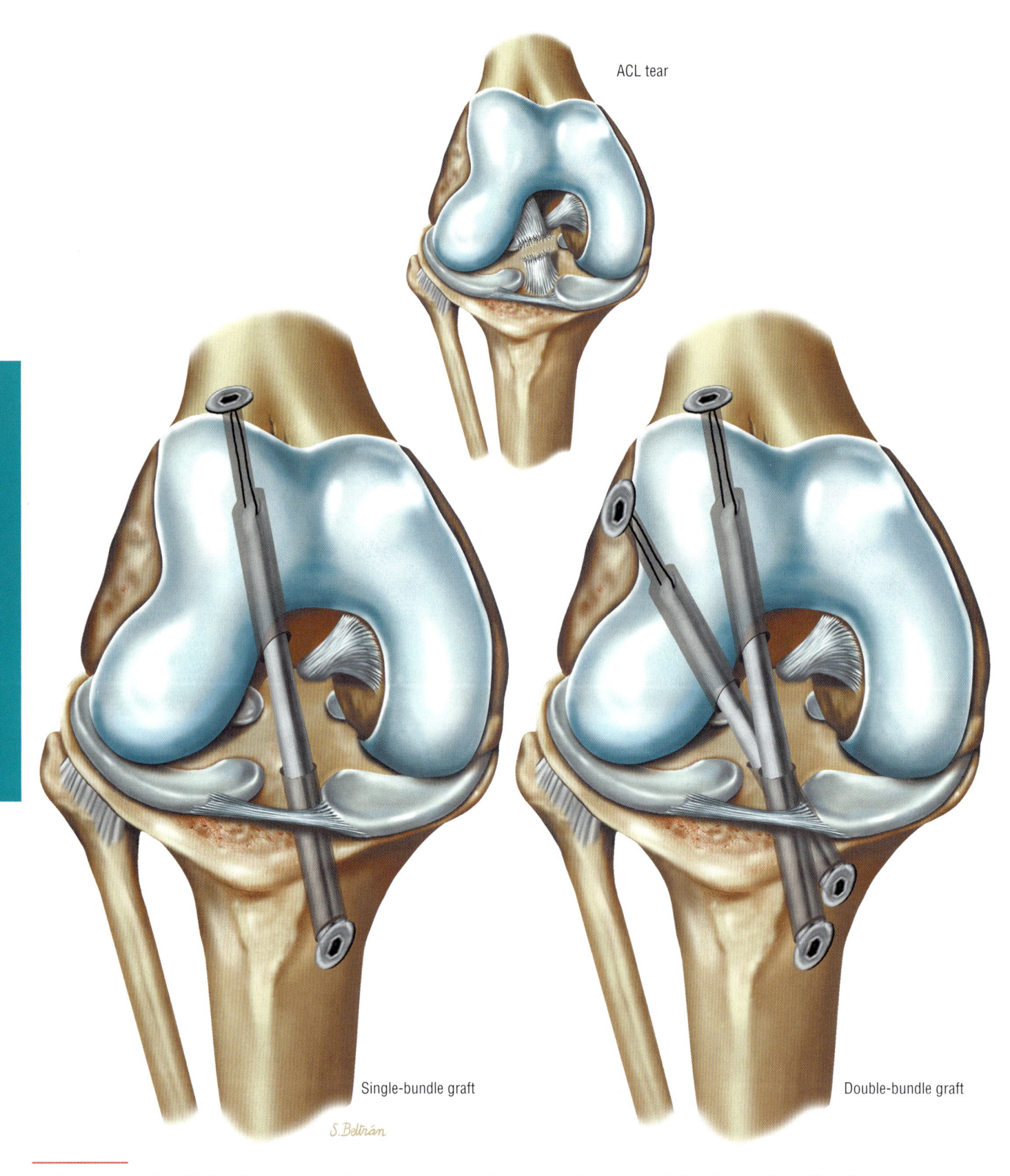

FIGURE 5.97 Double-bundle anatomic ACL reconstruction used to recreate the anteromedial and posterolateral bundles, resist combined rotary loads, and improve anteroposterior stability.

Cruciate Ligaments

ACL Graft Tunnel and Fixation

Roof of intercondylar notch

Correct position for tibial tunnel

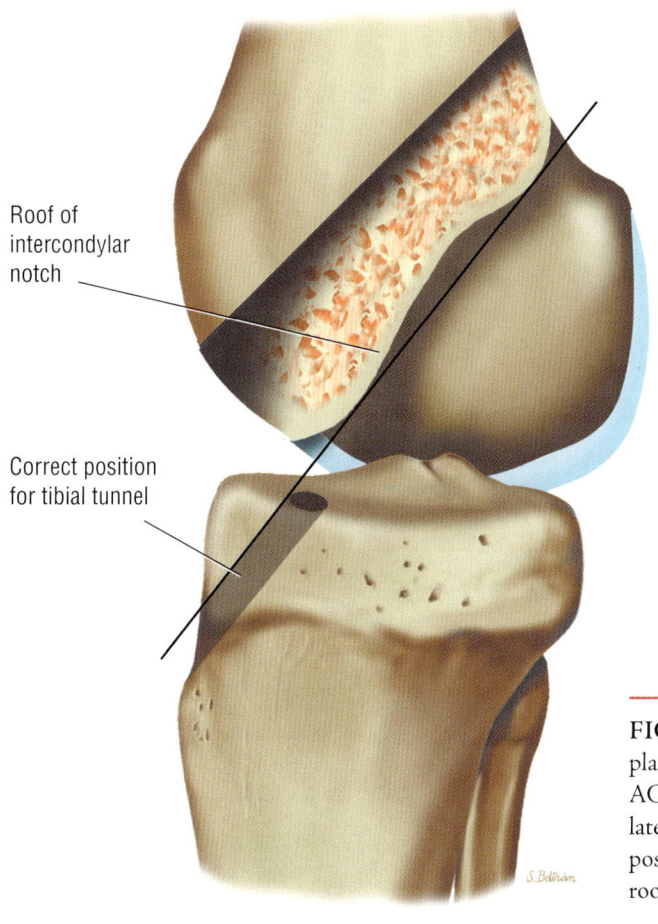

FIGURE 5.98 ACL graft tibial tunnel placement at the posterior portion of the ACL tibial insertion site (near the posterolateral bundle location). The tibial tunnel is posterior to the slope of the intercondylar roof (Blumensaat line).

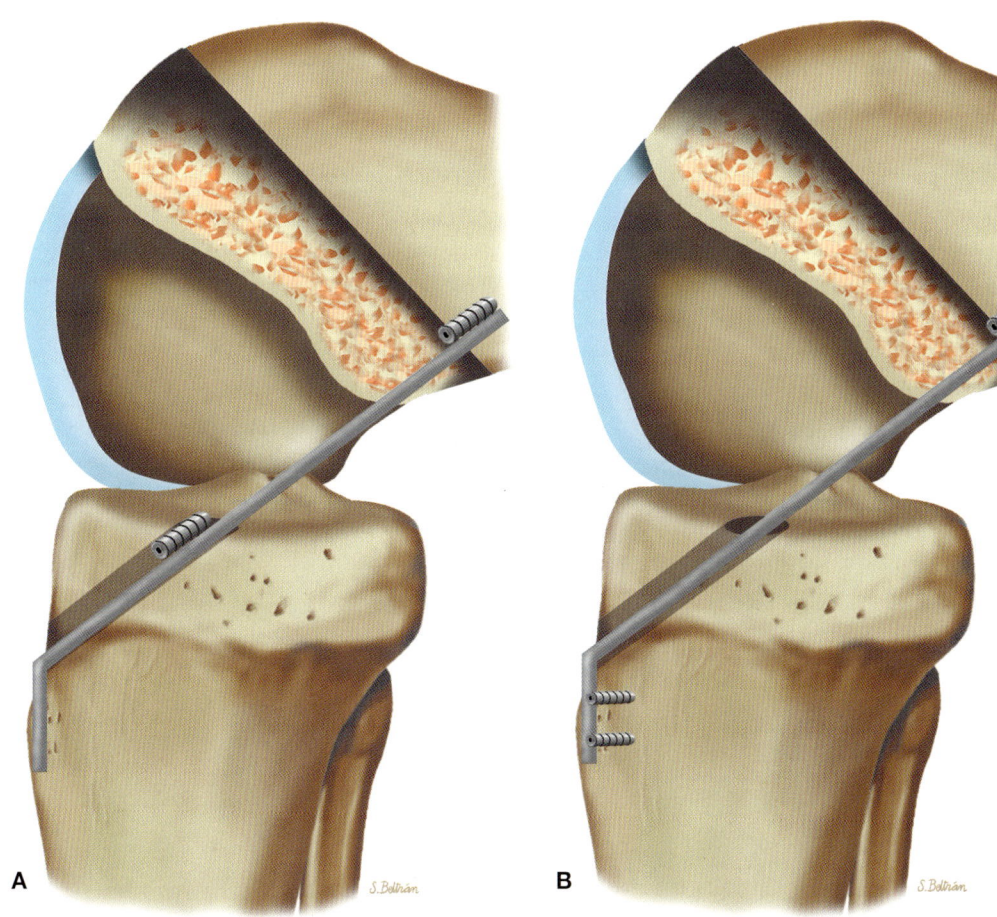

FIGURE 5.99 (**A**) Proximal fixation of an ACL graft. (**B**) Distal fixation of an ACL graft.

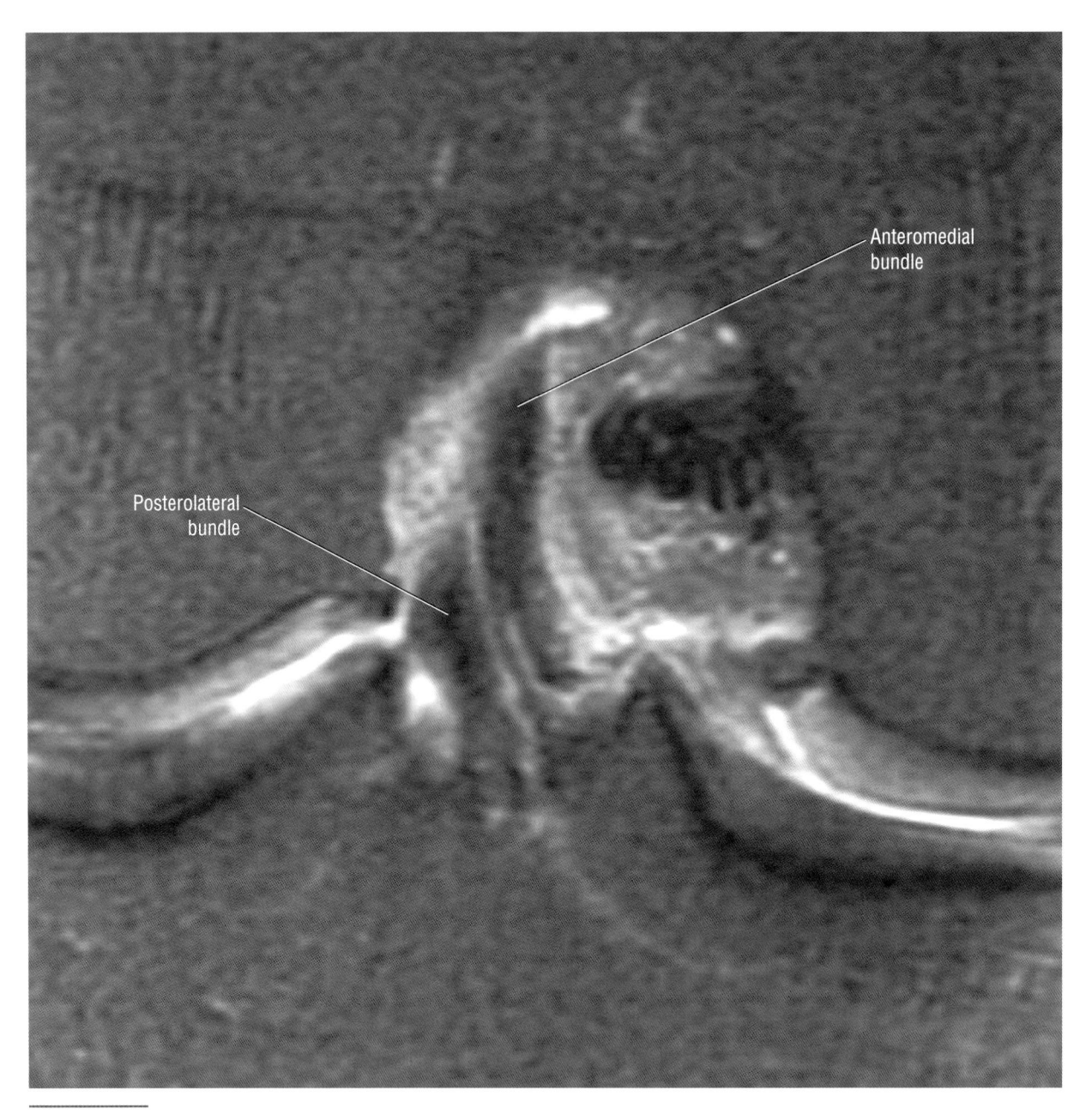

FIGURE 5.100 In a double-bundle reconstruction, the goal is to reconstruct the AM and PL bundles as shown in the coronal MR image of the normal ACL. The PL bundle of the ACL has a predominant role in rotatory control.

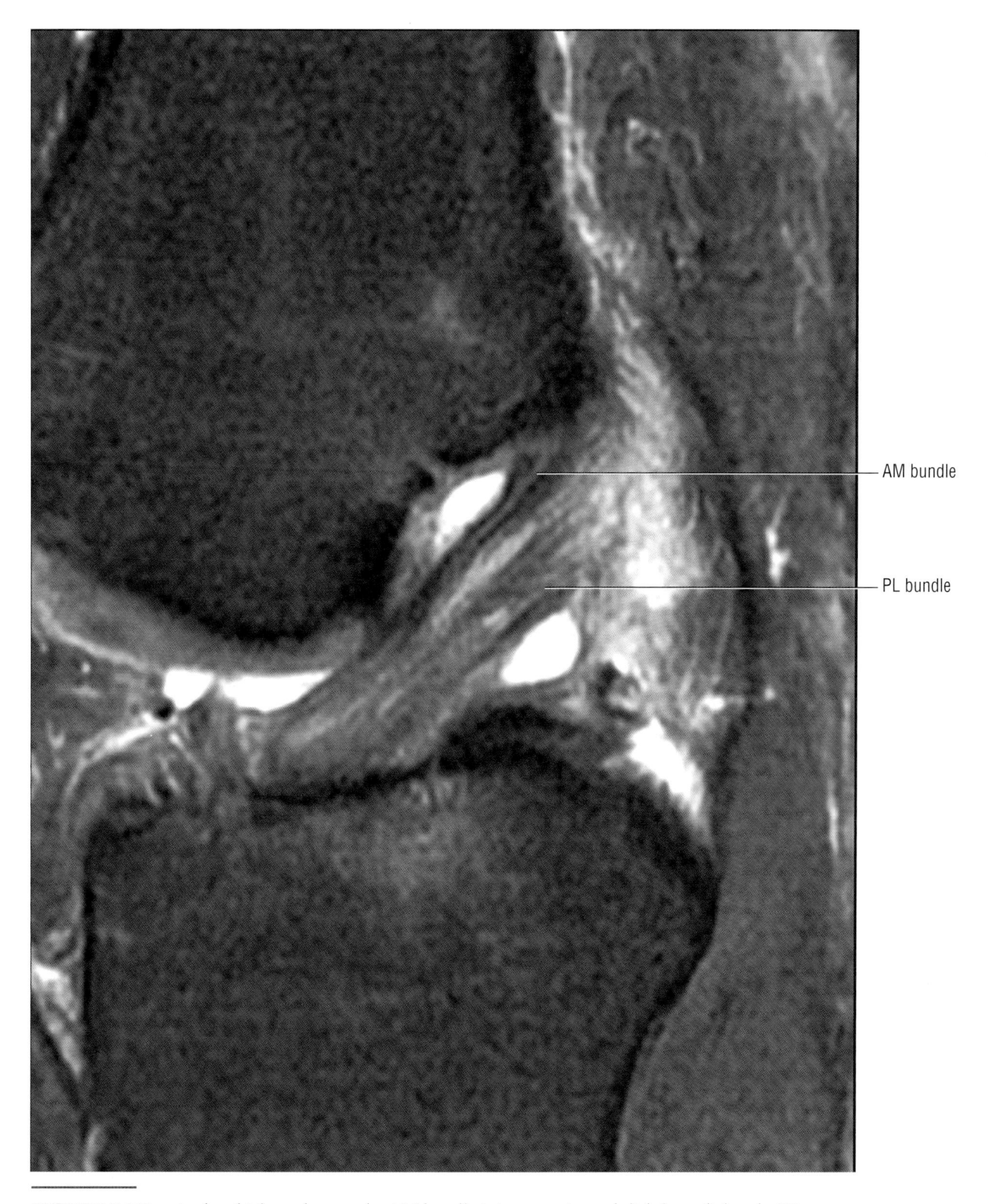

FIGURE 5.101 At the tibial attachment, the AM bundle is just anterior and slightly medial to the PL bundle. The AM fibers are more anterior and proximal to the PL bundle at the femoral footprint in the position of extension. In an ACL tear, the axis of rotation (normally central and close to the tibial spines) is medialized and is associated with increased anterior tibial translation and internal rotation of the lateral tibial plateau. Sagittal FS PD FSE image.

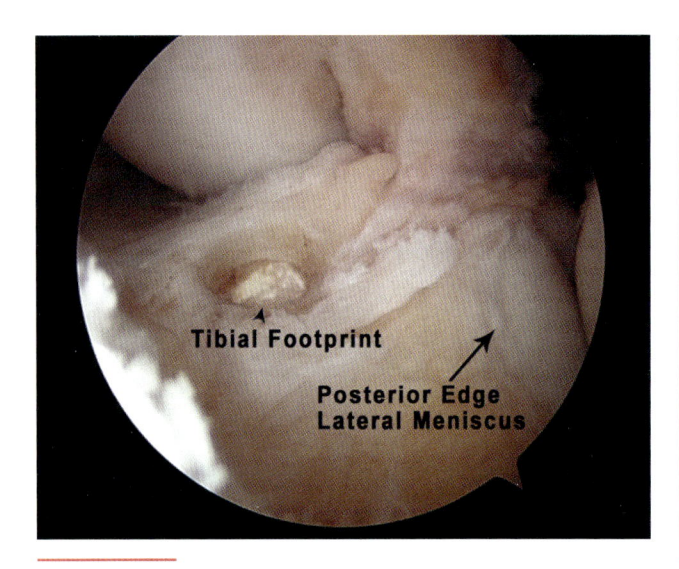

FIGURE 5.102 Tibial footprint of native ACL marked by electrocautery. (Reprinted from Fu FH. *Master Techniques in Orthopaedic Surgery: Sports Medicine*. Philadelphia, PA: Lippincott Williams & Wilkins; 2010, with permission.)

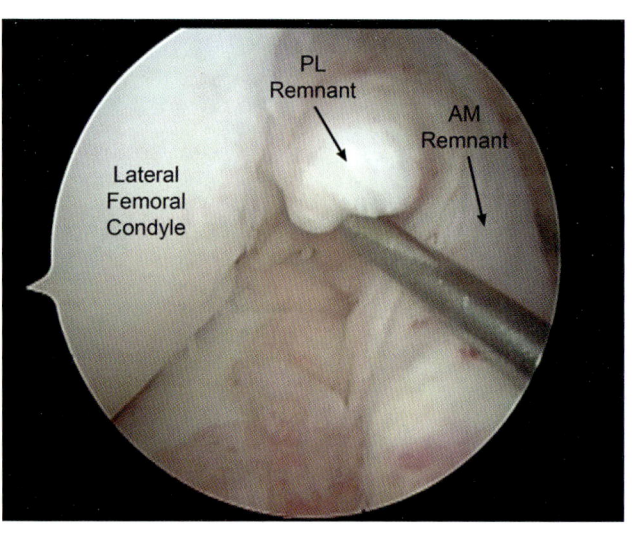

FIGURE 5.103 Diagnostic arthroscopy. View from the AL portal demonstrates an ACL rupture with both the AM and PL bundles identified. An ACL tear can be classified by location as femoral, mid-substance, or tibial. ACL ruptures can also be described as partial versus full thickness and isolated single AM or PL bundle versus combined double-bundle tears. (Reprinted from Fu FH. *Master Techniques in Orthopaedic Surgery: Sports Medicine*. Philadelphia, PA: Lippincott Williams & Wilkins; 2010, with permission.)[147]

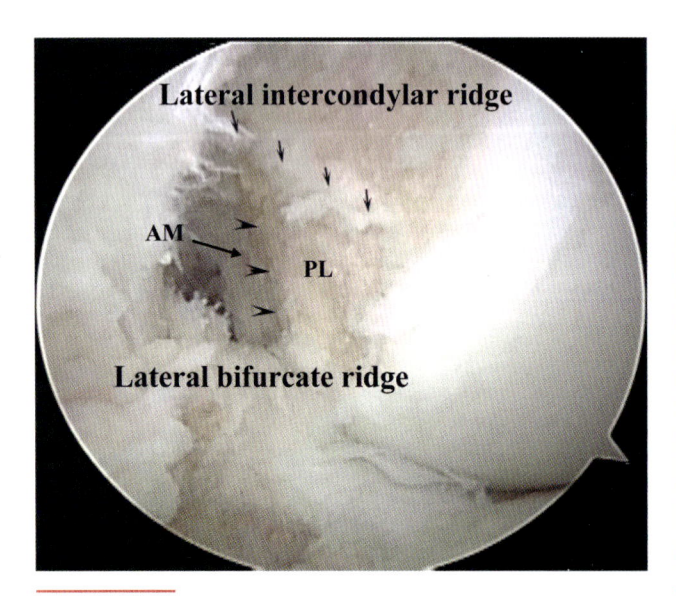

FIGURE 5.104 Bony landmarks for native ACL. The lateral intercondylar ridge demonstrates the anterior border of the femoral ACL footprint. The lateral bifurcate ridge separates the femoral insertion sites of the AM and PL bundles. (Reprinted from Fu FH. *Master Techniques in Orthopaedic Surgery: Sports Medicine*. Philadelphia, PA: Lippincott Williams & Wilkins; 2010, with permission.)

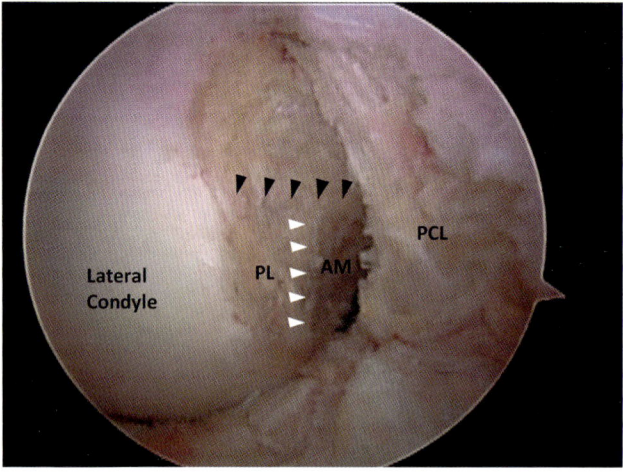

FIGURE 5.105 Arthroscopic landmarks. The ACL footprint has been identified with the knee in 90 degrees of flexion. The lateral intercondylar ridge (*black arrowheads*) and the lateral bifurcate ridge (*white arrowheads*) are identified. View from accessory anteromedial portal (AAM). (Reprinted from Fu FH. *Master Techniques in Orthopaedic Surgery: Sports Medicine*. Philadelphia, PA: Lippincott Williams & Wilkins; 2010, with permission.)

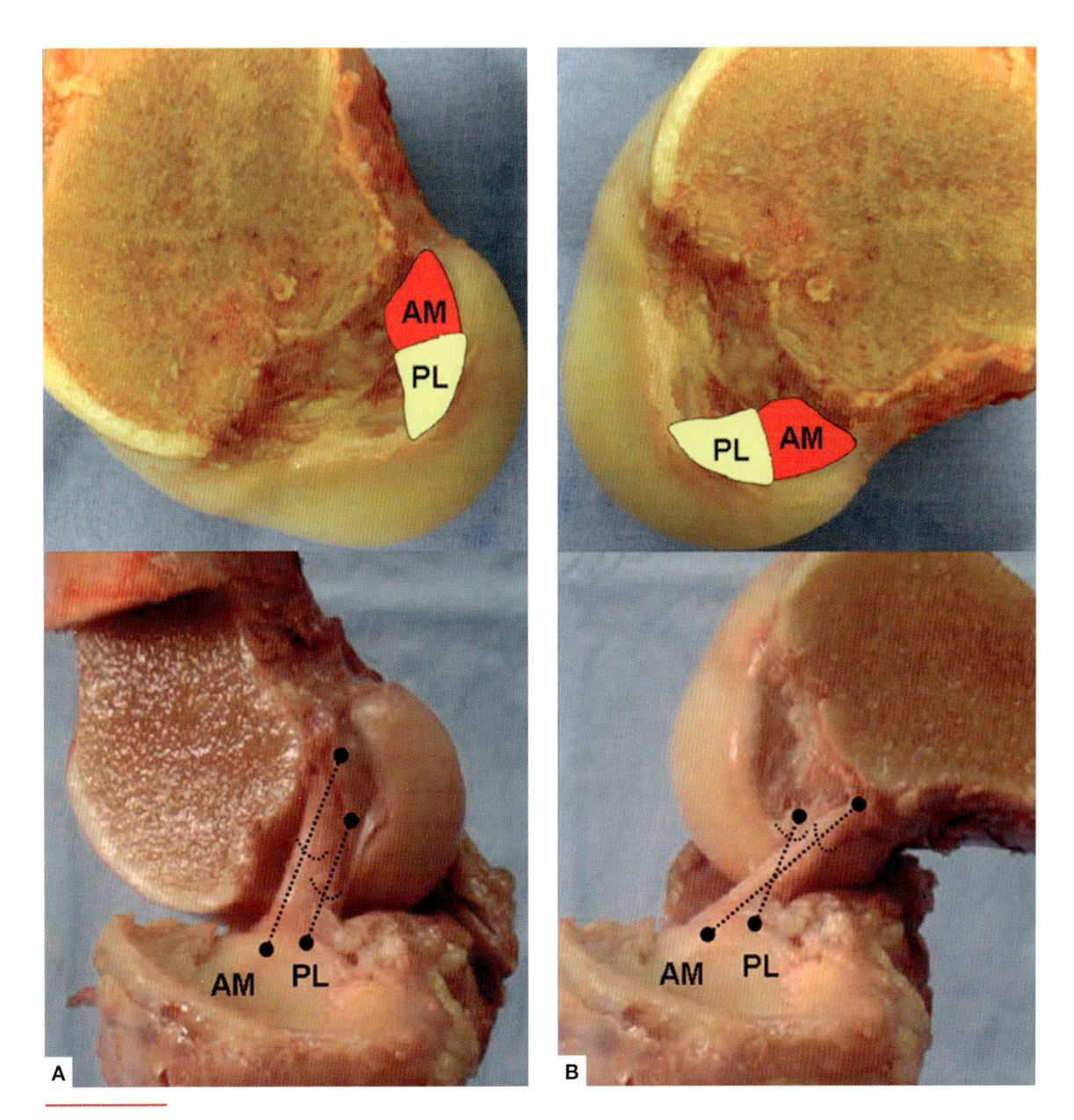

FIGURE 5.106 Cadaveric dissection of ACL double-bundle footprint. The positions of both the AM and PL bundles are shown in full extension (**A**) and 90 degrees of flexion (**B**). In knee full extension, the femoral insertion of the PL bundle is distal and posterior to the AM femoral insertion. In flexion of the knee, the PL arcs around the AM femoral insertion to be located anterior to the AM bundle in 30 to 40 degrees of knee flexion. (Reprinted from Chhabra A, Starman JS, Ferretti M, et al. Anatomic, radiographic, biomechanical, and kinematic evaluation of the anterior cruciate ligament and its two functional bundles. *J Bone Joint Surg Am*. 2006;88:2–10, with permission.)[40,147]

Anatomic Double-Bundle ACL Reconstruction

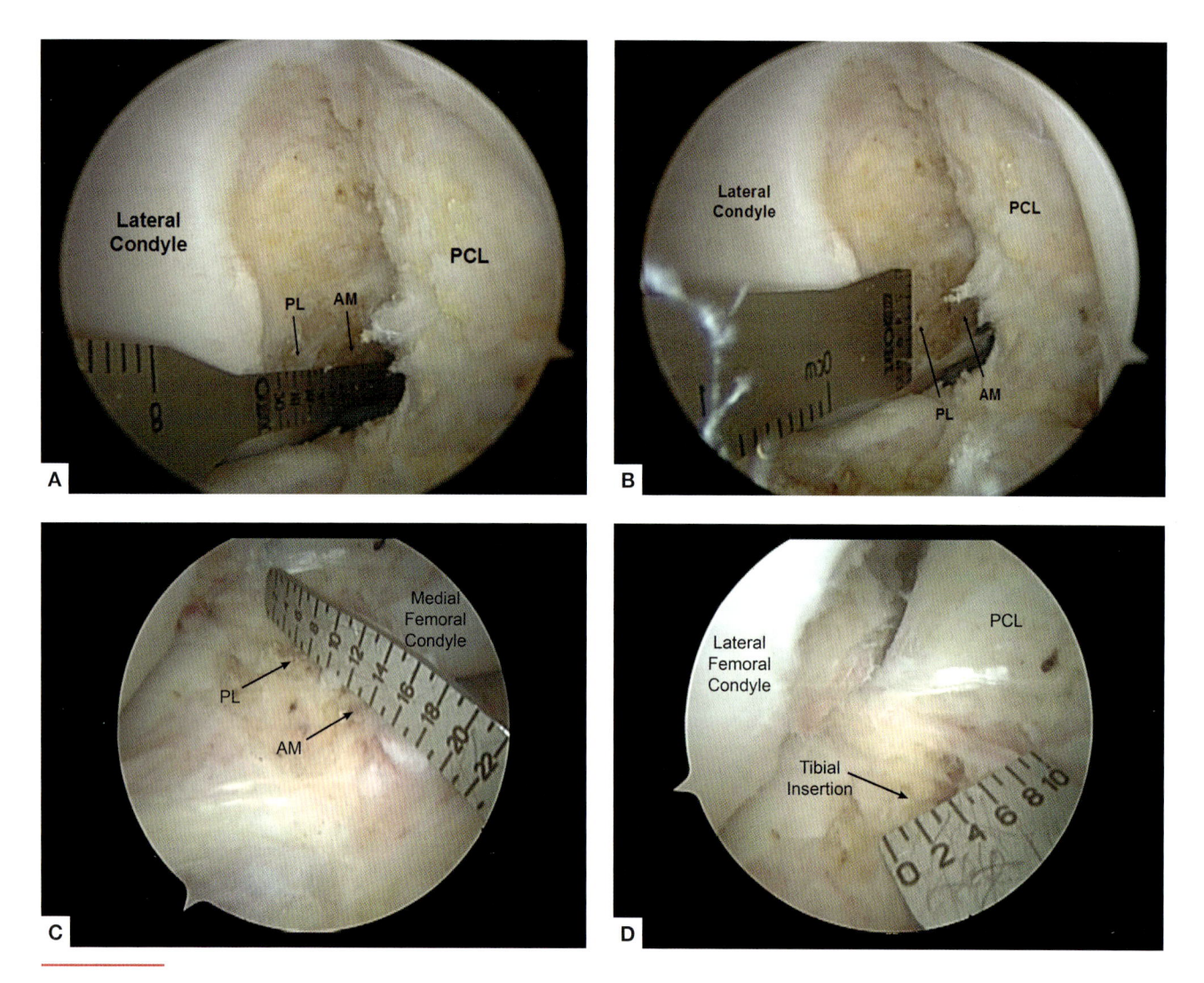

FIGURE 5.107 Measurement of the ACL footprint. (**A**) Length of the total femoral footprint. (**B**) Anterior-posterior length of both the AM and PL footprints. (**C**) Total tibial footprint length. (**D**) Width of tibial AM and PL footprints. (Reprinted from Fu FH. *Master Techniques in Orthopaedic Surgery: Sports Medicine.* Philadelphia, PA: Lippincott Williams & Wilkins; 2010, with permission.)

- The principles of anatomic double-bundle reconstruction involve:
    - Anatomic tunnel placement
    - Restoration of the two functional bundles
    - Proper tensioning of the AM and PL bundles
    - Individualized reconstruction to replicate the native structure

Cruciate Ligaments

Anatomic Double-Bundle ACL Reconstruction

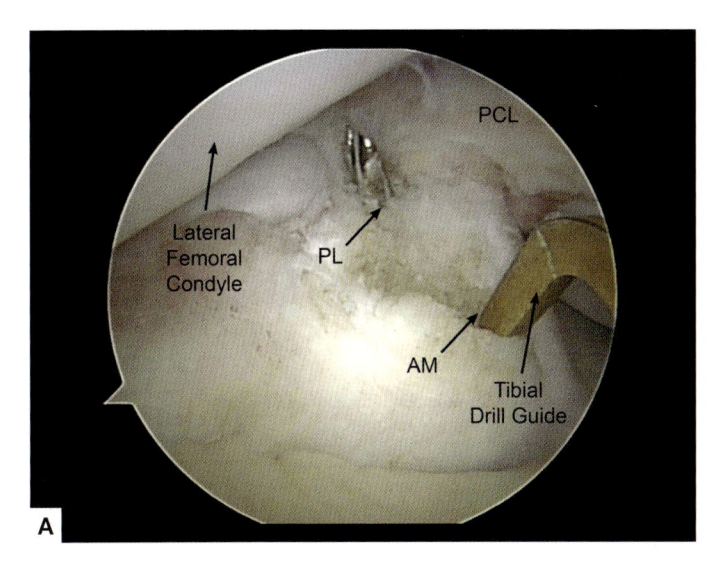

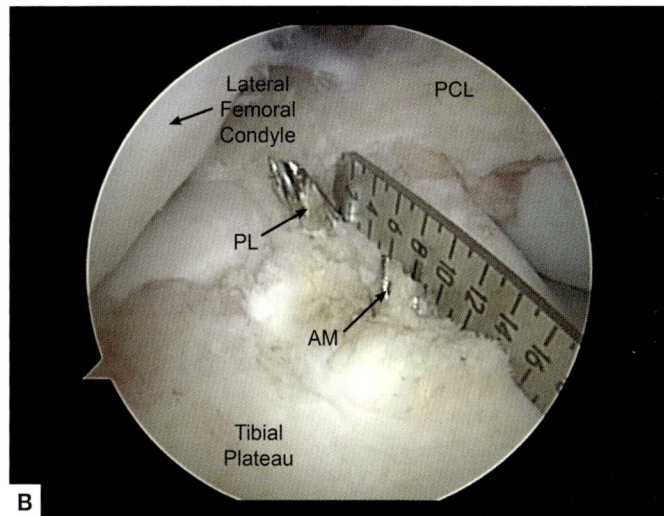

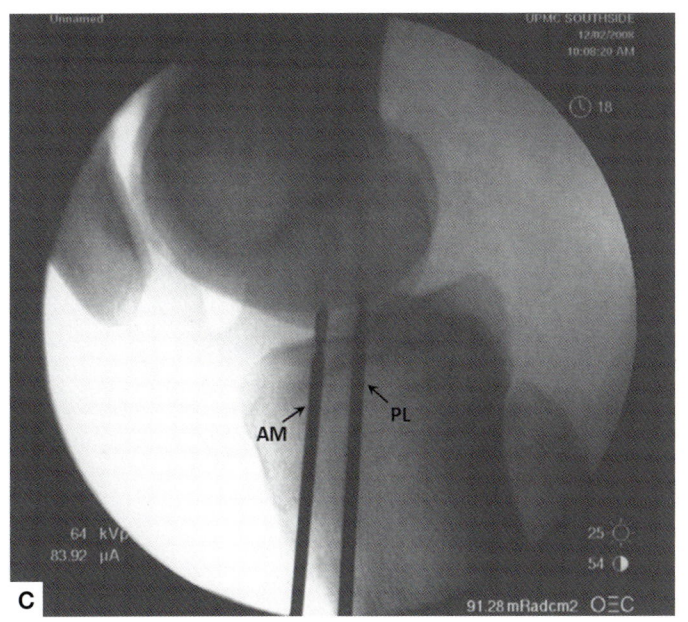

FIGURE 5.108 Preparation of tibial tunnels after the AM and PL footprints are established. View from AL portal. Instrumentation placed through AM portal. (**A**) The PL tunnel guide pin has been placed, and the ACL guide tip is centered in the AM tibial footprint. (**B**) Both the PL and the AM guide pins are in place. (**C**) Lateral radiograph verifying guide pin placement and trajectory. (Reprinted from Fu FH. *Master Techniques in Orthopaedic Surgery: Sports Medicine*. Philadelphia, PA: Lippincott Williams & Wilkins; 2010, with permission.)

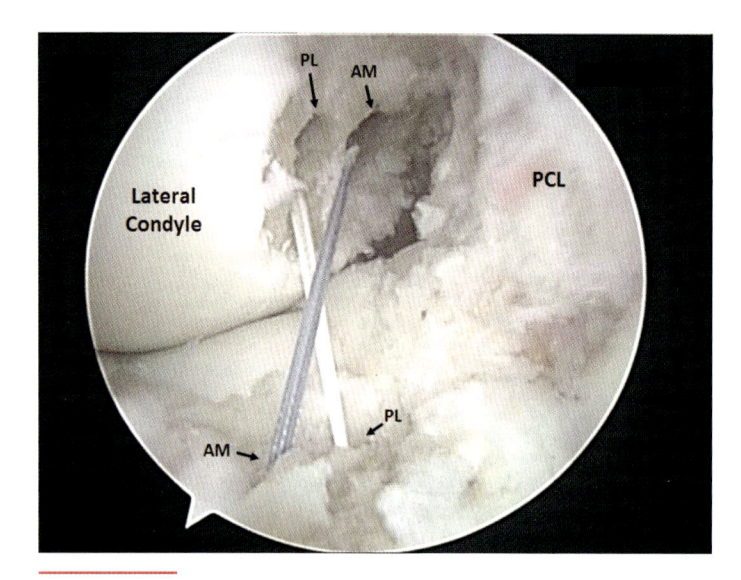

FIGURE 5.109 The tunnels are loaded with shuttle suture for graft placement. Both tunnels should be loaded with suture prior to individual graft placement in order to avoid interference. (Reprinted from Fu FH. *Master Techniques in Orthopaedic Surgery: Sports Medicine*. Philadelphia, PA: Lippincott Williams & Wilkins; 2010, with permission.)

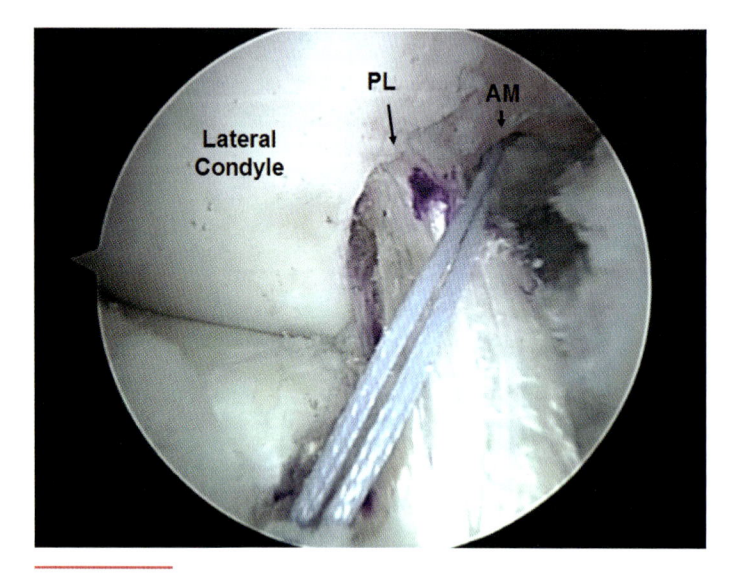

FIGURE 5.110 The PL graft is advanced into the femoral tunnel. The PL graft is tensioned in full knee extension and the AM graft is tensioned with the knee at 45 degrees of flexion. (Reprinted from Fu FH. *Master Techniques in Orthopaedic Surgery: Sports Medicine*. Philadelphia, PA: Lippincott Williams & Wilkins; 2010, with permission.)

Cruciate Ligaments 513

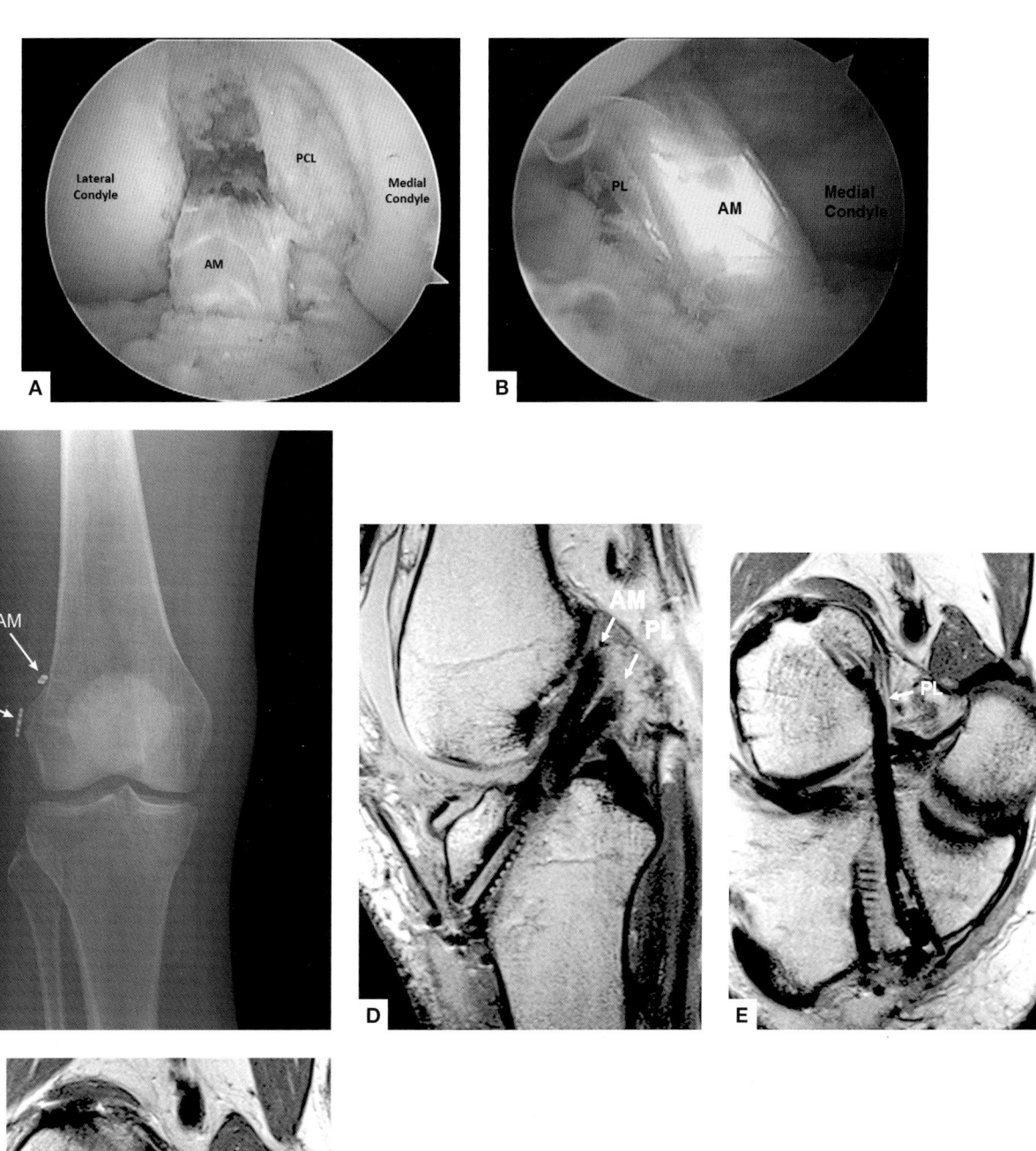

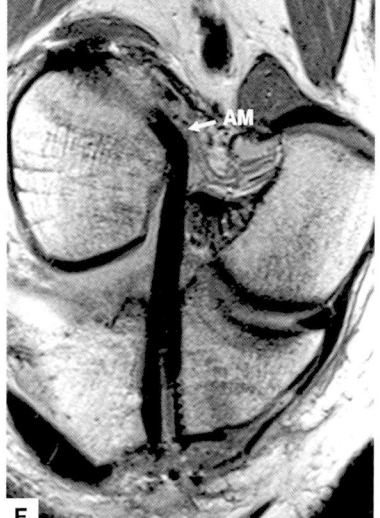

FIGURE 5.111 Double-bundle ACL reconstruction (anatomic). (**A**) View from AM portal. (**B**) View from AL portal. (**C**) Radiographic (anteroposterior view). (**D**) Postoperative sagittal MR image. (**E**) Postoperative coronal MR image of PL bundle. (**F**) Postoperative coronal MR of AM bundle. (Reprinted from Fu FH. *Master Techniques in Orthopaedic Surgery: Sports Medicine*. Philadelphia, PA: Lippincott Williams & Wilkins; 2010, with permission.)

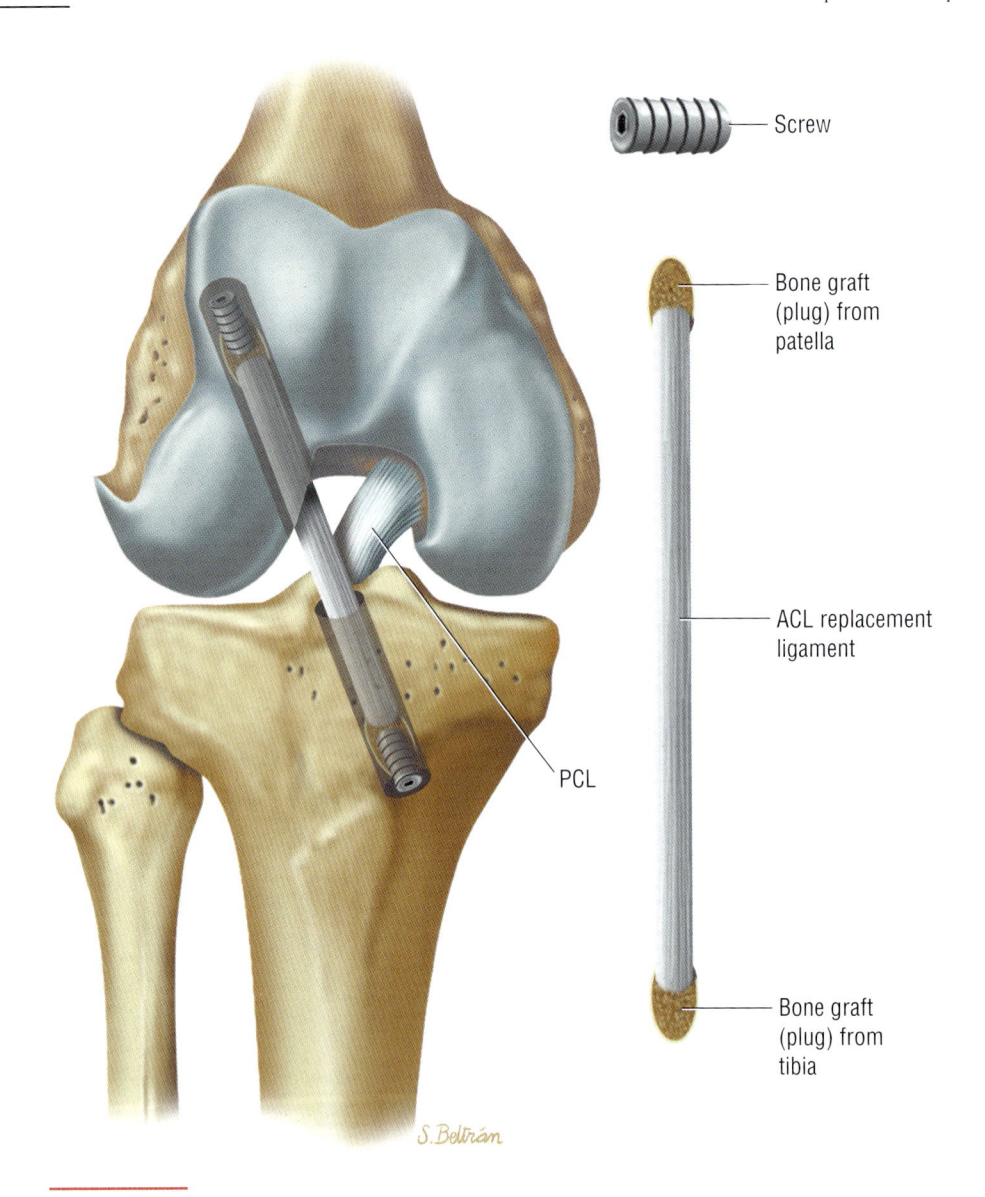

FIGURE 5.112 Bone–patellar tendon–bone graft reconstruction components for ACL replacement. The tibial tunnel is at least 3cm distal to the joint line and about 1.5cm medial to the tibial tuberosity.

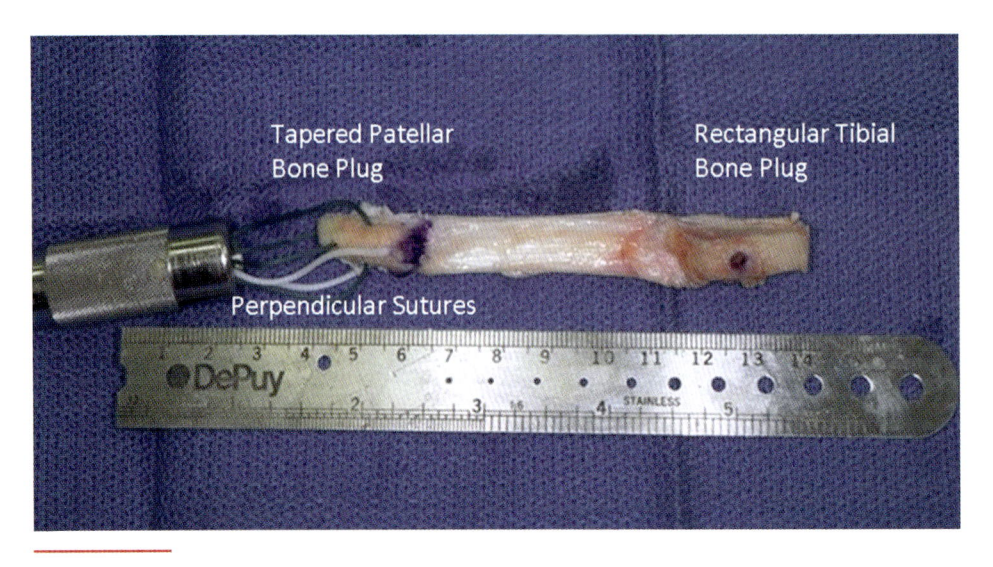

FIGURE 5.113 Bone–patellar tendon–bone graft with bone plugs. (Reprinted from Fu FH. *Master Techniques in Orthopaedic Surgery: Sports Medicine*. Philadelphia, PA: Lippincott Williams & Wilkins; 2010, with permission.)

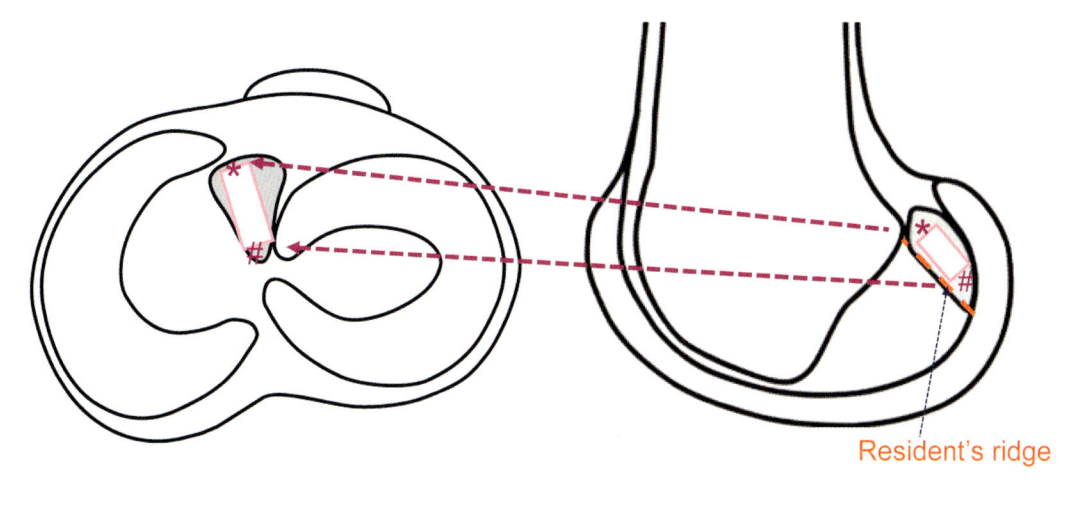

FIGURE 5.114 Proper placement and orientation of BTB graft showing corresponding femoral and tibial attachment points. The resident's ridge is a landmark (on the lateral notch wall) for femoral tunnel drilling in ACL reconstruction. (Reprinted from Fu FH. *Master Techniques in Orthopaedic Surgery: Sports Medicine*. Philadelphia, PA: Lippincott Williams & Wilkins; 2010, with permission.)

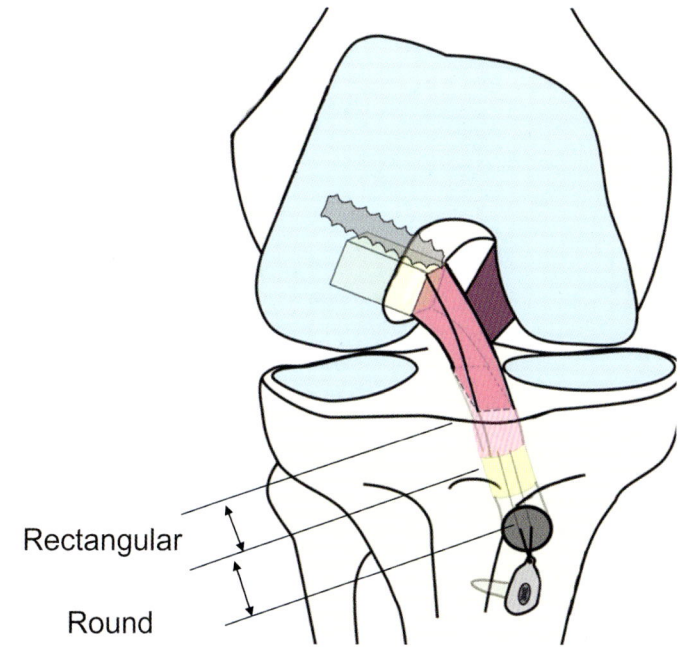

FIGURE 5.115 Rectangular tunnel ACL reconstruction with bone-patellar tendon-bone graft. Rectangular tunnel technique maximizes the graft tunnel contact area in the femur and tibia. (Reprinted from Fu FH. *Master Techniques in Orthopaedic Surgery: Sports Medicine*. Philadelphia, PA: Lippincott Williams & Wilkins; 2010, with permission.)

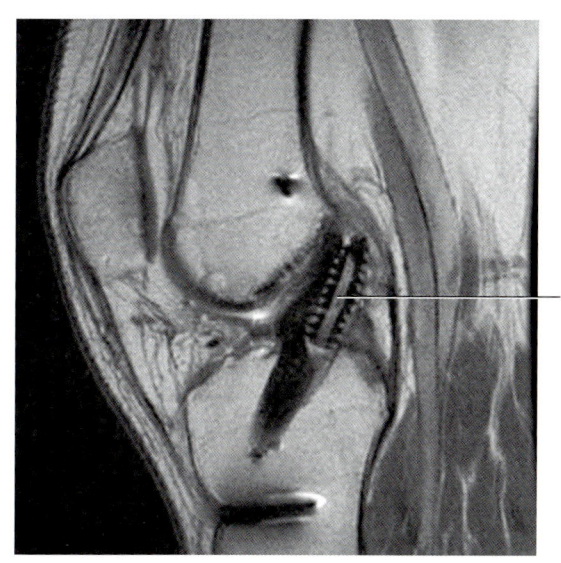

FIGURE 5.116 A dislodged tibial interference screw seen posterior to the intraarticular course of the graft. The interference screw was used to wedge the bone plug in the tunnel (sagittal PD FSE image).

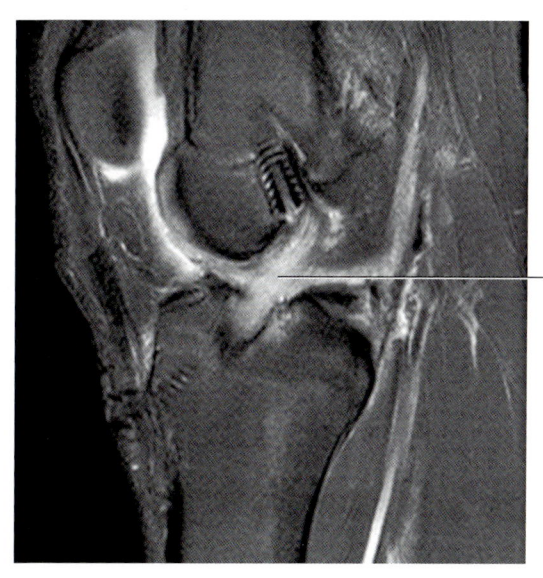

FIGURE 5.117 Postligament replacement. FS PD image shows an intact ACL graft of intermediate to hyperintense signal intensity.

- Excessive lateral positioning of the tunnel also likely to result in impingement
- If entire articular opening of tibial tunnel is anterior to slope of the intercondylar roof (as seen on lateral roentgenogram or sagittal MR) → severe roof impingement[197]
- If a portion of articular opening of tibial tunnel is anterior to slope of the intercondylar roof → moderate graft impingement
- Optimal placement of tibial tunnel
    - Centering 2 to 3mm posterior to the center of the ACL insertion helped avoid roof impingement.
    - Tunnel with distal opening inferior to tibial tubercle and extending posterosuperiorly immediately anterior to the anterior tibial spine on flat tibia[105]
    - Center is 42% of the sagittal distance from the anterior aspect of the tibial plateau.
- Roof impingement occurs in grafts that are only 30% of anterior-to-posterior distance of the tibial plateau.[105,197]
- Entire articular opening of tibial tunnel is posterior to slope of the intercondylar roof.
- Slope of intercondylar roof may change with flexion; thus, tibial tunnel should be placed parallel to the slope of the intercondylar roof with knee in full extension[194]
- Opening of properly placed tibial tunnel into the joint is centered on intercondylar eminence on coronal MR images.[105]
- Exit sites do not correspond to location or position of interference screws, staples, or bone plugs used for ACL reconstruction.
- Unimpinged ACL graft has no discernible blood supply for as long as 2 years after implantation.[196]
- Periligamentous soft tissues are vascularized (enhance on MR contrast studies) and cover the graft by 1 month.
- Synovial diffusion and not revascularization may be more important in viability of unimpinged ACL graft.
- Unimpinged grafts show low signal on T1, PD, and T2 (including FSE T2) images.

- Unimpinged and impinged ACL reconstructions with bone–patellar tendon–bone grafts, hamstring tendons, and Achilles tendons have similar imaging characteristics (except for MR changes at donor sites).[105]
- Normal hypovascular appearance of postoperative ACL graft characterized by low signal intensity, similar to PCL, including portions of graft within osseous tunnels[16,105]
- 10% of clinically normal or stable grafts may show intermediate signal intensity.[105]
- Intermediate signal does not indicate retear of the graft, especially in the absence of associated signs of impingement (e.g., an anteriorly positioned tibial tunnel).
- Accuracy of MR in evaluating ACL allograft reconstructions
    - Excellent (92%) correlation between MR findings and clinical examination for patellar tendon autografts (3-mm sections)[380]
    - 100% correlation between MR findings and second-look arthroscopy in ACL reconstructions using patellar bone–tendon–tibial bone autografts
- Buckling of PCL associated with ACL laxity in these cases
- Less satisfactory MR results reported in a review of ACL reconstructions performed with fascia latae from the ITB and a MacIntosh lateral substitution over-the-top repair.[296,329]
- 84% accuracy for carbon fiber ligament augmentation of the ACL with intraarticular and extraarticular grafts[136]
- MR useful in identifying intact, partially torn, and complete tears of ACL autografts, as correlated with results of clinical examination and arthroscopy[308]
- Imaging of ACL autograft in its anatomic plane and use of T2 weighting were necessary to determine graft integrity and to differentiate partial from complete tears.
- Increased signal intensity of ACL grafts
    - Temporal changes in unimpinged grafts may be due to process of ligamentization, including development of a synovial envelope.
    - May also represent earliest signs of clinically occult roof impingement
    - May be seen in ACL reconstructions using hamstring tendons in children with open physes despite clinical stability[354,367]
    - Best appreciated on T1- or PD-weighted images

ACL Graft Tunnel Motion

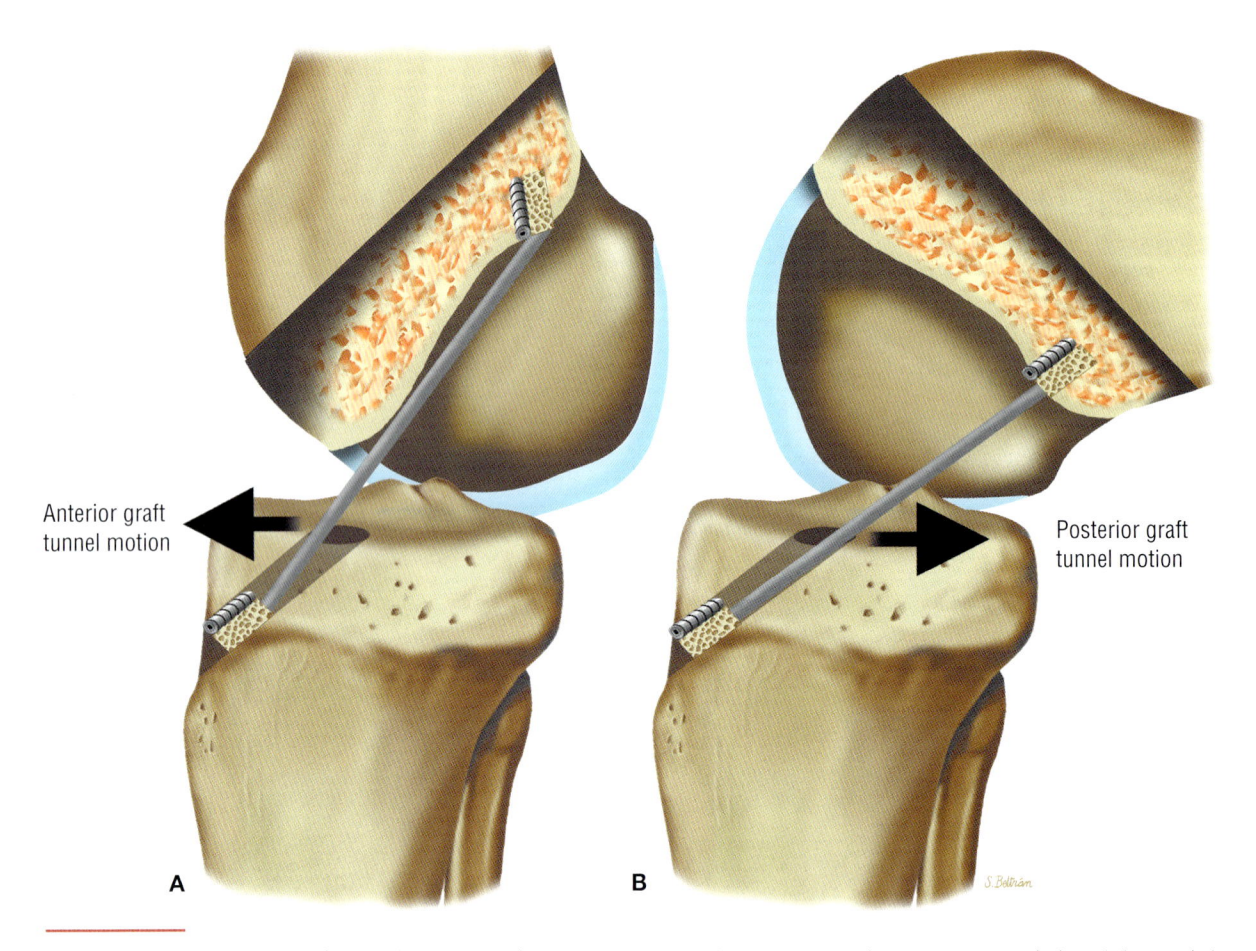

FIGURE 5.118 ACL graft tunnel motion in the anteroposterior plane occurring during extension (**A**) and flexion (**B**). A windshield wiper effect predominates at the tibial tunnel side of the ACL graft. If the bone block is placed distally, the windshield wiper effect is increased as a function of increased distance of the graft fixation relative to the joint line.

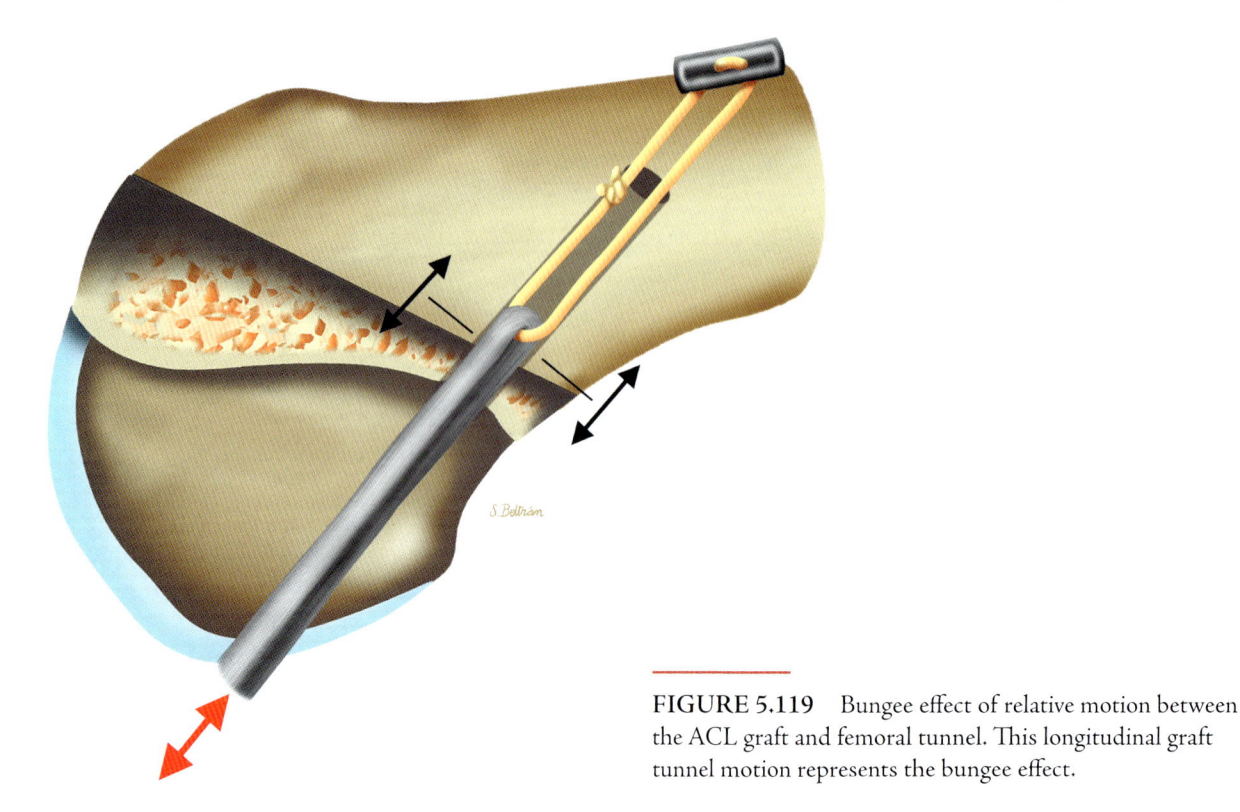

FIGURE 5.119 Bungee effect of relative motion between the ACL graft and femoral tunnel. This longitudinal graft tunnel motion represents the bungee effect.

Cruciate Ligaments

ACL Graft Revision

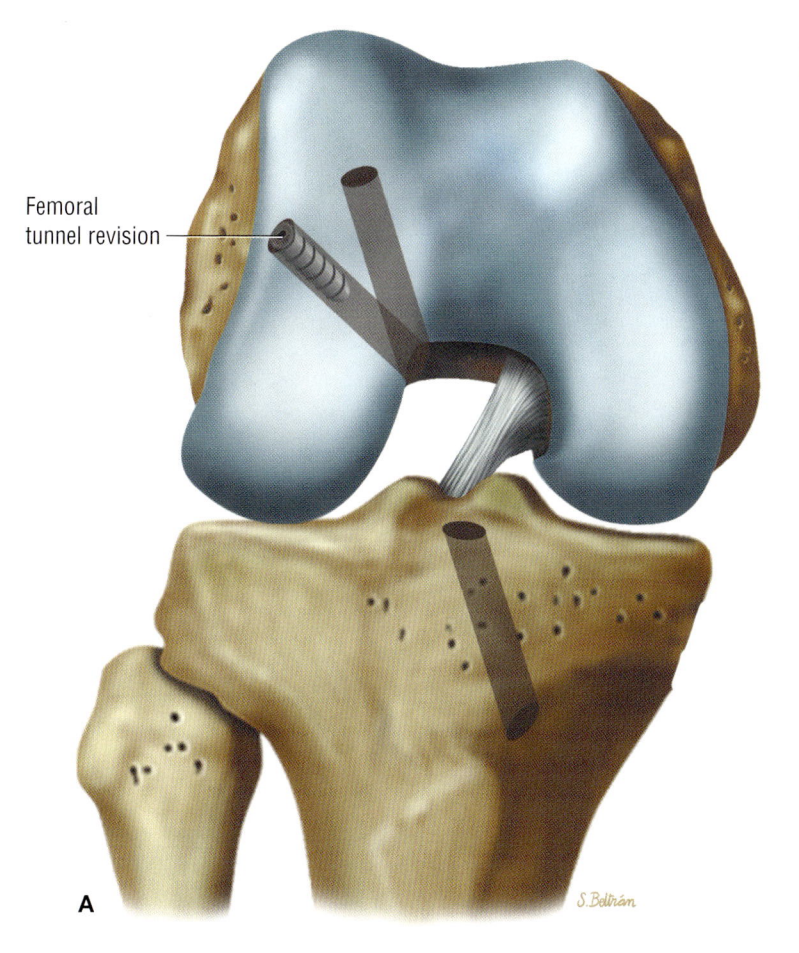

FIGURE 5.120 (**A**) Revision of a vertically oriented ACL graft with a divergent tunnel technique. The femoral tunnel is realigned to the relative 10 o'clock position. (**B**) Improper anterior femoral tunnel placement in lateral perspective. (**C**) Posterior femoral tunnel revision after initial improper anterior femoral tunnel placement.

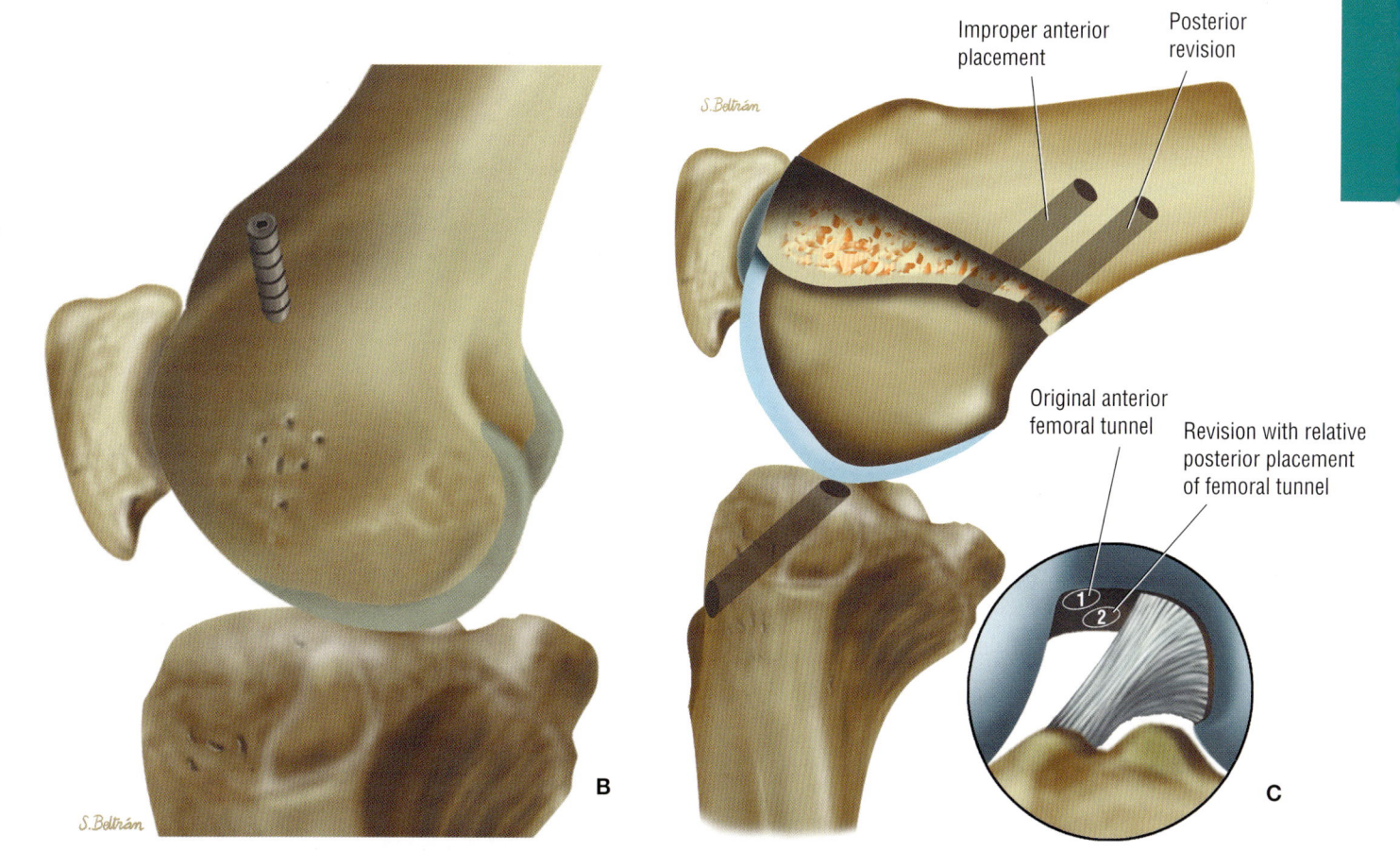

Femoral tunnel revision

A

B

Improper anterior placement

Posterior revision

Original anterior femoral tunnel

Revision with relative posterior placement of femoral tunnel

C

Roof Impingement

- Clinical findings suggestive of roof impingement
    - Knee joint effusion
    - Extension deficit
    - Recurrent instability
    - Anterior knee pain
    - Combination of above findings[511]
- MR findings in roof impingement
    - Regionally increased signal intensity in distal two thirds of the graft
    - Posterior bowing of graft caused by direct contact with intercondylar roof
    - Placement of a portion of tibial tunnel anterior to the slope of intercondylar roof in a fully extended knee (confirms roentgenographic diagnosis)[511]
    - Arthroscopic patterns of graft injury associated with roof impingement
    - Development of fibrocartilaginous nodule or cyclops lesion anterior to distal third of ACL graft
    - Fractured graft bundles
    - Guillotined fibers at entrance into notch
    - Parallel fragmentation of graft fibers (lax bundles)
    - Extrusion or molding of graft by distal end of the notch[511]
    - Dislodged bone plugs
    - Localized fibrocartilaginous nodule or cyclops lesion may limit knee extension.
        - Cyclops lesions graded 1, 2, or 3 depending on anterior extent along the femoral condyle[384]
        - Low to intermediate signal intensity on T1, T2, and FS PD FSE images
        - Best visualized in sagittal plane, between Hoffa's fat pad and leading edge of distal ACL graft[43]
    - Fractured bundles involving anterior portion of graft are the most common injury in graft impingement.

- Consistent with intercondylar roof impingement affecting anterior surface of graft before extension of damage to posterior fibers

- Ruptured anterior bundle identified on MR as separate from the intact but impinged posterior bundle fibers

- Process of graft rupturing removes site of impingement on that portion of the graft; thus, ruptured portion may show lower signal intensity than impinged fibers.

- Identification of dislodged bone plugs may require use of T1, PD, or GRE contrast.

- Improves visualization of low-signal-intensity osseous components or osseous ends of ruptured ACL graft within or anterior to intercondylar notch

- May have associated graft angulation and elongation from impingement by intercondylar roof

- Increased signal intensity observed in distal two thirds of ACL graft may persist for 1 to 3 years after implantation.[195]

- Enlargement of roof can alleviate signs of graft impingement, including return to normal low-signal-intensity appearance within 12 weeks.

- Increased signal intensity may occur in ACL graft with roof impingement but without initial evidence of clinical instability; however, patients with an impinged graft who subsequently regain a complete range of extension do become clinically unstable.[197]

- Gradual graft elongation secondary to roof impingement precedes development of instability.

Side Wall Impingement

- Indentation of graft as it curves over medial aspect of lateral femoral condyle on coronal MR images
- May be associated with low positioning of femoral tunnel opening in intercondylar notch
- Usually apparent at arthroscopy
- Gadolinium contrast studies confirm synovial envelope vascularity and improve conspicuity of ACL graft
- Anterior and posterior borders of graft enhance relative to synovial envelope.
- Intraligamentous enhancement of graft thought to represent occult or unrecognized roof impingement (this is not present in normal unimpinged grafts)[15]
- Enhancement in impinged graft may be related to intrinsic revascularization or replacement of injured graft tissue by vascularized periligamentous tissue.[196]
- Most common cause of failed ACL reconstruction is anteriorly placed femoral tunnel (nonisometric graft elongates with flexion).
- Graft failure demonstrated by discontinuity of fibers or dysfunction of graft (excessive anterior displacement tibial displacement greater than 7mm).
- MR arthrography provides another technique for accurate assessment of ACL graft integrity.[310]
- Fibrosis of scar tissue may be assessed in sagittal plane and involve patellar tendon and Hoffa's fat pad.

MR Evaluation of Postoperative Patellar Tendon

- MR changes in patellar tendon seen immediately after ACL reconstruction[81]
- Initially: increased signal intensity on T1, PD, and FS PD FSE images with associated thickening in anteroposterior plane
- At 12 months: uncomplicated donor sites show normal low signal intensity or residual line of higher signal intensity parallel to tendon at harvest site; residual thickening of tendon
- Symptomatic patellar tendons measure greater than 10mm in anteroposterior dimension at 12 months.[105]
- Patella baja, secondary to adhesion and fibrosis, may be seen during first 6 months postoperatively.
- Patellar tendon donor site complications: patellar fracture, tendinitis, tendon rupture, patellar entrapment, and reflex sympathetic dystrophy (all can be evaluated by MR)

Cruciate Ligaments

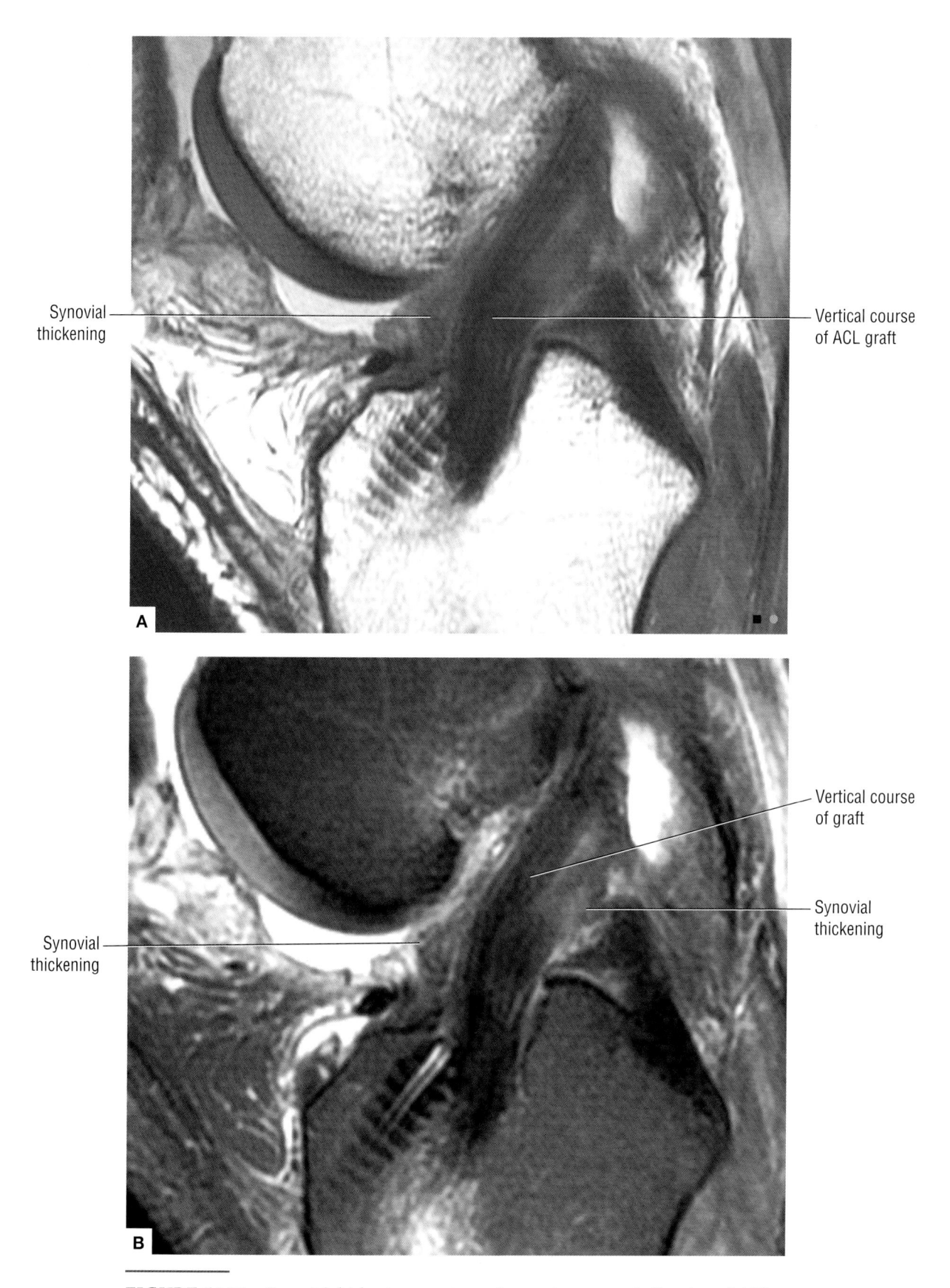

FIGURE 5.121 Synovial thickening anterior and posterior to a vertically oriented ACL graft. Synovial thickening is also present along the free edge of Hoffa's fat pad. Sagittal PD (**A**) and FS PD (**B**) images.

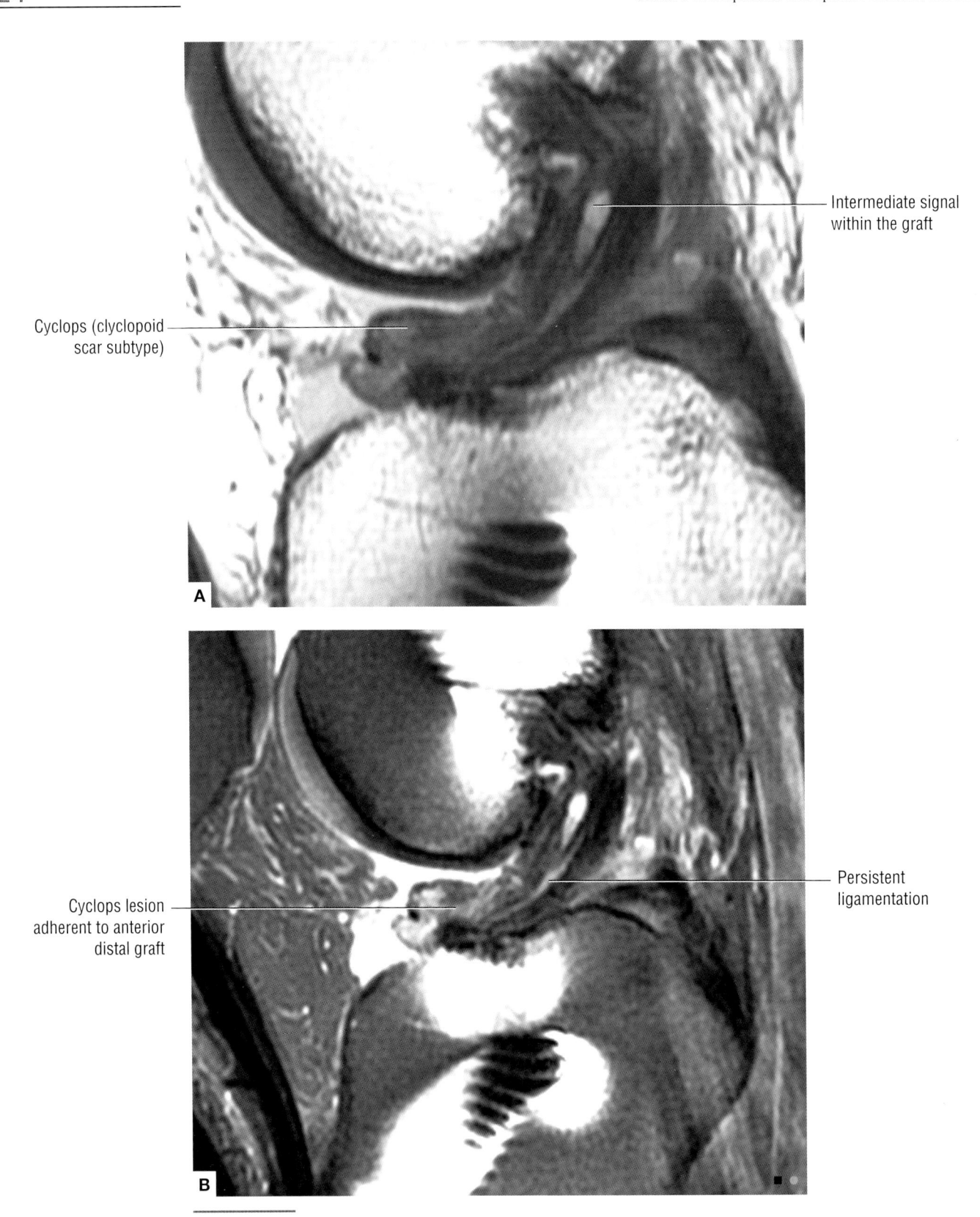

FIGURE 5.122 Teardrop-shaped cyclops fibrocartilaginous lesion in the anterior intercondylar notch, which in this case is adherent to the anterior distal fibers of the ACL graft. The morphology of the cyclops lesion, which follows the anterior contour of the distal ACL, is consistent with a soft cyclopoid scar subtype (histologic correlate). The cyclopoid scars consist of fibroproliferative tissue and can be compressed without terminal loss of knee extension. Graft signal with maintenance of graft continuity may be seen in the normal process of ligamentization or between individual bundles in multistrand hamstring graft material. Sagittal PD (**A**) and FS PD (**B**) images.

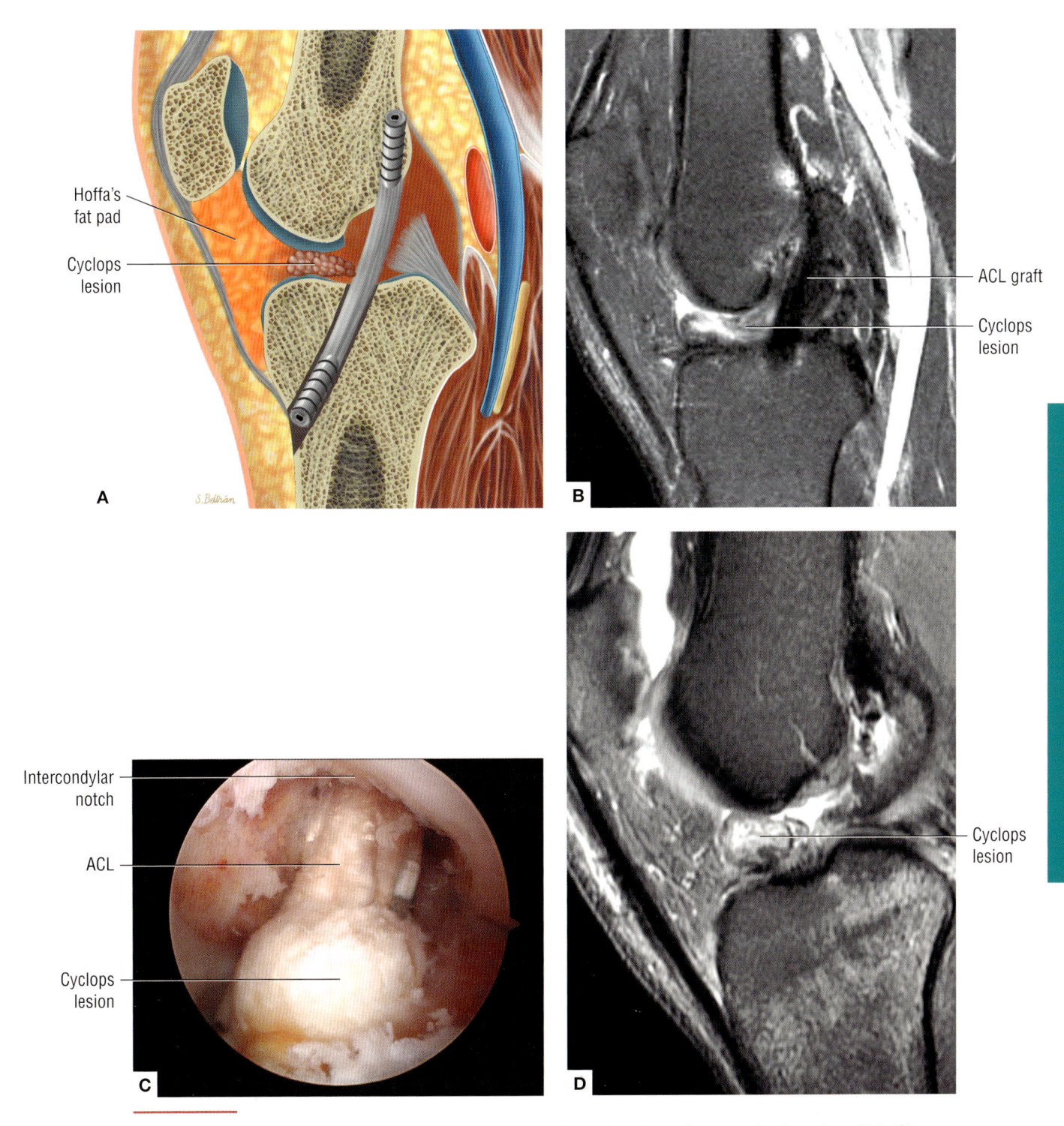

FIGURE 5.123 (**A**) Sagittal section color illustration of a cyclops lesion between the free edge of Hoffa's fat pad and the anterior surface of the distal ACL graft. (**B**) Sagittal FS PD FSE image with intermediate-signal-intensity soft tissue cyclops lesion producing a loss of knee extension. (**C**) The anterior location of a hard nodular cyclops. These lesions may contain osseous or cartilaginous tissue and lead to clinical entrapment. (**D**) A separate case showing a large nodular cyclops lesion associated with a failed ACL graft. Note the more nodular subtype does not conform to the contour of the adjacent tissues.

FIGURE 5.124 Extensive scarring of the anterior interval as a complication of ACL reconstruction. True arthrofibrosis would be associated with complete replacement of fat signal in Hoffa's fat pad with hyperintense scar tissue.

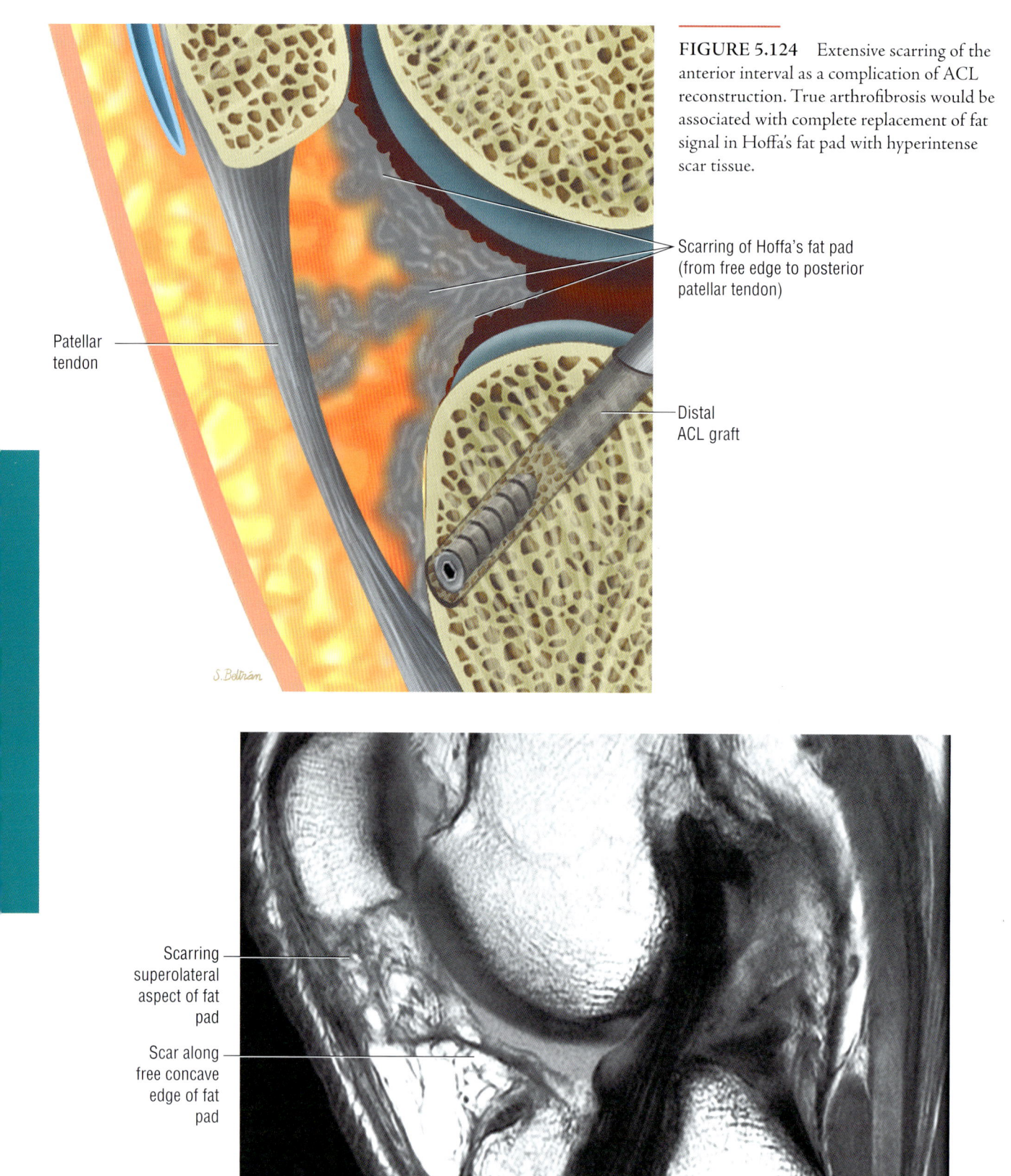

FIGURE 5.125 Scar tissue may be located along the free edge of the fat pad or replace the fat signal within Hoffa's fat pad. Scar tissue may also tether the deep surface of the patellar tendon. Arthrofibrosis usually implies massive scar tissue replacement and resultant decreased range of motion. Sagittal PD FSE image.

Cruciate Ligaments

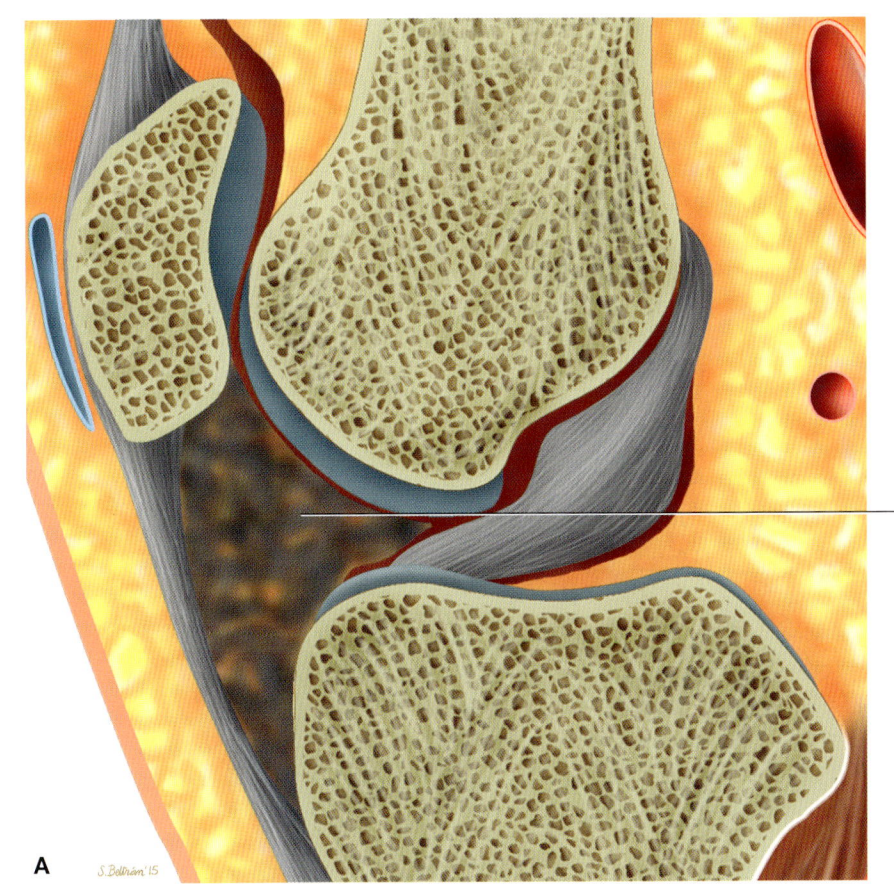

Diffuse scarring as seen in arthrofibrosis

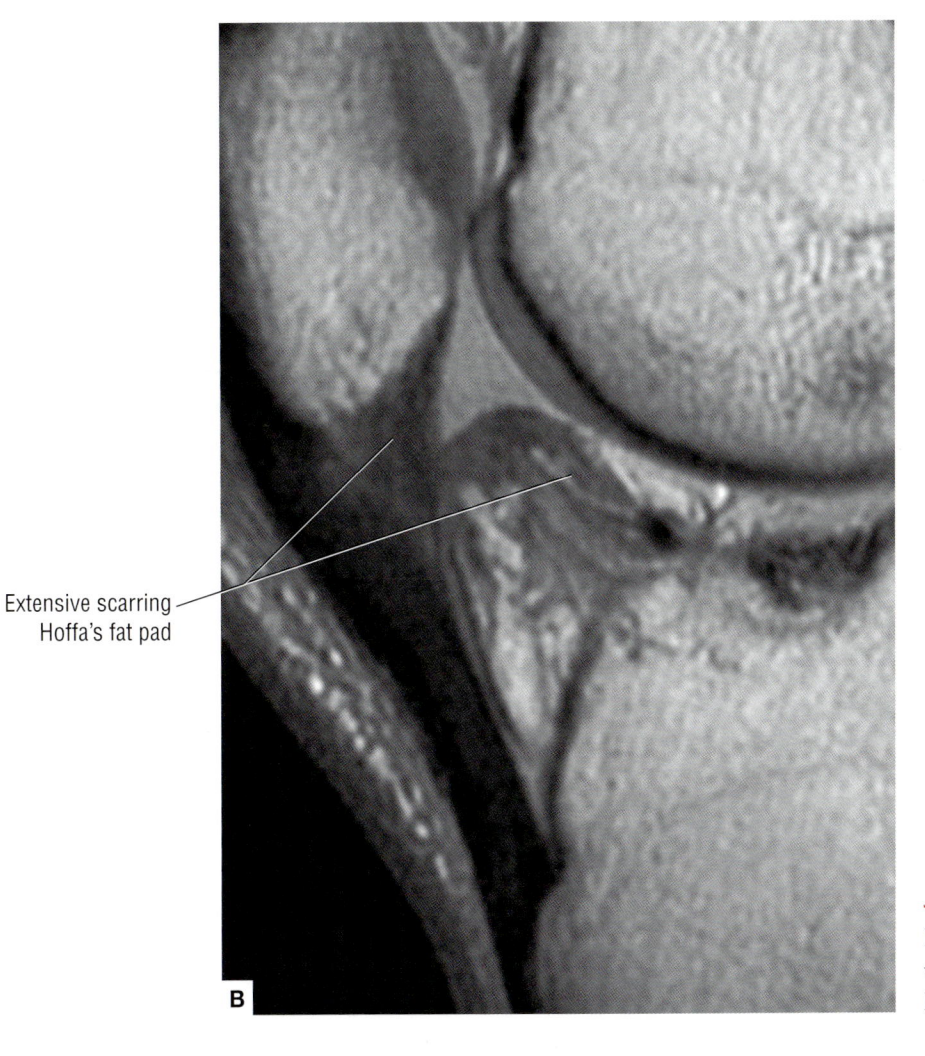

Extensive scarring Hoffa's fat pad

FIGURE 5.126 Arthrofibrosis is associated with a diffuse, not localized, scarring reaction. Illustration (**A**) and sagittal PD FSE image (**B**).

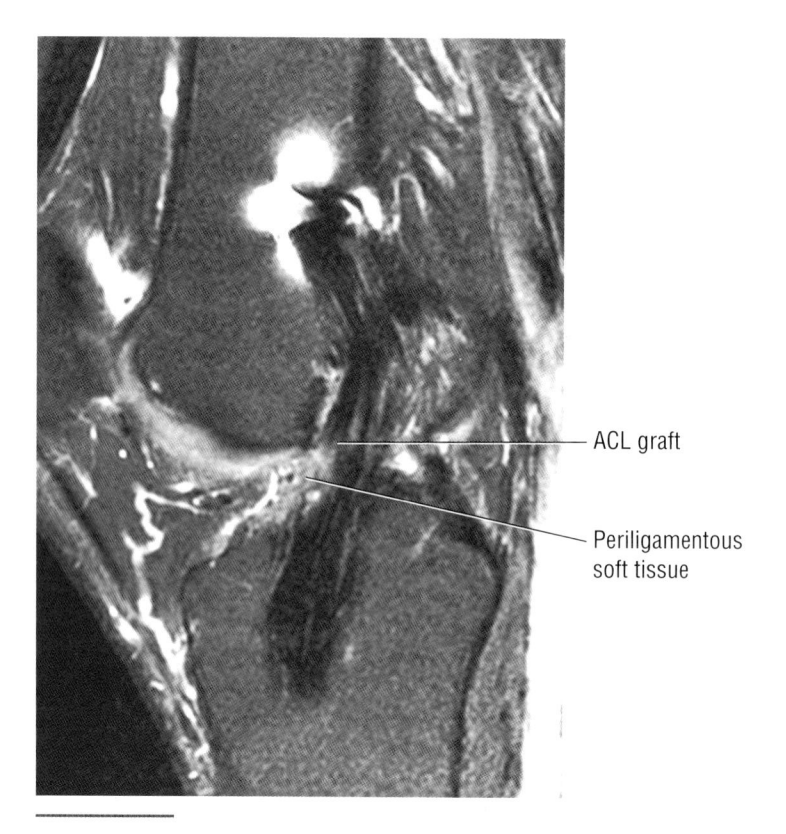

FIGURE 5.127 Intermediate-signal-intensity periligamentous soft tissue anterior to an unimpinged ACL graft (sagittal FS PD FSE image).

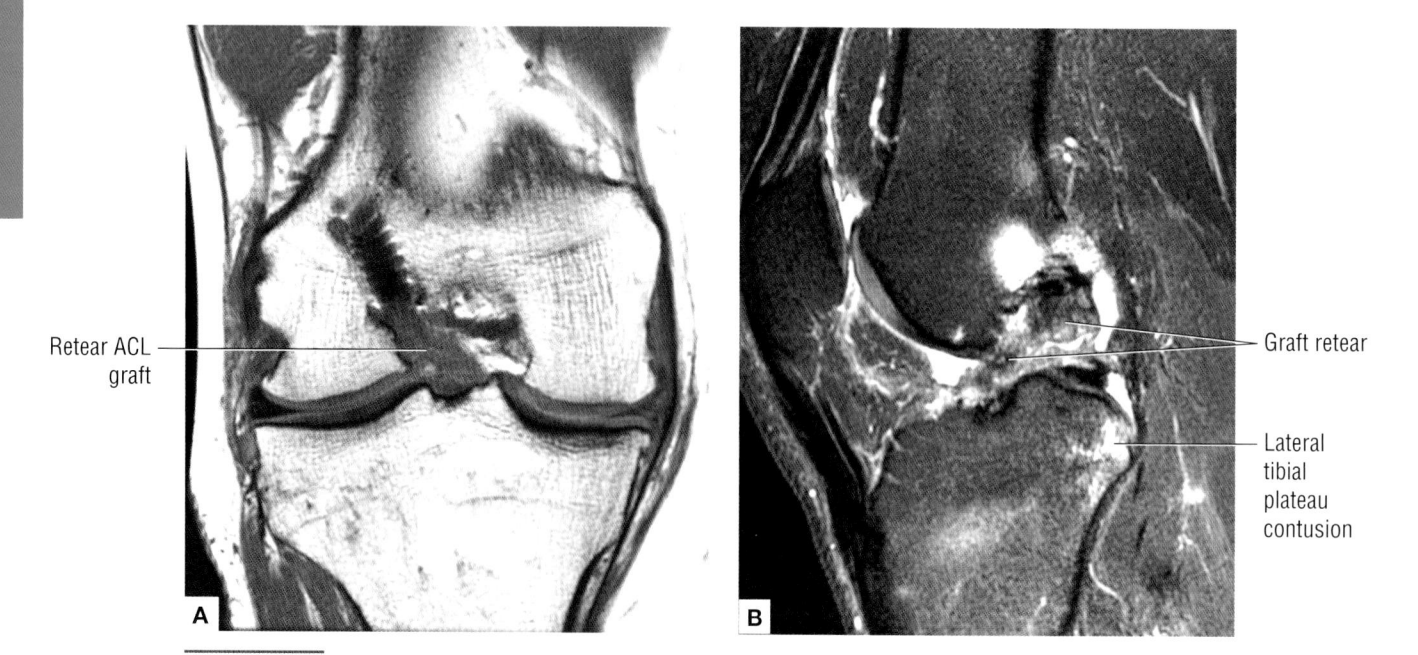

FIGURE 5.128 Acute retear of an ACL graft. A hyperintense posterior lateral tibial plateau contusion, as well as diffuse ligament hyperintensity and discontinuity, can be seen on coronal T1-weighted FSE (**A**) and sagittal FS PD FSE (**B**) images.

Cruciate Ligaments

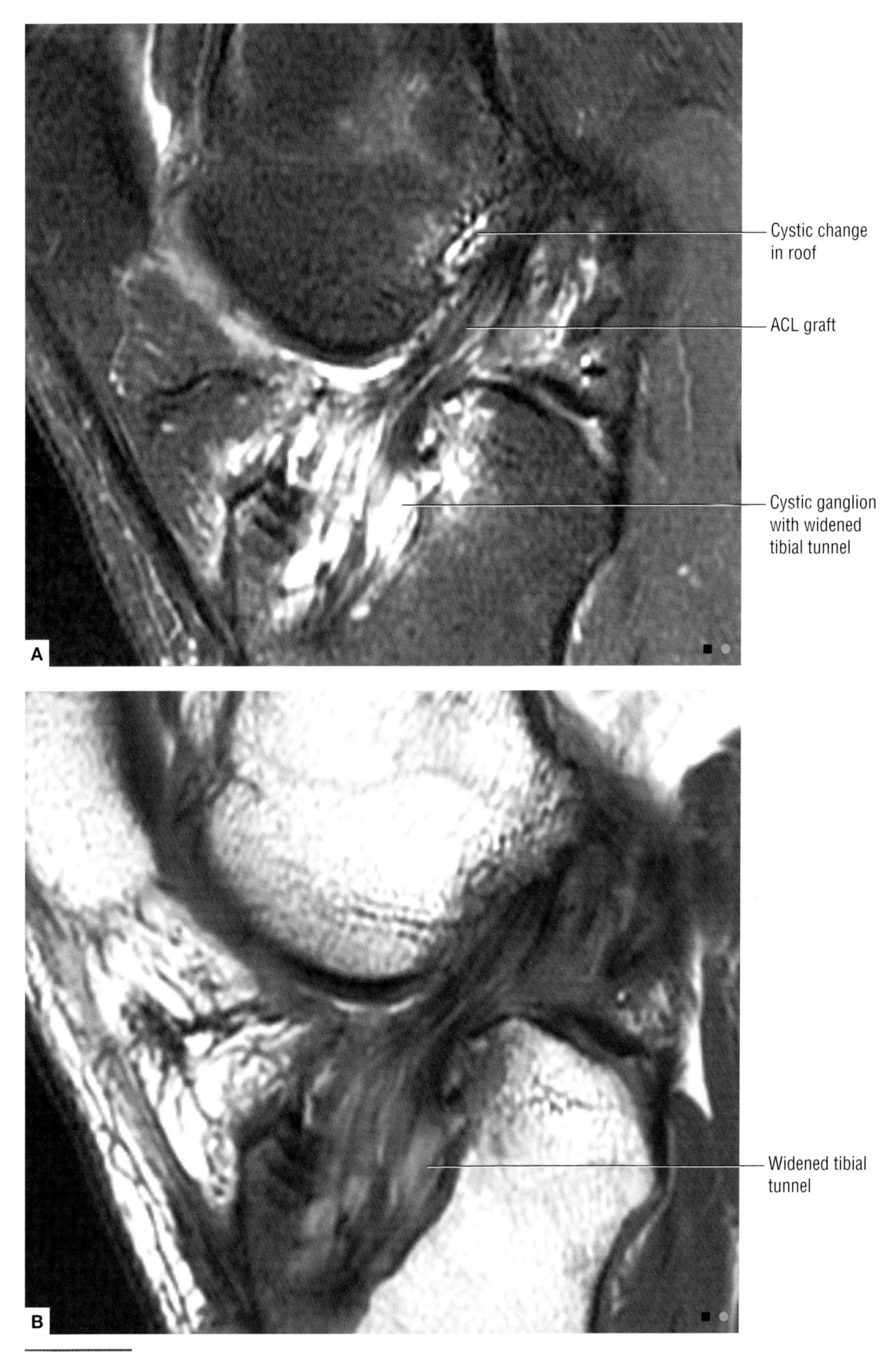

FIGURE 5.129 Tibial tunnel ganglion cyst resulting in tunnel enlargement. Associated mucoid degeneration may be associated with notch cysts as well. Sagittal FS PD (**A**) and PD (**B**) images.

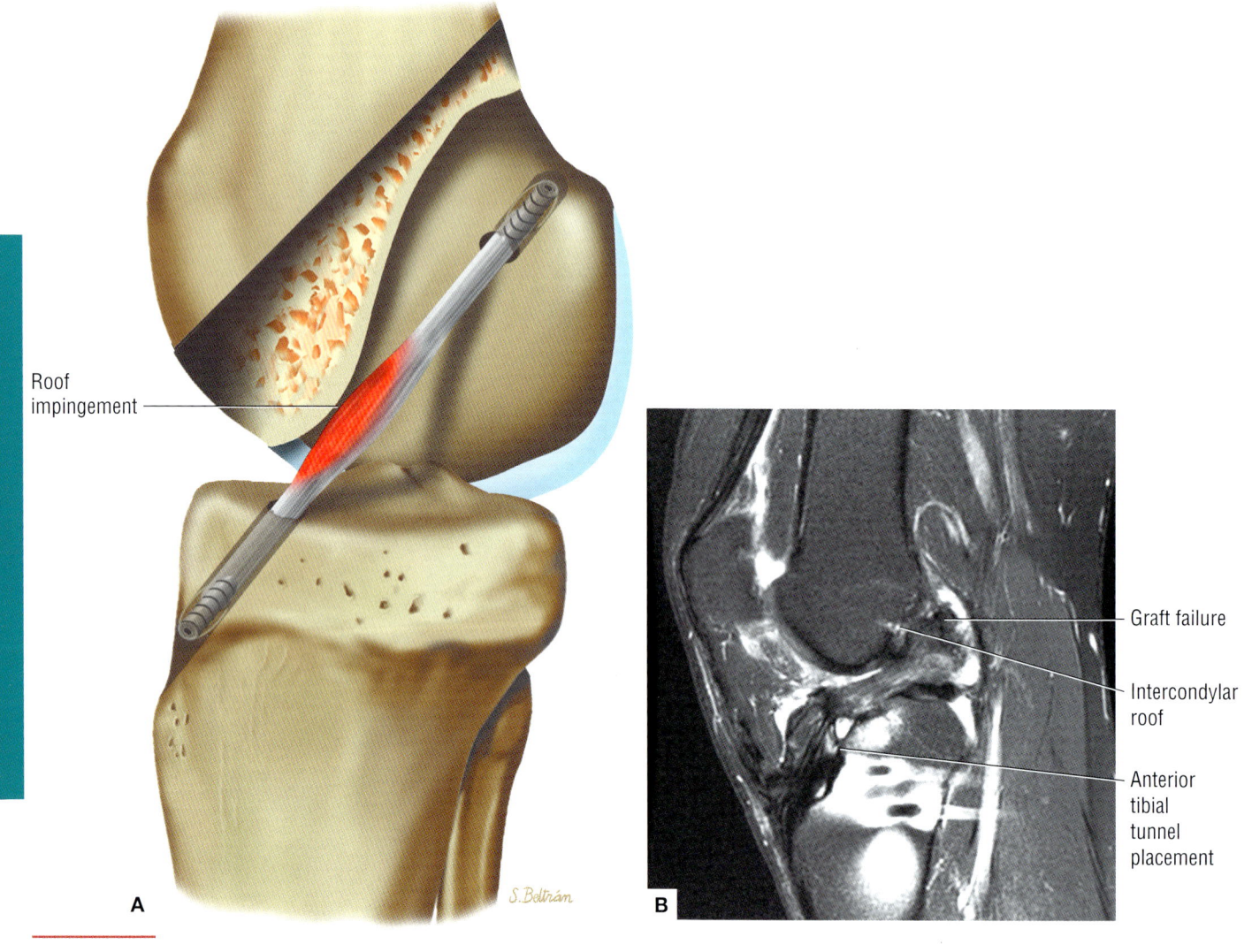

FIGURE 5.130 (**A**) Distal ACL graft impingement at the intercondylar roof. The normal or unaltered intercondylar notch forms a 35- to 40-degree angle with the long axis of the femoral diaphysis. Internal notchplasty and proper tunnel placement are required to prevent impingement. (**B**) Graft failure and roof impingement. The tibial tunnel is anterior to the projected slope of the intercondylar roof. The hyperintense ACL graft has failed proximally (sagittal FS PD FSE image).

Partial ACL graft tear involving anterior fibers

Displaced anterior fibers of ACL graft

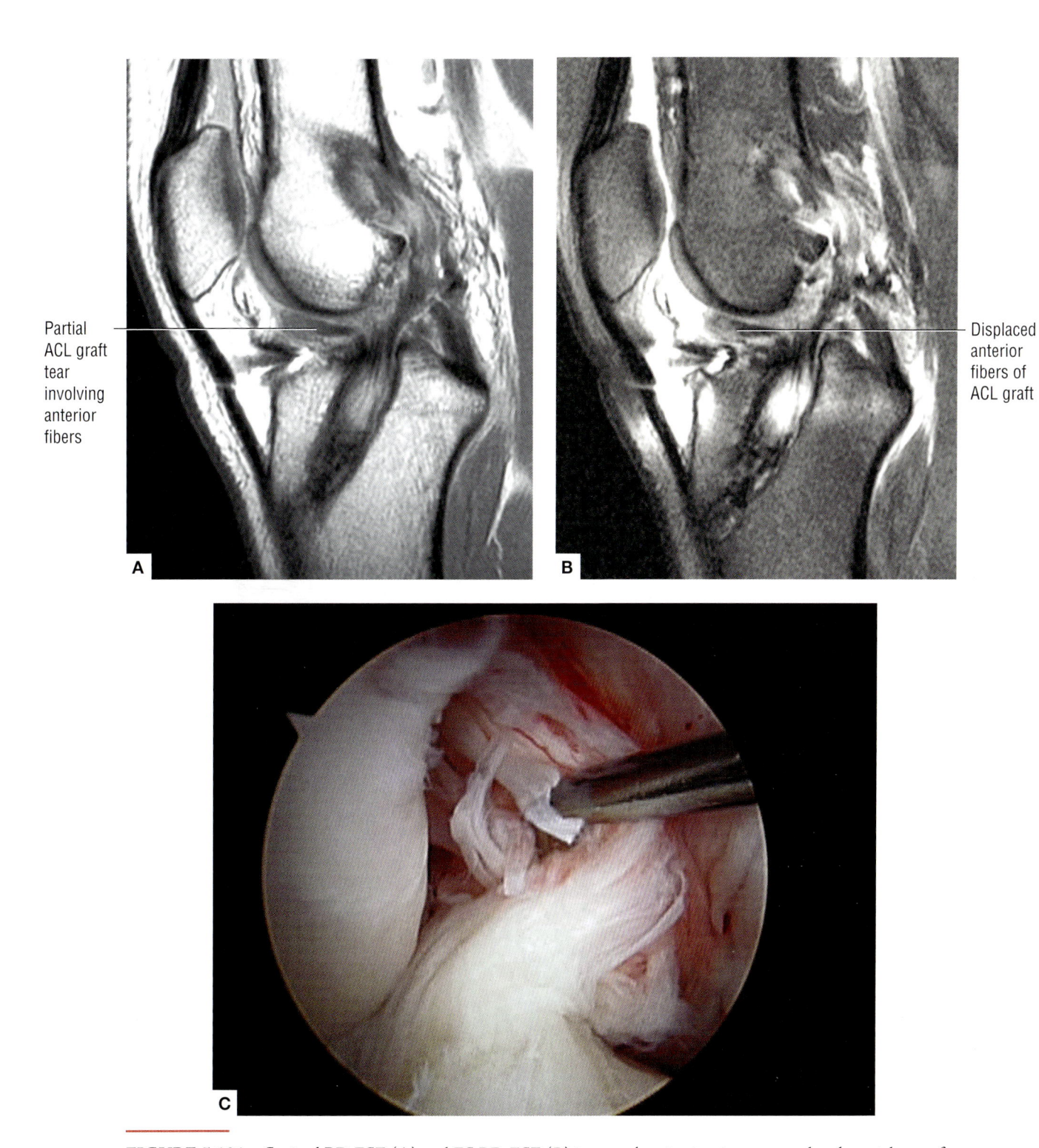

FIGURE 5.131 Sagittal PD FSE (**A**) and FS PD FSE (**B**) images showing impingement-related partial tear of the anterior fibers of an ACL graft. (**C**) Arthroscopic view of lax ACL graft fibers. The tibial tunnel does intersect the intercondylar roof and is thus anterior to the intersection of Blumensaat line with the tibia.

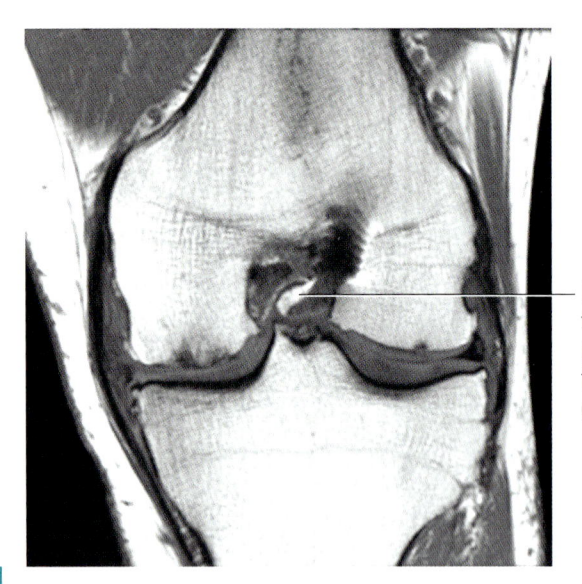

FIGURE 5.132 Dislodged femoral bone in failed ACL graft. Coronal PD FSE image.

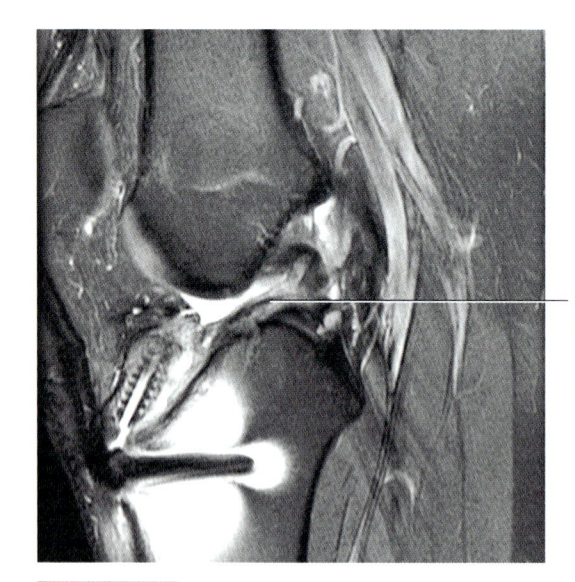

- Dislodged femoral plug in failed ACL graft

FIGURE 5.133 Complete discontinuity in ruptured ACL graft. Residual fibers are oriented horizontally and scarred to the PCL (sagittal FS PD FSE image).

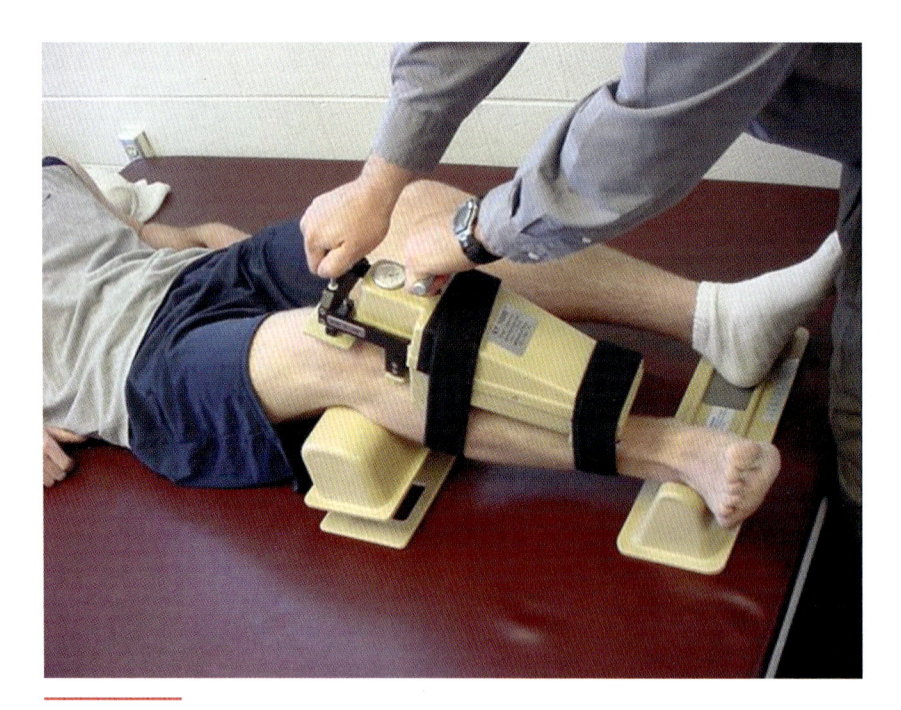

- Horizontal orientation of ACL graft remnant

FIGURE 5.134 KT-1000. KT-1000 was developed to provide objective measurements of sagittal plane motions of the tibia relative to the femur. The KT-1000 and its second iteration, the KT-2000, measure anterior tibial translation. The knee is tested in approximately 20 to 30 degrees of flexion. The maximum anterior displacement test with the arthrometer clinically approximates the Lachman test. (Reprinted from Fu FH. *Master Techniques in Orthopaedic Surgery: Sports Medicine*. Philadelphia, PA: Lippincott Williams & Wilkins; 2010, with permission.)

Cruciate Ligaments

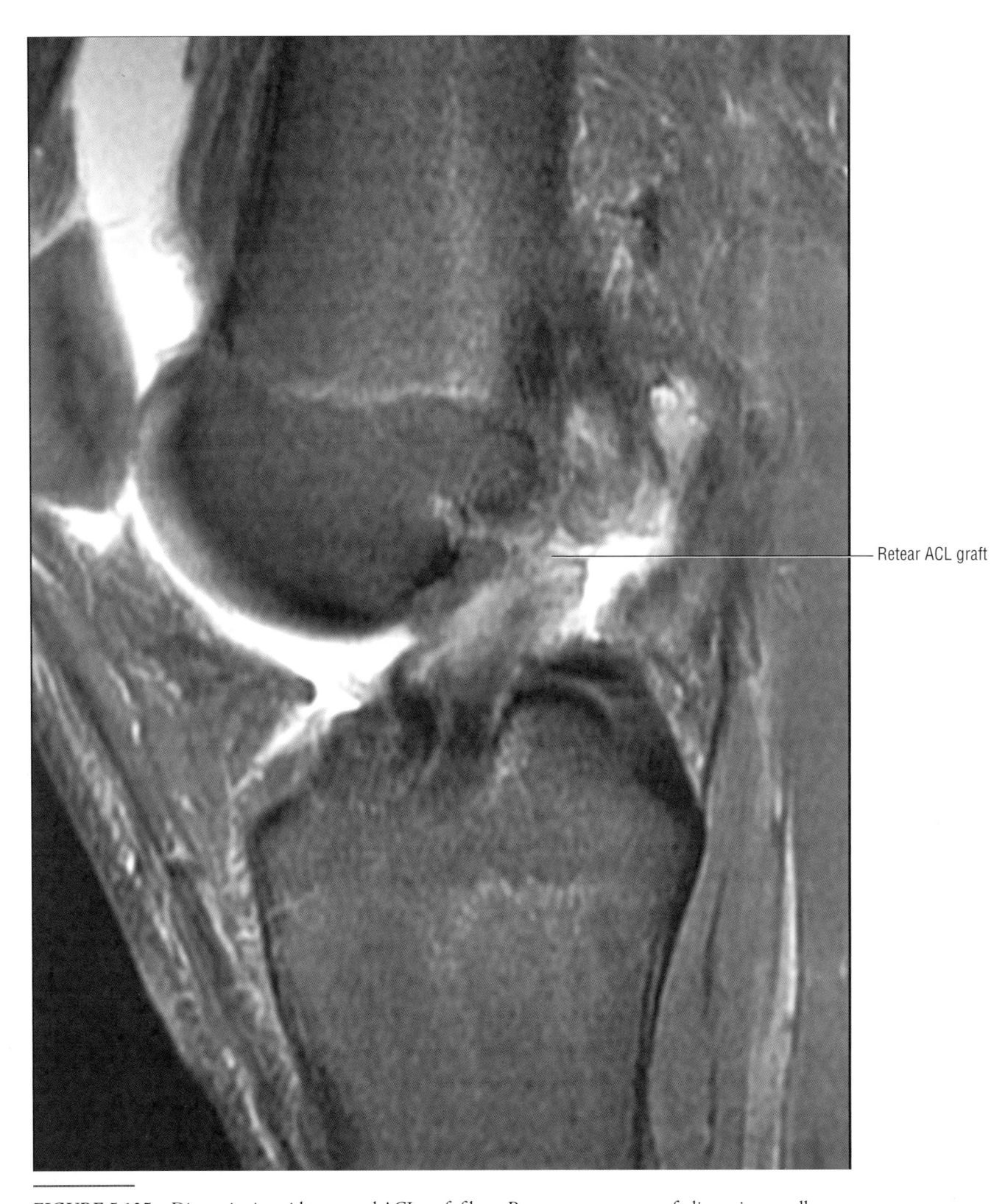

Retear ACL graft

FIGURE 5.135 Discontinuity with retracted ACL graft fibers. Retear or recurrent graft disruption usually requires evaluation of both coronal and sagittal images. Direct and indirect imaging findings are similar to that of a native ACL tear.

Ruptured ACL graft with complete loss of fiber striations

Disruption of ACL graft

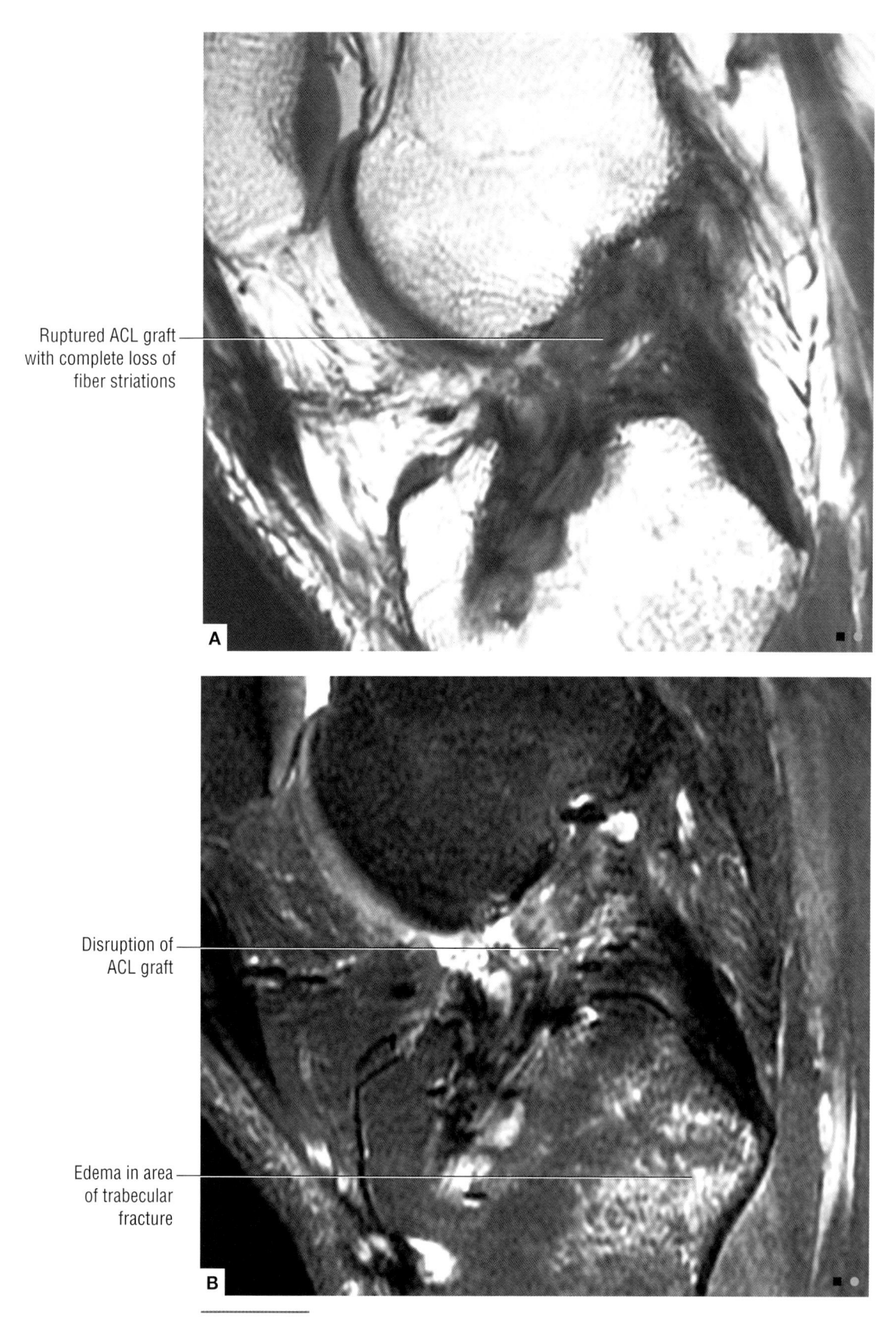

Edema in area of trabecular fracture

FIGURE 5.136 ACL graft disruption with acute lateral compartment trabecular edema. Sagittal PD FSE (**A**) and FS PD FSE (**B**) images.

Cruciate Ligaments

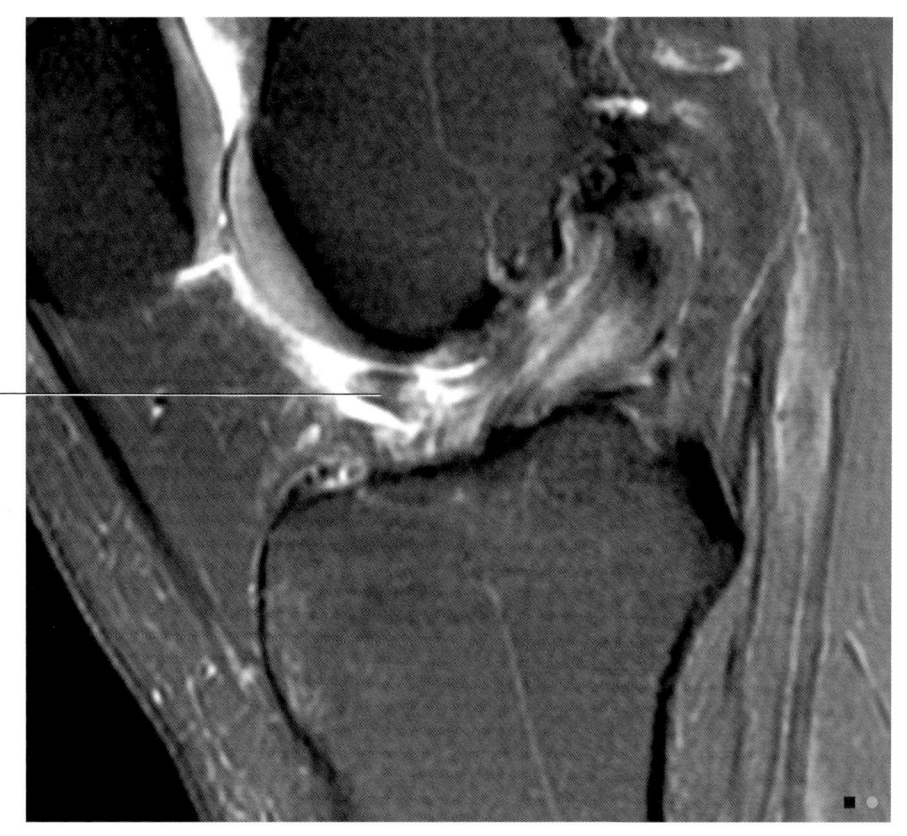

Displaced anterior graft fixation debris

FIGURE 5.137 Bone plugs and bioabsorbable interference screws may displace into the joint posterior to Hoffa's fat pad. Sagittal FS PD FSE image.

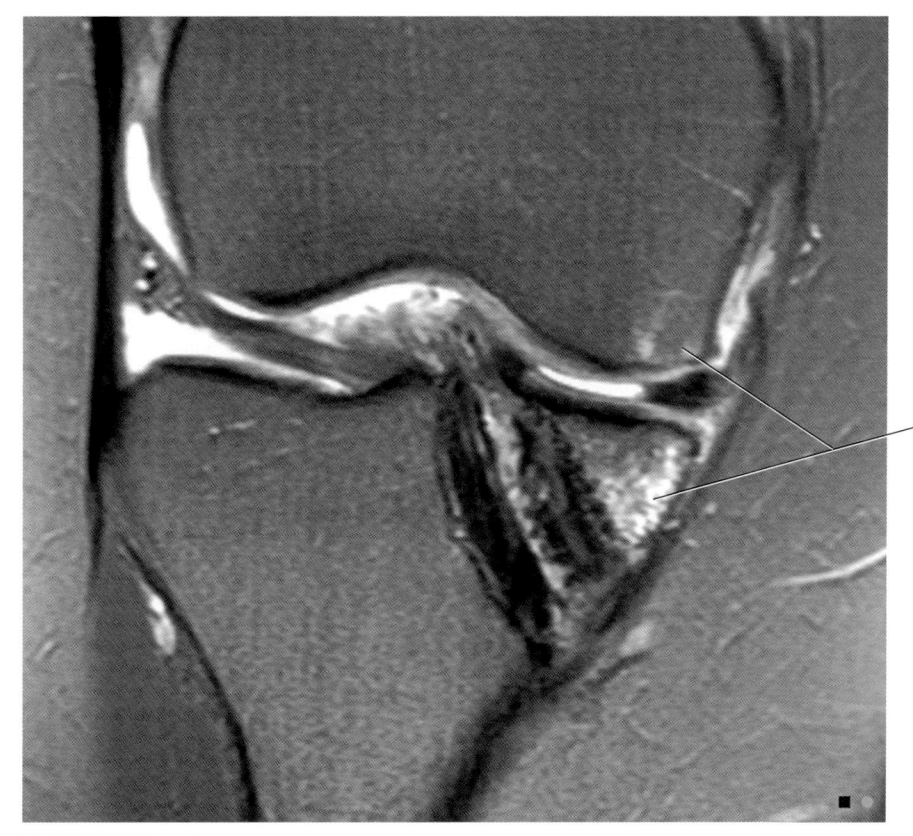

Subchondral edema anterior medial compartment

FIGURE 5.138 Medial compartment degenerative change associated with subchondral marrow edema independent of the ACL graft. Coronal FS PD FSE image.

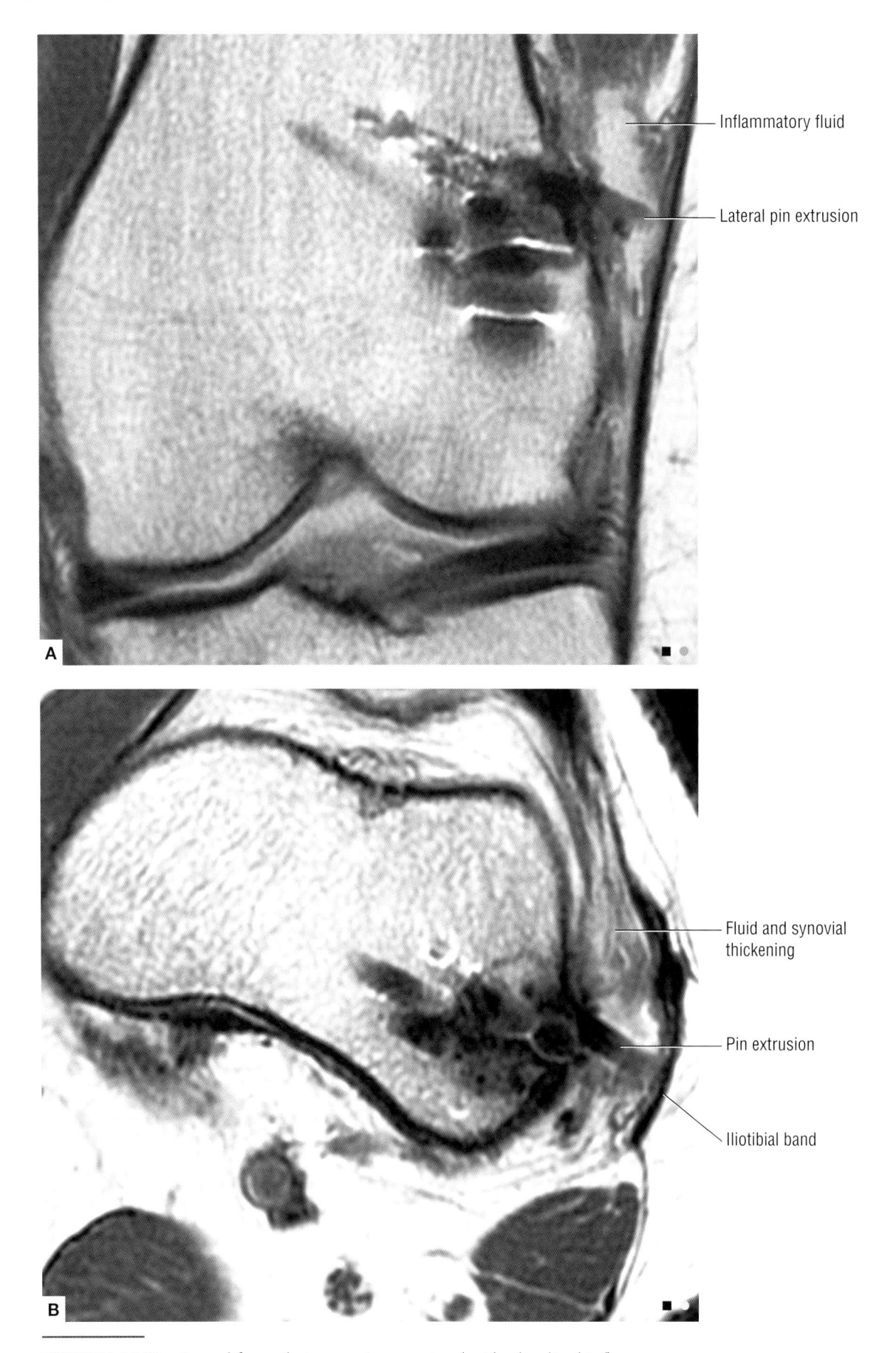

FIGURE 5.139 Lateral femoral pin extrusion associated with a localized inflammatory reaction resulting in iliotibial band syndrome. Coronal (**A**) and axial (**B**) PD FSE images.

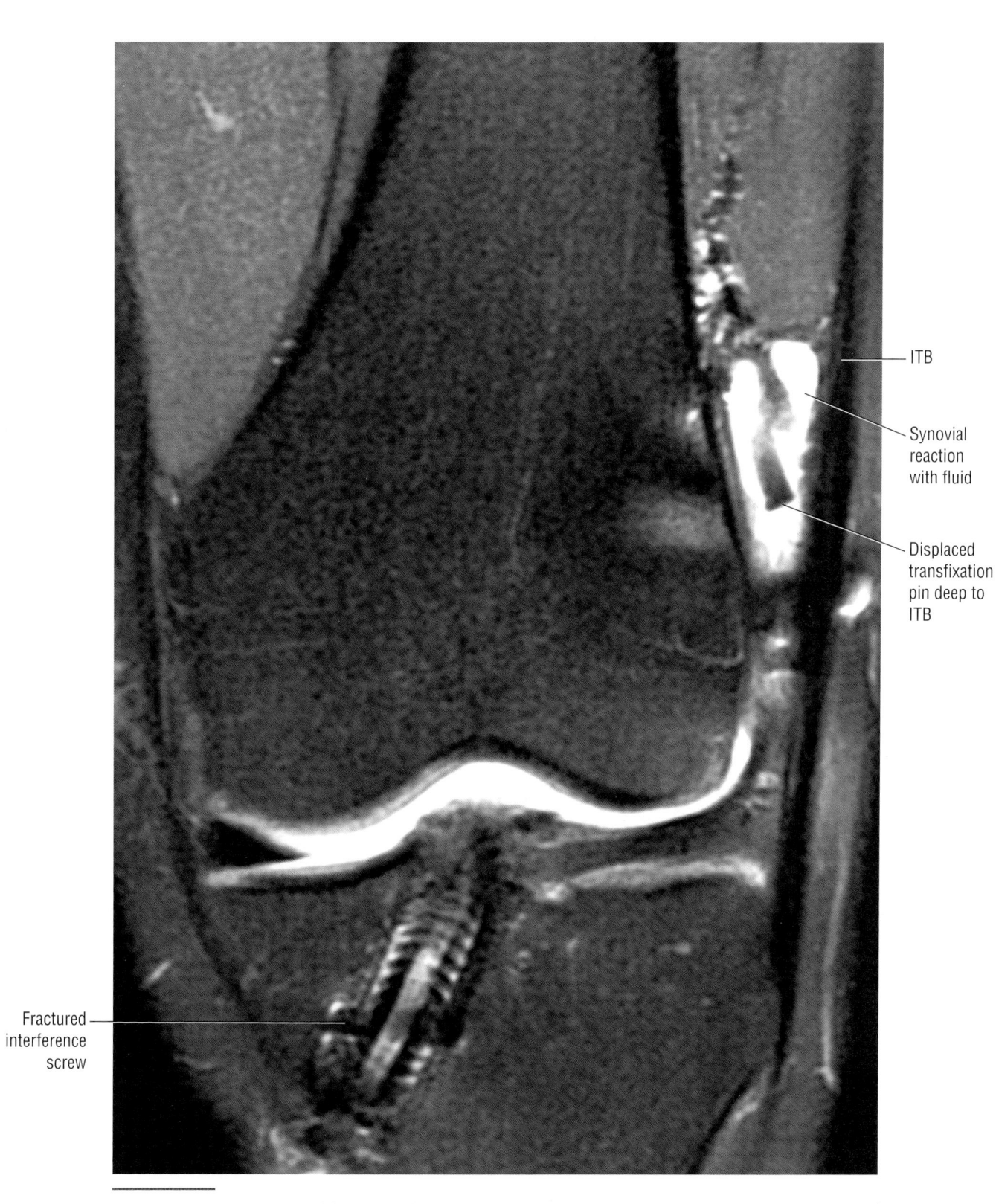

FIGURE 5.140 Fractured fragment of transfixation pin deep to iliotibial band. Fractured tibial interference screw. Bioabsorbable interference screws have complications including cyst formation, tunnel widening, effusions, fracture, and intraarticular migration. Coronal FS PD FSE image.

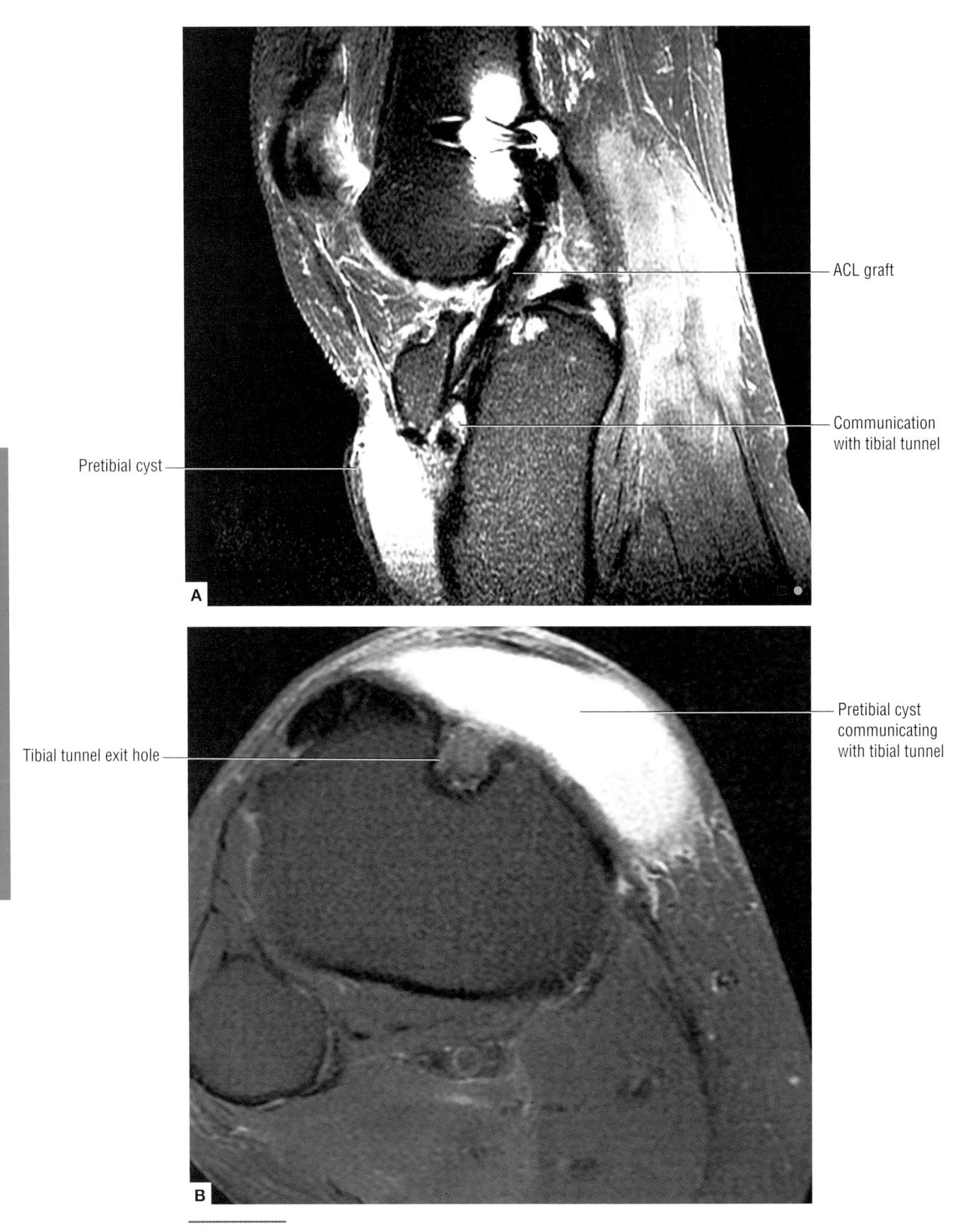

FIGURE 5.141 Tunnel (tibial tunnel) and pretibial cysts are uncommon complications of ACL reconstruction. They usually occur at 1 to 5 years postoperatively. Determine if there is joint communication. Presence of the cyst does not imply that the graft is unstable. Sagittal (**A**) and axial (**B**) FS PD images.

Cruciate Ligaments

ACL Allograft with Stem Cells

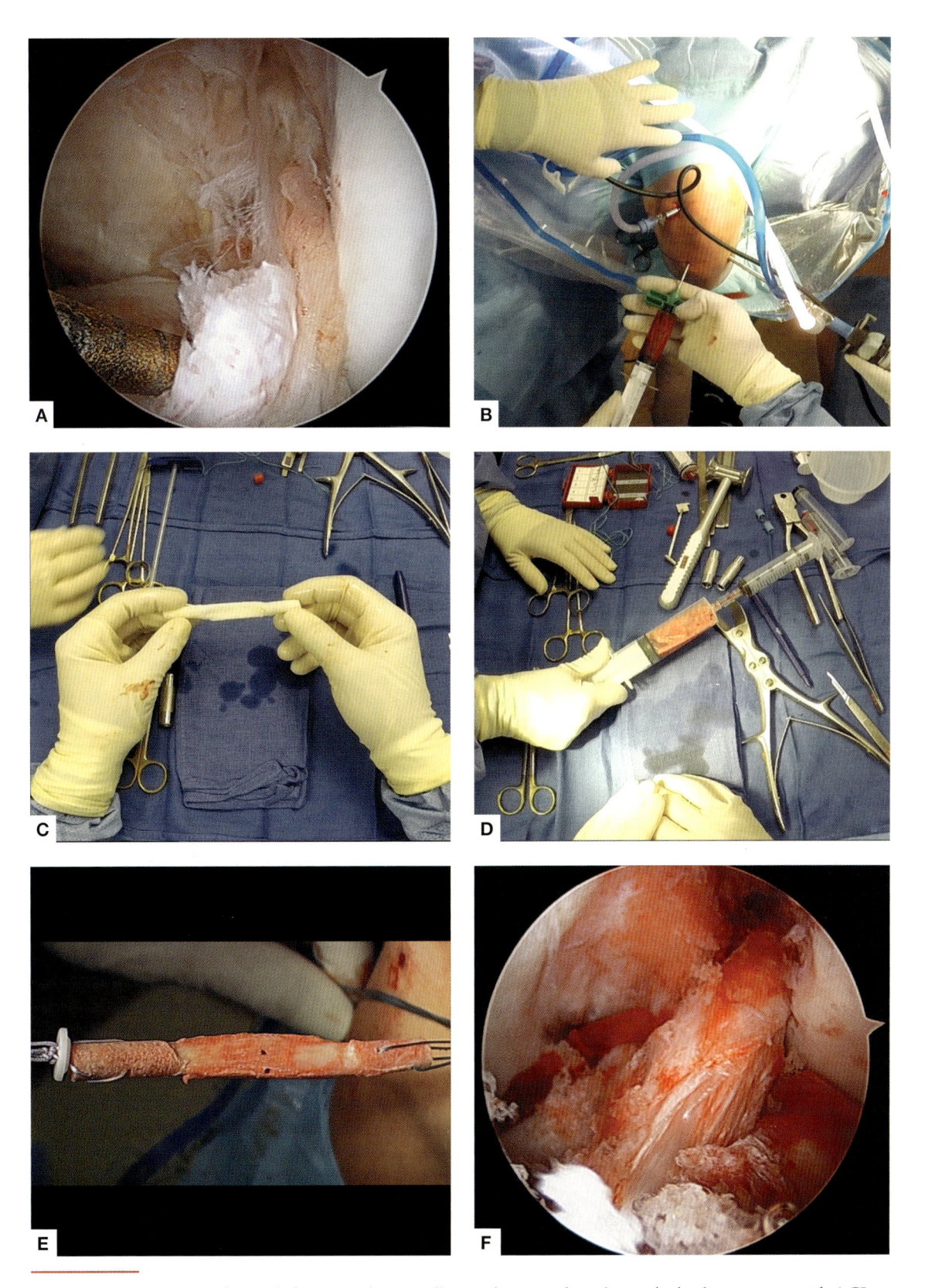

FIGURE 5.142 Use of growth factors and stem cells to enhance and accelerate the healing process with ACL ligament grafting. (**A**) Ruptured ACL. (**B**) Aspiration of marrow for stem cell concentration. (**C**) ACL allograft preparation. (**D**) Vacuum aspiration of stem cells into ACL allograft. (**E**) Bone–patellar tendon–bone allograft infused with stem cells and prepared for placement. (**F**) Placement of graft in the knee. (Courtesy of The Stone Clinic, San Francisco, California.)

Posterior Cruciate Ligament (PCL)

Key Concepts

- PCL injuries include reverse Segond fractures, arcuate sign, and anterior compartment osseous contusions.

- MR findings of partial or interstitial tears of the PCL are more common than complete ruptures.

Functional Anatomy

- PCL has greater length and is stronger than the ACL.

- PCL originates in lateral aspect of medial femoral condyle, crosses ACL, and attaches to posterior intercondyloid fossa of the tibia.[81,202]

- Averages 38mm in length and 13mm in width at midportion[83]

- Cross-sectional area of PCL decreases from proximal to distal attachments.
    - PCL footprints on femoral tibia are three times larger than mid-substance cross-sectional area.

- Smaller tibial insertion attaches onto inclined recessed shelf, posterior and inferior to articular plateau of tibia.

- Large femoral origin on the lateral wall of medial femoral condyle, where PCL attaches to flat upper border and convex lower border that parallels articular surface of medial femoral condyle.

- Intraarticular but extrasynovial and enveloped by fold of synovium reflected from posterior capsule

- Composed of anterolateral and posteromedial bands (or bundles) that tighten on flexion and extension, respectively (PCL anatomy is complex and represents a continuum of up to four geographical fiber regions)

- With progressive knee flexion, posteromedial band passes anterior to and under anterolateral band.

- Larger anterolateral band tightens with knee flexion and relaxes with knee extension.

- Smaller posteromedial band is lax in flexion and tightens in extension.

- A smaller posterior oblique band or bundle has also been described.

Posterior Cruciate Ligament

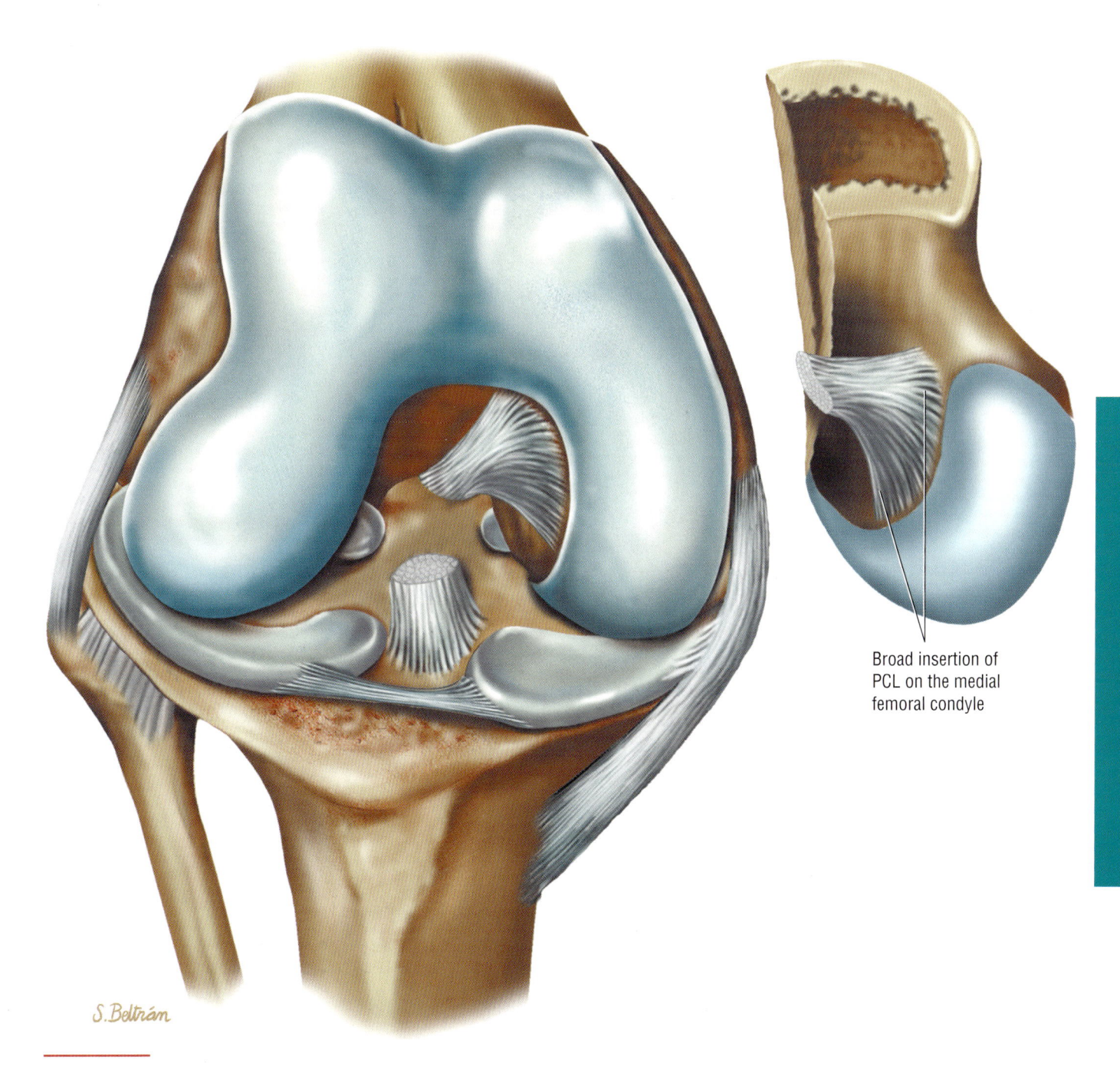

FIGURE 5.143 A coronal color illustration from the anterior perspective shows the broad insertion of the PCL on the medial femoral condyle with horizontal orientation of fibers in extension. This contrasts to the vertical femoral attachment of the ACL. The PCL has traditionally been described as having a long, thick anterolateral bundle and a shorter posteromedial bundle. The anterolateral bundle tightens with knee flexion, and the posteromedial bundle tightens with knee extension. The PCL exists as a fiber continuum and is not made up of morphologically distinct bands. The PCL has been further described as having anterior, central, posterior longitudinal, and posterior oblique fiber regions.

- Functional and morphologic descriptions divide PCL into an anterior and central portion (constitutes bulk of the ligament) and posterior longitudinal and posterior oblique components (10% to 15% of the ligament).

- Central stabilizer of the knee, restraining posterior tibial displacement on the femur

- Stabilizes against excessive varus or valgus angulation

- Resists internal rotation of tibia on the femur

- Isolated PCL (rare) has little effect on tibial rotational laxity or varus and valgus angulation in absence of associated injury of extraarticular restraints.

- Combined injury of PCL and posterolateral (arcuate) complex results in significant increase in both varus angulation and tibial external rotation, maximal at 90 degrees of knee flexion.

- Most PCL fibers are not isometric, except in posterior oblique region at the posterosuperior margin of the anterior femoral PCL attachment.

- Meniscofemoral ligaments

    - Ligament of Humphrey: anterior to PCL; taut in flexion

    - Ligament of Wrisberg: posterior to PCL; connects posterior horn of lateral meniscus to lateral aspect of medial femoral condyle near PCL origin; taut in extension

    - Either meniscofemoral ligament found in 80% of knee joint specimens[524]; both present in 6% to 88% of knees[179]

    - Both meniscofemoral ligaments tighten with internal rotation of tibia (posterior drawer test should be performed in neutral or external tibial rotation).[69,75]

    - Considered stabilizers of posterior horn of lateral meniscus

    - During knee flexion, meniscofemoral ligament increases in congruence between meniscotibial socket and lateral femoral condyle and may function as secondary restraint to posterior tibial translation after PCL rupture.[83]

Cruciate Ligaments

Meniscofemoral Ligaments

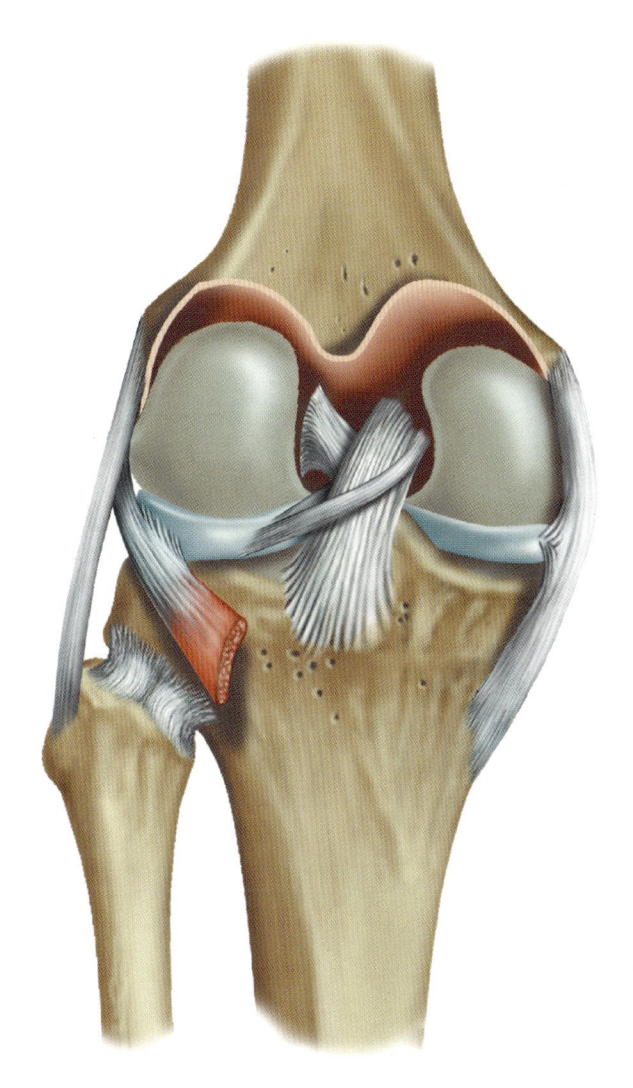

FIGURE 5.144 Posterior view of color illustration (coronal perspective) of the ligaments of Humphrey and Wrisberg.

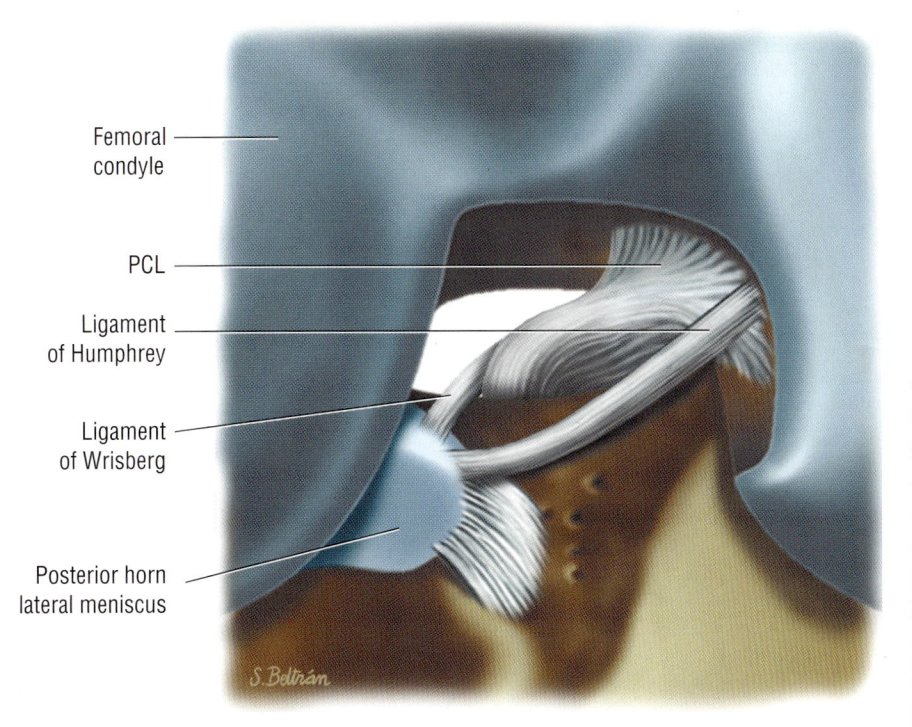

FIGURE 5.145 An illustration from the anterior perspective directed posteriorly shows both meniscofemoral ligaments at their attachment to the posterior horn of the lateral meniscus. The ligament of Humphrey courses anterior to the PCL, and the ligament of Wrisberg passes posterior to the PCL.

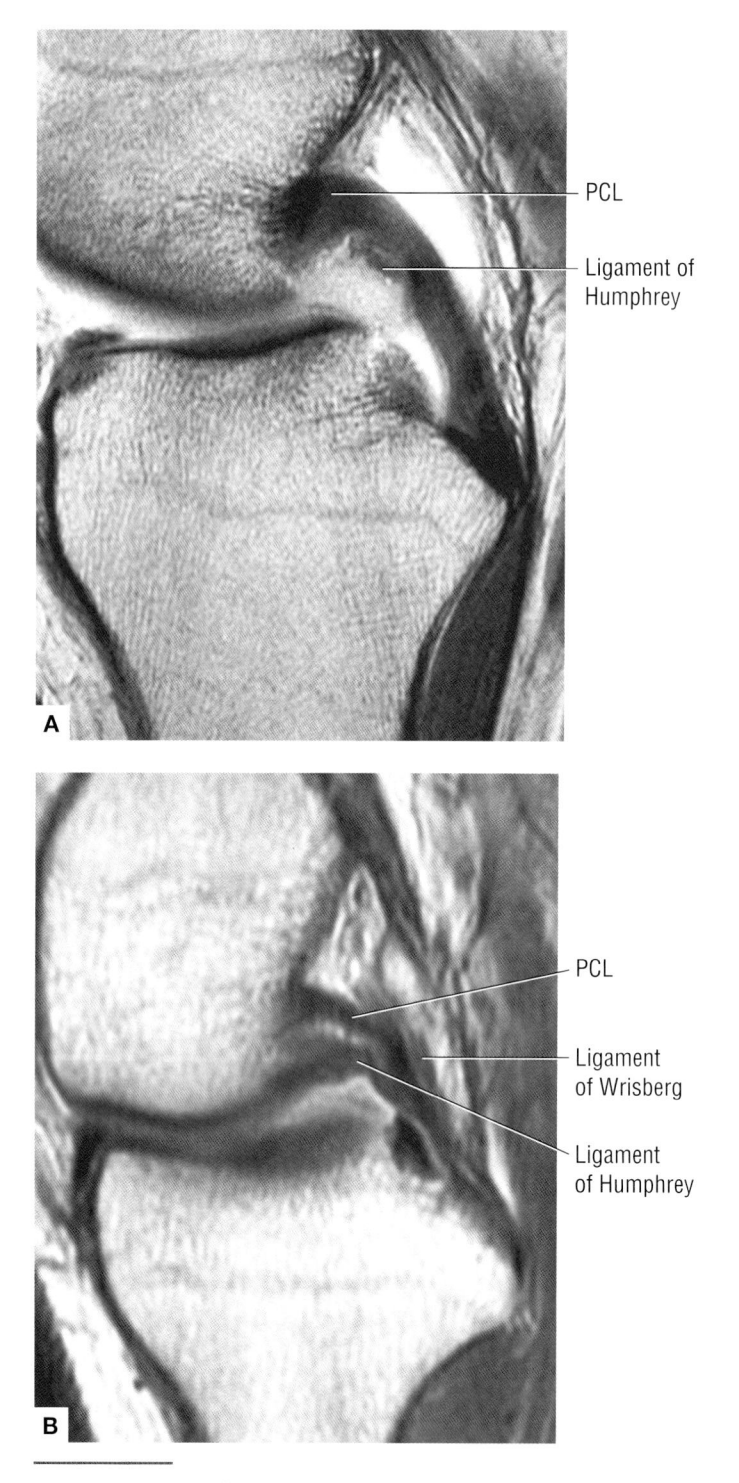

FIGURE 5.146 (**A**) The ligament of Humphrey in the sagittal plane. There are two normal variants of the meniscofemoral ligaments. They may be present as a single ligament, or both Humphrey's and Wrisberg's ligaments may be present. (**B**) Prominent ligament of Humphrey simulating a double PCL on a sagittal PD FSE image. This normal variant should not be mistaken for the double PCL sign of the displaced fragment of a bucket-handle tear.

Cruciate Ligaments

FIGURE 5.147 The distal PCL attaches to the posterior intercondylar area and posterior tibial surface in a central fovea 1.5cm distal to the joint line (coronal T1-weighted FSE image).

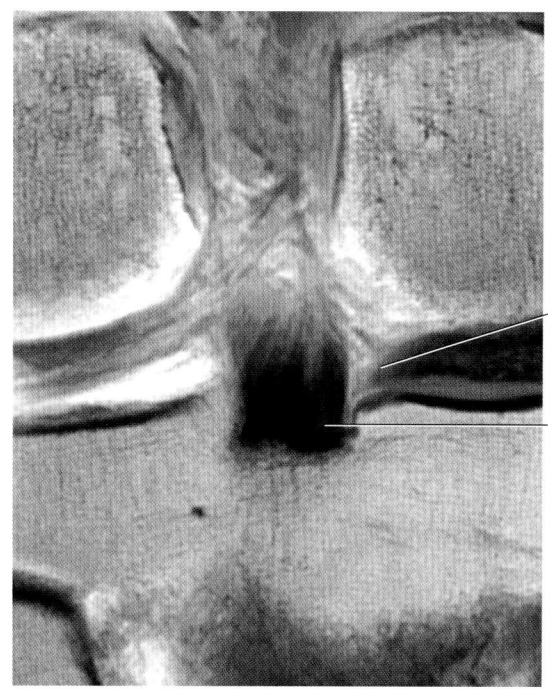

Root attachment of medial meniscus

Tibial foveal attachment of PCL

ACL
PCL
Ligament of Humphrey

Ligament of Wrisberg
Ligament of Humphrey
PCL

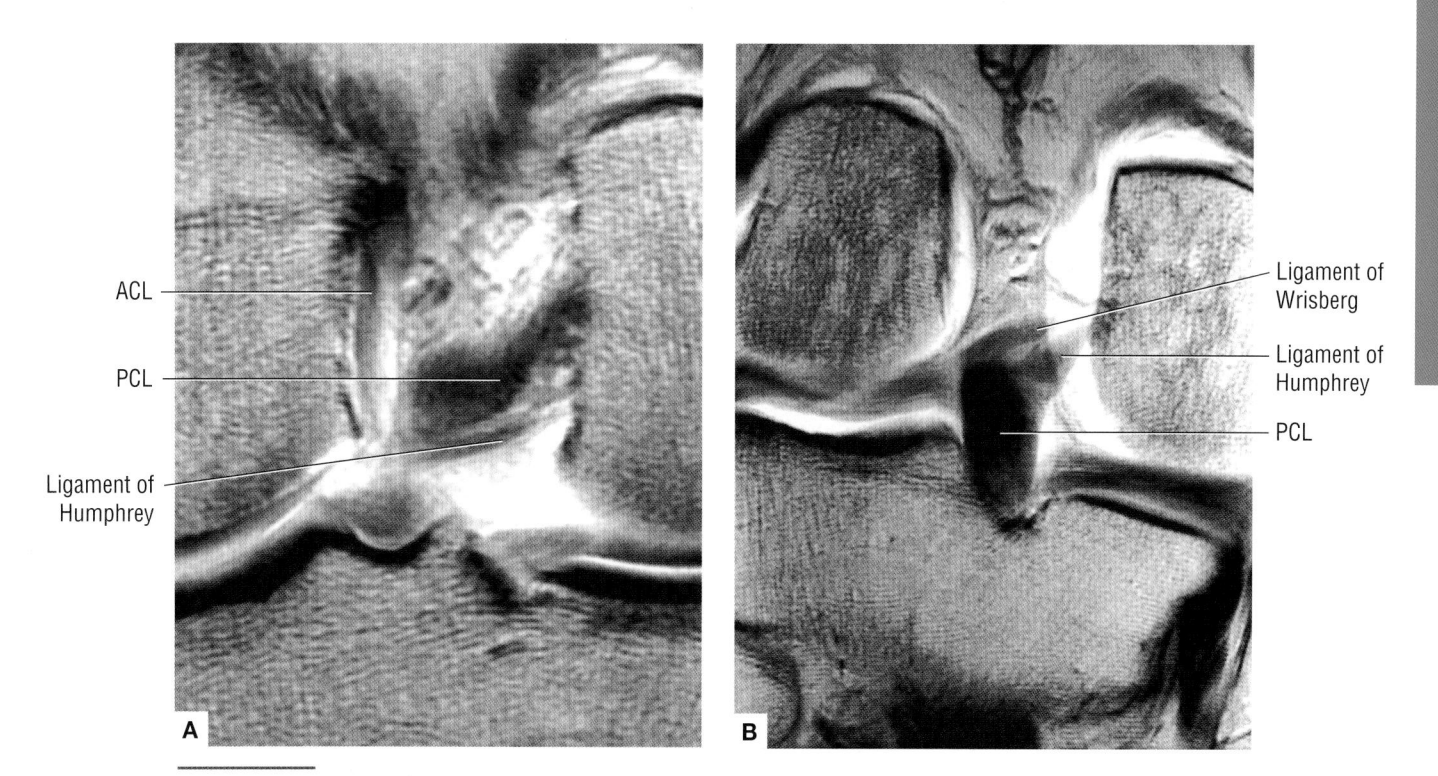

FIGURE 5.148 (A) Coronal T1-weighted image with the ligament anterior and inferior to the PCL. (B) On this coronal image, the meniscofemoral ligaments of Humphrey and Wrisberg are both seen to arise from the posterior horn of the lateral meniscus and to insert on the posterolateral aspect of the medial femoral condyle.

Extension (fibers relaxed)   ## Flexion (fibers taut)

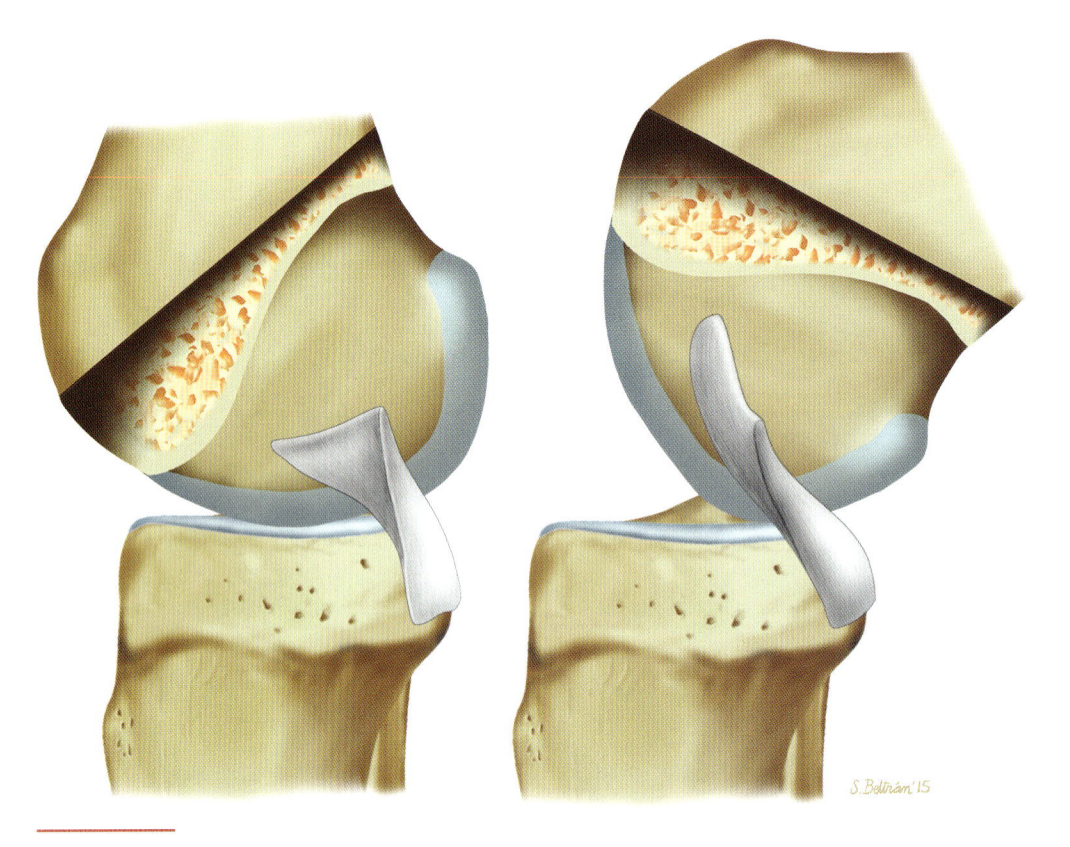

FIGURE 5.149 Posterior cruciate ligament biomechanics between lax fibers in extension and taut fibers in flexion. The PCL limits posterior tibial translation. The anterolateral (AL) bundle represents the primary restraint to the posterior tibial drawer from 30 to 120 degrees of flexion. The postero-medial (PM) bundle resists 50% of the load of the AL bundle during the same range of motion. At 120 degrees or greater in knee flexion, the PM becomes the dominant structure in the PCL. In knee extension, the PM bundle also has the capacity to carry larger loads than the AL bundle, although it still does not contribute significantly to resist posterior tibial translation.

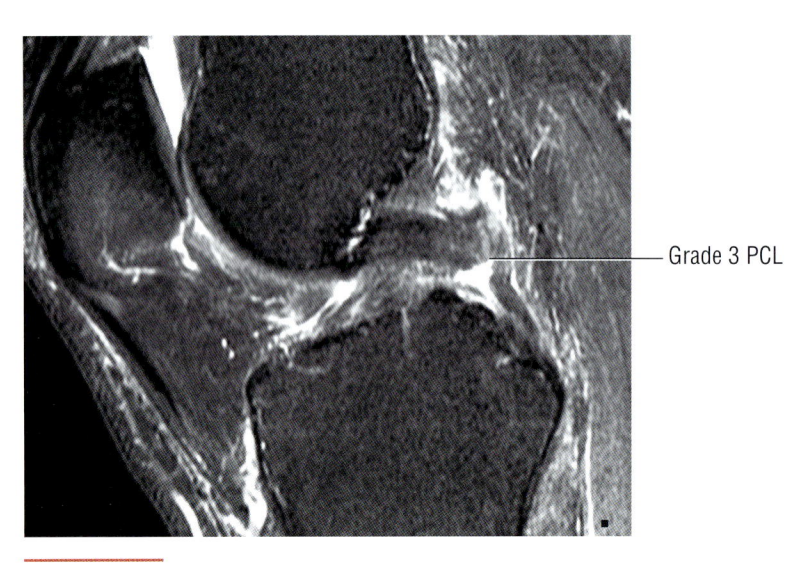

Grade 3 PCL

FIGURE 5.150 Grade 3 mid-substance tear of the PCL. The sagittal plane is the best plane to determine the location of the tear as femoral, mid-substance, or tibial. Sagittal FS PD FSE image.

Location and Mechanism of Injury of the PCL

- PCL is twice as strong as ACL, with larger cross-sectional area and higher tensile strength.

- Lower incidence of rupture of PCL[69,241,242]

- PCL injuries represent only 5% to 20% of all knee ligament injuries.[219]

- PCL tears most common in midportion (76%), followed by avulsions from the femur (36% to 55%) and tibia (22% to 42%)[202,291,488]

- Mechanism of injury
    - Rupture may be caused by excessive rotation, hyperextension, dislocation, or direct trauma while knee is flexed.[319,423]
    - Motor vehicle accidents (dashboard injuries) and injuries sustained in contact sports (such as football) are most common causes of damage to PCL.[82,319]
    - Isolated PCL injuries represent approximately 30% of cases.

- Associated injuries
    - Tears of ACL, meniscus, collateral ligaments, or posterolateral structures[75,204]
    - Lateral compartment pathology or patellar articular cartilage injury[159]
    - Posterolateral instability (posterolateral capsule and popliteus complex are secondary restraints to posterior tibial displacement)
    - Posteromedial instability less common (MCL makes less important contribution as secondary restraint to posterior tibial displacement)[69]
    - Acute hemarthrosis not as severe as with ACL injuries[356]
    - Frequent lack of soft tissue swelling may lead to delay in clinical diagnosis.
    - Relatively uncommon meniscal abnormalities (unlike ACL-deficient knee)[322]
    - Incidence of meniscal tears and articular cartilage injuries in medial compartment increases in chronic PCL injuries.[159]
    - PCL insufficiency may lead to articular cartilage degeneration in medial compartment when there is lateral shift of the normal center of the axis of rotation of the joint.

- Occult knee dislocation may be associated with disruption of both ACL and PCL or any multiligament injury.[82]

- Clinical diagnosis
    - Positive posterior drawer sign (posterior tibial displacement) seen in up to 60% of cases[69]
    - Posterior sag sign seen in complete tears of the PCL
    - Tibia sags into posterior subluxation relative to femur with patient supine and knee flexed at 90 degrees.[82]
    - Other clinical tests for PCL injury include the quadriceps active test, which results in anterior tibial translation during quadriceps contraction, and various versions of the reverse pivot-shift test.
    - In combined injuries with knee dislocation, it is important to conduct neurovascular evaluation.

Arthroscopic Evaluation

- Direct arthroscopic findings include mid-substance and interstitial tears, ligament stretching, and avulsion of bony insertions.

- Indirect arthroscopic findings include degenerative changes of patellofemoral joint and medial compartment.

- Sloppy ACL sign: relatively increased laxity of ACL secondary to posterior tibial drop-back

- Posterior tibial drop-back: phenomenon of gravity-assisted posterior tibial subluxation produced by absence of restraining function of the PCL[12]

- Limitations
    - Poor visualization of PCL in presence of intact ACL
    - Misinterpretation of normal ligament of Humphrey (meniscofemoral ligament) as an injury
    - Location of arthroscopic portals selected to visualize the PCL (the inferolateral patellar portal and occasionally the posteromedial arthroscopic portal should allow complete visualization of the entire PCL)[130]

Posterior Cruciate Ligament: Mechanism of Injury

Direct pretibial trauma

Forced hyperflexion

Hyperextension

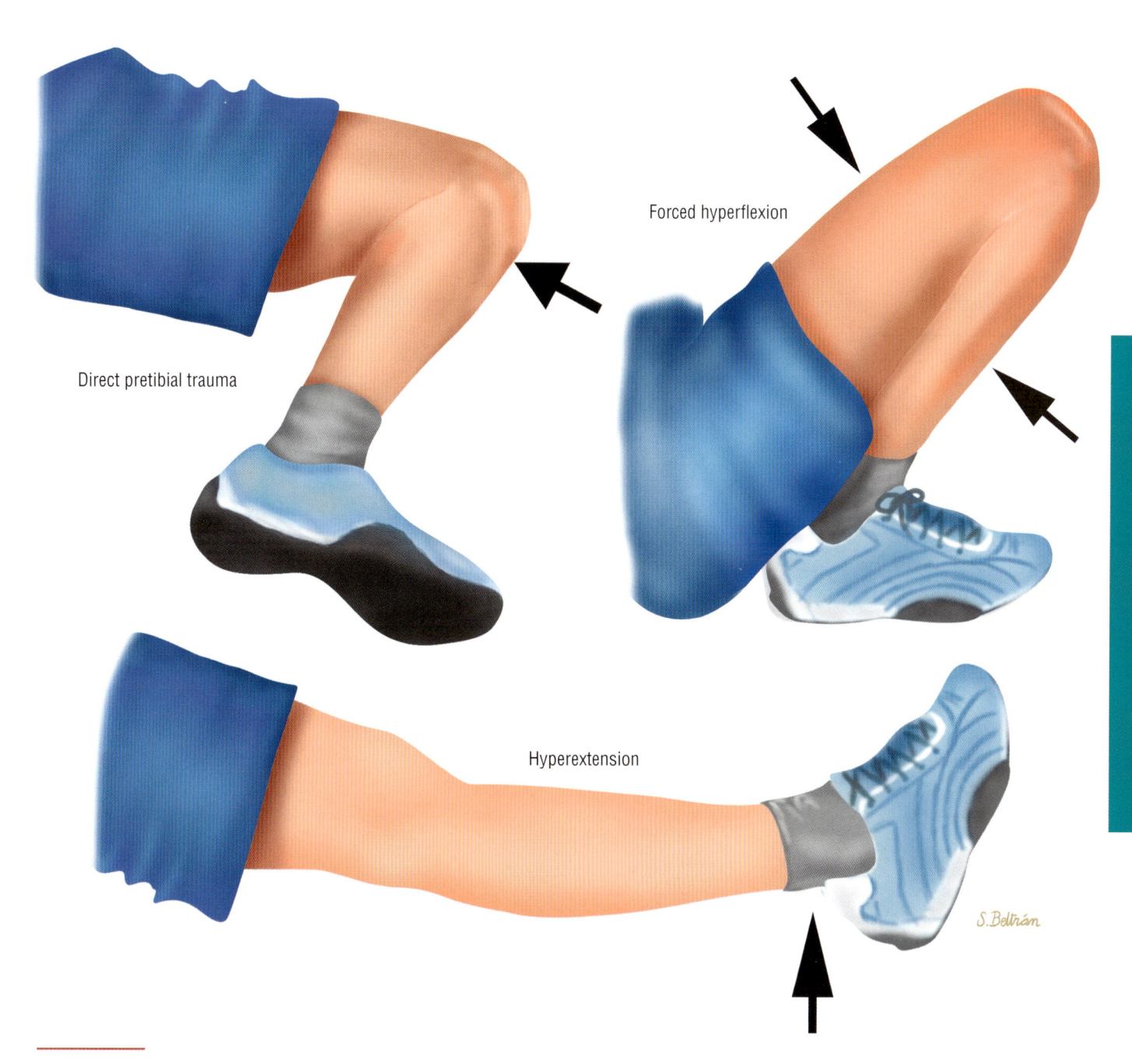

FIGURE 5.151 Mechanisms of posterior cruciate ligament injury. The most common mechanism of injury is an anterior blow to the proximal tibia. In sports-related trauma, hyperflexion is the most common mechanism of injury. The PCL is also injured in different knee dislocation mechanisms.[40]

PCL Hyperextension Injury

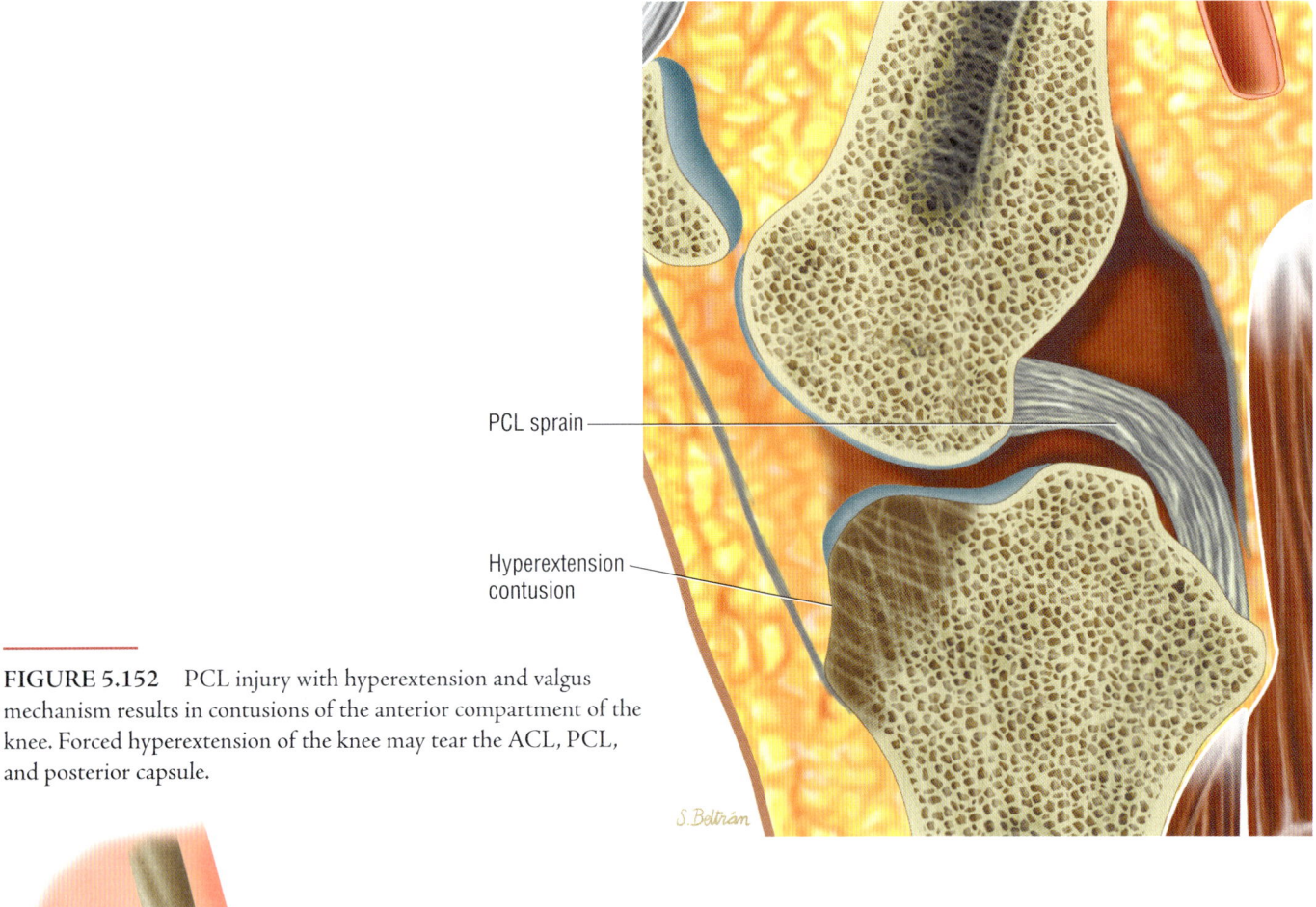

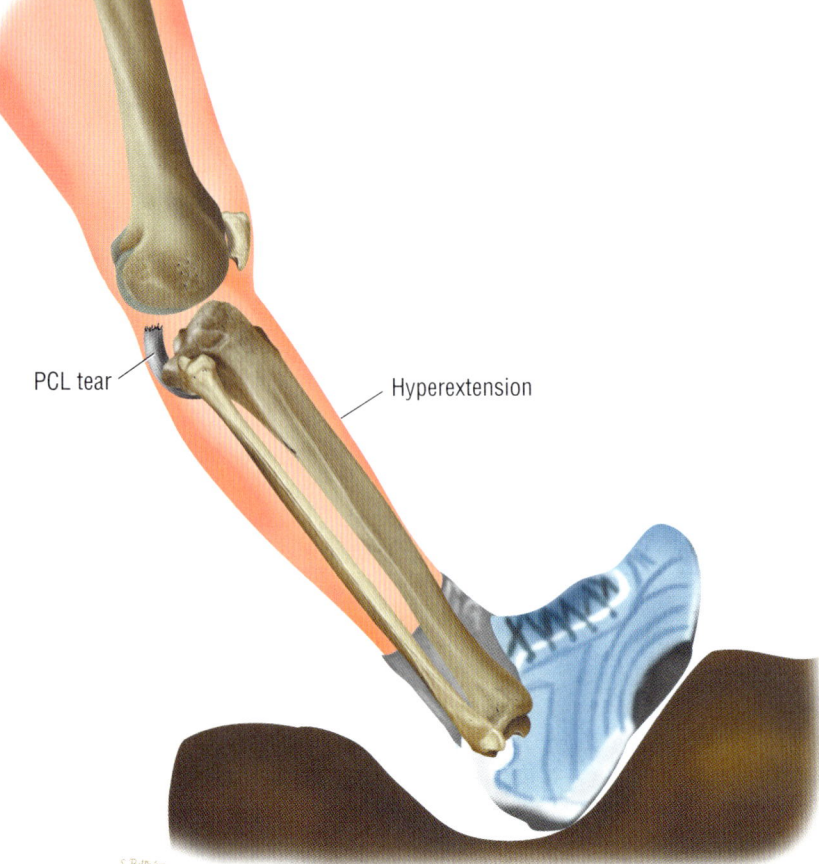

FIGURE 5.152 PCL injury with hyperextension and valgus mechanism results in contusions of the anterior compartment of the knee. Forced hyperextension of the knee may tear the ACL, PCL, and posterior capsule.

FIGURE 5.153 PCL rupture associated with hyperextension injury.

MR Imaging

- **Normal PCL**
    - Uniform low-signal-intensity band
    - Morphology and signal intensity routinely evaluated on axial, coronal, and sagittal images
    - In sagittal plane, PCL has arcuate shape with knee positioned in neutral or minimal flexion[393] and is visualized in its entire length on one or two consecutive images.
    - Becomes taut with knee flexion and more lax with hyperextension
    - In posterior coronal plane, PCL demonstrates a more vertical orientation as it is sectioned in the downward slope of its curved arc.
    - Mid- and anterior-coronal images display more circular cross-section of the ligament.
    - Axial images can be used to follow the ligament from posterior tibia to broad anterior medial femoral condyle attachment.
    - Magic-angle effect could produce inhomogeneity of signal intensity in an arthroscopically normal PCL, based on orientation of the PCL to the magnetic field.

- **Meniscofemoral ligaments**
    - Low-signal-intensity structures identified in up to 60% of MR examinations
    - More commonly seen on sagittal images (midportion of PCL), but often identified on coronal and axial images
    - Visualization may improve in presence of edema and hemorrhage associated with torn PCL.

- **Protocols**
    - Same protocols for evaluation of PCL and ACL injuries; combination of T1- and FS T2-weighted FSE images in all three planes (axial, coronal, and sagittal)
    - Excellent MR depiction of both normal PCL morphology and tears, confirmed by arthroscopy and arthrotomy[172]
    - Findings of increased signal intensity with normal PCL morphology on T1- or PD-weighted images require addition of conventional T2-, T2*-, or FS T2-weighted FSE images to identify the sites of pathology.

- Hemorrhage and edema (acute injuries) are bright on T2- (including FSE) and T2*-weighted images, and cause less distortion or mass effect than seen with ACL tears.

- Coronal images can be used to confirm regions of signal abnormality on sagittal images.

- Linear intrasubstance splits and regions of hyperintensity are displayed in cross-section.

- PCL injuries

    - Any increase in PCL signal intensity on T1-, PD-, T2-, T2*-, or FS PD-weighted FSE images is abnormal.

    - In a retrospective review by Sonin et al.,[451] 38% of patients with PCL injuries had complete tears, 55% had partial tears, and 63% had mid-substance injuries.

    - 20% of PCL injuries were proximal and 3% were distal.

    - Isolated PCL injuries were found in 24% of patients.

    - Tibial insertion avulsion injuries were found in 7% of patients.

- Interstitial tears

    - Entire ligament or a long segment may be difficult to identify because of diffuse widening and increased signal intensity.

    - Long segment of interstitial tear may produce division into separate fiber bundles.

- Partial tears

    - Increased signal intensity with discernible fibers identified

    - Chronic partial tear may be difficult to identify on MR, even in presence of clinically positive posterior sag sign.[82]

    - Easier to assess ligament morphology on FS PD-weighted FSE images than on GRE (greater degree of hyperintensity in regions of edema and hemorrhage)

- Complete tears

    - Amorphous high signal intensity without definable ligamentous fibers[451]

    - Alternatively, focal discontinuity or a gap may be seen at the site of tear.

- **Chronic tears**
    - Result in abnormal ligamentous morphology with intermediate signal intensity on T1- and T2-weighted images
    - May see apparent continuity across an area of ligamentous scarring
    - May also be indicated by abnormal laxity of fibers or failure of PCL to become taut during flexion
- **Associated osseous injuries**
    - Bone contusions in anterolateral tibia and posterior lateral femoral condyle consistent with forced posterior displacement of tibia in flexed knee[450]
    - Hyperextension injuries may demonstrate contusions of anterotibial articular surface and the anterior aspect of the femoral condyle and may have associated ACL rupture.
    - Avulsion tear off tibial plateau may be associated with high-signal-intensity ligamentous hemorrhage and bone fragment containing marrow.
    - Subchondral marrow edema and hemorrhage between avulsed fragment and tibia frequently seen on FS PD-weighted FSE and STIR images.
    - Reverse Segond fracture: avulsion fracture fragment on medial aspect of medial tibial plateau associated with deep portion of MCL[128]
    - Seen with PCL disruption and tears of peripheral medial meniscus
    - Anteromedial capsular expansion of the semimembranosus tendon may also play a role in this injury, similar to the role of the posterior fibers of the iliotibial tract in the lateral Segond fracture.
    - Arcuate sign: avulsion fracture of the posterosuperior apex of the fibular styloid process
    - High predictive value for associated PCL tears
    - Usually mid-substance PCL injury or distal tibial avulsions
    - Posterolateral corner injuries and associated ACL pathology should also be evaluated.

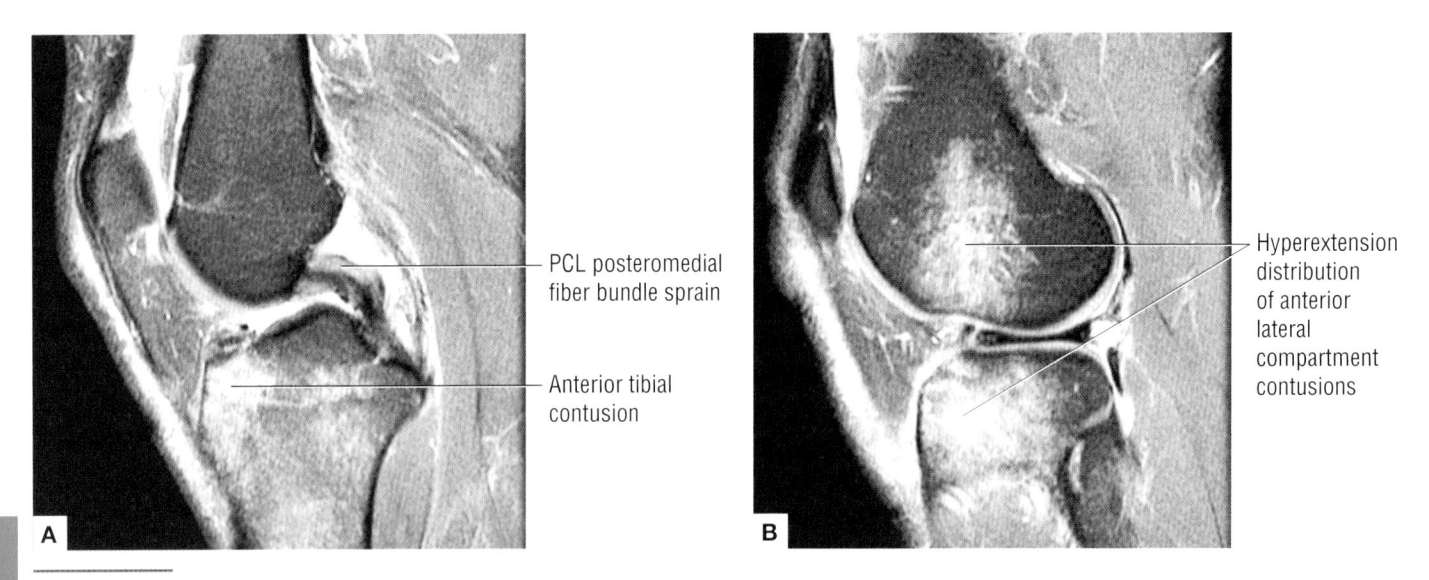

FIGURE 5.154 (**A**) Sagittal FS PD FSE image showing PCL sprain with anterior tibial contusion and posteromedial fiber bundle involvement. (**B**) Lateral sagittal FS PD FSE image with anterior lateral compartment contusions.

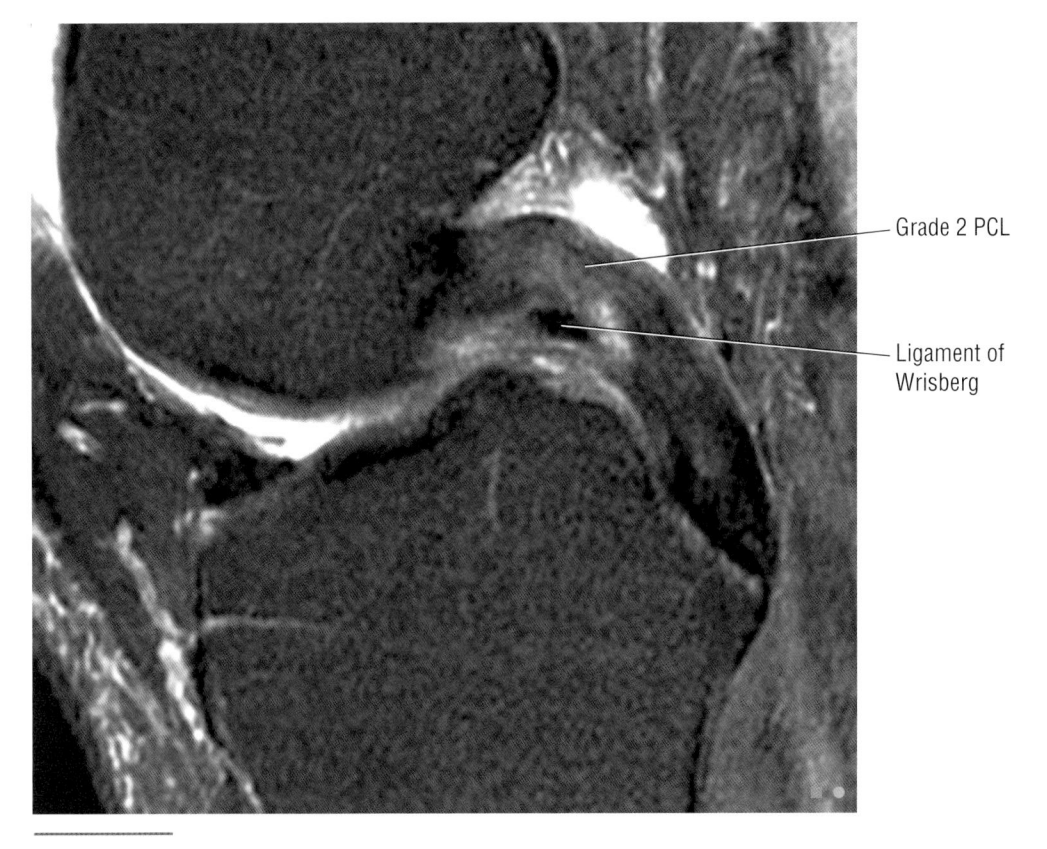

FIGURE 5.155 A partial PCL rupture/tear implies continuity of remaining fibers. The retention of the remaining fibers resists a posterior load applied to the knee. MR is associated with cross-section diameter reduction or loss of parallel fiber architecture in grade 2 injuries. Sagittal FS PD FSE image.

Cruciate Ligaments

PCL Flexion Injury

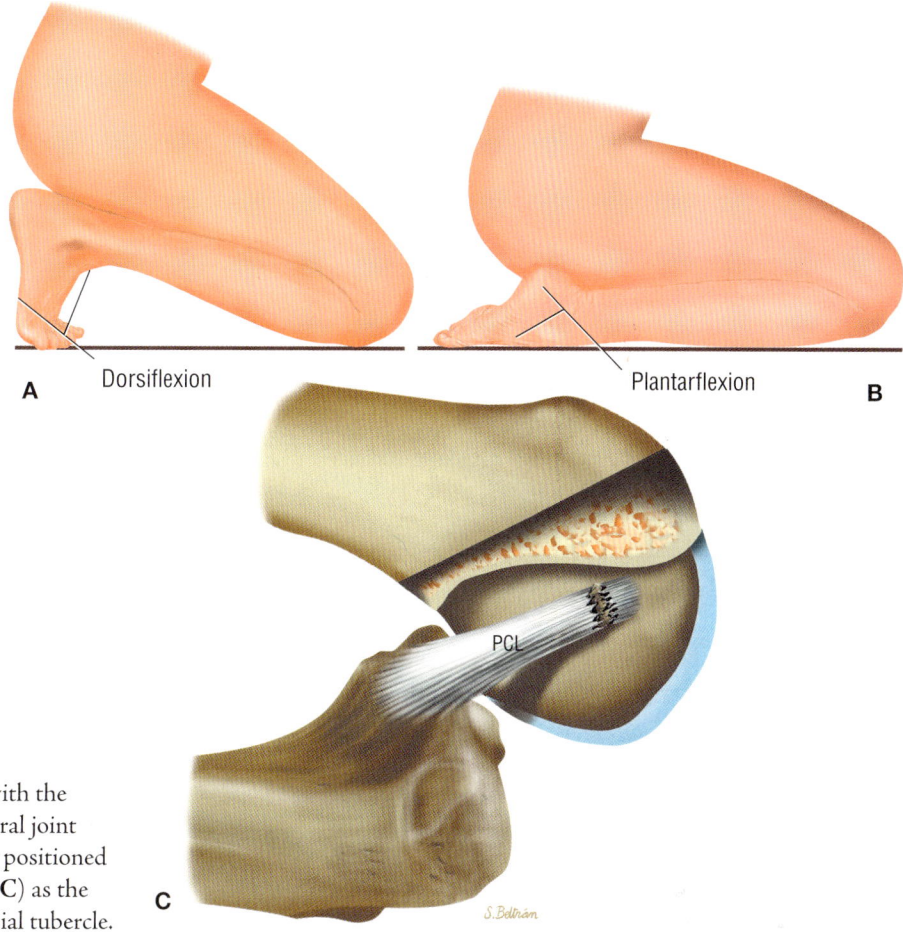

FIGURE 5.156 A fall onto a flexed knee with the foot in dorsiflexion (**A**) results in patellofemoral joint injury. In contrast, a fall landing with the foot positioned in plantarflexion (**B**) results in a PCL injury (**C**) as the posterior force vector is transmitted to the tibial tubercle.

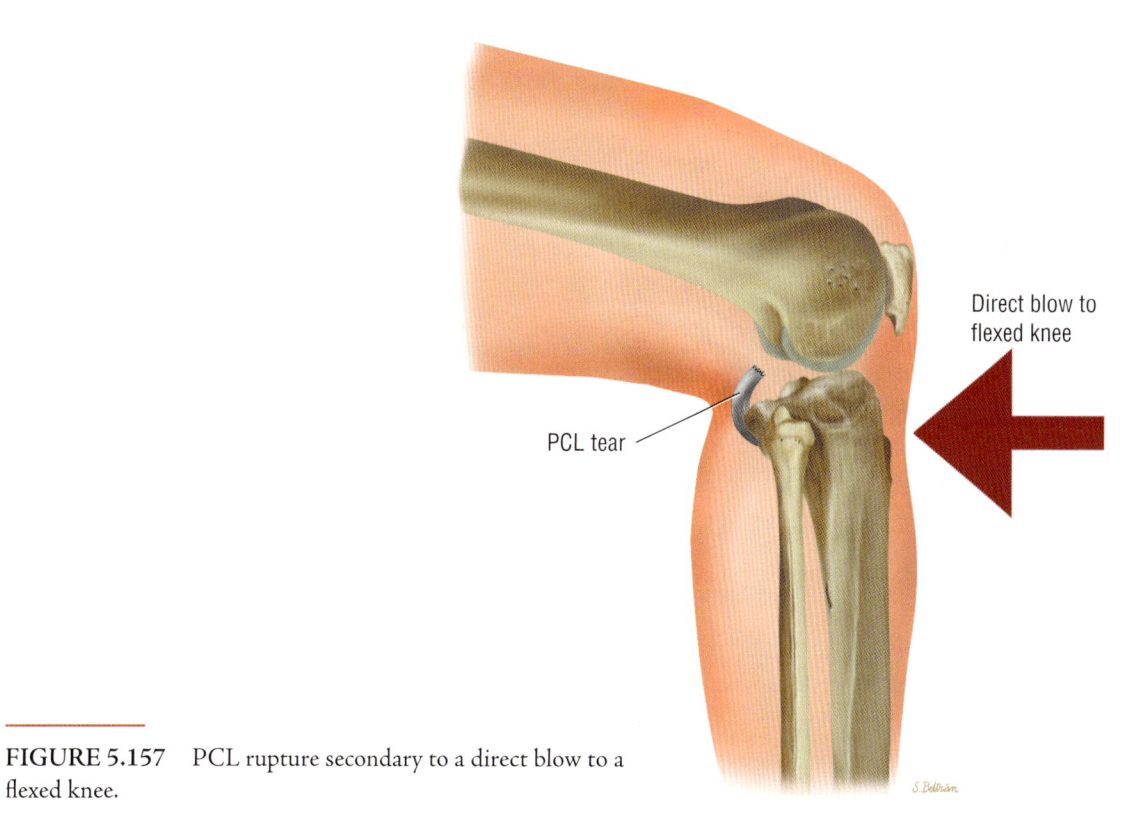

FIGURE 5.157 PCL rupture secondary to a direct blow to a flexed knee.

- Other associated injuries
    - Associated findings include involvement of MCL more often than LCL and of medial meniscus more commonly than lateral meniscus.[451]
    - Abnormally high arc or buckling of the PCL may indicate ACL tear with secondary forward tibial displacement.
    - Relatively small joint effusions in most patients[451]
    - Avulsion of fibular head or Gerdy's tubercle in severe posterolateral disruptions
    - Osteoarthritis of the medial, lateral, and patellofemoral compartments in chronic injuries
    - Sensitivity and specificity of MR in identifying complete PCL tears of the PCL have been reported to be 100%.[322]

Treatment

- Nonoperative
    - Acute isolated PCL injuries (except when posterior tibial drop-back is greater than 10 to 15mm)

- Surgical treatment
    - PCL tears with tibial plateau avulsions require direct repair.
    - Mid-substance and femoral avulsions require augmentation and reconstruction with free or vascularized grafts from patellar tendon or semitendinosus and gracilis tendons or allografts.[69,75]
    - Symptomatic chronic PCL injuries, acute bony avulsions, and acute combined injuries[322]
    - PCL tears associated with ACL tears or extensive capsular disruptions

- Complications
    - Serious complication associated with PCL reconstruction is neurovascular injury during tibial tunnel preparation.
    - Delayed complications related to PCL reconstruction include loss of motion, avascular necrosis involving medial femoral condyle, and recurrent laxity.[322]
    - PCL grafts show revascularization phenomenon similar to ACL grafts, accounting for increased intraligamentous signal on MR during first postoperative year.[439]

Cruciate Ligaments

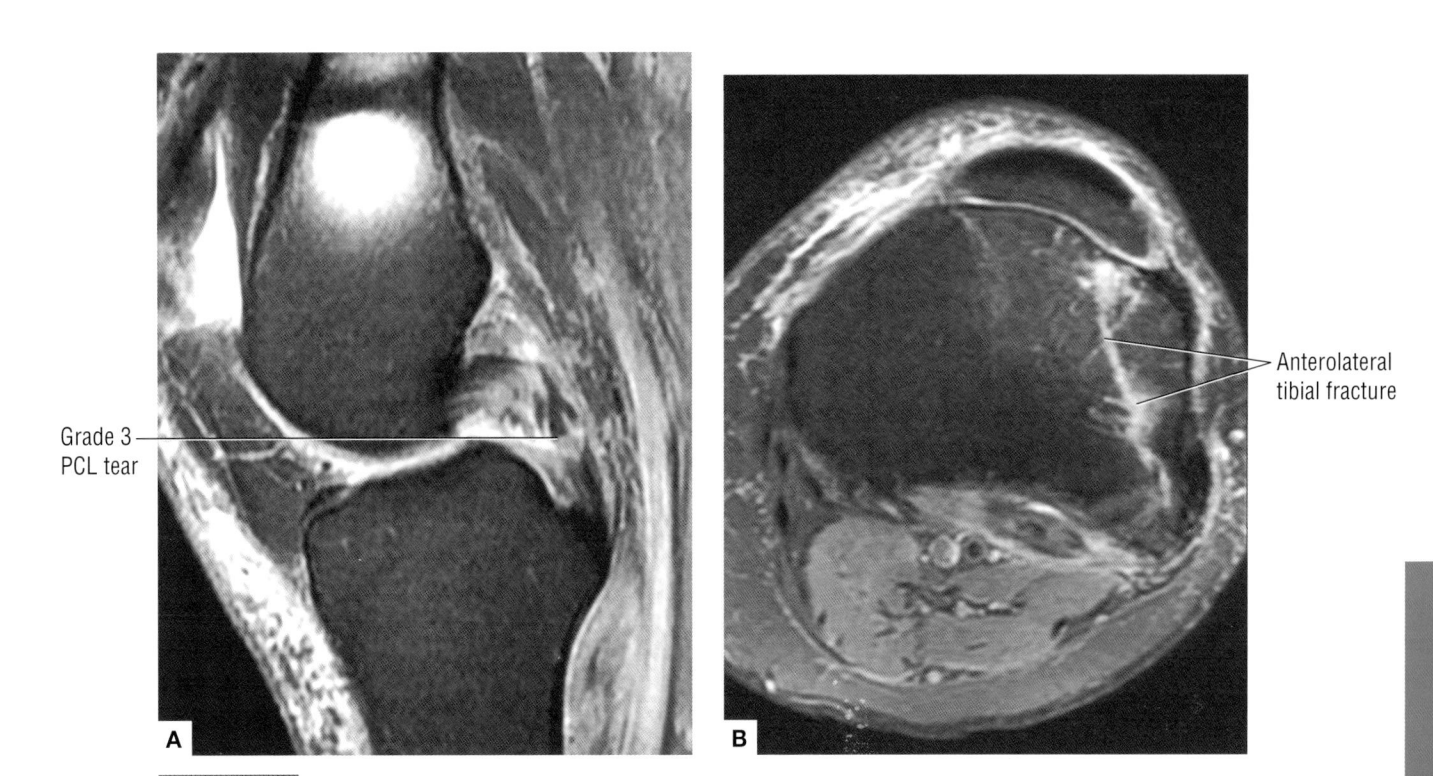

FIGURE 5.158 (**A**) Dashboard injury caused by a posteriorly directed force applied to the proximal tibia with the knee in 90 degrees of flexion. This sagittal FS PD FSE image shows complete loss of PCL continuity secondary to a complex interstitial PCL tear. (**B**) Axial FS PD FSE image showing an anterolateral fracture resulting from direct trauma by the dashboard during impact.

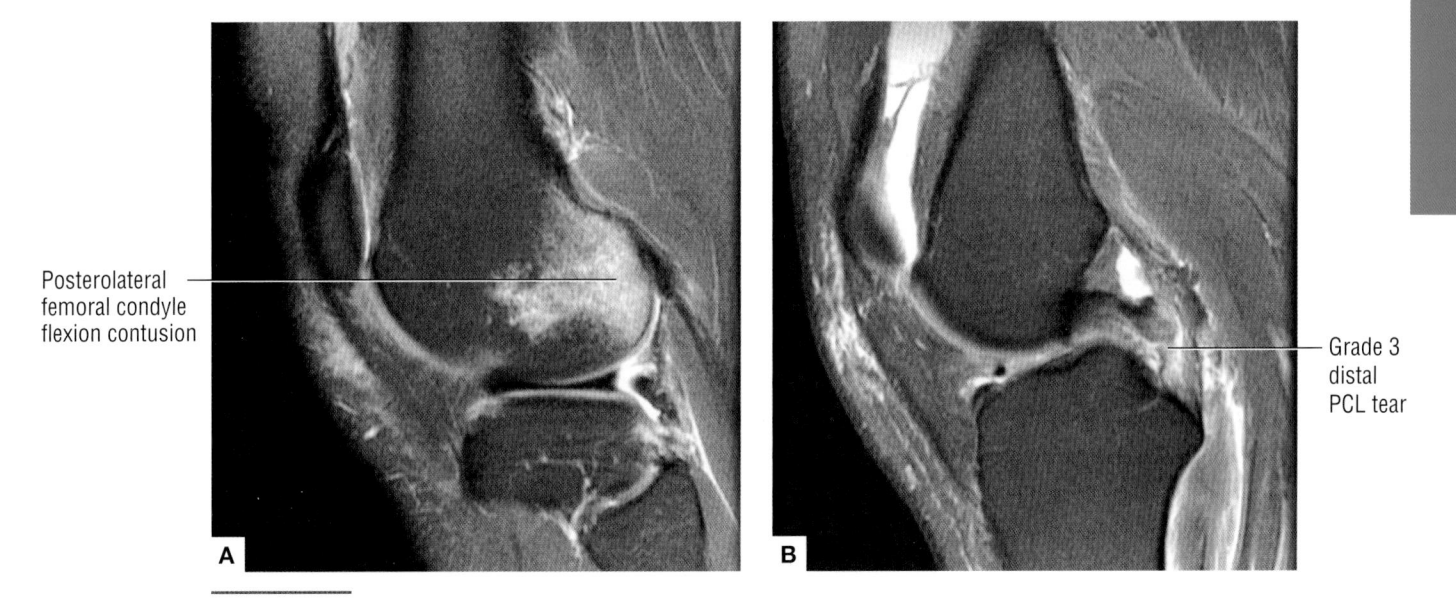

FIGURE 5.159 At least one of the meniscofemoral ligaments is intact in either acute or chronic PCL injuries. Grade 3 PCL distal tear is shown with posteriorly located lateral femoral condyle flexion-related contusion. PCL reconstruction is considered for cases of grade 3 laxity with combined ligament injuries (e.g., posterolateral corner injuries) or meniscal, chondral, or osseous avulsions. (**A, B**) Sagittal FS PD FSE images.

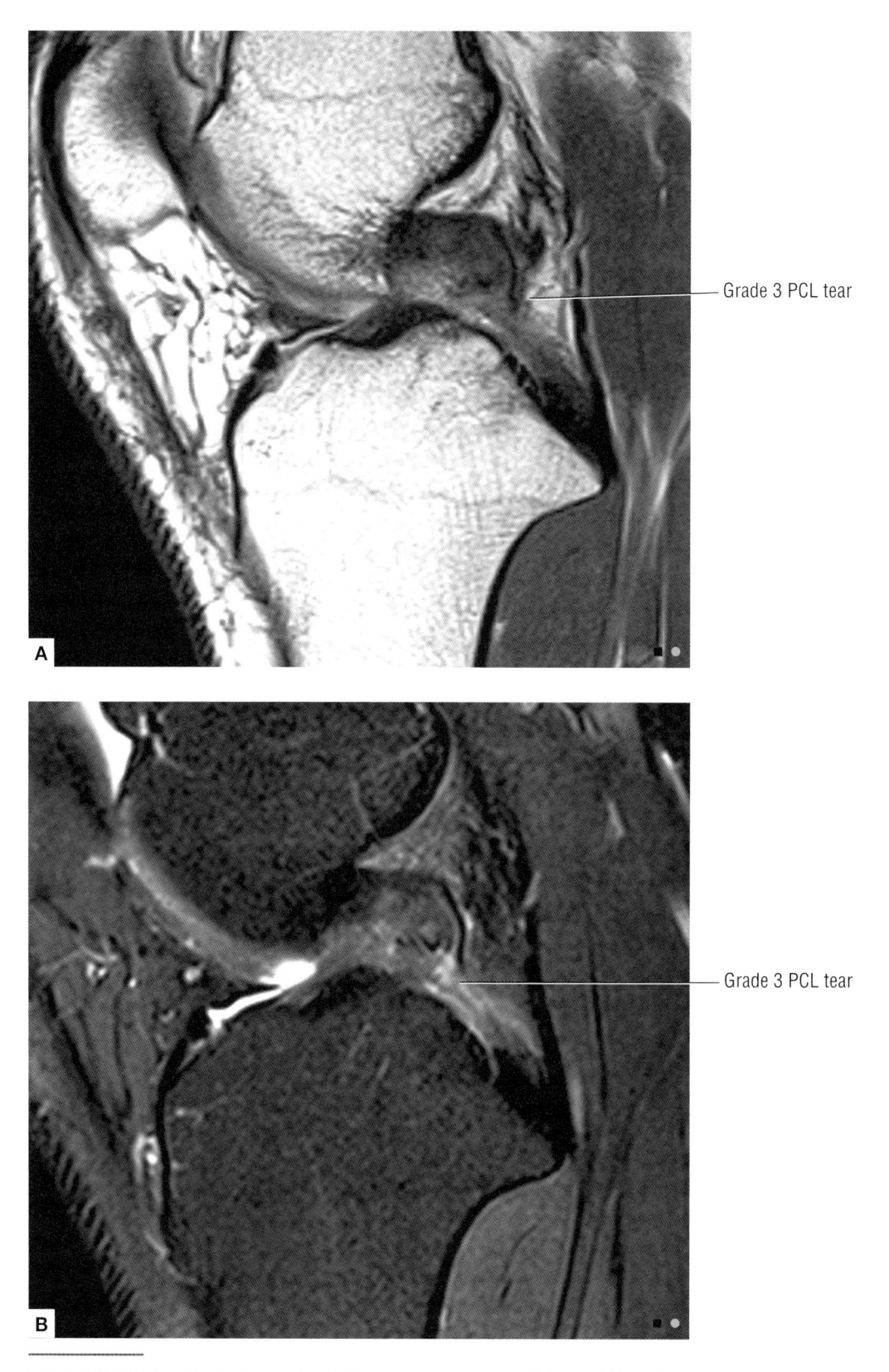

FIGURE 5.160 Grade 3 chronic PCL tear at the junction of the middle and distal thirds. Sagittal PD (**A**) and FS PD (**B**) images.

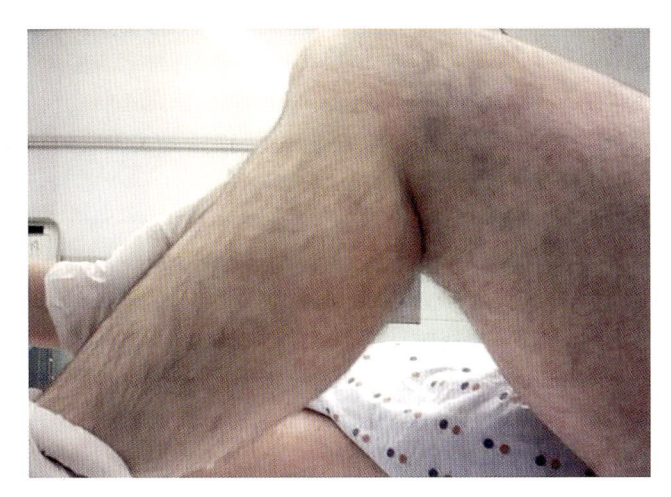

FIGURE 5.161 The posterior drawer exam (most sensitive to PCL injury) is performed with the patient supine, the knee flexed to 90 degrees, and the foot supported on the table. The examiner's thumbs are placed on top of the medial and lateral tibial plateaus, and a posterior force is applied to the proximal tibia. Posterior tibial translation compared to contralateral side results in a positive test. Grade 1, 0 to 5mm; grade 2, 5 to 10mm; grade 3, >10mm. (Reprinted from Fu FH. *Master Techniques in Orthopaedic Surgery: Sports Medicine.* Philadelphia, PA: Lippincott Williams & Wilkins; 2010, with permission.)

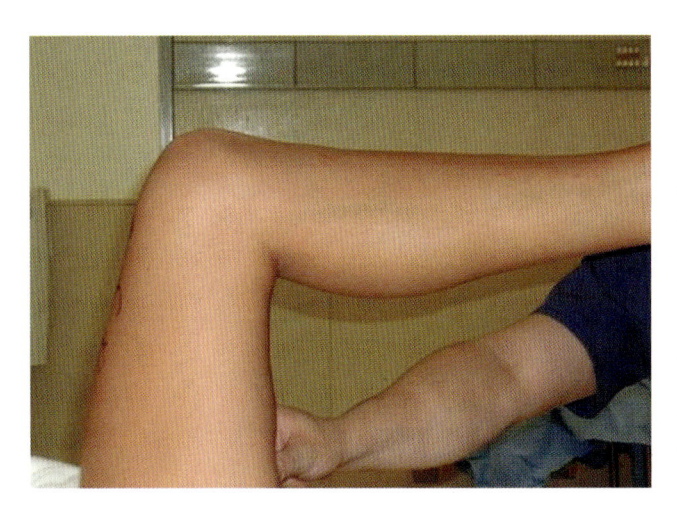

FIGURE 5.162 Godfrey test (posterior sag) is performed with the patient supine, the hip and knee flexed to 90 degrees, and the foot supported by the examiner. Abnormal posterior sag of the tibia relative to the femur results in positive test. (Reprinted from Fu FH. *Master Techniques in Orthopaedic Surgery: Sports Medicine.* Philadelphia, PA: Lippincott Williams & Wilkins; 2010, with permission.)

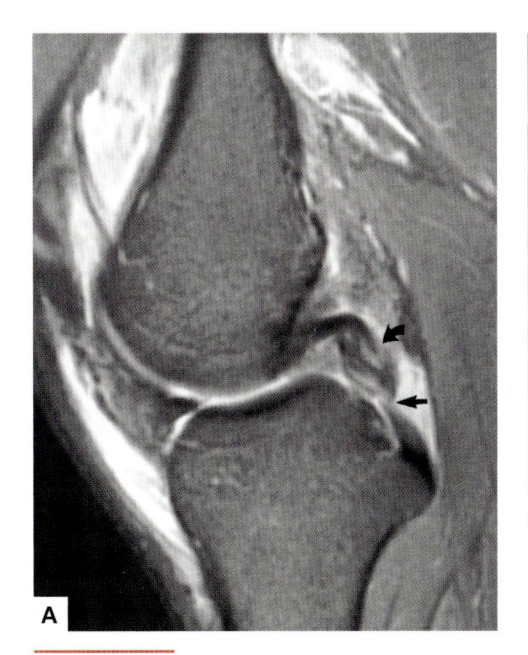

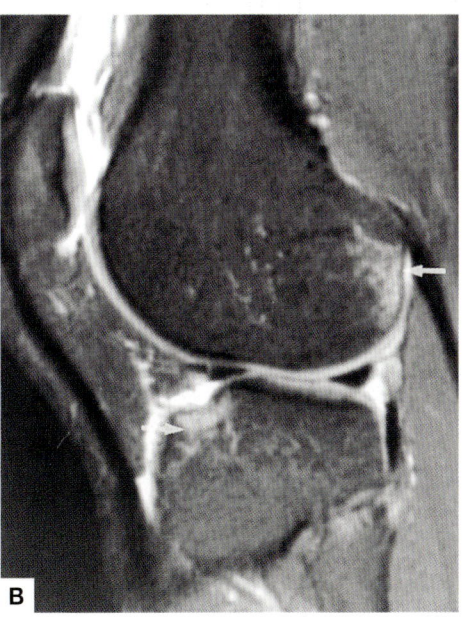

FIGURE 5.163 (**A**) FS PD-weighted FSE sagittal image of a PCL tear with focal discontinuity (*straight arrow*). Note the enlarged end of the torn proximal segment (*curved arrow*), which has associated interstitial tearing. The identification of a discrete gap or ligament discontinuity is a less common presentation of a ruptured PCL. (**B**) Associated bone contusions (*arrows*) involve the anterior lateral tibia and posterior lateral femoral condyle.

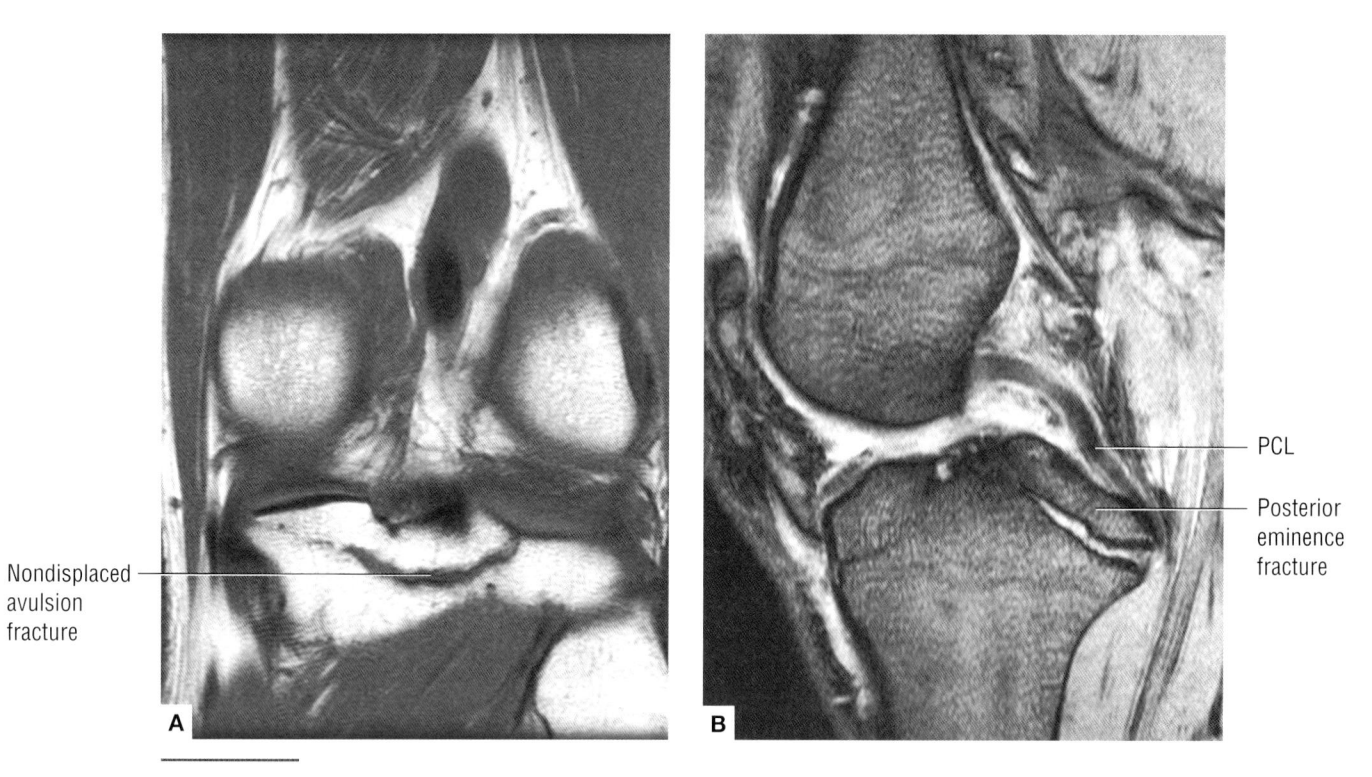

FIGURE 5.164 Isolated and nondisplaced avulsion fractures involving the PCL can be treated with immobilization. (**A**) Coronal T1-weighted FSE image. (**B**) Sagittal T2* GRE image.

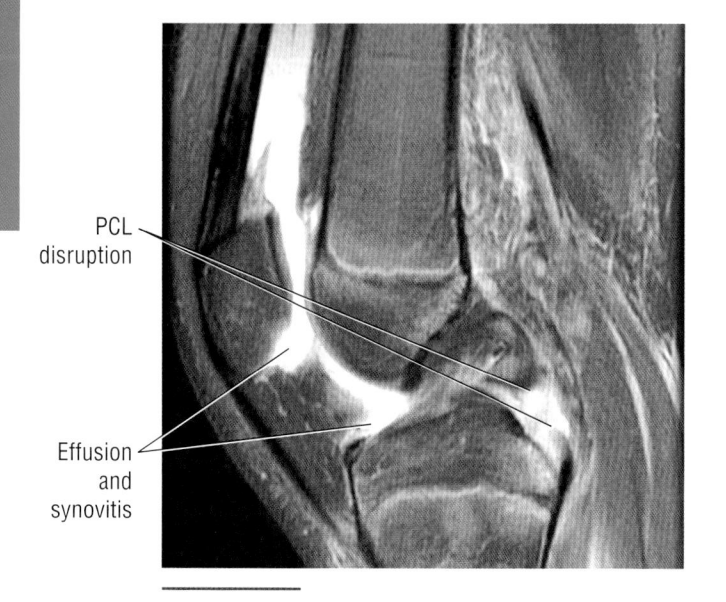

FIGURE 5.165 In the dashboard mechanism of injury, the posterior capsule is lax and the anterolateral bundle of the PCL is taut in 90 degrees of knee flexion. This produces either an isolated PCL rupture or an avulsion fracture of the tibial attachment site, as is seen in this case. Displaced avulsion fractures of the PCL require operative management (sagittal FS PD FSE image).

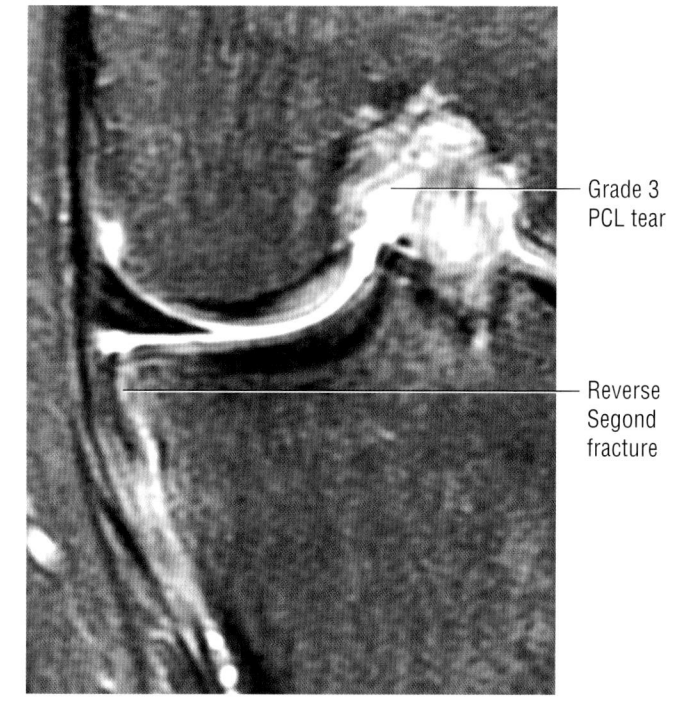

FIGURE 5.166 Reverse Segond fracture associated with grade 3 proximal PCL tear. The reverse Segond fracture of the medial tibial plateau is associated with the deep capsular portion of the MCL and occurs adjacent to the anteromedial capsular expansion of the semimembranosus tendon (coronal FS PD FSE image).

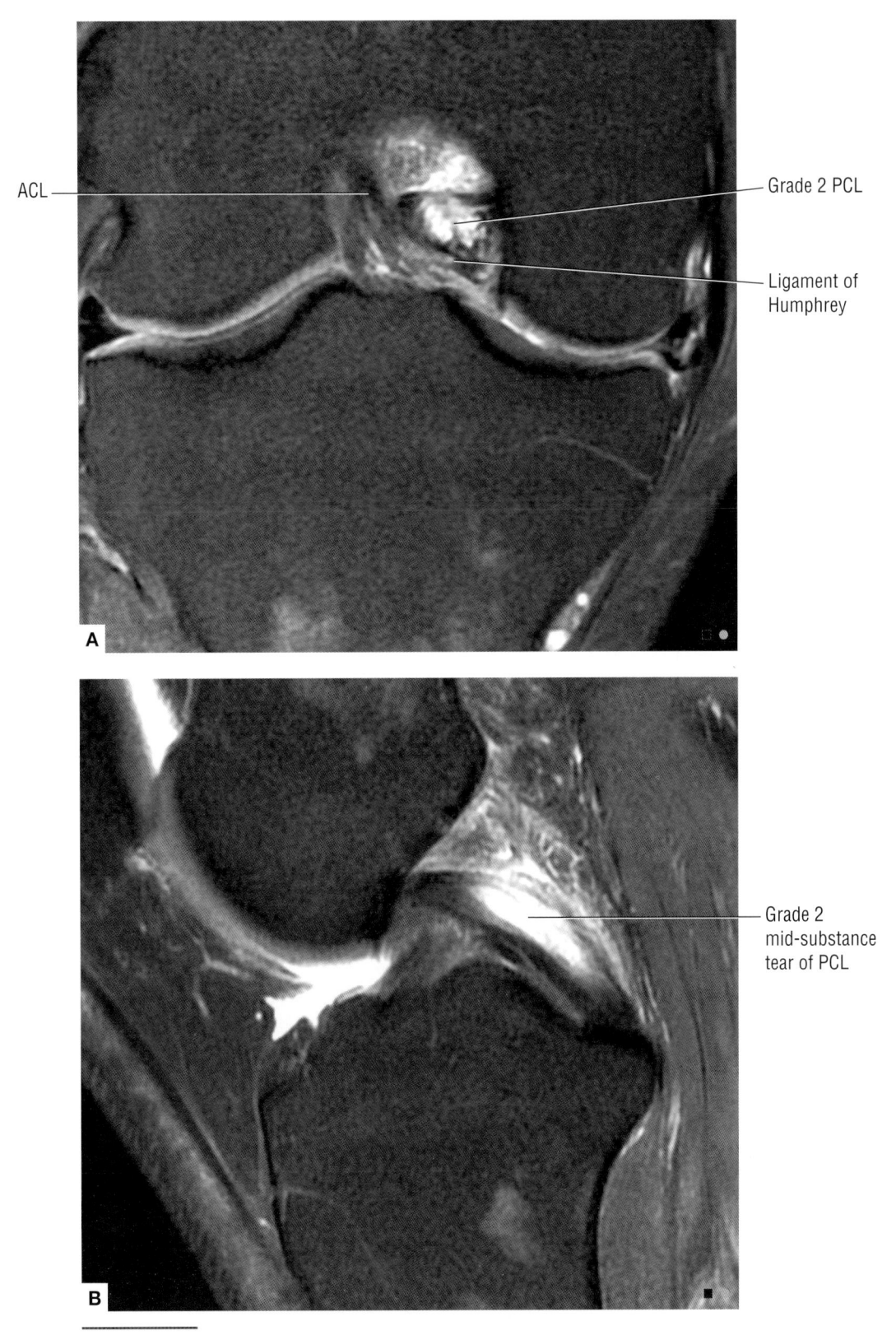

FIGURE 5.167 Acute mid-substance grade 2 injury involving posteromedial bundle fibers. Coronal (**A**) and sagittal (**B**) FS FSE images.

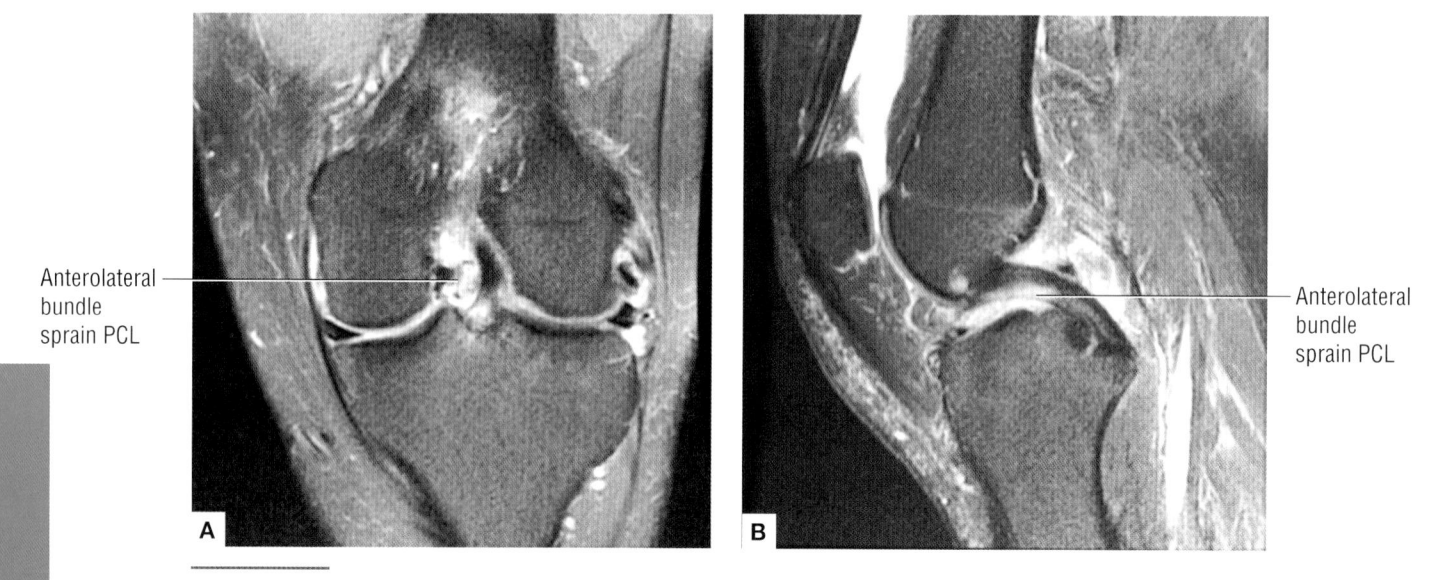

FIGURE 5.168 As the PCL tightens with flexion, forced hyperflexion produces excessive strain on the anterolateral bundle of the PCL. This type of sprain may lead to interstitial failure of the PCL. (**A**) Coronal FS PD FSE image. (**B**) Sagittal FS PD FSE image.

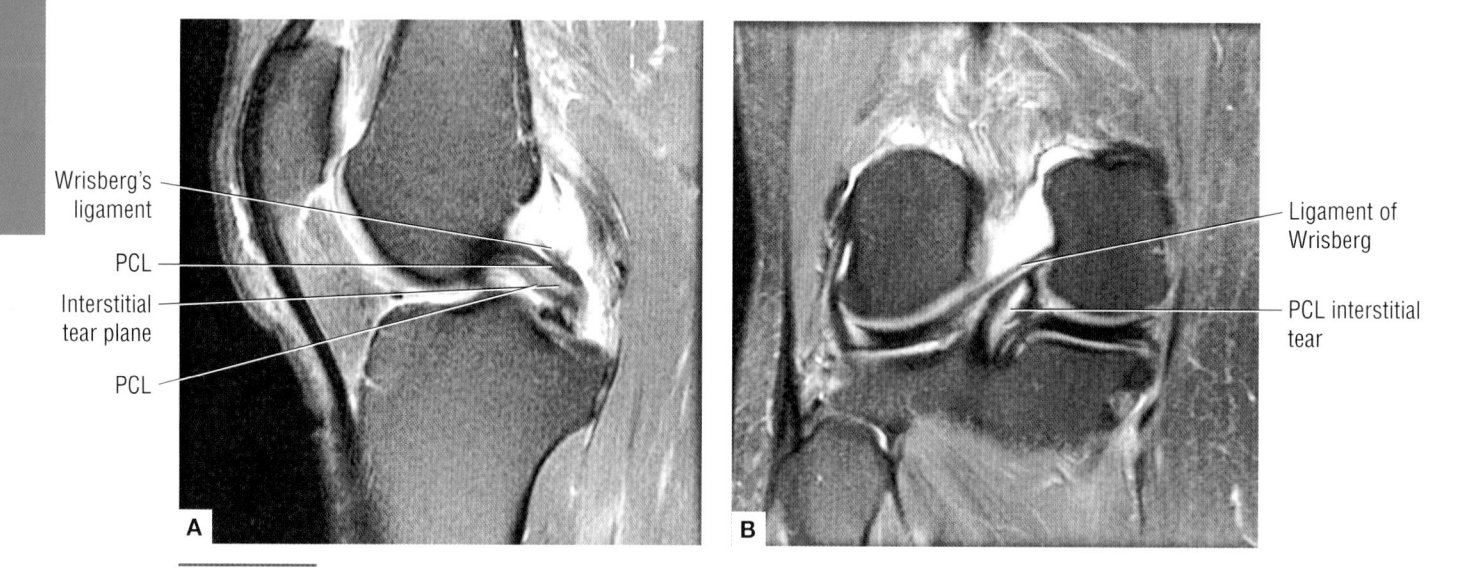

FIGURE 5.169 Interstitial PCL tear producing two segments of torn ligament separate from and anterior to the ligament of Wrisberg as seen on sagittal (**A**) and coronal (**B**) FS PD FSE images.

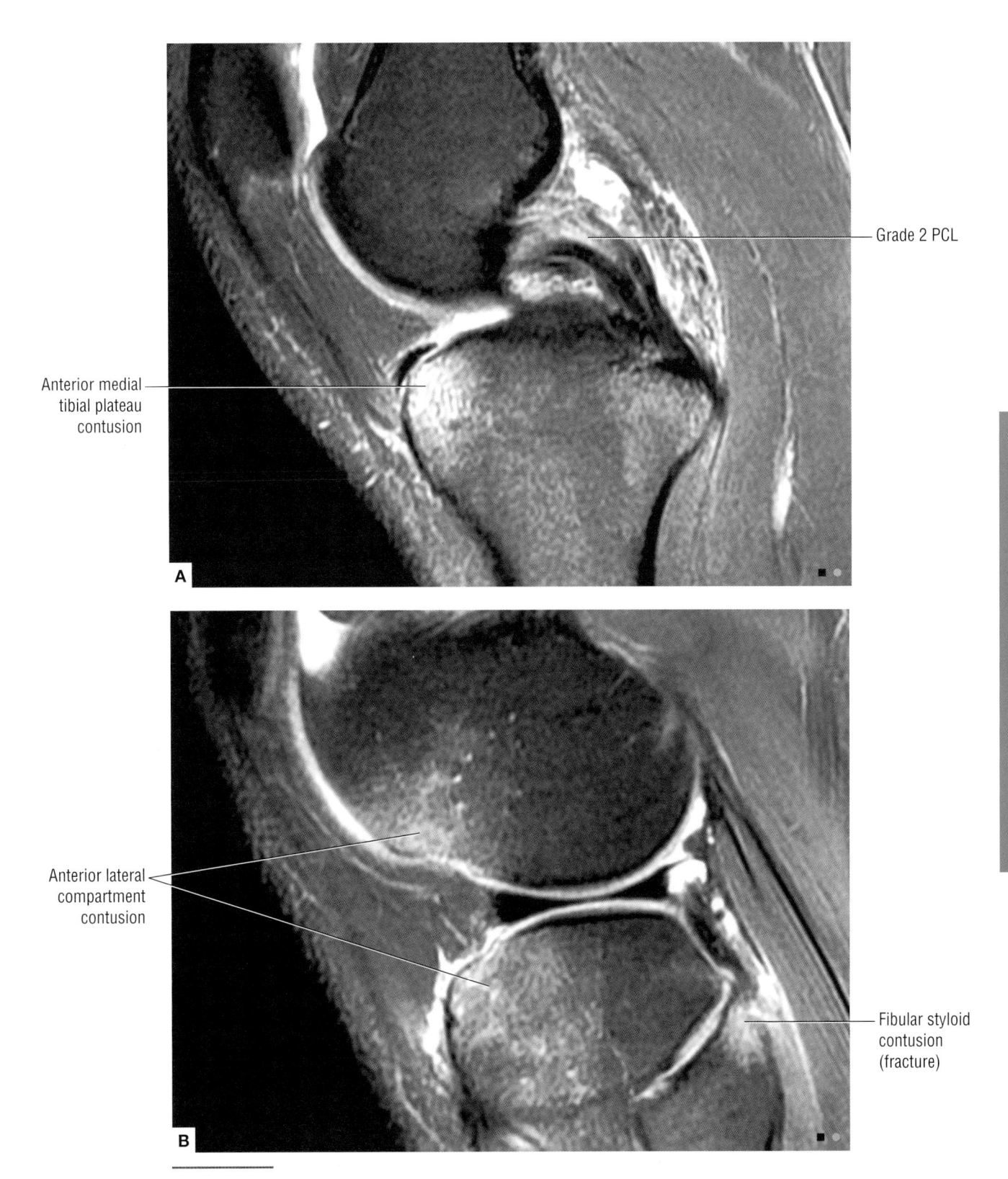

FIGURE 5.170 Grade 2 PCL injury with associated posterolateral injury with a nondisplaced fibular styloid fracture at the attachment of the popliteofibular ligament. Sagittal (**A–C**) and coronal (**D**) FS PD FSE images. (*Continued*)

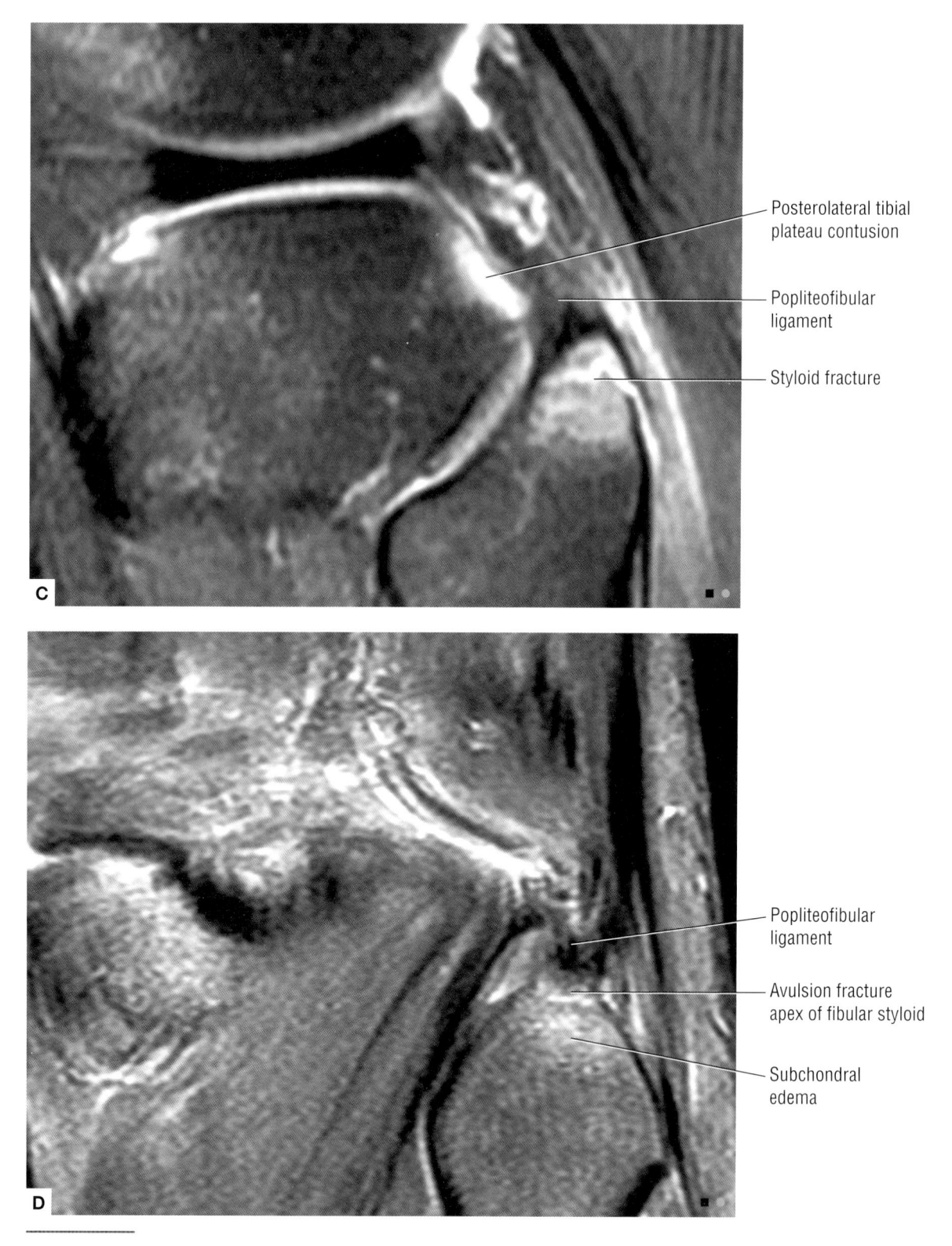

FIGURE 5.170 *(Continued)* Grade 2 PCL injury with associated posterolateral injury with a nondisplaced fibular styloid fracture at the attachment of the popliteofibular ligament. Sagittal (**A–C**) and coronal (**D**) FS PD FSE images.

Cruciate Ligaments

Grade 3 PCL

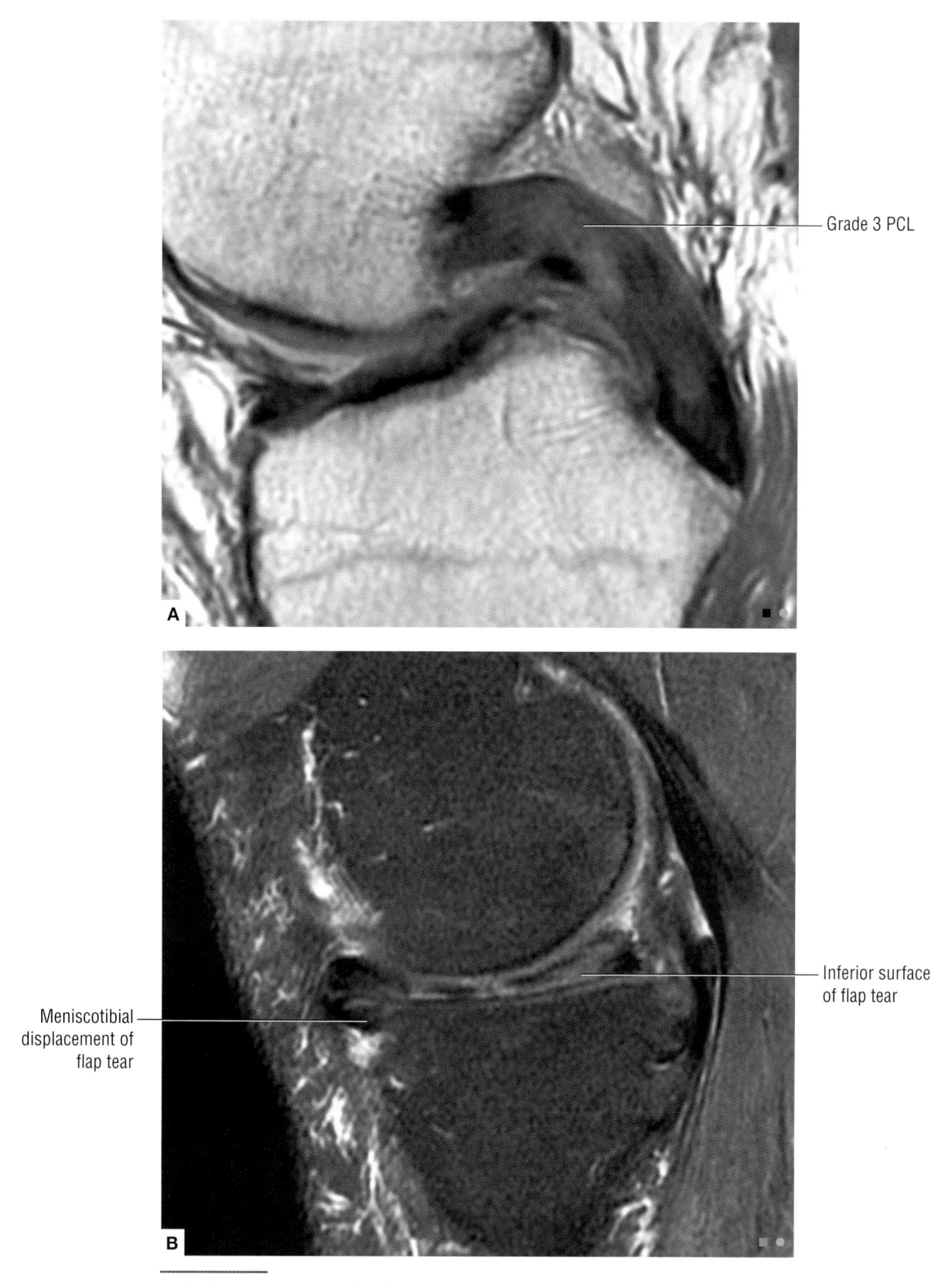

Meniscotibial displacement of flap tear

Inferior surface of flap tear

FIGURE 5.171 Complex flap tear associated with a grade 3 PCL. Sagittal PD (**A**) and FS PD (**B**) images.

Displaced segment of meniscus

Free edge of superior surface

Free edge of foreshortened inferior meniscal surface

A

Normal medial meniscus

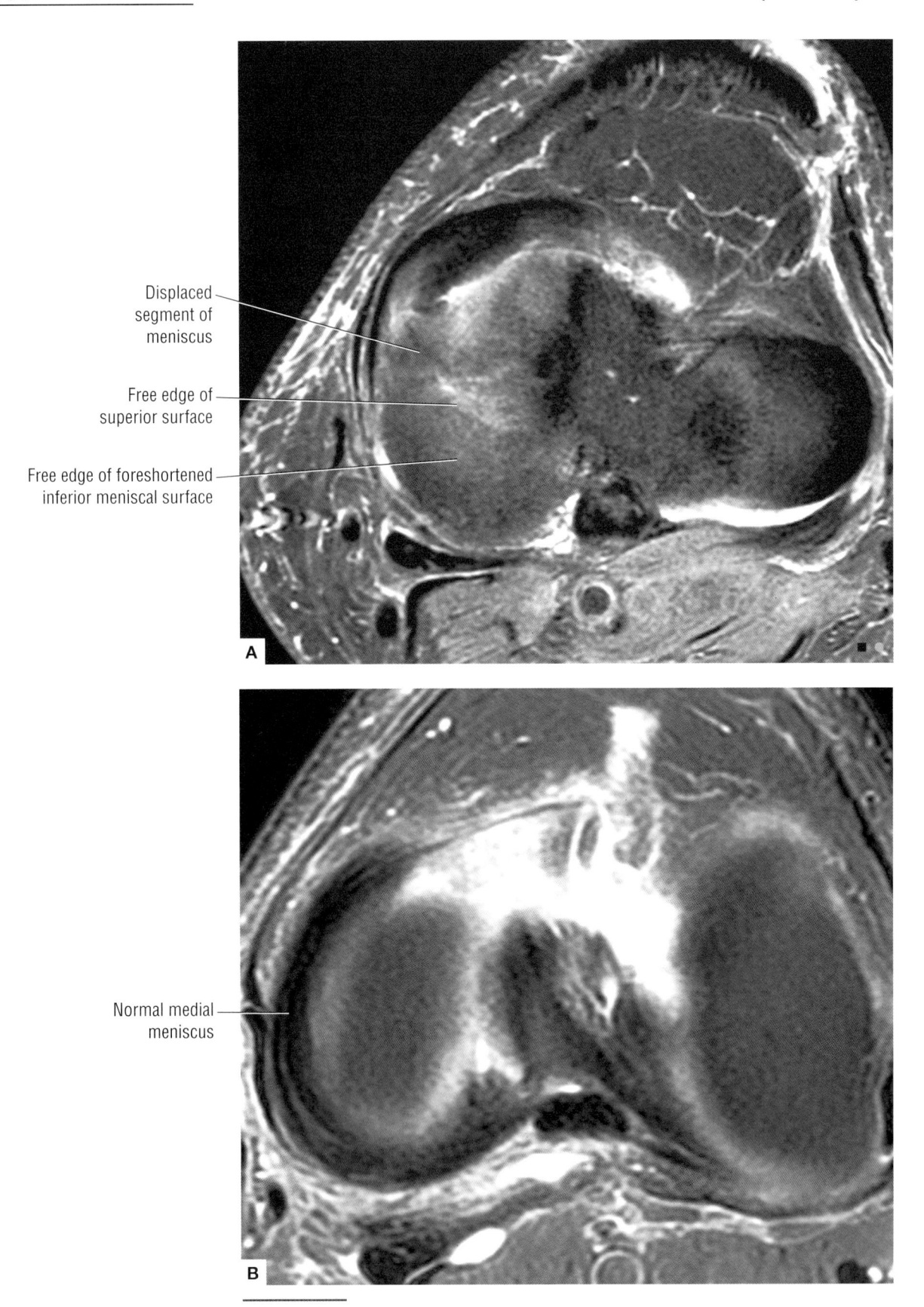

B

FIGURE 5.172 Trauma-related (compared to sports athletes) PCL injuries involve high energy as the tibia is forced posteriorly. Associated injuries include the postero-lateral corner, ACL (hyperextension mechanism), medial meniscus, medial collateral ligament, and chondral impaction. Displaced flap tear of the medial meniscus is associated with trauma from a grade 3 PCL tear (**A**). Nondisplaced medial meniscus flap tear shown for comparison (**B**). Axial FS PD FSE images (**A, B**).

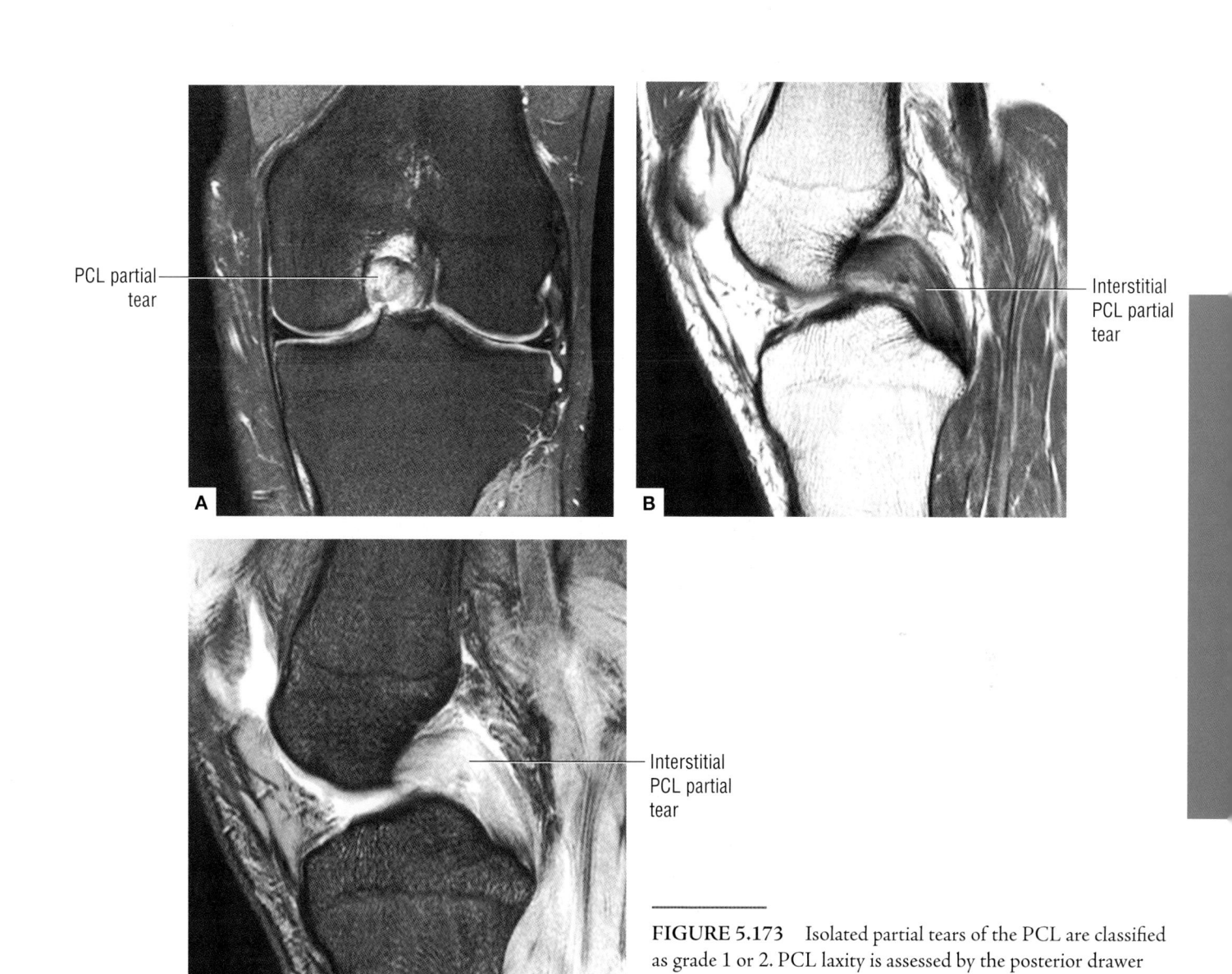

FIGURE 5.173 Isolated partial tears of the PCL are classified as grade 1 or 2. PCL laxity is assessed by the posterior drawer test (step-off between the medial tibial plateau and the medial femoral condyle). **(A)** Coronal FS PD FSE. **(B)** Sagittal PD FSE. **(C)** Sagittal T2* GRE.

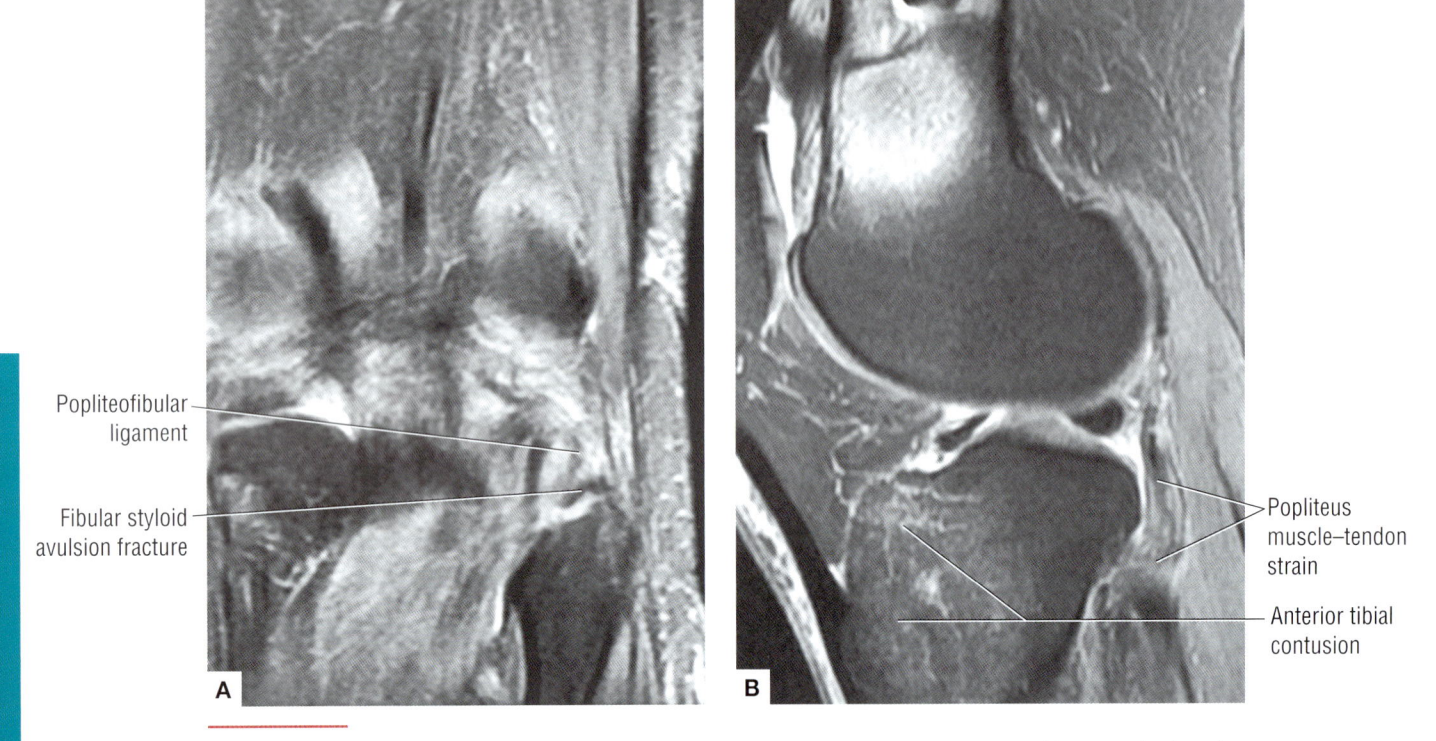

FIGURE 5.174 (**A**) PCL-associated pattern of posterolateral complex injury with fibular styloid avulsion at the attachments of the popliteofibular and arcuate ligaments. (**B**) The popliteus muscle and tendon are also involved with a muscle–tendon unit strain (sagittal FS PD FSE image).

- 50-90% of PCL injuries are combined with injuries to other knee structures
- 60% of PCL injuries are associated with lesions involving the posterolateral corner structures (PLSs)
- Combined PCL and PLS injuries compromise the restraints to both posterior tibial translation and external rotation.
    - Associated with chondral overload and accelerated articular cartilage degeneration[40]

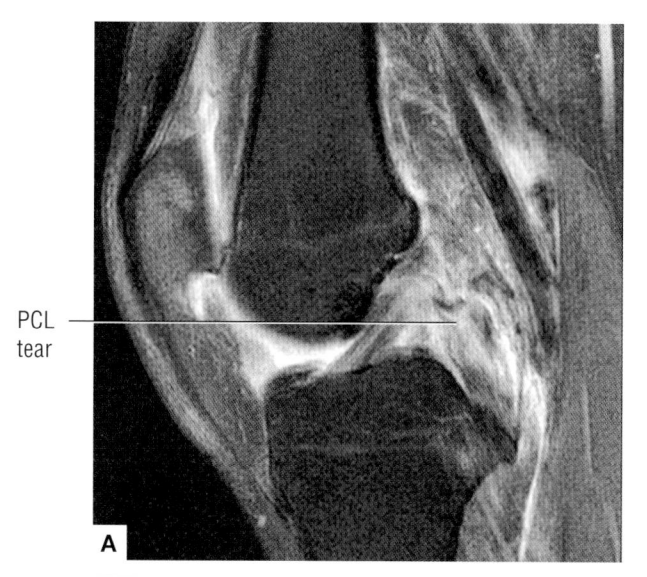

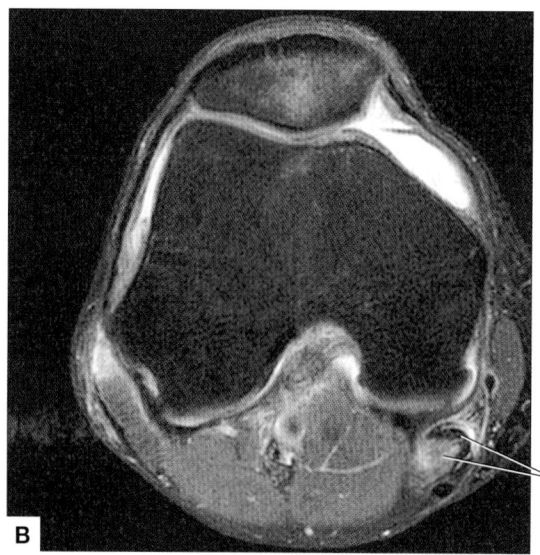

FIGURE 5.175 PCL tear in association with strain of the distal biceps femoris muscle–tendon unit. The popliteofibular ligament and arcuate ligaments were spared because the instability was primarily varus and not posterolateral. The LCL provides varus stability and does not play a role in assisting the PCL in preventing posterior tibial translation. In contrast, the popliteal complex, including the popliteofibular and arcuate ligaments, represents the primary restraint to posterolateral rotatory instability and a secondary restraint to posterior tibial translation. (**A**) Sagittal FS PD FSE image. (**B**) Axial FS PD FSE image.

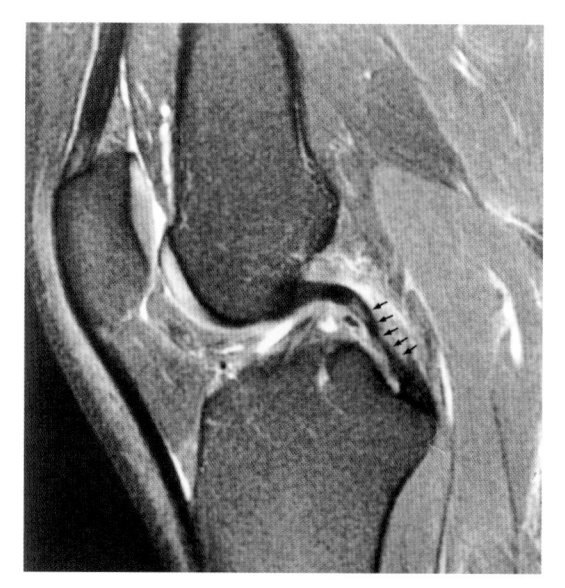

FIGURE 5.176 A chronic PCL tear with irregular ligament morphology and contour (*arrows*) on a FS PD-weighted FSE sagittal image. PCL continuity, however, is partially maintained. Both fibrous scar tissue and the normal PCL may display hypointensity on T1- and T2-weighted sequences. Contour irregularities, including ligamentous redundancy or tapering, are associated with chronic PCL disruptions. The intact PCL is taut in partial knee flexion.

PCL Tear and Reconstruction

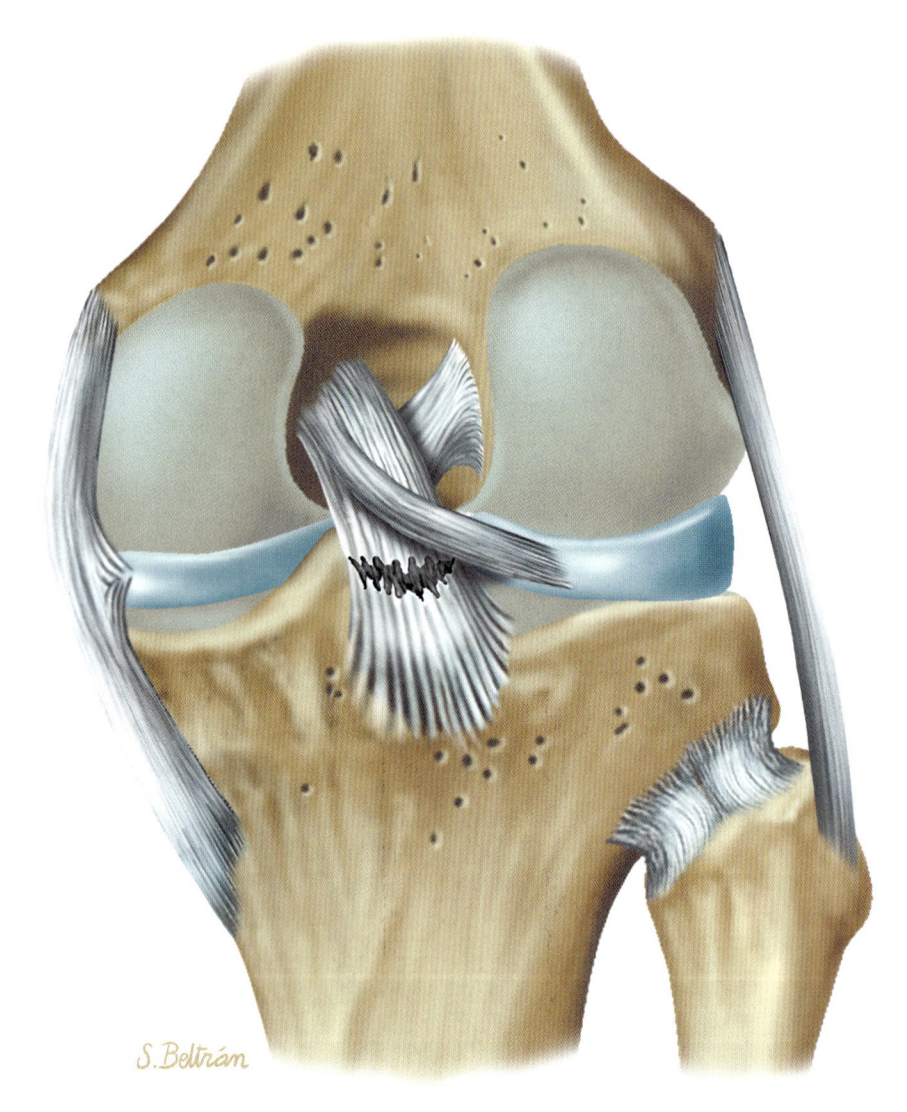

FIGURE 5.177 At least one of the meniscofemoral ligaments is intact in either acute or chronic PCL injuries. Grade 3 PCL distal tear is shown with posteriorly located lateral femoral condyle flexion-related contusion. PCL reconstruction is considered for cases of grade 3 laxity with combined ligament injuries (e.g., posterolateral corner injuries) or meniscal, chondral, or osseous avulsions.

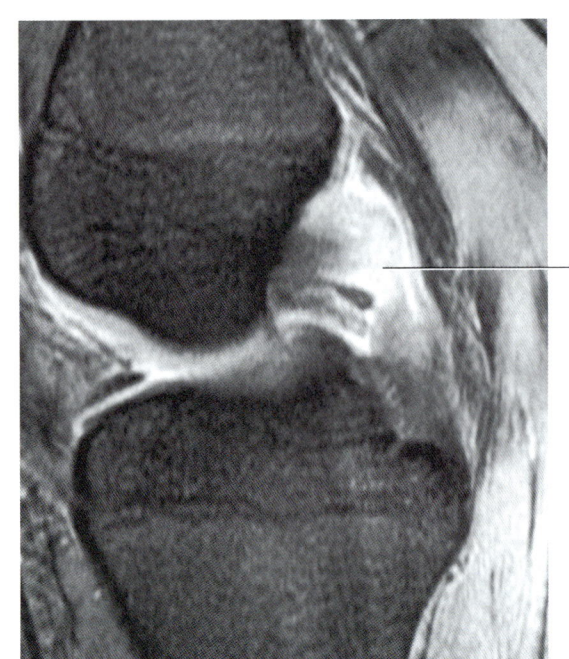

Middle third PCL tear

FIGURE 5.178 A complete PCL interstitial tear involving the middle third of the ligament on a FS PD-weighted FSE sagittal image. A hyperintense fluid signal is insinuated between the planes of the torn fibers. The intact hypointense ligament of Humphrey is present.

Cruciate Ligaments

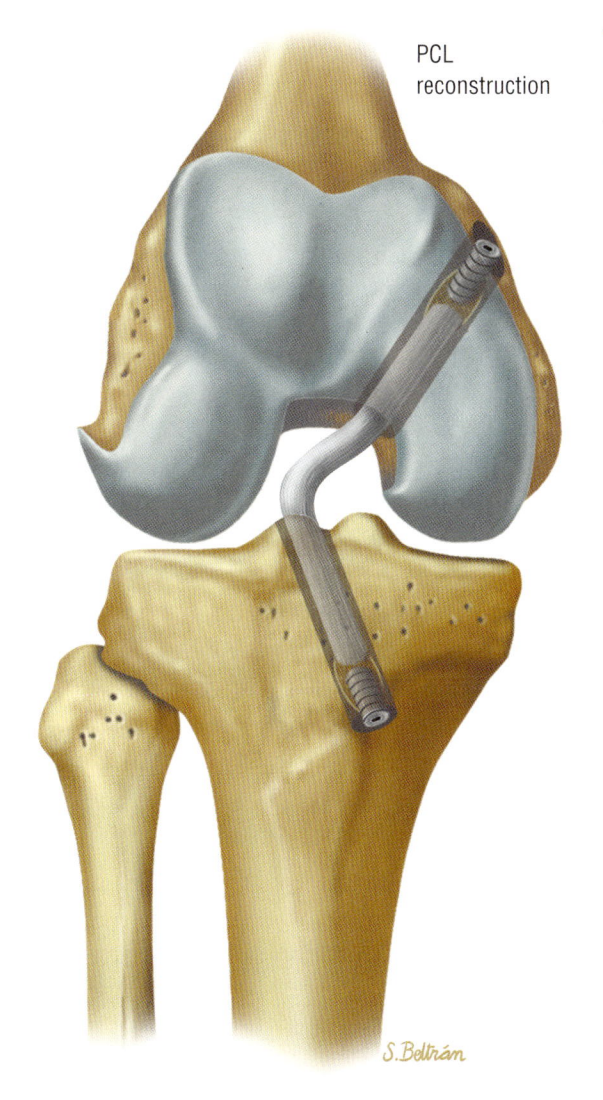

FIGURE 5.179 Bone–patellar tendon–bone and Achilles tendon are allografts commonly used for PCL reconstruction. The double-bundle technique offers the advantage of less posterior tibial translation compared to single-bundle reconstruction (coronal color illustration, anterior perspective).

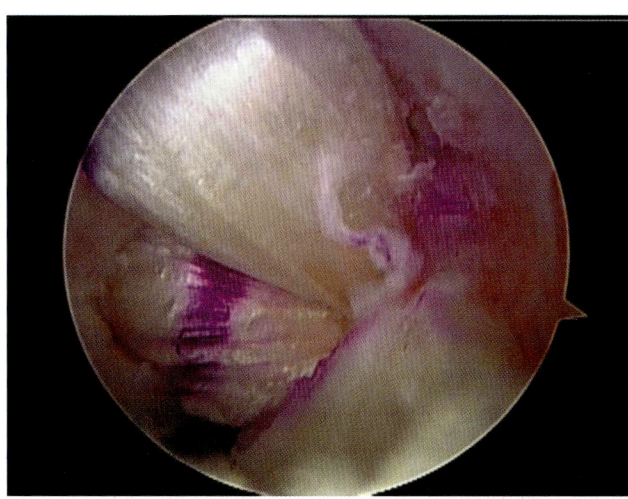

FIGURE 5.180 PCL grafts in the double-bundle technique. Single-bundle repair is commonly used for acute injuries. An intact bundle of a native PCL is preserved, and the PCL is treated with an augmentation technique. The double-bundle technique is useful in the chronic setting, especially when remaining structures are incompetent. (Reprinted from Fu FH. *Master Techniques in Orthopaedic Surgery: Sports Medicine.* Philadelphia, PA: Lippincott Williams & Wilkins; 2010, with permission.)

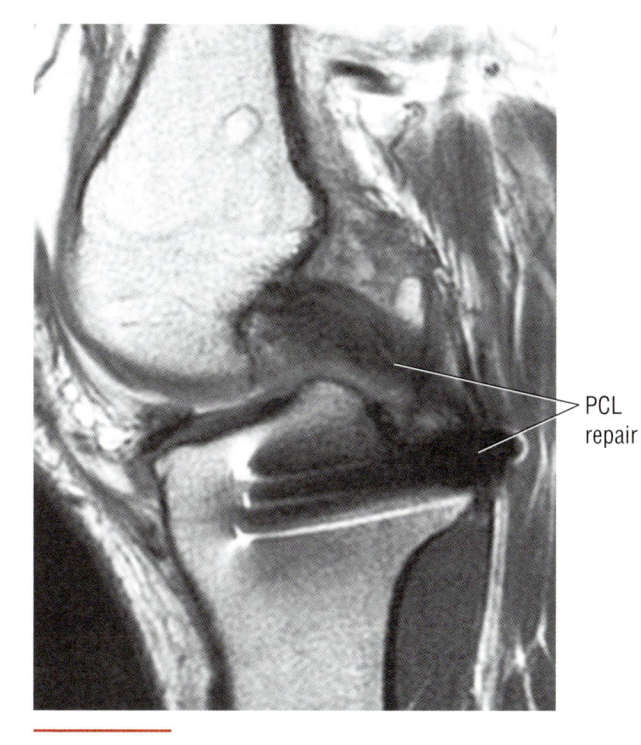

FIGURE 5.181 Repaired distal PCL tear on sagittal PD FSE image. Chronic PCL injuries are associated with chondrosis of the patellofemoral joint and the medial femoral condyle and an increased incidence of meniscal tears with posterior tibial translation. The tibiofemoral contact shifts anteriorly, unloading the posterior horn of the medial meniscus and increasing articular cartilage wear.

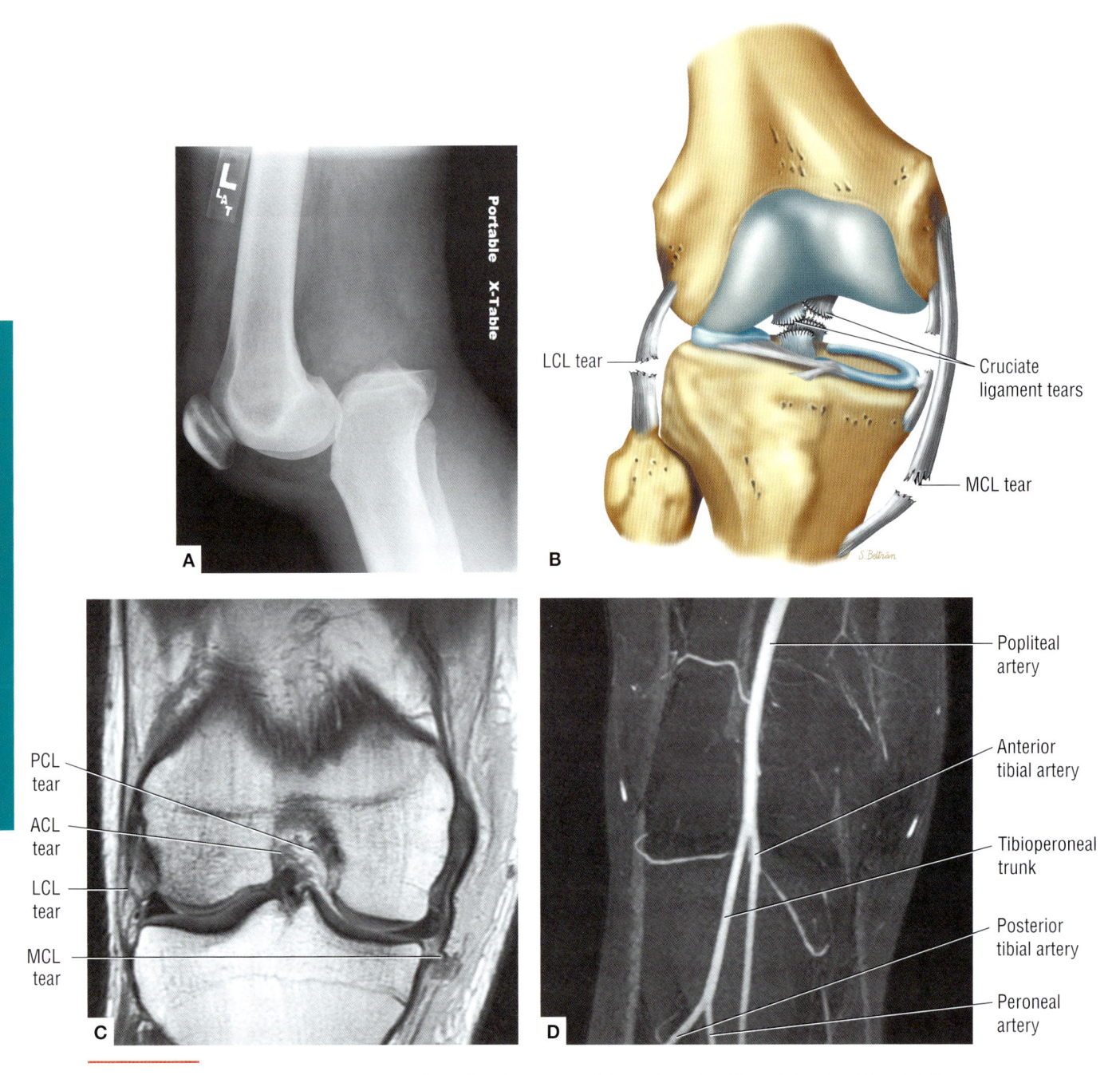

FIGURE 5.182 Multiligament injury with grade 3 disruption of the ACL and PCL and distal MCL and LCL tears in the knee dislocation. Although the popliteal vessels were patent, the incidence of the injury to the popliteal vessels and peroneal nerve is between 15% and 49%. (**A**) Lateral radiograph prior to reduction. (**B**) Coronal illustration of knee dislocation injuries. (**C**) Coronal PD FSE image. (**D**) MR angiogram of normal popliteal vessels.

Cruciate Ligaments 573

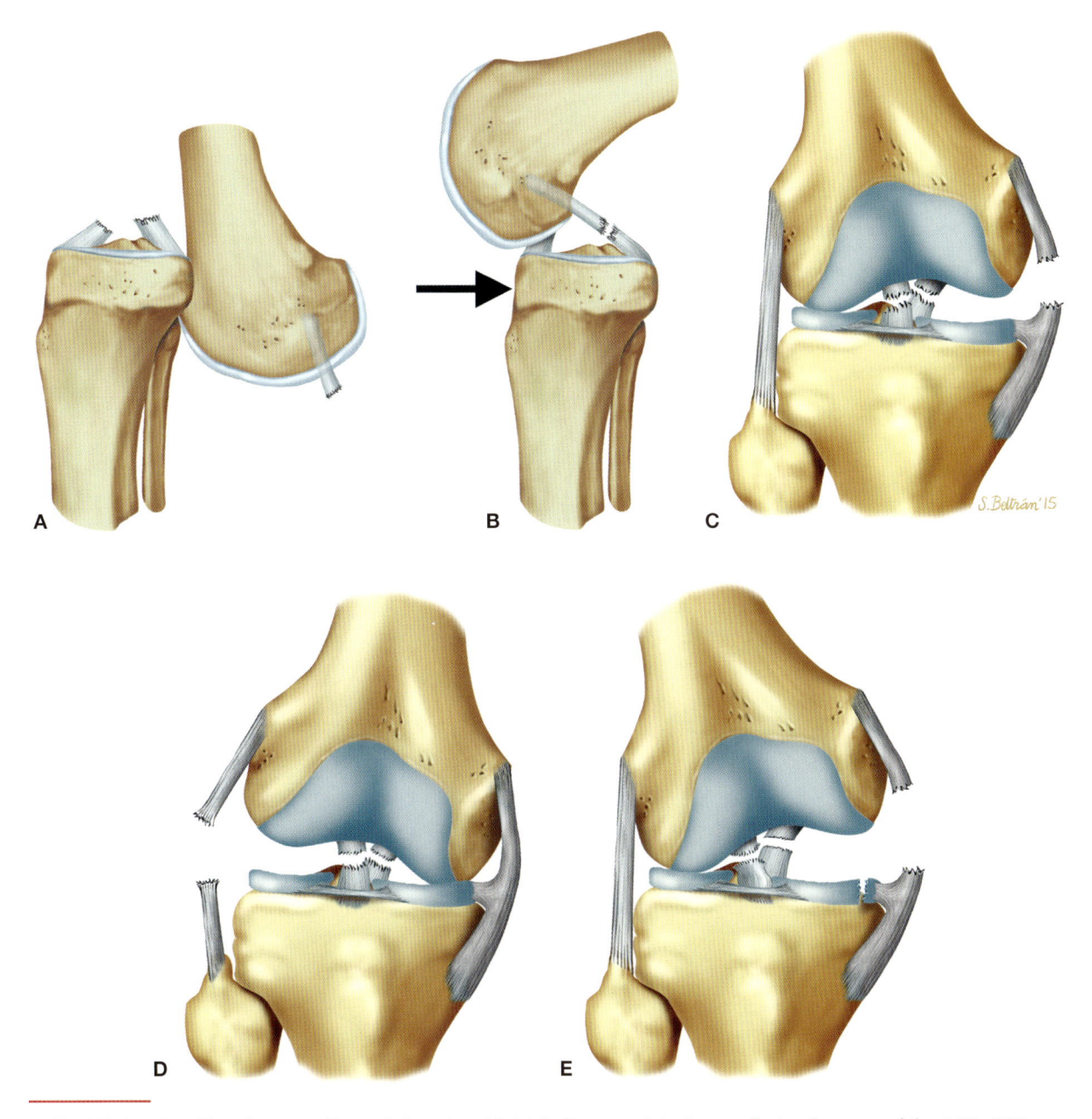

FIGURE 5.183 Classification of knee dislocation. Multiple-ligament injuries usually involve tears of the ACL, PCL, and at least one collateral ligament complex. In knee dislocation, there is a complete loss of contact between tibial and femoral aticular surfaces. Injuries (dislocations with bicruciate disruption) can be classified as:[12] (**A**) Pure anterior. (**B**) Pure posterior. (**C**) Medial combined. (**D**) Lateral combined. (**E**) Complex.

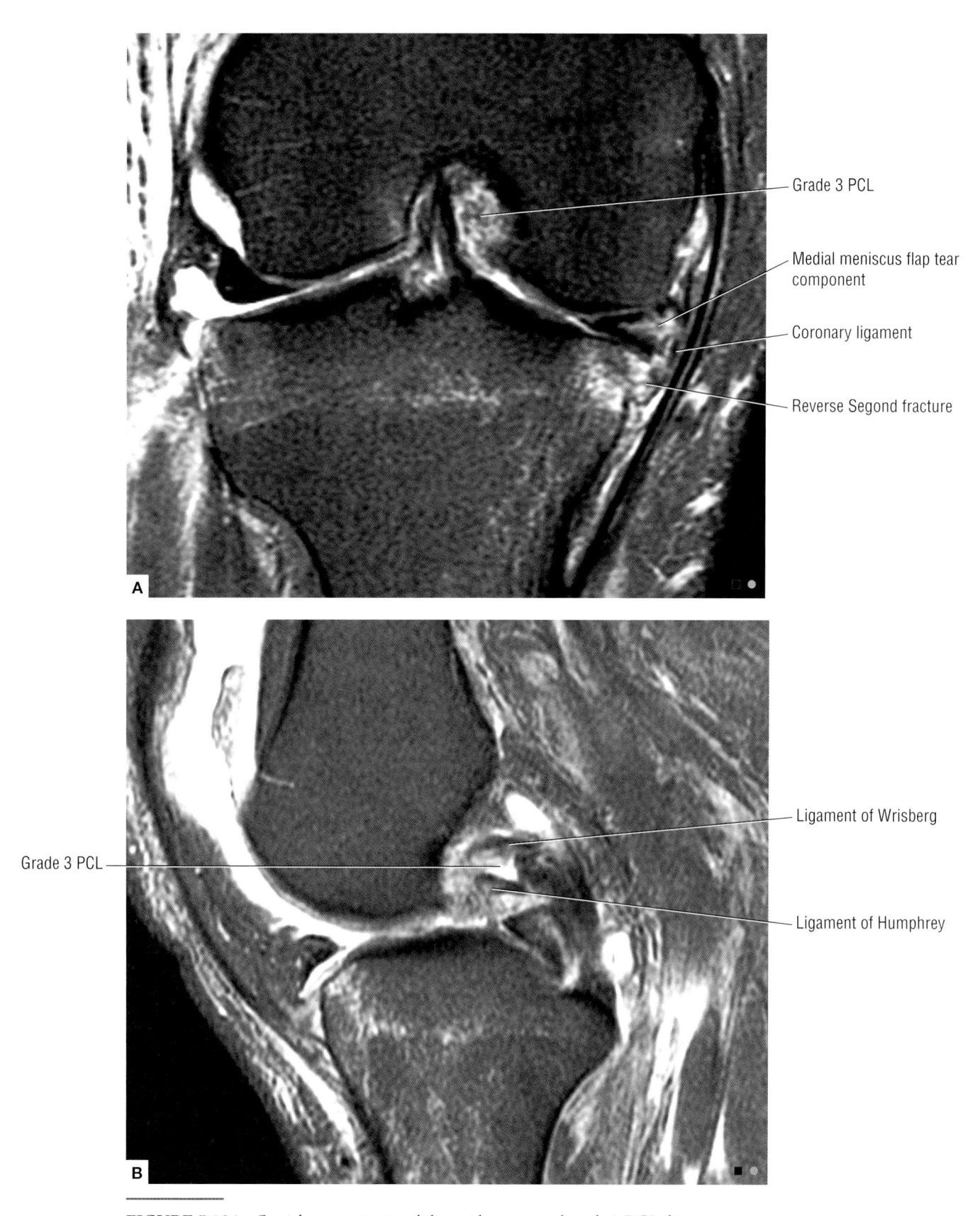

FIGURE 5.184 Straight posterior instability with a proximal grade 3 PCL disruption. The ACL and collateral ligaments are intact. The avulsion of the PCL is from its femoral attachment. The reverse Segond fracture involves an avulsion fracture of the medial tibial plateau. The reverse Segond fracture is associated both with a tear of the PCL and medial meniscus. Coronal (**A**) and sagittal (**B**) FS PD FSE images.

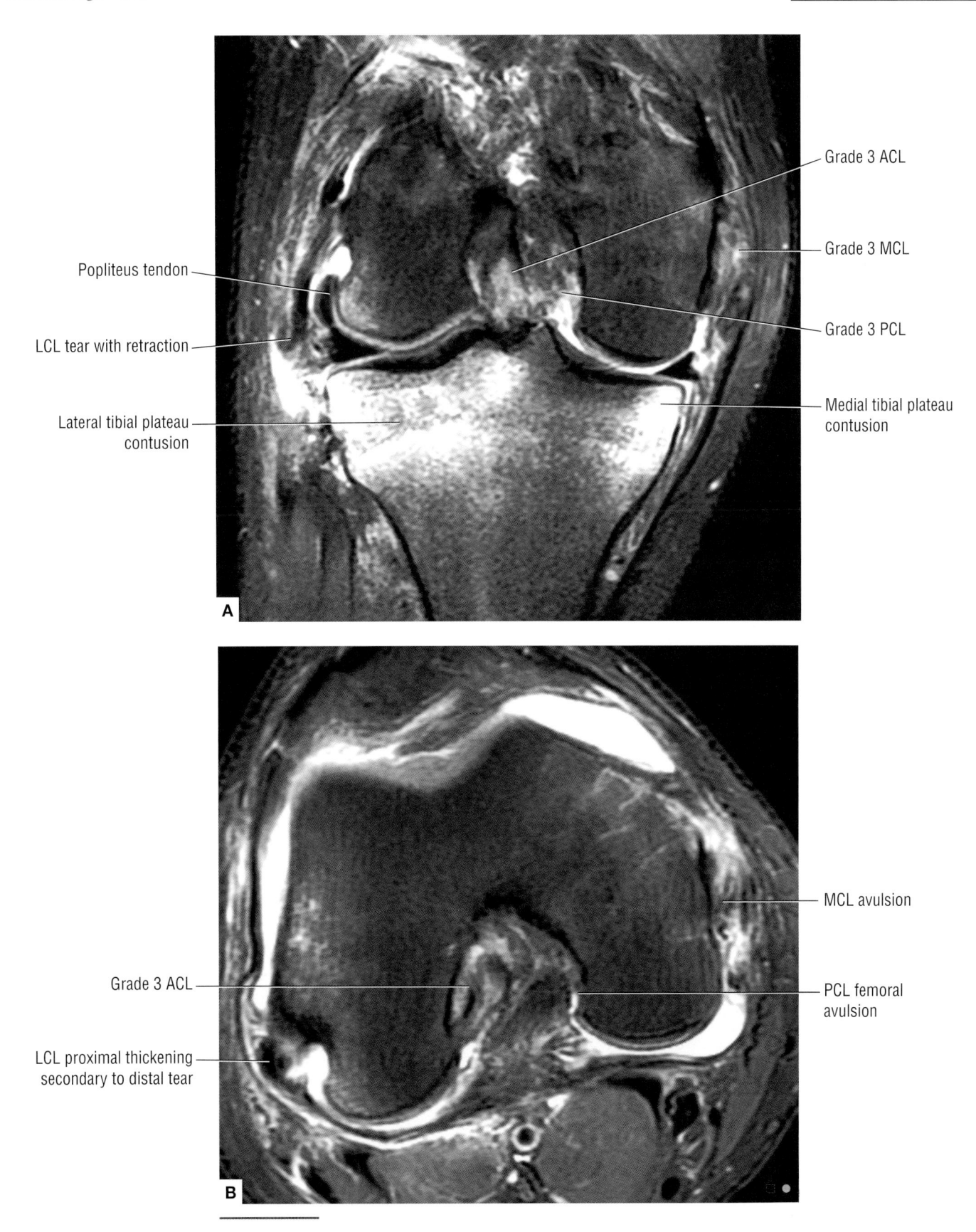

FIGURE 5.185 Multiligament injury with grade 3 distal ACL tear and grade 3 proximal PCL disruption. The LCL is torn distally and is retracted proximally. The medial epicondylar attachment of the MCL is torn. Trabecular bone contusions exist in both femoral condyles and tibial plateaus. Coronal (**A**) and axial (**B**) FS PD FSE images.

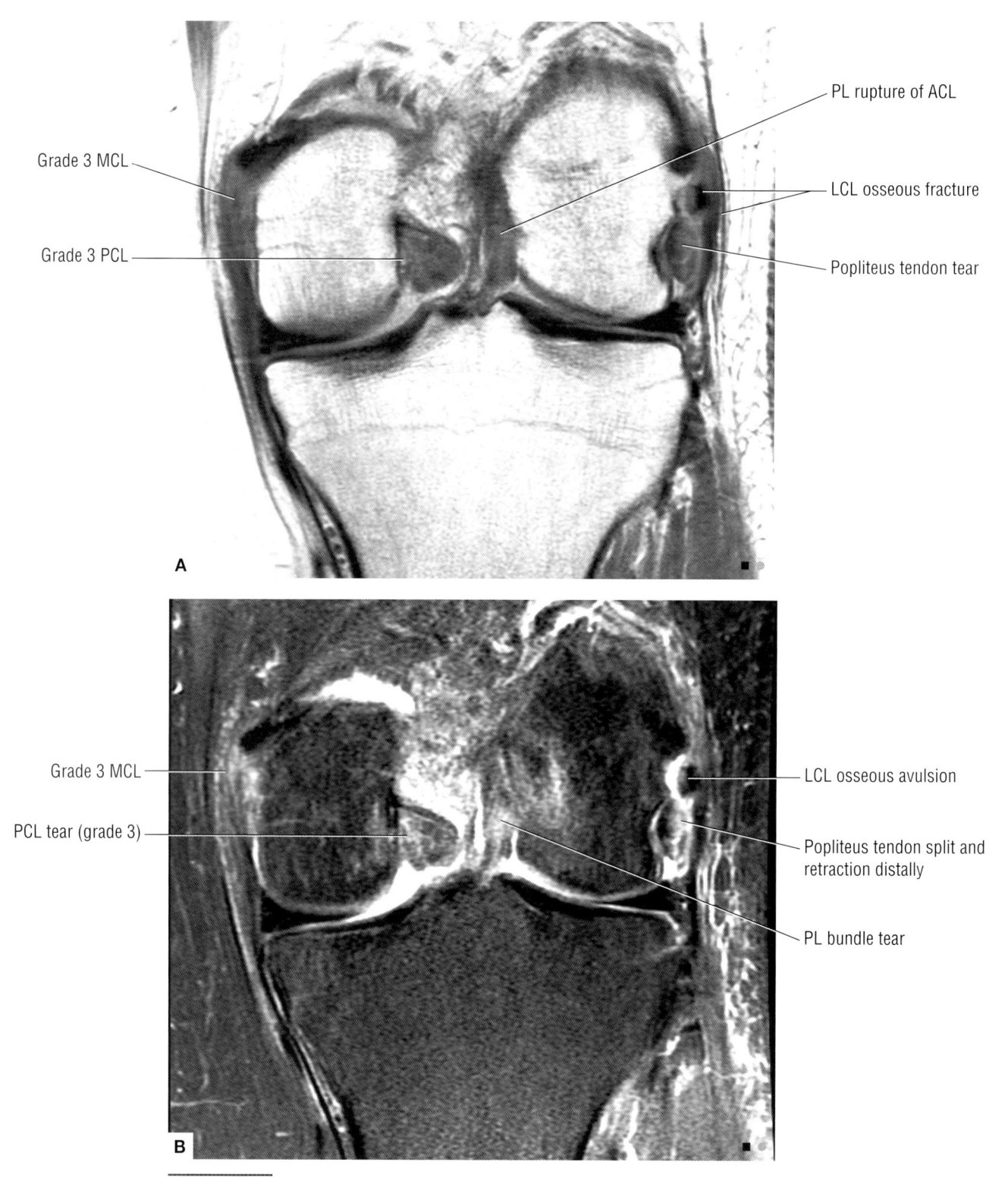

FIGURE 5.186 Posterolateral corner multiligament injury with grade 3 MCL, grade 3 LCL with osseous avulsion, grade 3 PCL, and ACL posterolateral bundle tear. The distal LCL and popliteofibular ligament attach to the retracted popliteus tendon where intact. Coronal (**A, B**) and sagittal (**C, D**) FS PD FSE images.

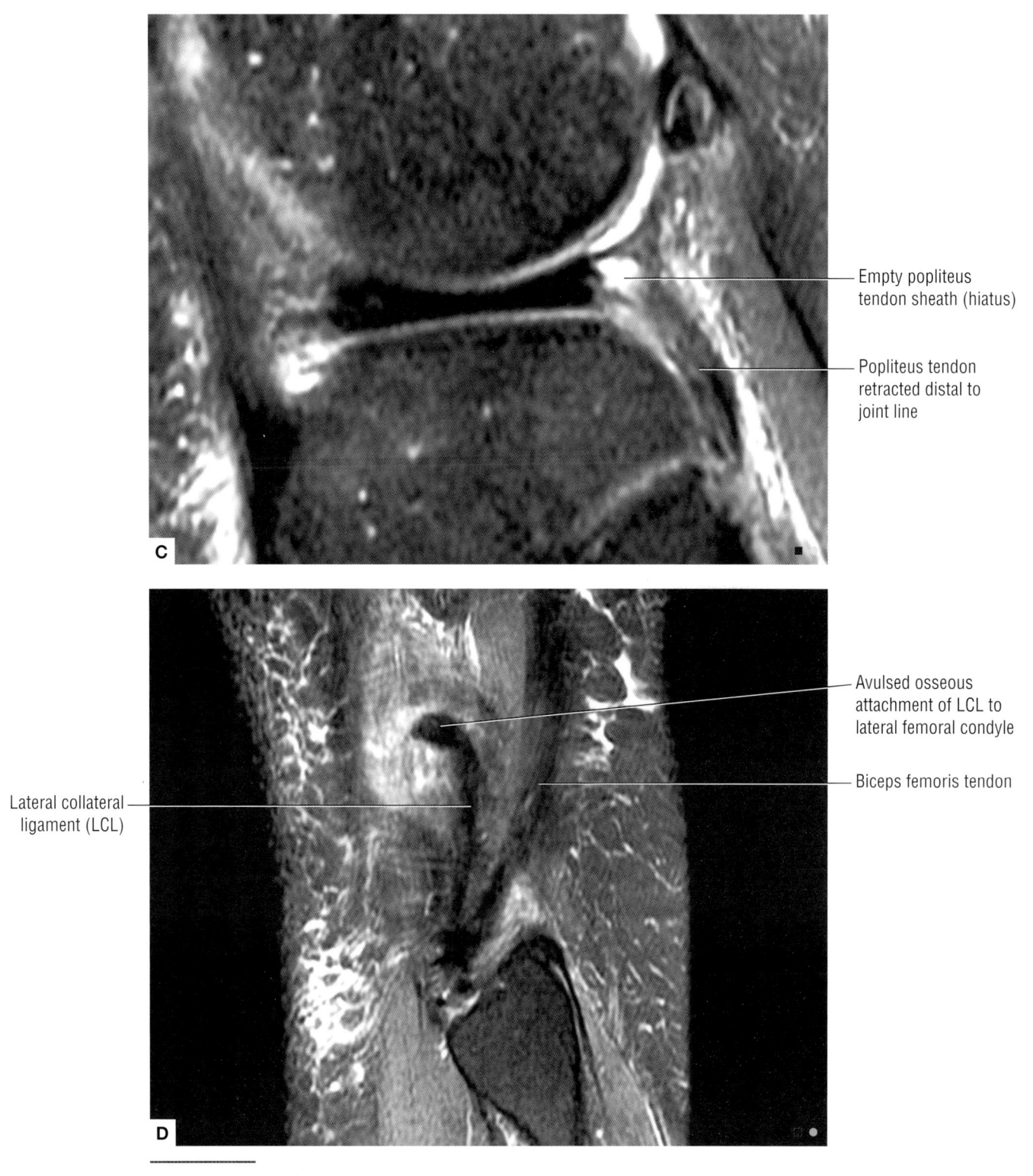

FIGURE 5.186 *(Continued)*

6
Collateral Ligaments

Medial Collateral Ligament (MCL) (pages 581–635)

Lateral Collateral Ligament (LCL) and Posterolateral Corner (PLC) (pages 636–693)

Collateral Ligaments

Medial Collateral Ligament (MCL)

Key Concepts

- Three key medial and posteromedial structures
    - MCL
        - Superficial MCL (sMCL)
        - Deep MCL (dMCL [meniscofemoral/meniscotibial attachments])
    - Posteromedial capsule (PMC)[40]
- Laxity of MCL is associated with distal MCL tears

Functional Anatomy

- Medial aspect of the knee divided into three layers from superficial to deep, according to Warren and Marshall[70]
    - Layer 1: deep fascia
        - Sartorius fascia anteriorly and thin fascia posteriorly
    - Layer 2: sMCL
    - Layer 3: joint capsule
        - Anterior third: attaches to anterior horn of medial meniscus, reinforced by medial retinaculum
        - Middle third: dMCL or medial capsular ligament
        - Posterior third: posterior oblique ligament (formed by fusion of layers 2 and 3 and composed of three arms—superficial, tibial, and capsular) and oblique popliteal ligament

- MCL itself composed of two layers[95]
    - Deep fibers, corresponding to layer 3, that attach to the capsule and medial meniscus peripherally
    - Superficial fibers, corresponding to layer 2
    - 8 to 11 cm long
    - Extends from origin on medial epicondyle (center of insertion is 3mm proximal and 5mm posterior to the medial epicondyle)
        - 15-mm diameter ellipse footprint anterior and distal to adductor tubercle[40]
    - Attaches 5 to 7cm inferior to tibial plateau and posterior to pes anserinus insertion
    - MCL insertion on the tibia covered by pes anserinus muscles
    - Remains taut across range of knee motion (represents the isometry of the sMCL)
- sMCL
    - In general, the term "MCL" refers to layer 2, the sMCL.
        - Extracapsular
    - Further divided into anterior and posterior portions
        - Anterior fibers tighten with knee flexion of 70 to 105 degrees[126]
    - In extension, MCL is taut and limits hyperextension.
    - In flexion, MCL remains taut and provides primary valgus stability (from 0 to 90 degrees of flexion).
        - Anterior sMCL fibers stretched in flexion
        - Posterior fibers become more lax.
        - dMCL and PMC are secondary restraints to valgus stress.[40]
    - Separated from underlying capsular ligament and medial meniscus by a bursa that reduces friction during flexion
    - Functionally tested with applied valgus stress in partial knee flexion with tibia in external rotation (allowing relaxation of the cruciate ligaments)
    - MCL function more important as flexion increases and posterior capsular structures become lax

- MCL function less important with increased valgus movement and rotation, as posteromedial aspect of the capsule becomes more involved[30]
- Primary valgus restraint relative to the deep capsular ligament[69]
    - If MCL fails at 10 to 15mm of joint opening, cruciate ligaments become primary restraints to valgus stress.

- Medial capsular ligament or dMCL (layer 3)
    - Represents a capsular ligament
        - The femoral attachment is immediately distal to the epicondylar attachment of the sMCL
        - The tibial attachment is to the medial aspect of the medial rim of the tibial plateau near the joint line and proximal to the attachment of the anterior arm of the semimembranosus expansion.
    - Composed of meniscofemoral and meniscotibial attachments to the meniscus
        - Firmly attached to periphery of medial meniscus at joint line
    - In anterior cruciate ligament (ACL)-deficient knee, sMCL and medial capsule function as secondary restraints to anterior tibial translation.
    - Meniscotibial component, when ruptured, is associated with pathologic mobility of the medial meniscus.
        - The medial meniscus lifts away from the tibial plateau when stressed by an abduction moment.
        - Rupture of the meniscotibial part of the dMCL mobilizes the medial meniscus and results in greater anterior laxity.
    - The anterior edges of the dMCL and sMCL are parallel and close to each other.
    - Posterior edge of dMCL blends with posterior edge of sMCL.
        - The posteromedial corner represents structures posterior to this junction.
        - Junction of larger layer 2 and 3 come together to blend as one capsular layer referred to as layer 3.
    - The dMCL is tightened by tibiofemoral motion.
        - Its fibers are shorter than other medial-sided structures.
        - Role in limiting tibial external rotation and anterior drawer in external rotation[40]

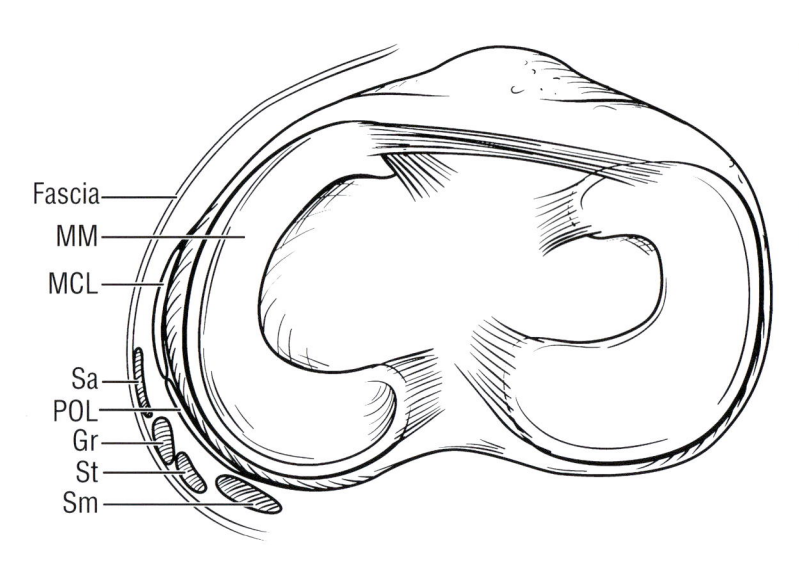

FIGURE 6.1 Cross-section view of the medial layers of the knee. Gr, gracilis; MM, medial meniscus; POL, posterior oblique ligament; Sa, sartorius; Sm, semimembranosus; St, semitendinosus. (Reprinted from Fu FH. *Master Techniques in Orthopaedic Surgery: Sports Medicine*. Philadelphia, PA: Lippincott Williams & Wilkins; 2010, with permission.)

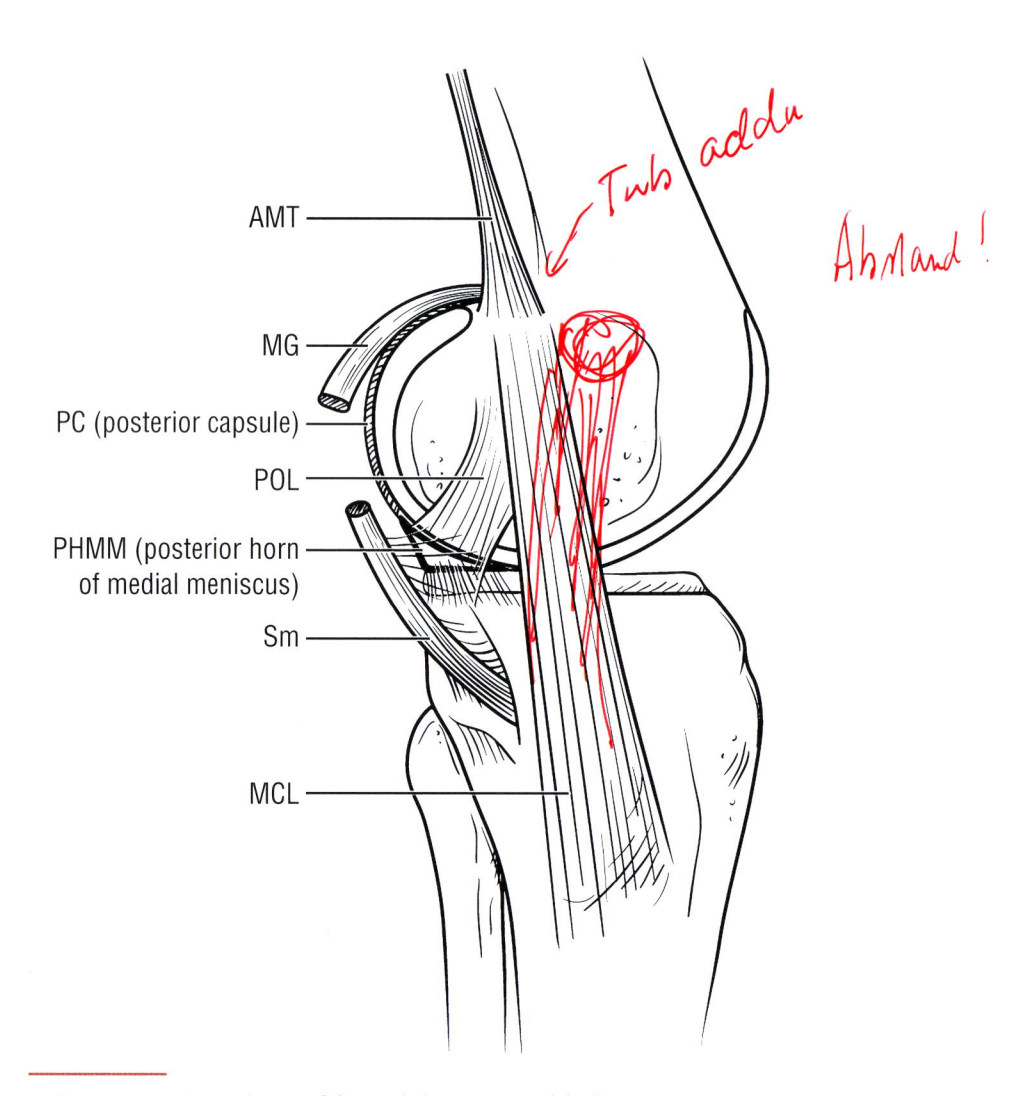

FIGURE 6.2 Sagittal view of the medial structures of the knee. AMT, adductor magnus tendon; MG, medial gastrocnemius; POL, posterior oblique ligament; Sm, semimembranosus. (Reprinted from Fu FH. *Master Techniques in Orthopaedic Surgery: Sports Medicine*. Philadelphia, PA: Lippincott Williams & Wilkins; 2010, with permission.)

Collateral Ligaments 585

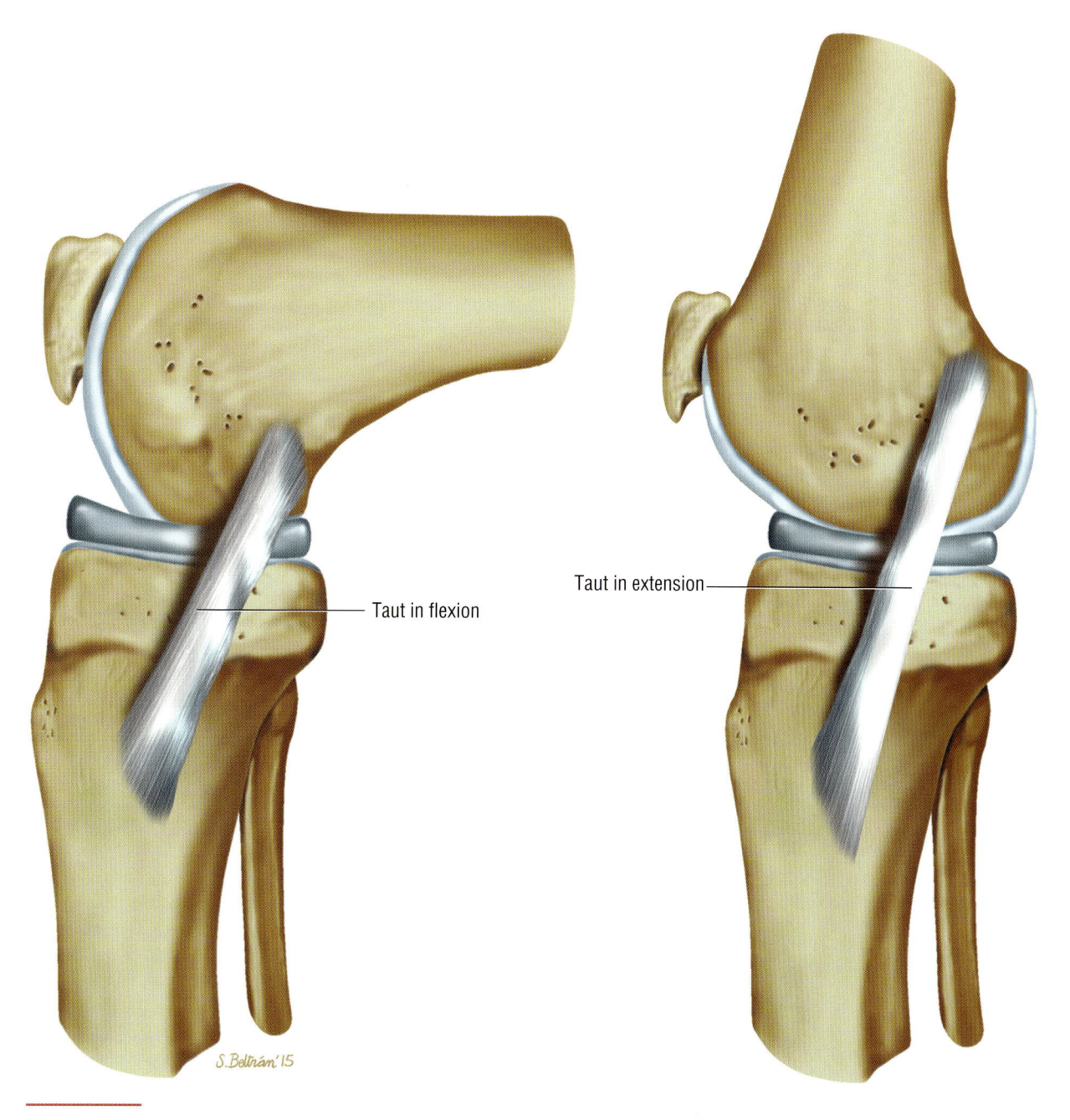

FIGURE 6.3 Anterior border of the superficial medial collateral ligament is taut in flexion while the posterior is taut in extension.

MCL and Posterior Oblique Ligament (POL)

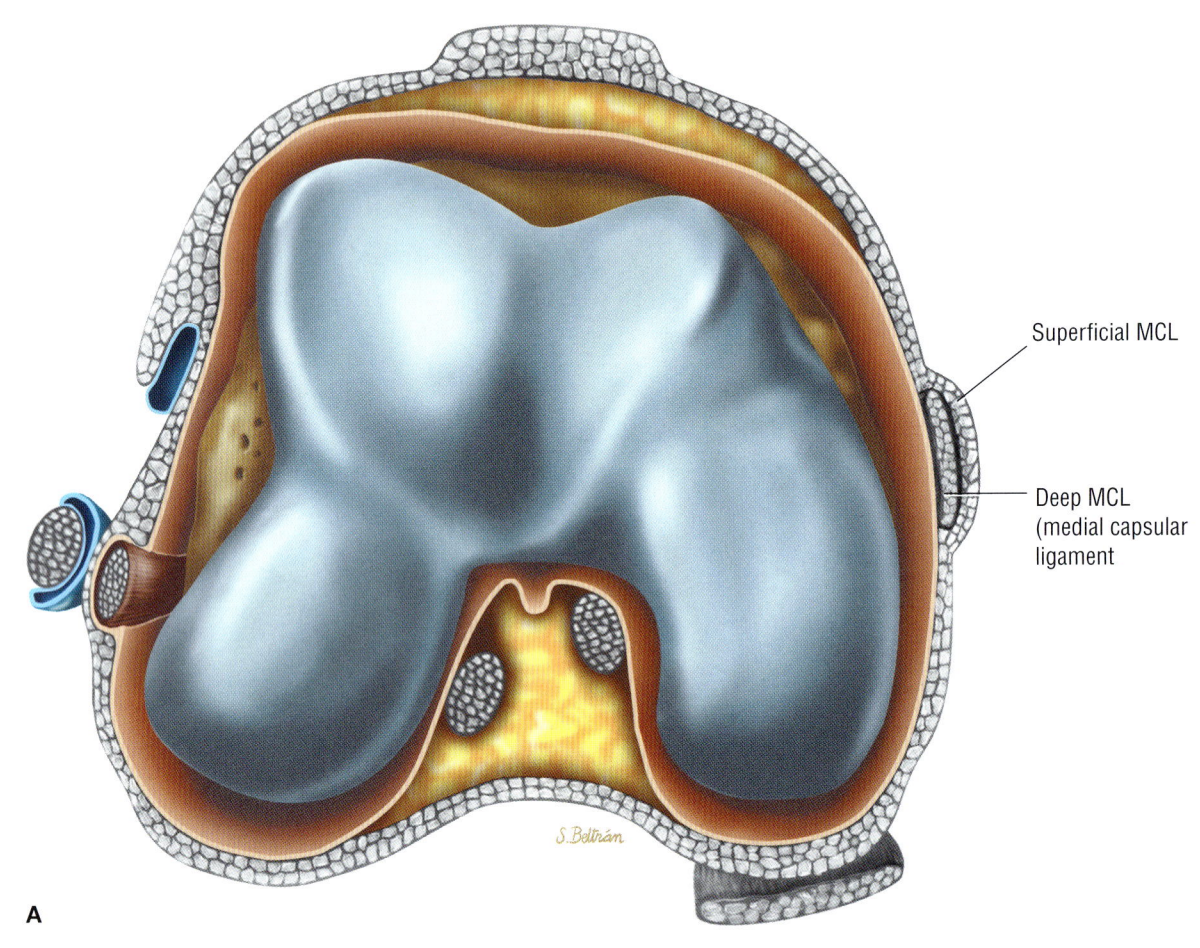

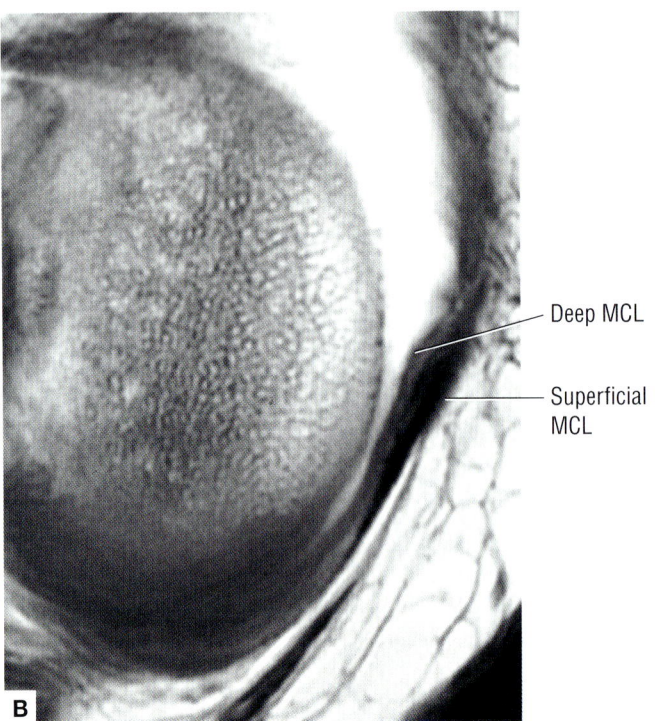

FIGURE 6.4 (**A**) Axial three-dimensional section demonstrating the superficial and deep MCL as well as the popliteus tendon and lateral collateral ligament. There are three layers that stabilize the medial aspect of the knee. MCL trauma may affect any or all of these layers. Layer 1 is the deep investing fascia, which merges with the posteromedial capsule and hamstring muscle group. Layer 2 contains the superficial MCL. Layer 3 is the joint capsule, which can be divided into three parts. The anterior third is attached to the anterior horn and is reinforced by the medial retinaculum. The middle third is the deep MCL, and the posterior third contains the posterior oblique ligament (POL) and oblique popliteal ligament (OPL). The POL component represents fused layers 2 and 3. (**B**) The MCL has an average thickness of 4.3mm at the femoral attachment and 2.3mm at the tibial attachment. The deep medial collateral ligament fuses with the superficial medial collateral ligament proximally but can be separated from the superficial MCL distally (axial T1-weighted MR arthrogram).

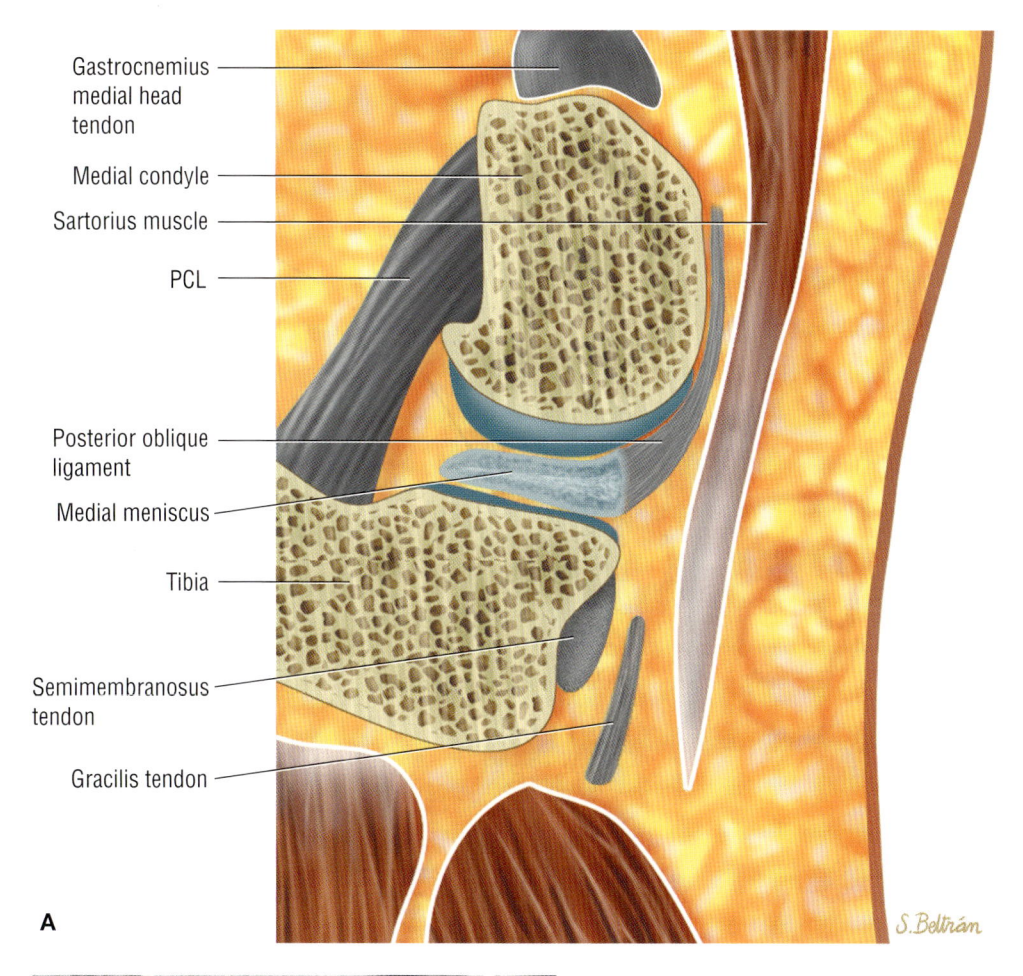

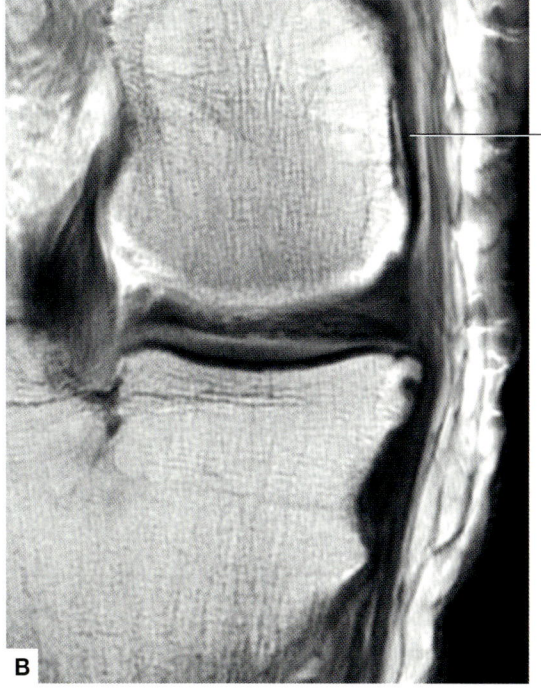

Collateral Ligaments 587

FIGURE 6.5 (**A**) Posteromedial coronal illustration showing the posterior oblique ligament (POL). The POL helps maintain medial stability and resists anteromedial tibial subluxation. It is tight in knee extension and lax in knee flexion. Sports-related injuries commonly occur between 45 and 90 degrees of knee flexion. The semimembranosus assists in flexion by pulling the medial meniscus posteriorly to avoid entrapment and also engages the POL through its expansion below the joint line. (**B**) Coronal T1-weighted MR arthrogram displays the POL as a thickened triangular capsular ligament originating posterior to the proximal superficial MCL. Distally, the POL is attached to both the posterior horn medial meniscus and the tibia immediately below the joint line.

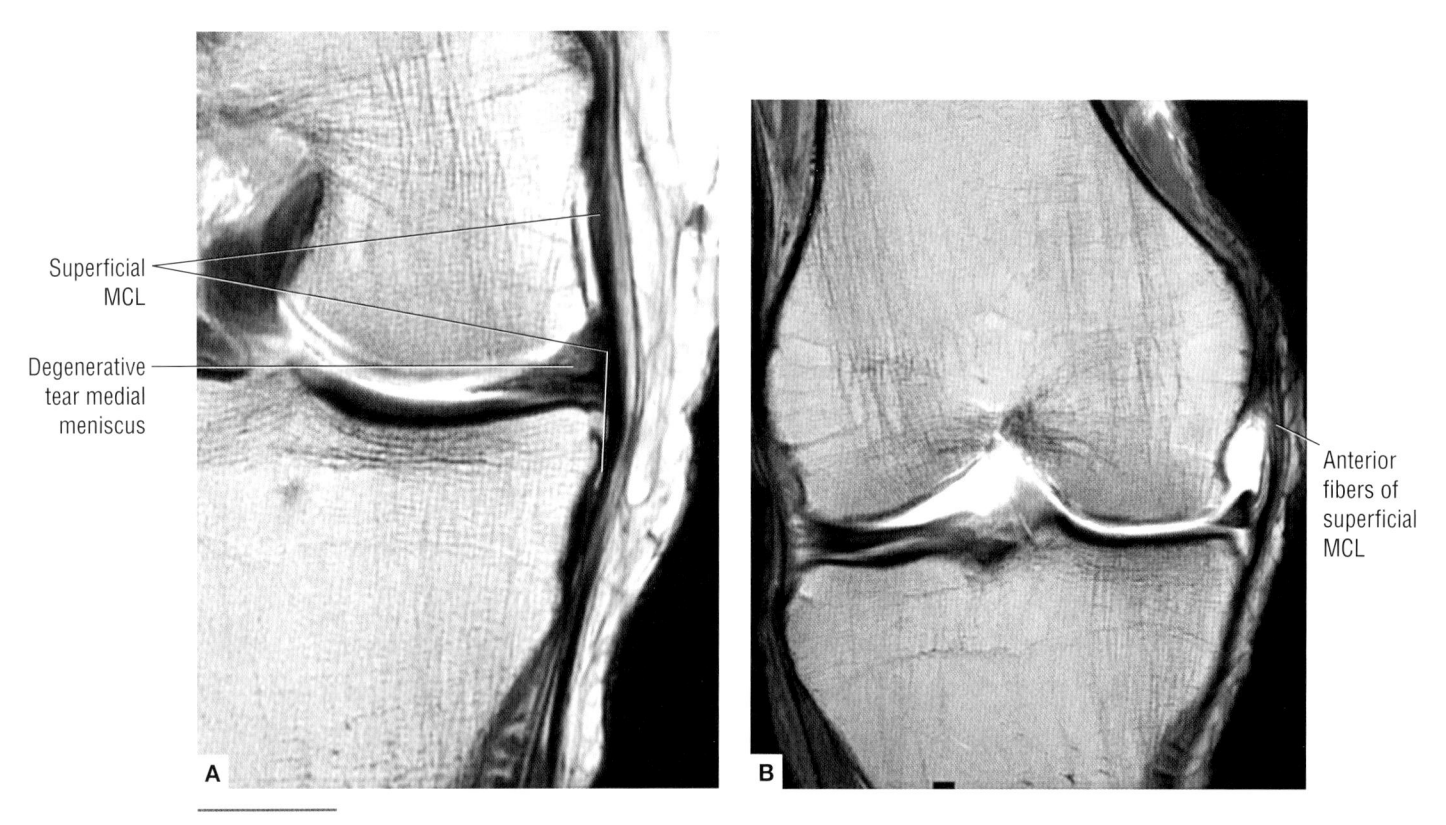

FIGURE 6.6 (**A**) The superficial MCL is 8 to 11cm long and 1.0 to 1.5cm wide. The distal attachment of the MCL is 5 to 7cm distal to the joint line on the anteromedial tibia deep to the pes insertion. (**B**) Tears of the MCL may be overestimated if they are assessed along its anterior border. The MCL should be assessed more posteriorly in the coronal plane of section, where the femoral condyles fuse or bridge together. This plane of section accurately depicts the long parallel fibers of the MCL attributed to primary restraint of abduction and external rotatory loads. In contrast, the posterior oblique ligament represents a secondary restraint to abduction loads, as do the cruciate ligaments. T1-weighted MR arthrograms.

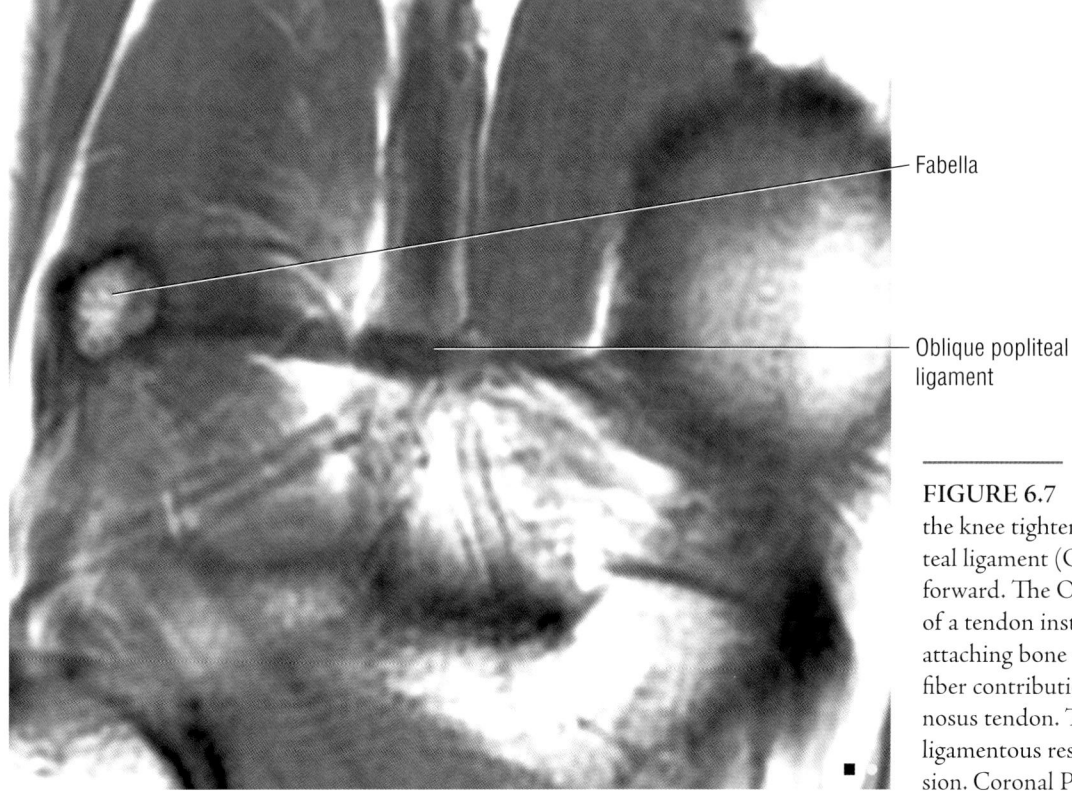

FIGURE 6.7 The posterior capsule of the knee tightens when the oblique popliteal ligament (OPL) is pulled medially and forward. The OPL may be considered more of a tendon instead of a ligament as it is not attaching bone to bone. The OPL receives fiber contribution from the semimembranosus tendon. The OPL provides primary ligamentous restraint to knee hyperextension. Coronal PD FSE image.

Collateral Ligaments 589

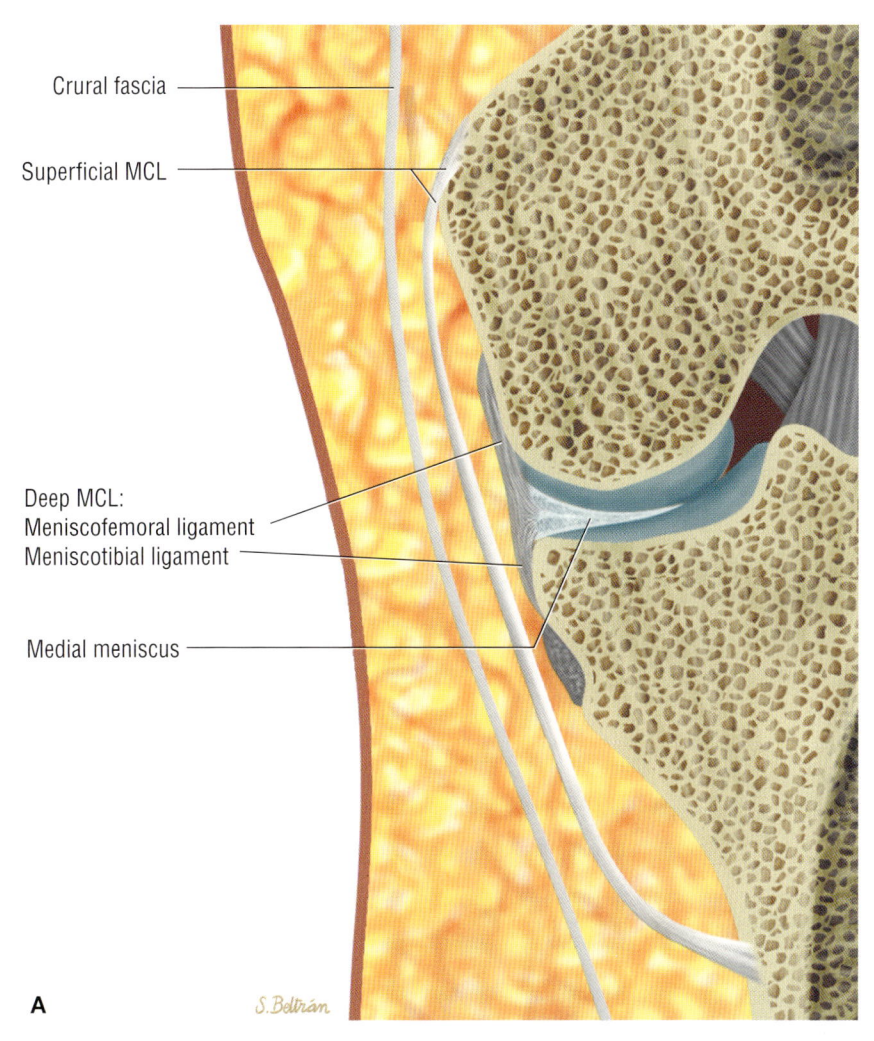

FIGURE 6.8 (**A**) The static medial stabilizers include the superficial medial collateral ligament (MCL), the posterior oblique ligament, and the deep capsular (meniscofemoral and meniscotibial) ligaments. Dynamic support is provided by the semimembranosus insertions and the vastus medialis. Layer 2 (superficial MCL) medial to layer 3 (deep capsular layer) on coronal (**B**) FS PD FSE images.

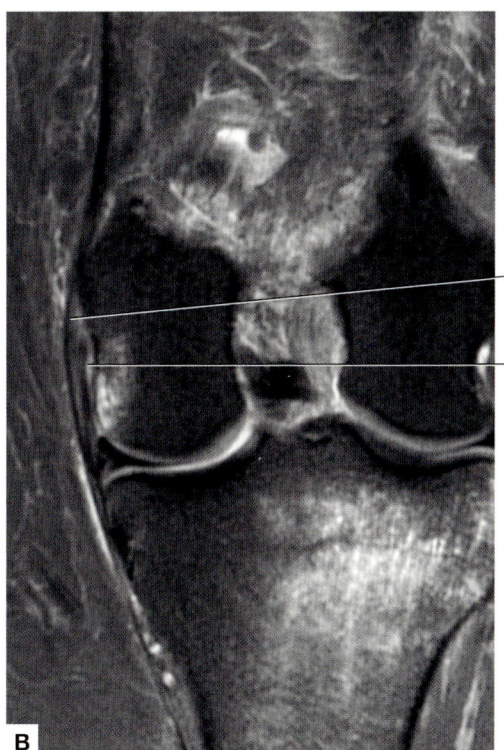

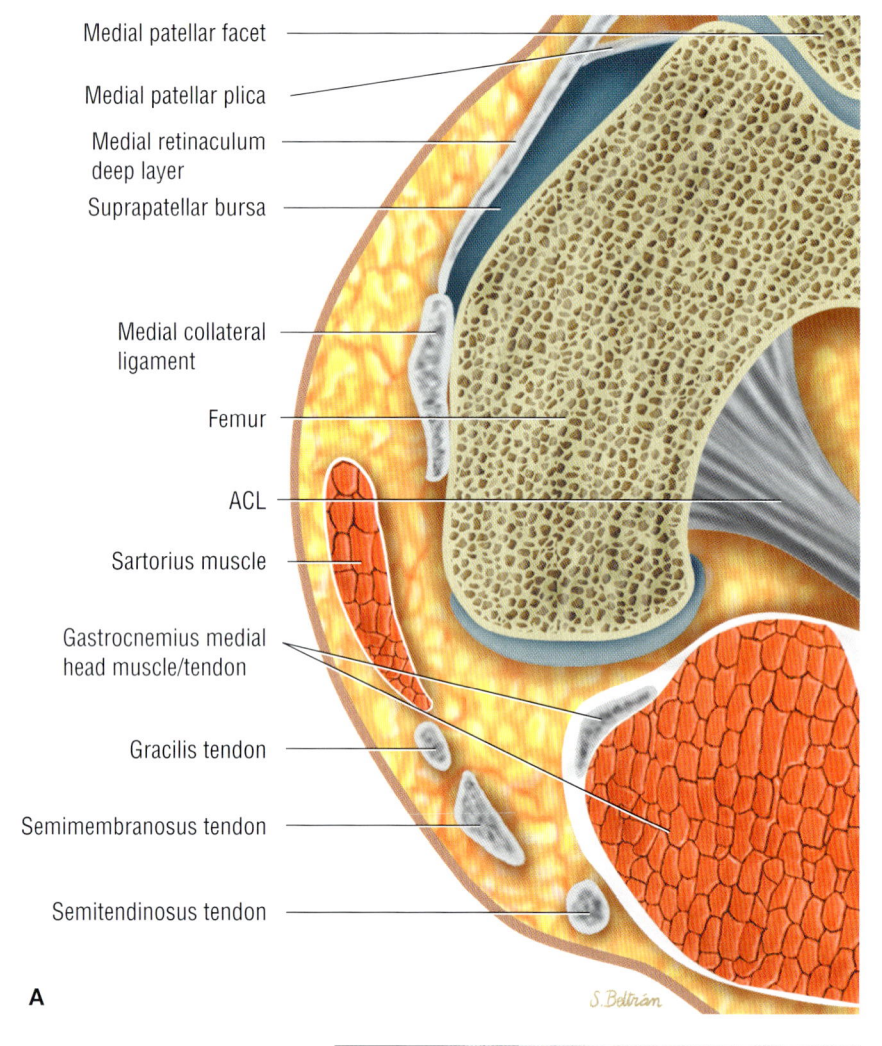

FIGURE 6.9 Posteromedial structures above the joint line on (**A**) a color axial cross-section and (**B**) an axial T1-weighted MR arthrogram.

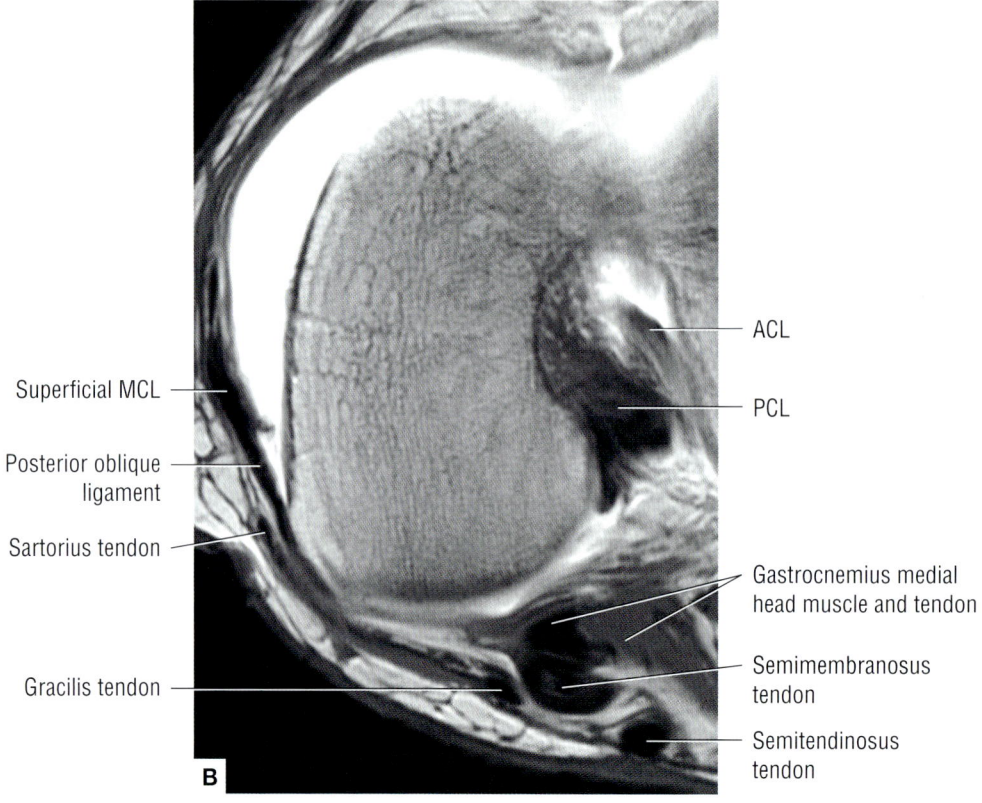

Collateral Ligaments

Posteromedial Corner

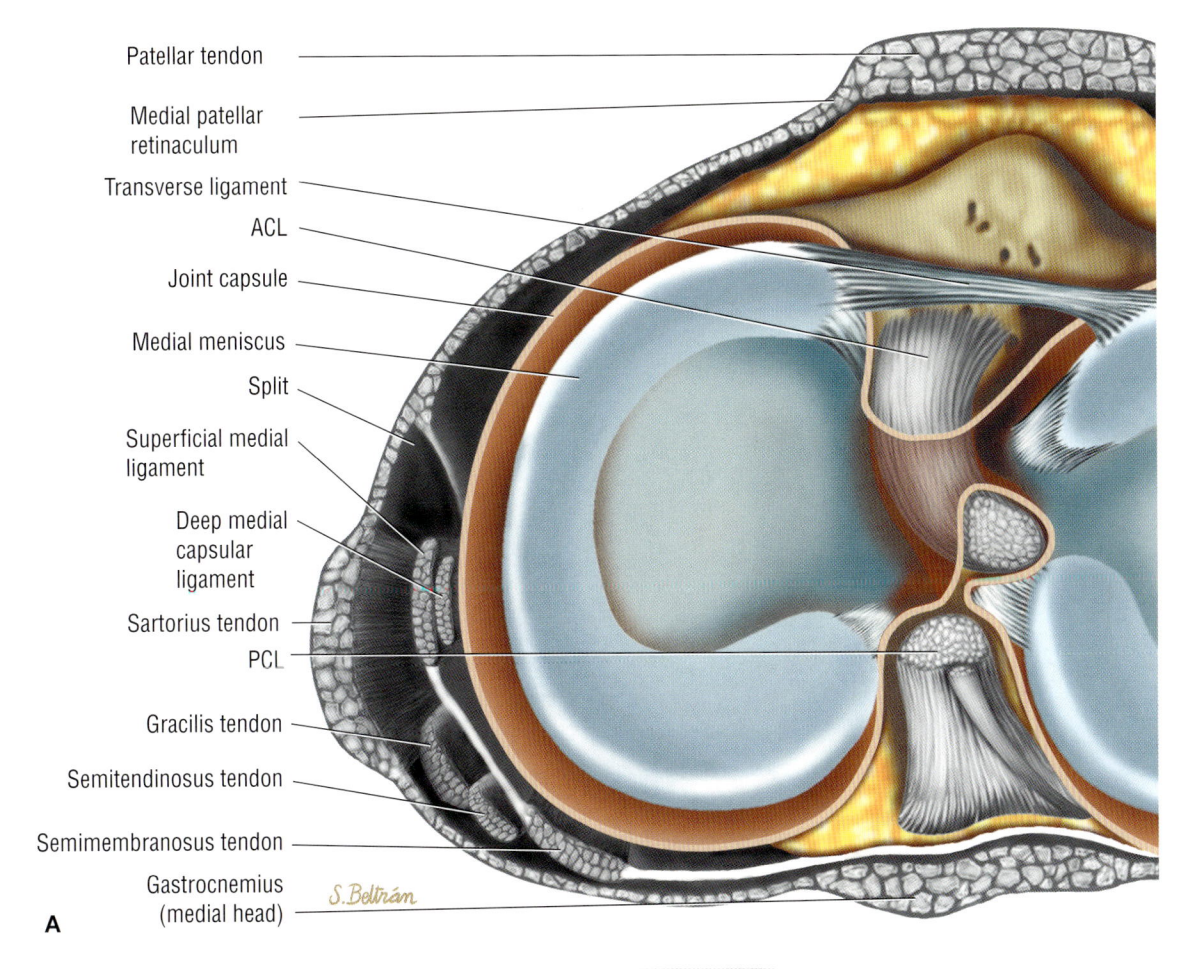

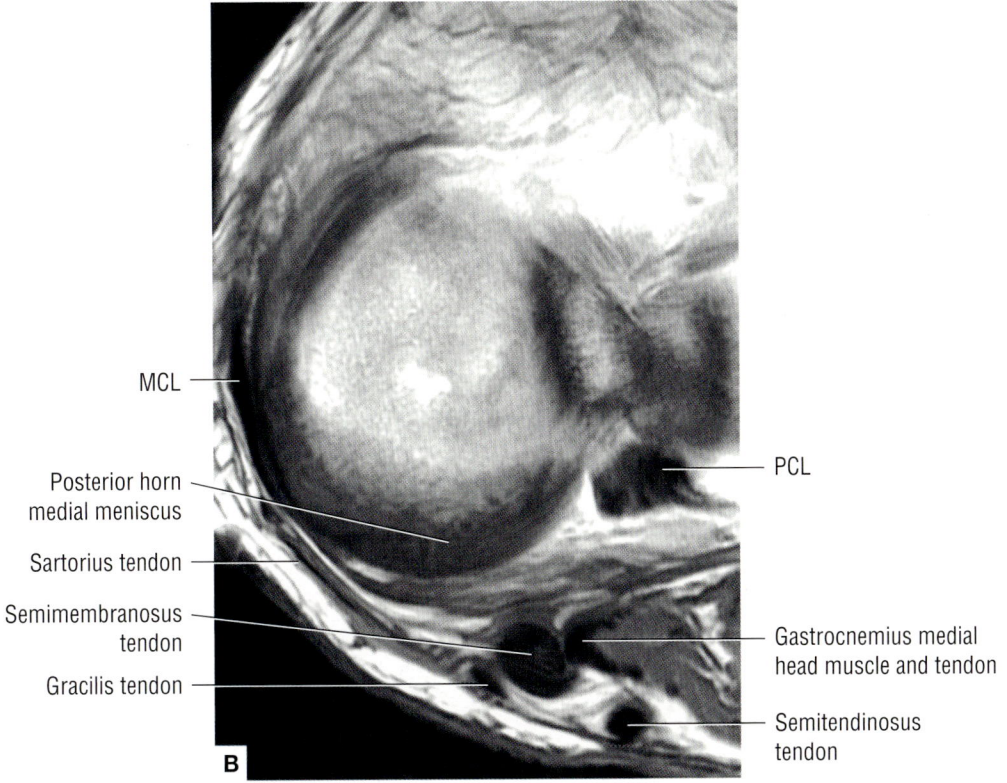

FIGURE 6.10 Posteromedial corner at the level of the joint line on (**A**) a superior view illustration and (**B**) an axial T1-weighted MR arthrogram. In addition to the medial capsuloligamentous complex, abduction stability is also provided by the vastus medialis extensor aponeurosis and pes anserine tendons.

FIGURE 6.11 Posteromedial corner at the level of the proximal tibia on (**A**) a cross-section illustration below the joint line and (**B**) an axial T1-weighted image at the level of the semimembranosus.

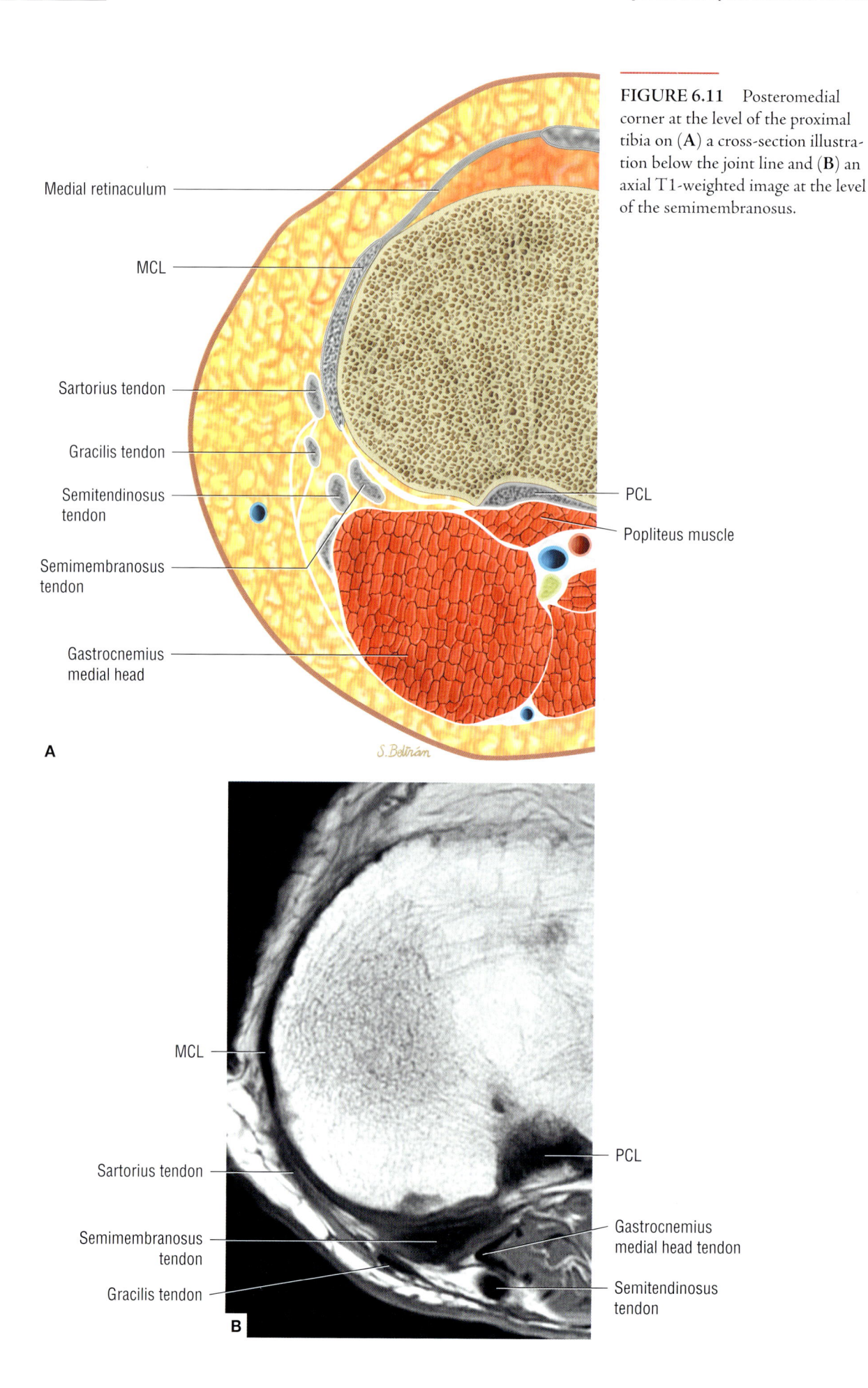

Collateral Ligaments

Pes Tendons and MCL

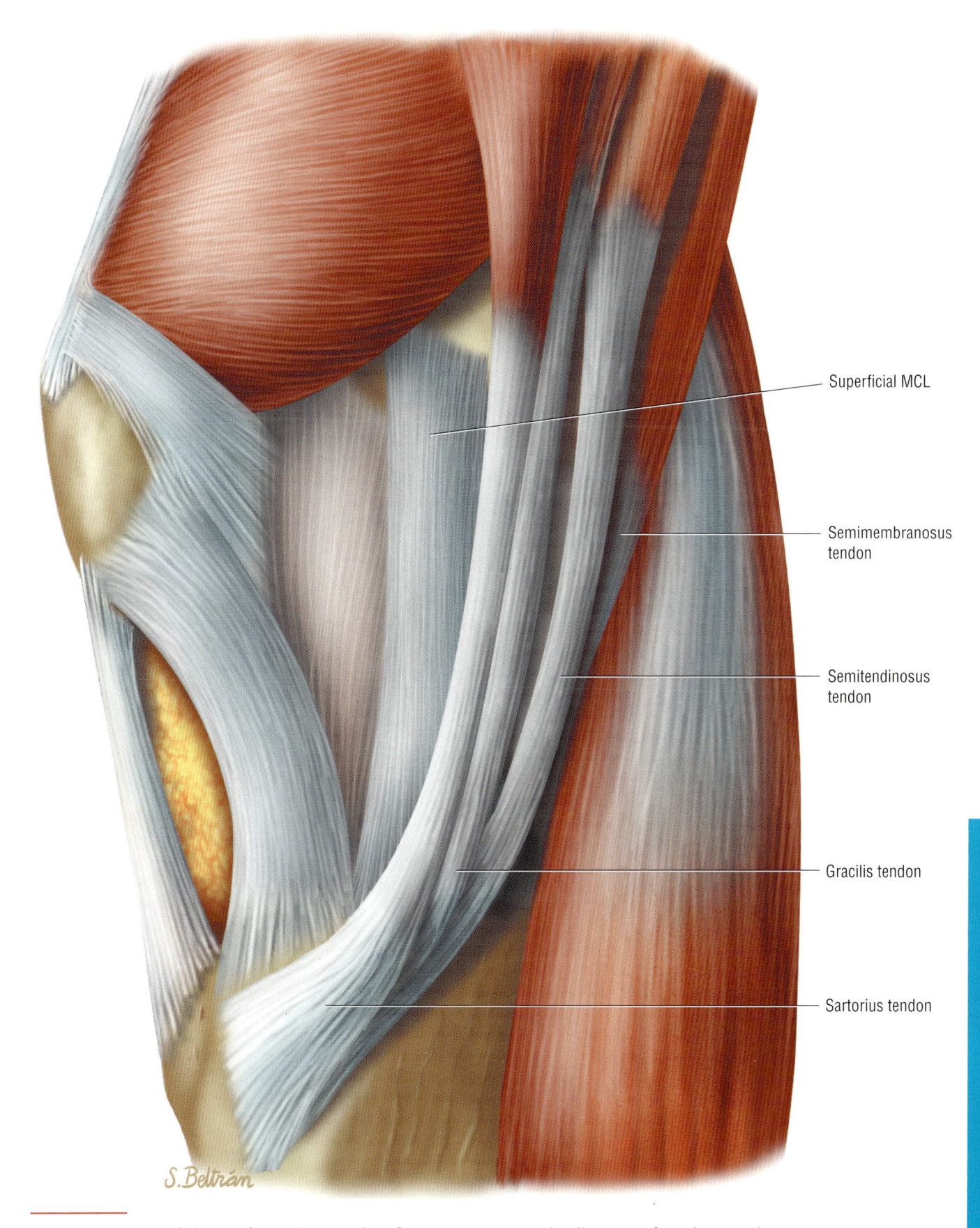

- Superficial MCL
- Semimembranosus tendon
- Semitendinosus tendon
- Gracilis tendon
- Sartorius tendon

FIGURE 6.12 Medial view of normal pes tendons for comparison on a color illustration from the sagittal perspective.

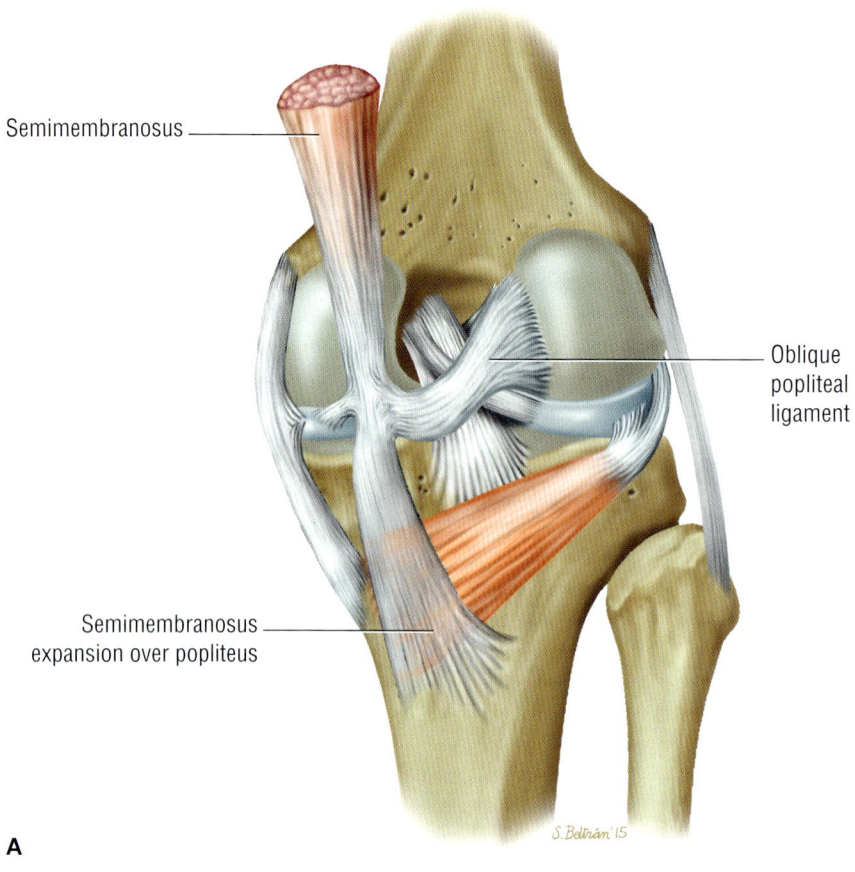

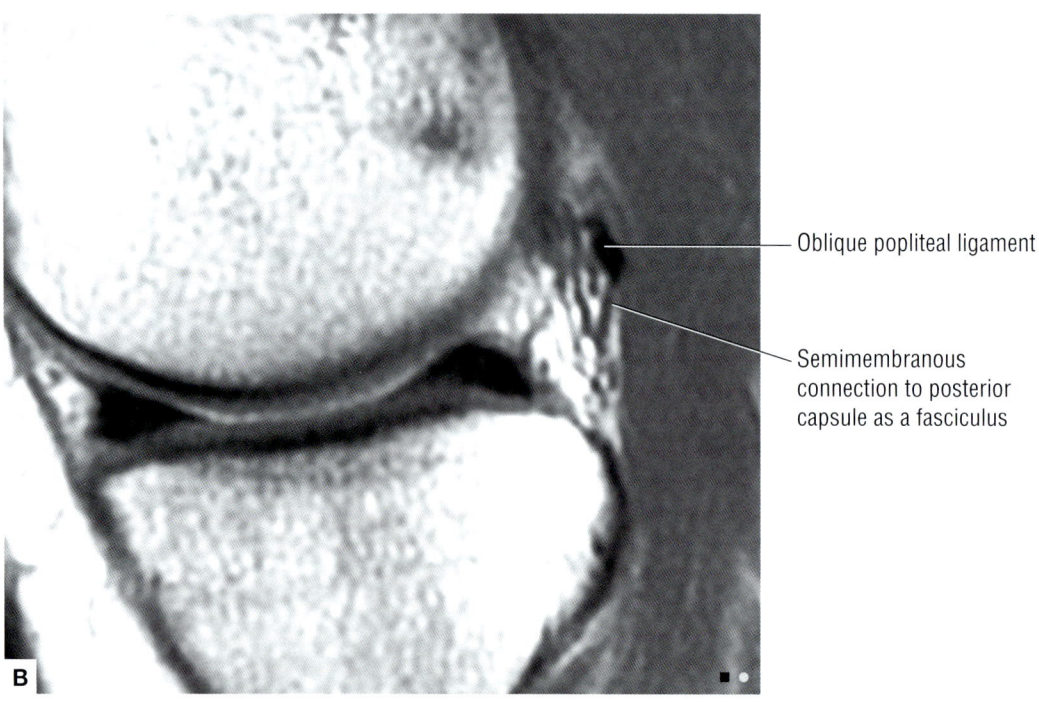

FIGURE 6.13 Medial course of the oblique popliteal ligament in the sagittal plane. The oblique popliteal ligament is a stabilizing structure for the posterior capsule in addition to the arcuate popliteal ligament. The oblique popliteal ligament contributes to the floor of the popliteal fossa immediately deep to the popliteal artery. Coronal posterior perspective (**A**) and PD FSE image (**B**).

Collateral Ligaments 595

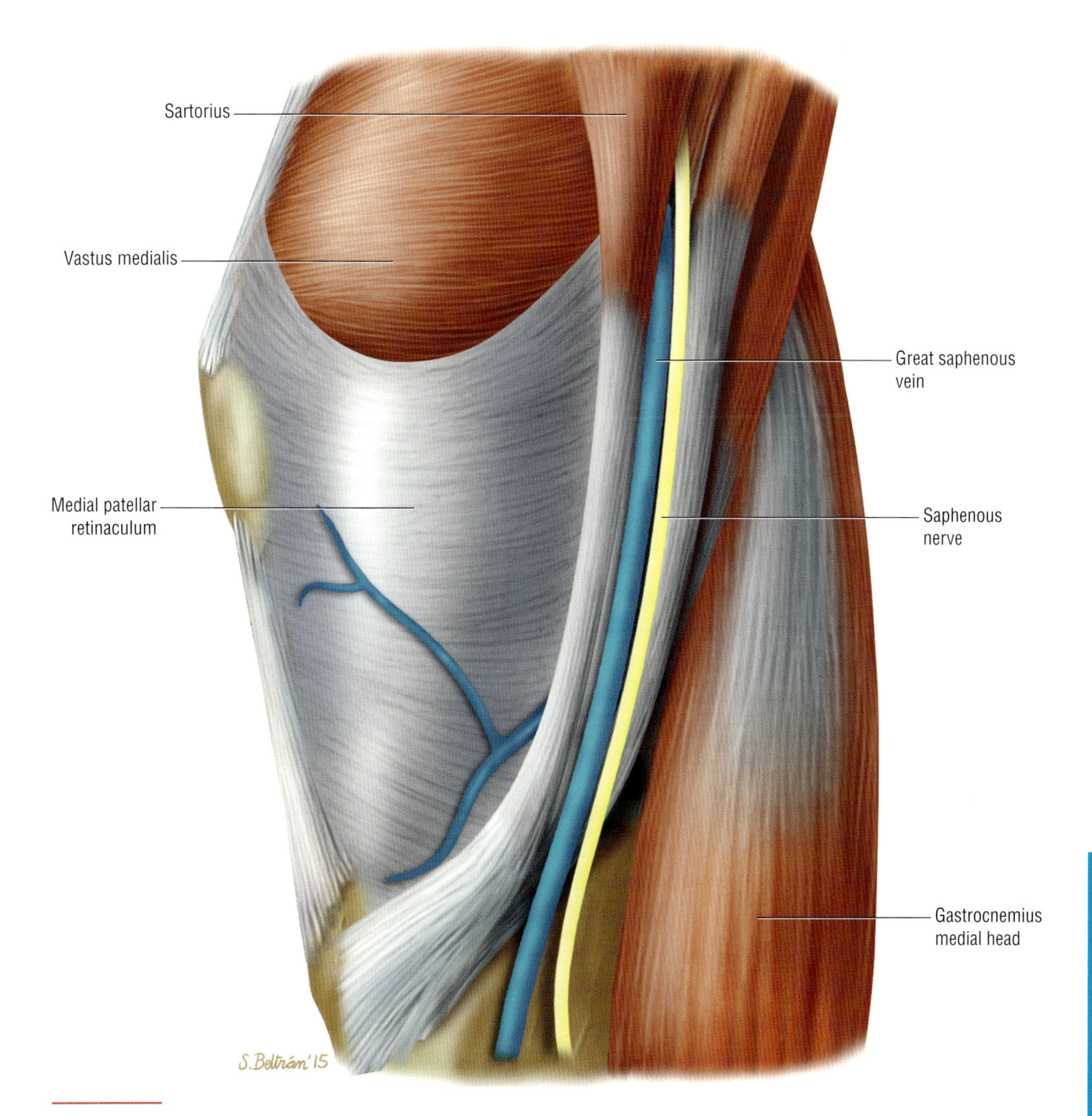

FIGURE 6.14 Layer 1 of the medial side. A deep fascial layer invests the sartorius muscle. Anteriorly, layers 1 and 2 fuse to form the medial patellar retinaculum.

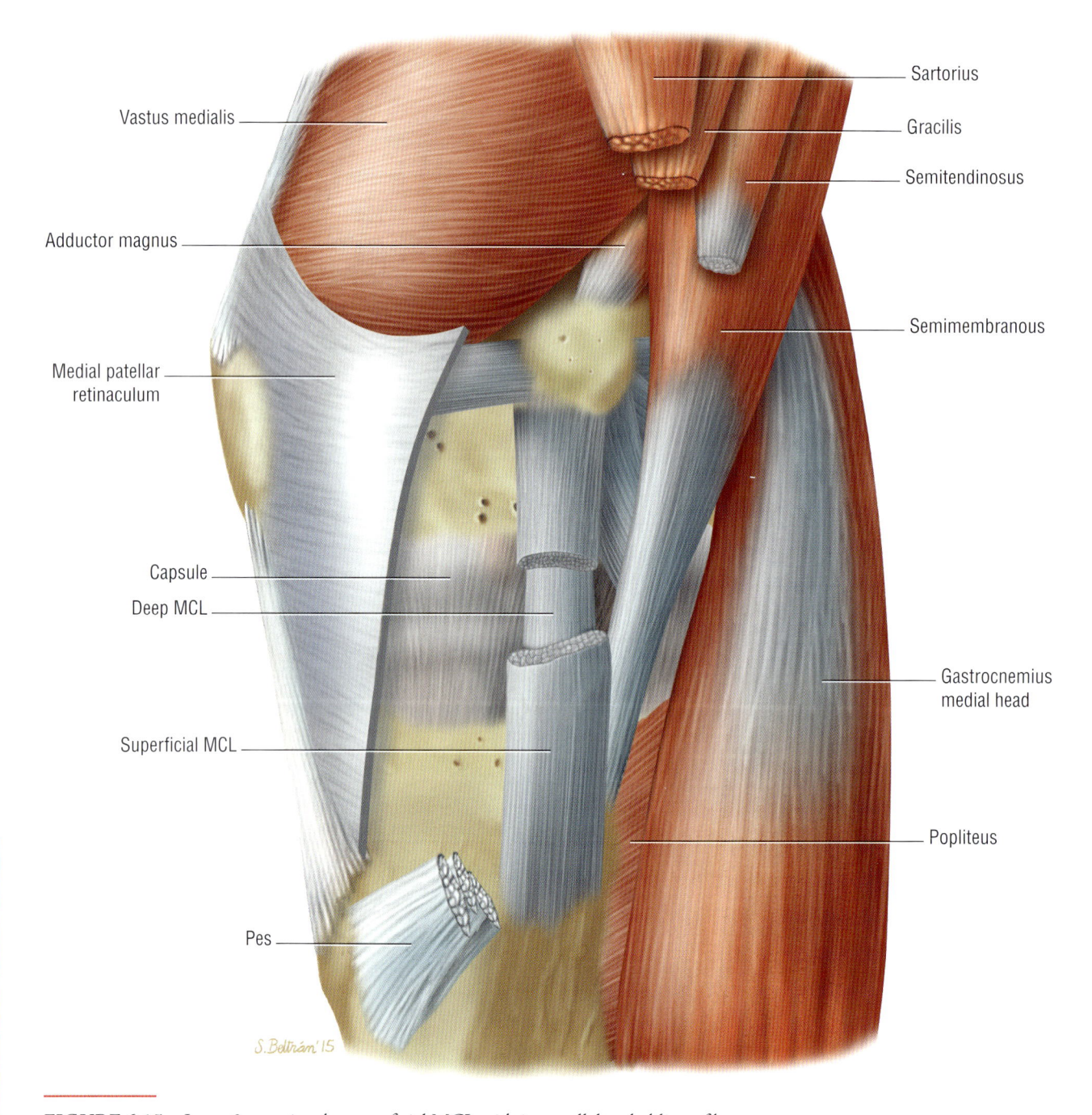

FIGURE 6.15 Layer 2 contains the superficial MCL with its parallel and oblique fibers.

Collateral Ligaments

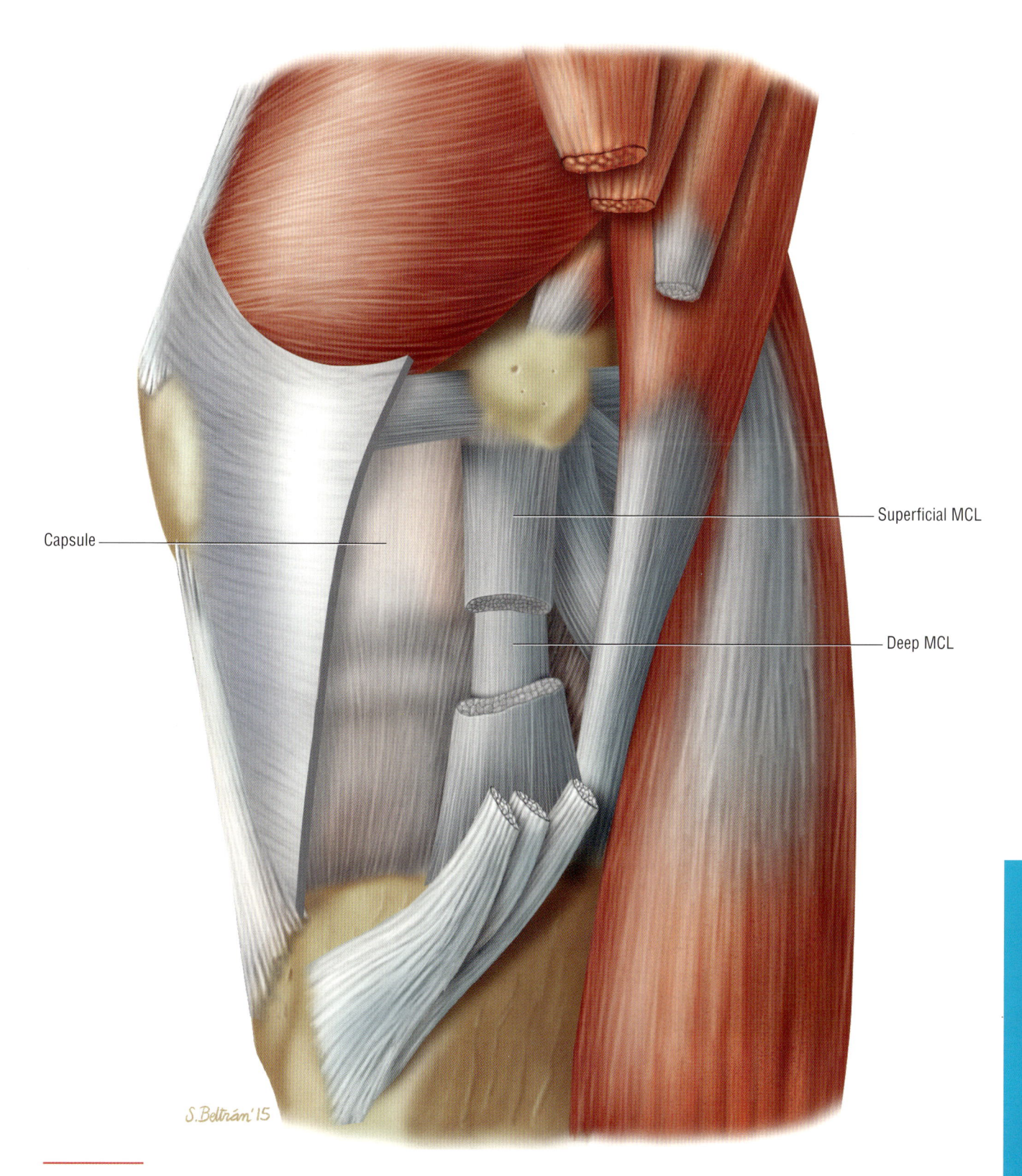

FIGURE 6.16 Layer 3 (joint capsule) is the deep MCL. Anteriorly, the anterior border of the deep MCL can be separated from the superficial MCL (sMCL). Posteriorly the deep MCL bends with the sMCL.

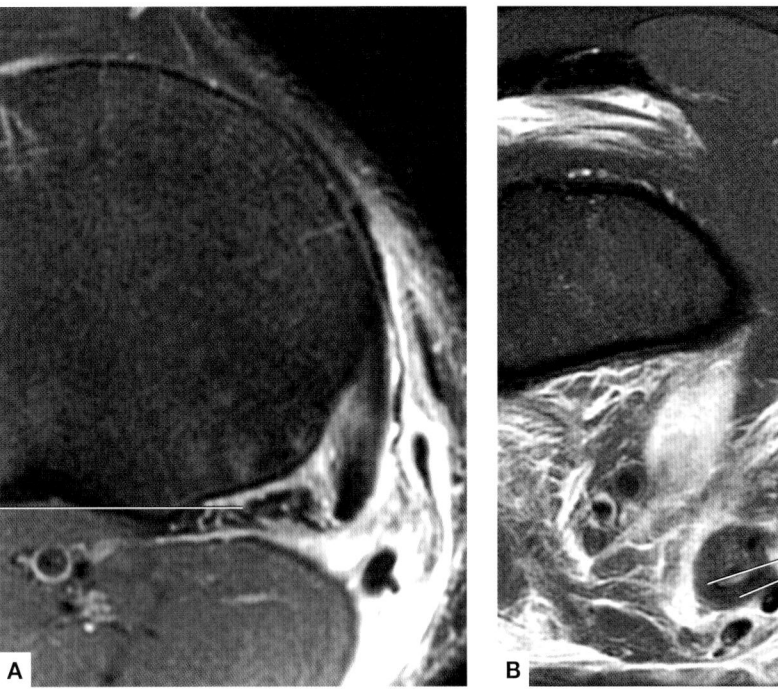

FIGURE 6.17 (**A**) The normal distal semimembranosus expansion on the posteromedial tibia as seen on an axial FS PD FSE image. (**B**) Axial FS PD FSE image in a separate case shows a torn retracted semimembranosus muscle–tendon junction.

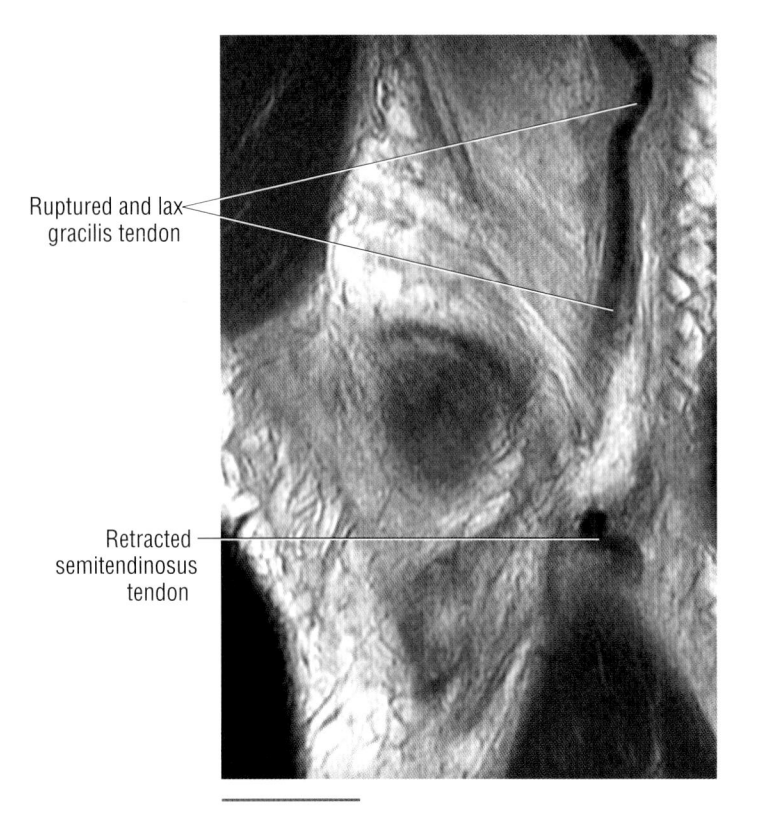

FIGURE 6.18 Ruptured gracilis and semitendinosus tendons on a sagittal PD FSE image.

Location and Mechanism of Injury of the MCL, Including the Posteromedial Corner

- Mechanism of injury
    - Usually a valgus force applied to flexed knee
- Associated injuries
    - Partial ruptures or sprains frequently involve fibrous attachments to medial femoral condyle.
    - Complete MCL rupture may be associated with tears of medial and posterior capsule, ACL, and medial meniscus.[487]
    - Peripheral medial meniscal tears more common with isolated MCL injury
    - Meniscal substance tears more frequently seen with combined MCL and ACL injuries[134]
    - Contusion or fracture from impact of lateral femoral condyle on lateral tibial plateau during valgus injury

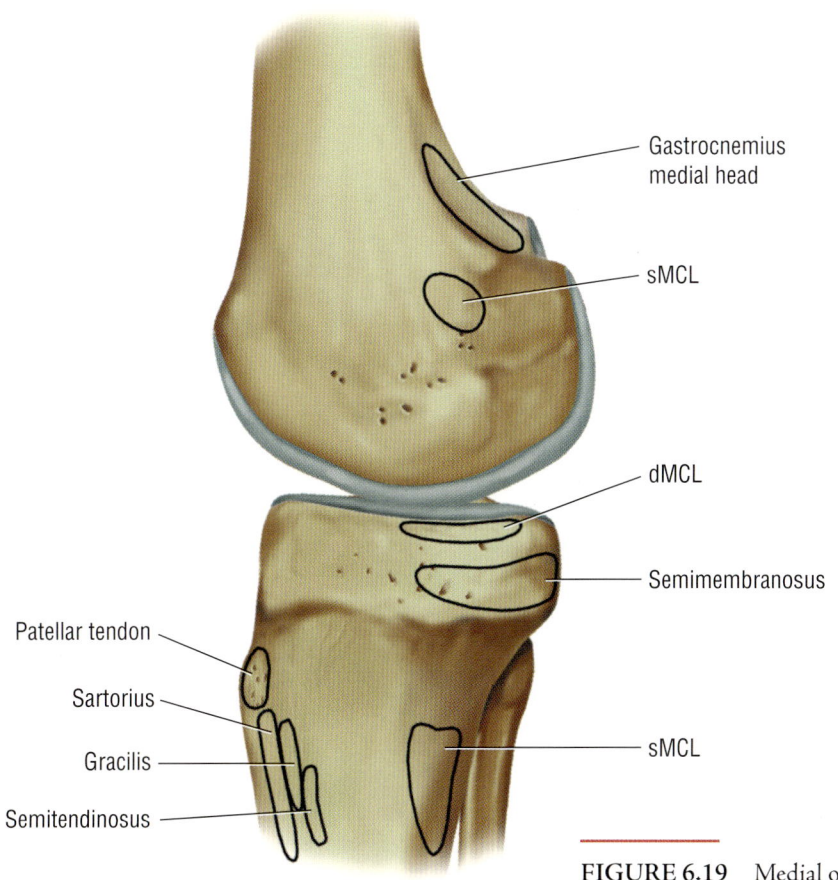

FIGURE 6.19 Medial osseous landmarks.

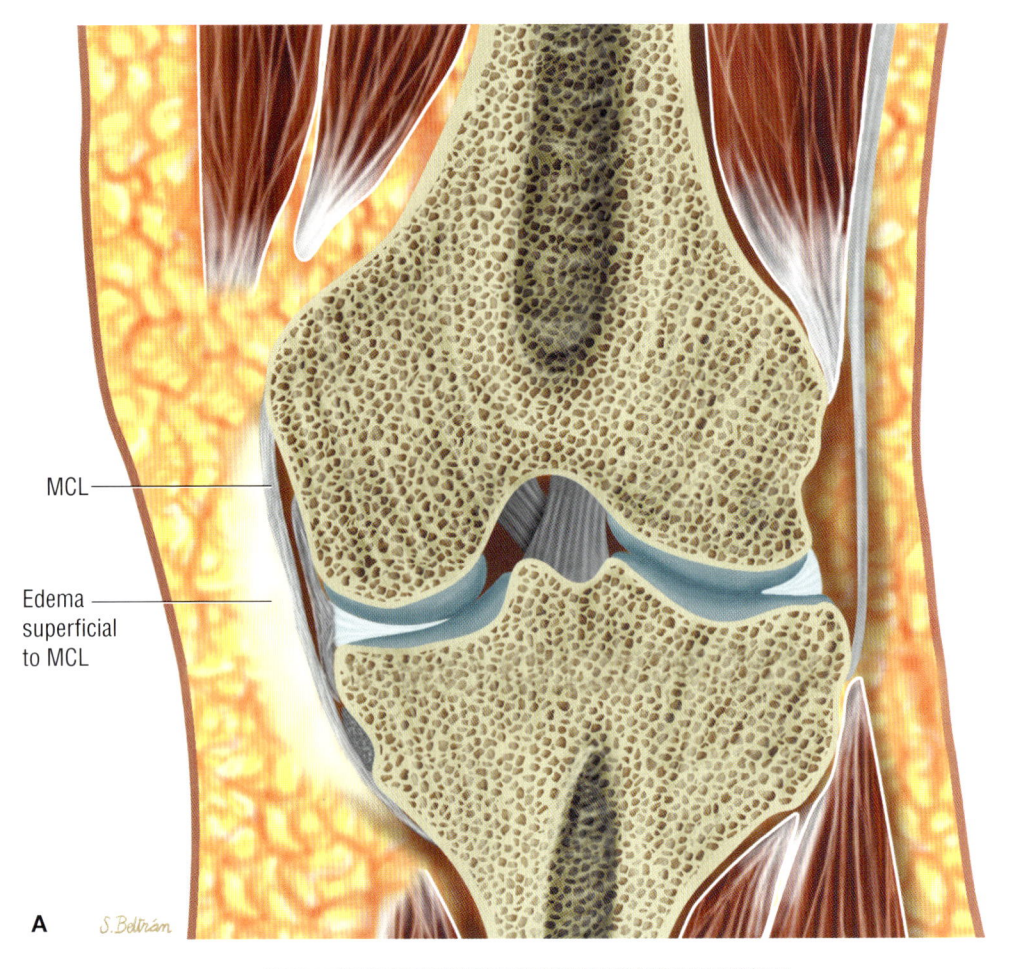

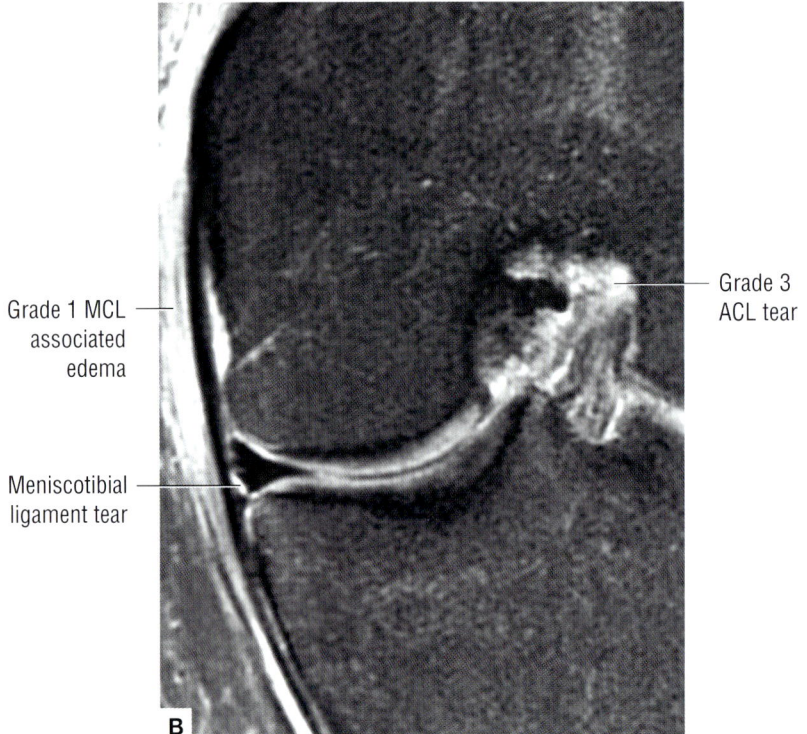

FIGURE 6.20 (**A**) A coronal color section showing a grade 1 MCL sprain with edema superficial to the ligament. Although there may be a few torn fibers, there is no loss of ligamentous integrity. (**B**) Coronal FS PD FSE image showing MCL grade 1 sprain and meniscotibial ligament tear in association with a tear of the ACL.

Classification of MCL Injuries

- Grade 1: minimal tear without instability
- Grade 2: partial tear with increased instability
- Grade 3: complete rupture with gross instability[69]
- Additional classification system for partial tears or sprains, based on quantification of joint space opening:
    - Grade 1: 0 to 5mm
    - Grade 2: 6 to 10mm
    - Grade 3: 11 to 15mm
    - Grade 4: 16 to 20mm
- Stress testing in extremity coil should be performed with knee in partial flexion to produce maximum medial joint space opening.
    - If knee opens with both valgus stress (>10mm for a complete MCL injury) and in full extension → second ligamentous injury, usually involving PCL
- Posteromedial corner or posteromedial capsule (PMC) of knee
    - Important and anatomically complex region
        - Identify most important load-bearing tissue bands relevant during surgical reconstruction/repairs.
        - PMC represents the joint capsule itself with dense fibers arrayed within that course from femoral to tibial attachments.[40]
    - Frequently injured in association with other medial supporting structures and the medial meniscus[393]
    - Receives important contribution from semimembranosus tendon, which has five arms at its insertion
        - Attachment to posteromedial aspect of tibia just distal to joint line
        - More anterior attachment to tibia deep to sMCL
        - Attachment of tendon sheath to PMC
        - Oblique popliteal ligament attachment
        - Distal attachment to fascia of popliteus muscle
        - Femoral attachment of PMC marks the limits of the synovial capsule of the medial condyle.

- Posterior oblique ligament
    - Formed by merging of previously described layers 2 and 3
        - Thicker band that courses in a posterior-distal direction
        - Passes from attachment distal/posterior to adductor tubercle to rim of the posterior medial tibial plateau
    - Represents connection between capsular attachment of semimembranosus tendon and oblique fibers of sMCL
- Functionally, posteromedial corner resists valgus laxity in knee extension.
    - Since PMC is attached posterior to femoral axis of flexion, it slackens or becomes lax with knee flexion.
    - The medial structures, including the PMC, function as important secondary restraints against tibial posterior drawer with the knee at or near full extension. The PMC is tightened in knee extension and tibial internal rotation (restraint to both internal rotation and posterior drawer).[40]
- Posteromedial corner injuries frequently involve the posterior horn of medial meniscus (peripheral aspect), popliteal oblique ligament, and MCL.
- Although semitendinosus tendon does not directly contribute to posteromedial corner, semitendinosus injuries may present with posteromedial knee pain.

Biomechanics of the MCL

- sMCL is not significantly stronger than PMC.
    - Both structures are stronger than the dMCL.
- sMCL has higher tensile stiffness than the dMCL or PMC.
    - sMCL can resist a greater load with an applied abduction (valgus) moment.
- dMCL fails at a lower elongation stress than the sMCL or PMC.
- Failure loads are higher in younger and more active population.[40]
    - Failure of sMCL by avulsion of the femoral attachment[40]

Magnetic Resonance (MR) Appearance of the MCL

- MR evaluation of MCL injuries best accomplished with coronal images
  - Demonstrate low-signal MCL and attachment points
  - Separation of deep and superficial layers distinguished on FS PD FSE-weighted images
- Intraligamentous bursa
  - Thin band of intermediate signal intensity between layers 2 and 3, originally thought to be fat
  - Often seen between anterior portion of MCL and deep medial capsular ligament complex[11]
  - Bursa may extend proximal and distal to the level of the joint line medially.
  - Increased signal intensity above or below the level of the meniscus may represent pathologic change, especially if it is seen where layers 2 and 3 fuse posteriorly.
- Separation of meniscofemoral and meniscotibial components of medial capsular ligament usually displayed on routine orthogonal coronal images
- Peripheral sagittal and axial images also used to identify course of oblique popliteal ligament at level of distal femoral condyle and joint line
  - Oblique popliteal ligament visualized as linear area of low signal intensity often appearing at same level as arcuate ligament complex
- Acute MCL sprain and tear
  - Grade 1 MCL injury (sprain)
    - Edema and hemorrhage identified parallel to sMCL and extending into subcutaneous fat
    - MCL remains normal in thickness and closely applied to underlying cortical bone.
  - Grade 2 MCL injury (partial tear)
    - Displacement of ligament fibers from adjacent cortical bone
    - High-signal-intensity edema and/or hemorrhage superficial and deep to MCL fibers.[421]

- Ligamentous attenuation or areas of fluid separating partially torn fibers
- Intraligamentous hyperintensity and thickening
- Segmental or focal ligamentous thickening
- Contusions of either medial femoral condyle or lateral tibial plateau may be associated with grade 2 or 3 sprains.

- **Grade 3 MCL injury (complete tear)**
  - Complete loss of continuity of ligamentous fibers with or without extension into capsular layer
  - Complete biomechanical failure of MCL is associated with disruption of medial capsular layer or ligament.[206,240]

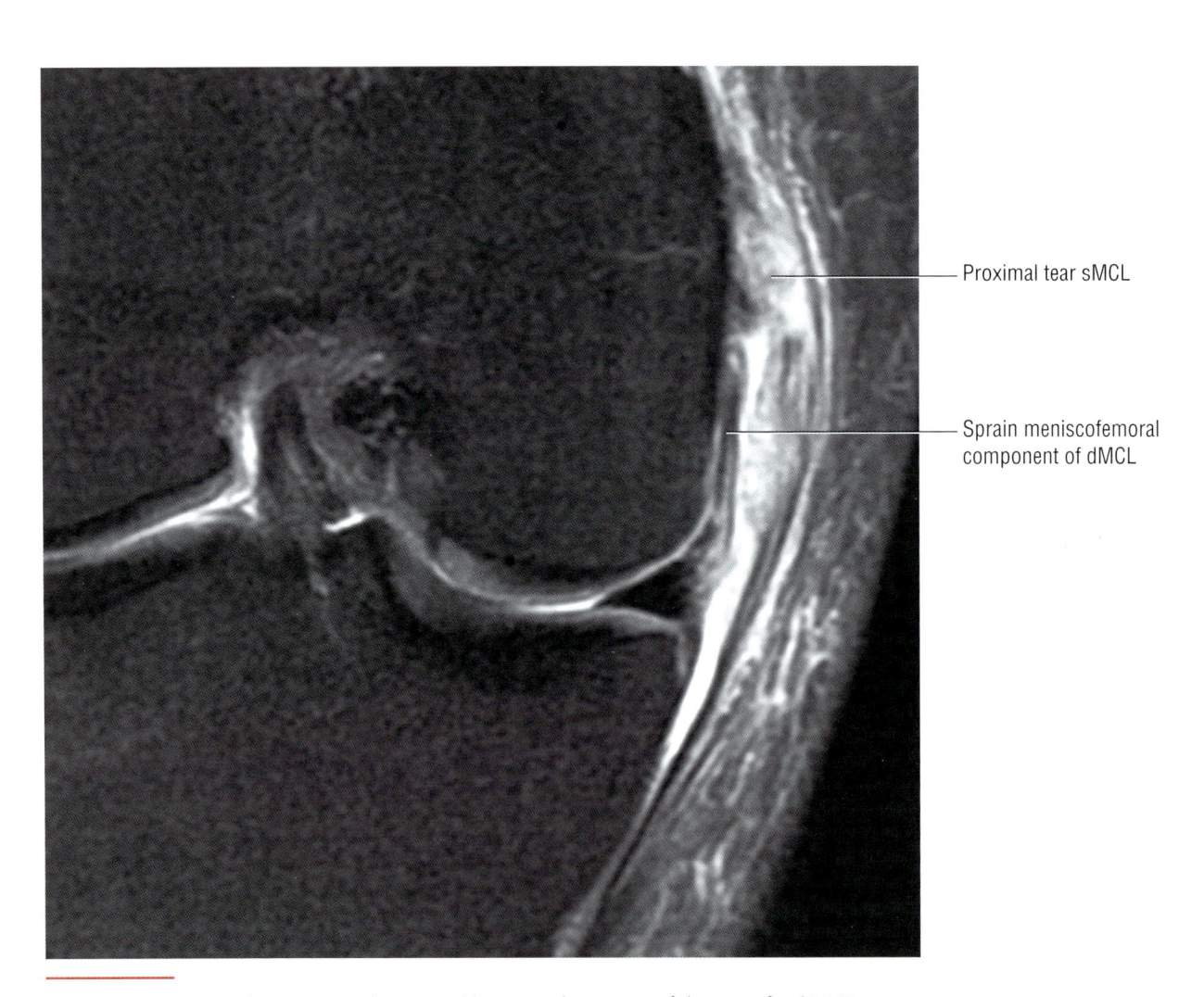

FIGURE 6.21 Grade 3 MCL with proximal ligament disruption of the superficial MCL (sMCL) and thickened sprained deep MCL (dMCL). Coronal FS PD FSE image.

Collateral Ligaments 605

MCL Sprain

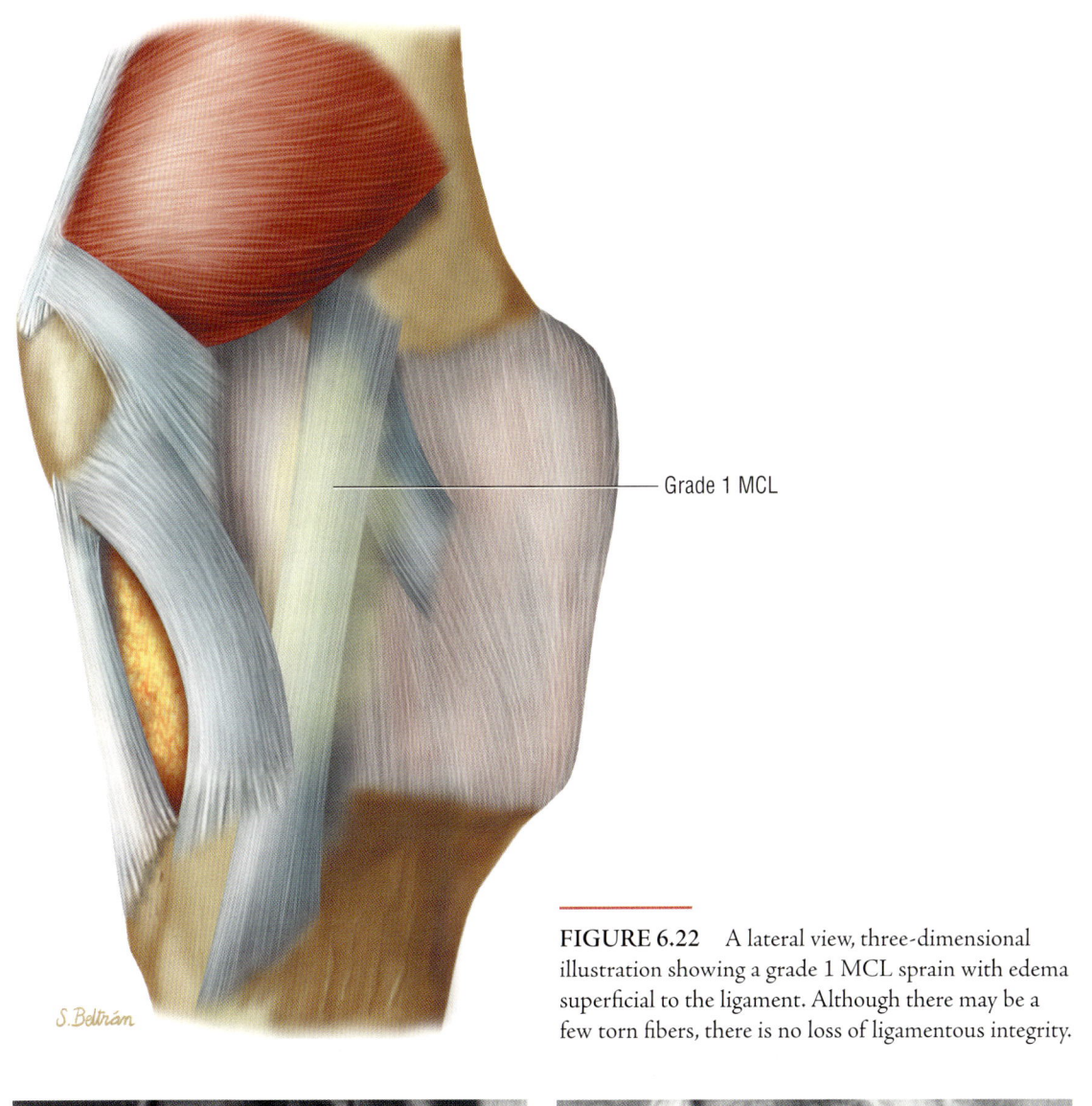

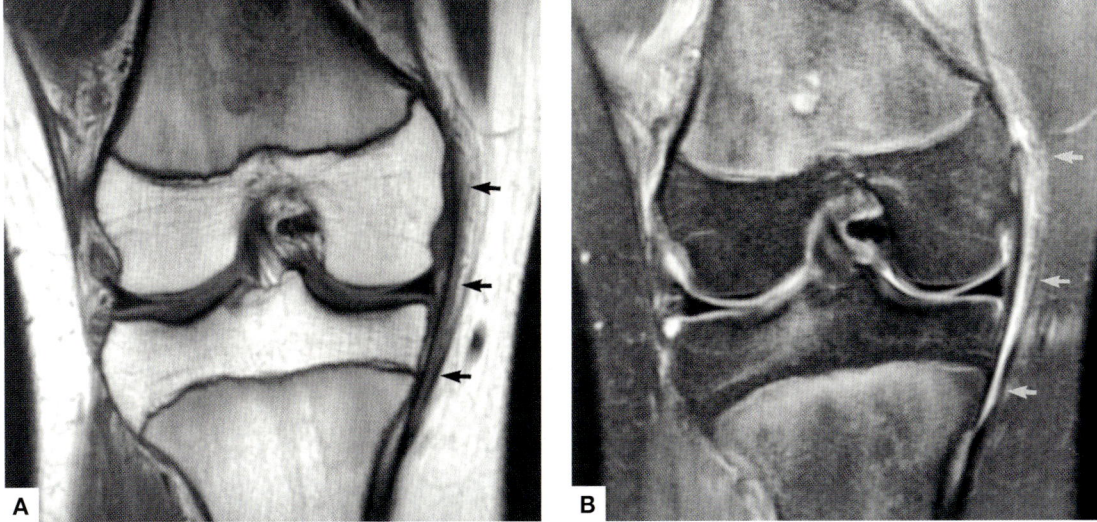

FIGURE 6.22 A lateral view, three-dimensional illustration showing a grade 1 MCL sprain with edema superficial to the ligament. Although there may be a few torn fibers, there is no loss of ligamentous integrity.

FIGURE 6.23 Grade 1 MCL sprain with fluid (*arrows*) superficial to the MCL is hypointense on a T1-weighted coronal image (**A**) and hyperintense on an FS PD-weighted FSE coronal image (**B**). There is no displacement or thickening of the low-signal-intensity ligament. A grade 1 tear is primarily a periligamentous injury with associated microscopic tearing of ligament fibers. Edema superficial to the MCL may in fact be related to a medial retinaculum sprain.

MCL Sprain

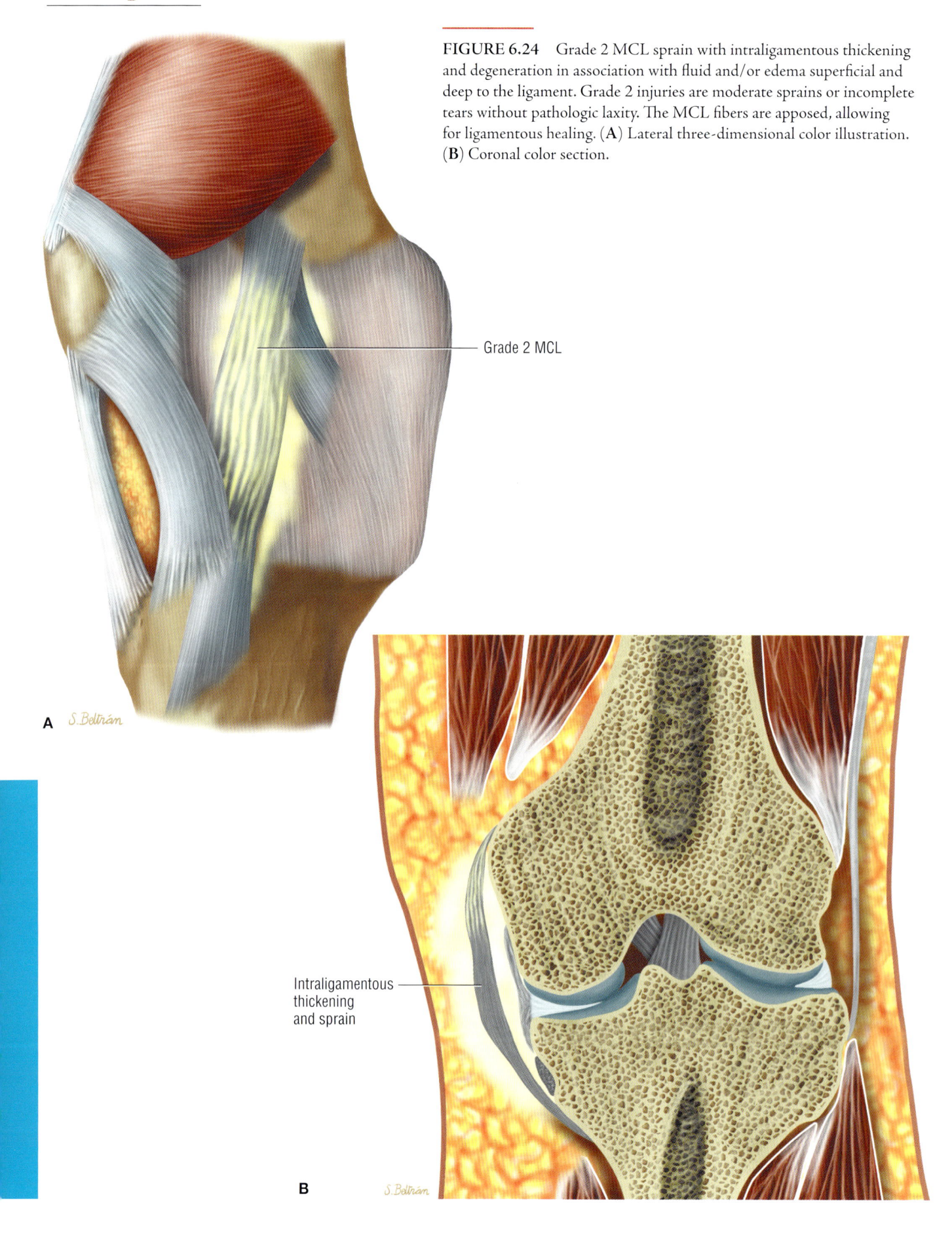

FIGURE 6.24 Grade 2 MCL sprain with intraligamentous thickening and degeneration in association with fluid and/or edema superficial and deep to the ligament. Grade 2 injuries are moderate sprains or incomplete tears without pathologic laxity. The MCL fibers are apposed, allowing for ligamentous healing. (**A**) Lateral three-dimensional color illustration. (**B**) Coronal color section.

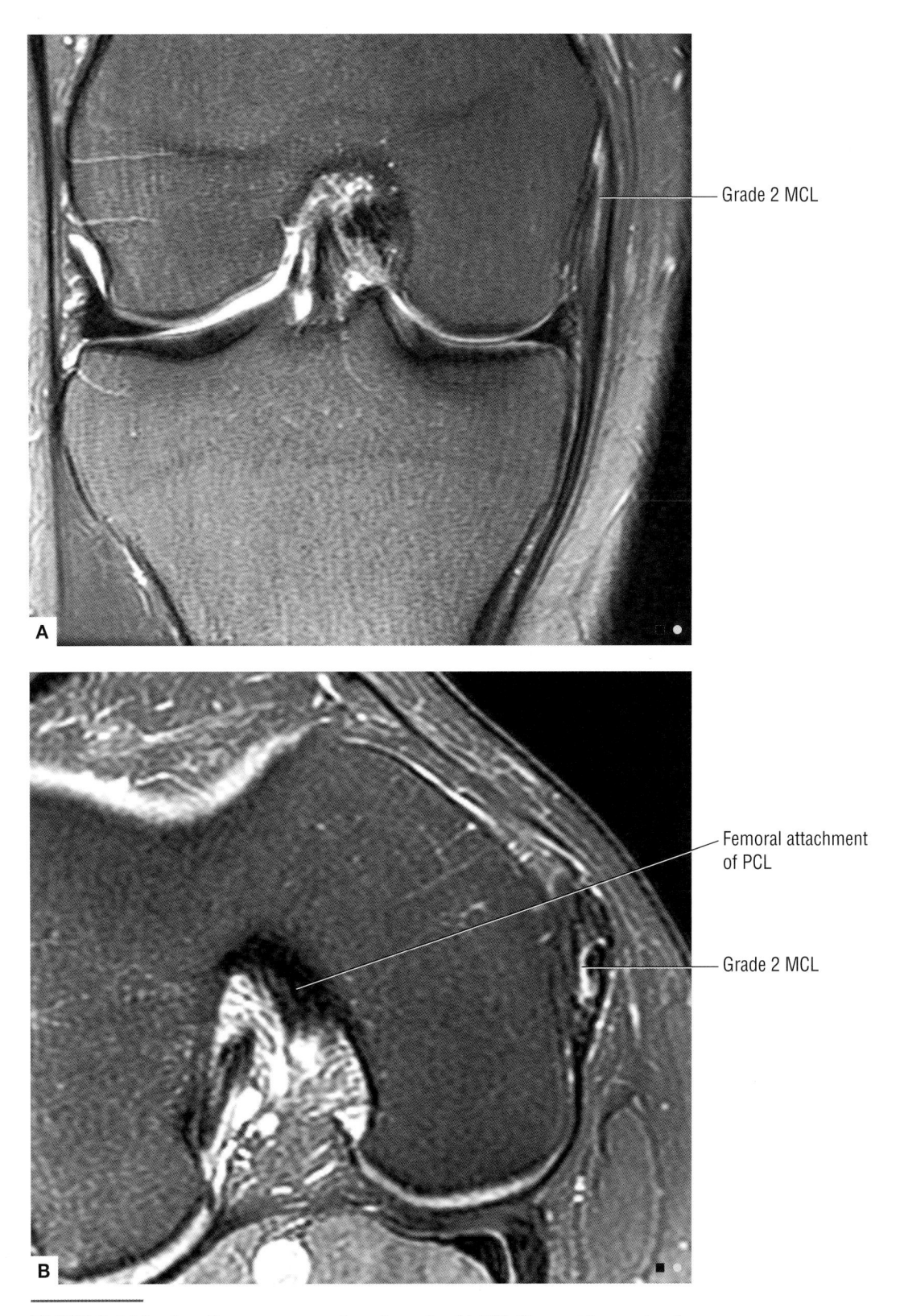

FIGURE 6.25 Intraligamentous tearing of proximal MCL fibers with associated ligament thickening. Coronal (**A**) and axial (**B**) FS PD FSE images.

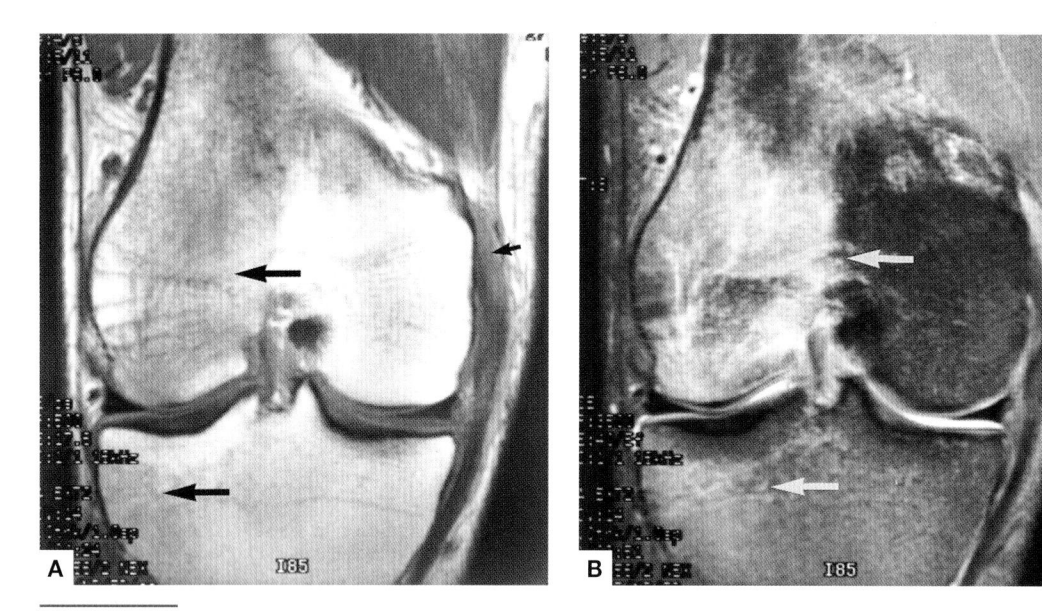

FIGURE 6.26 T1 (**A**) and FS PD-weighted FSE (**B**) coronal images of a grade 2 MCL tear. The tear is characterized by ligamentous thickening, intraligamentous hyperintensity (*small arrows*), and edema superficial and deep to the ligament. There is no loss of MCL continuity. The valgus mechanism of injury is associated with lateral compartment bone contusions (*large arrows*). Because the distinction between grade 2 and grade 3 tears may be difficult, these injuries often are classified as a grade 2/3 sprain.

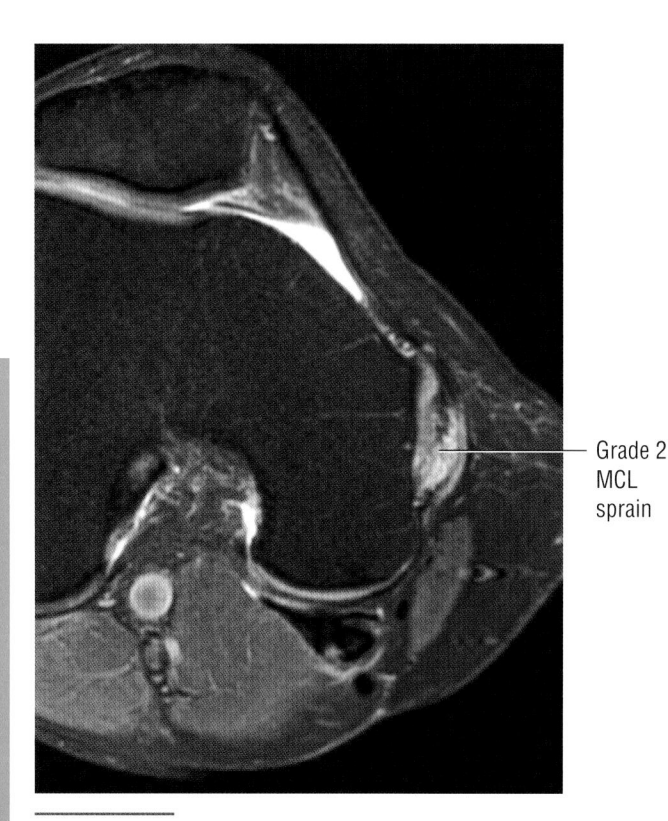

FIGURE 6.27 Grade 2 MCL sprain with thickened hyperintense fibers without loss of taut ligament (axial FS PD FSE image).

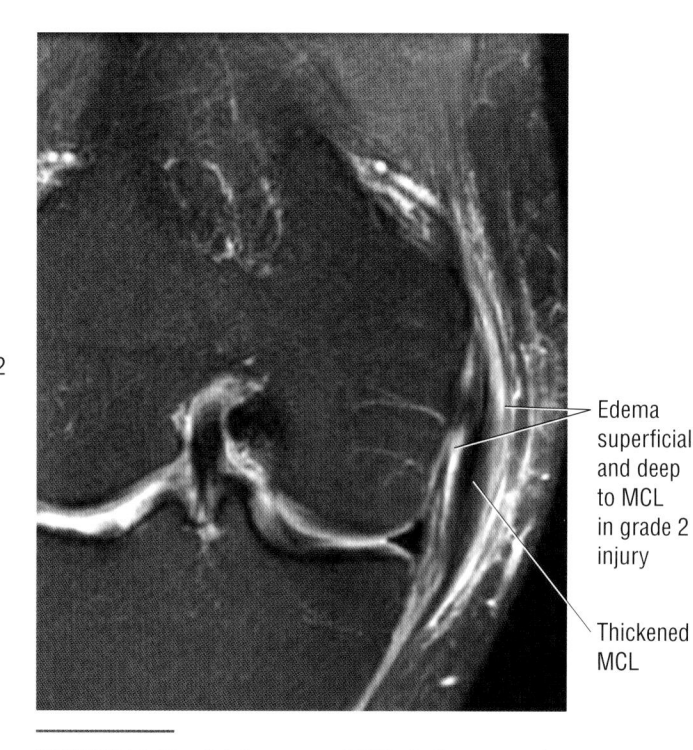

FIGURE 6.28 Mid-segment MCL thickening without loss of continuity. Edema is superficial and deep to this grade 2 sprain (coronal FS PD FSE image).

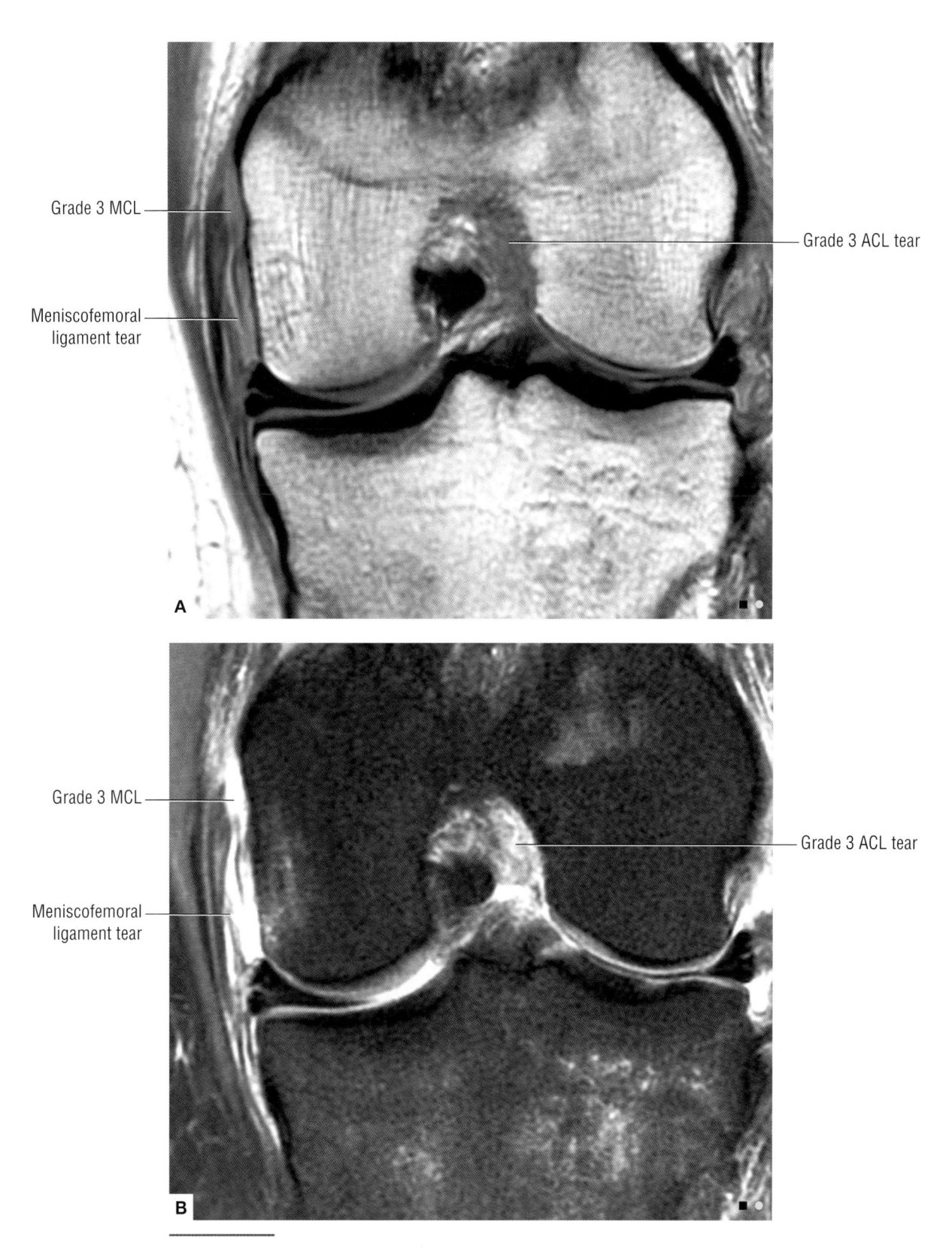

FIGURE 6.29 Grade 3 tear of proximal MCL femoral attachment with associated disruption of the meniscofemoral ligament. Coronal PD (**A**) and FS PD (**B**) images. Meniscofemoral failure occurs more easily than meniscotibial failure.

MCL Sprain

Proximal MCL tear (grade 3)

Thickened and edematous MCL fibers

S. Beltrán

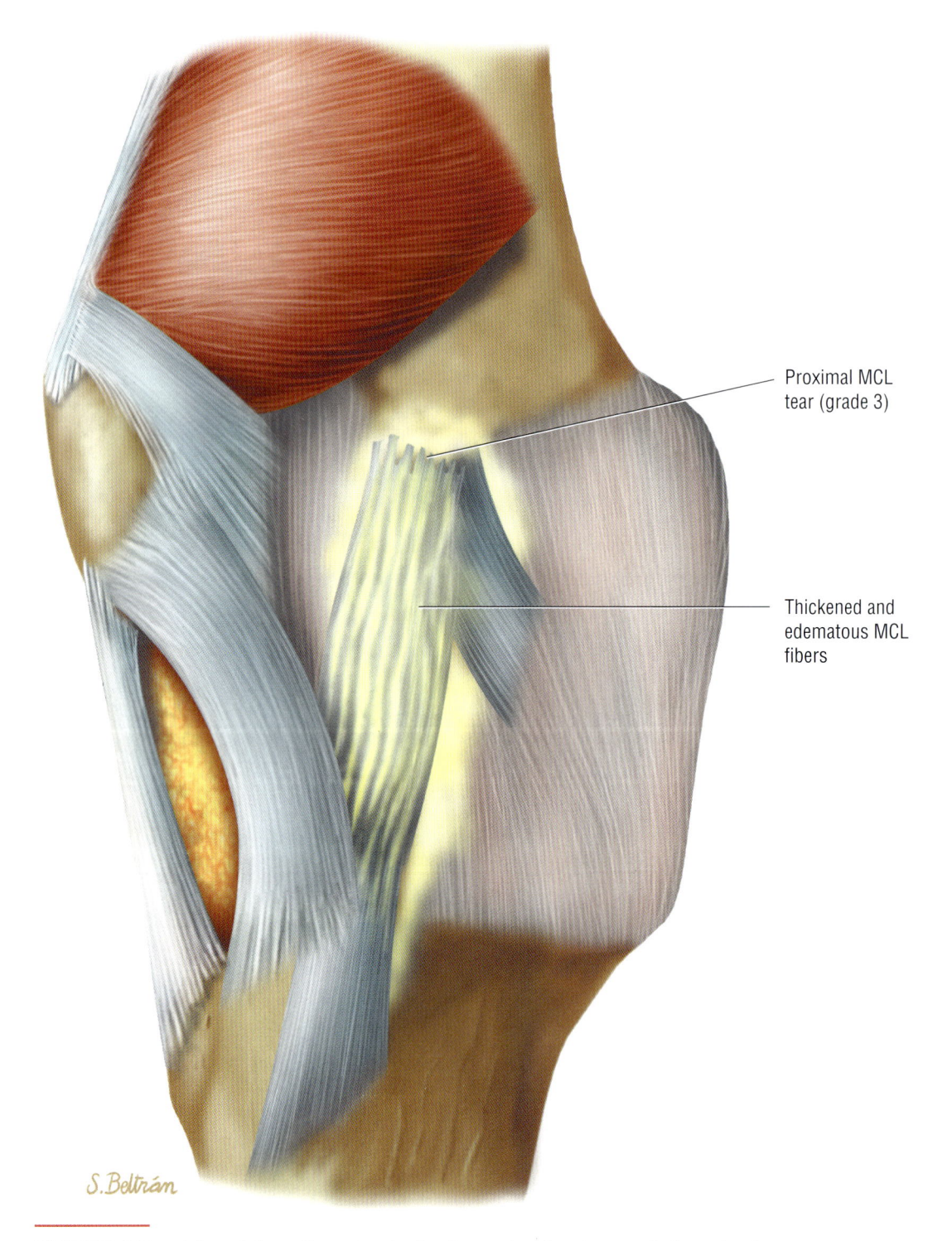

FIGURE 6.30 A lateral three-dimensional color illustration showing a grade 3 proximal sprain or tear with loss of ligament integrity. Swelling and ecchymosis are common, and there is associated pathologic laxity. Grade 3 tears may have no endpoint to abduction stress.

Associated MR Findings of the MCL

- Extensive joint effusion/hemarthrosis and extravasation of joint fluid (which tracks along ligament fibers)
- Associated capsular disruption
    - May result in diminished or absent joint swelling
    - May be associated with peripheral meniscal tear and widening of medial joint space
- Focal hemorrhage at femoral epicondylar attachment in complete ligamentous avulsions
    - May see subchondral marrow hyperemia or hemorrhage in adjacent bone
    - Subacute hemorrhage demonstrates increased signal intensity on T1- and T2-weighted images.
- Tear of distal or tibial attachment
    - May be associated with wavy or serpiginous ligamentous contour due to ligamentous laxity
    - Retracted distal MCL tear may have more serpiginous morphology and requires surgical repair.
    - May be associated with pes tendon sprains, although a pes tendon rupture can occur without MCL tear
    - FS PD-weighted FSE images useful in documenting interval healing with reattachment of torn MCL
    - Process of religamentization or healing may be associated with intermediate signal in region of increased ligament thickness.
- Chronic MCL tear
    - Thickened ligament without increased signal intensity
        - Axial images particularly useful in identifying separation of distal MCL fibers from underlying tibia and, in conjunction with coronal images, evaluating extent of injury and involvement of either anterior or posterior portions of sMCL
        - Coronal images also used to quantify proximal retraction or laxity associated with distal MCL tears
    - *Pellegrini-Stieda disease*
        - Ossification of the femoral epicondylar or proximal attachment of the MCL

- Thought to be result of chronic trauma
- Areas of ossification may demonstrate marrow fat signal intensity or may be hypointense if sclerotic.
- Thickened ligamentous healing may be demonstrated at same time that calcification or periarticular ossification is detected.
- Ossification may affect MCL, adductor magnus tendon, or both.
- Acute MCL avulsions may also be associated with low-signal-intensity fractured cortical fragment.

- **Osseous injuries**
    - Nondisplaced compression fractures of lateral tibial plateau secondary to valgus injury
    - Contusions in lateral femoral condyle
    - Fractures or bone contusions demonstrate low signal intensity on T1-weighted images and increased signal intensity on T2-weighted, FS FSE, and STIR images.
    - MR is sensitive for identification of these injuries, even when radiographic findings are normal.[469]

- **MCL (tibial collateral ligament) and pes anserinus bursitis**
    - Patients present with medial joint pain.
    - MCL bursitis
        - Hyperintense signal between layer 2 (sMCL) and layer 3 (medial capsular ligament) on T2- or FSE PD-weighted scans
        - Well-defined, elongated collection of fluid extending predominantly inferior to the joint line
        - May be observed without associated pathology in medial meniscus, capsular ligament, or MCL[94]
    - Pes anserinus bursitis
        - Characterized by fluid anterior to conjoined sartorius, semitendinosus, and gracilis tendons
        - Demonstrates low signal intensity on T1-weighted images and hyperintensity on FS PD FSE images
        - May see septation or hemorrhage within the bursa[142]
        - Pes bursa overlies the pes tendons and is located distal to the MCL bursa.
        - Associated with athletic activity or degenerative arthritis

Collateral Ligaments

Retracted MCL fibers (sMCL)

Meniscotibial ligament tear (dMCL)

MCL tear (sMCL)

Retracted meniscotibial ligament

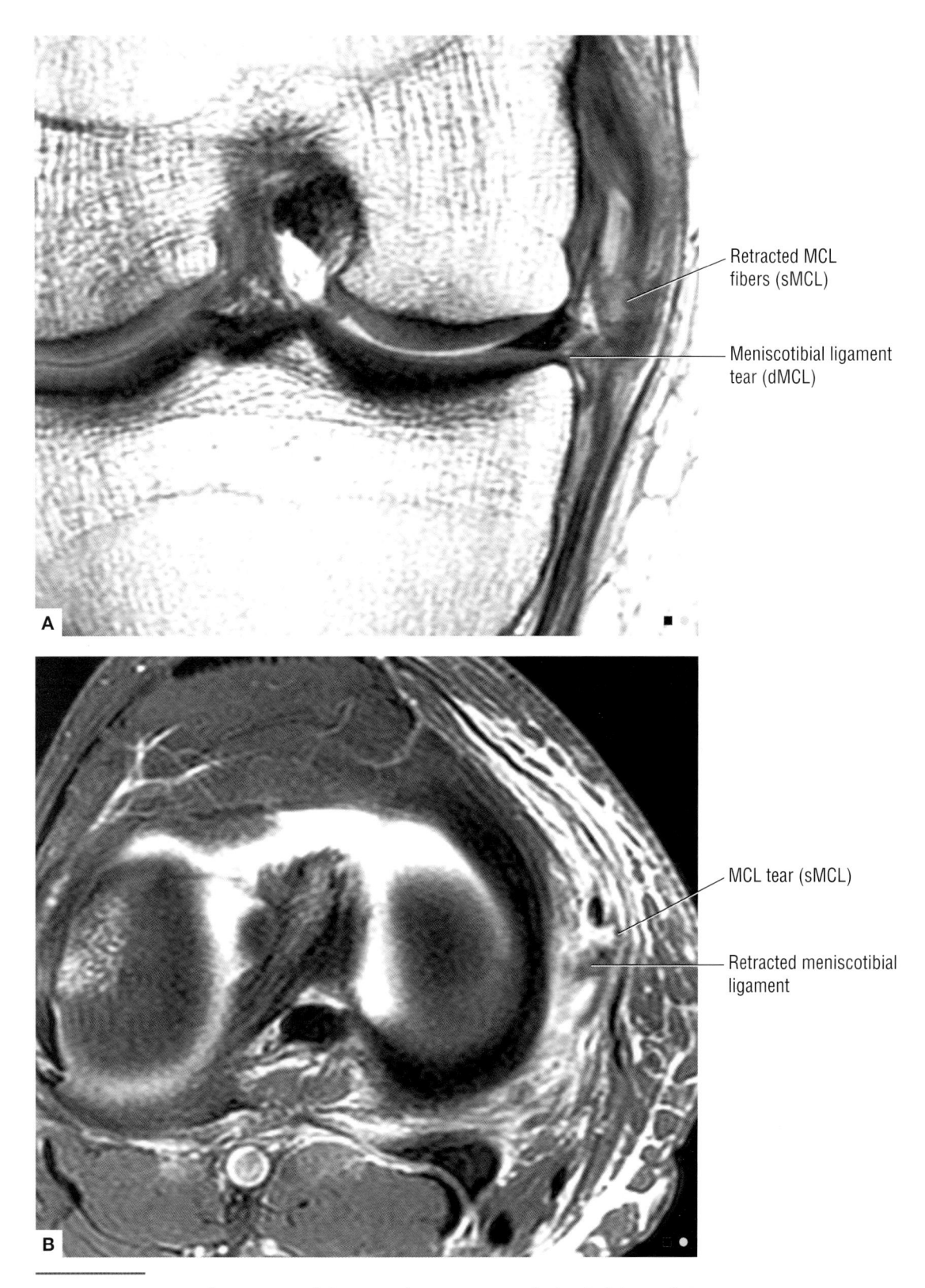

FIGURE 6.31 Grade 3 MCL with ligament discontinuity at the level of the medial joint line. Potential incarceration of interposed deep MCL (dMCL) into tear site of the superficial MCL (sMCL). Coronal PD (**A**) and axial FS PD (**B**) images.

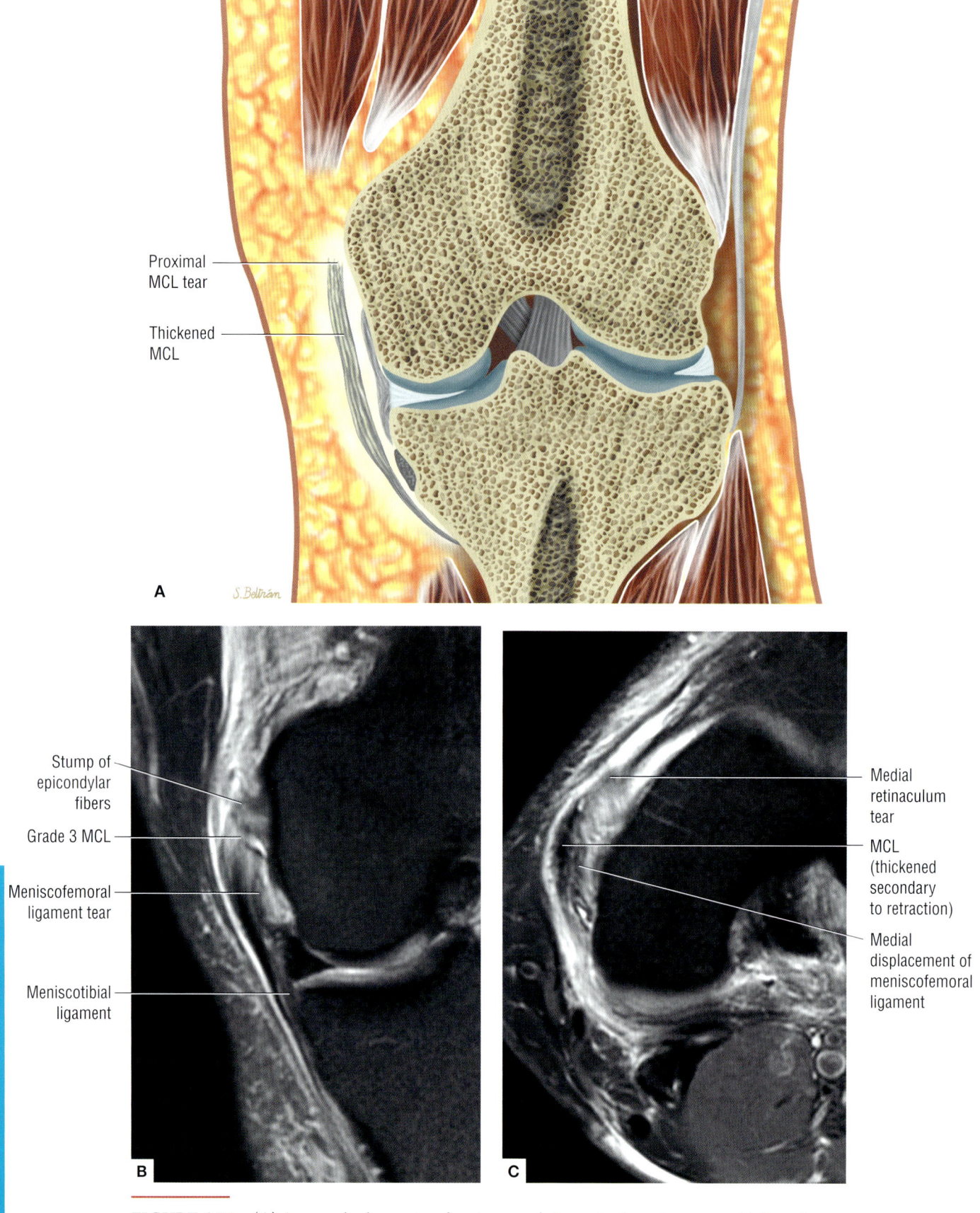

FIGURE 6.32 (**A**) A coronal color section showing a grade 3 proximal sprain or tear with loss of ligament integrity. Swelling and ecchymosis are common, and there is associated pathologic laxity. Grade 3 tears may have no endpoint to abduction stress. Coronal (**B**) and axial (**C**) FS PD FSE images of a grade 3 proximal MCL tear. A small stump of proximal epicondylar fibers remains (**B**). The meniscofemoral ligament is torn, whereas the meniscotibial ligament is intact. The associated tearing of the medial retinaculum is shown in the axial plane (**C**). Note the increased thickness of the partially retracted MCL.

Collateral Ligaments

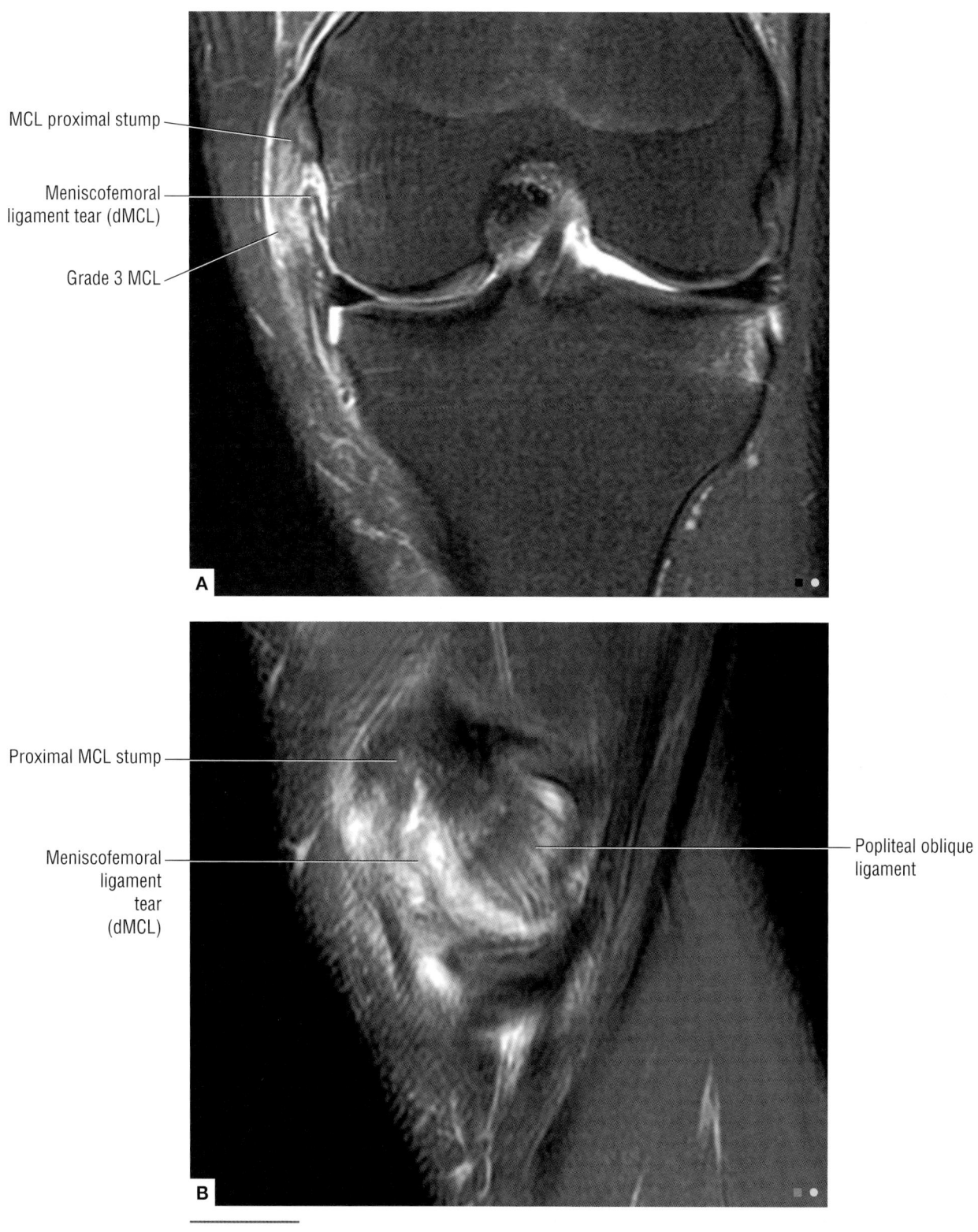

FIGURE 6.33 Grade 3 MCL with femoral ligamentous stump and disrupted meniscofemoral ligament (deep MCL). Coronal (**A**) and sagittal (**B**) FS PD FSE images.

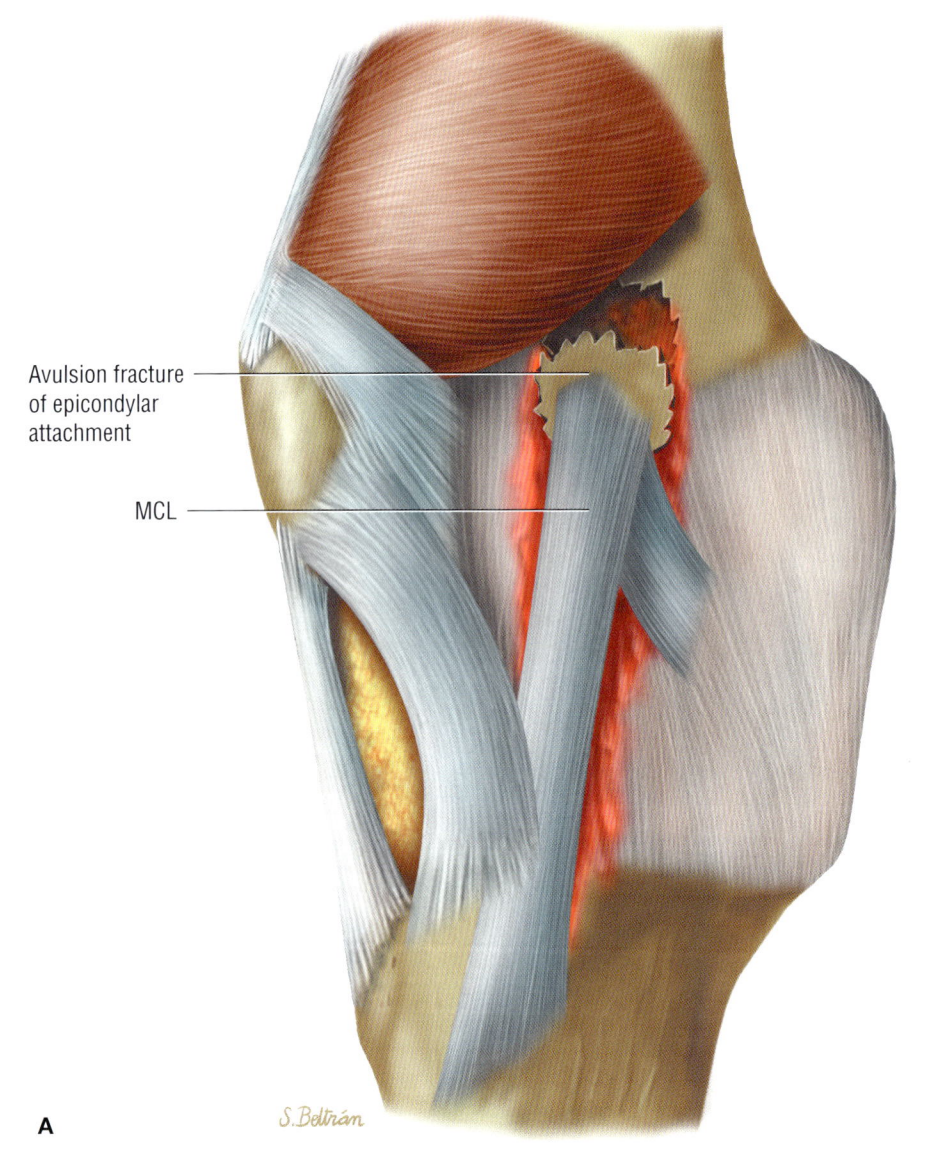

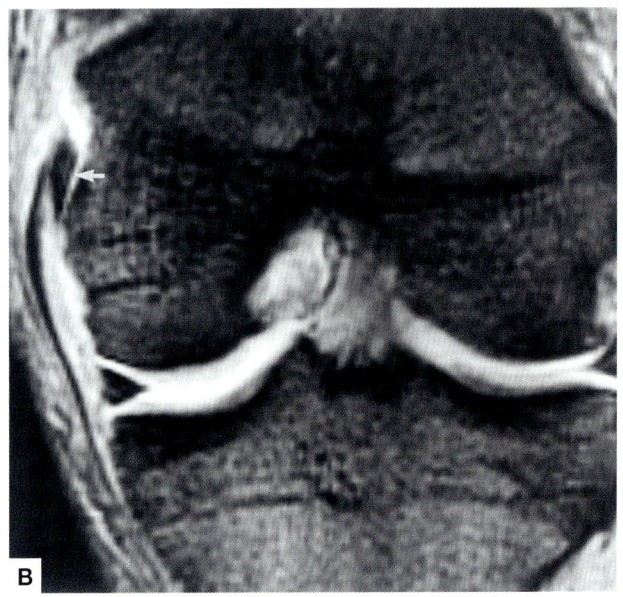

FIGURE 6.34 (A) Lateral view, three-dimensional color illustration of an avulsion fracture of the epicondylar attachment of the MCL. (B) A grade 3 MCL tear with an avulsed bone fragment (*arrow*) from the femoral epicondyle is seen on this T2*-weighted coronal image. The associated extracapsular hemorrhage is hyperintense.

Collateral Ligaments 617

Medial epicondylar avulsion fracture
MCL attachment to avulsed fragment

Medial epicondylar avulsion fracture

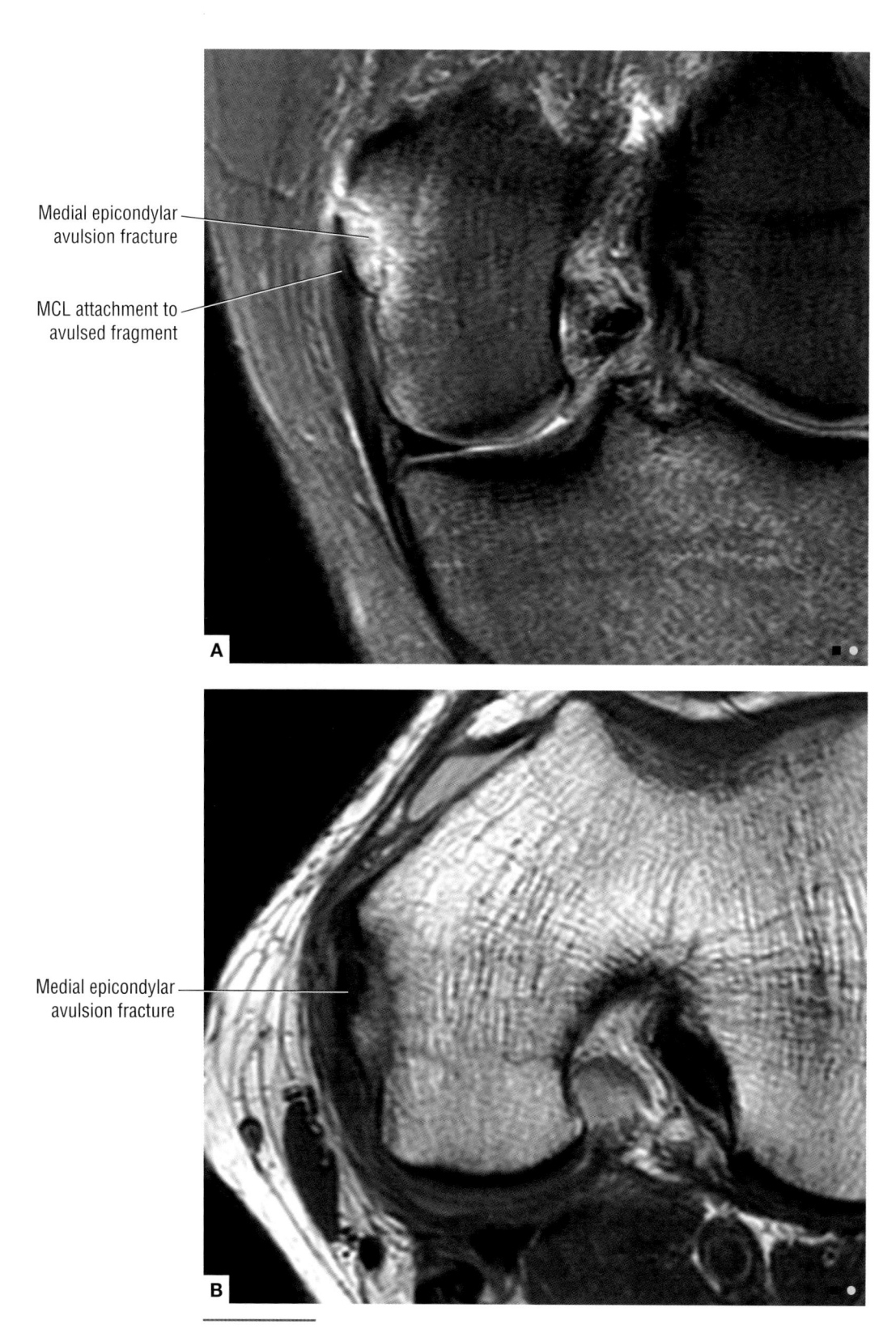

FIGURE 6.35 Proximal MCL avulsion fracture from the medial epicondyle. Coronal FS PD (**A**) and axial (**B**) PD FSE images.

618

Stoller's Orthopaedics and Sports Medicine: The Knee

Retracted and lax MCL with distal avulsion

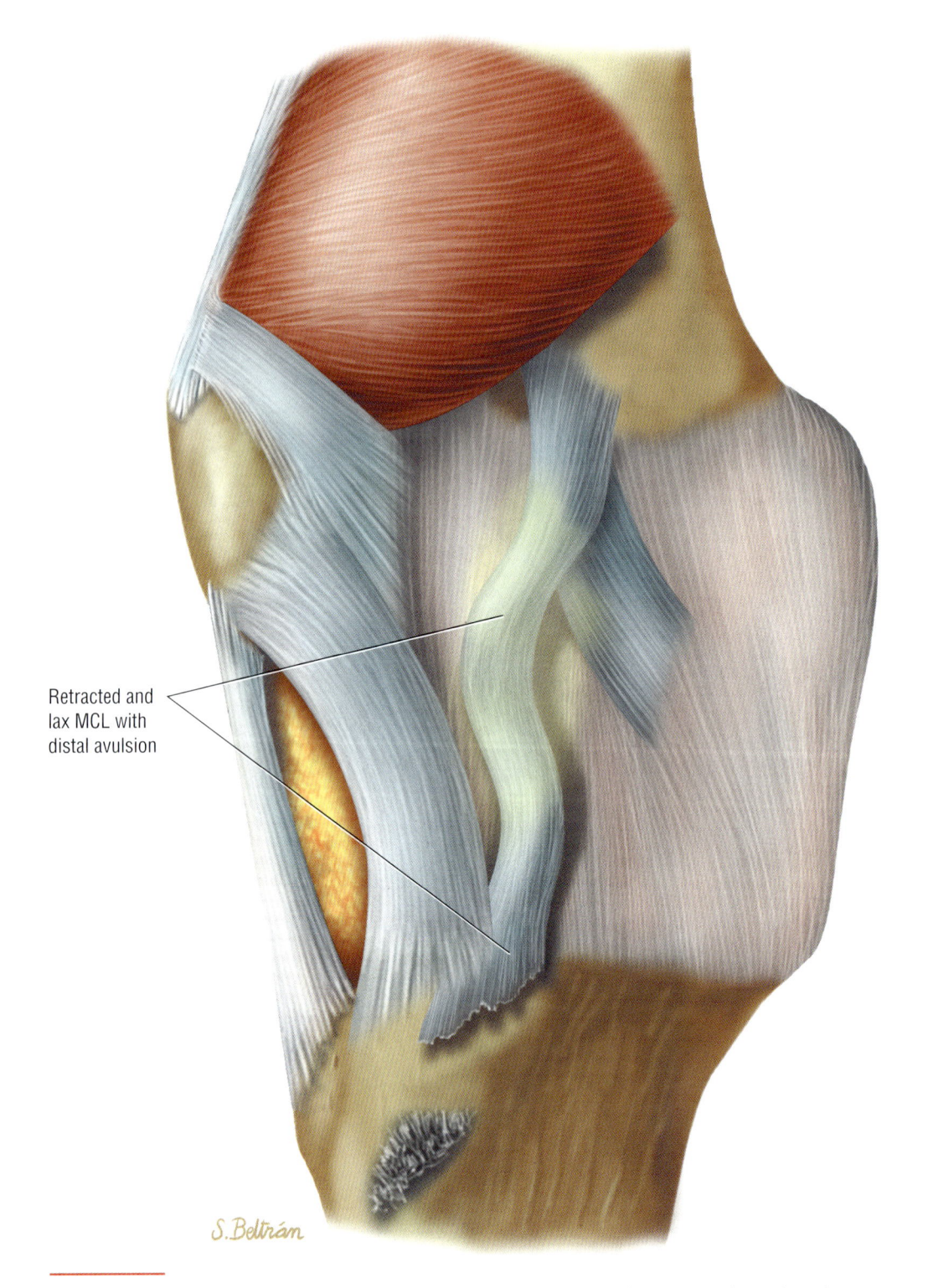

FIGURE 6.36 Retracted distal MCL tear with ligamentous folding demonstrated on a lateral three-dimensional color illustration.

Collateral Ligaments

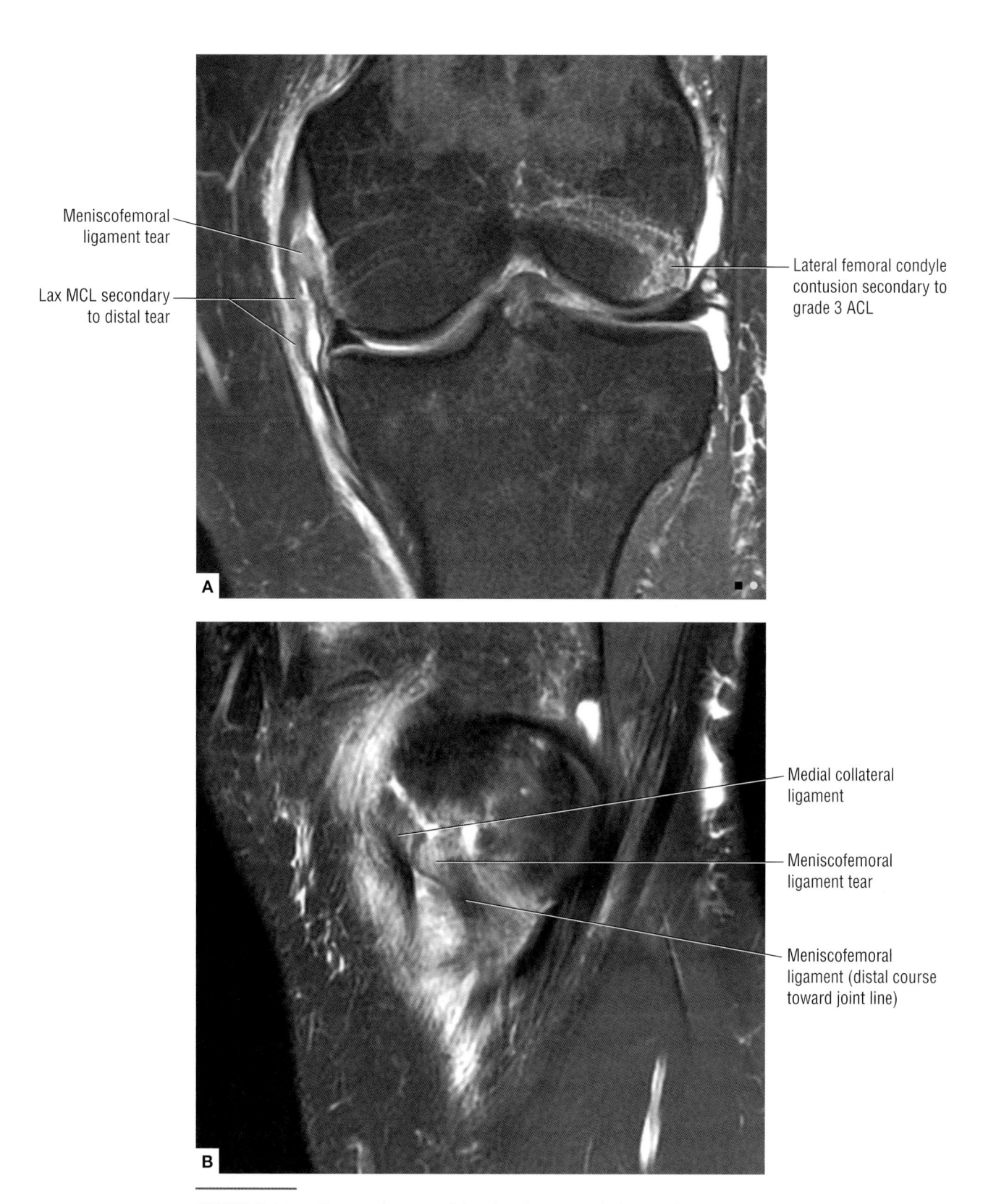

- Meniscofemoral ligament tear
- Lax MCL secondary to distal tear
- Lateral femoral condyle contusion secondary to grade 3 ACL
- Medial collateral ligament
- Meniscofemoral ligament tear
- Meniscofemoral ligament (distal course toward joint line)

FIGURE 6.37 Proximal retracted distal MCL tear with disrupted meniscofemoral ligament. Coronal (**A**) and sagittal (**B**) FS PD FSE images.

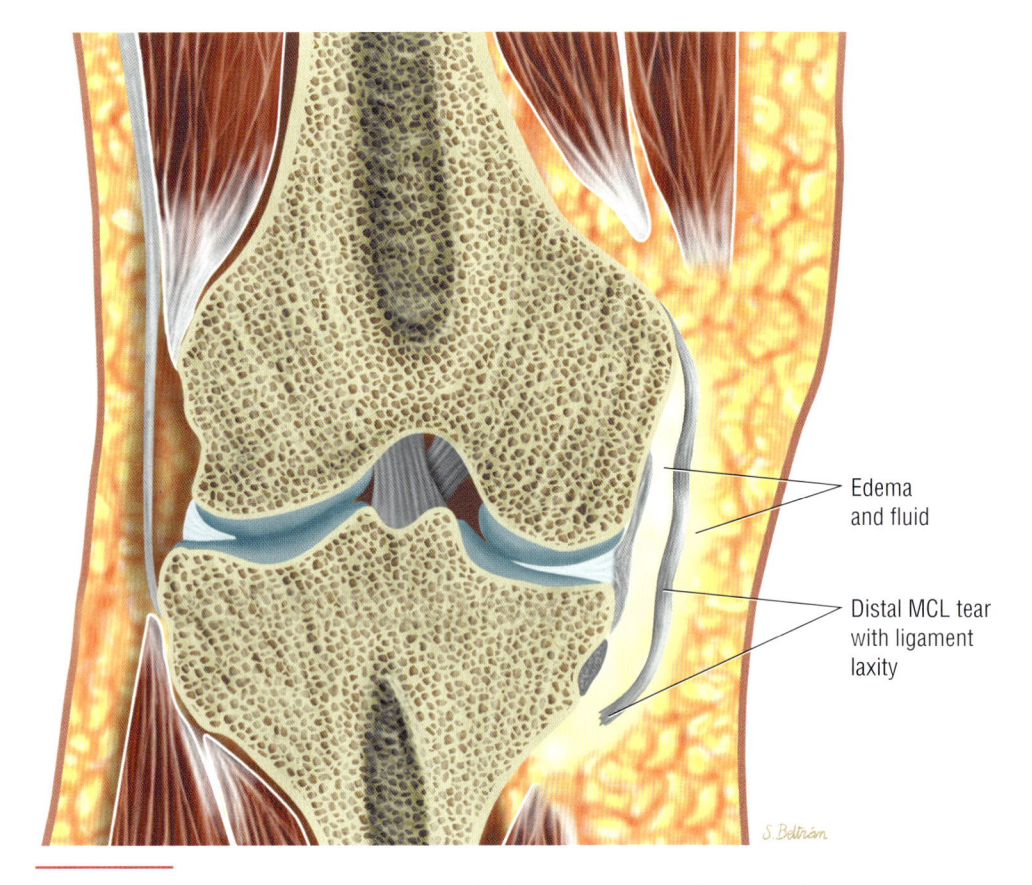

FIGURE 6.38 Coronal color illustration of a distal MCL tear without significant retraction.

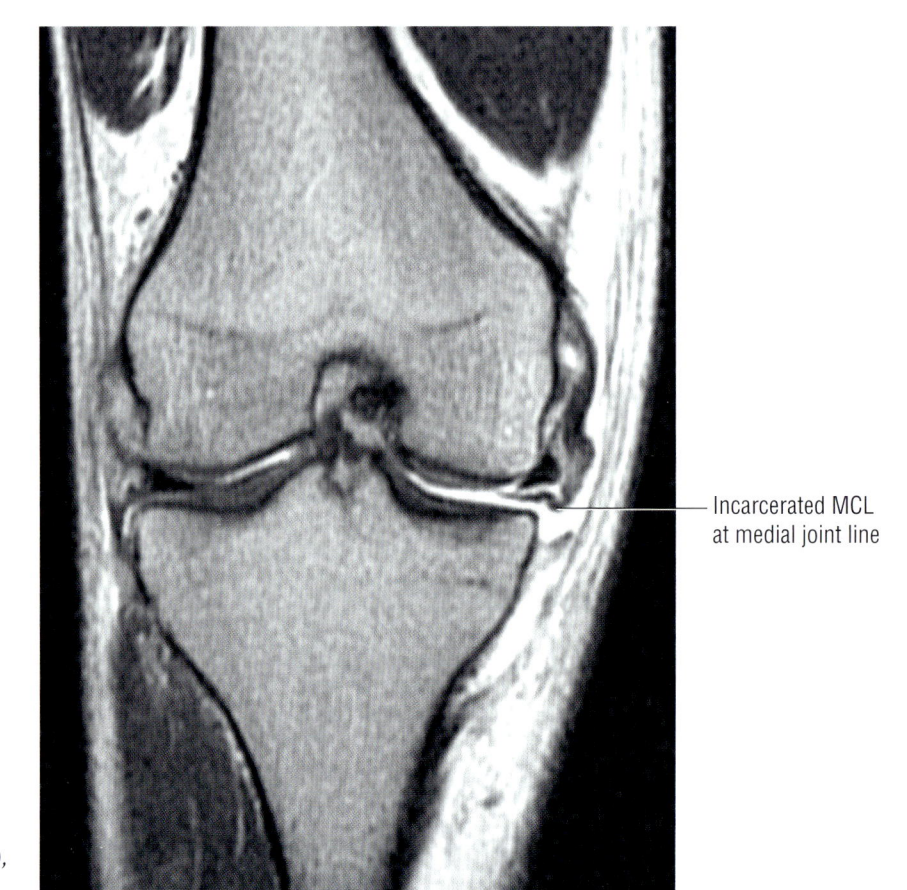

FIGURE 6.39 MR image demonstrating incarceration of the MCL into the medial compartment, mandating operative reduction of the MCL. (Reprinted from Fu FH. *Master Techniques in Orthopaedic Surgery: Sports Medicine.* Philadelphia, PA: Lippincott Williams & Wilkins; 2010, with permission.)

Collateral Ligaments

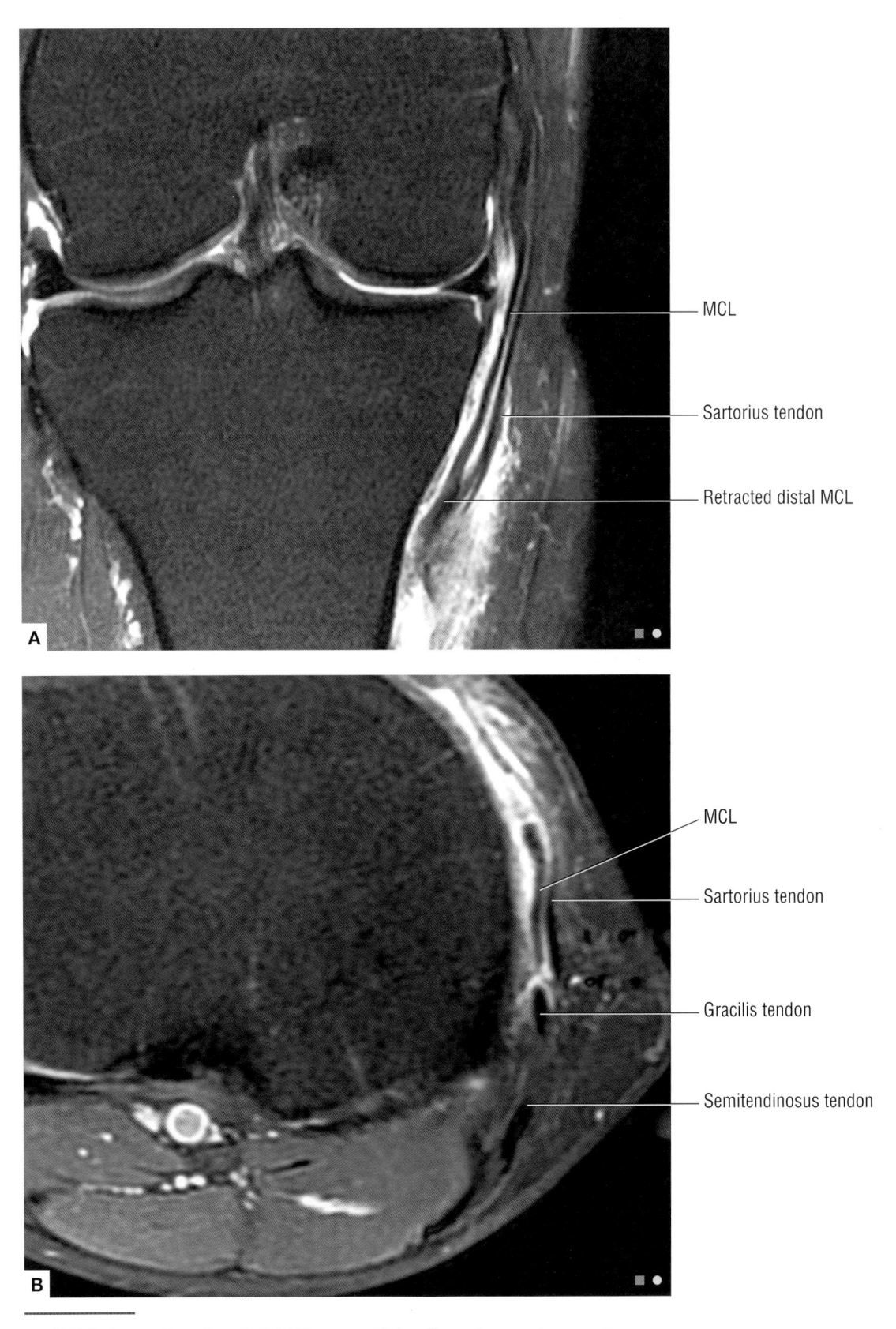

FIGURE 6.40 Distal grade 3 MCL tear with lax fibers deep to the sartorius component of the pes tendon group. Coronal (**A**) and axial (**B**) FS PD FSE images.

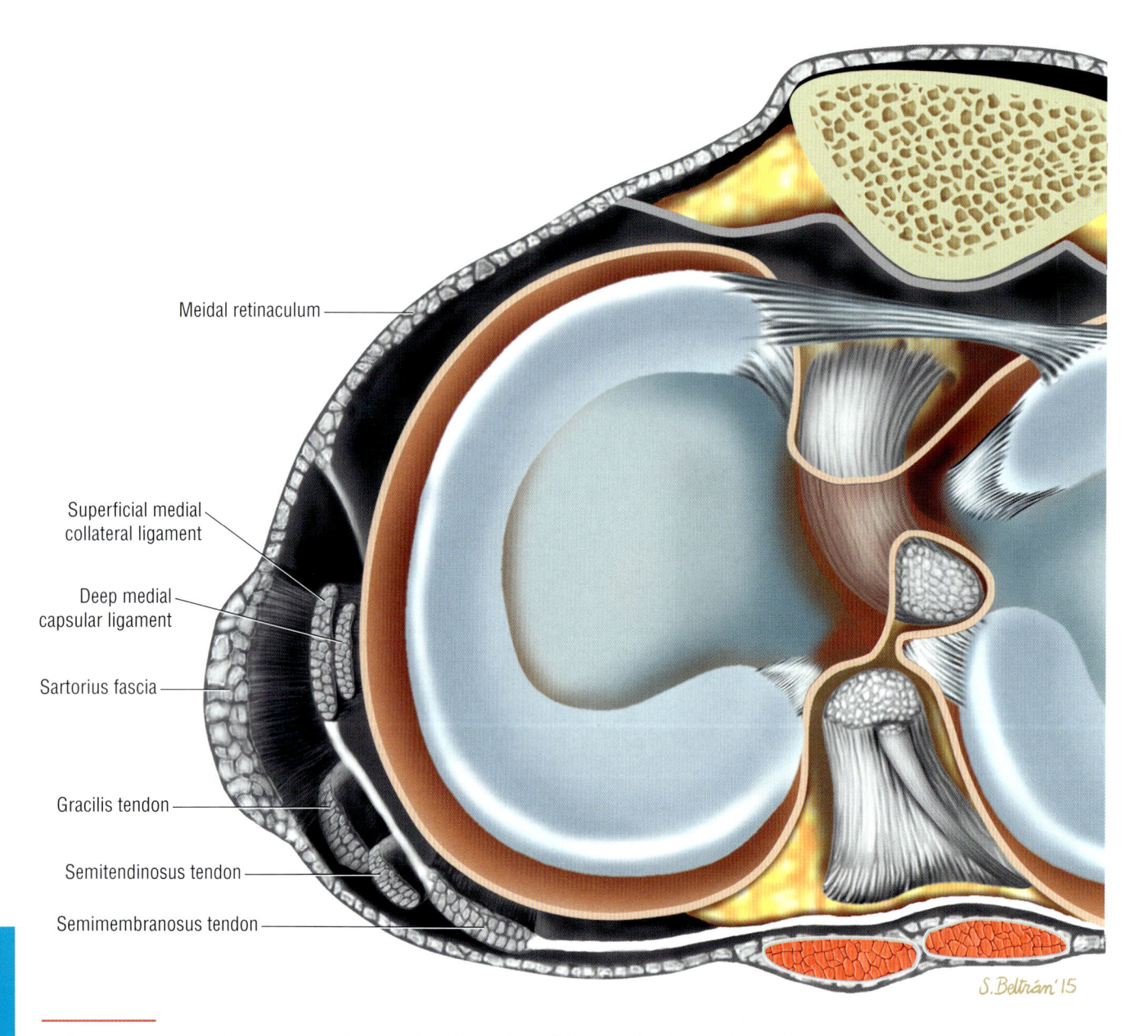

FIGURE 6.41 Axial cross-section showing the relationship of the superficial MCL (layer 2) to the pes tendons. The pes tendons are between layers 1 and 2.

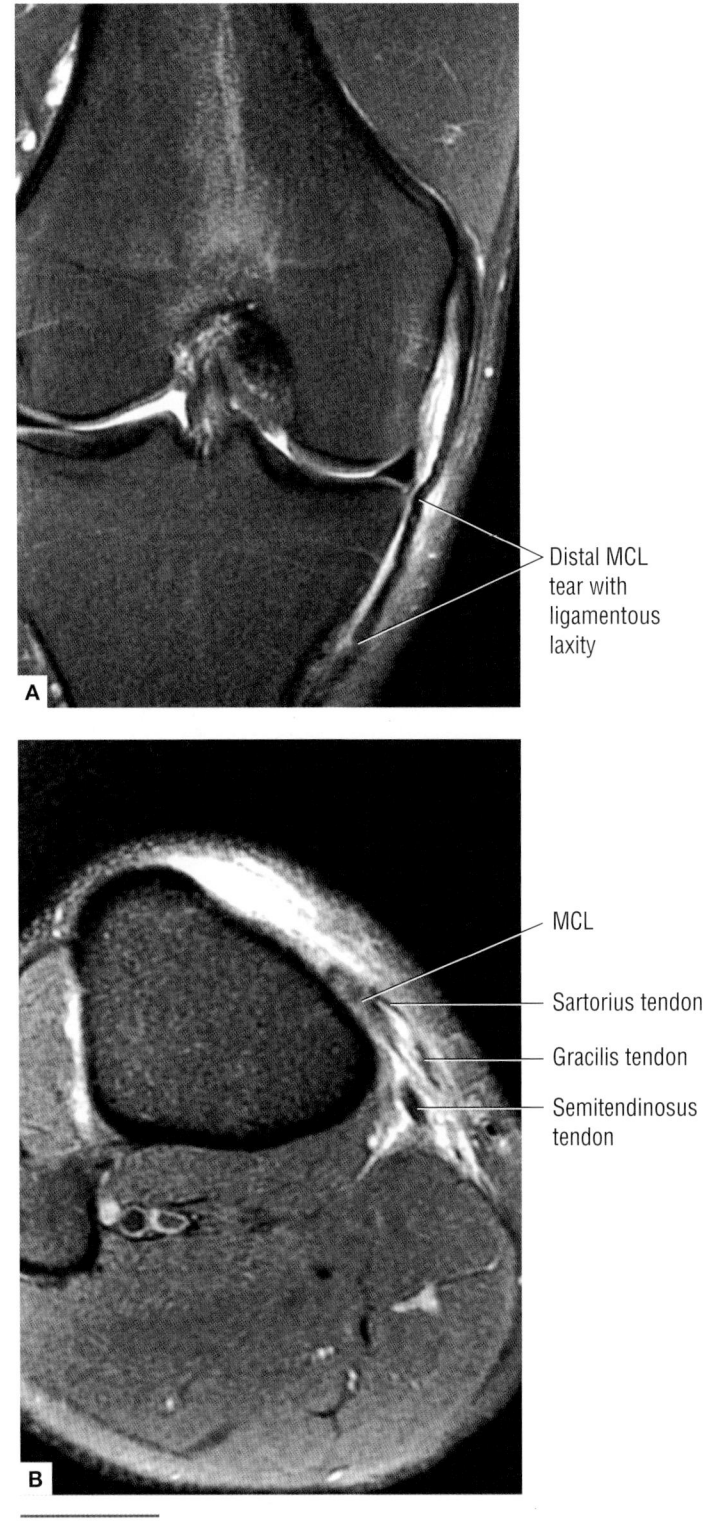

FIGURE 6.42 (**A**) Coronal FS PD FSE image of a distal MCL tear with mild ligamentous laxity and minimal retraction. (**B**) Distal thickened MCL on corresponding axial FS PD FSE. The distal pes tendons remain superficial to the torn MCL.

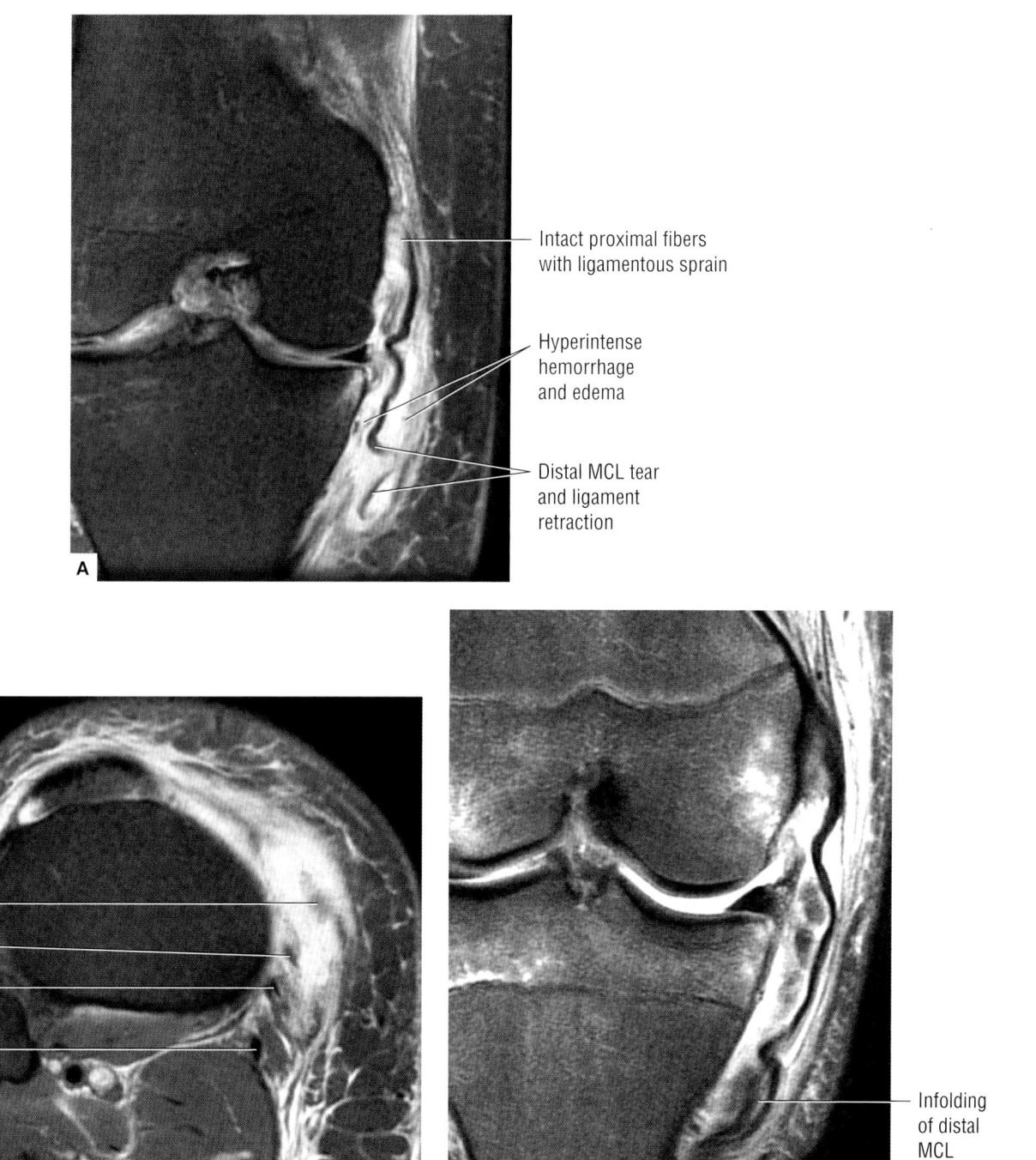

FIGURE 6.43 Retracted distal MCL tear with ligamentous folding demonstrated on a coronal FS PD image (**A**) and an axial FS PD FSE image (**B**). The distal MCL is medially displaced superficial to the pes tendons. (**C**) On a coronal FS PD FSE image in a separate case, there is infolding of the avulsed distal MCL, which is retracted medial to the pes tendons.

Collateral Ligaments 625

Grade 3 ACL

Subchondral edema from valgus impaction of lateral compartment

Distal MCL tear with ligament laxity

A

Distal MCL tear

Sartorius

Gracilis

Semitendinosus

B

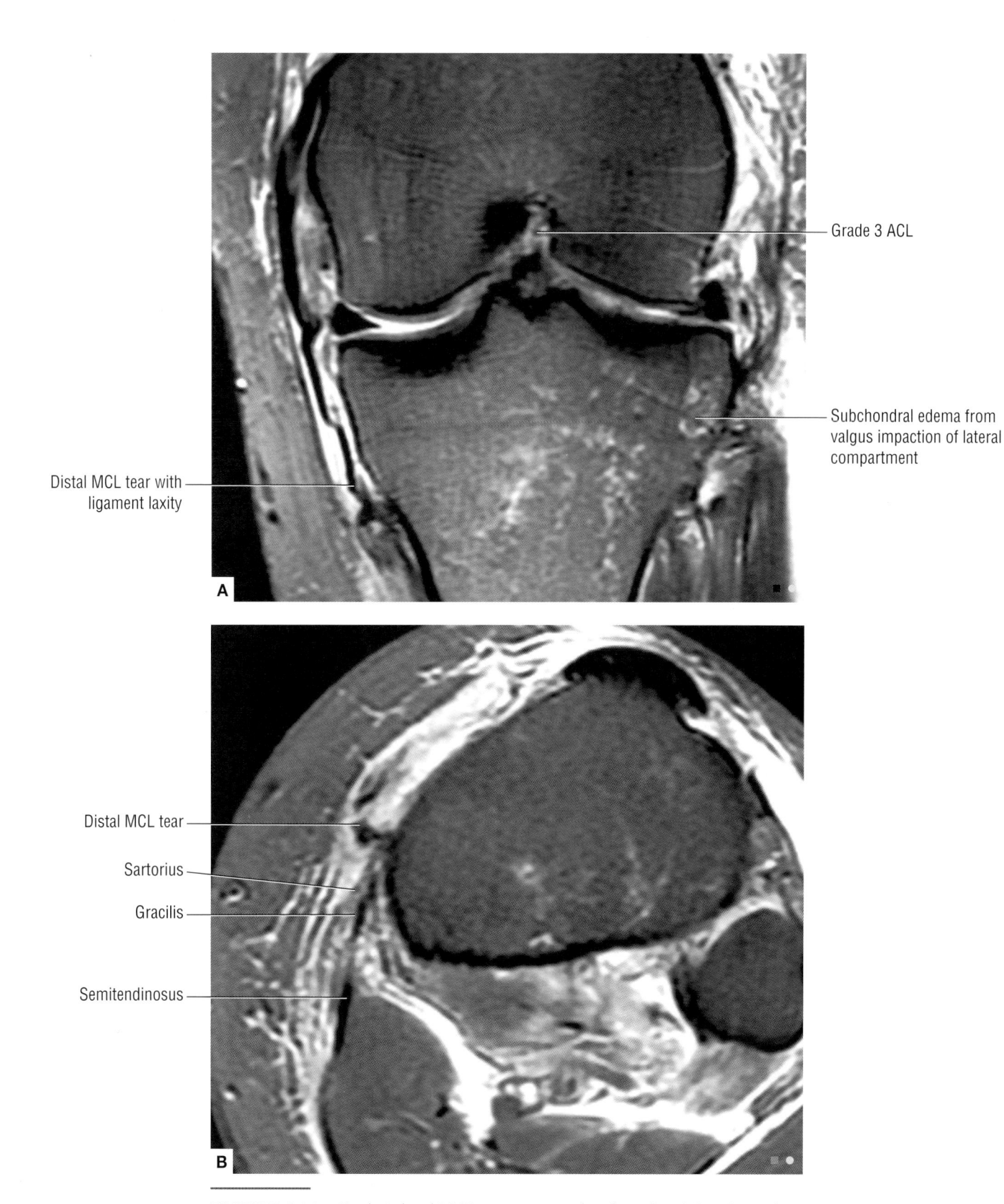

FIGURE 6.44 Grade 3 distal MCL tear associated with grade 3 ACL. Coronal (**A**) and axial (**B**) FS PD FSE images.

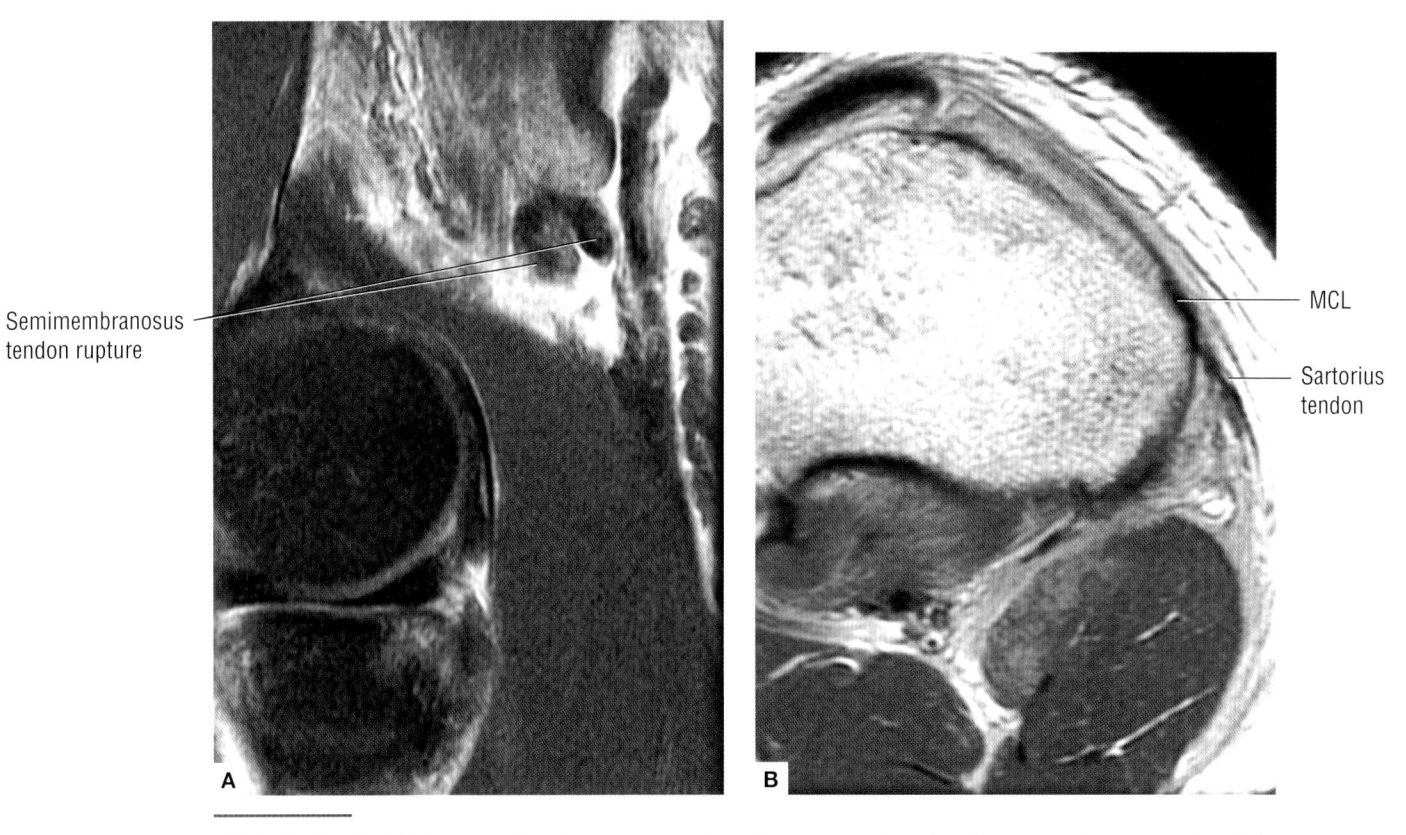

FIGURE 6.45 (**A**) Ruptured and retracted semimembranosus and semitendinosus tendons on an FS PD FSE sagittal image. (**B**) Axial PD FSE image showing an absent gracilis and the semitendinosus below the joint line. The MCL and sartorius are intact distally.

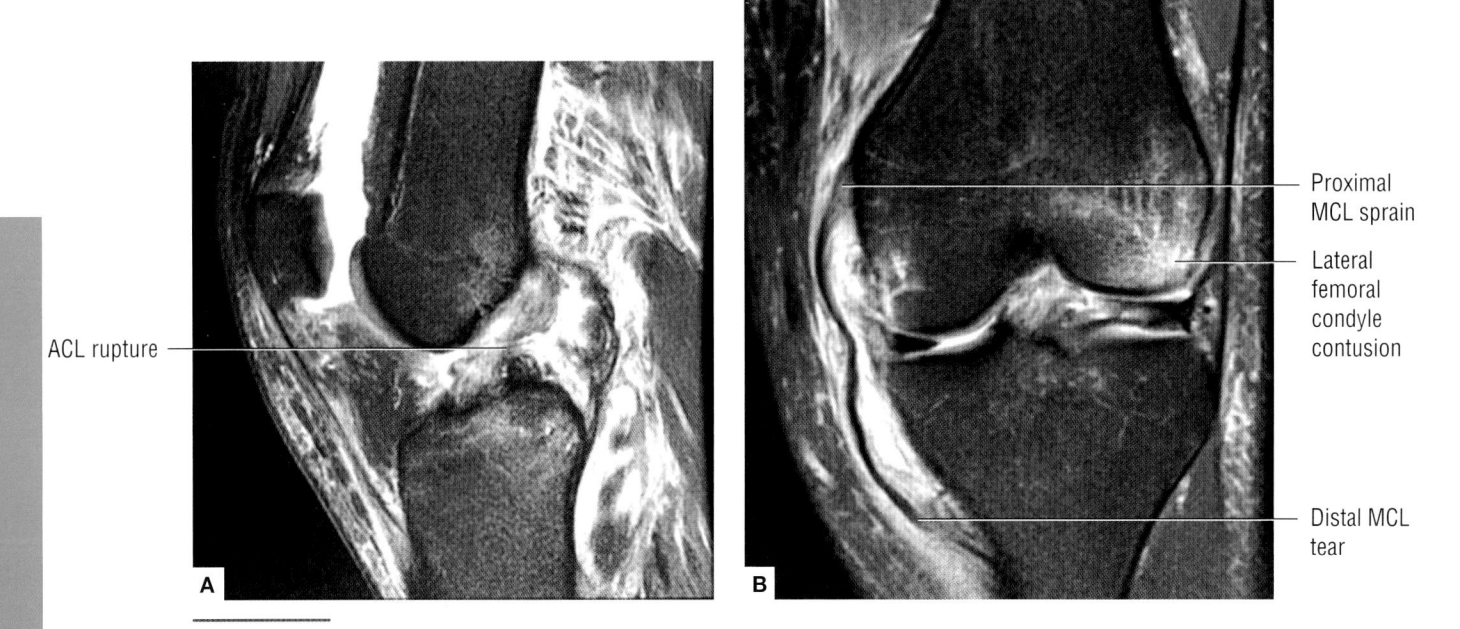

FIGURE 6.46 Grade 3 ACL disruption (**A**) associated with a grade 3 distal MCL tear (**B**). Both menisci were torn. ACL–MCL injuries are a common combination knee ligament injury. Associated meniscal tears are frequently seen. ACL–MCL injuries demonstrate increased anterior displacement and increased valgus angulation at both 0 degrees and 30 degrees of flexion. Isolated MCL injuries may only demonstrate valgus angulation at 30 degrees of flexion. There is also increased internal rotation.

Collateral Ligaments 627

Ossification MCL femoral attachment

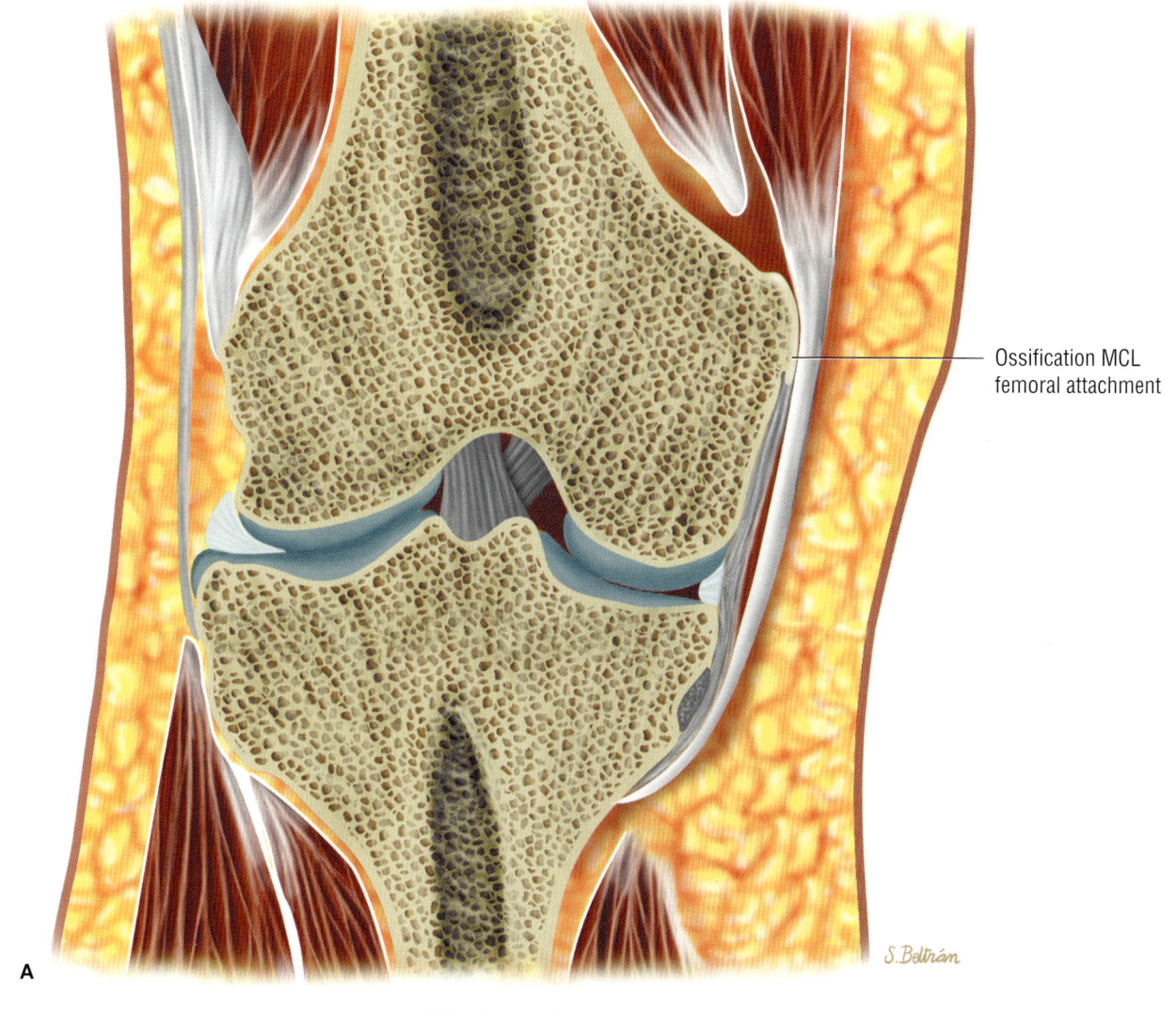

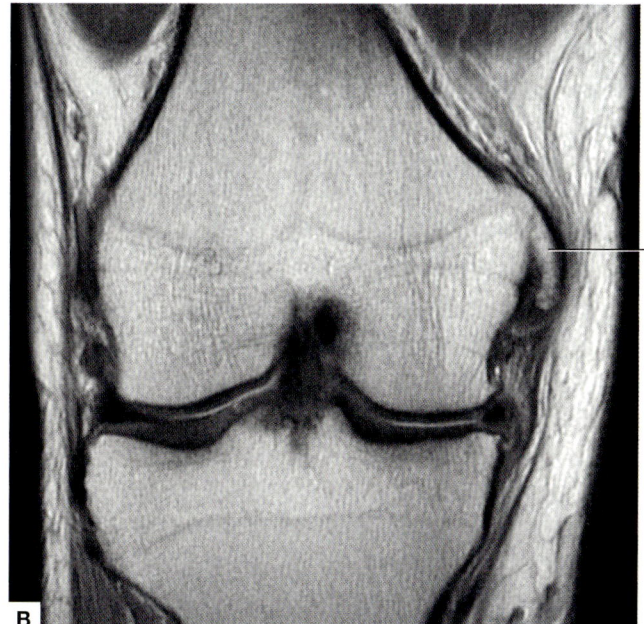

Ossification of MCL femoral attachment

FIGURE 6.47 Pellegrini-Stieda syndrome with ossification of the femoral attachment of the MCL. (**A**) Coronal color illustration. The ossification is directed along the long axis. (**B**) Coronal PD FSE image.

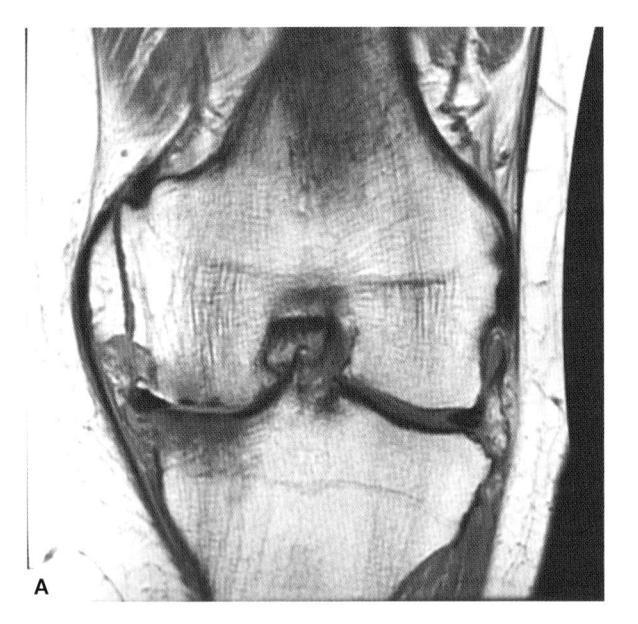

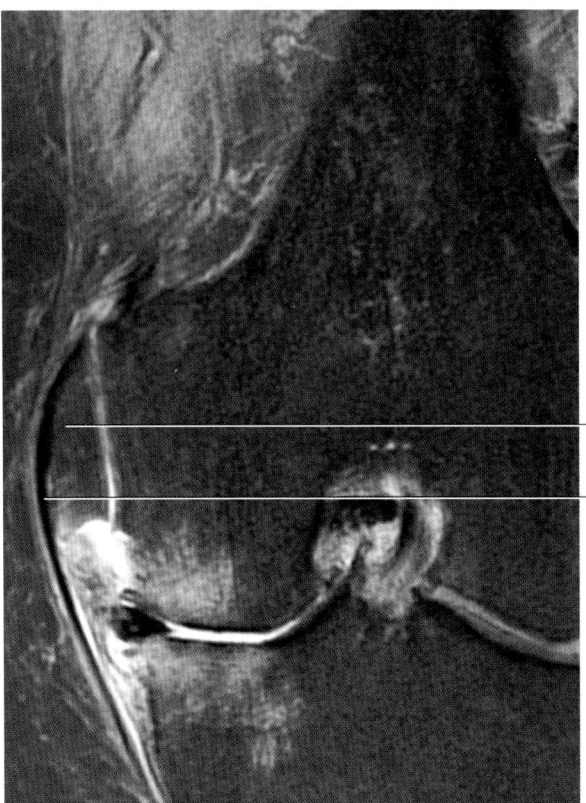

FIGURE 6.48 (**A**) Pellegrini-Stieda ossification of the proximal portion of the superficial MCL with marrow fat signal on a coronal PD FSE image. (**B**) Chronic disruption of the meniscofemoral ligament and degenerative medial compartment changes are identified on this coronal FS PD FSE image. The areas of chronic ossification show uniform fat suppression.

Collateral Ligaments

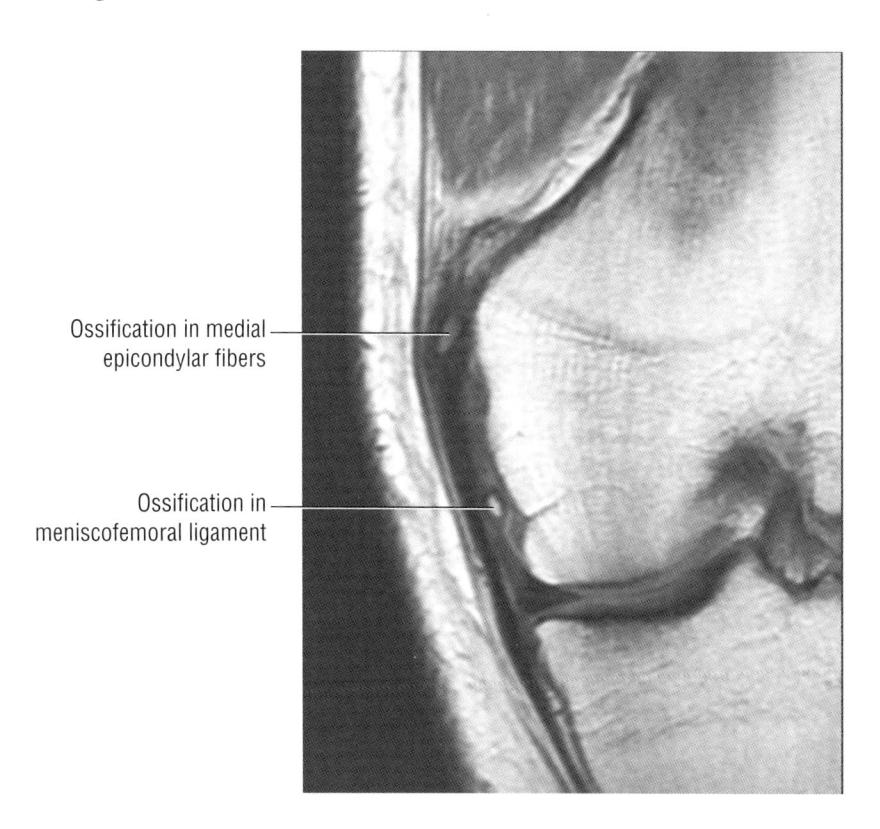

FIGURE 6.49 Pellegrini-Stieda ossification in the proximal MCL and in the meniscofemoral component of the deep capsular layer. Coronal PD FSE image.

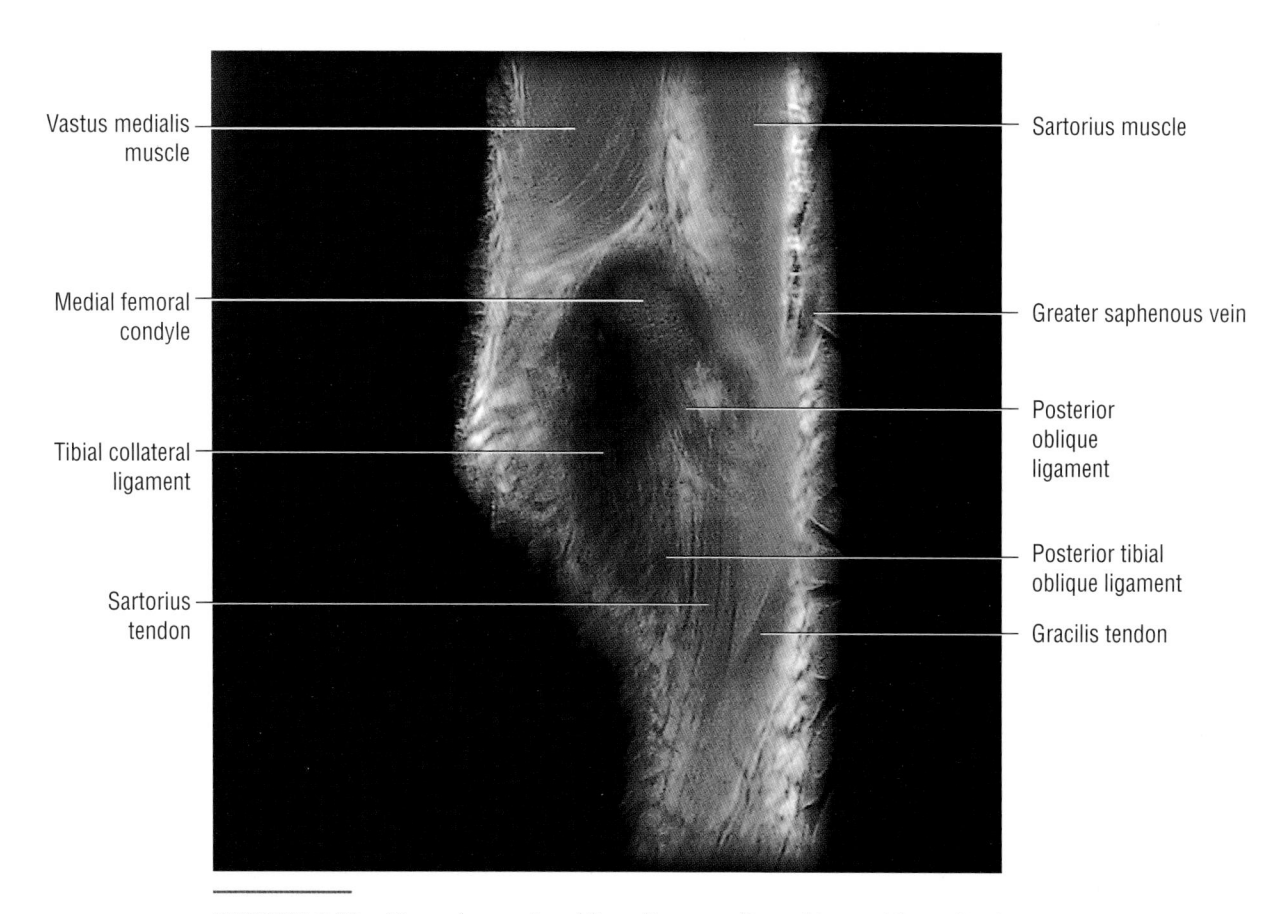

FIGURE 6.50 Normal posterior oblique ligament directed in an oblique distal course posterior to the superficial medial collateral (tibial collateral) ligament.

FIGURE 6.51 (**A**) The bursa of Voshell is located between the superficial and deep MCL distally and is a potential site for inflammation. Medial or tibial collateral ligament bursitis is seen between the superficial MCL and meniscotibial ligament of the deep capsular layer (layer 3). (**B**) Coronal FS PD FSE image. (**C**) Axial FS PD FSE image.

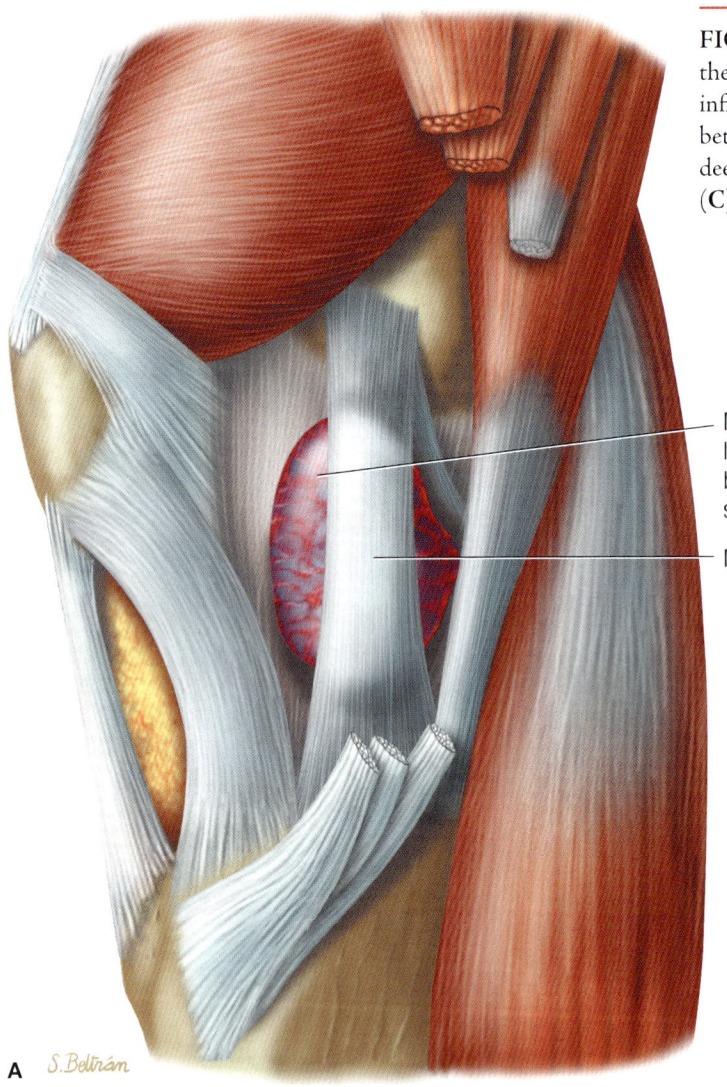

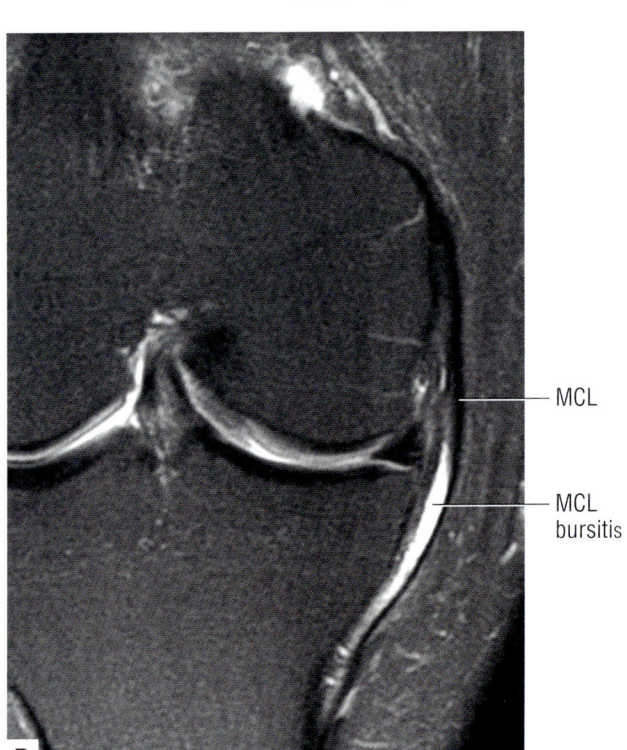

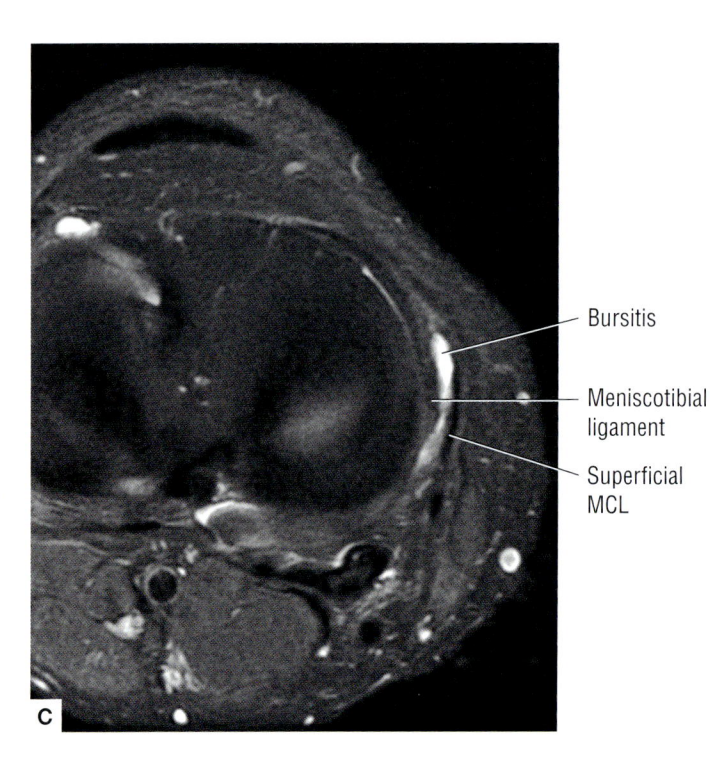

Collateral Ligaments

Tibial collateral ligament bursitis

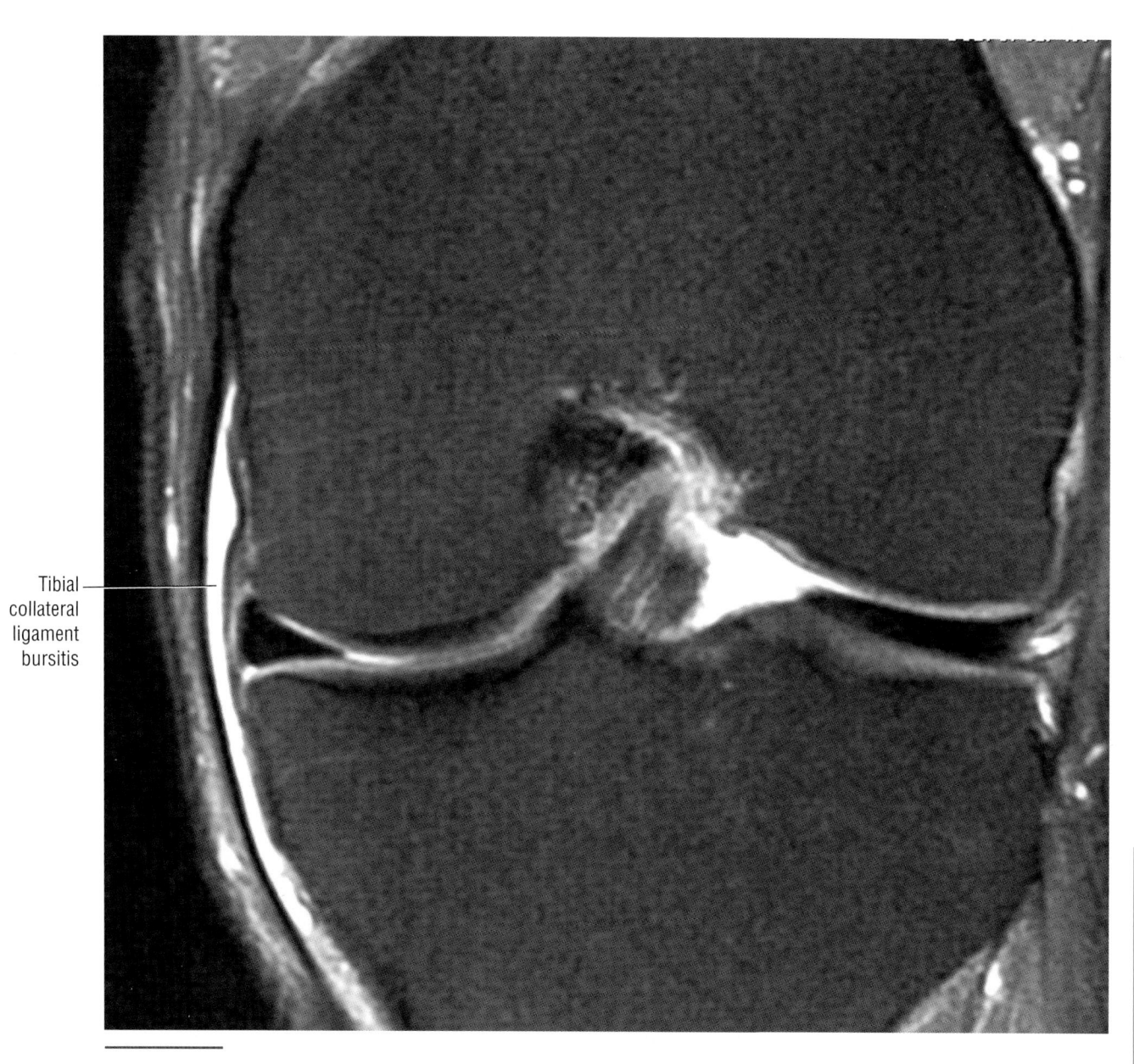

FIGURE 6.52 Linear hyperintense fluid collection deep to the superficial medial (tibial) collateral ligament. Coronal FS PD FSE image.

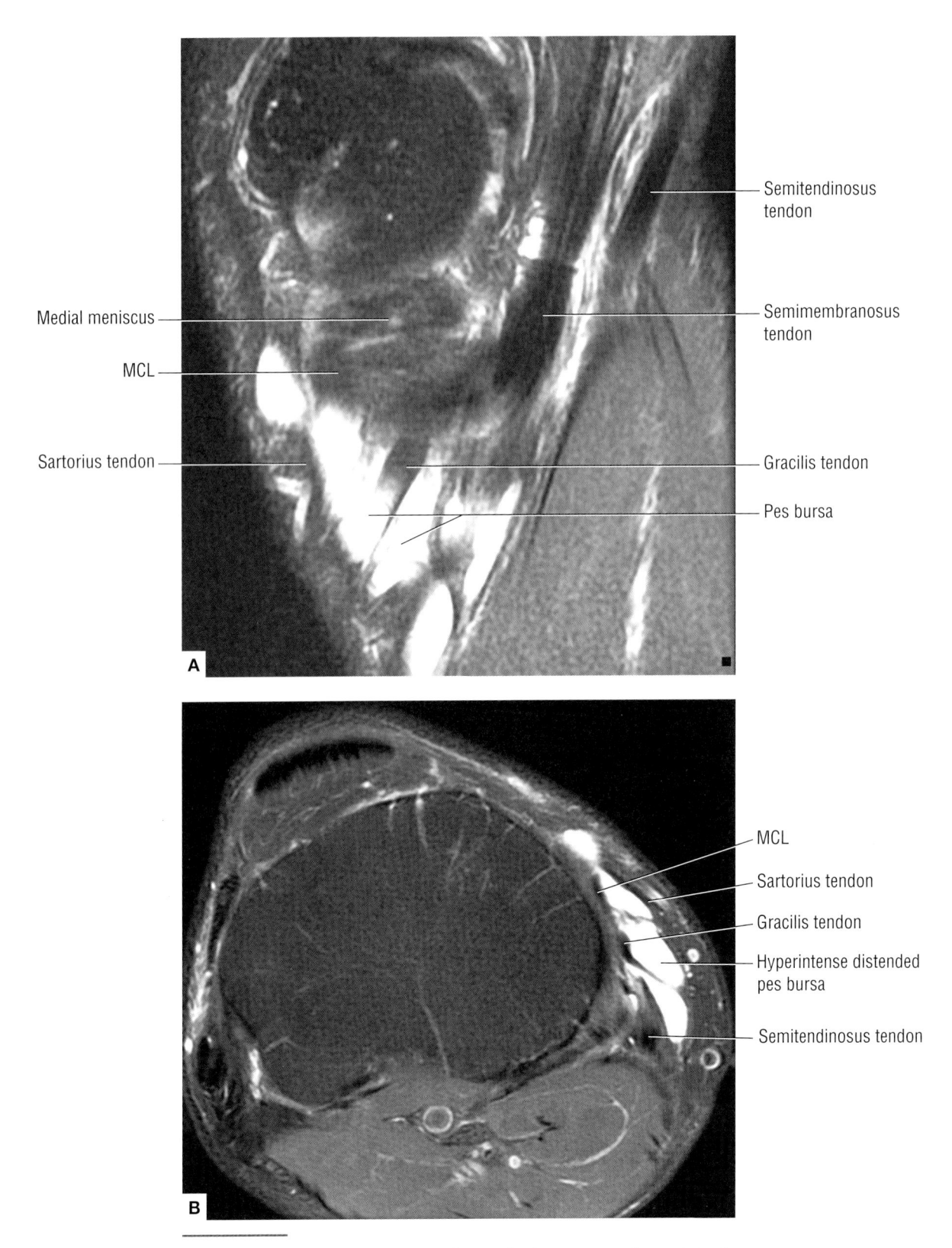

FIGURE 6.53 The pes anserinus (goose foot) represents the conjoined tendons of the sartorius, gracilis, and semitendinosus. Sagittal (**A**) and axial (**B**) FS PD FSE images.

Collateral Ligaments 633

Gracilis tendon

Semitendinosus tendon

Pes bursa inflammation

Sartorius tendon

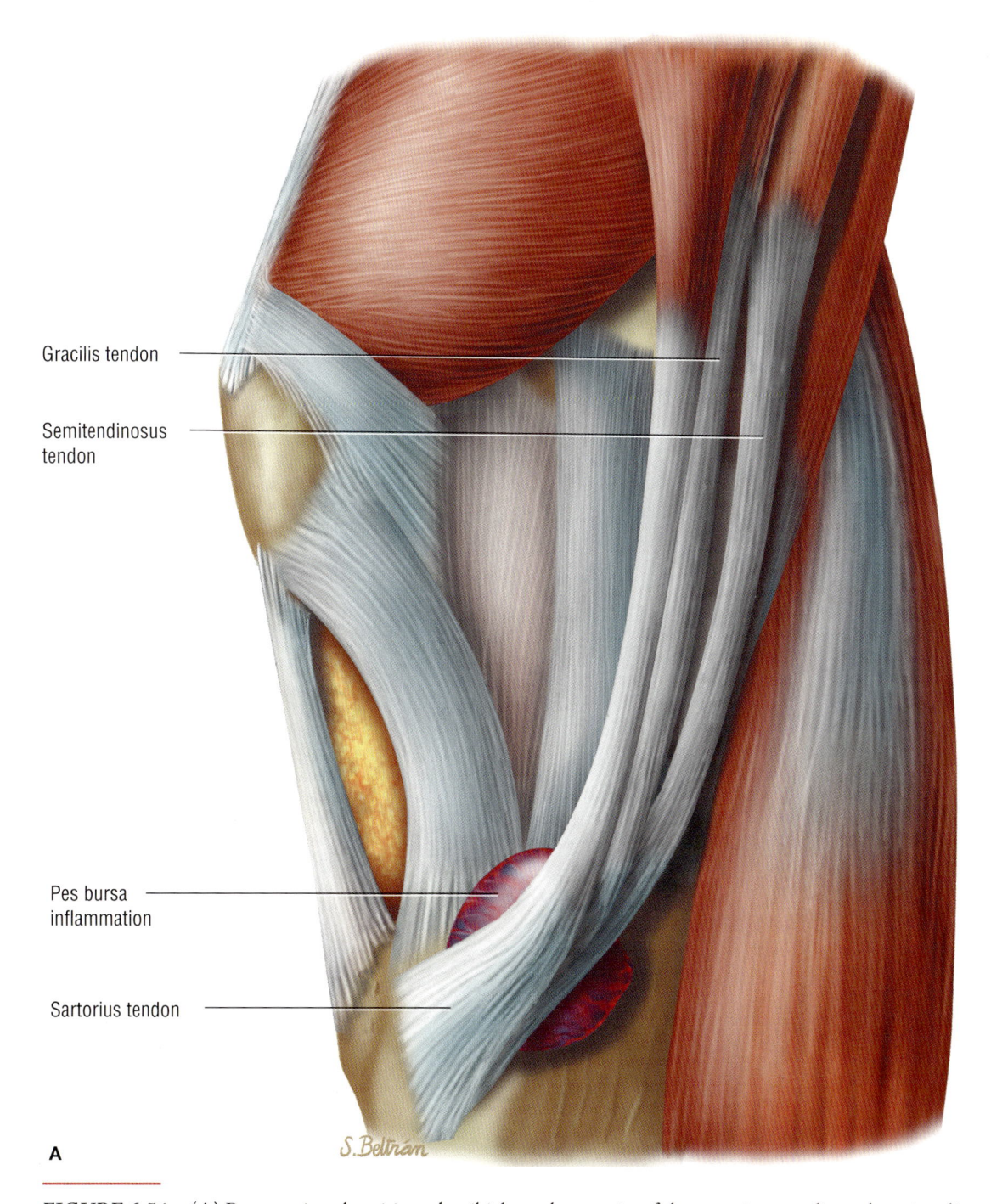

FIGURE 6.54 **(A)** Pes anserinus bursitis at the tibial attachment site of the sartorius, gracilis, and semitendinosus tendons. The pes bursa can be injured by direct trauma or contusion, and pes bursitis may be associated with excessive pronation (lateral three-dimensional color illustration). *(Continued)*

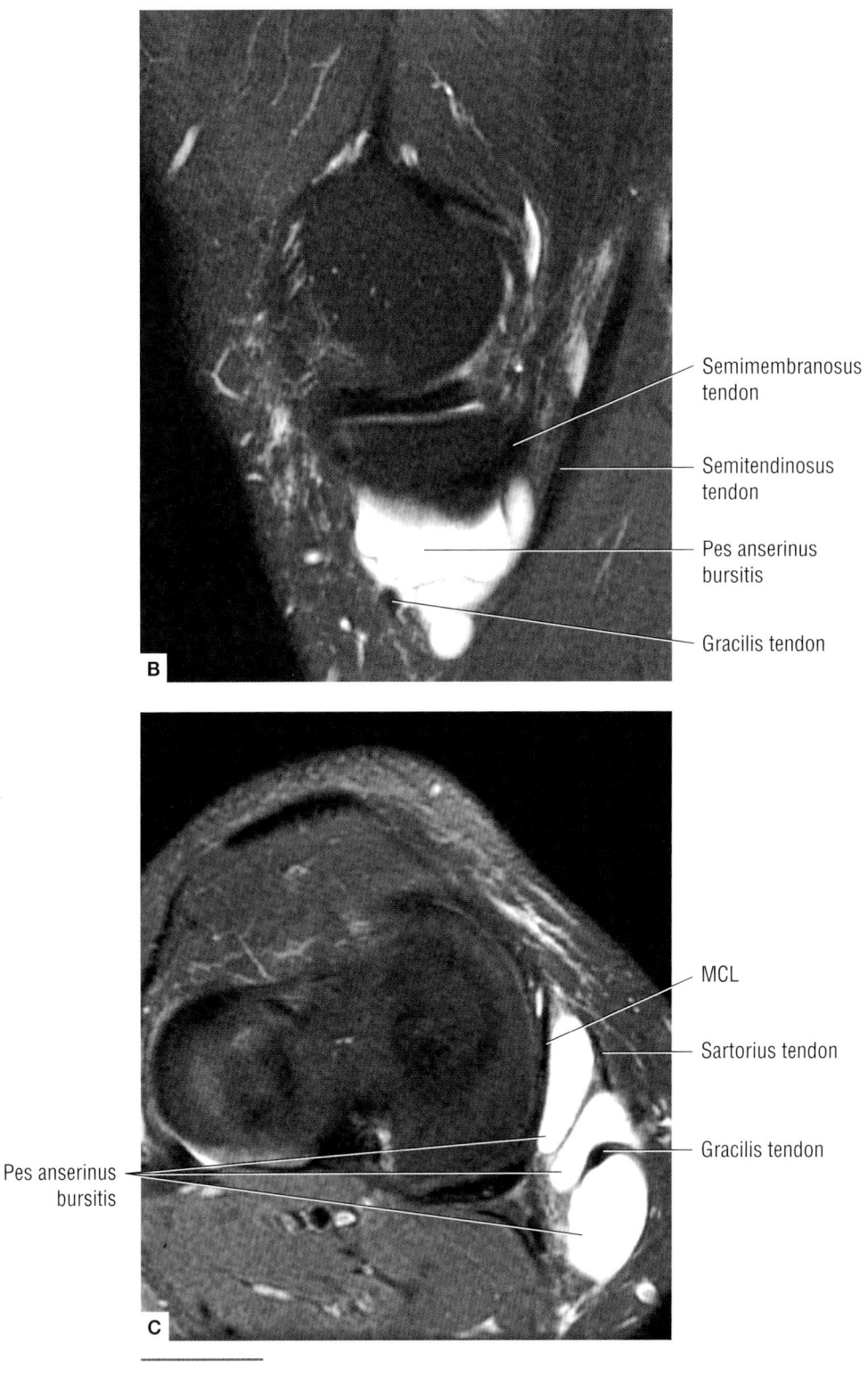

FIGURE 6.54 *(Continued)* **(B)** Pes bursa fluid anterior to the semitendinosus tendon below the medial joint line (sagittal FS PD FSE image). **(C)** Septated presentation of pes bursitis with the distended pes bursa superficial to the MCL and deep to the sartorius and gracilis tendons at the level of the proximal tibia (axial FS PD FSE image).

Healing and Treatment

- Healing of the MCL occurs best when disrupted ends of ligament are in direct contact or proximity.
    - Size of gap between torn ends affects ability of ligament to heal.
    - Tension has positive effect on ligament healing.
- Ligament recovers only 50% of original modulus and tensile strength after 12 months.
    - Load and stiffness of MCL–bone complex may still be normal, as the healed tissue is thickened, with a larger cross-sectional area.[126]
- MCL injuries, even grade 3 disruptions, heal unless associated with damage to other supporting structures.[470]
    - Valgus stress test
        - Medial compartment evaluated at 30-degree flexion with applied valgus stress
        - When performed in knee extension, this test can check the status of posterior cruciate ligament (PCL) and posteromedial compartment.[40]
- MCL scar (hypointense and thickened on MR images) is biomechanically inferior to the native ligament because of increased cellularity and decreased total collagen.
- Grades 1, 2, and 3 isolated MCL sprains treated with early functional rehabilitation
    - In isolated grade 3 MCL tears, operative treatment and nonoperative treatment equally effective
- Combined MCL and ACL injuries usually treated with surgical repair of only the ACL
    - Posterior oblique ligament assists MCL in resisting valgus and external rotation forces in extension and flexion.

Lateral Collateral Ligament (LCL) and Posterolateral Corner (PLC)

Key Concepts

- LCL tears are associated with injury to other posterolateral structures.

- Popliteus muscle or myotendinous unit strains represent extraarticular injuries; intraarticular popliteus tears (less common) involve the hiatus or popliteus femoral attachment.

- LCL and biceps femoris attach to lateral margin of fibular head (not the styloid), accounting for reduced likelihood of avulsion injury compared to popliteofibular, fabellofibular, and arcuate ligaments.

Lateral Collateral Ligament and Posterolateral Corner

- Lateral aspect of knee also divided into three structural layers[69,423]:
    - Layer 1: most superficial
        - Fascia lata
        - Iliotibial tract with its anterior expansion
        - Superficial portion of biceps femoris with its posterior expansion
    - Layer 2:
        - Quadriceps retinaculum anteriorly
        - Two patellofemoral ligaments or retinacula posteriorly
        - Layers 1 and 2 merge at lateral aspect of patella.
    - Layer 3: deepest layer
        - Lateral joint capsule, including attachments to lateral meniscus
        - Lateral capsular ligament with meniscofemoral and meniscotibial components
        - Lateral collateral ligament located posteriorly between superficial and deep divisions of layer 3
        - Fabellofibular ligament, arcuate ligament, popliteus, and popliteofibular ligament[40]

- Lateral collateral ligament (also called the *fibular collateral ligament*)
    - Layer 3 structure
    - Axial plane anatomy demonstrates relationships of LCL and biceps femoris and popliteus tendons at the level of the lateral femoral condyle and joint line.
        - Popliteus tendon is located just medial to the LCL at level of lateral meniscus.
        - Insertion of popliteus tendon onto popliteus fossa of lateral femoral condyle is distal and anterior to the proximal LCL (popliteus tendon crosses deep to the LCL).
- Posterolateral (arcuate) complex includes:
    - LCL
    - Popliteus tendon
    - Lateral head of gastrocnemius muscle
    - Arcuate ligament[341,535]
    - Popliteofibular ligament
    - Fabellofibular ligament
- Arcuate ligament
    - Layer 3 structure
    - Spans posterolateral joint and is attached to apex of the fibular head deep to the fabellofibular ligament (when present)
    - Y-shaped with medial (arcuate) and lateral (upright) limbs
    - Medial limb runs from posterior capsule at level of distal femur and extends medially on popliteus muscle to oblique popliteal ligament.
        - Oblique popliteal ligament is formed by reflected portion of semimembranosus tendon and makes up primary portion of the posterior capsule.
    - Lateral (upright) limb extends from posterior capsule and courses laterally over popliteus muscle and tendon to insert on posterior aspect of the fibula.[504]

- Popliteofibular ligament
    - Layer 3 structure
    - Deep to lateral limb of arcuate ligament
    - Takes origin from posterior aspect of fibula (posterior to biceps insertion)
    - Extends toward junction of popliteus muscle and tendon[177]
    - Joins the popliteus tendon proximal to the musculotendinous junction of the popliteus, thus connecting the fibula to the femur through the popliteus tendon
- Fabellofibular or short lateral ligament
    - Courses parallel to LCL from fabella to fibula
    - Inserts posterior and medial to biceps femoris tendon
    - In absence of fabella, lateral limb of the arcuate ligament is known as short lateral ligament.
        - If fabella absent, short lateral ligament may be attenuated or absent
    - Possible inverse relationship between size of fabellofibular and arcuate ligaments
        - In presence of large fabella, fabellofibular ligament is prominent, while arcuate ligament is attenuated or absent.
        - Fabellofibular ligament (when present) functions as the lateral limb of arcuate ligament.[227]
- Fabellopopliteal ligament
- Superior and inferior popliteomeniscal fascicles
    - Attachments of popliteus tendon to the PHLM
    - Contribute to roof and floor of the popliteal hiatus
- Biceps femoris muscle has tendinous attachments to fibular head.
    - Direct arm of the short head
    - Direct and anterior arms of long head

Collateral Ligaments

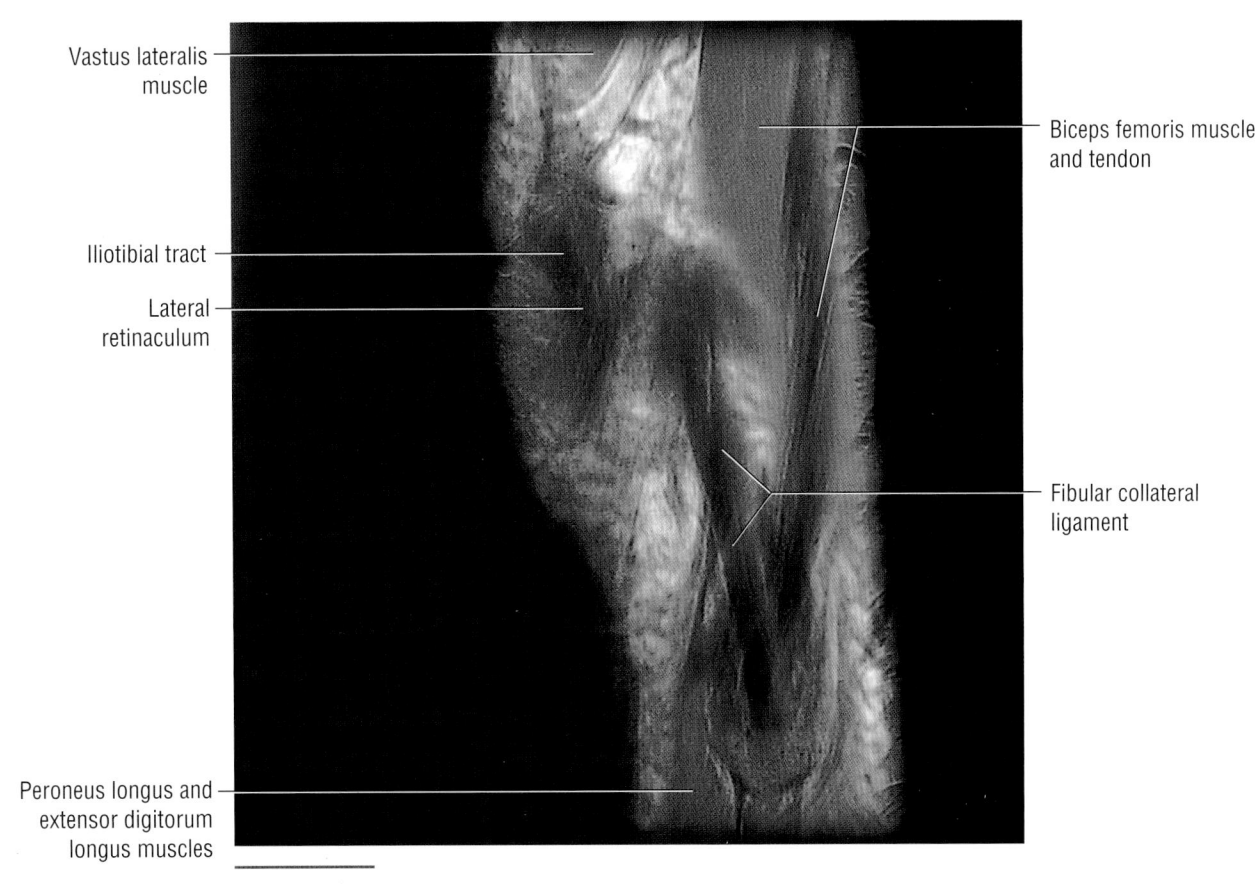

FIGURE 6.55 Superficial lateral structures of the knee on peripheral sagittal image.

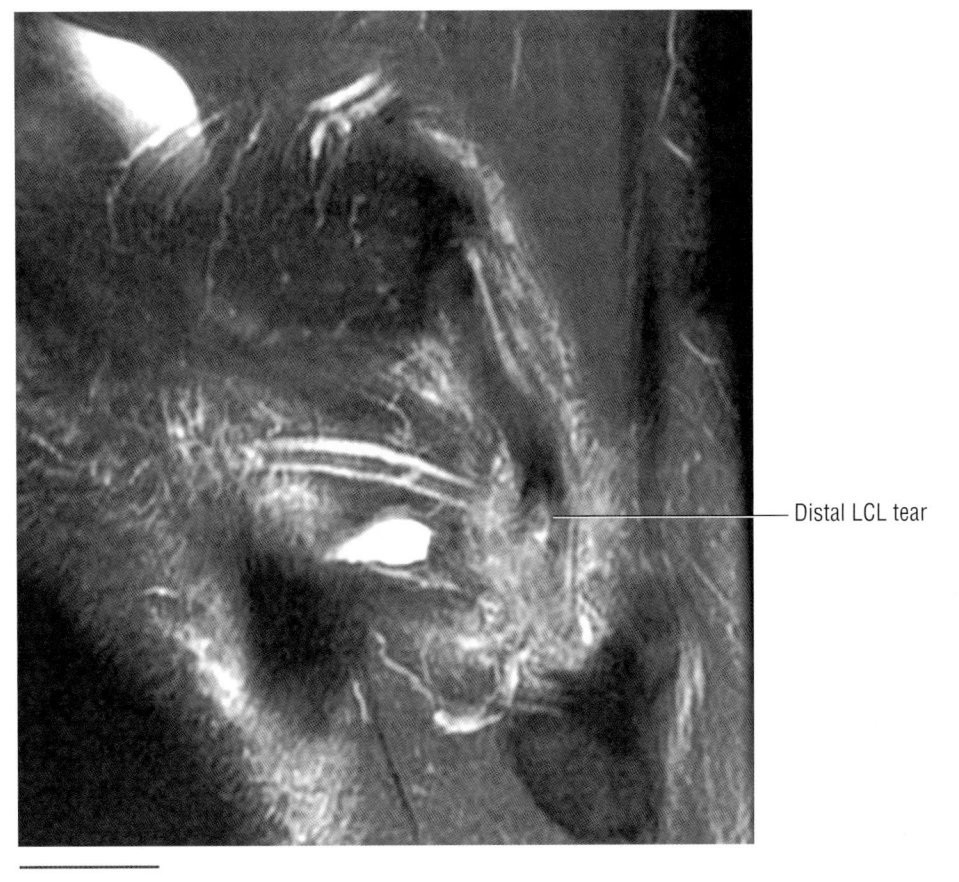

FIGURE 6.56 Disruption of distal third of LCL with avulsion from the lateral fibular head. Sagittal FS PD FSE image.

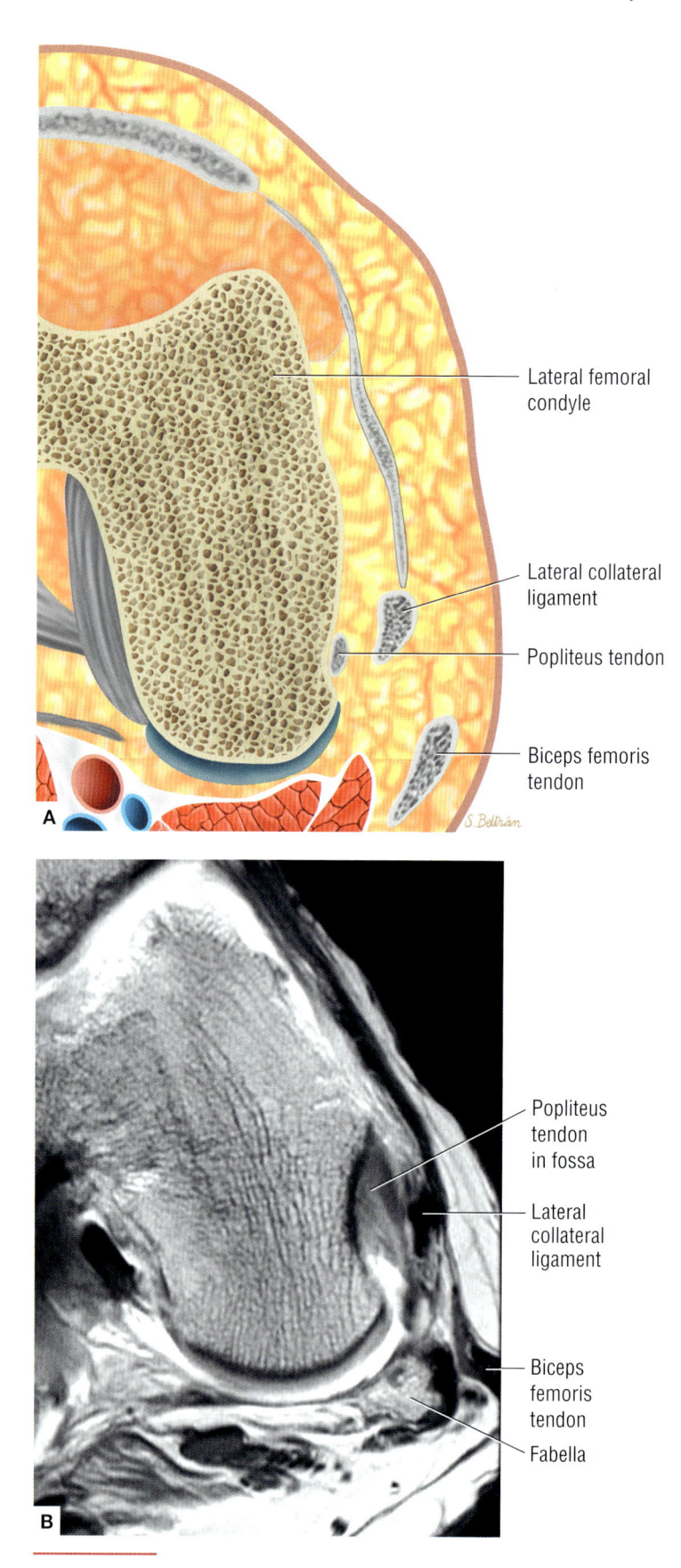

FIGURE 6.57 **(A)** Color axial cross-section at the level of the lateral femoral condyle. The popliteus tendon courses deep to the lateral collateral ligament proximally and is overlapped by the biceps femoris in its distal extent (not noted in text). **(B)** Axial T1-weighted MR arthrogram.

Collateral Ligaments 641

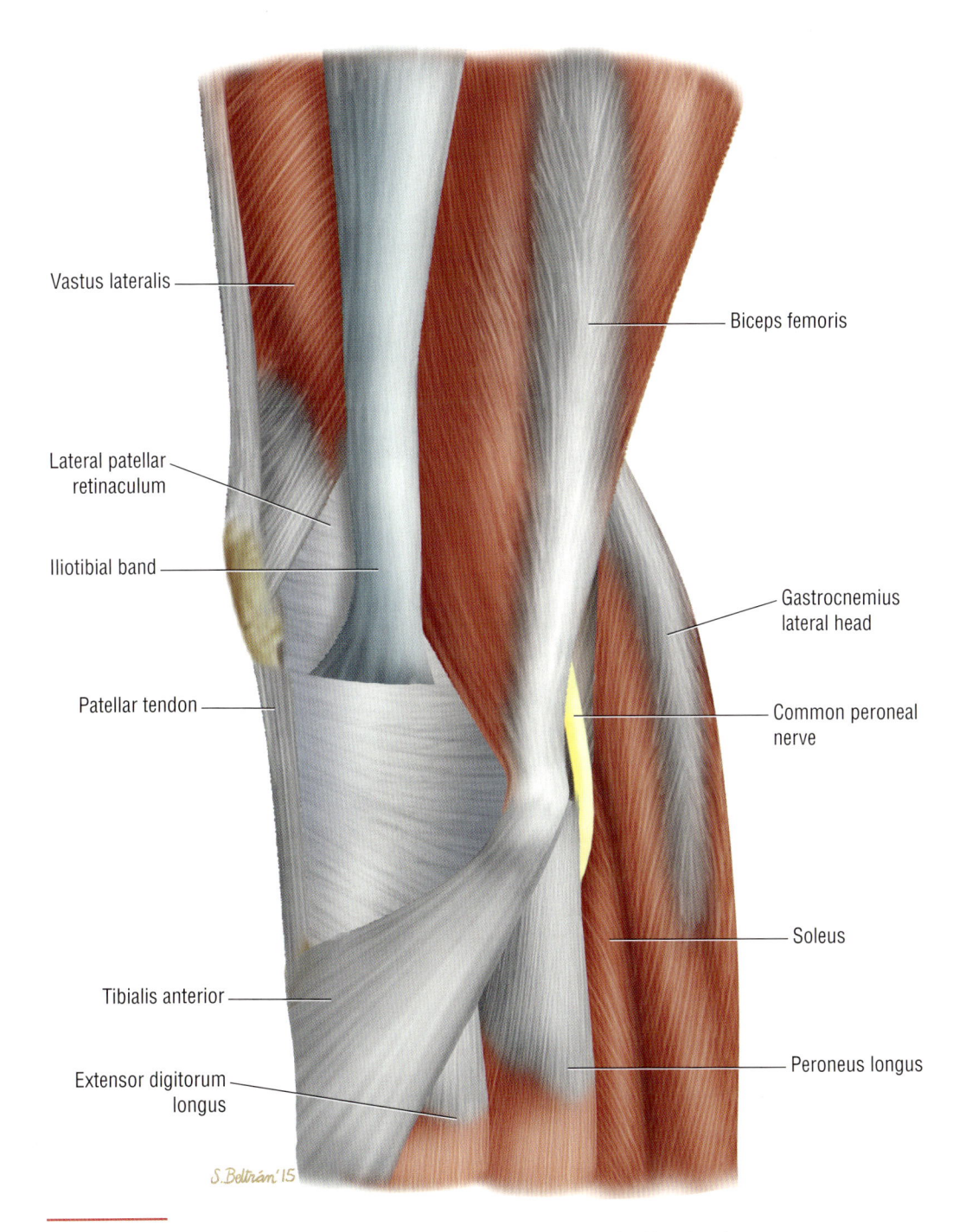

FIGURE 6.58 Layer 1 of the lateral aspect of the knee. The iliotibial band and its anterior expansion and the biceps femoris and its posterior expansion make up layer 1. Fascia interconnects these structures.

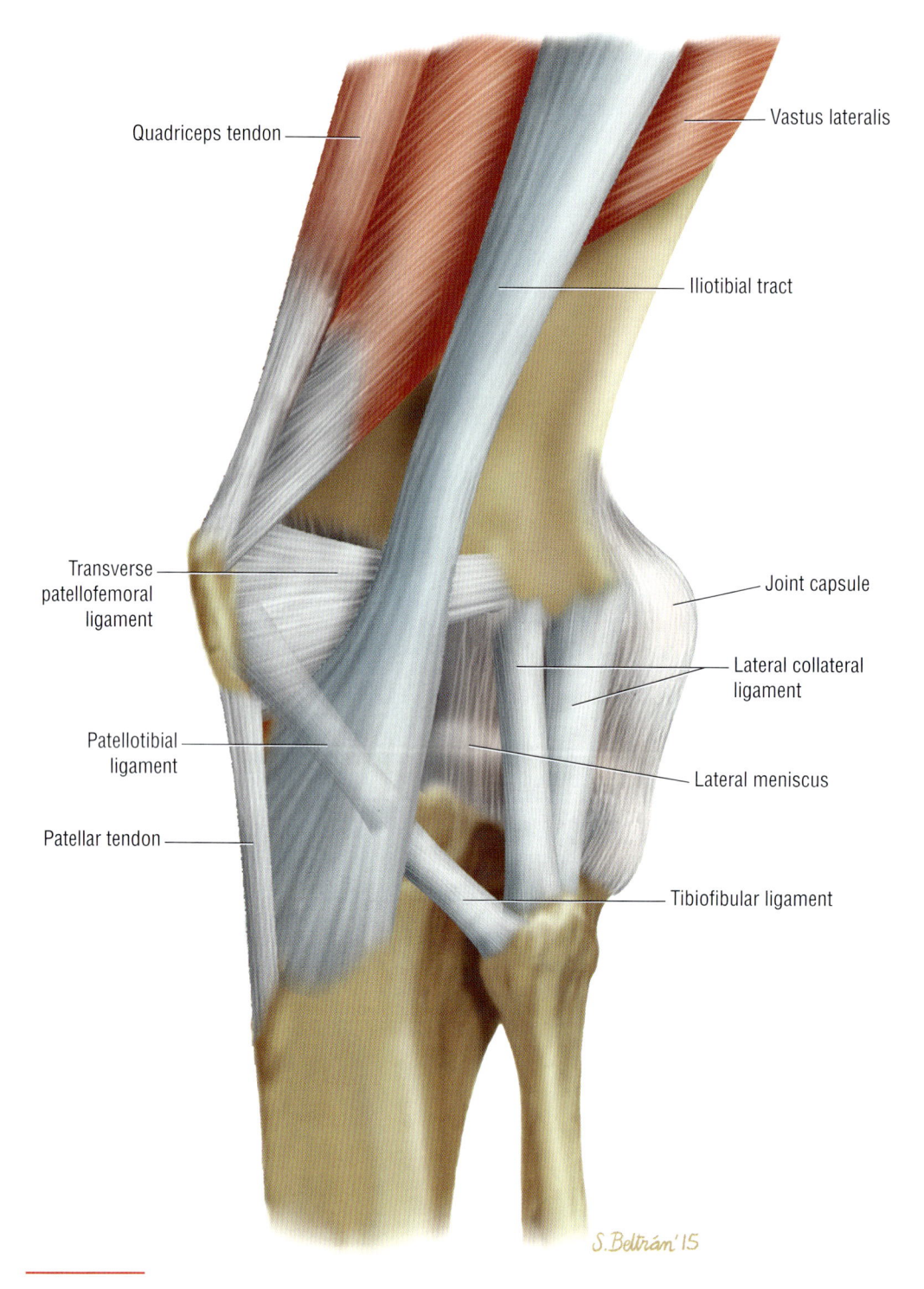

FIGURE 6.59 In layer 2, the lateral retinaculum consists of two major components: the superficial oblique retinaculum and the deep transverse retinaculum.

Collateral Ligaments

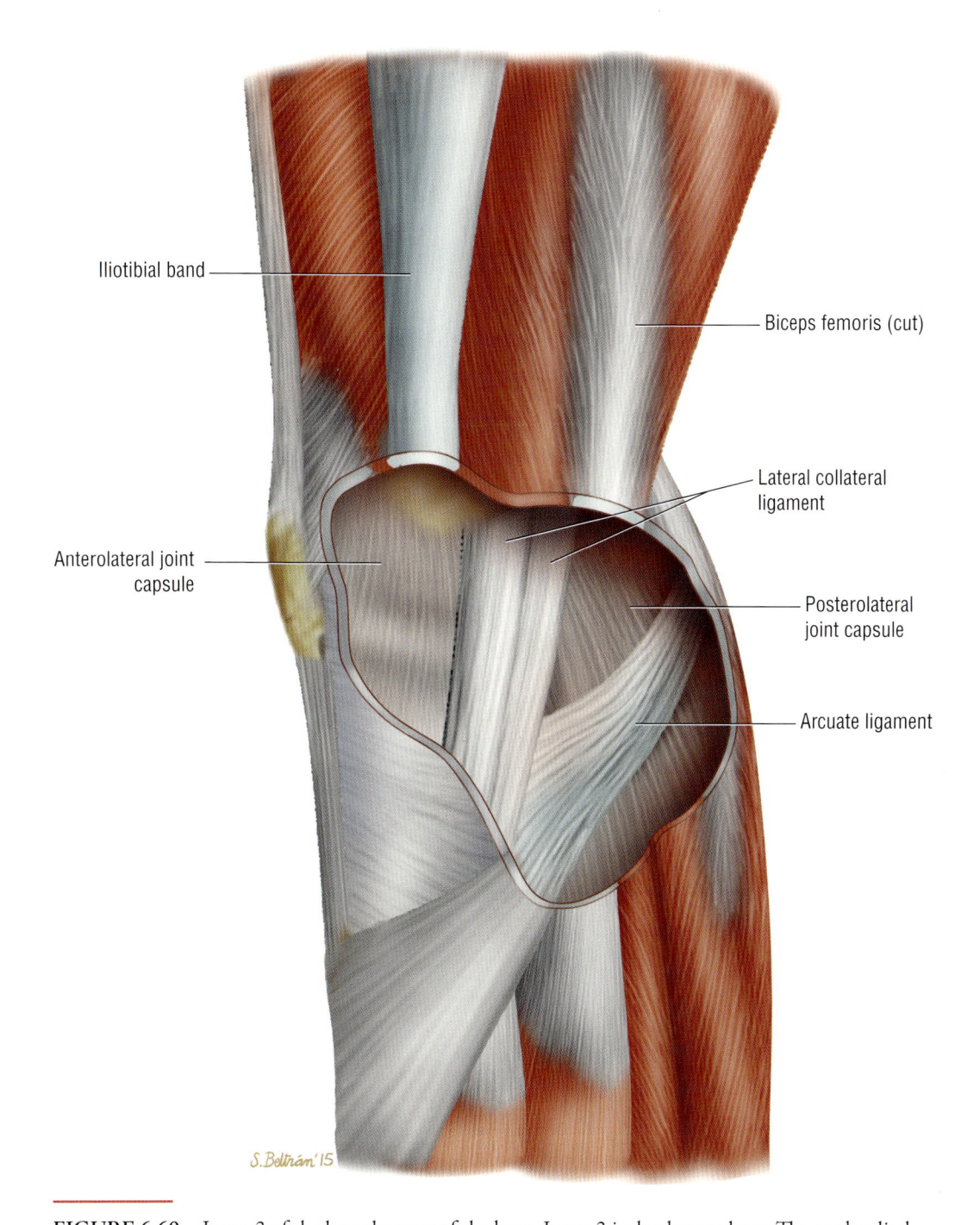

FIGURE 6.60 Layer 3 of the lateral aspect of the knee. Layer 3 is the deepest layer. The weaker limb of the arcuate ligament arches superiorly superficial (posterior) to the popliteus muscle and merges with the oblique popliteal ligament (OPL). The medial limb of the arcuate ligament is commonly torn in association with ACL tears and is not biomechanically significant.

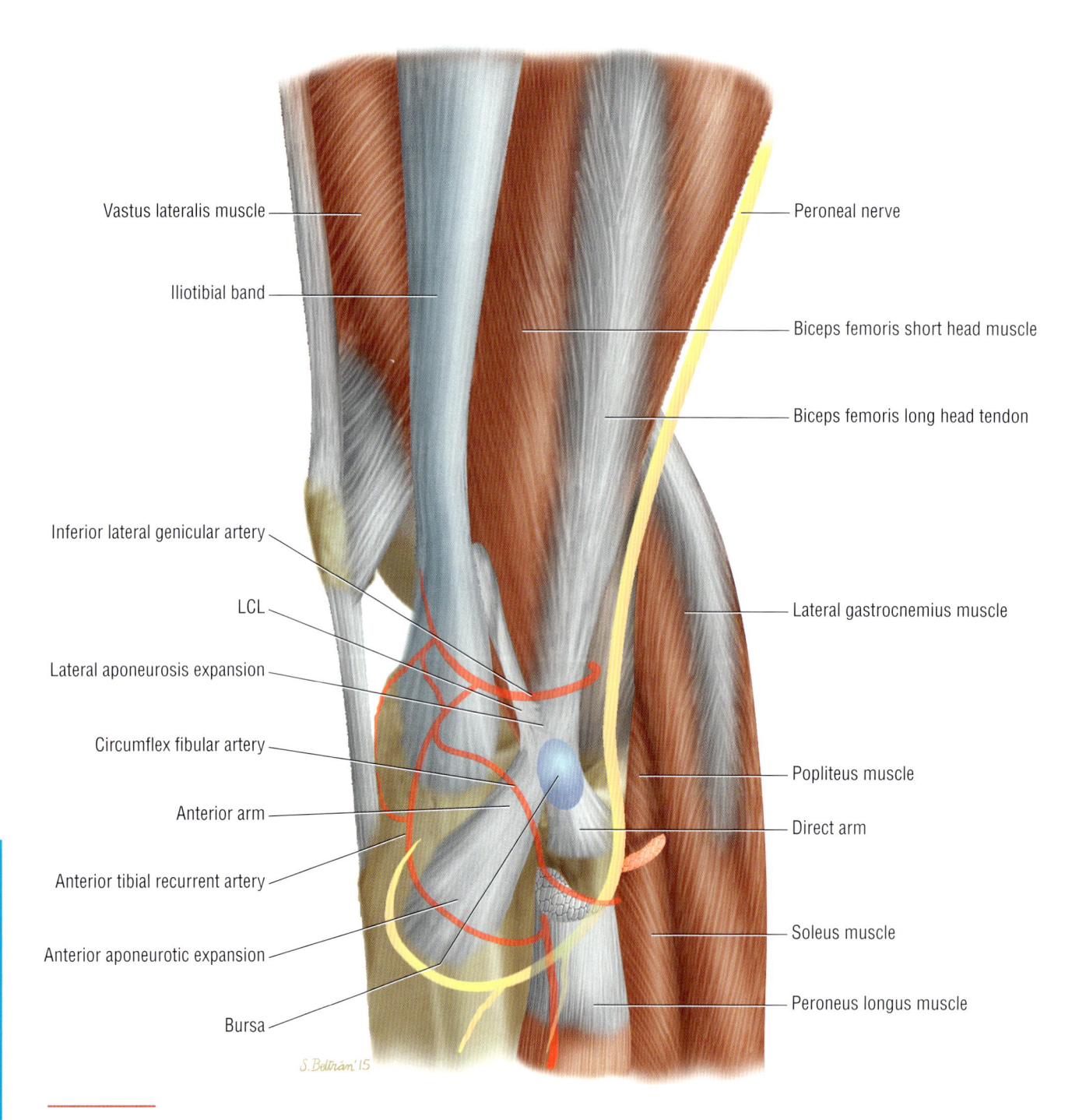

FIGURE 6.61 Long head of the biceps with multiple insertions.

Collateral Ligaments

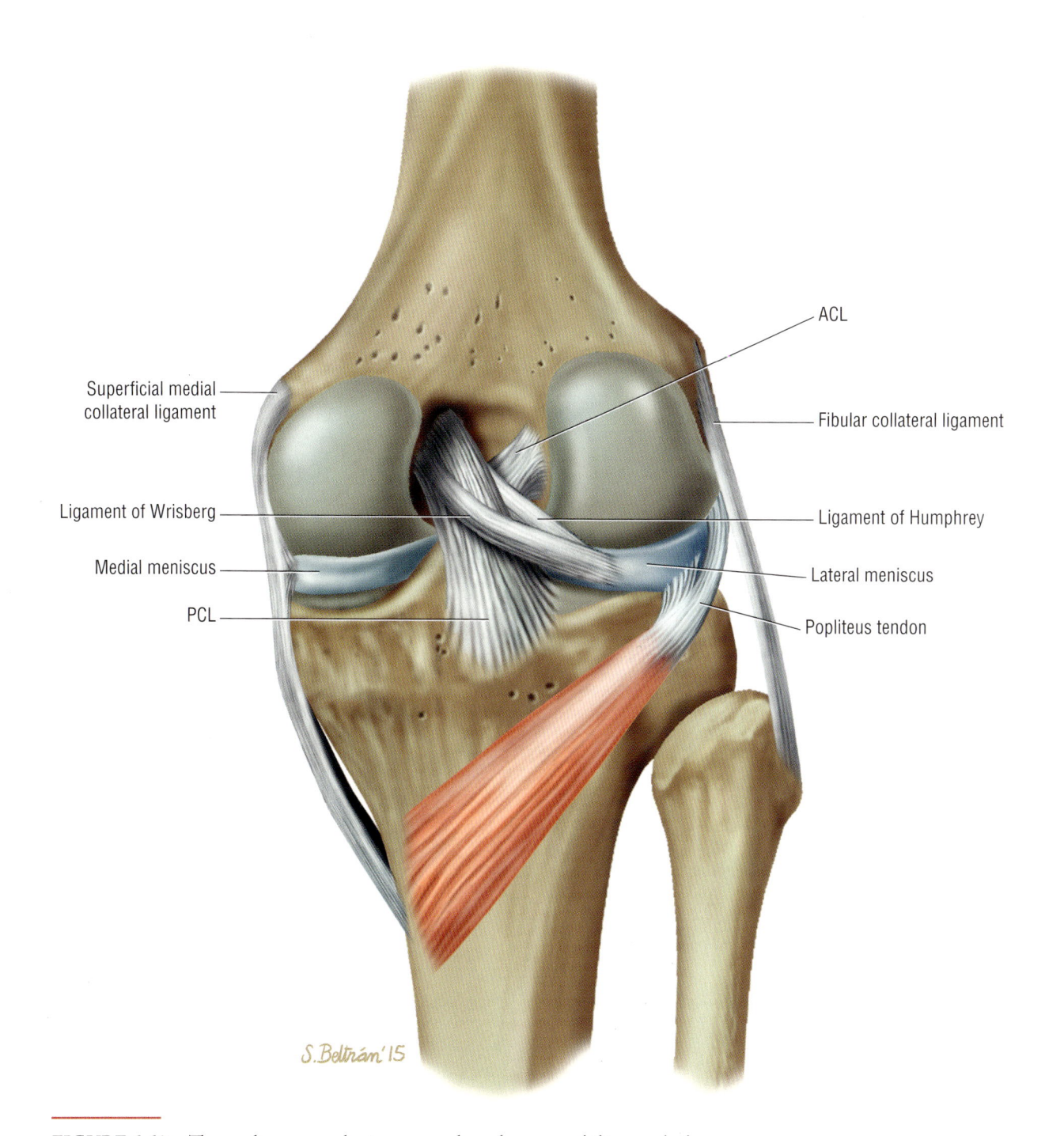

FIGURE 6.62 The popliteus complex is a posterolateral rotary stabilizer to the knee.

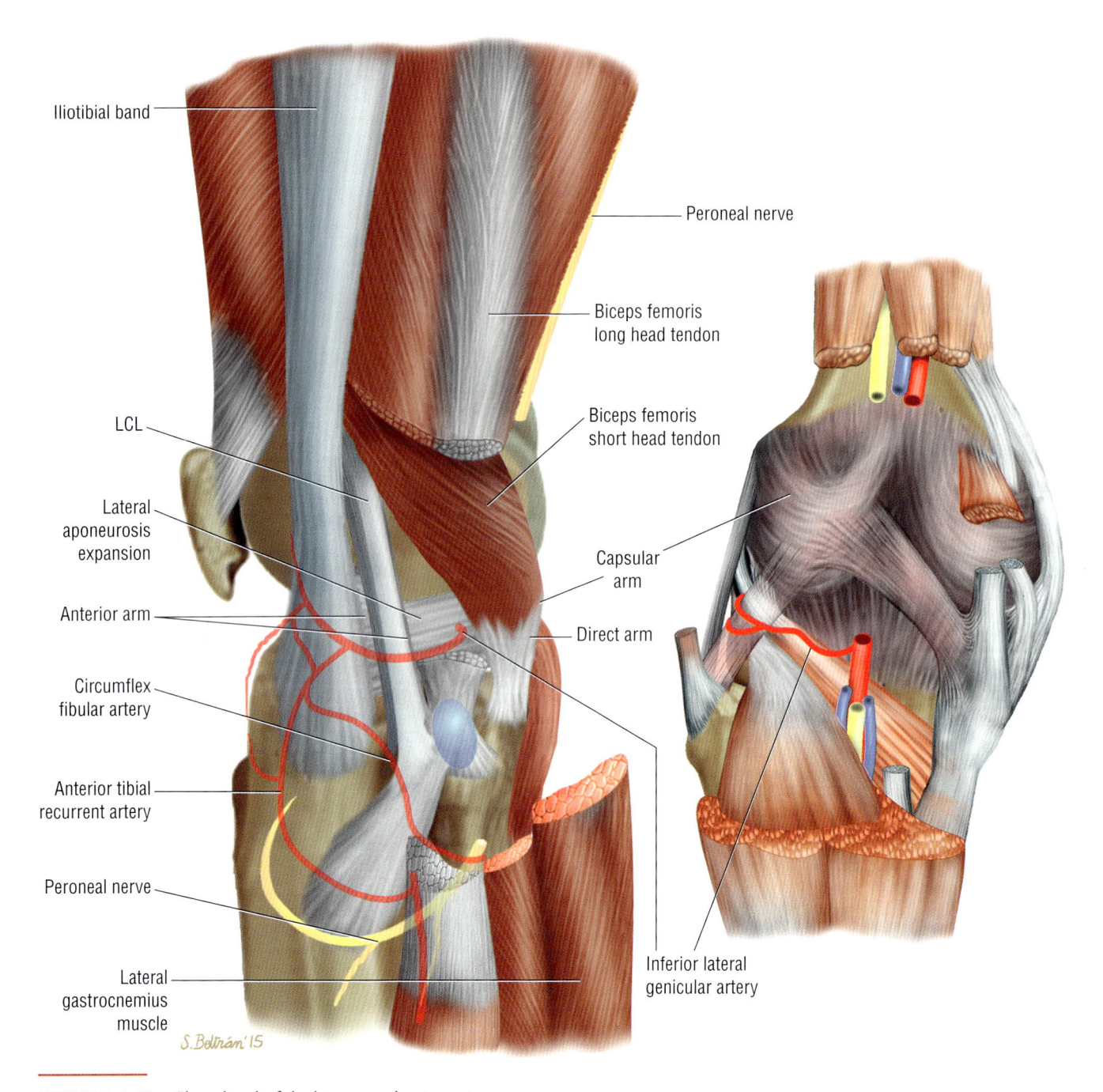

FIGURE 6.63 Short head of the biceps tendon insertion.

Collateral Ligaments

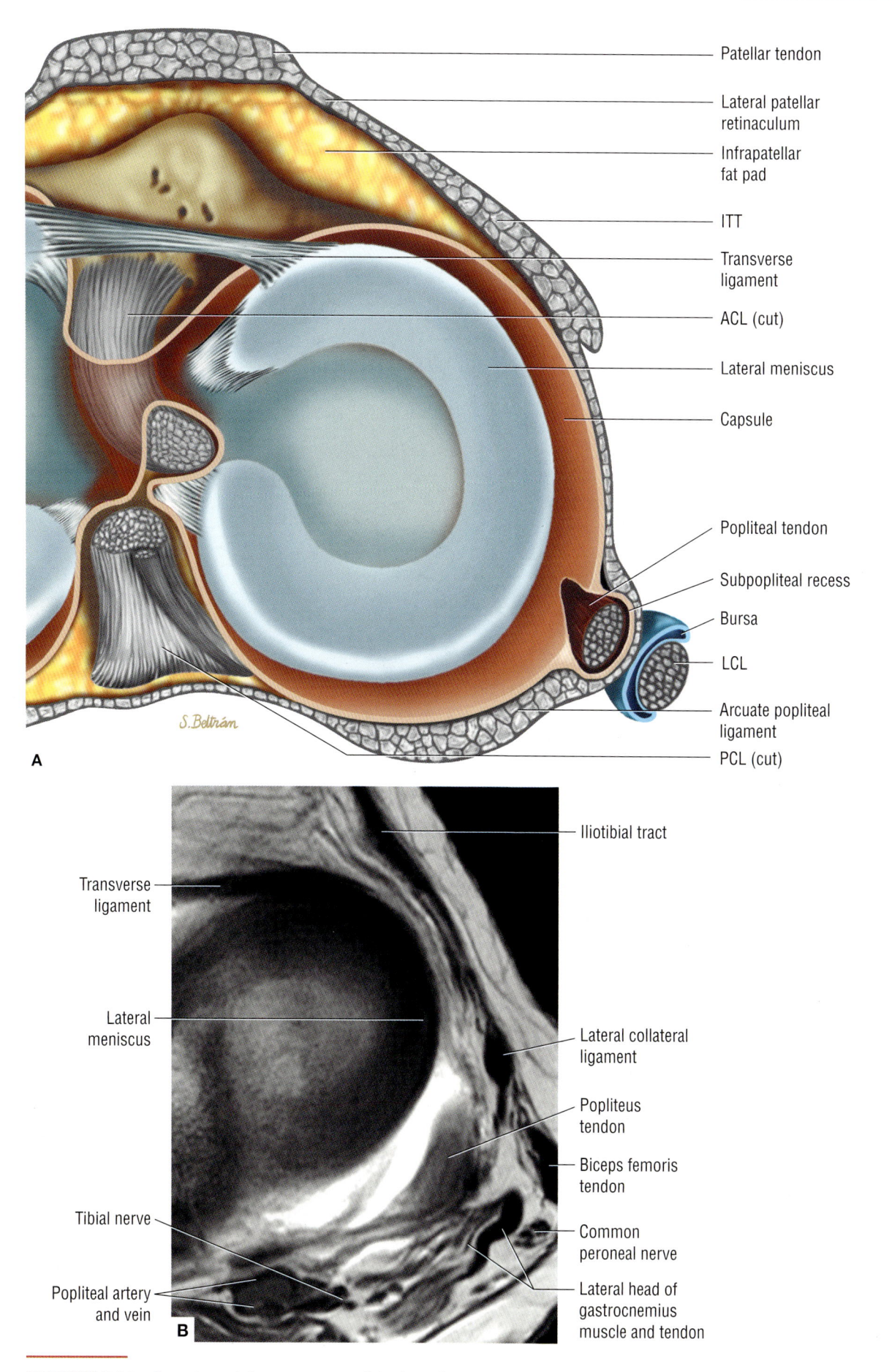

FIGURE 6.64 Superior axial cross-section of the lateral compartment at the level of the lateral meniscus on (**A**) a three-dimensional color illustration and (**B**) an axial T1-weighted MR arthrogram. ITT, iliotibial tract.

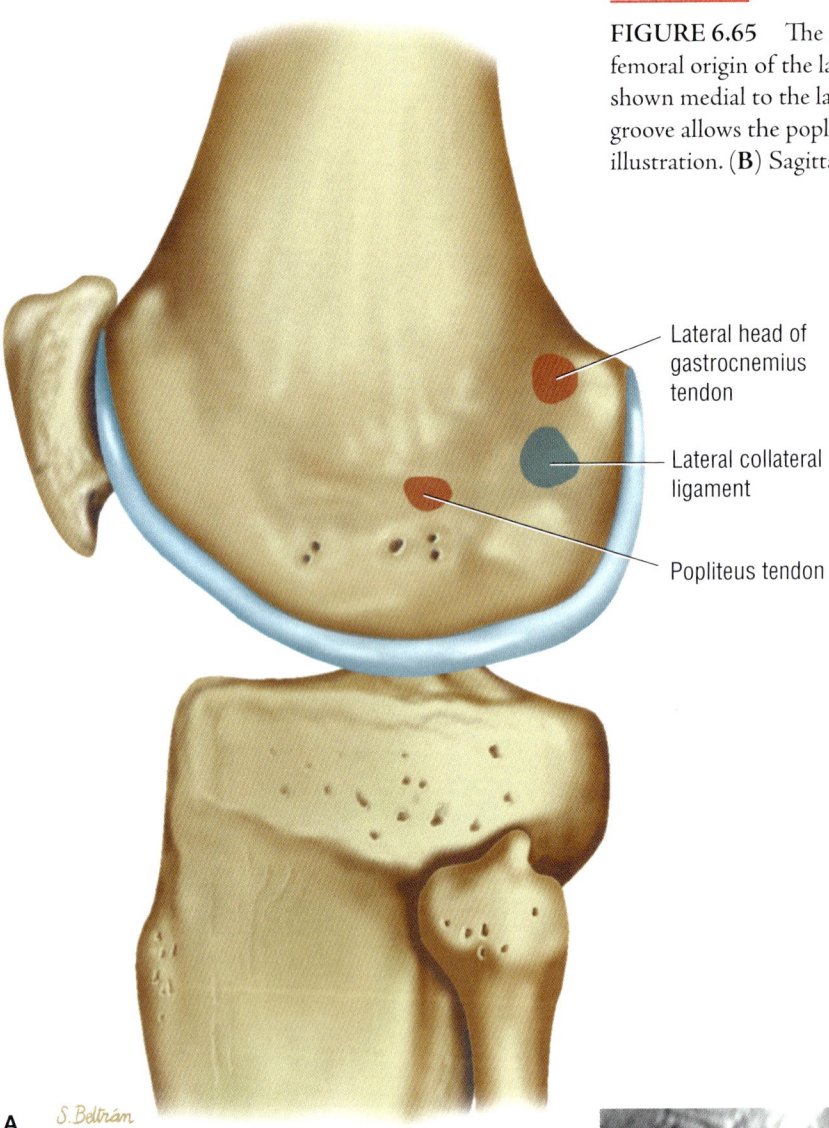

FIGURE 6.65 The popliteus tendon attaches anterior and distal to the femoral origin of the lateral collateral ligament. The popliteus tendon is shown medial to the lateral collateral ligaments. The lateral femoral condylar groove allows the popliteus tendon to course posteriorly. (**A**) Lateral color illustration. (**B**) Sagittal PD FSE image.

- Lateral head of gastrocnemius tendon
- Lateral collateral ligament
- Popliteus tendon

- Lateral head gastrocnemius tendon
- Lateral collateral ligament
- Popliteus tendon

Collateral Ligaments

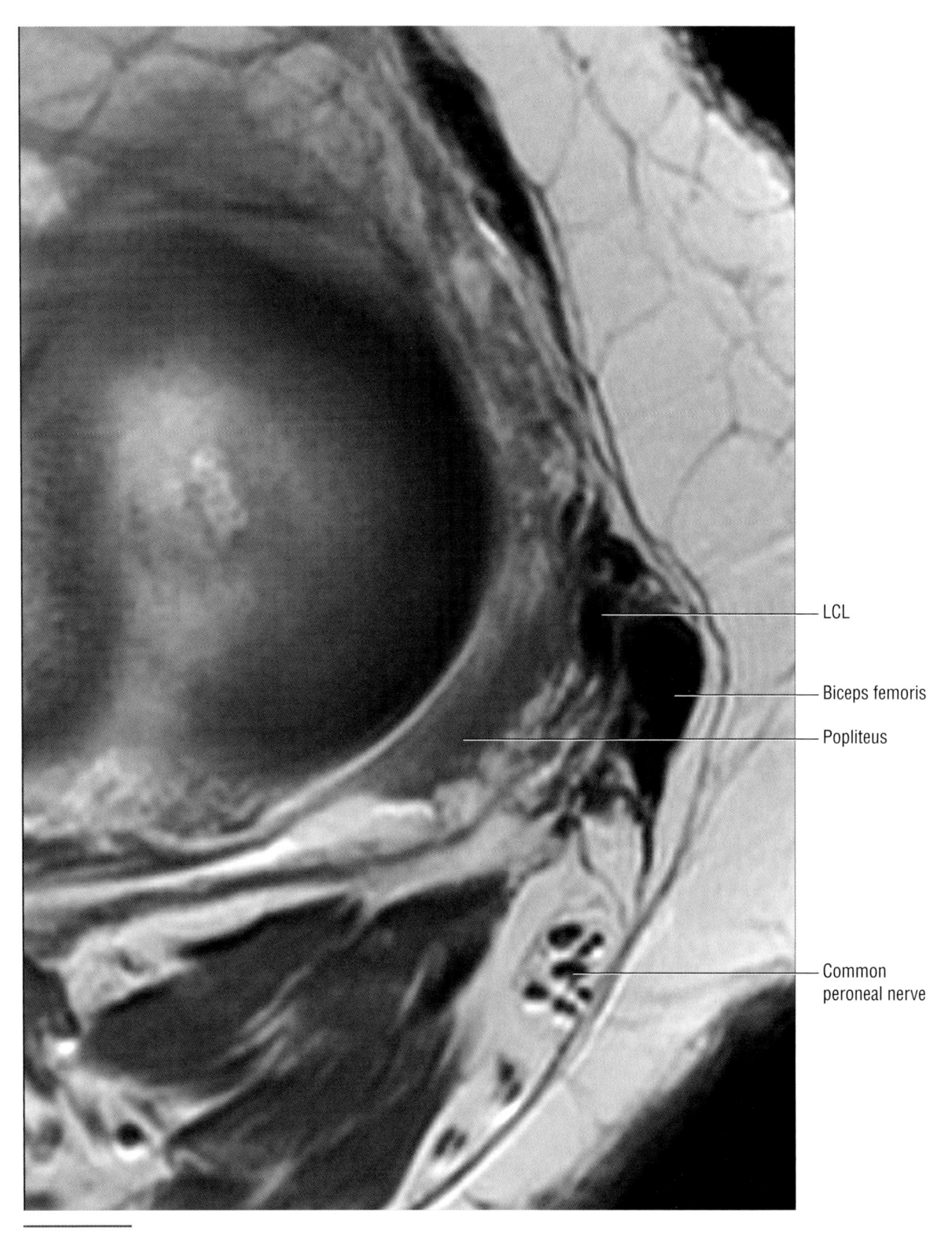

- LCL
- Biceps femoris
- Popliteus
- Common peroneal nerve

FIGURE 6.66 Layer 3 (deepest layer) of the lateral side of the knee contains the lateral capsule, LCL, fabellofibular ligament, arcuate ligament, popliteus tendon, and popliteofibular ligament (PFL). The LCL is located directly lateral to the popliteus tendon at the lateral joint line.

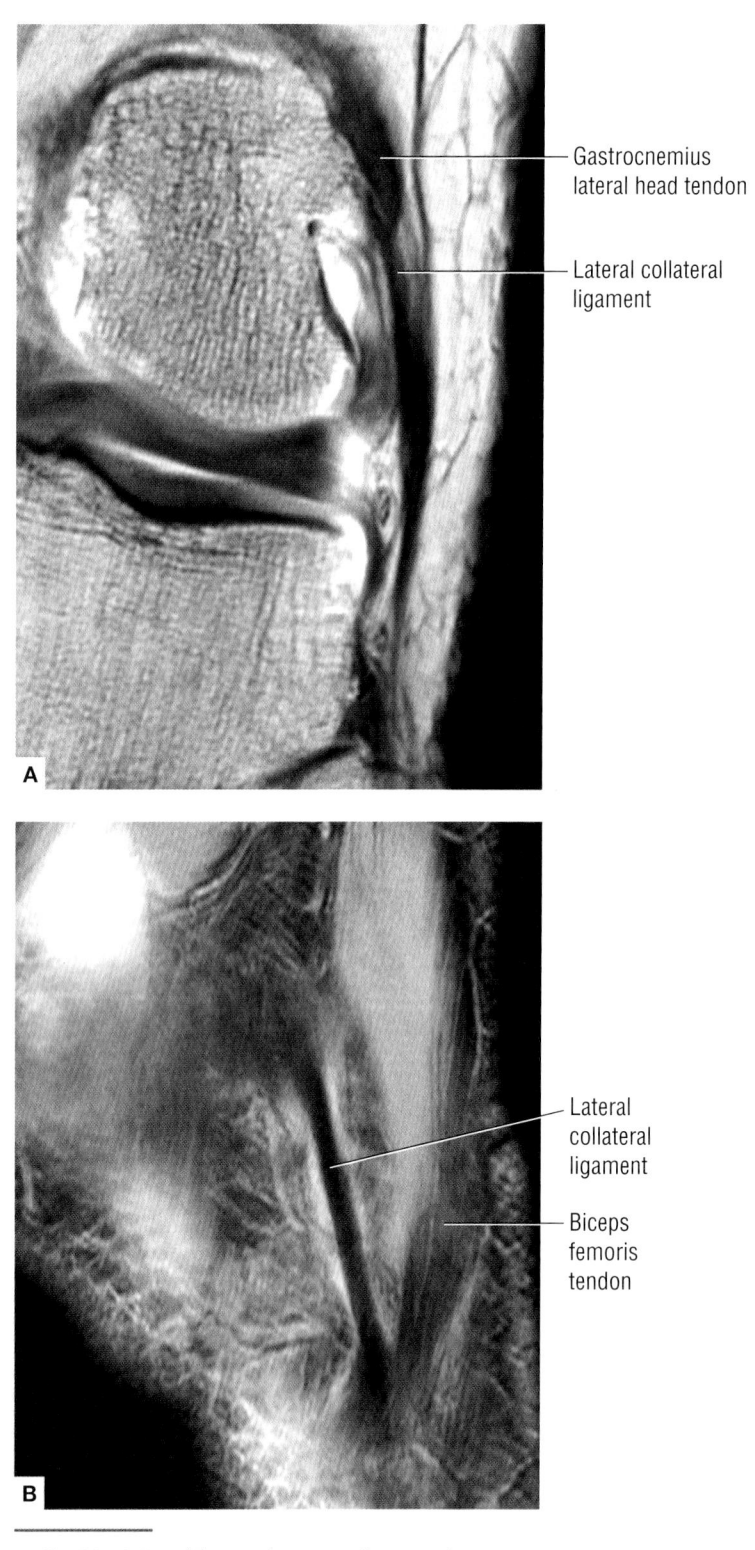

FIGURE 6.67 The popliteus tendon attaches anterior and distal to the femoral origin of the lateral collateral ligament. The lateral femoral condylar groove allows the popliteus tendon to course posteriorly. (**A**) Coronal T1 MR arthrogram. (**B**) Hypointense lateral collateral ligament coursing obliquely from the lateral femoral condyle distally and posteriorly to attach to the fibular head.

Collateral Ligaments

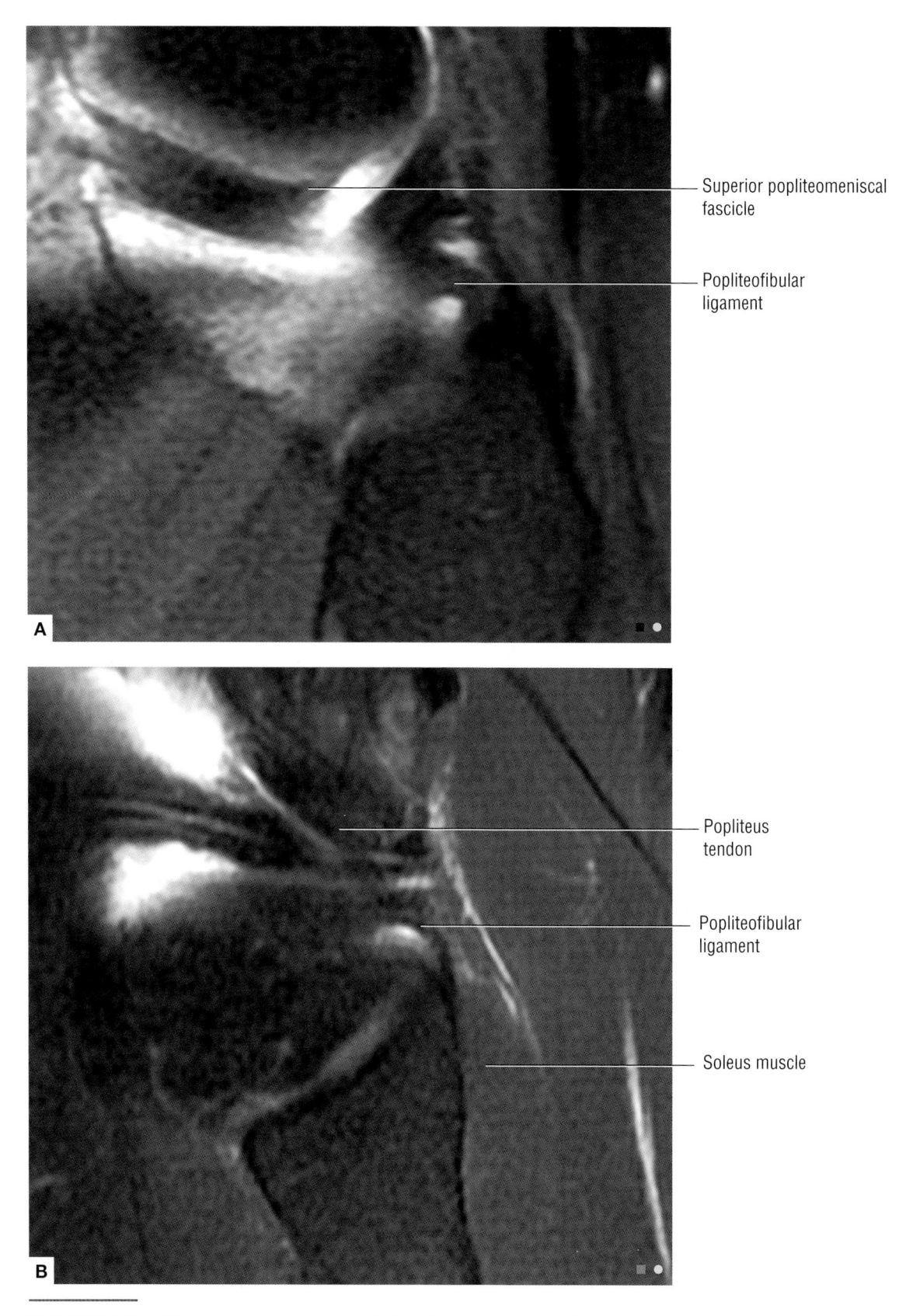

FIGURE 6.68 The superior (posterosuperior) and inferior (anteroinferior) popliteomeniscal fascicles can be identified in the coronal and sagittal planes. A third or posteroinferior popliteomeniscal fascicle is a medial aponeurotic extension from the popliteus musculotendinous area to the inferomedial aspect of the posterior horn of the lateral meniscus. Sagittal FS PD FSE images.

Popliteofibular Ligament

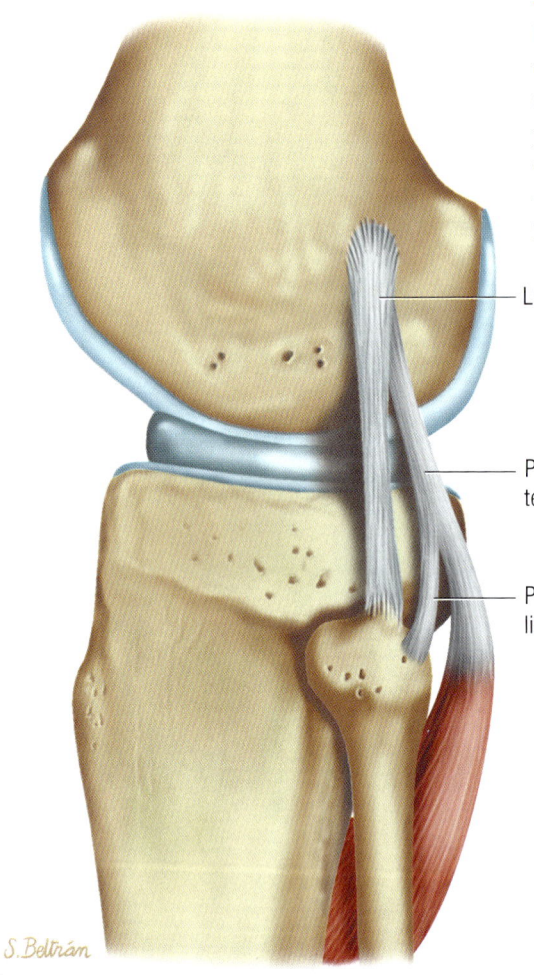

FIGURE 6.69 (**A**) The popliteofibular ligament originates from the posterior aspect of the fibula and extends toward the junction of the popliteus muscle and tendon. The popliteus tendon attachments to the tibia and the popliteofibular ligament help resist posterior translation and varus and external rotation. (**B**) Popliteofibular ligament attaching to the upper facet of the apex of the fibular head. The upper facet is just medial to the highest point of the apex.

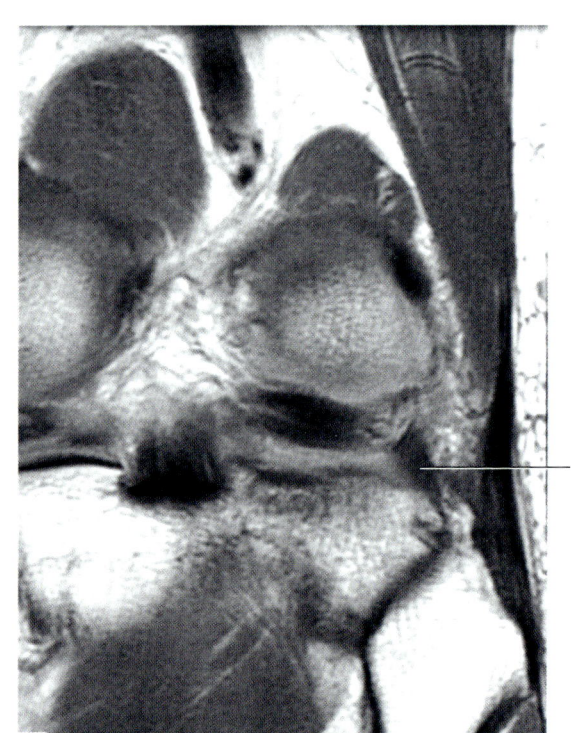

Anatomy of the Lateral Collateral Ligament

- One of three key structures of the posteromedial corner
- 5 to 7cm long and 4 to 5mm in width[40]
- Extracapsular
- Courses extraarticularly
- Free from meniscal attachment
- Courses from lateral femoral epicondyle to conjoined insertion with biceps femoris tendon on the fibular head[138]
    - Proximal attachment to femur is 1.4mm proximal and 3.1mm posterior to lateral epicondyle.
    - Some fibers expand over a portion of the lateral epicondyle directly.
    - Main attachment is a depression just proximal and posterior to lateral epicondyle.
    - Runs under superficial layer of iliotibial band and aponeurosis of long head biceps femoris to attach to lateral aspect of fibular head[40]
- Intracapsular popliteus tendon passes medial to LCL.
- Posterior fibers of LCL blend with deep capsule, which contributes to arcuate ligament.
- The proximal-distal attachment of the distal LCL on the lateral fibular head is longer than its proximal femoral osseous attachment.

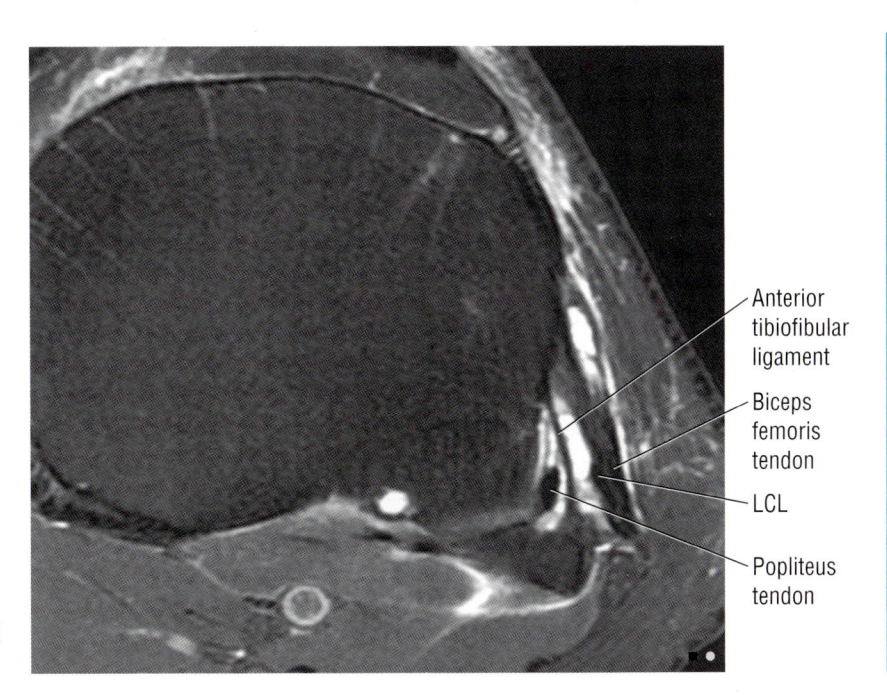

FIGURE 6.70 LCL and biceps femoris proximal to their lateral fibular head attachment. Axial FS PD FSE image.

Anatomy of the Iliotibial Band

- Iliotibial band (ITB) = iliotibial tract
- Important landmark of PLC since ITB is rarely injured
- Four main components
    - Superficial layer
        - Covers to posterior aspect of vastus lateralis
        - Courses inferiorly (distal) to attach to Gerdy's tubercle
    - Iliopatellar band
    - Deep fibers or Kaplan's fibers
        - Attach ITB to femur in region of intermuscular septum
    - Capsulo-osseous layer
        - Fascial sling attaches to ITB
        - Distal attachment to tibia in area of meniscotibial attachment of the mid-third of the lateral capsular ligament
        - Also referred to as retrograde tract fibers
        - Forms sling over PLC
            - Contributes to reduction in the pivot shift
- Intraoperative landmark for other PLC structures because of low rate of injury of ITB (approximately 3% of PLC injuries)[40]
    - ITB only involved in the most severe of PLC injuries

Anatomy of the Mid-Third Capsular Ligament

- Thickening of the lateral capsule
- Courses from femur to tibia analogous to dMCL on the medial side
- Femoral attachment immediately anterior to popliteus tendon attachment on femur
- Posterior femoral attachment is anterior to lateral gastrocnemius tendon attachment.
- Attaches to lateral meniscus[40]

Anatomy of Lateral Gastrocnemius Tendon

- Lateral gastrocnemius tendon[40]
    - Tendinous thickening lateral aspect gastrocnemius
    - Blends into meniscofemoral portion of posterolateral capsule at level of fabella or cartilaginous fabella
    - A bony or cartilaginous fabella is always present.
    - Lateral gastrocnemius tendon rarely involved in PLC injuries
        - Femoral attachment close to supracondylar process lateral landmark or reference point since intact even in severe injuries of PLC
            - Reference for acute PLC repairs or chronic reconstructions

Anatomy of the Long Head of the Biceps Femoris

- Six different anatomic components
- Two tendinous components that attach to fibular head
    - Direct arm
        - Attaches to lateral aspect of fibular styloid
    - Anterior arm
        - Crosses lateral to fibular head
        - Fascial attachment to aponeurosis that covers anterior compartment
        - Forms a bursa where it crosses the distal quarter of the LCL
            - Bursa surrounds LCL in a 270-degree arc.
            - Inclusion through the biceps bursa is used to perform repairs or reconstructions of PLC.
- Fascial attachments as other component parts of biceps femoris
    - Proximally, a reflected arm attaches to posterior border of ITB.
    - Lateral aponeurosis attaches to posterolateral aspect of LCL.
        - Creates dynamic control of LCL through the action of the biceps femoris complex
    - Distal aponeurosis from long head of biceps femoris to lateral gastrocnemius complex[40]

Anatomy of the Short Head of the Biceps Femoris

- Disrupted with osseous or soft tissue Segond avulsions[40]
- Five major components
  - Main muscle belly
    - From posterolateral distal femur to its attachment on medial aspect of long head of common tendon
  - Tendinous attachment with main common tendon
    - Becomes direct arm of short head
    - Attaches lateral to tip of fibular styloid
  - Capsular arm
    - Thick and stout and located proximal to its tendinous attachment
    - Courses to posterolateral joint capsule and lateral gastrocnemius tendon
    - Distal capsular arm attaches to tip of fibular styloid and proximally to region of fabella on lateral gastrocnemius tendon.
      - Represents, in fact, the fabellofibular ligament
      - The fabellofibular ligament is tight in extension and lax in flexion.
      - Fabellofibular ligament is variable in its thickness but not the actual presence of this structure because it is always defined by the distal edge of the capsular arm of the short head and thus must be present whether or not there is a visible fabella.
  - Fine aponeurosis distal to capsular arm called the short biceps lateral aponeurosis[40]
    - Courses from short-head biceps tendon to posterolateral aspect of LCL
    - Anterior arm
      - Courses medial to LCL
      - Attaches posterior to meniscotibial portion of mid-third lateral capsular ligament

Anatomy of Popliteus Complex

- Posterolateral rotary stabilizer with static and dynamic function
- Main tendinous attachment of popliteus muscle in upper popliteal sulcus of popliteus
    - Center of attachment is 18.5mm anterior to LCL femoral attachment[40]
- Distally, popliteus has three popliteomeniscal fascicles that attach lateral meniscus to popliteus tendon
    - Level of popliteal hiatus
    - Anteroinferior popliteomeniscal fascicle
        - Strongest and most stability to lateral meniscal motion
    - Posterosuperior popliteomeniscal fascicle
    - Posteroinferior popliteomeniscal fascicle
- Popliteofibular ligament
    - At level of popliteus musculotendinous junction
    - Courses from popliteus tendon to posteromedial aspect of fibular styloid
        - Two divisions of popliteofibular ligament
            - Anterior
            - Posterior (larger and stronger)
    - Proximal aspect of popliteofibular ligament blends with distal aspect of popliteomeniscal fascicles.
- Popliteal aponeurosis
    - From proximal aspect of popliteus muscle to the posterior horn of lateral meniscus[40]

Anatomy of Coronary Ligament to the Lateral Meniscus

- Meniscotibial portion of posterior capsule
- Courses laterally from popliteomeniscal fascicles to root attachment of lateral meniscus
  - Originates medially and just lateral to posterior cruciate ligament
  - Lateral border is at the edge of the popliteal hiatus
  - Stability to posterior horn of lateral meniscus[40]

Biomechanics of LCL and Posterolateral Structures

- Preventing varus and valgus rotation
  - LCL is the primary restraint to varus motion.
  - Secondary varus stability
    - Popliteus tendon
    - ACL and PCL
- Preventing anterior tibial translation
  - Isolated PCL sectioning is not associated with increased anterior tibial translation.
  - ACL and posterolateral structure sectioning results in anterior tibial translation.
  - PLC thus has important secondary role in preventing anterior tibial translation with an associated ACL tear.
  - Patients who present with increased anterior tibial translation (positive Lachman's test) should be evaluated for concurrent PLC structure injury.
- Preventing posterior translation of the tibia
  - PLC structures have primary and secondary role in providing posterior stability.
  - Minor primary role in preventing abnormal posterior tibial translation that occurs at extension
  - Significant secondary role in preventing posterior tibial translation in PCL-deficient knees
  - Patients with a 3+ positive drawer test should be evaluated for an associated PLC injury plus the PCL tear.[40]

- Preventing internal rotation
    - Minor role of PLC structures in preventing primary internal rotation
    - Secondary restraint to internal rotation in the ACL-deficient knee near full extension
- Preventing external rotation
    - Important role of PLC in preventing external rotation
    - Greatest external rotation occurs at 30 degrees of knee flexion
    - In the presence of either an ACL or PCL injury, the amount of external rotation at 90 degrees of flexion will be similar to the external rotation that occurs at 30 degrees of flexion with isolated PLC sectioning.[40]
- Popliteomeniscal fascicle stabilizing role to the lateral meniscus
    - Sectioning popliteomeniscal fascicles resulted in increased anterior motion of the loaded lateral meniscus.
    - Anteroinferior popliteomeniscal fascicle
        - Larger
        - Greater stability compared with the thinner posterosuperior popliteomeniscal fascicle
    - Popliteomeniscal fascicle disruption
        - Increased meniscal motion
        - Mechanical symptoms
- PLC injury and knee joint contact forces
    - Increase in joint contact pressure with PCL injury
        - Patellofemoral joint
        - Medial compartment of knee
        - Highest increase occurs in joint contact pressures with PCL and PLC injury.
        - Osteoarthritis increased risk with combined PCL and PLC knee injuries.[40]

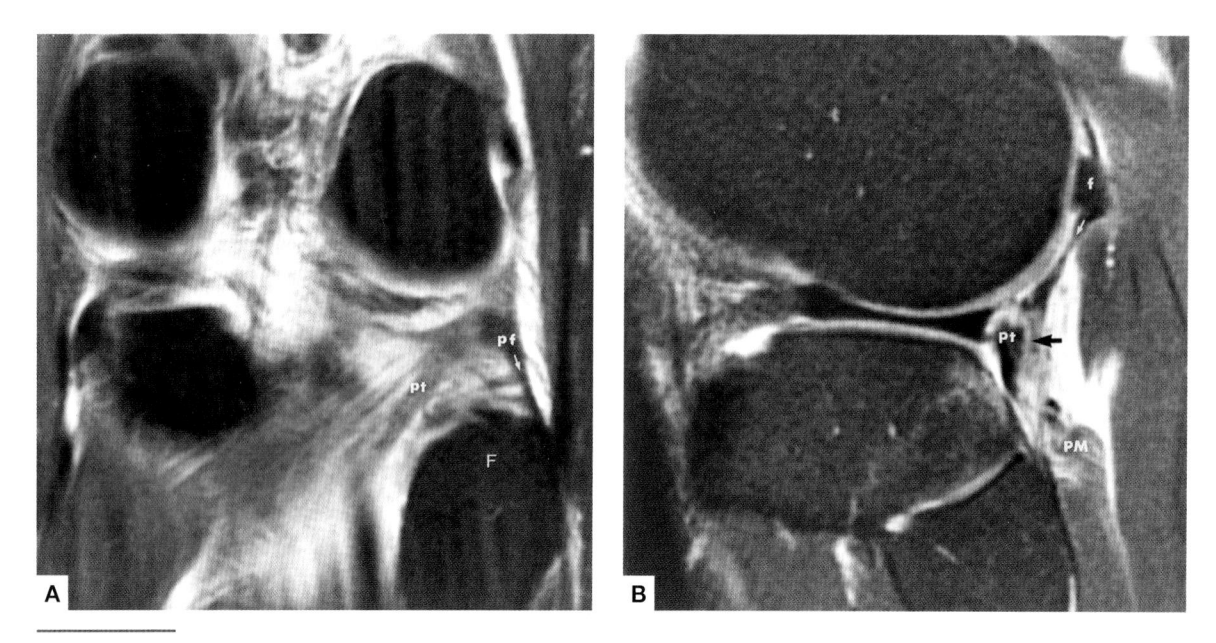

FIGURE 6.71 Posterolateral capsular structures on FS T2-weighted FSE coronal (**A**) and sagittal (**B**) images. As a normal variant, the arcuate ligament may not be visualized in the presence of a fabellofibular ligament. (**A**) F, fibula; Pf and *arrow*, popliteofibular ligament; Pt, popliteus tendon. (**B**) f, fabella; PM, partial torn popliteus muscle; Pt, popliteus tendon; *small arrow*, fabellopopliteal ligament; *large arrow*, torn arcuate ligament.

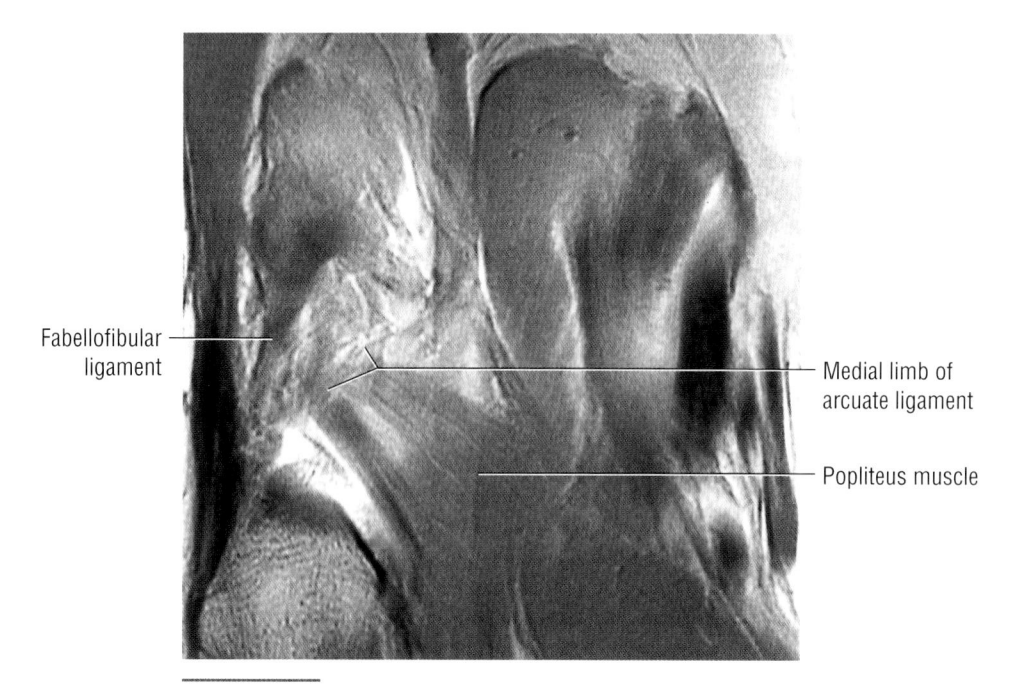

FIGURE 6.72 Proximal course of the fabellofibular ligament on a coronal T1-weighted MR arthrogram.

Collateral Ligaments

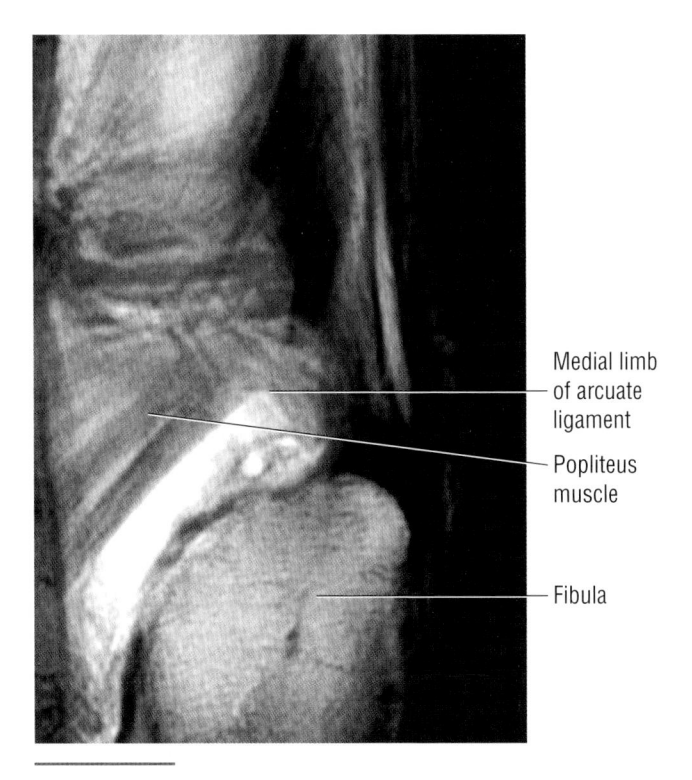

FIGURE 6.73 Medial limb of arcuate ligament on posterior coronal T1-weighted MR arthrogram.

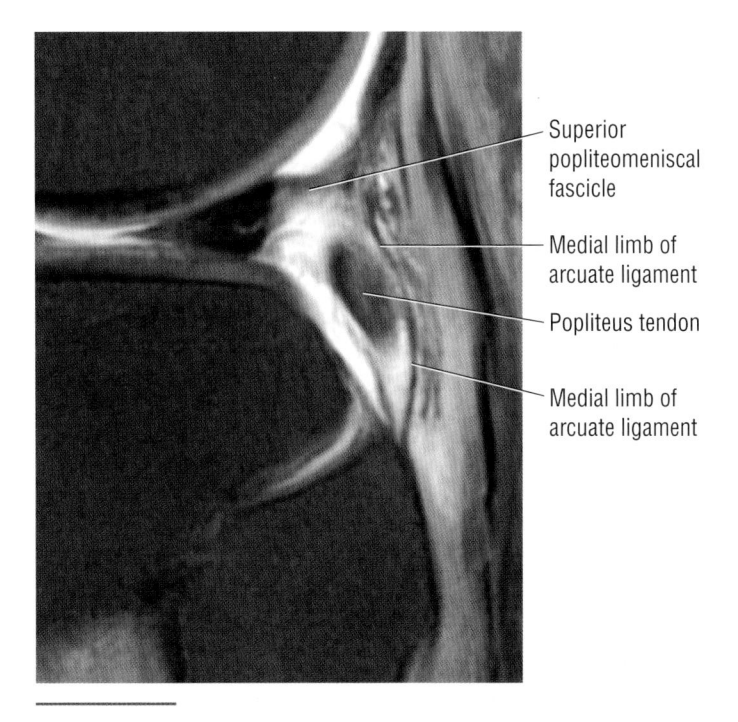

FIGURE 6.74 Medial limb of the arcuate ligament identified posterior to the popliteus tendon. The medial limb is best visualized on the sagittal images, which show the posterior horn of the lateral meniscus immediately medial to the body of the lateral meniscus. At this location, the attachment of the medial limb to the apex of the fibular head is shown, as is the normal deficiency of the inferior popliteomeniscal fascicle (sagittal FS PD FSE image).

Location and Mechanism of Injury of the LCL and Posterolateral Structures

- Mechanism of LCL injury
    - Applied varus force with the leg in internal rotation can cause injury to the LCL and capsule.
    - Arcuate ligament and complex stabilize the posterolateral aspect of the knee against varus and external rotation.[504]
    - LCL injury or disruption significantly less common than MCL injury
- PLC injury
    - Can result from direct or noncontact forces that cause knee hyperextension or hyperextension and external rotation
        - Direct blow to tibia with knee flexed or extended
        - Twisting injury
    - May be seen in conjunction with either ACL or PCL injury
        - Combined PCL and posterolateral capsular injuries often missed at initial clinical presentation
        - Posterolateral pain, buckling into hyperextension with weight bearing, and instability
- Cruciate and lateral meniscal tears may be associated with lateral compartment ligament tears.
    - MR imaging may reveal joint space widening, fracture of fibular head, and Segond fracture, in association with ACL injuries.[69]
- *Posterolateral instability* classified into three types:
    - Type A
        - Increased external rotation without varus instability
        - Injury to popliteofibular ligament and popliteus tendon
    - Type B
        - Increased external rotation with moderate varus laxity
        - Injury to popliteofibular ligament, popliteus tendon, and LCL
    - Type C
        - Increased external rotation plus complete varus laxity
        - Injury to popliteofibular ligament, popliteus tendon, LCL, lateral capsule, and cruciate ligament

MR Appearance of the LCL

- Normal LCL
    - Best seen on posterior coronal images
    - Appears as band of low signal intensity
    - Located at level of popliteus tendon and lateral meniscus
    - Attaches proximally to popliteal fossa and distally to lateral aspect of fibular head
    - Peripheral sagittal images demonstrate LCL anatomy at level of fibular head.

- LCL injury
    - Edema and hemorrhage less frequent compared to medial injuries
    - Ligamentous thickening with increased signal intensity on T2- or FSE PD-weighted images (with FS)
    - Signal intensity not as high in LCL injuries compared to MCL disruptions, perhaps because normal capsular separation of LCL excludes accumulation of extravasated joint fluid
    - In complete disruptions, LCL demonstrates wavy or serpiginous contour and loss of ligamentous continuity.
        - May be proximal migration of avulsed ligament from fibular attachment
    - FS PD FSE axial images important in diagnosing LCL tears when course of entire ligament cannot be visualized on coronal images
    - LCL injuries graded by system similar to that described for MCL injuries

- Associated injuries
    - Biceps femoris injuries
        - Biceps femoris muscle also plays important role as lateral stabilizer.
    - Popliteofibular ligament or combined popliteofibular, fabellofibular, and arcuate ligament avulsions
        - More commonly associated with fibular styloid avulsion fractures compared to the more lateral LCL avulsions[201,469]

- Tears of ITB
    - Association among LCL tears, popliteus tendon ruptures (at the fossa), and iliotibial tract disruptions
    - Inclusion of ITB on anterior coronal images is important if this structure is to be used to reconstruct the LCL.
- Popliteus muscle and tendon
    - Areas of muscle edema and hemorrhage best displayed on FS PD-weighted FSE or STIR sagittal and axial images
    - Focal enlargement of popliteus muscle may be secondary to hemorrhage or tearing of muscle fibers.
    - Areas of increased signal intensity visualized at muscle–tendon junction on sagittal images in conjunction with ACL and PLC injuries
    - Associated with concomitant injuries to posterolateral complex
    - Isolated popliteus tendon rupture is rare.[518]
    - Normally, popliteus tendon resists external rotation of the tibia, acting as both static and active restraint.
- Deep venous thrombosis as posttraumatic complication of significant ACL/PLC trauma
    - Medial head of the gastrocnemius should be evaluated for collateral venous flow.

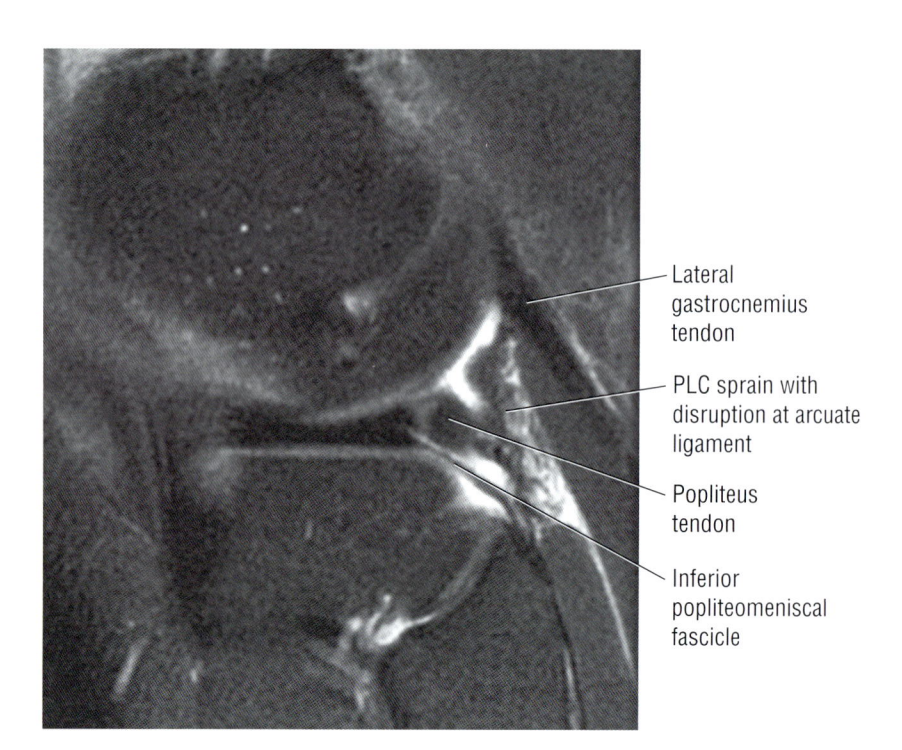

FIGURE 6.75 Mild posterolateral corner sprain with tear of the arcuate ligament (medial limb).

Collateral Ligaments

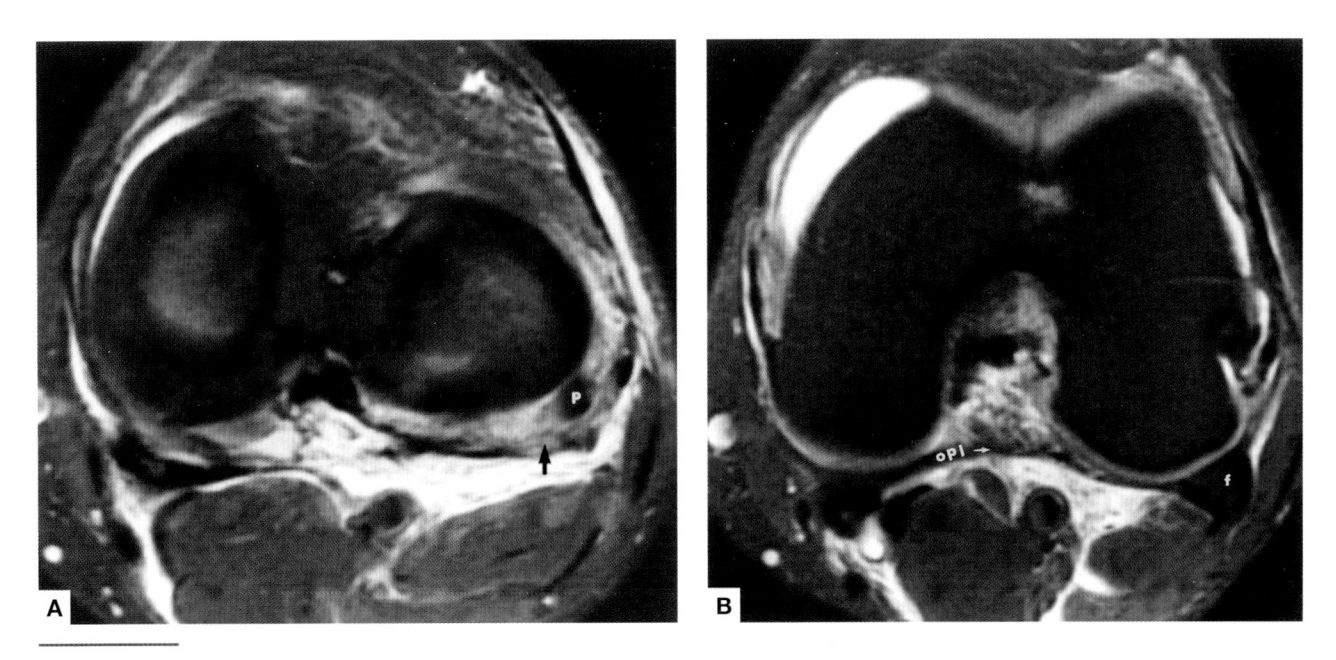

FIGURE 6.76 FS PD-weighted FSE axial images showing the relation of the popliteus tendon (P) and arcuate ligament sprain (*arrow*) at the level of the joint line (**A**) and the normal visualization of the oblique popliteal ligament (opl and *arrow*) on a more superior axial image at the level of the femoral condyles (**B**). f, fabella.

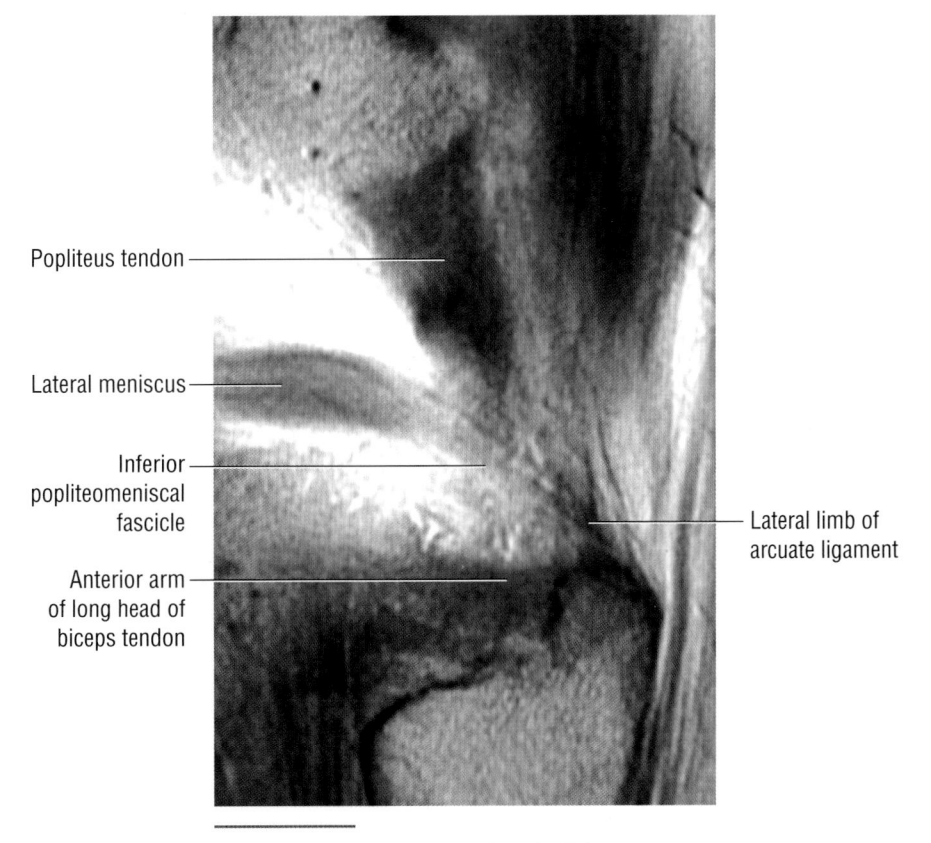

FIGURE 6.77 The lateral limb of the arcuate complex. The entire arcuate ligament may be attenuated or absent in the presence of a fabellofibular ligament.

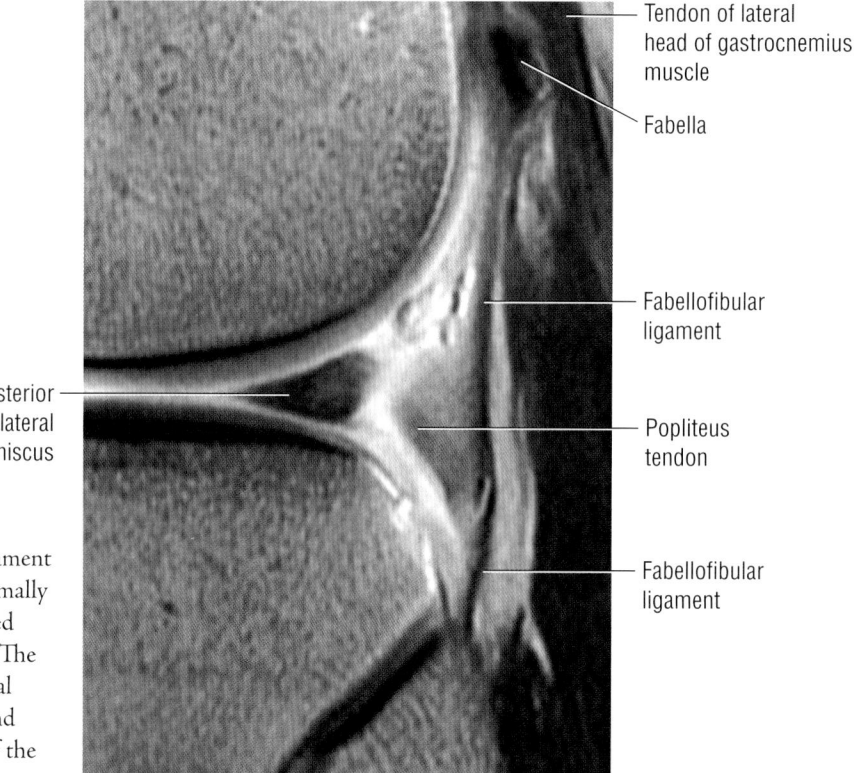

FIGURE 6.78 Prominent fabellofibular ligament with the attachments to both the fabella proximally and the fibular styloid process distally identified on this sagittal T1-weighted MR arthrogram. The fabellofibular ligament is posterior to the lateral limb of the arcuate ligament and anterior to and separate from the tendon of the lateral head of the gastrocnemius muscle.

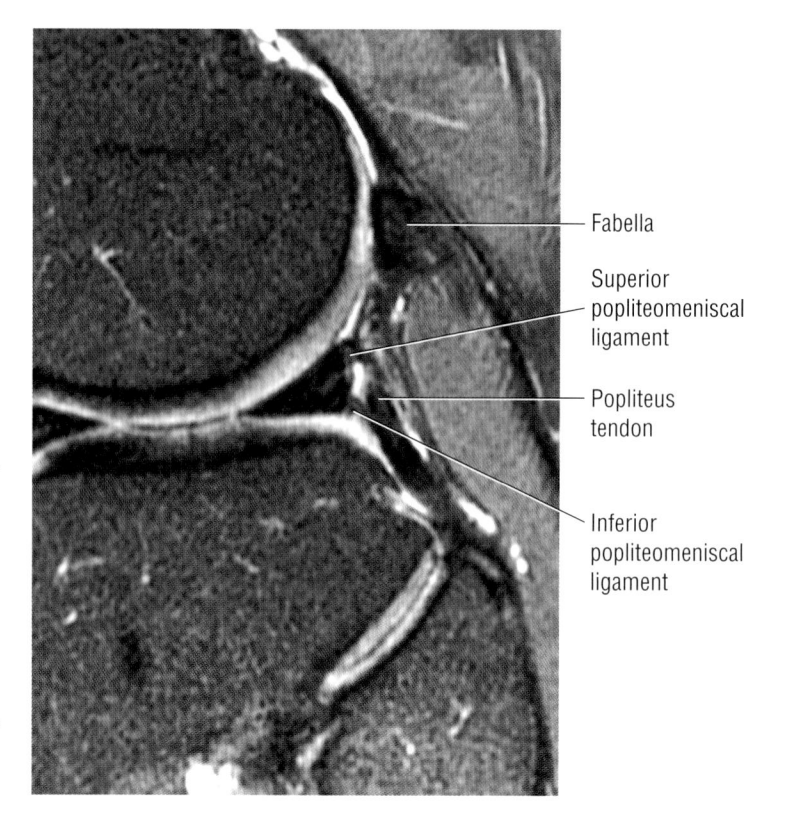

FIGURE 6.79 The popliteus tendon courses through the popliteal hiatus and is bound anteroinferiorly and posterosuperiorly by popliteomeniscal fascicles. There is also a direct attachment to the lateral meniscus by both the superior and inferior popliteomeniscal fascicles. The popliteus tendon is covered by synovial membrane on its medial side. This sagittal FS PD FSE image shows the superior and inferior meniscal fascicles allowing the passage of the popliteus tendon and forming the hiatus posterolaterally. A smaller or absent arcuate ligament may exist in the presence of a bony fabella.

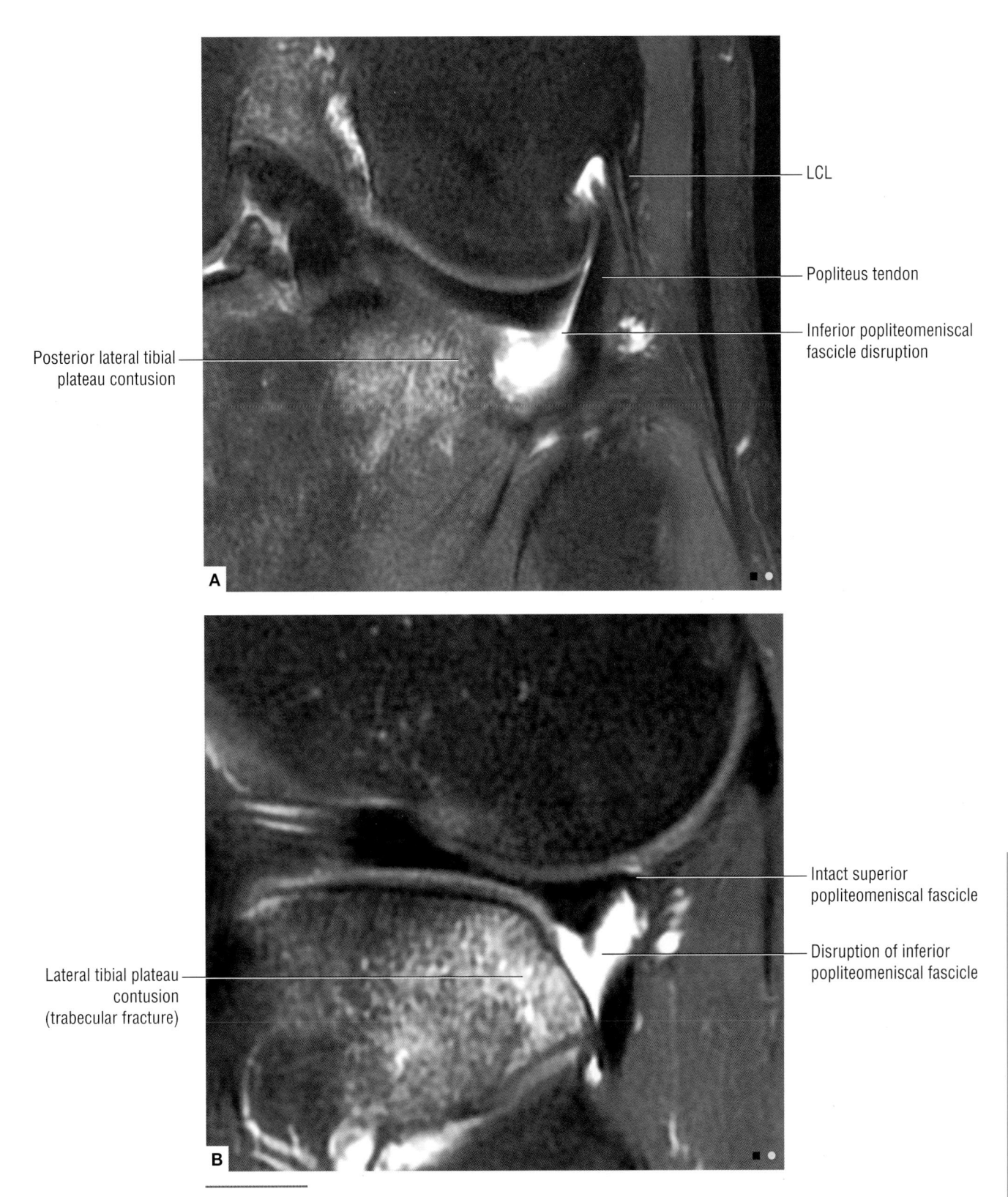

FIGURE 6.80 Tear of inferior (anteroinferior) popliteomeniscal fascicle associated with a grade 3 ACL tear. Coronal (**A**) and sagittal (**B**) FS PD FSE images.

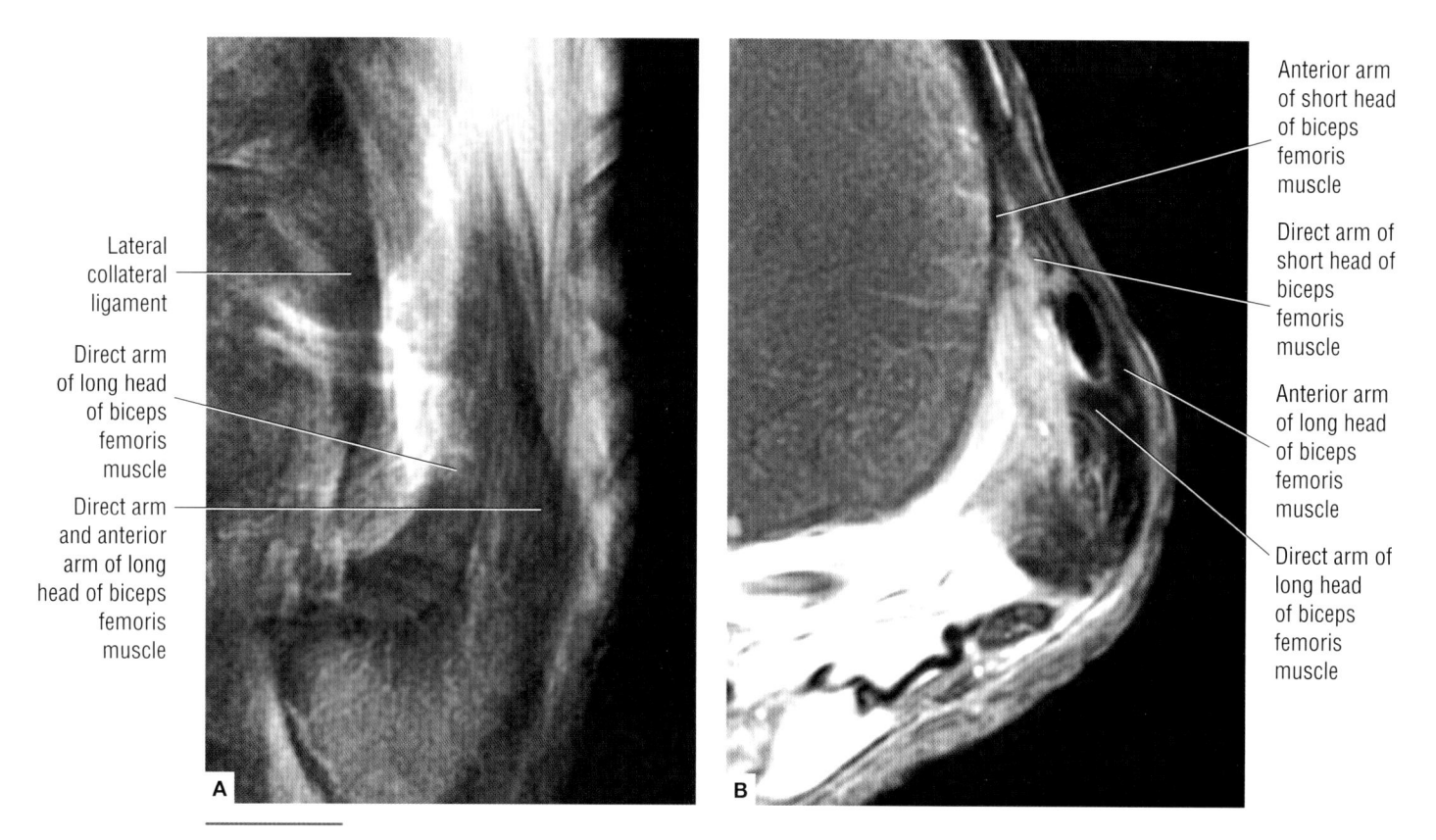

FIGURE 6.81 (**A**) Lateral collateral ligament anterior to the fibular attachment of the anterior and direct arms of the long head of the biceps femoris tendon. Sagittal FS PD FSE image. (**B**) The long head of the biceps femoris tendon is divided into an anterior and direct arm, both of which are superficial and posterior to the lateral collateral ligament. Axial T1-weighted image.

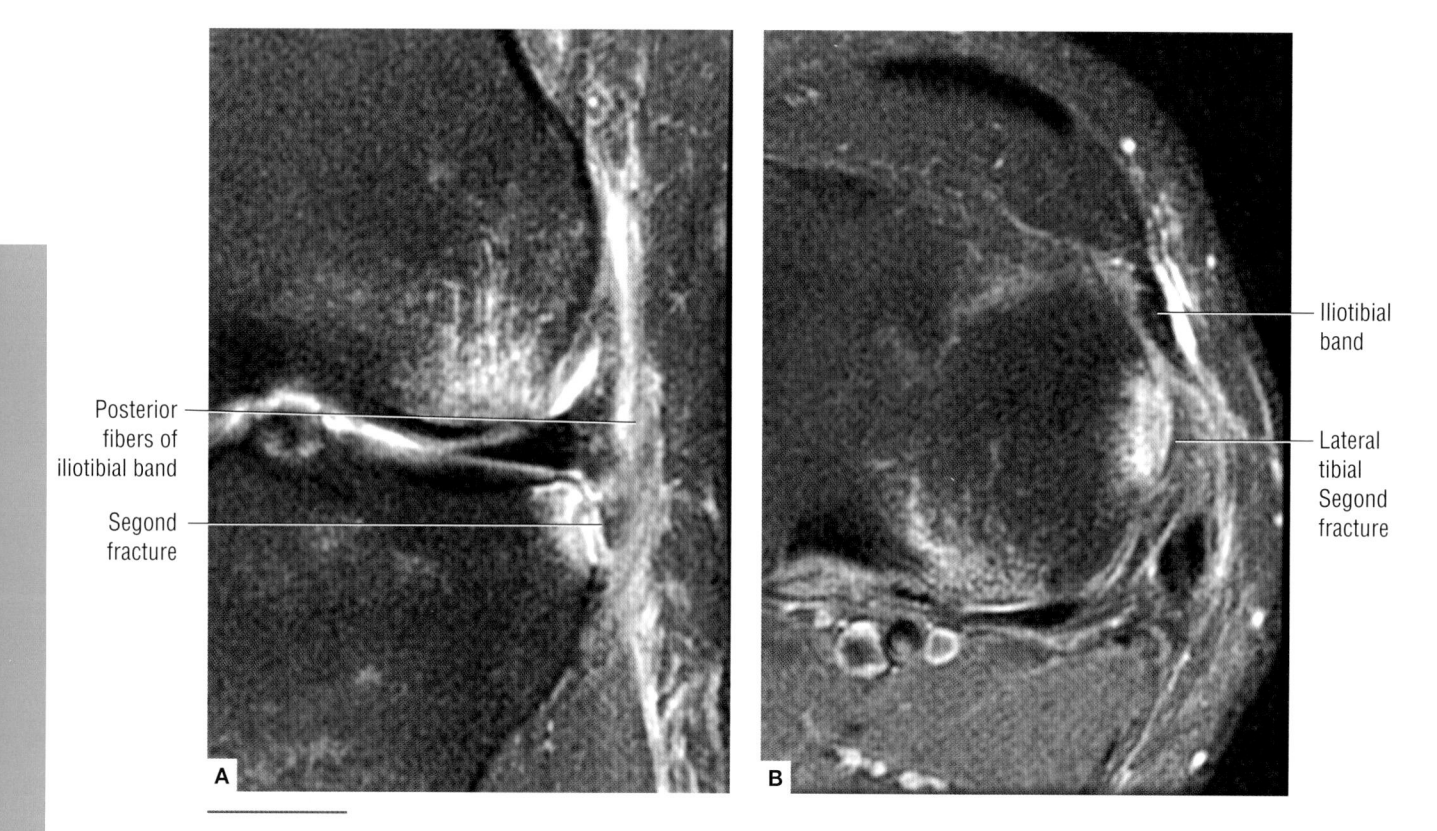

FIGURE 6.82 Acute Segond fracture with osseous avulsion secondary to the pull of the posterior fibers of the ITB on coronal (**A**) and axial (**B**) FS PD FSE images.

Collateral Ligaments

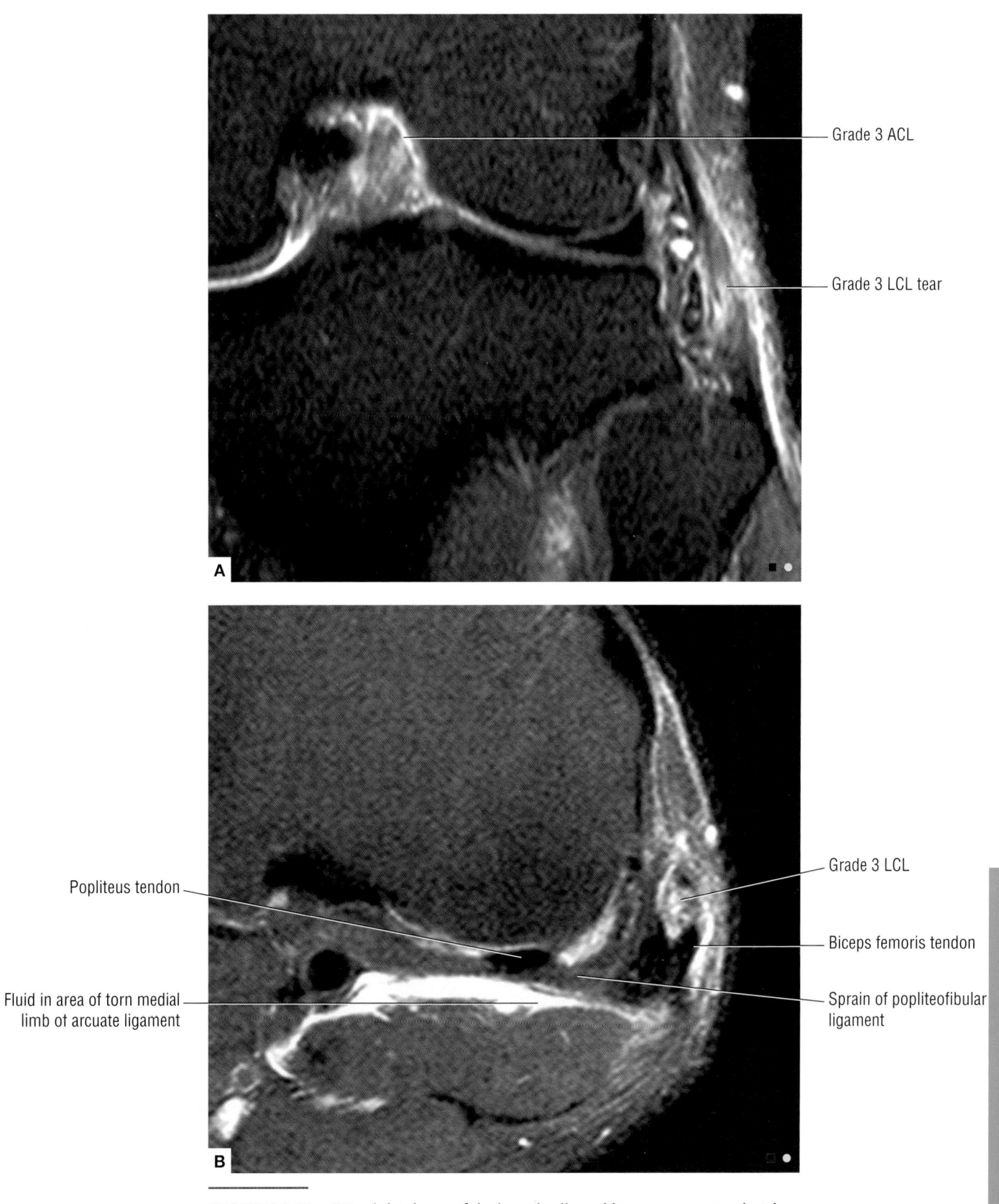

FIGURE 6.83 Distal third tear of the lateral collateral ligament associated with a grade 3 ACL tear. The popliteus tendon and the popliteofibular ligament are intact. Coronal (**A**) and axial (**B**) FS PD FSE images.

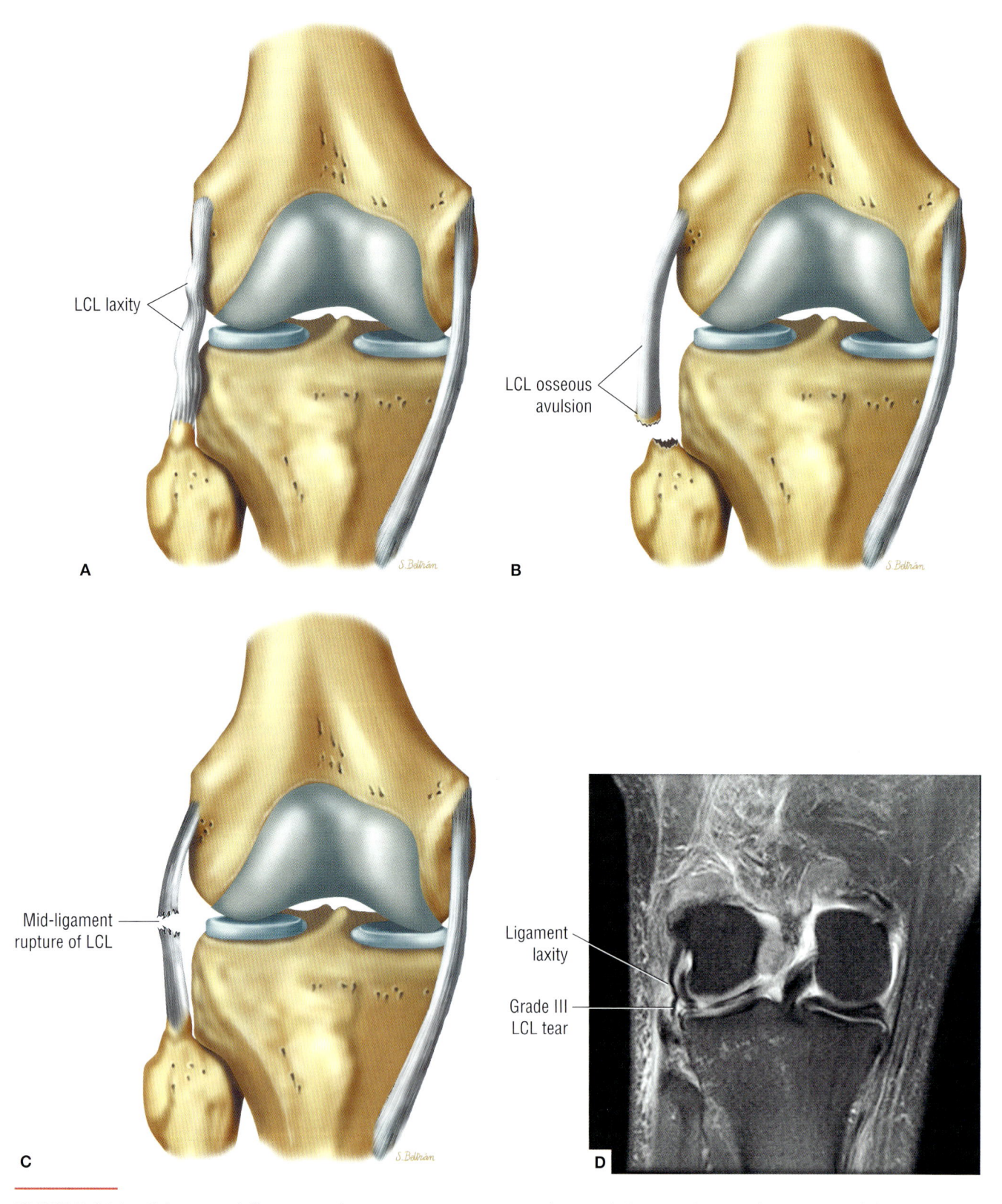

FIGURE 6.84 Color coronal illustrations from an anterior perspective showing (**A**) a partial tear with LCL laxity, (**B**) a grade 3 distal LCL osseous avulsion, and (**C**) a grade 3 middle third rupture of the LCL. (**D**) Distal LCL tear with proximal ligament laxity on a coronal FS PD FSE image.

Treatment of LCL Injuries

- Avulsion LCL injury from femur or fibula can be treated with suture repair.

- Interstitial LCL injury can be treated by augmentation with the biceps tendon.

- Associated PLC injuries, with either acute or chronic posterolateral instability, are often associated with cruciate ligament injuries.
    - Best treated with surgical reconstructions that initially address the cruciate ligaments
    - Subsequent operative repair of posterolateral structures[210]
    - Surgical repair of LCL may be necessary when there are associated acute ACL injuries.[69]

- Surgery also used to treat grade 3 tears without associated ACL tear when both primary (i.e., LCL) and secondary (i.e., posterolateral or arcuate complex) restraints are injured
    - Results of surgical reconstructions in acute posterolateral instability are superior to the results of those performed in cases of chronic posterolateral instability.[503]

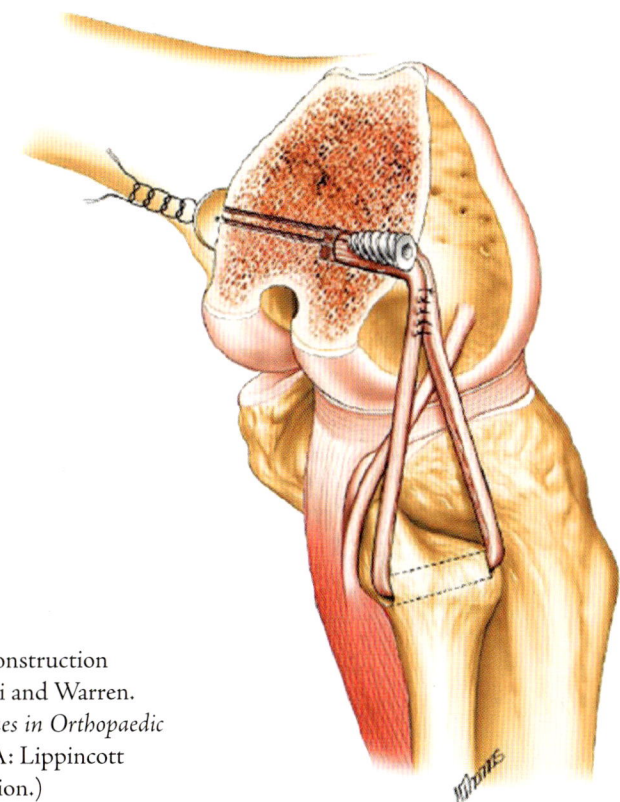

FIGURE 6.85 Technique for LCL reconstruction using biceps tendon as described by Veltri and Warren. (Reprinted from Fu FH. *Master Techniques in Orthopaedic Surgery: Sports Medicine*. Philadelphia, PA: Lippincott Williams & Wilkins; 2010, with permission.)

Posterolateral Corner Attachments and Injury

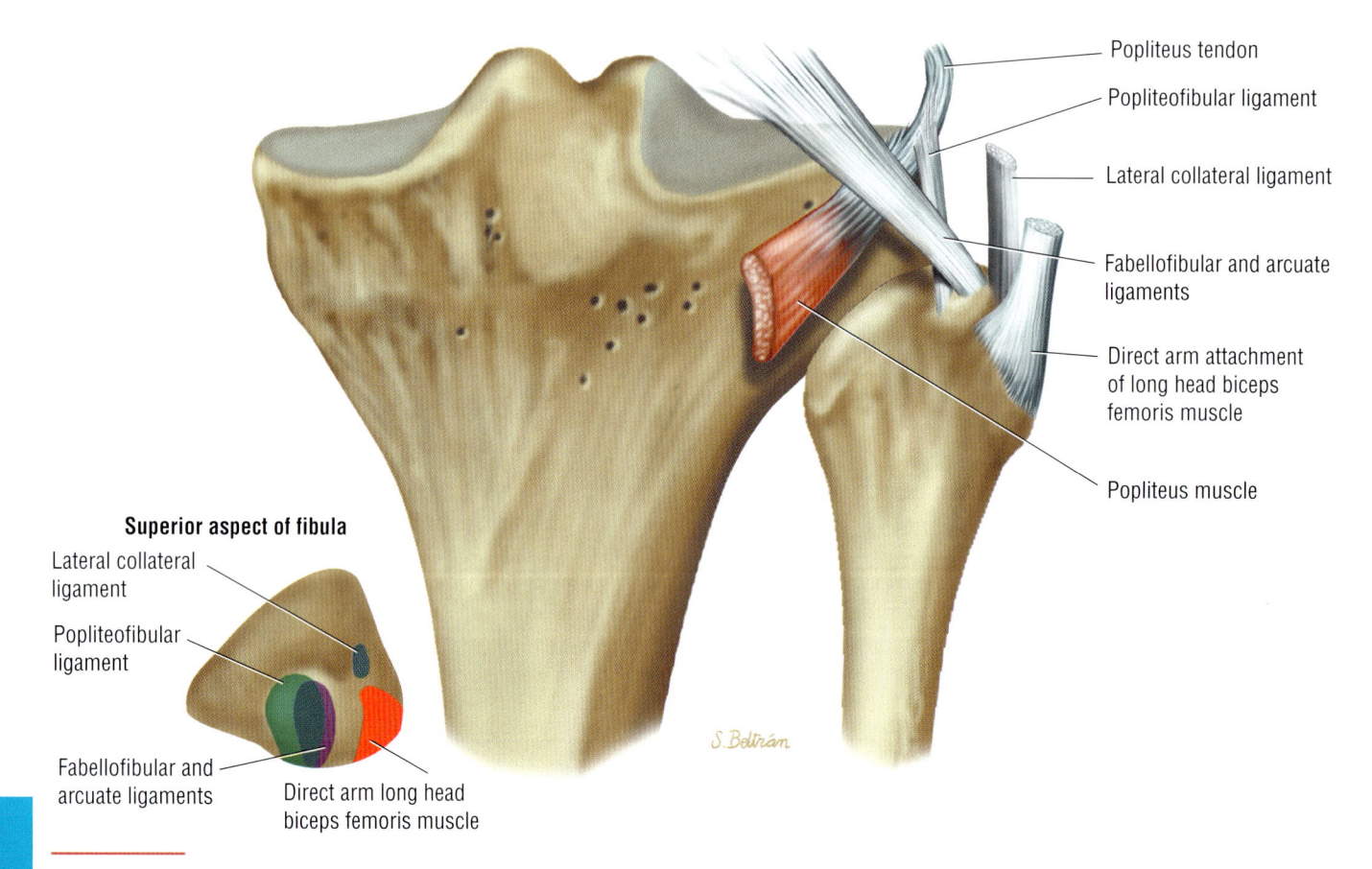

FIGURE 6.86 The popliteofibular ligament attaches to the upper facet of the apex of the fibular head medial to the insertions of the fabellofibular and arcuate ligaments. The lateral collateral ligament and the direct arm of the long head of the biceps femoris tendon are attached more peripherally to the lateral margin of the fibular head.

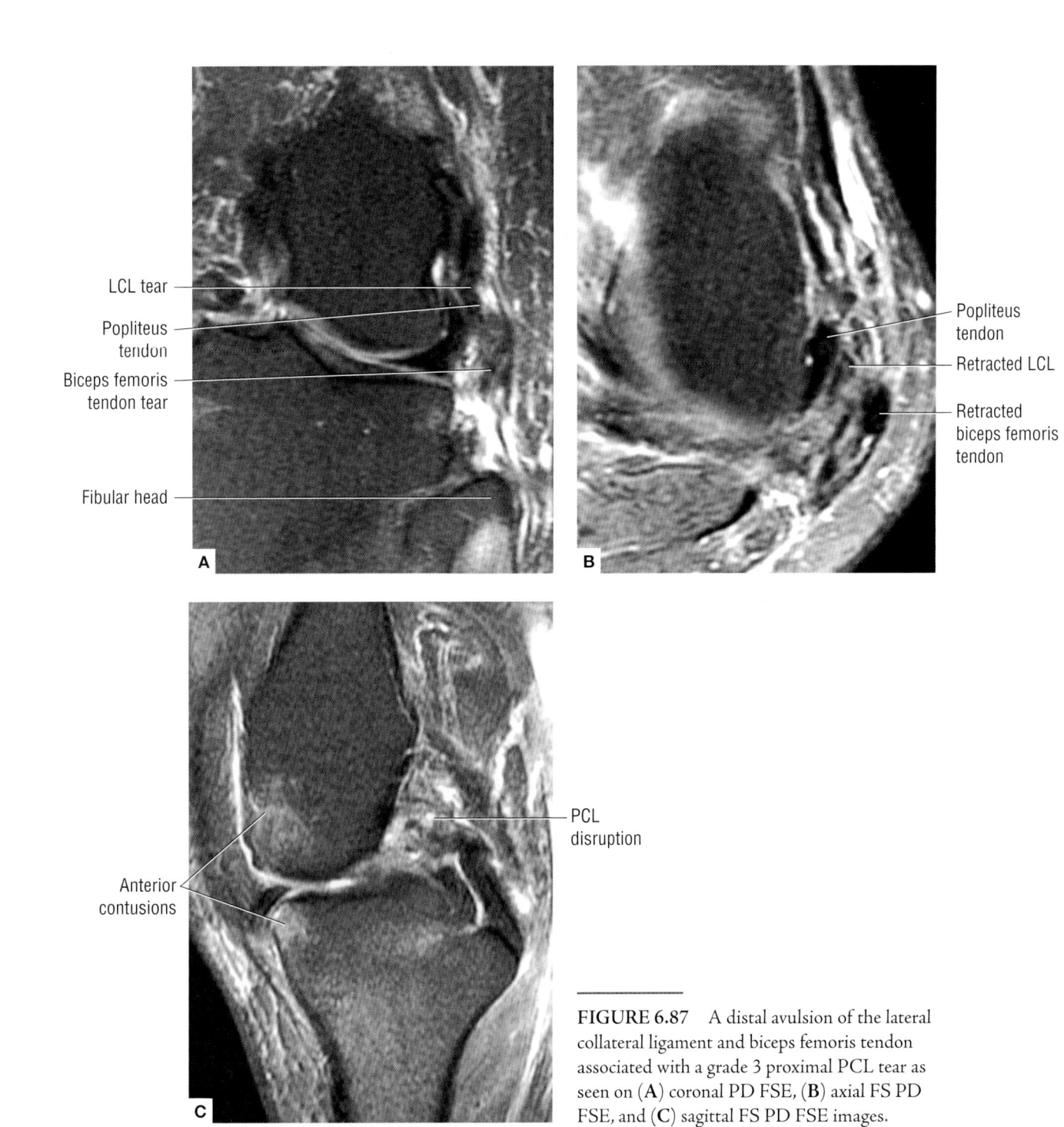

Collateral Ligaments 673

FIGURE 6.87 A distal avulsion of the lateral collateral ligament and biceps femoris tendon associated with a grade 3 proximal PCL tear as seen on (**A**) coronal PD FSE, (**B**) axial FS PD FSE, and (**C**) sagittal FS PD FSE images.

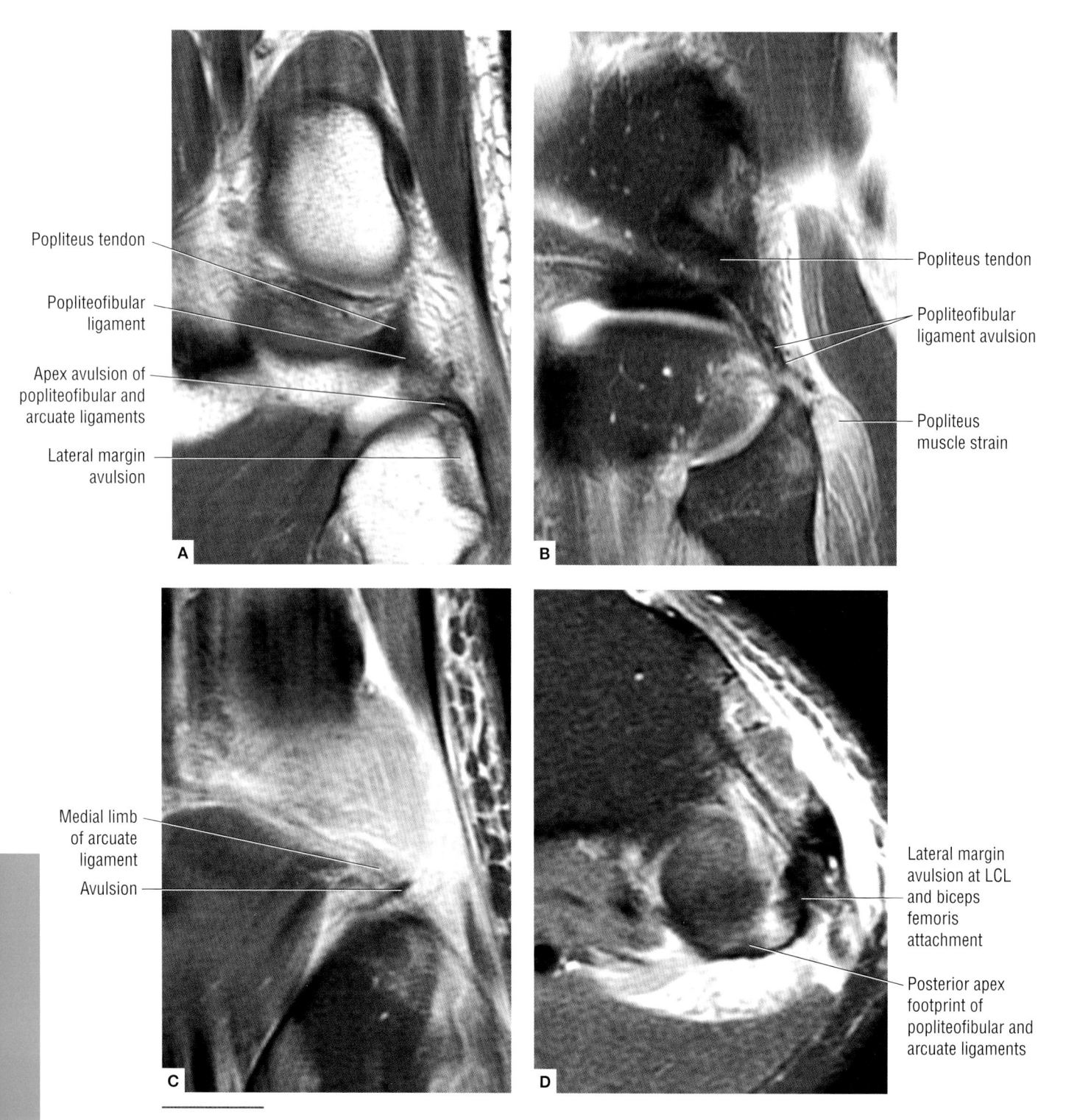

FIGURE 6.88 Popliteofibular and arcuate ligament avulsion at the fibular apex with lateral collateral ligament and biceps femoris avulsion at the lateral margin of the fibular head. (**A**) Coronal PD FSE image. (**B**) Sagittal FS FSE image. (**C**) Coronal FS PD FSE image. (**D**) Axial FS PD FSE image.

Collateral Ligaments

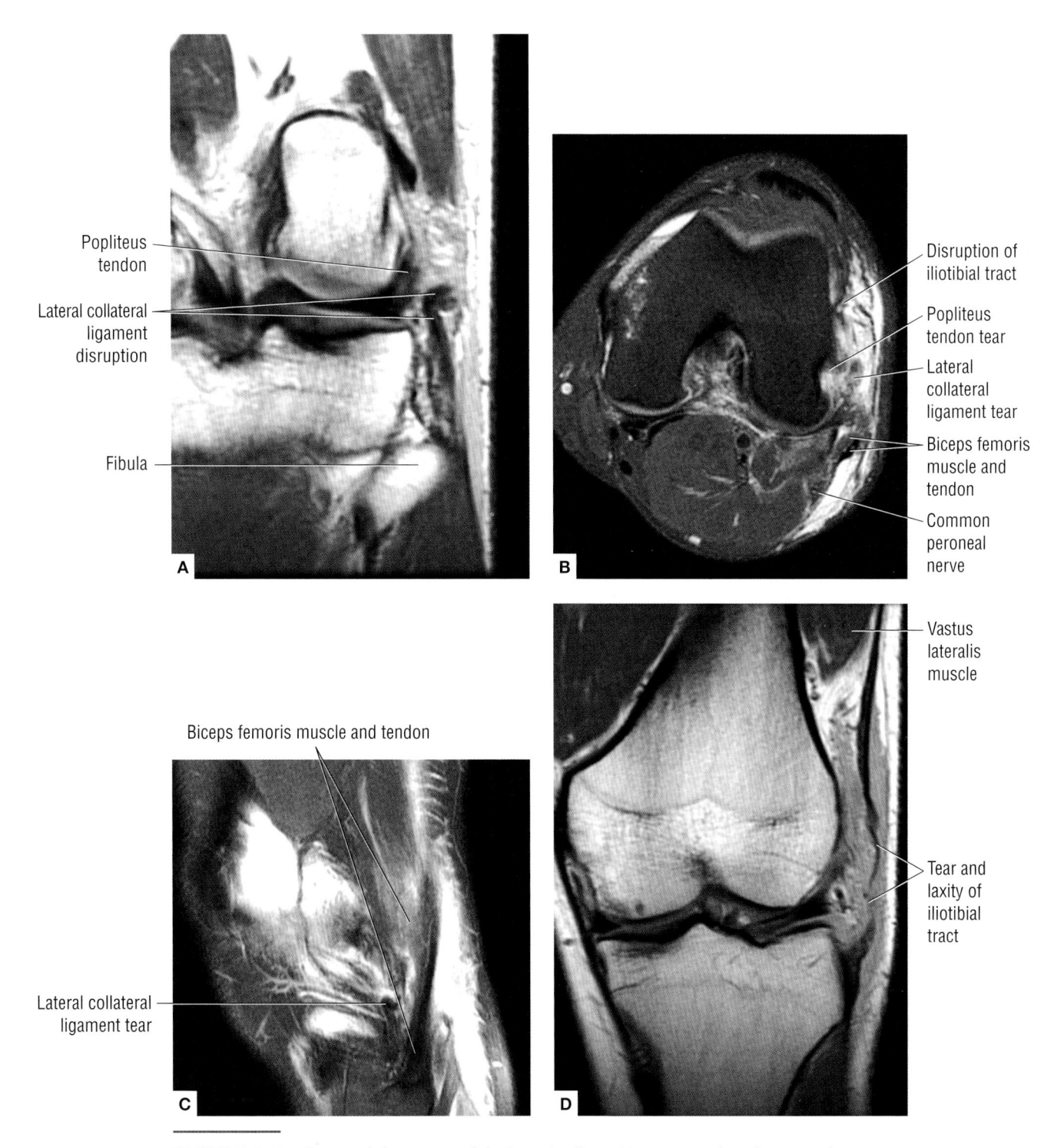

FIGURE 6.89 Proximal disruption of the lateral collateral ligament and popliteus tendon associated with distal iliotibial tract tear. A biceps femoris muscle sprain is shown proximally. (**A**) Coronal PD FSE image. (**B**) Axial FS PD FSE image. (**C**) Sagittal FS PD FSE image. (**D**) Coronal FS PD FSE image.

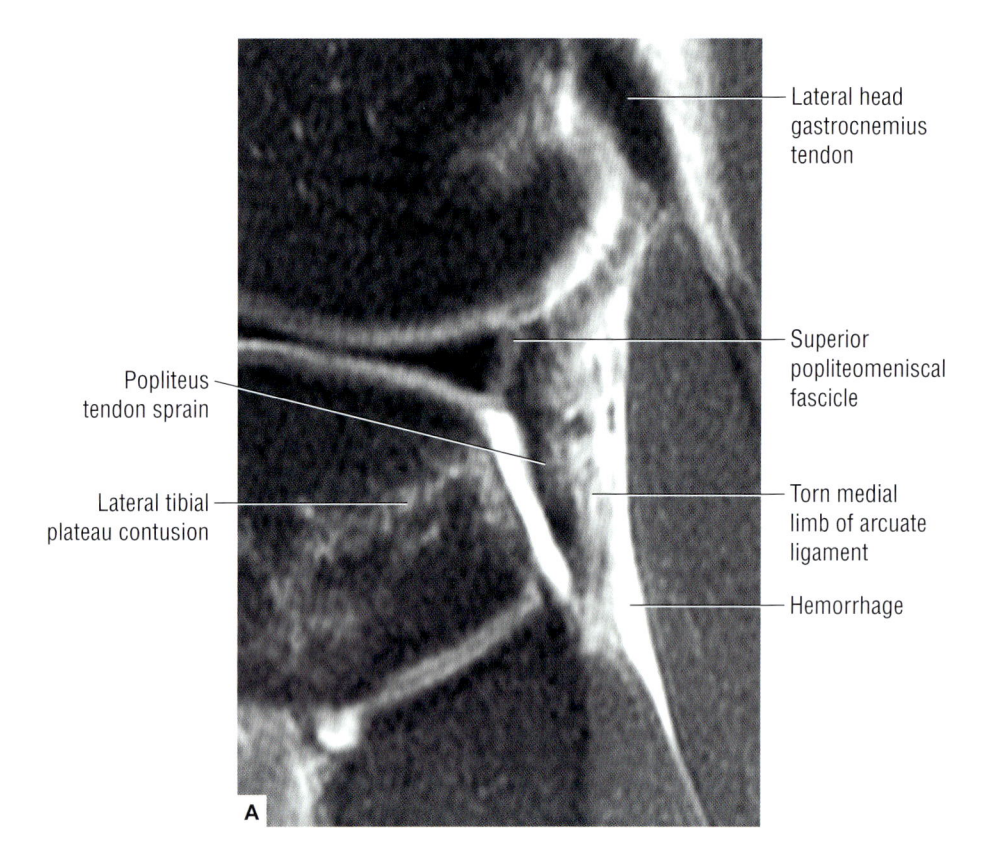

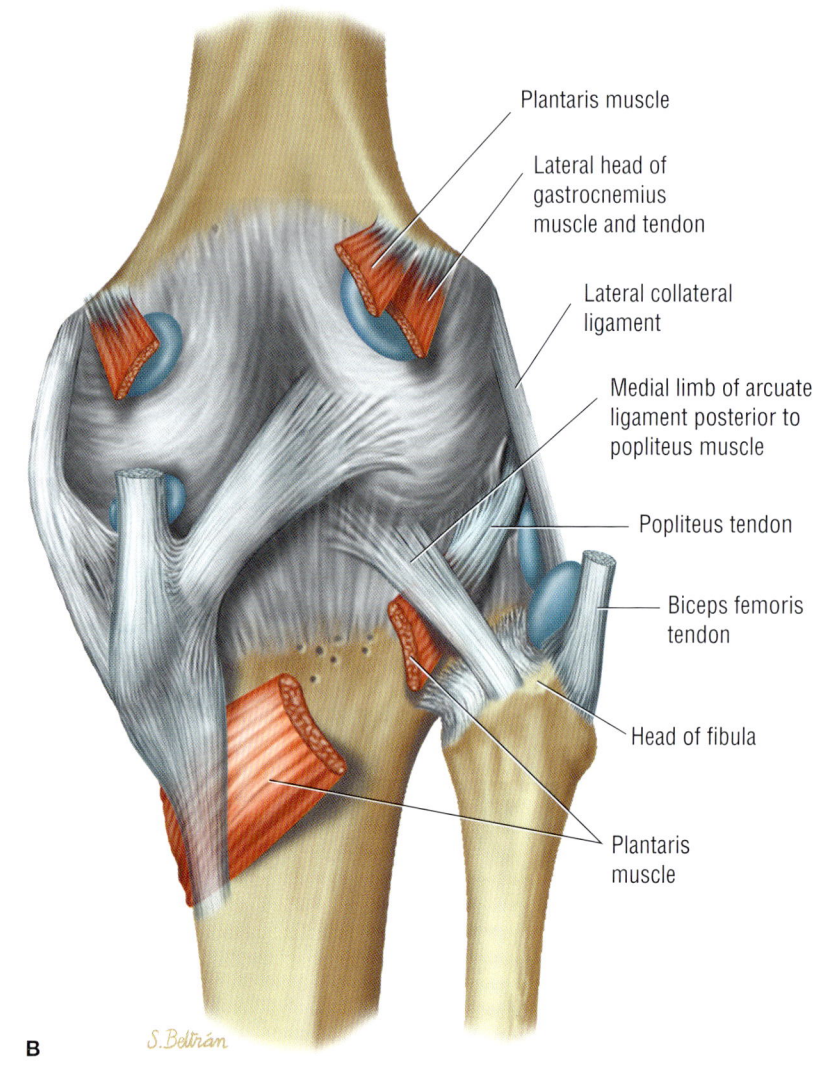

FIGURE 6.90 (**A**) Sagittal FS PD FSE image of a posterolateral corner injury. The torn medial limb of the arcuate ligament can be identified posterior to the popliteus tendon. The medial and lateral limbs of the arcuate ligament normally attach to the apex of the fibular head. The medial limb of the arcuate ligament is usually identified at the plane of section, where there is a complete superior popliteomeniscal fascicle and deficiency of the inferior popliteomeniscal fascicle. The lateral limb of the arcuate ligament can be demonstrated in a more lateral or peripheral sagittal plane, where the popliteomeniscal fascicle and normal deficiency of the superior popliteomeniscal fascicle are seen. This corresponds to a sagittal image through the body of the lateral meniscus. (**B**) Color illustration showing the posterior view of the normal posterior capsule and posterolateral corner for reference.

Collateral Ligaments

Arcuate and Fabellofibular Ligament

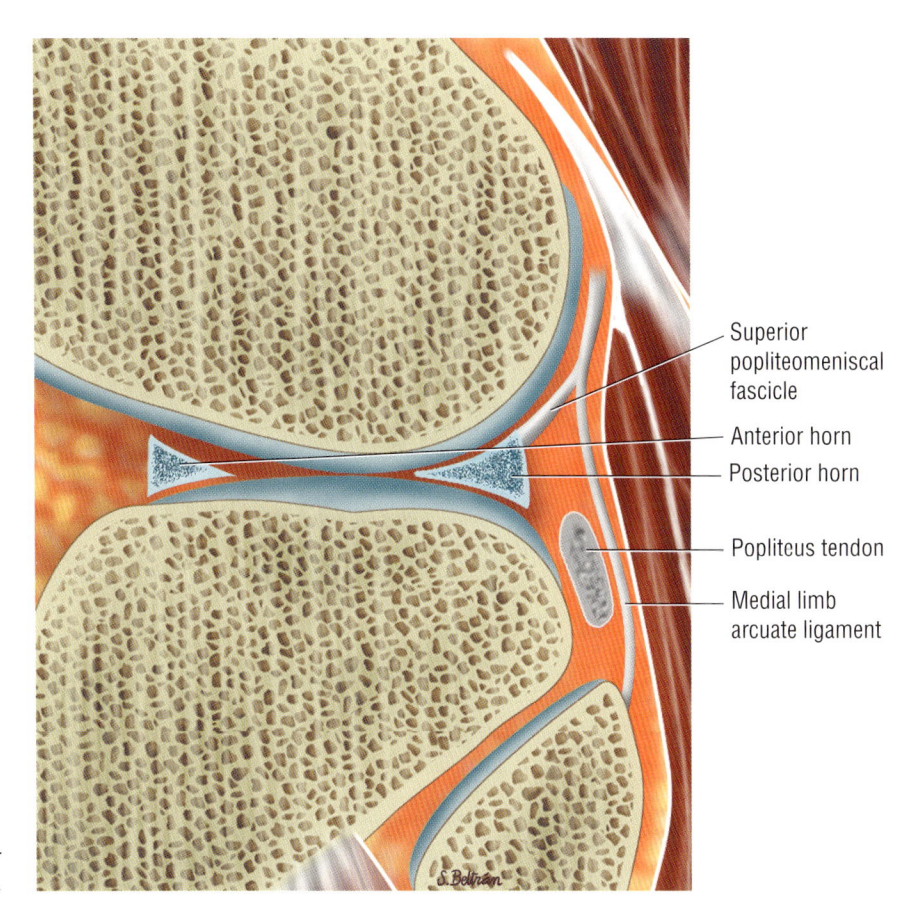

FIGURE 6.91 Medial limb of the arcuate ligament identified posterior to the popliteus tendon.

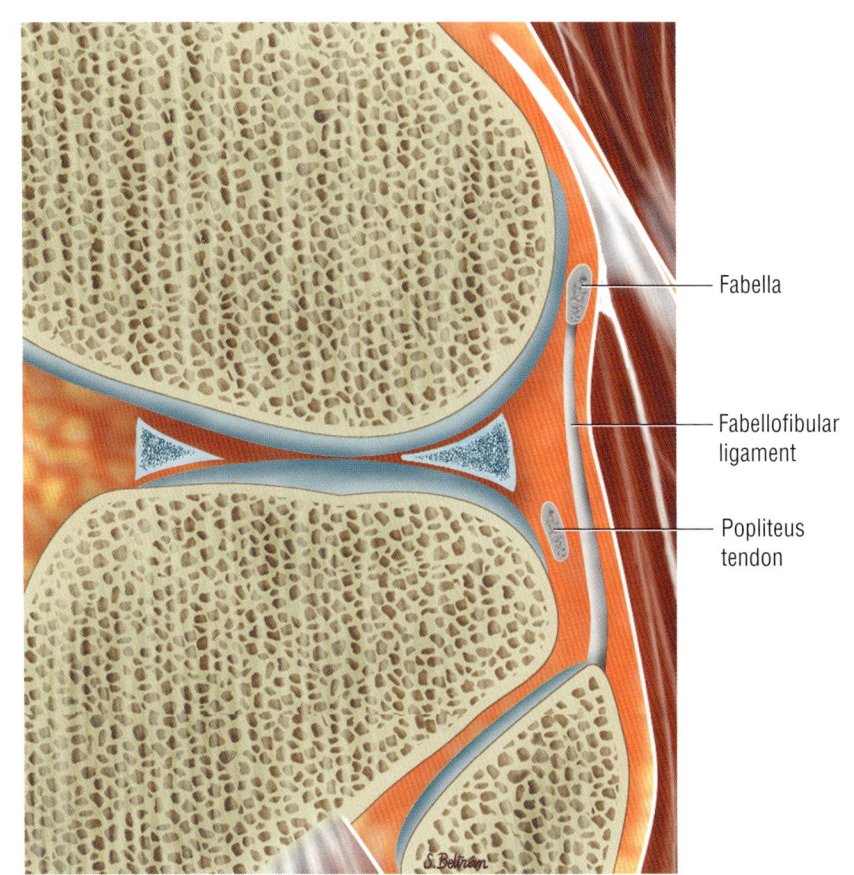

FIGURE 6.92 Prominent fabellofibular ligament with the attachments to both the fabella proximally and the fibular styloid distally.

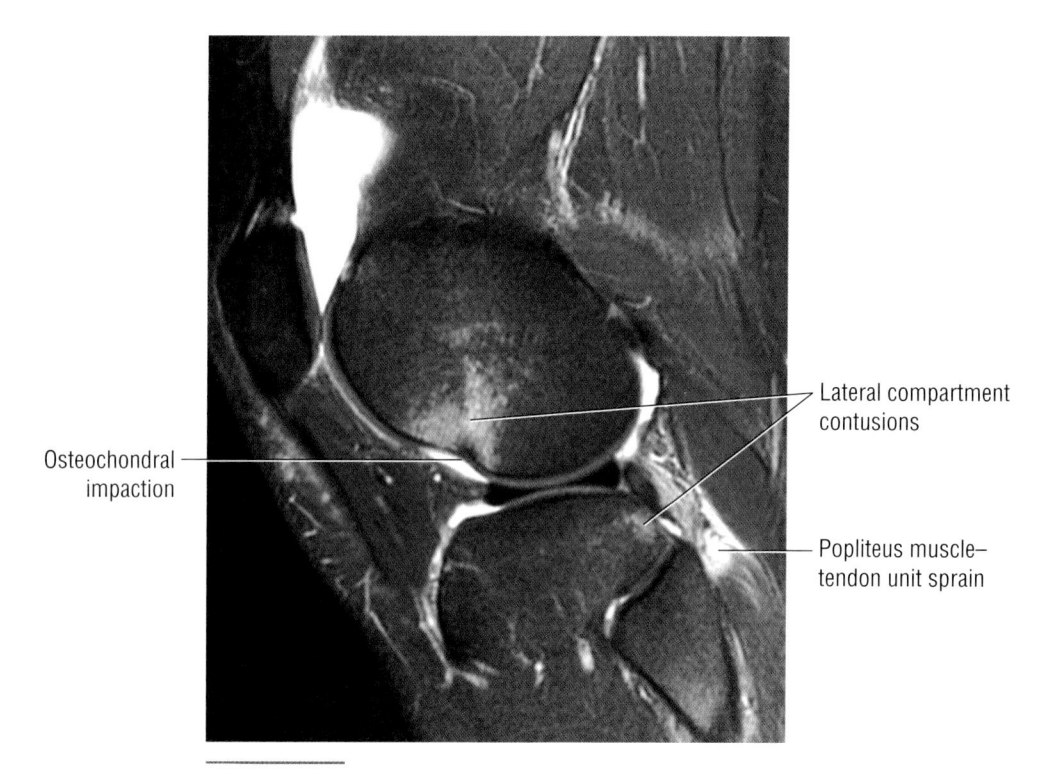

FIGURE 6.93 Popliteus muscle tendon sprain in ACL-related posterolateral corner injury on a sagittal FS PD FSE image.

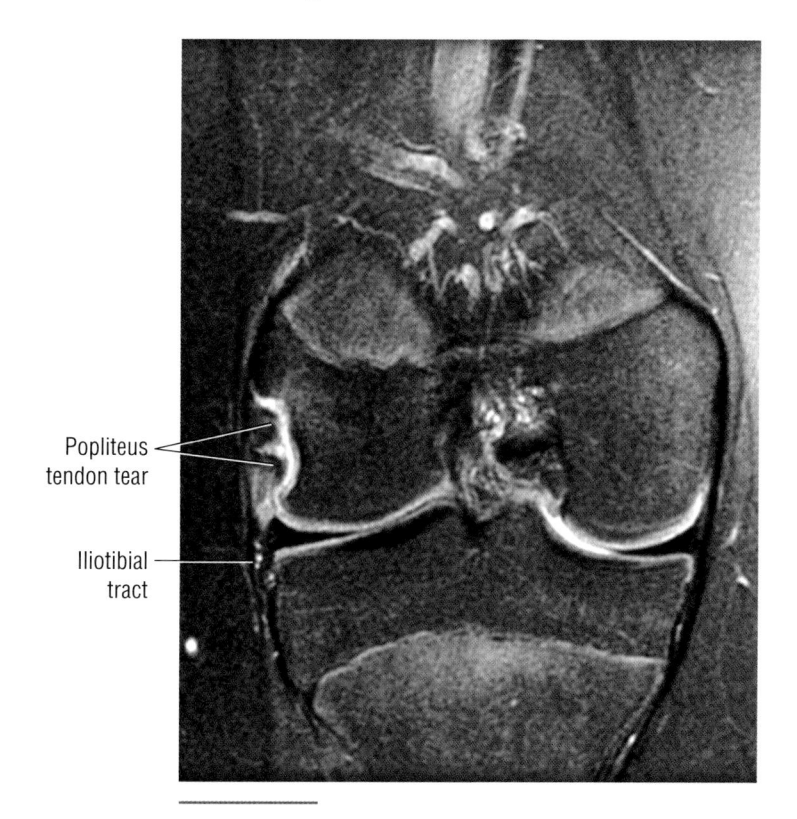

FIGURE 6.94 Isolated proximal popliteus tendon tear on a coronal FS PD FSE image.

Collateral Ligaments

- Displaced flap from posterior horn lateral meniscus
- Truncated posterior horn lateral meniscus (flap tear)
- Depressed lateral tibial plateau osseous fragment

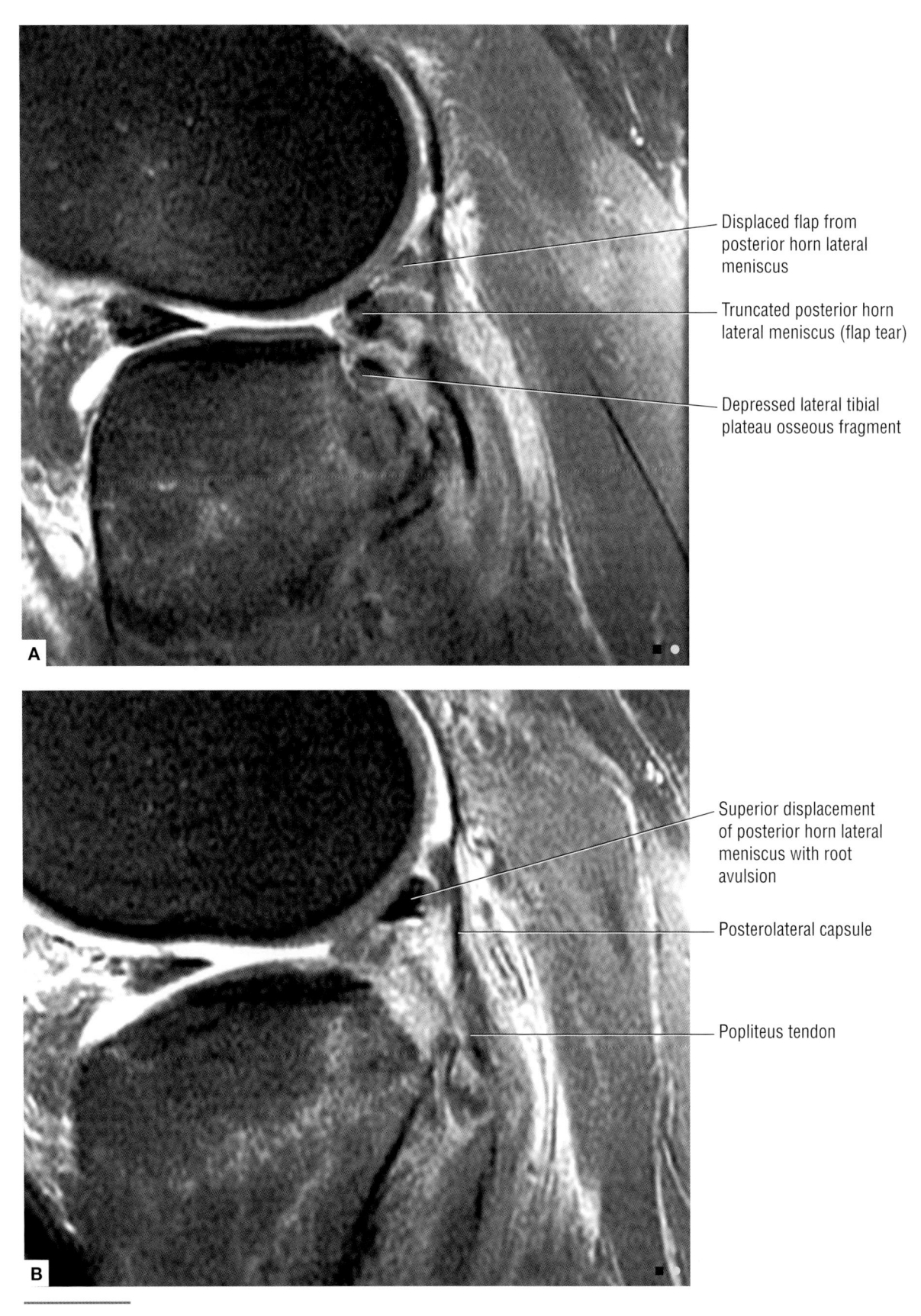

- Superior displacement of posterior horn lateral meniscus with root avulsion
- Posterolateral capsule
- Popliteus tendon

FIGURE 6.95 Distal posterior horn of the lateral meniscus (LM) in a post-fall posterolateral corner injury associated with an ACL tear and comminuted lateral tibial plateau fracture. (**A, B**) Sagittal FS PD FSE images. (*Continued*)

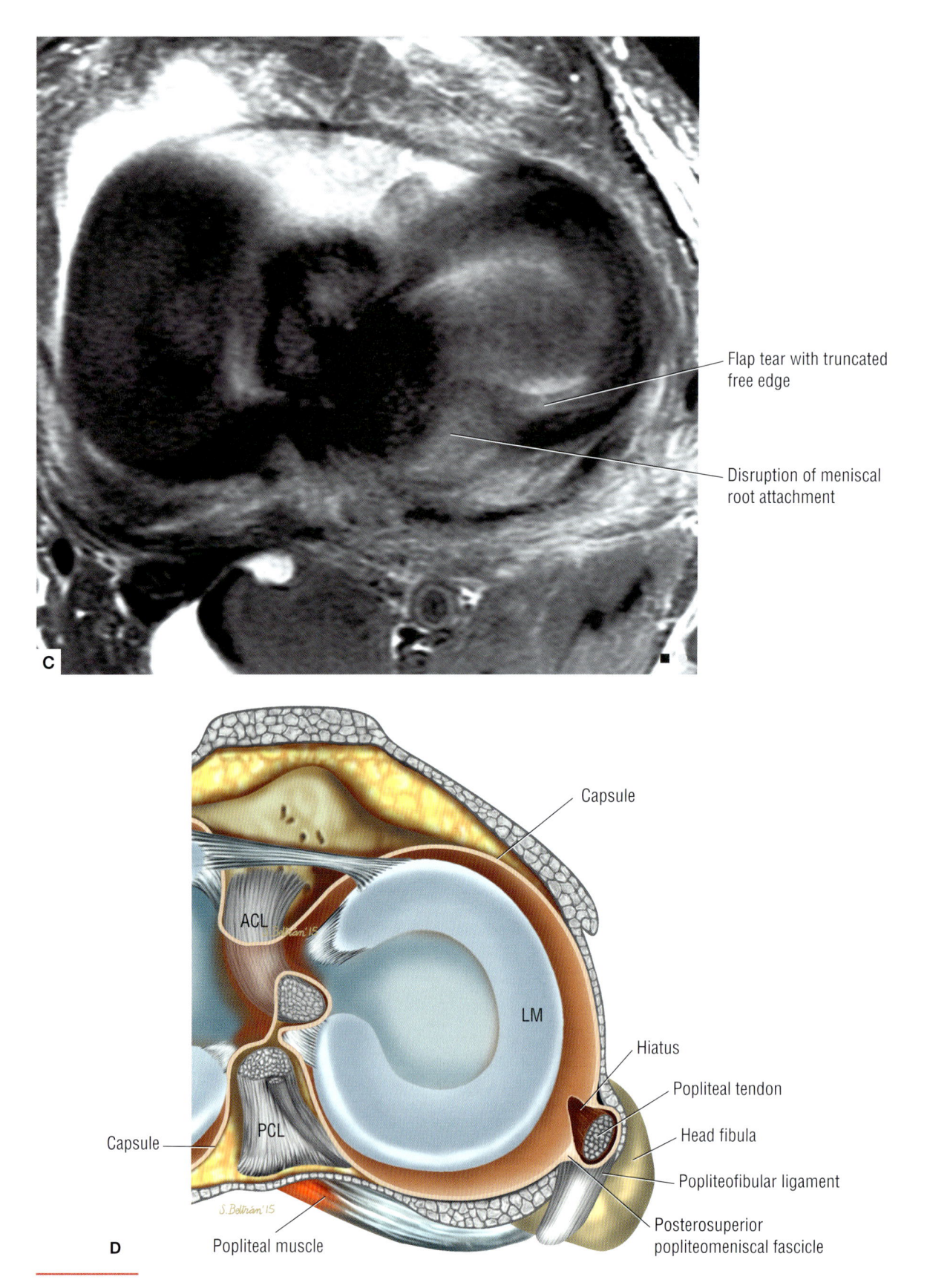

FIGURE 6.95 *(Continued)* Axial FS PD FSE image (**C**) and axial cross-section (**D**) of the popliteal hiatus region of the posterolateral corner.

Collateral Ligaments 681

Popliteofibular ligament avulsion with styloid edema

Disrupted popliteofibular ligament posterior to lateral aspect of tibiofibular joint

FIGURE 6.95 *(Continued)* Coronal (**E**) and sagittal (**F**) images at the level of the upper facet avulsion of the popliteofibular ligament.

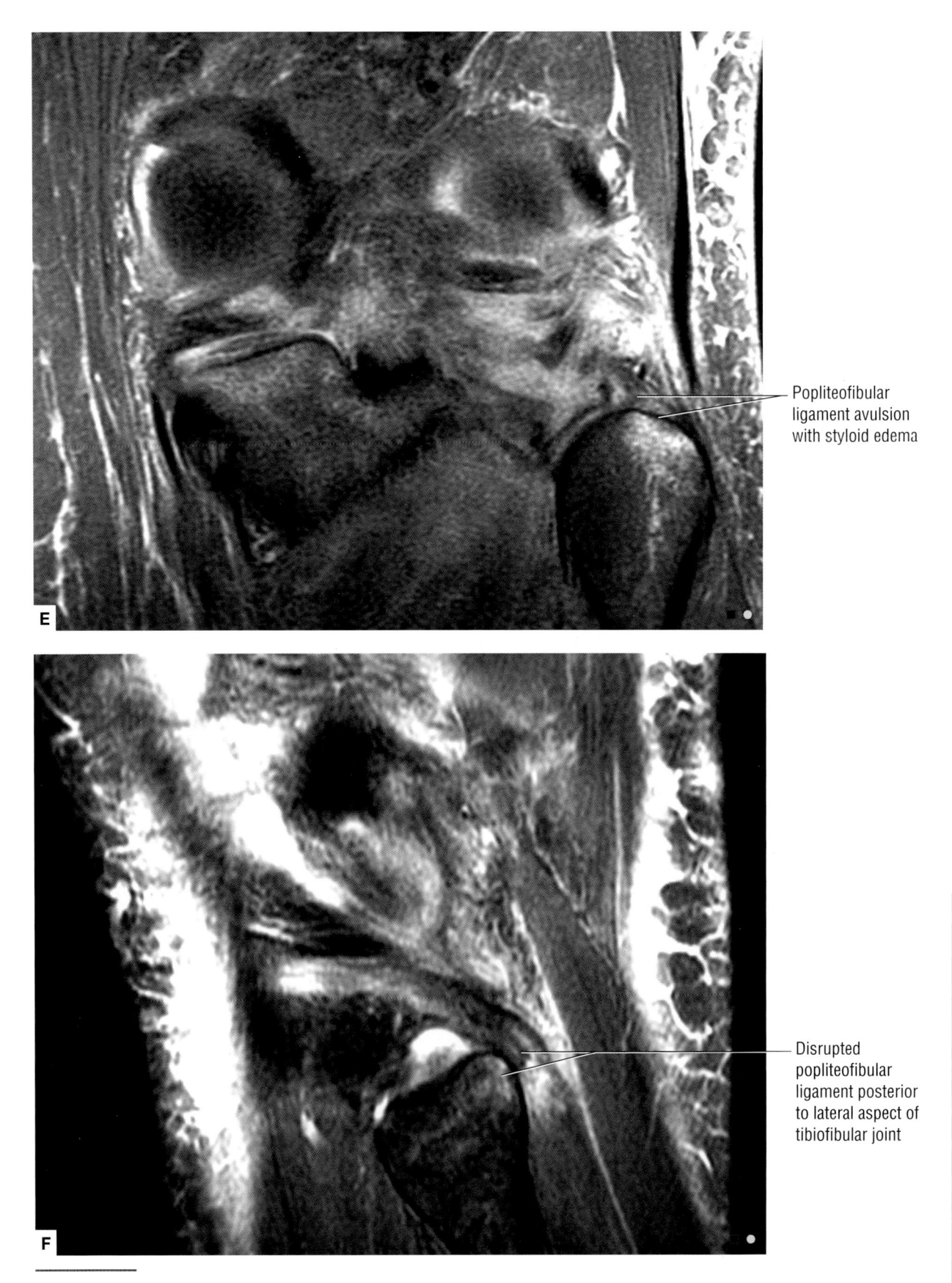

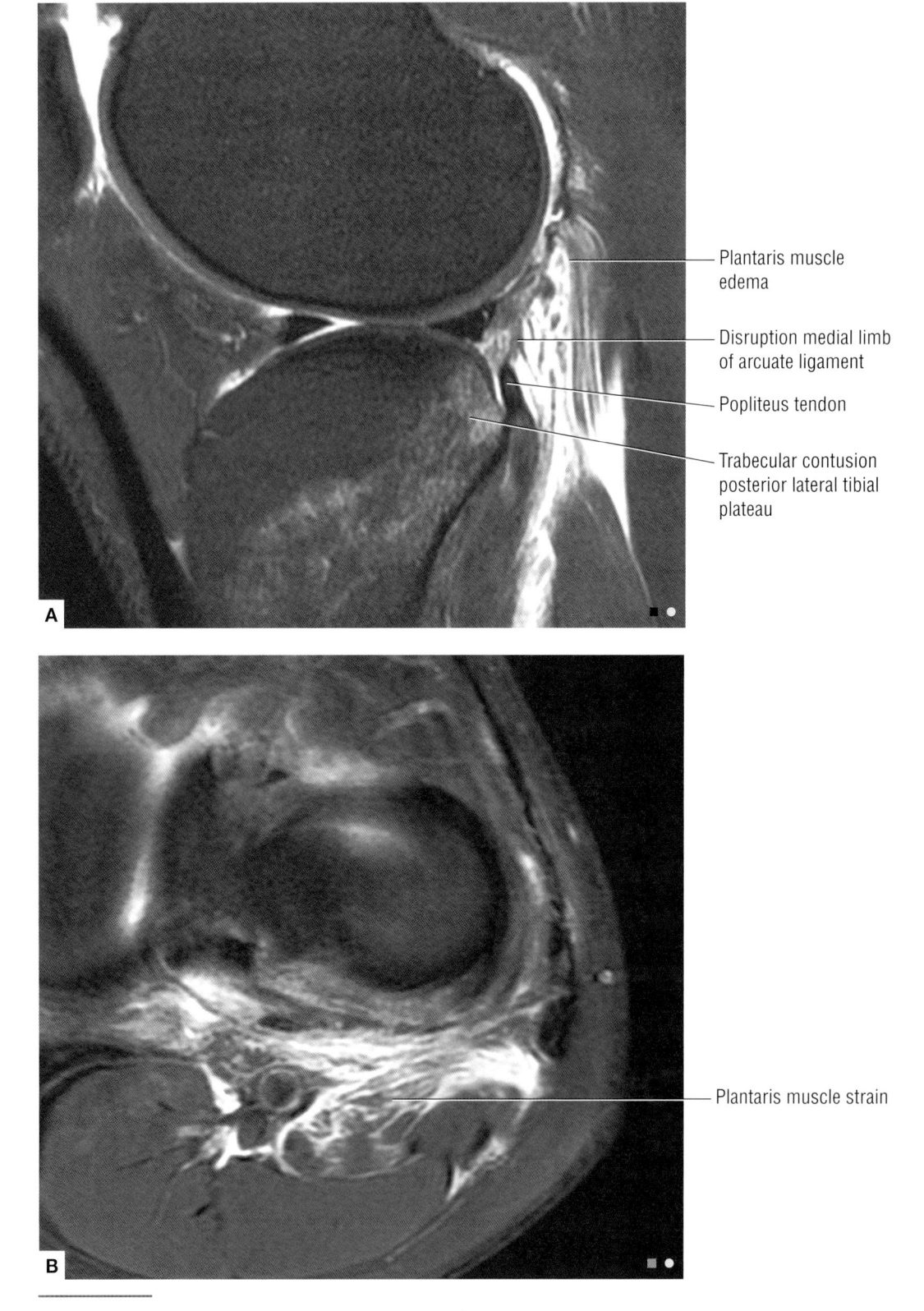

FIGURE 6.96 Plantaris muscle strain in association with an ACL-related (grade 3 ACL) posterolateral corner injury. Sagittal (**A**) and axial (**B**) FS PD FSE images.

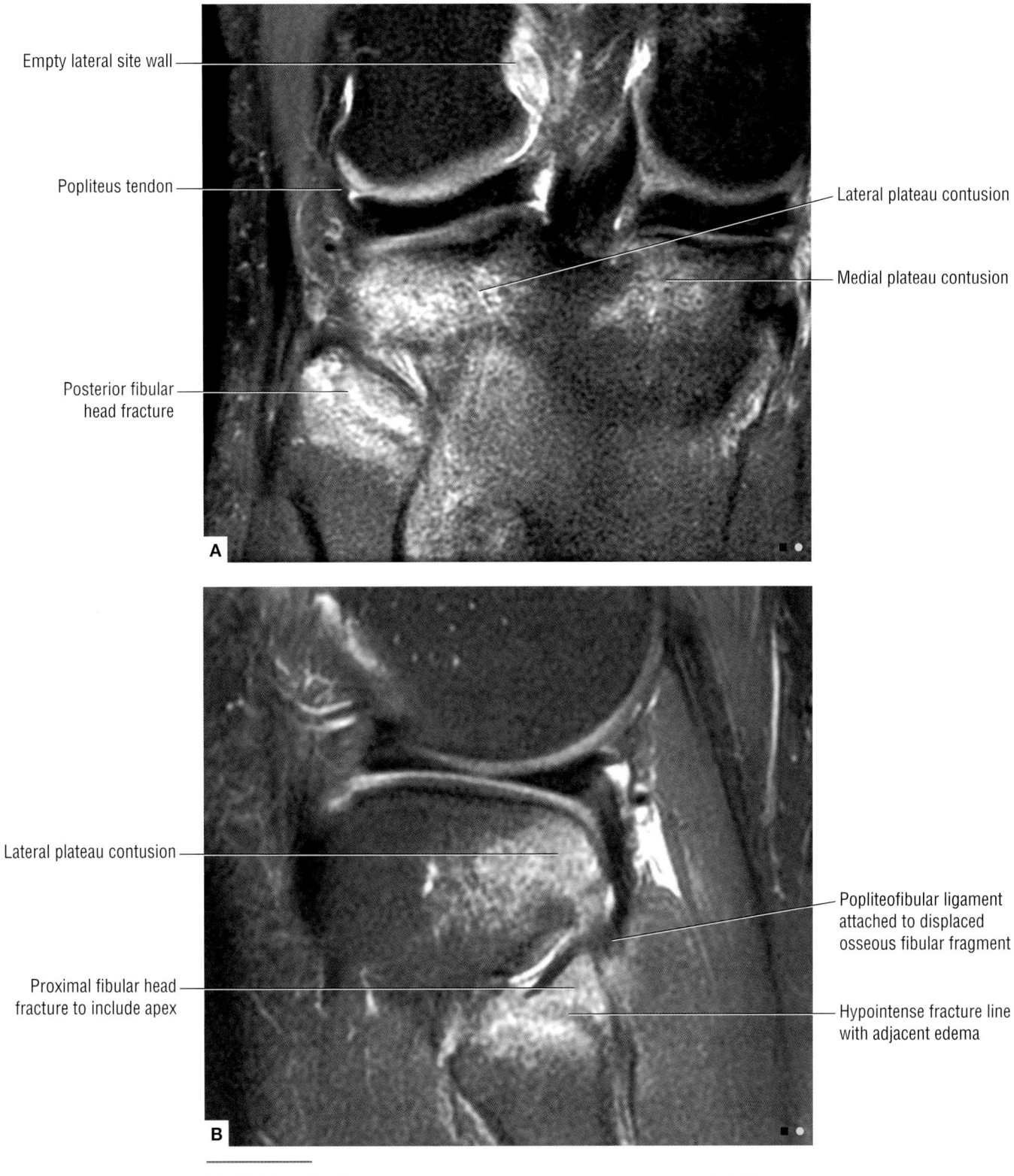

FIGURE 6.97 Posterolateral corner motorcycle injury with grade 3 ACL tear and displaced fibular head fracture involving the apex area of the popliteofibular ligament attachment. Coronal (**A**) and sagittal (**B**) FS PD FSE images.

Rupture of the popliteomeniscal fascicles

Popliteofibular ligament

Popliteus tendon

Contusion of lateral femoral condyle at sulcus terminalis

Torn superior popliteomeniscal fascicle

Capacious hiatus

Popliteus tendon

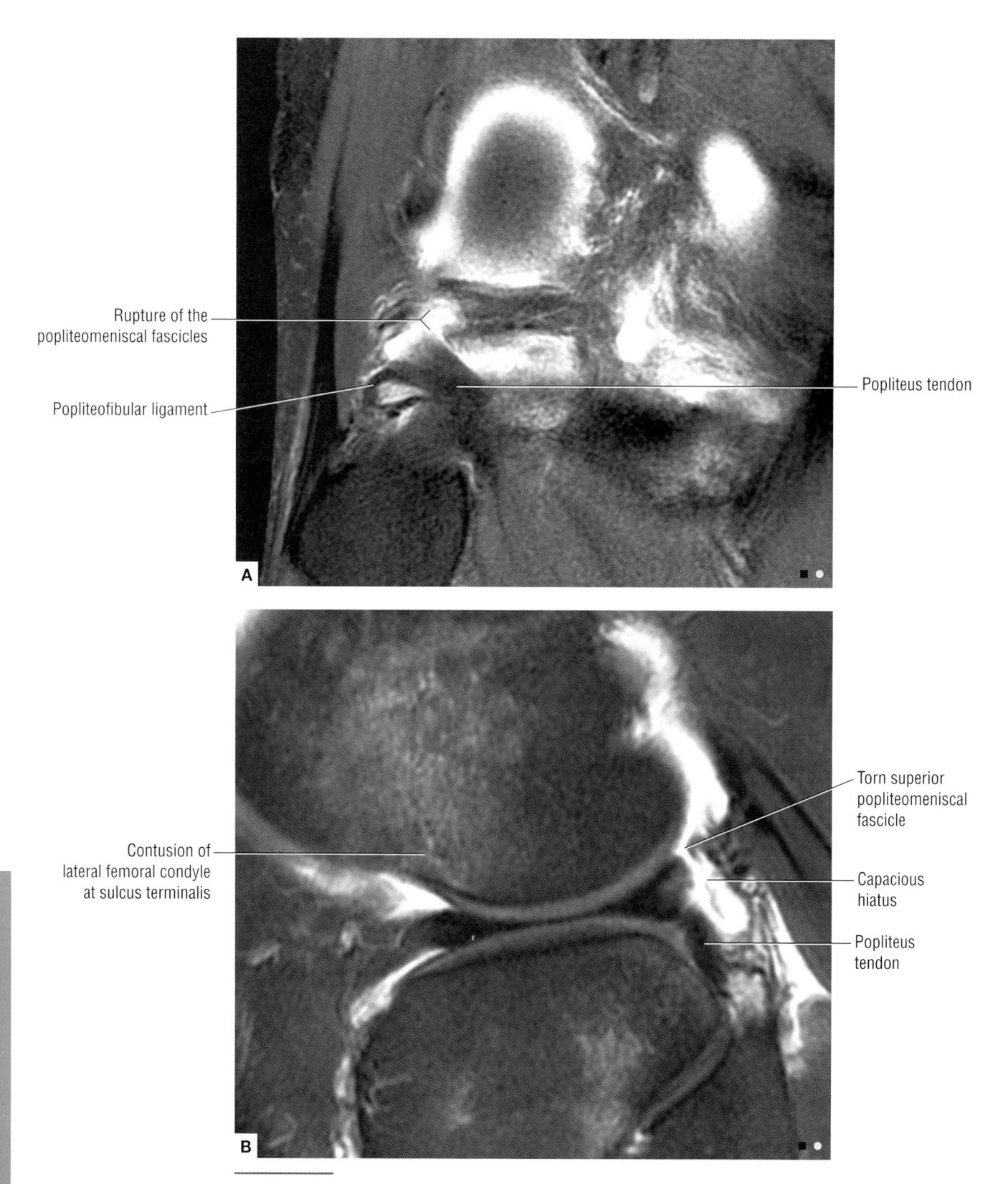

FIGURE 6.98 Lateral compartment contusions associated with a grade 3 ACL tear and disruption of the popliteomeniscal fascicles. Coronal (**A**) and sagittal (**B**) FS PD FSE images.

Collateral Ligaments

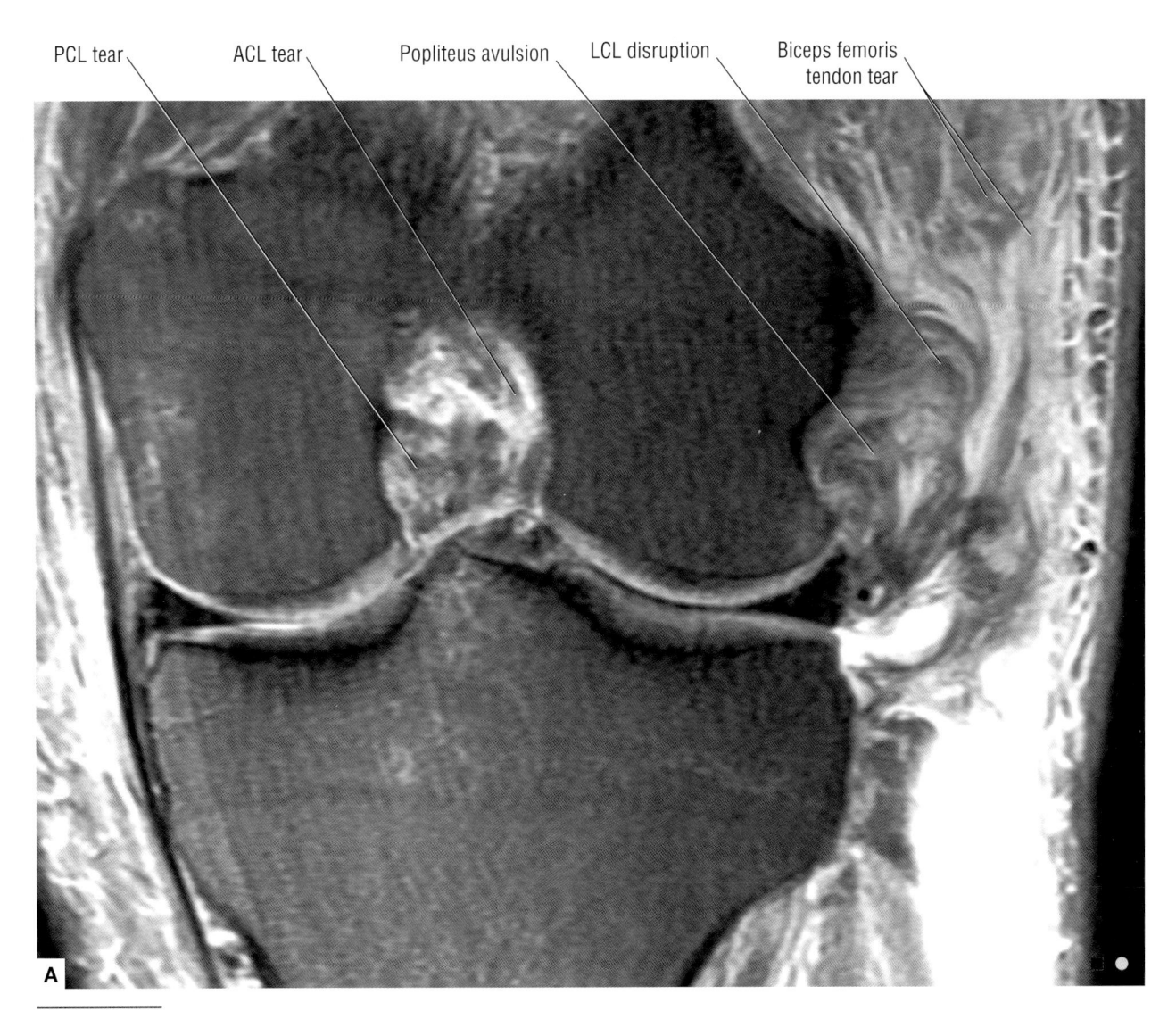

FIGURE 6.99 ACL, PCL, LCL, biceps femoris, popliteus tendon, and cruciate ligament disruption in a multiple-ligament injured knee. The popliteofibular ligament is attached to the posterolateral fibular fracture fragment. (**A**) Coronal FS PD FSE image. (*Continued*)

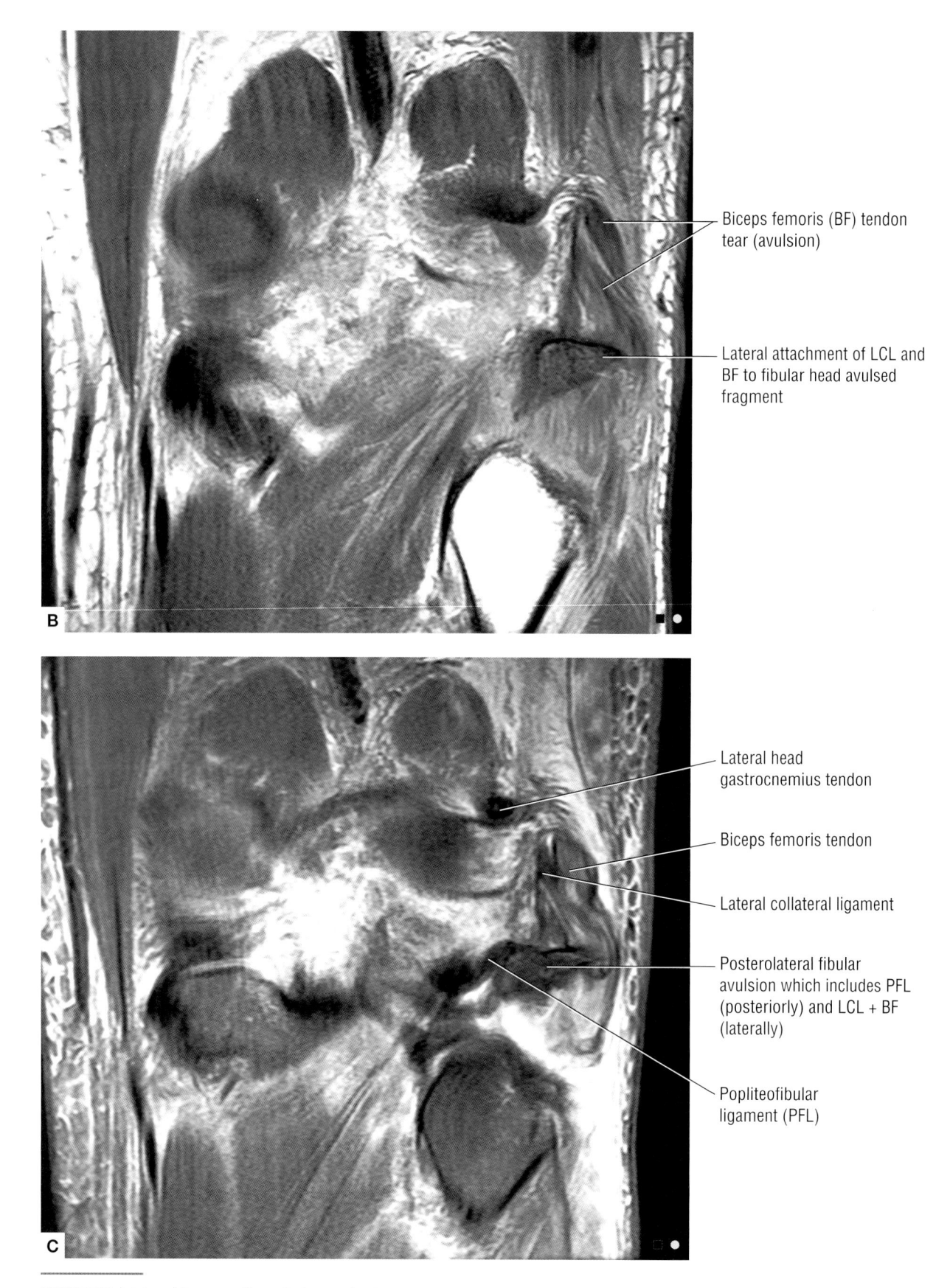

FIGURE 6.99 *(Continued)* **B, C.** Coronal FS PD FSE images.

Collateral Ligaments

- Medial retinacular sprain
- Intact MCL
- Grade 3 PCL
- Iliotibial tract
- Lateral capsular rupture
- Grade 3 ACL
- Posterior capsule rupture

- Popliteofibular ligament (PFL)
- PFC attached to proximally displaced posterior fibular head fragment

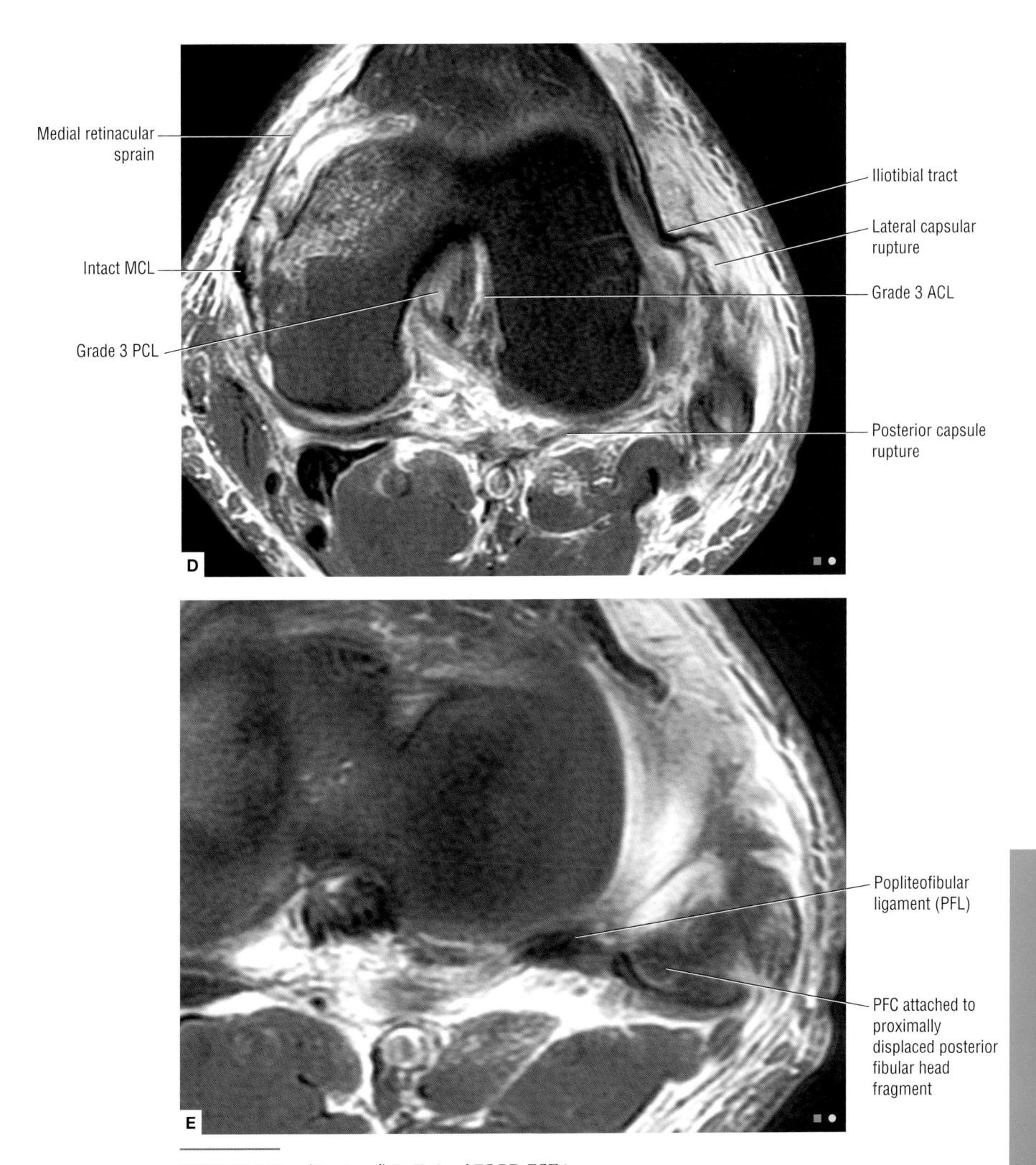

FIGURE 6.99 *(Continued)* **D, E.** Axial FS PD FSE images.

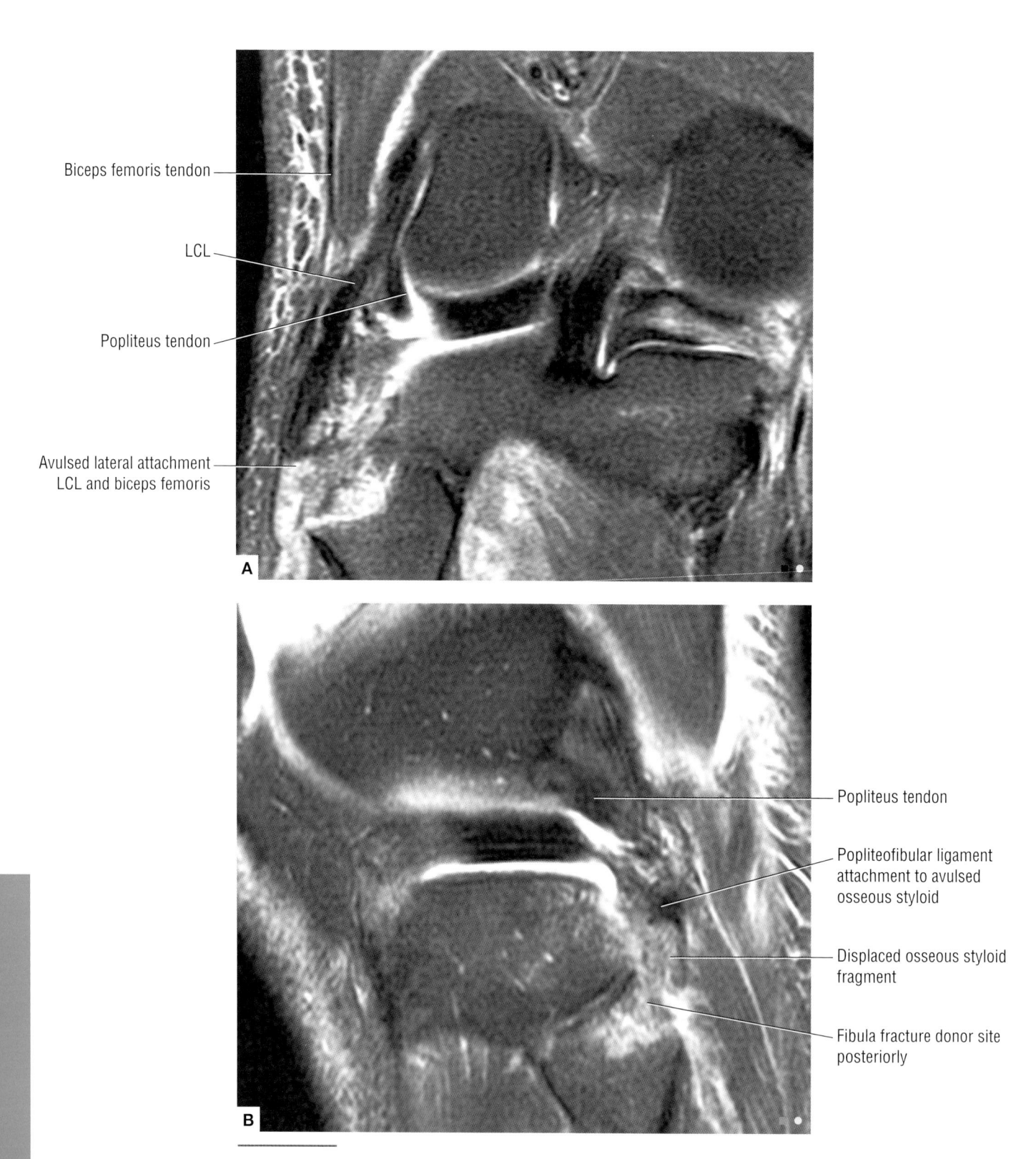

FIGURE 6.100 High-energy trauma with posterolateral corner complex injury involving an osseous avulsion of the lateral collateral ligament and biceps femoris tendon. Multiligamentous injuries are associated with severe posterolateral complex injuries and knee dislocations. Coronal (**A**) and sagittal (**B**) FS PD FSE images.

Collateral Ligaments

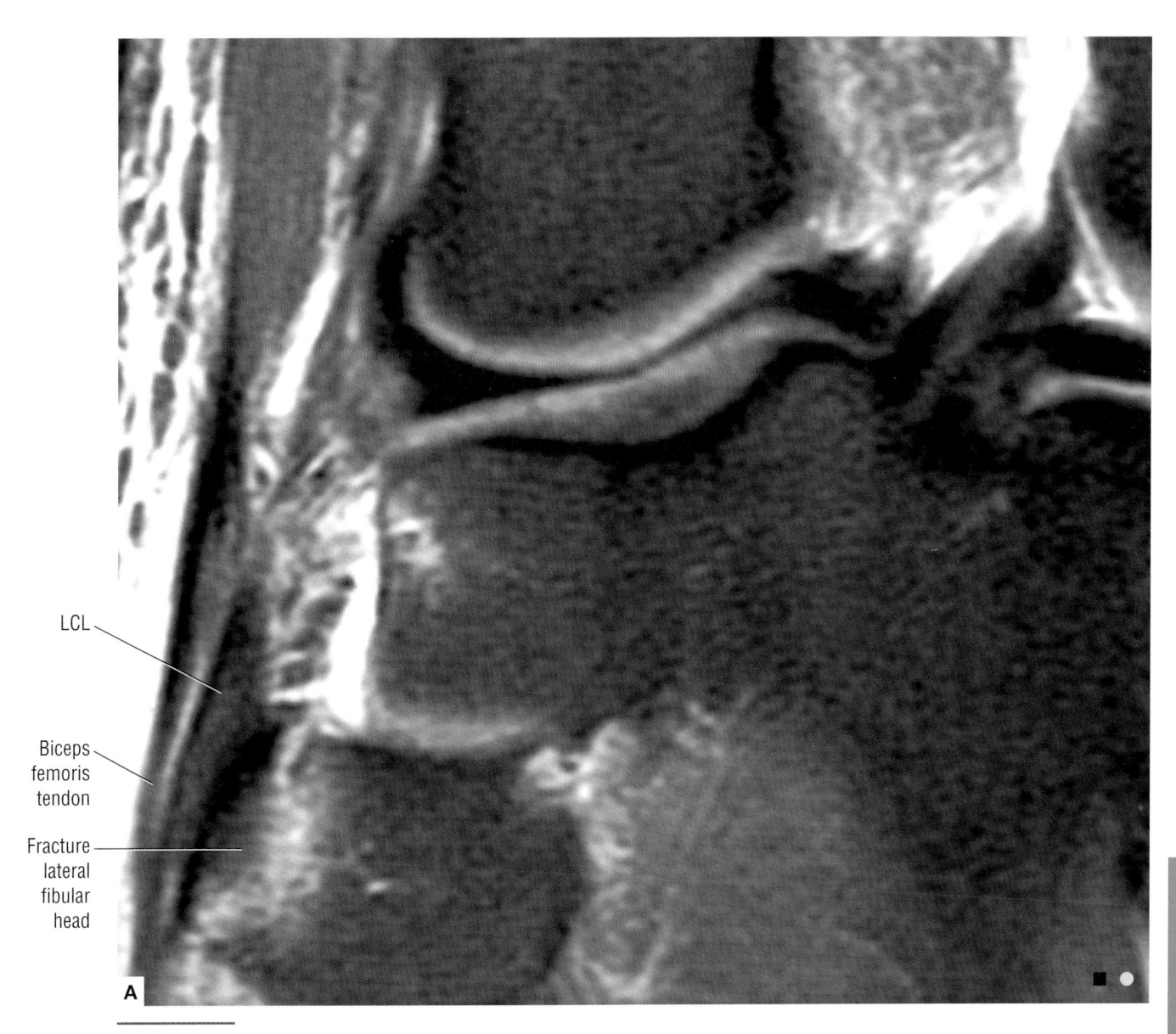

FIGURE 6.101 Fracture avulsion of the lateral fibular head attachment of the lateral collateral ligament (LCL) and biceps femoris tendon. The proximal fibular fracture also extends posteriorly to involve the attachment site of the popliteofibular ligament (PFL). Coronal (**A, B**) and axial (**C**) FS PD FSE images. (*Continued*)

Popliteofibular ligament (PFL)

Lateral fibular head avulsion of LCL and biceps femoris attachment

Avulsion of upper facet attachment of PFL

Lateral fibular head fracture

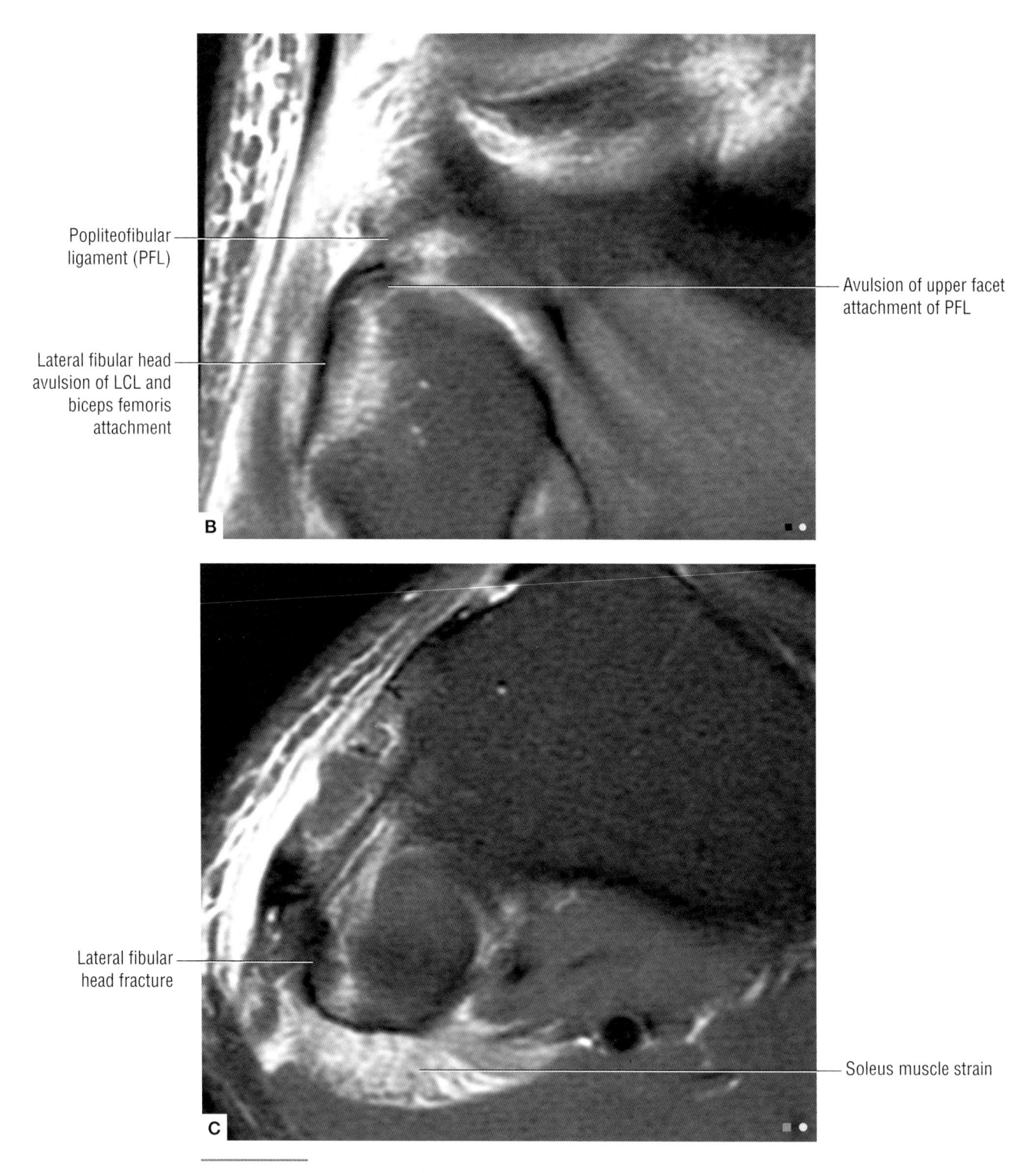

Soleus muscle strain

FIGURE 6.101 (*Continued*)

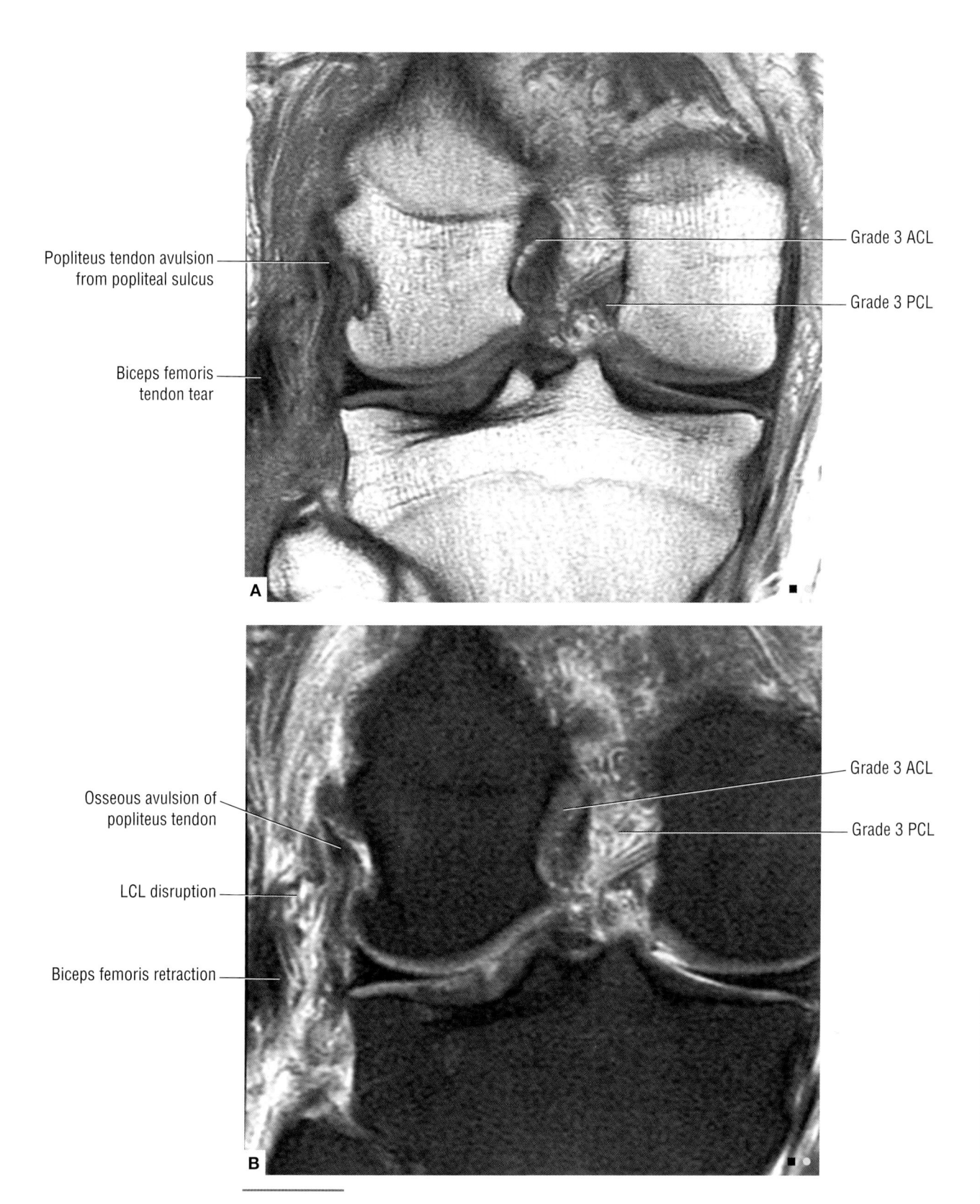

FIGURE 6.102 Posterolateral corner injury with osseous avulsion of popliteus tendon, disruption of the distal course of the lateral collateral ligament (LCL) and biceps femoris, and tear of the popliteofibular ligament from the upper facet of the posterosuperior fibular head. There is a grade 3 ACL and PCL injury. The posterolateral corner findings are a component of this multiple-ligament injury. Most cases of knee dislocation involve the ACL, PCL, and at least one collateral ligament. Coronal PD (**A**) and FS PD (**B**) images. (*Continued*)

FIGURE 6.102 (*Continued*) (**C**) Sagittal FS PD image.

- Stripped fibular attachment of PFL
- Soleus muscle strain

- Lateral collateral ligament
- Biceps femoris graft
- Biceps femoris muscle

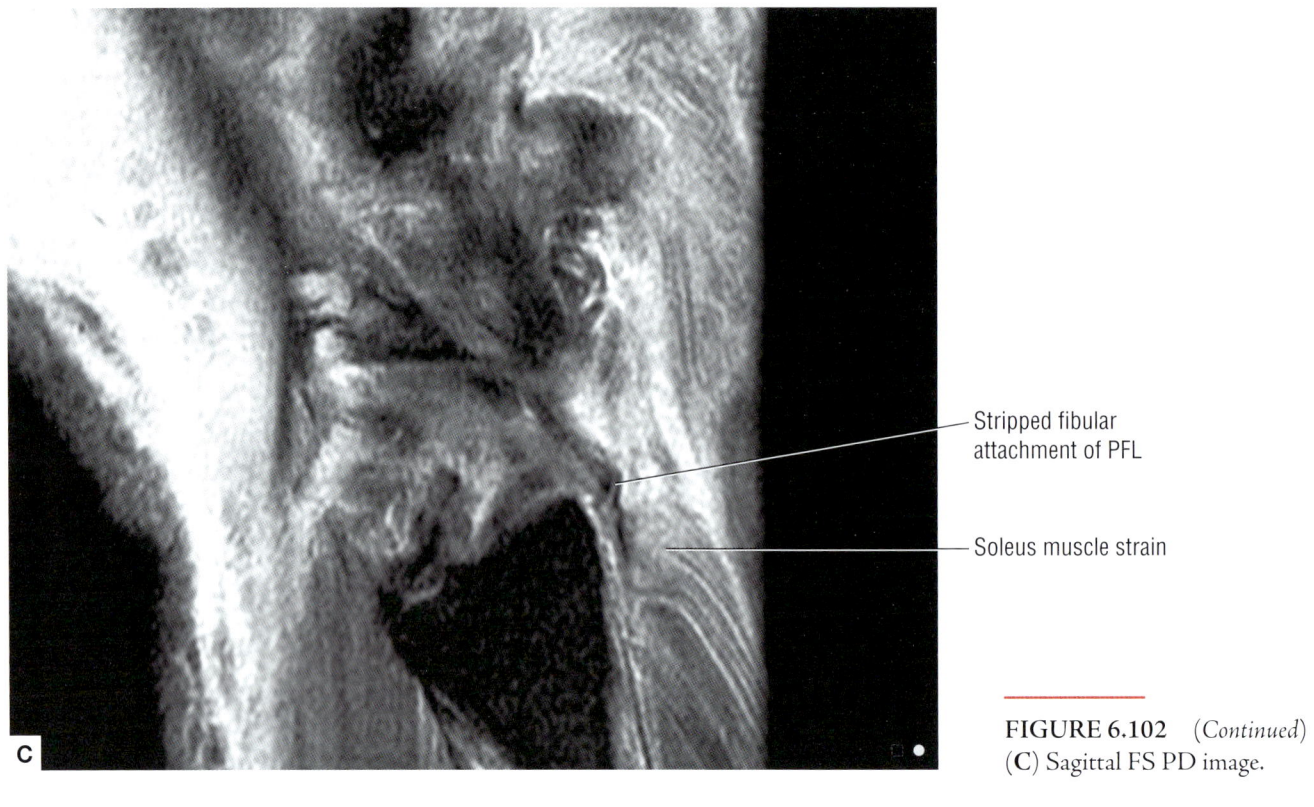

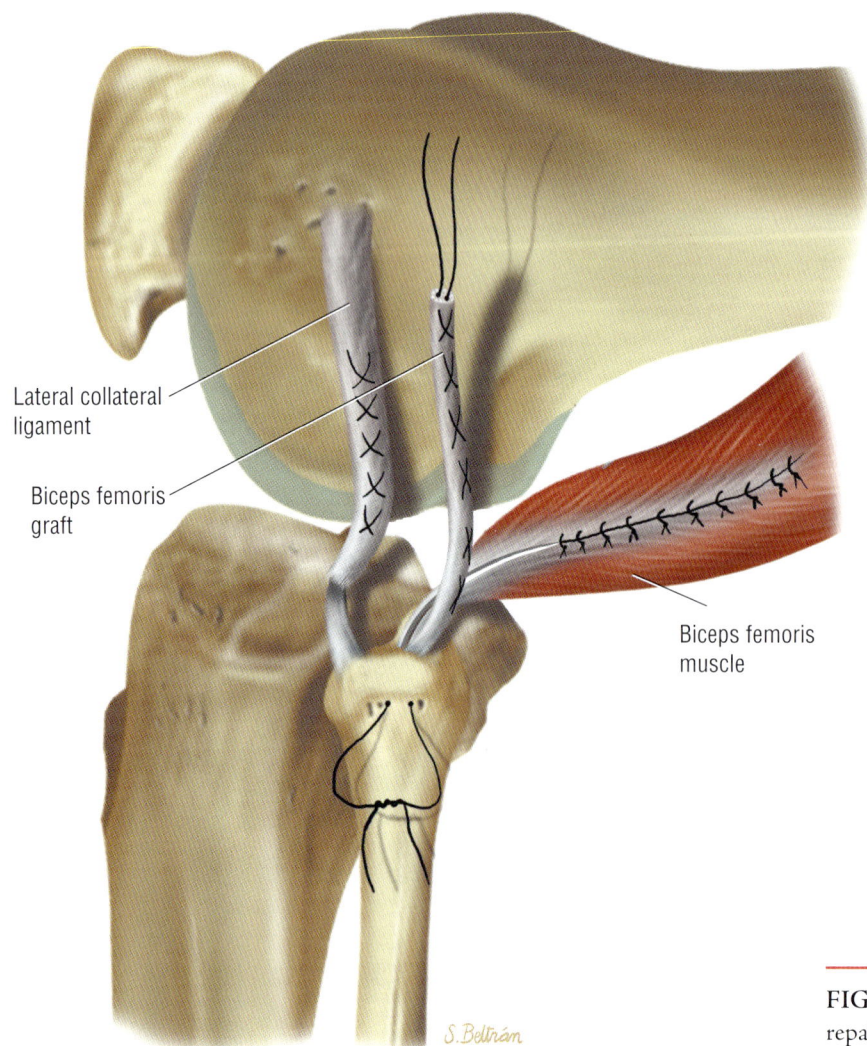

FIGURE 6.103 Posterolateral corner primary repair supplemented with biceps femoris graft reinforcement of the LCL.

Collateral Ligaments

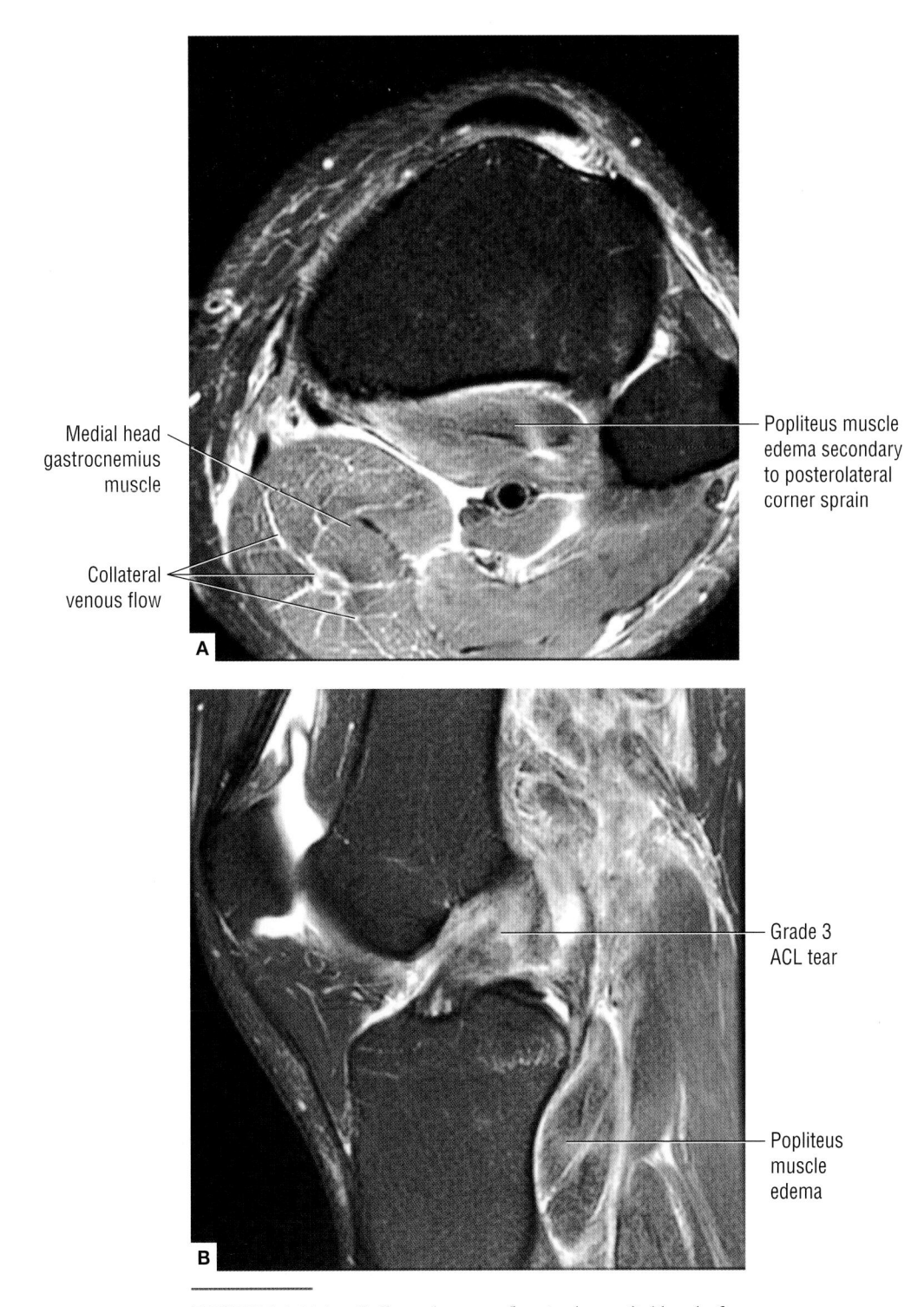

FIGURE 6.104 Collateral venous flow in the medial head of the gastrocnemius after ACL/posterolateral corner injury as seen on (**A**) axial FS PD FSE and (**B**) sagittal FS PD FSE images.

7
Patellofemoral Joint and the Extensor Mechanism

Classification of Patellofemoral Disorders (page 697)

Anatomy of the Patellofemoral Joint (page 699)

Chondromalacia (pages 706–750)

Medial and Lateral Retinacula (pages 751–786)

Iliotibial Band Syndrome (pages 787–797)

Extensor Mechanism and Patellar Tendon Abnormalities (pages 798–824)

Patellar Bursae (pages 825–829)

Selected Patellofemoral Surgical Procedures (pages 830–832)

Quadriceps Tendon and Muscle Tears (pages 833–841)

Patellofemoral Joint and the Extensor Mechanism

Key Concepts

- Medial patellar facet has convex articular surface, whereas lateral patellar facet has concave articular surface.

- Medial patellar facet is divided into medial odd facet and lateral middle facet; middle facet is thus located between lateral and odd patellar facets.

- Excessive lateral pressure syndrome is associated with lateral patellar facet chondromalacia and edema of the superolateral aspect of Hoffa's fat pad.

Patellofemoral Joint and the Extensor Mechanism

- Axial images required to characterize patellofemoral articulation
    - Obliquely oriented lateral and medial facets cannot be accurately characterized on sagittal or coronal images.
    - Patellar facets, trochlear groove, and retinaculum.

Classification of Patellofemoral Disorders

- *Insall's classification*: patellofemoral disorders divided into groups based on presence or absence of articular cartilage damage[210]
    - Disorders with cartilage damage: chondromalacia, osteoarthritis, osteochondral fractures, and osteochondritis dissecans
    - Variable cartilage damage: malalignment syndrome and plicae
    - Without cartilage damage: prepatellar bursitis, tendinosis, overuse syndromes, and reflex sympathetic dystrophy

Patellar Malalignment and Abnormal Tracking

- Patellofemoral joint disorders are primary source of anterior knee pain and occur with frequency comparable to meniscal lesions.[88,302,468,510]

- Patellar malalignment and abnormal tracking
  - Typically produced by incongruence between patella and femoral trochlear groove
  - Result in instability of patellofemoral joint[88,302,468,510]
  - Produce significant shearing forces and excessive contact stresses, leading to lesions and eventual degeneration of the articular cartilage[409,458]
  - Even in absence of detectable cartilage defect, a chronically malaligned patella may change load distribution in patellofemoral joint and cause clinical symptoms.[88,468,510,467]

- Clinical diagnosis[3,88,302,328,458,467,468,510]
  - Abnormalities of patellar alignment and tracking appear during earliest portion of range of motion as patella enters and articulates with femoral trochlear groove.[14,16,17,88,90,234,377,467,468,510,525]
    - As flexion increases, patella moves deeper into femoral trochlear groove.
    - Patellar displacement less likely to occur at this point because femoral trochlear groove buttresses and stabilizes patella[88,302,467,468]

- Imaging diagnosis
  - Diagnostic imaging techniques that show the joint in initial degrees of flexion are best suited for identification of abnormalities.[3,14,16,88,90,328,389]
  - Patellar malalignment and abnormal tracking not consistently or reliably identified when imaging performed at flexion angles greater than 30 degrees (i.e., most radiographic methods)[16,17,90,234,389]

Anatomy of the Patellofemoral Joint

- Congruence of shapes of patella and femoral trochlear groove is important for proper function of patellofemoral joint.[65,137,150,262,270]
    - Dysplastic bony anatomy and/or abnormal soft tissue structures commonly seen in conjunction with patellofemoral instability[137,150,208,262,270]
    - Normal patellar alignment and tracking may exist even with abnormal morphology.[137,150,208,262,270]
- Evaluation of patellofemoral joint anatomy best accomplished with sequential axial section images with joint positioned in extension[104,432,434]

Anatomy of the Patella

- Sesamoid bone contained within quadriceps tendon
    - Functions both to protect femoral articular surface and to increase efficiency of the quadriceps mechanism via fulcrum effect
- Width (51 to 57mm) and height (57 to 58mm) of patella are remarkably constant, although thickness (midequatorial plane) is variable.
- Anterior patellar surface (convex)
    - Rough cribriform surface that provides attachment for quadriceps tendon in its upper third
    - Inferior third V-shaped point enveloped by patellar tendon.
- Posterior patellar surface
    - Inferior portion
        - Usually nonarticular, representing nearly 25% of height
    - Superior portion
        - Upper three-fourths of posterior surface covered by hyaline cartilage
- Articular surface of patella
    - Roughly oval and divided into medial and lateral facets by a vertical ridge oriented along the long axis of the patella

- Medial facet
    - Considerable anatomic variation, usually flat or convex with articular cartilage of varying thickness
    - Subdivided by a small vertical ridge (the *secondary ridge*) into medial facet proper and smaller *odd facet* along its medial border
    - Secondary ridge runs in longitudinal oblique direction and is closer to midline proximally than distally.
    - Odd facet is concave or flat and may be in same plane as medial facet or may be oriented at as much as a 60-degree angle to it.
- Lateral facet
    - Both longer and wider than medial facet
    - Concave in both vertical and transverse planes
    - Two transverse ridges divide patella into upper, middle, and lower thirds; most constant of these separates the middle and lower thirds of the lateral facet.

- Wiberg classification: three-part scheme to describe majority of patellar facet configurations, based on configuration of subchondral bone of facets on tangential conventional radiographs[522]
    - Type 1: both facets gently concave, symmetrical, and nearly equal in size
    - Type 2: medial facet is smaller than lateral
        - Medial facet is flat or convex; lateral facet remains concave.
        - Most common configuration (65% of patellae)
        - Differences between type 1 and type 2 patellae represent a continuum and may be subtle.
    - Type 3: medial facet distinctly smaller with marked lateral predominance
        - Accounts for 25% of patellae[77,270,427,434]

- Ficat and Hungerford classification: alternative classification scheme based on angle subtended by two major facets on conventional radiographs[137]
    - Angle greater than 140 degrees: *pebble-shaped patella*
    - Angle 90 to 100 degrees: most closely corresponds to Wiberg type 3
    - Angle of 90 degrees: hemipatella with one articular facet (*Alpine hunter's cap deformity*)
        - Commonly observed in patients with lateral instability
        - Associated with hypoplasia of vastus medialis and decreased depth of femoral trochlear sulcus
    - Acute angle with a single articular facet: *half-moon patella*

Anatomy of the Femoral Trochlear Groove

- Femoral trochlear groove provides mechanical restraint that helps stabilize and serves as a guide for the patella during joint flexion.[77,104,137,150,262,270,427]
- Normal femoral trochlear shape
    - Deep sulcus with well-defined medial and lateral facets that are either equal in size or with a slightly larger lateral facet[65,137,150,262]
    - Most important aspect of groove shape is that it conforms to shape of the patella for proper articulation.[137,150,262,270]
- Wide variety of abnormal shapes of femoral trochlear groove
    - Hypoplastic or dysplastic medial or lateral aspects
    - Shallow or flattened femoral trochlear groove or sulcus may be associated with patellofemoral joint instability.[104,137,150,262,270]

FIGURE 7.1 Normal trochlear groove and sulcus angle. The thick articular cartilage and orientation of the patellar facets optimize the axial plane for evaluating patellar facet chondral surfaces and cartilage stratification. The trochlear groove, however, is best evaluated in the sagittal plane because of the dramatic change in curvature of the femoral condylar surface and partial volume issues with adjacent fat; resultant axial plane heterogeneity favors primary assessment of trochlear cartilage. Axial PD FSE image.

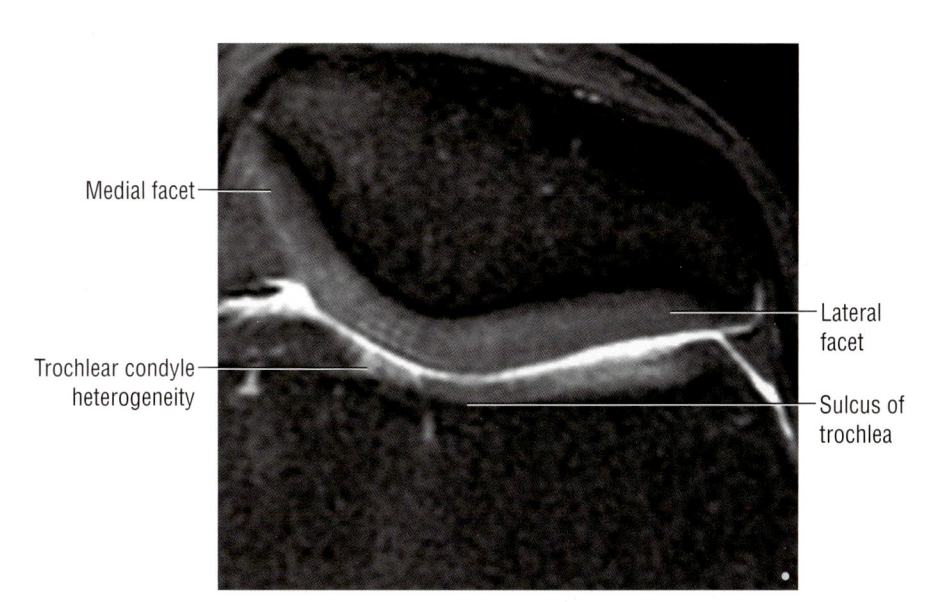

Patella Alta and Patella Baja

- Height of patella relative to femoral trochlear groove is biomechanically important for proper function of the patellofemoral joint.[104,260,420]

- Contact points between cartilaginous surfaces of patella and femoral trochlear groove during joint flexion are drastically altered if patella is positioned too high or too low.

- Abnormal patellar height may be partially responsible for patellar malalignment and abnormal tracking.[137,208,260,262,270,420,459]

- Normal patellar height
    - Inferior pole of patella is positioned in superior aspect of femoral trochlear groove.[104,420,427]

- *Patella alta*
    - Abnormally high position of patella
    - Diagnosed when inferior pole of patella is positioned above superior aspect of femoral trochlear groove with joint extended

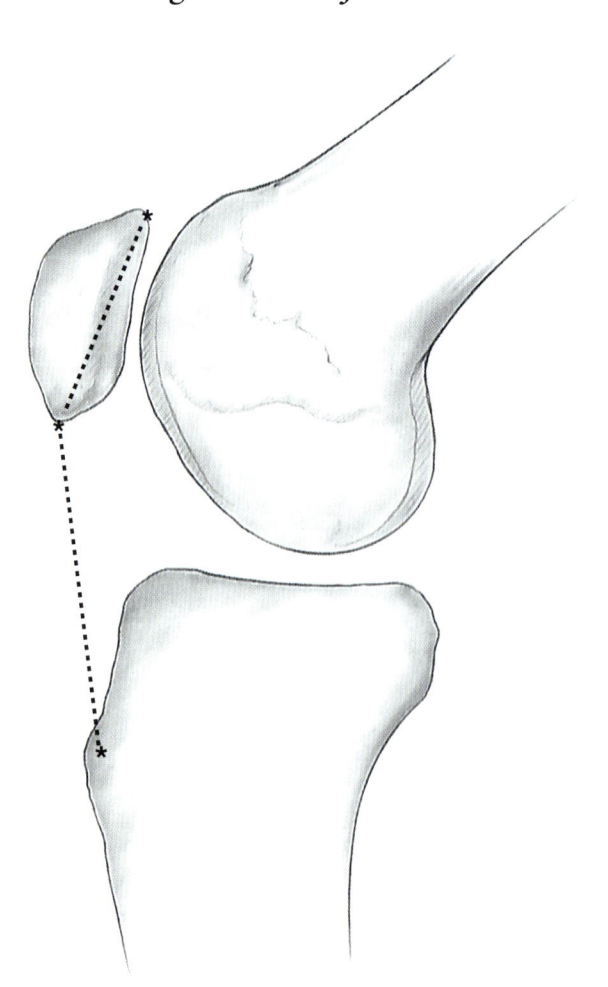

FIGURE 7.2 Insall and Salvati's ratio (P/PT). Normal values with the knee in 30 degrees of flexion range from 0.8 to 1.2. (Reprinted from Jackson DW. *Master Techniques in Orthopaedic Surgery: Reconstructive Knee Surgery*, 3rd ed. Philadelphia, PA: Lippincott Williams & Wilkins; 2008, with permission.)

- Associated with patellofemoral joint instability, patellar dislocation, and chondromalacia patellae[59,245,514]

■ *Patella baja*
- Abnormally low position of patella
- Patella positioned in or below the femoral trochlear groove with joint extended
- In conjunction with Osgood-Schlatter disease[268]
- May also be found after patellar realignment procedures that involve repositioning or shortening of the patellar tendon[104,268,427,432]

Kinematic MR Imaging of the Patellofemoral Joint

■ Extension of the patellofemoral joint
- Essentially no forces acting on patella
- Patella may be situated medially, laterally, or in a central position relative to femoral trochlear groove.
- "Pseudo-subluxation" of the patella during extension is considered a normal variant, since it may be found in any of above positions.
- Images obtained in extension useful for determining position of patella as it enters femoral trochlear groove

■ Flexion of patellofemoral joint[436]
- Normal alignment and tracking dependent on interaction of:
  - Dynamic stabilizers (primarily the quadriceps muscles)
  - Static stabilizers (patellar tendon, lateral patellofemoral ligament, lateral patellar ligament, medial retinaculum, lateral retinaculum, and fascia lata)
  - Bony structures (congruence between shapes of patella and femoral trochlear groove)
  - Alignment of femur and tibia[65,137,210,262,420,436]

■ In normal patellar alignment and tracking, patellar ridge is positioned directly in the center of the femoral trochlear groove.[48,420,434]

Pathokinematics

- Lateral Subluxation of the Patella
    - Common form of patellar malalignment and abnormal tracking
    - Either ridge of patella is laterally displaced relative to femoral trochlear groove or centermost part of femoral trochlea.
    - Lateral facet of patella overlaps lateral aspect of femoral trochlea.
    - Occurs with varying degrees of severity
    - Typically caused by unbalanced forces from lateral soft tissue structures, possibly combined with insufficient counterbalancing forces from medial soft tissue structures
    - Dysplastic patella, dysplastic femoral trochlear groove, and/or patella alta may also be partially responsible.
    - Redundant lateral retinaculum in selective cases[431,433,436,437]
        - Indicates that subluxated patella not caused by excessive force from lateral retinaculum
- Lateral Patellar Tilt or Excessive Lateral Pressure Syndrome[137]
    - Clinically characterized by anterior knee pain
    - Radiologically illustrated by tilting of the patella with functional patellar lateralization, usually onto a dominant lateral facet[137,150]
    - Pathologic etiology is excessive force from lateral retinaculum.[150]
        - Patellar tilting with excessive lateral pressure syndrome may be either transient (centralization or correction of the patellar malalignment occurs during joint flexion) or progressive (there is additional tilting with increasing increments of joint flexion).[104,270,432,434]
    - Underlying hyperpressure in excessive lateral pressure syndrome can produce significant destruction of the articular cartilage.[137,150]

- May produce lateral joint line narrowing as a result of decreased cartilage thickness or even gross cartilage degeneration along the median ridge and lateral patellar facet[137,150]
- Dysplastic patella and/or femoral trochlear groove
  - More likely if excessive lateral pressure syndrome is present during growth and development of patellofemoral joint (final shapes of patella and femoral trochlea are modified by use)[150]
- Surgical release of the lateral retinaculum is usually effective.[150,270]

Medial Subluxation of the Patella (Patella Adentro)

- Medial displacement of patellar ridge relative to femoral trochlear groove or centermost part of femoral trochlea[126,429,434]
- Frequently found in symptomatic patients after surgical patellar realignment procedures due to overcompensation of lateral tethering or stabilizing mechanisms of the patellofemoral joint[126,205,429,434]
- Various causative factors, existing either separately or in combination
  - Excessively tight medial retinaculum
  - Insufficient lateral retinaculum
  - Abnormal patellofemoral anatomy
  - Quadriceps imbalance (extreme internal rotation of lower extremities and atrophy of vastus lateralis are common clinical findings)[48]

Lateral-to-Medial Subluxation of the Patella

- Patella is positioned in slight lateral subluxation during initial increments of joint flexion (5 to 10 degrees), moves into and across femoral trochlear groove or femoral trochlea as flexion increases, and displaces medially during higher increments of flexion.
- Typically found in association with patella alta and/or dysplastic bony anatomy where there is lack of stabilization by femoral trochlear groove[427,432]

Chondromalacia

Key Concepts

- Chondromalacia is commonly associated with patellofemoral overload or malalignment.
- FS PD FSE images identify basal, intrasubstance, and surface chondral defects.
- Patellar facets are evaluated on axial images, whereas trochlear groove articular cartilage is assessed on sagittal images.
- Patellar subchondral sclerosis is associated with chronic chondral injuries.

Chondromalacia Patellae

- Characterized by patellofemoral (retropatellar) joint pain, accentuated during knee flexion, and associated crepitus
- Softening, edema, or fissuring of articular cartilage
- Associated degenerative changes, including sclerosis or hyperemia of subchondral bone
- Most often affects adolescents and young adults and may be primary and idiopathic or occur subsequent to patellar trauma[392]
- Patella alta, increased valgus angle, and femoral condyle hypoplasia may predispose to cartilage changes involving medial and lateral facets.
- Causes of acute chondromalacia
    - Instability, direct trauma, and fracture
- Causes of chronic chondromalacia
    - Subluxation, increased quadriceps angle (Q angle), quadriceps imbalance, posttraumatic malalignment, excessive lateral pressure syndrome, late effects of direct trauma or pressure, posterior cruciate ligament (PCL) injuries, inflammatory arthritis, synovitis, and infection[69]

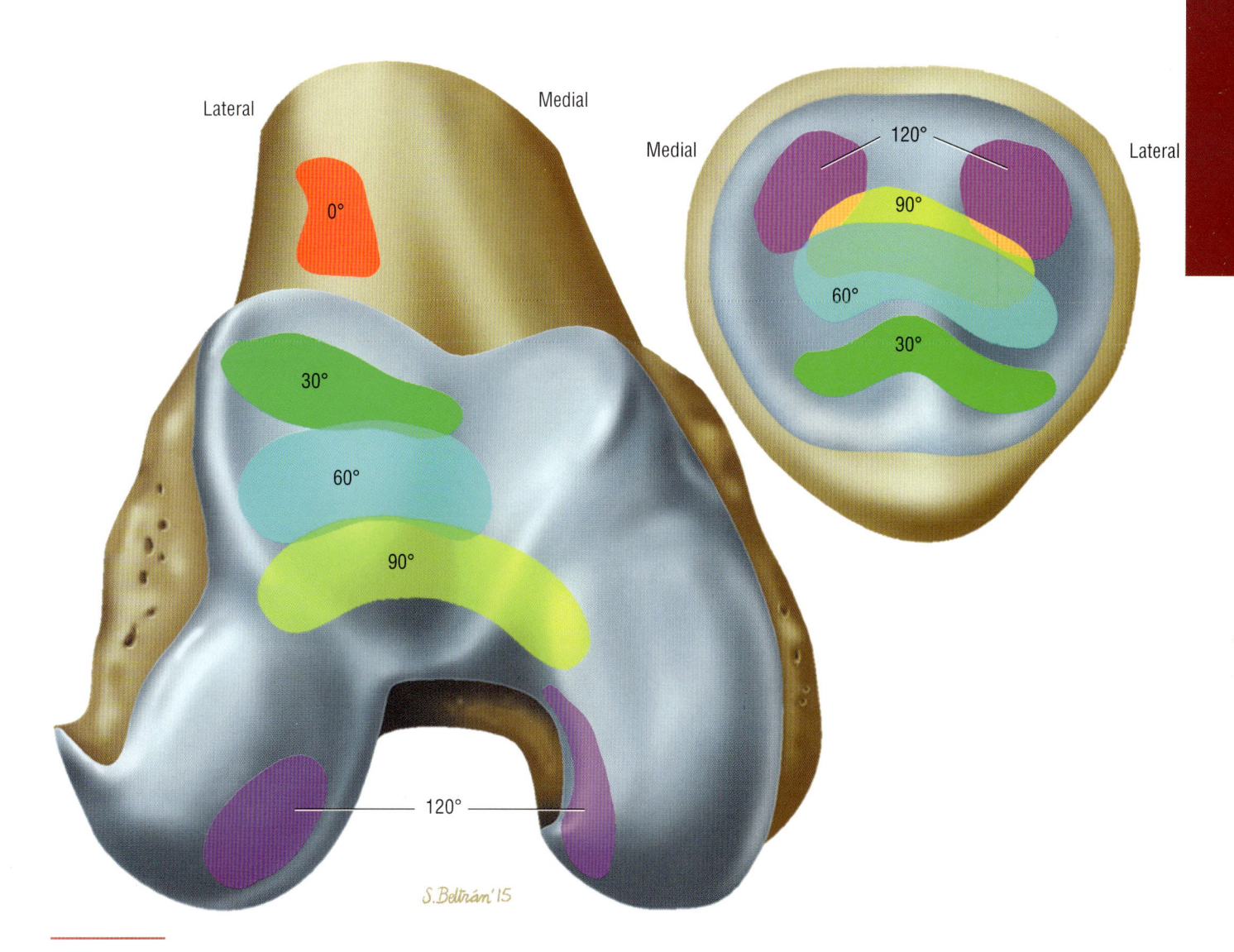

FIGURE 7.3 Patellofemoral joint contact areas based on the knee flexion angle. A normal medial patellar shift is produced when the patella engages and follows the trochlear groove. With an increased flexion angle, the patellar contact area progresses proximally, while the trochlear contact area progresses distally.

Lateral　　　　　　　　　　　　　　　　　　　　Medial

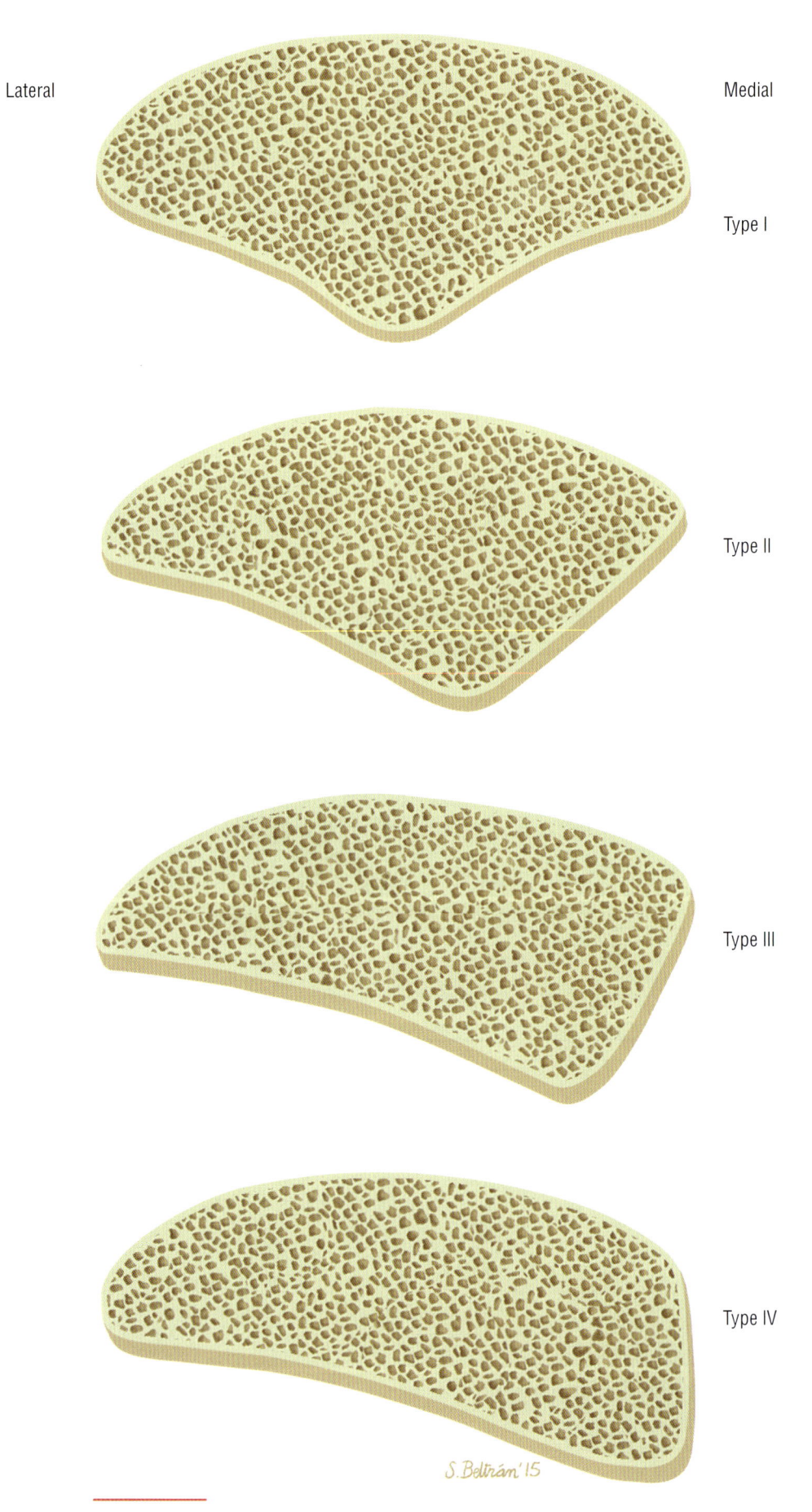

Type I

Type II

Type III

Type IV

FIGURE 7.4 Wiberg patella types. There is relative hypoplasia of the medial facet in type IV.

Patellar Chondromalacia

Grade 1

Grade 2

Grade 3

Grade 4

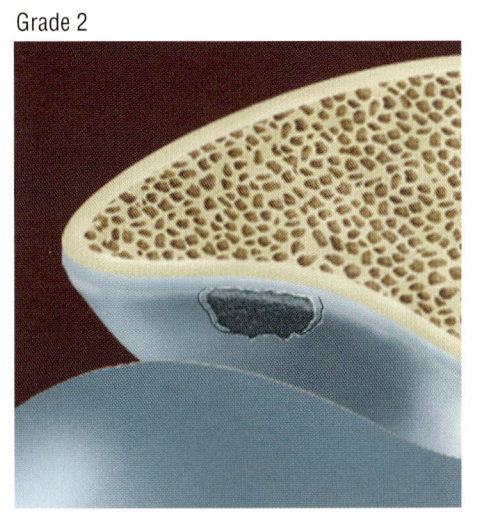

FIGURE 7.5 Outerbridge classification of chondromalacia. Grade 1 chondromalacia with softening of articular cartilage. Grade 1 represents closed chondromalacia, which includes softening and blistering. Grade 2 chondromalacia with fragmentation and fissuring less than 0.5 inch in diameter. Grade 3 chondromalacia with fragmentation and fissuring greater than 0.5 inch in diameter. Grade 4 with full thickness chondral erosion to exposed subchondral bone.

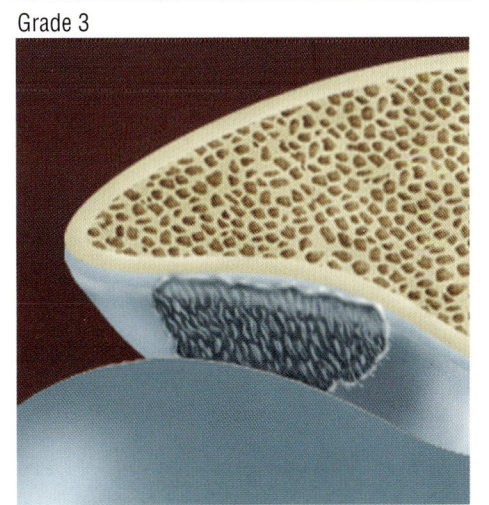

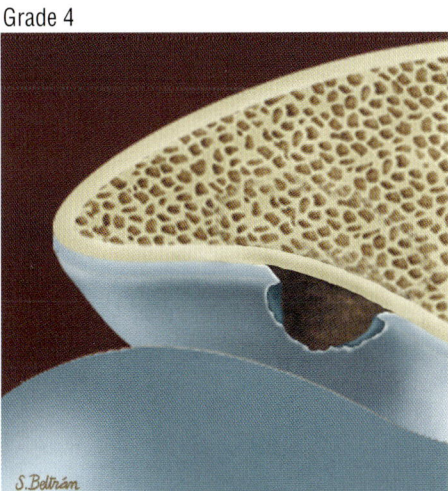

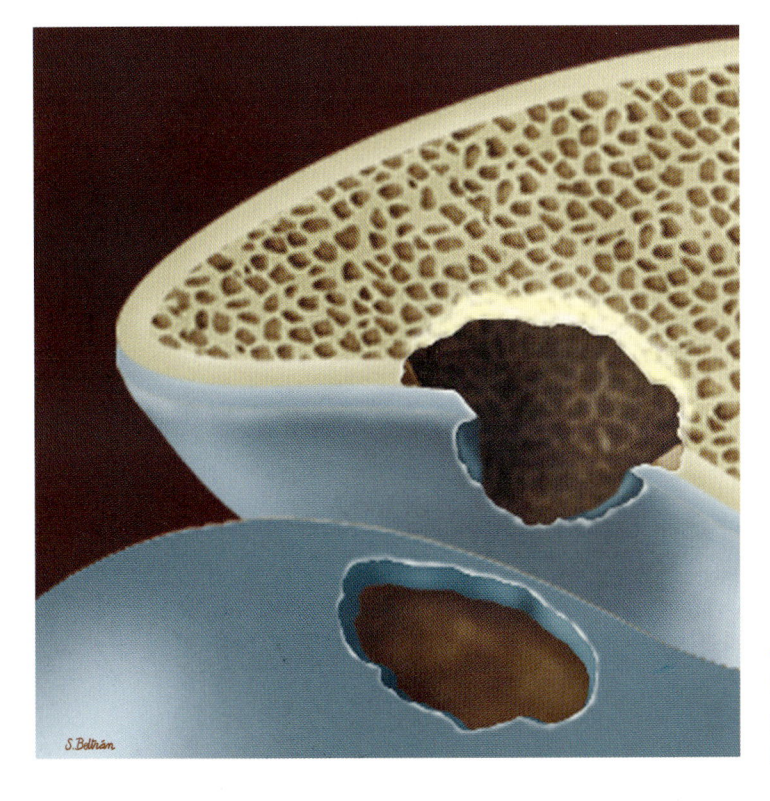

FIGURE 7.6 Patellofemoral arthrosis (arthritis) with progression of chondromalacia to involve subchondral erosion of the patella and erosion of the opposing femoral chondral surface.

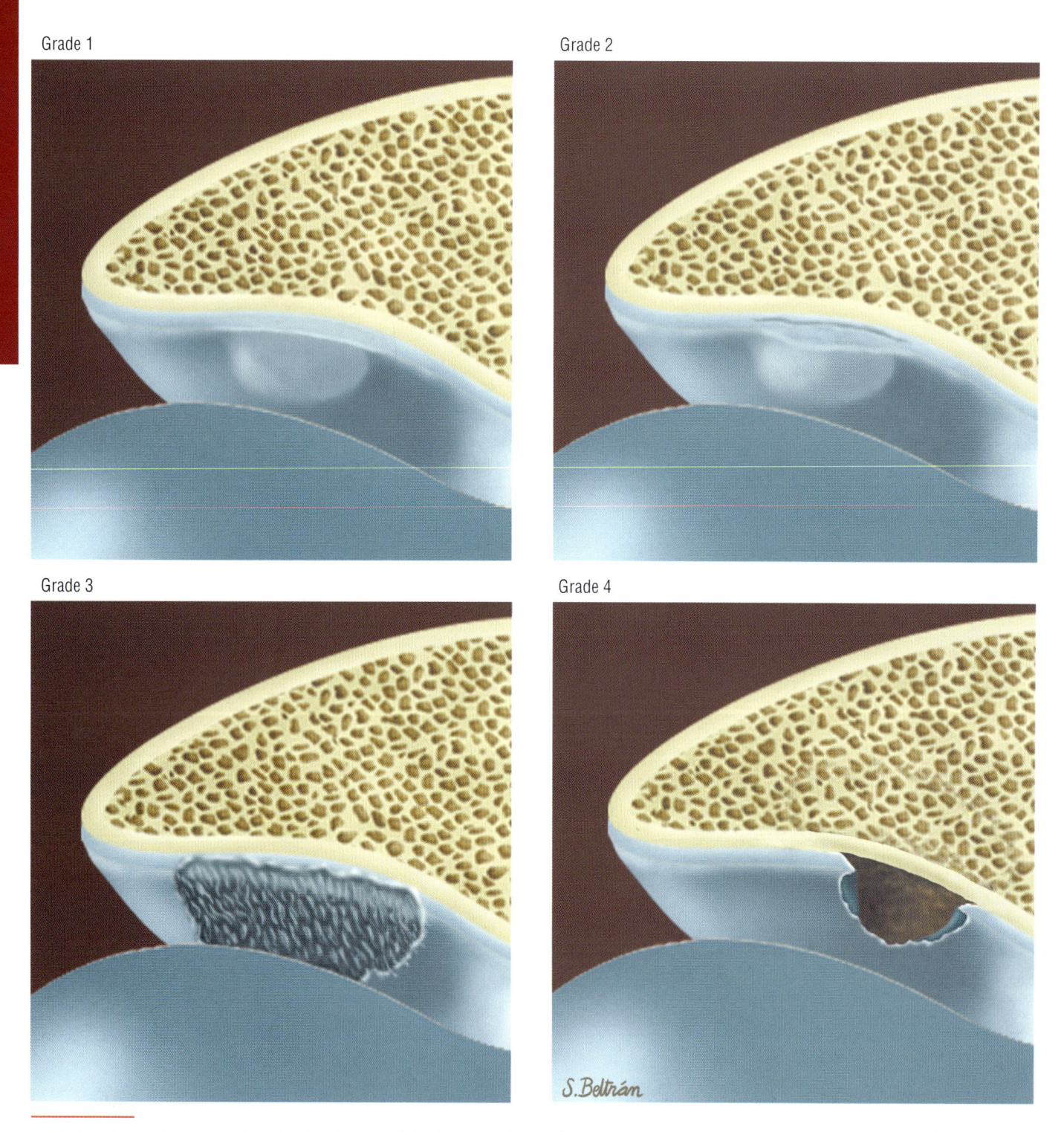

FIGURE 7.7 Alternative classification distinguishing between chondral softening in grade 1 and blistering in grade 2. Grade 3 still represents chondral fibrillation, and grade 4 is frank cartilage ulceration.

MR Appearance of Chondromalacia

- Outerbridge classification of chondromalacia into five arthroscopic grades[290,362]:
    - Grade 0: normal articular cartilage
    - Grade 1: discoloration of articular cartilage, sometimes accompanied by blistering, usually without fragmentation or fissuring
        - Blistering represents separation of superficial layer of articular cartilage.
        - Localized softening, swelling, and fibrillation limited to area of 0.5cm or less in diameter
    - Grade 2: fissuring and fibrillation within soft areas extending to depth of up to 1 to 2mm and area of 1.3cm or less in diameter
    - Grade 3: fissuring and fibrillation may involve more than half the depth of cartilage thickness and area greater than 1.3cm in diameter
        - Cartilage surface resembles crabmeat with fasciculation of multiple cartilaginous fragments attached to underlying subchondral bone.
        - No involvement of subchondral bone
    - Grade 4 (end-stage): complete loss or erosion of articular cartilage surface with exposed subchondral bone
- Advanced patellofemoral arthrosis (arthritis) and end-stage chondromalacia may have same appearance; however, subchondral erosions or cyst formation is better classified as patellofemoral arthritis
- Chondromalacia may also present with either basal or superficial degenerative pattern.[107]
    - Basal degeneration
        - Affects younger patients
        - Associated with posttraumatic disruption of basal collagen
        - Leads to cartilage softening and subsequent blisters, ulcers, and fragmentation

- - Superficial degeneration
    - Occurs in older patients
    - Begins with loss of ground substance or cartilage matrix and leads to fissuring, fragmentation, and eventual exposure of subchondral bone[401]

- Primary abnormality in chondromalacia is decrease in sulfated mucopolysaccharides within ground substance, leading to unstable collagen framework.[153]

- Arthroscopic grading system developed by Shahriaree incorporates both traumatic and nontraumatic types of chondromalacia.[107,153]

  - Grade 1: chondromalacia caused by trauma shows softening, whereas nontraumatic chondromalacia demonstrates fibrillation.
  - Grade 2: separation of superficial from deep layer of articular cartilage in a blister lesion
    - Fissures as vertical collagen fibers become exposed
  - Grade 3: ulceration, fragmentation, and cartilage fibrillation in larger areas of cartilage
  - Grade 4: frank cartilage ulceration with craters of exposed bone and progression to involvement of subchondral bone

MR Protocols

- Protocols used for evaluation of chondromalacia patellae
  - FS PD-weighted FSE images (routinely) or MR arthrography (optionally) to evaluate and define fluid–cartilage interface[153,452]
  - T2 mapping of cartilage heterogeneity in patients with chondromalacia
    - Based on T2 relaxation time of cartilage
    - Chondral degeneration associated with increase in T2 values due to increased chondral water content and decreased T2 shortening effects of the matrix relative to water[152]

- - - Increase in water content and mobility related to decrease in proteoglycan size and glycosaminoglycan (GAG) content, as well as alterations in collagen content
    - T2 mapping allows diagnosis prior to development of frank chondral erosions.
    - Continued improvements in three-dimensional (3D) articular pulse sequences, which demonstrate T2- and FS PD-like contrast, will be required to quantify early chondral degeneration in chondromalacia and osteoarthritis.
  - Delayed gadolinium-enhanced MR imaging of cartilage (dGEMRIC)
    - Technique to identify early chondral lesions by assessing amount of GAG in cartilage[54]
    - Contrast distributed in higher concentration in areas of low GAG content (since GAG abundant in negatively charged carboxyl and sulfate groups)
    - Contrast does not penetrate into areas rich in GAG.
  - MR arthrography with intraarticular contrast
    - Limited and used primarily in evaluation of surface chondral degenerations
- T2* gradient echo (GRE) images not used because of insufficient contrast resolution
  - High signal intensity of articular cartilage
  - Small fissures with imbibed synovial fluid may be missed.
- On FS axial or STIR images, fat signal intensity anterior to the trochlear groove may be mistaken for articular cartilage irregularities.
  - Corresponding T1- or PD-weighted axial or sagittal images better display cartilage.
- Sagittal images are less sensitive to cartilage erosions and may show straightening or loss of normal convex curve when viewed in profile.
- Subchondral low signal intensity (sclerosis) may be associated with irregular surface erosions.
- Patellar cysts may be seen in early stages of softening, before erosions occur.

Evaluation of Patellar Articular Cartilage

- Normal patellar articular cartilage
    - Homogeneous and smooth in contour
    - Low signal intensity on PD- and conventional T2-weighted images
    - Low to intermediate signal intensity or gray signal intensity on FS PD-weighted FSE images (similar to STIR sequences)
- Striations or zones of articular cartilage corresponding to collagen architecture have been shown on high-resolution T2-weighted images (using 80-μm in-plane resolution).
    - Superficial, or gliding, zone: forms articular surface of the joint
    - Transitional zone: larger than and deep to the superficial zone
    - Radial, or deep, zone: largest layer of articular cartilage
    - Calcified zone: deepest, thin; divides articular cartilage from underlying subchondral bone (including subchondral plate and deeper cancellous bone)
- Zonal architecture is distinguished by brighter-signal-intensity superficial zone with relative hypointensity of the deeper zones.
    - Bilaminar appearance may be due to either higher water content in superficial cartilage or anisotropic arrangement of collagen fibers.[153]
- Superficial Zone
    - Higher collagen-to-proteoglycan ratio and higher water content than deeper zones[153]
- Transitional Zone
    - Between superficial and radial zones
    - Collagen fibrils form arcades but may appear to be more randomly oriented when viewed at high magnification.[335]
    - Higher proteoglycan content and lower water and collagen content than superficial zone
    - More water and proteoglycan content than radial zone
    - Visualized with relative increased signal intensity (compared to deeper radial zone) on PD- or FS PD-weighted images.

Patellofemoral Joint and the Extensor Mechanism

- **Radial Zone**
  - Between transitional and calcified zones
  - Relatively hypointense compared to the transitional layer on FS PD FSE images
  - Collagen fibers preferentially arranged perpendicular to subchondral plate
  - Although anisotropic arrangement was considered the theoretical basis for magic-angle effect in articular cartilage, Mosher et al.[336] demonstrated that magic-angle effects do not account for regional differences in cartilage signal intensity.
    - Radial zone shows least orientation dependence.
    - The most superficial 20% of cartilage demonstrates the greatest change in T2 as related to orientation of collagen fibrils.

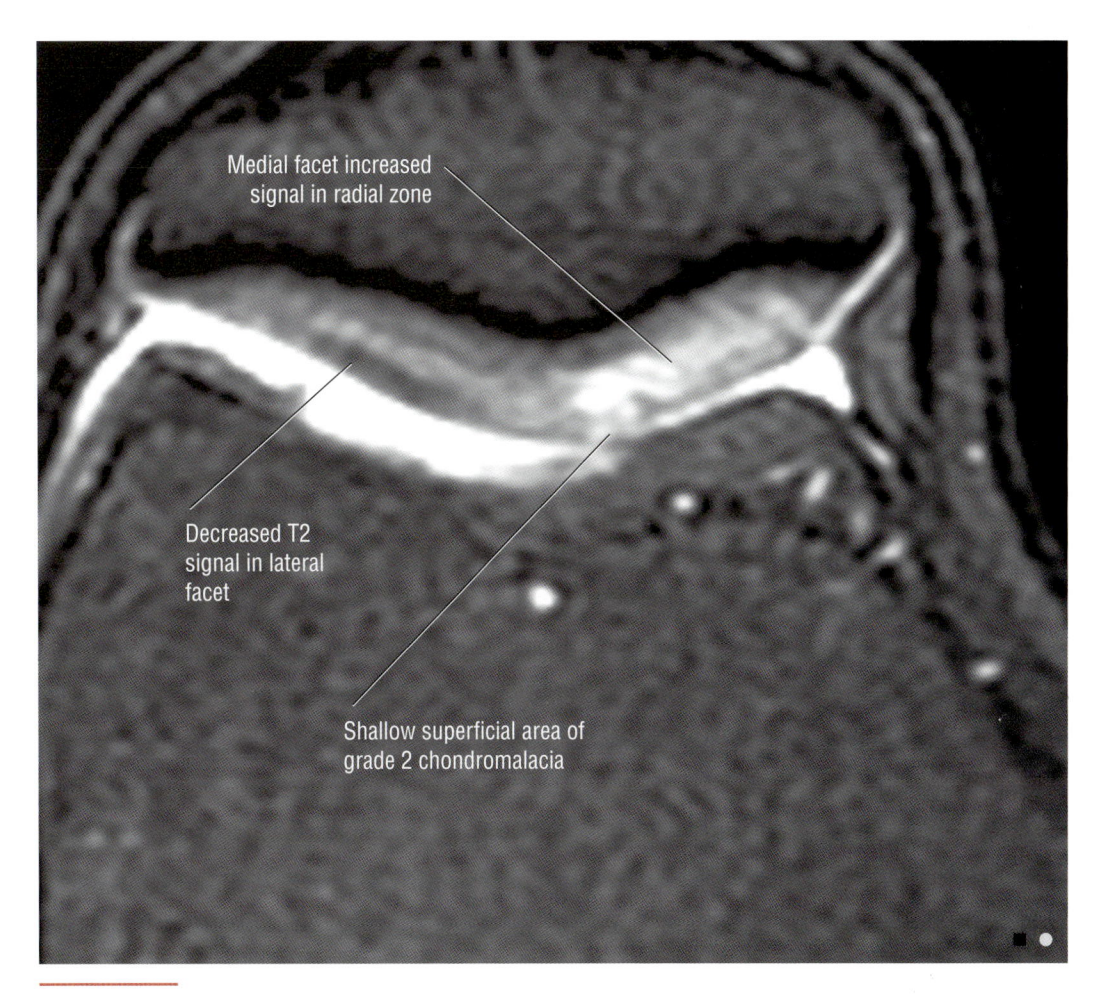

FIGURE 7.8 Medial facet articular cartilage hyperintensity is associated with altered organization of collagen matrix, which is also associated with an overlying shallow area of open chondromalacia (grade 2 degeneration). The decreased T2-weighted signal of the lateral facet reflects both fragmentation of collagen fibrils and hypertrophic healing response associated with an increased concentration of molecular water binding sites in the collagen matrix. Axial FS PD FSE image.

Cartilage Changes in Chondromalacia Patellae

- FS PD-weighted FSE images more sensitive than MR arthrography for evaluation of basal articular changes

- MR arthrography is better for detection of articular cartilage surface irregularity.

- MR Grading Classification

    - Arthroscopic grades of chondromalacia correlated with findings on MR imaging[77,537]

    - Early descriptions relied primarily on T1-weighted images without FS PD-weighted FSE, STIR techniques, or MR arthrography.

    - Correlation with pathologic specimens has demonstrated ability of MR to characterize cartilage morphology, particularly ulcerations of the cartilage surfaces (i.e., fibrillation).[182]

    - Grade 1

        - Focal areas of decreased T1 signal intensity without cartilage surface or subchondral bone extension

        - Focal areas of hyperintensity on FS PD-weighted FSE images without any discontinuity in smooth superficial cartilage contour

        - Early-stage blister formation with focal chondral convexity (considered a part of cartilage softening and swelling)

        - Small surface irregularities (<1mm) may be seen on FS PD-weighted FSE images, representing the earliest changes of softening and swelling.

        - Focal basal or deep layer hyperintensity

        - Chondral softening usually hyperintense on FS PD FSE images, although more chronic or stable intracartilaginous change may be hypointense

        - Histologic changes of articular cartilage softening (*closed chondromalacia*) occur in transitional zone.

        - Changes in collagen matrix include reorientation of collagen fibers into collapsed segments, associated with decrease in matrix proteoglycans.[107]

- **Grade 2**
  - Fissuring and fragmentation confined to small area (usually <1.3cm), in addition to blister-like swelling
  - Less than 50 percent thickness articular cartilage
  - Intracartilaginous hyperintensity with superficial and focal surface irregularity may also be seen.

- **Grade 3**
  - High-signal-intensity of imbibed fluid in surface articular cartilage defects
  - Focal ulcerations and "crabmeat" lesions (greater than half thickness of articular cartilage)

- **Grade 4**
  - Frank articular cartilage defects, exposed subchondral bone, and underlying fluid. Full thickness of chondral involvement.

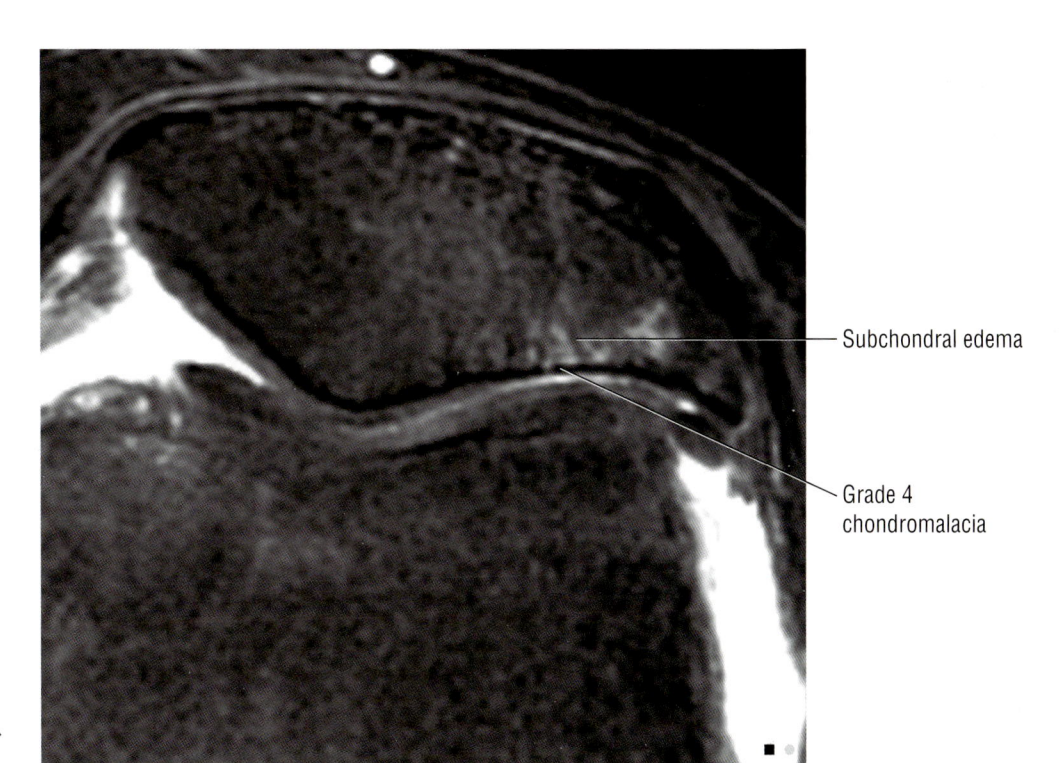

FIGURE 7.9 Grade 4 lesion of chondromalacia with full thickness loss of lateral facet articular cartilage. Increased T2-weighted subchondral signal is associated with this grade of chondral involvement. Axial FS PD FSE image.

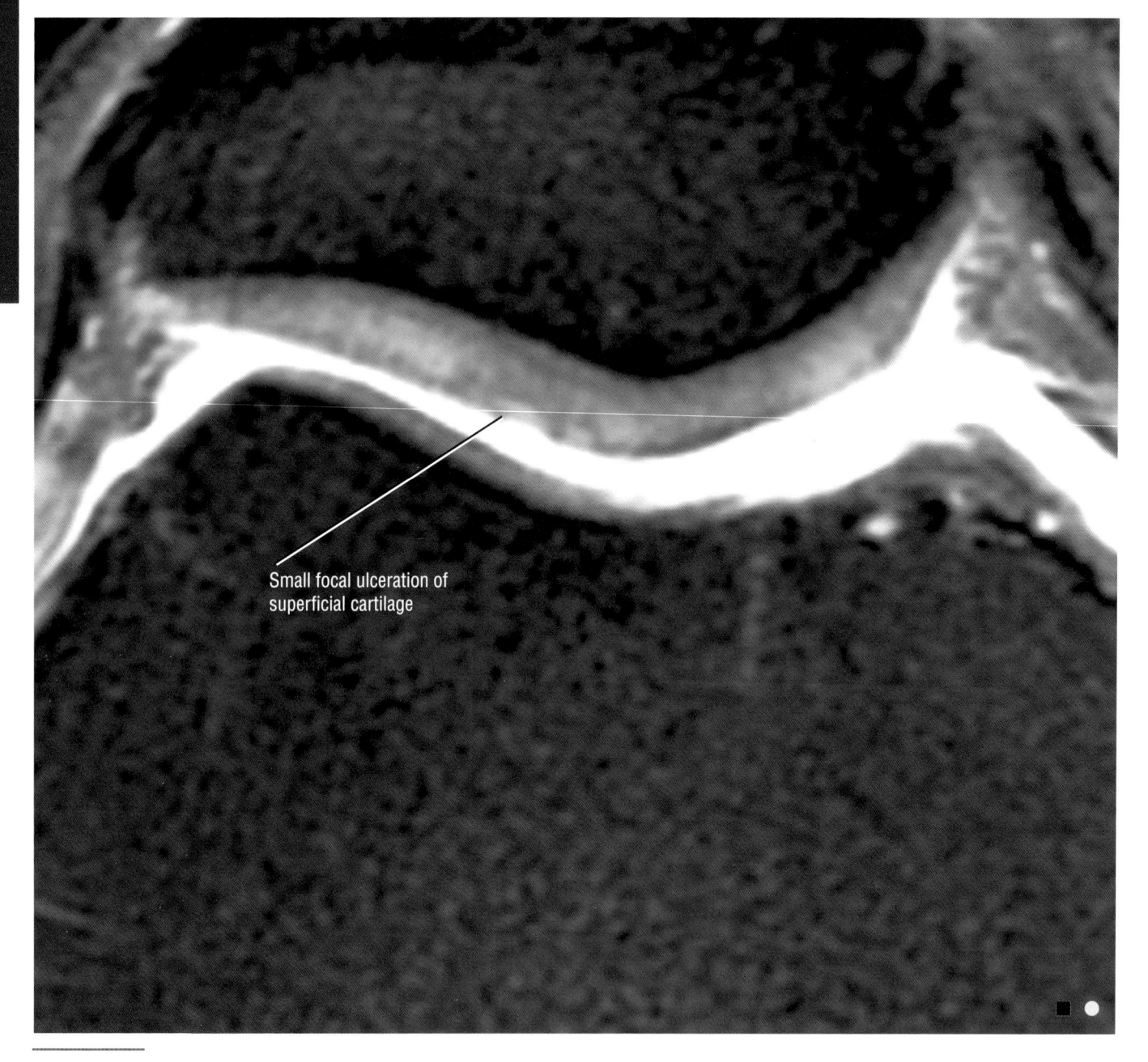

FIGURE 7.10 In contrast to linear articular cartilage fissures, this case demonstrates a small ulceration (lesions usually associated with breakdown of a superficial blister). Grade 2 chondromalacia on axial FS PD FSE image.

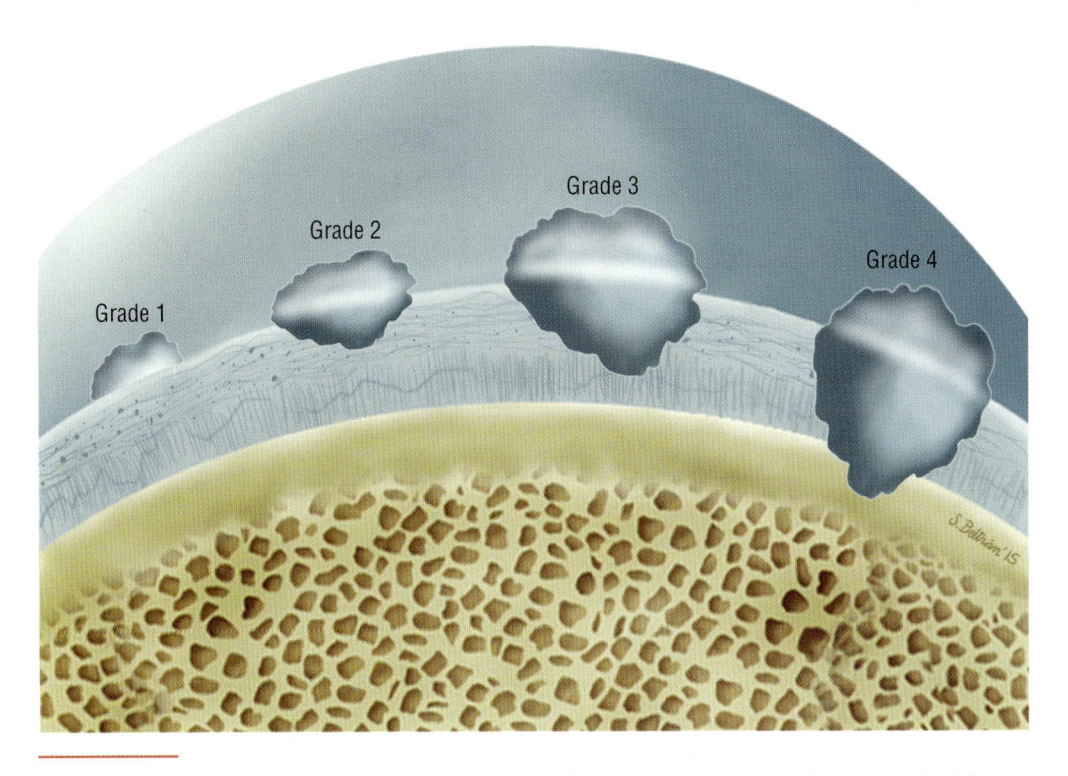

FIGURE 7.11 Grades of articular cartilage lesions from grade 1 chondral softening and/or blister to a full thickness fissure or defect in grade 4.

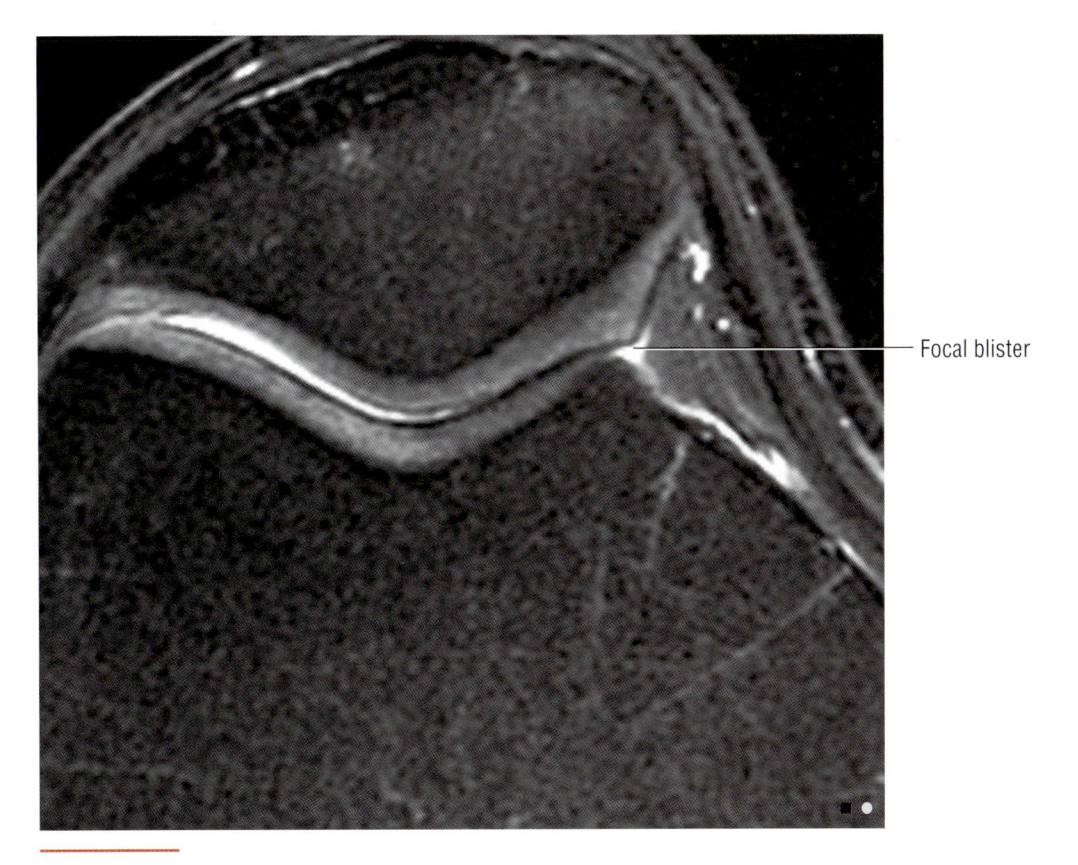

FIGURE 7.12 Grade 1 blister lesion of the medial patellar facet. There is a focal convexity of the chondral surface in the blister. Axial FS PD FSE image.

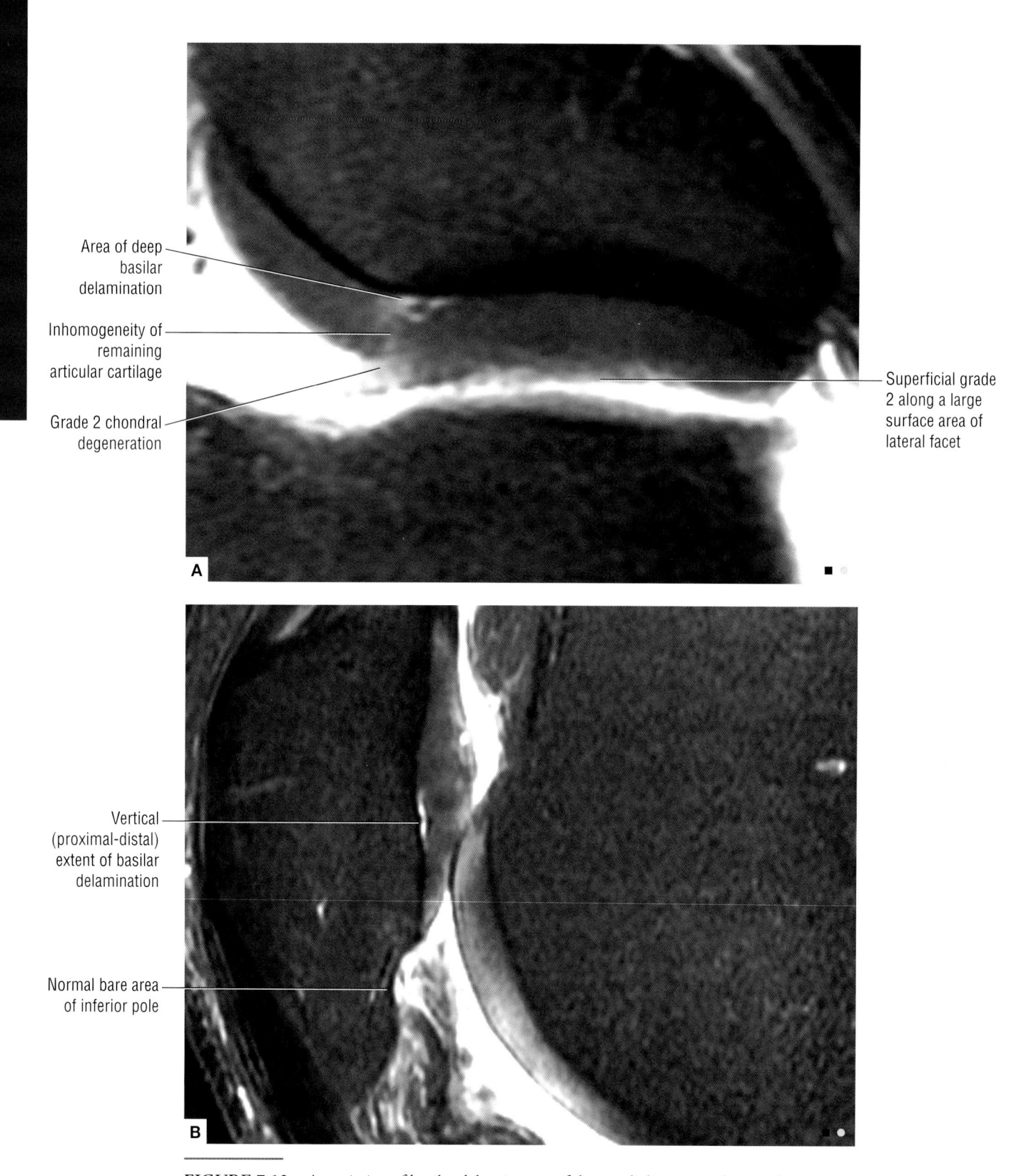

FIGURE 7.13 Association of basilar delamination of deep radial zone cartilage with opposing surface grade 2 chondral fissure. The inhomogeneity of the transitional and radial zone cartilage between the superficial zone and the basilar layer of the radial zone is shown as area of ill-defined intermediate/increased signal. Axial (**A**) and sagittal (**B**) FS PD FSE images.

Patellofemoral Joint and the Extensor Mechanism

Grade 4 chondral loss inferior pole lateral facet

Full-thickness chondral lesion with both exposure and extension to subchondral bone

Subchondral cysts

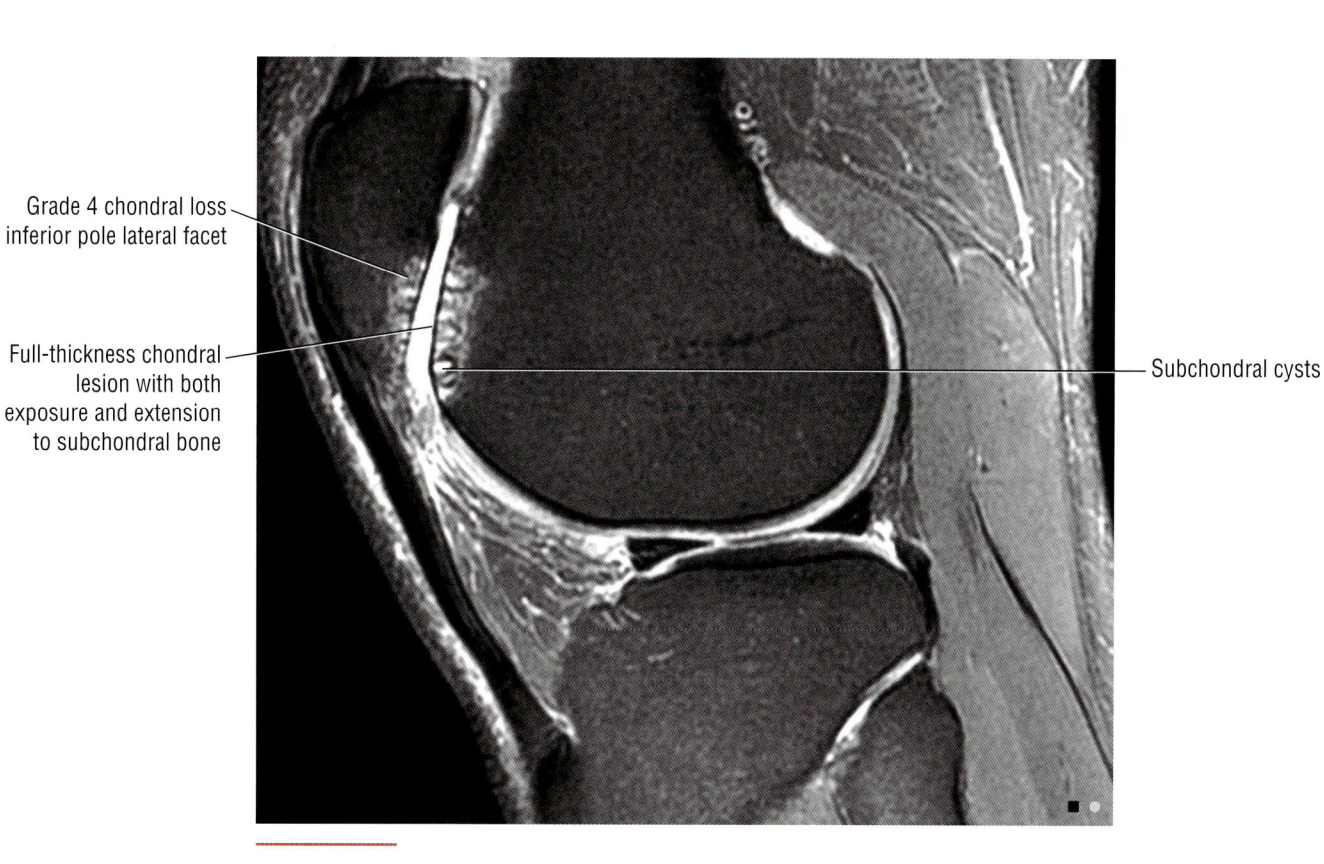

FIGURE 7.14 Grade 4 chondral loss between inferior pole lateral patellar facet and anterolateral femoral condyle of trochlear groove. Chondromalacia has progressed to patellofemoral osteochondritis (arthrosis) with subchondral cyst formation. Sagittal FS PD FSE image.

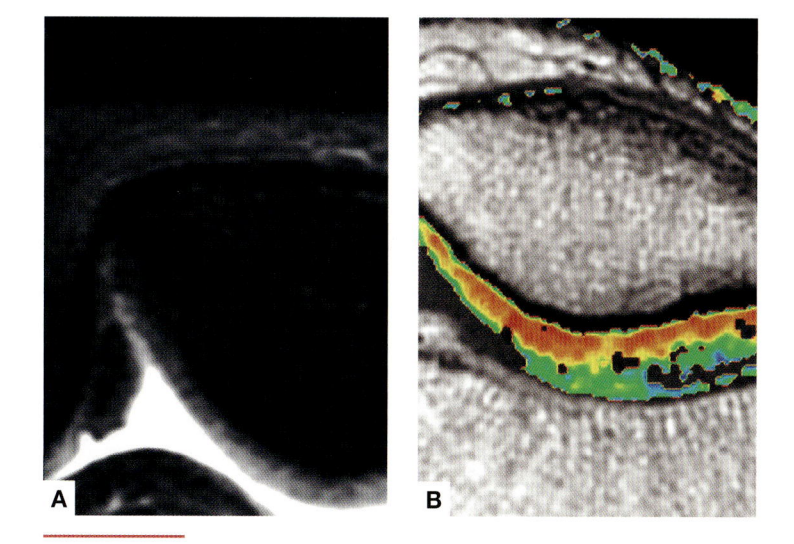

FIGURE 7.15 (**A**) Patellar facet articular cartilage displays intermediate signal intensity on this axial FS PD FSE image. (**B**) Relative T2 relaxation color map of patellar cartilage. Cartilage T2 ranges from 20 to a maximum of 80ms. *Orange* represents longer T2 values in the radial zone, corresponding to collagen fibrils, and *green* and *yellow* represent longer T2 values in the superficial and transitional zones. In the presence of chondromalacia, collagen fibril degradation causes a T2 increase not visible on conventional MR images.

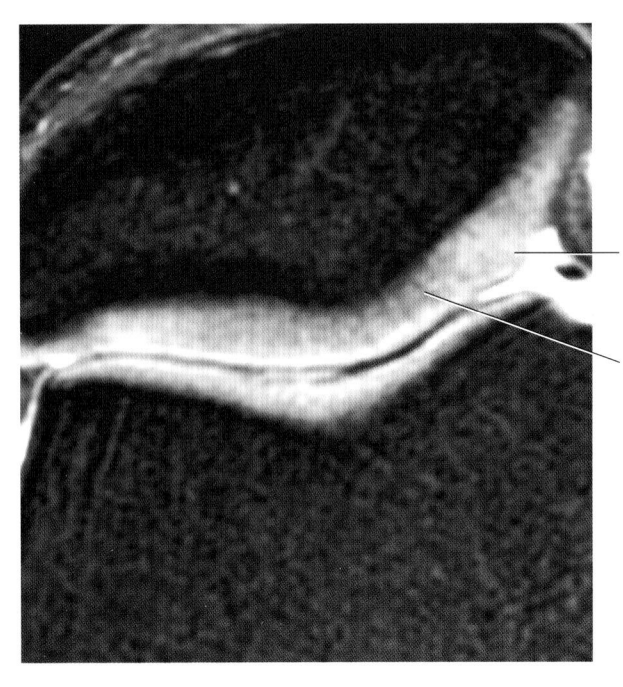

FIGURE 7.16 Axial FS PD FSE image showing hypointense signal intensity corresponding to the radial zone of articular cartilage collagen fibrils, which demonstrate an orientation perpendicular to the subchondral plate in the deep radial zone. The focal area of medial facet blister formation is visualized with increased signal intensity. The transitional zone and the deeper radial zone are responsible for the bilaminar appearance of articular cartilage on MR.

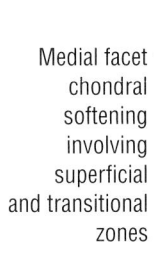

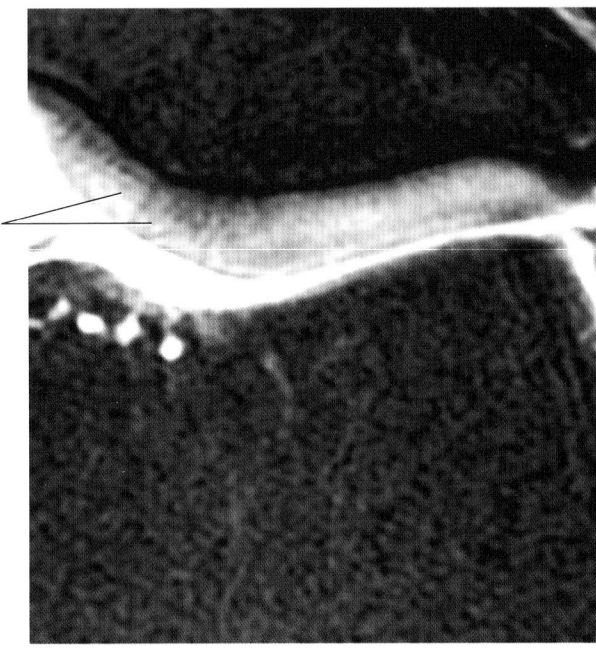

FIGURE 7.17 Early stage of chondral softening in the medial facet characterized by subtle discontinuity of a thin superficial hypointense band (corresponding to the superficial zone) and with increased or hyperintense heterogeneity without the transitional and upper radial zones. Axial FS PD FSE image.

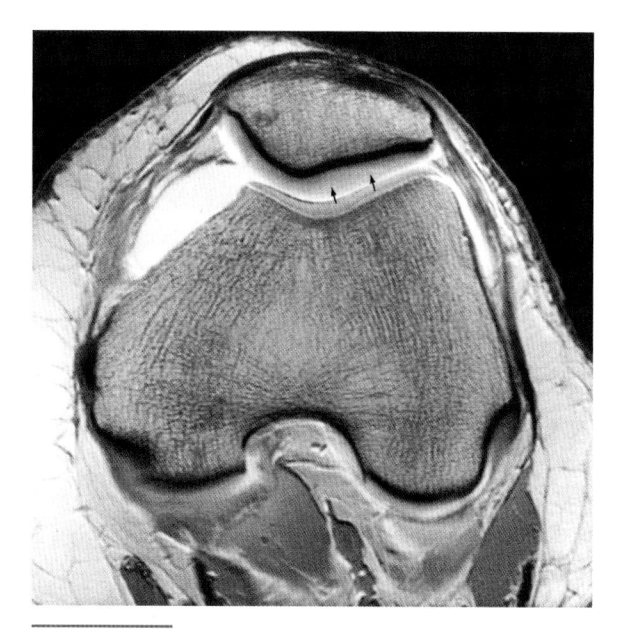

FIGURE 7.18 MR arthrography with intraarticular gadolinium–diethylene triamine pentaacetic acid outlines the articular cartilage surfaces of the patella and trochlear groove on a T1-weighted axial image. The MR arthrogram demonstrates the subtle bilaminar appearance of the lateral patellar facet articular cartilage, which shows higher signal intensity in the more superficial layer of cartilage (*arrows*). This technique is limited to evaluation of the superficial layer or surface of the articular cartilage and is less sensitive to intracartilaginous changes.

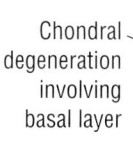

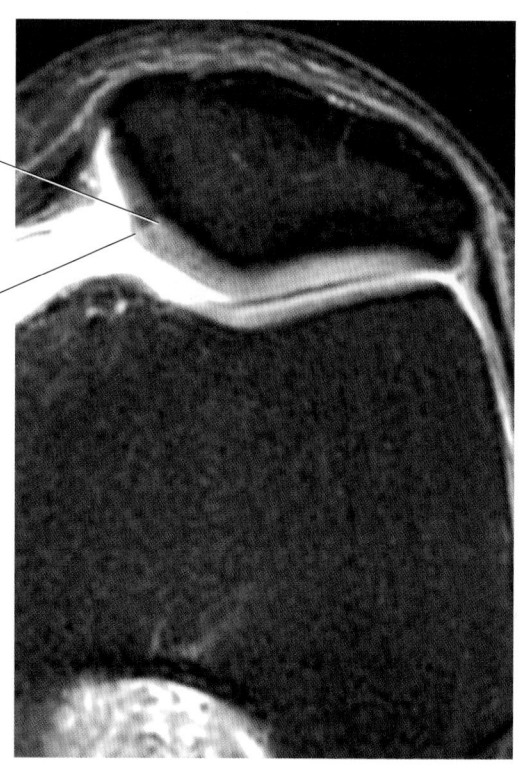

FIGURE 7.19 Grade 1 medial facet chondral softening with convex blister formation. Chondral softening can be demonstrated arthroscopically with a probe.

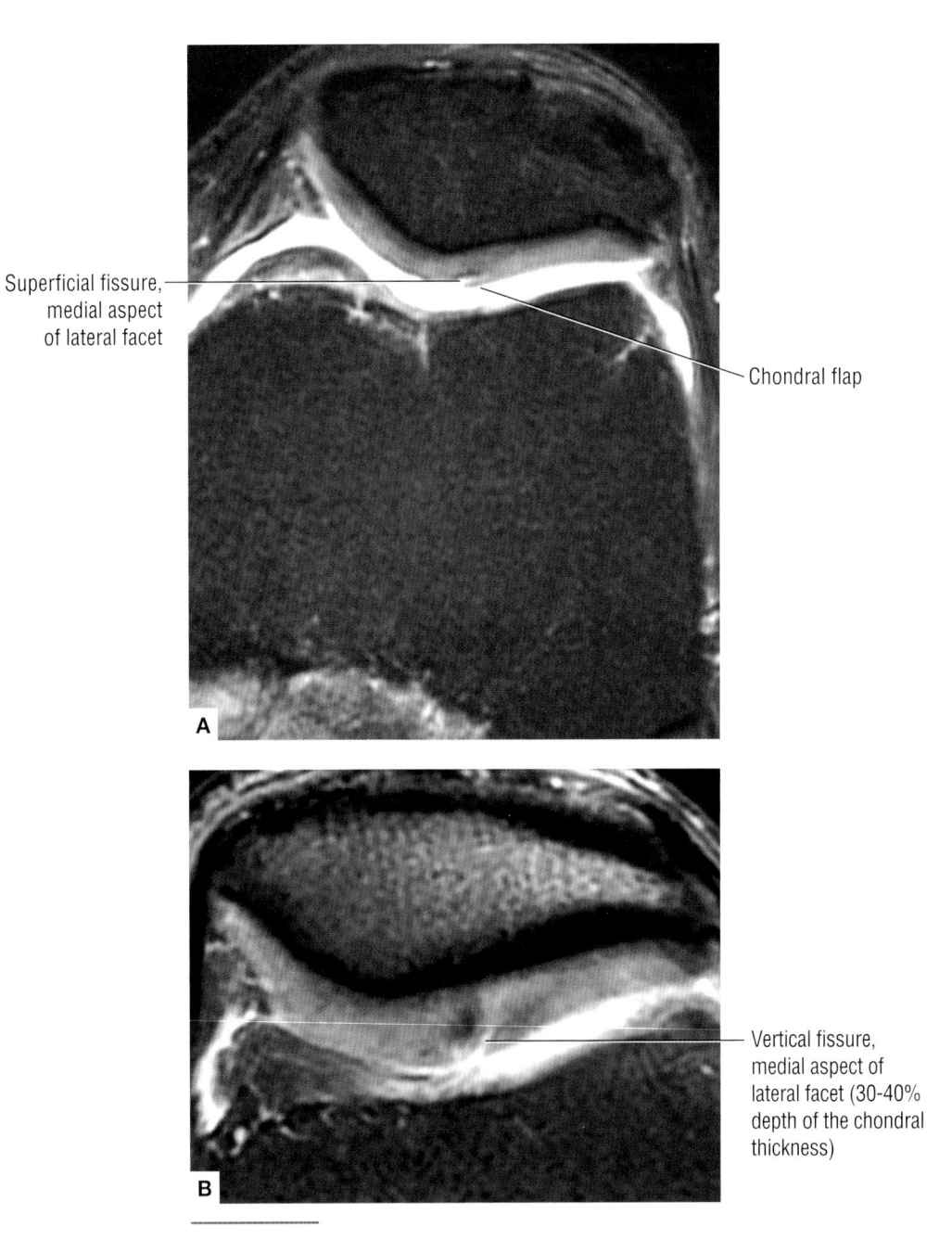

FIGURE 7.20 (**A**) Superficial fissure of the medial aspect of the lateral patellar facet in grade 2 chondromalacia. This fissure produces a small flap because its orientation is parallel or tangential to the articular cartilage surface. (**B**) Vertical fissure of the medial aspect of the lateral patellar facet. Axial FS PD FSE images.

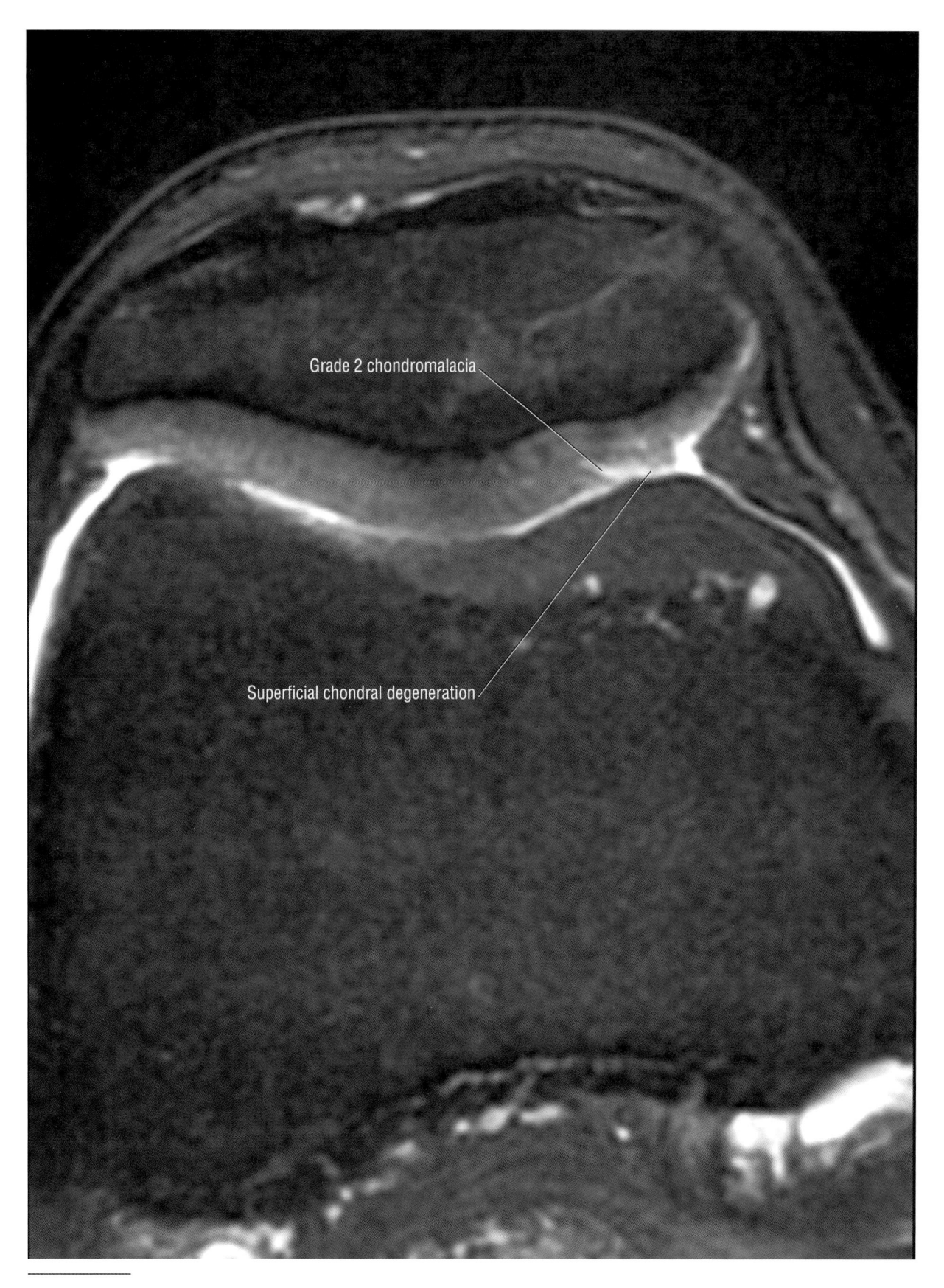

FIGURE 7.21 Grade 2 chondral fissure just less than half the thickness of the articular cartilage. More superficial grade 2 changes of the medial facet are contiguous. Axial FS PD FSE image.

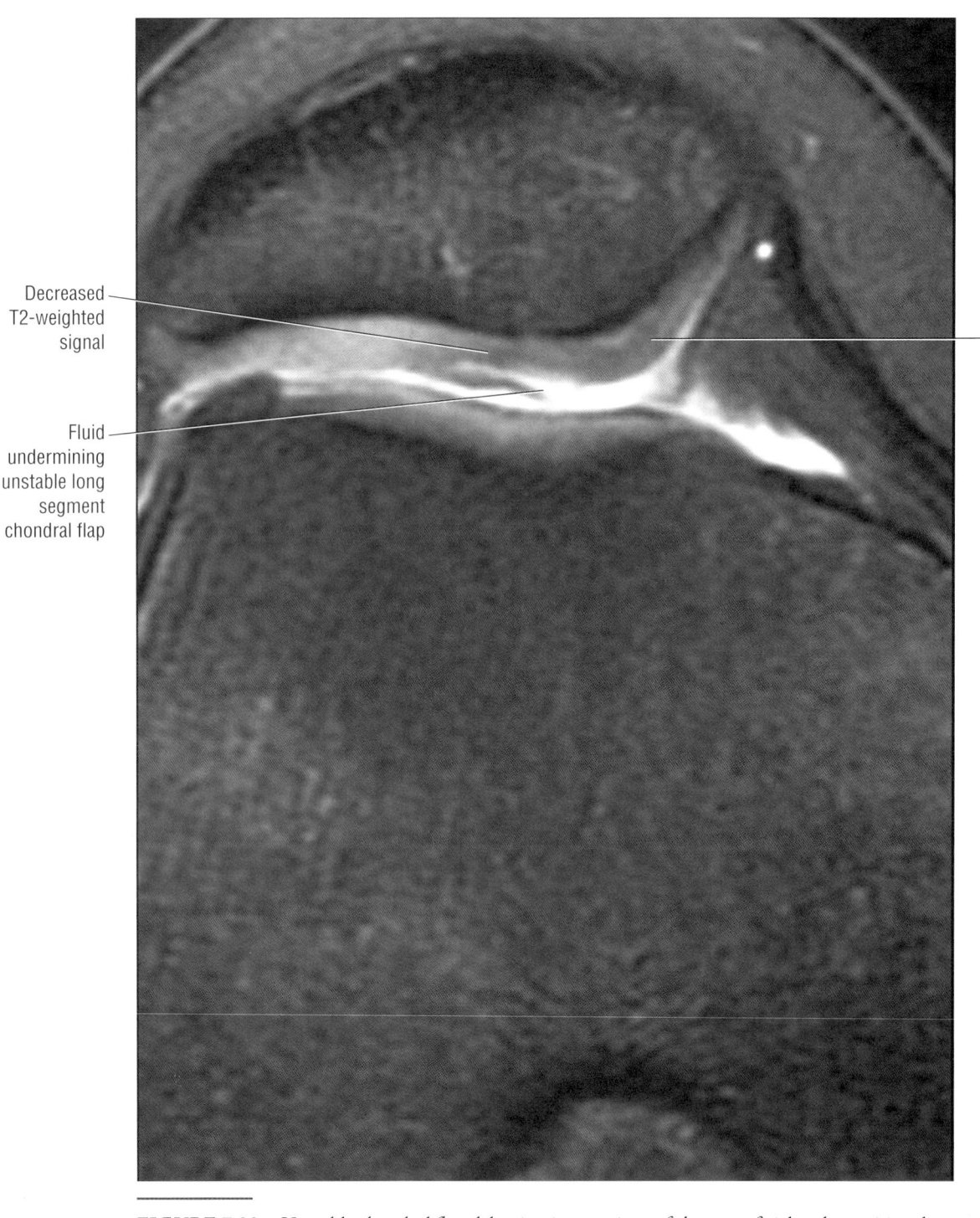

FIGURE 7.22 Unstable chondral flap delaminating portions of the superficial and transitional zone regions of the medial aspect of the lateral patellar facet. The decreased T2-weighted signal along the margins of the fissure and adjacent patellar ridge and medial facet is a more chronic finding and may be seen adjacent to areas of T2 hyperintensity. The decreased chondral signal (decreased T2-weighted signal) may reflect a hypertrophic attempt at a healing response of the cartilage or a process of collagen fibril fragmentation associated with a greater concentration of water-binding sites on the collagen. This intracartilaginous hypointense signal is not as frequently observed compared to the direct influx of fluid through chondral fissures, which results in the more characteristic hyperintensity associated with chondral fissures. Axial FS PD FSE image.

Patellofemoral Joint and the Extensor Mechanism

Medial fissure involving medial aspect lateral facet

Fissure of lateral aspect of medial facet

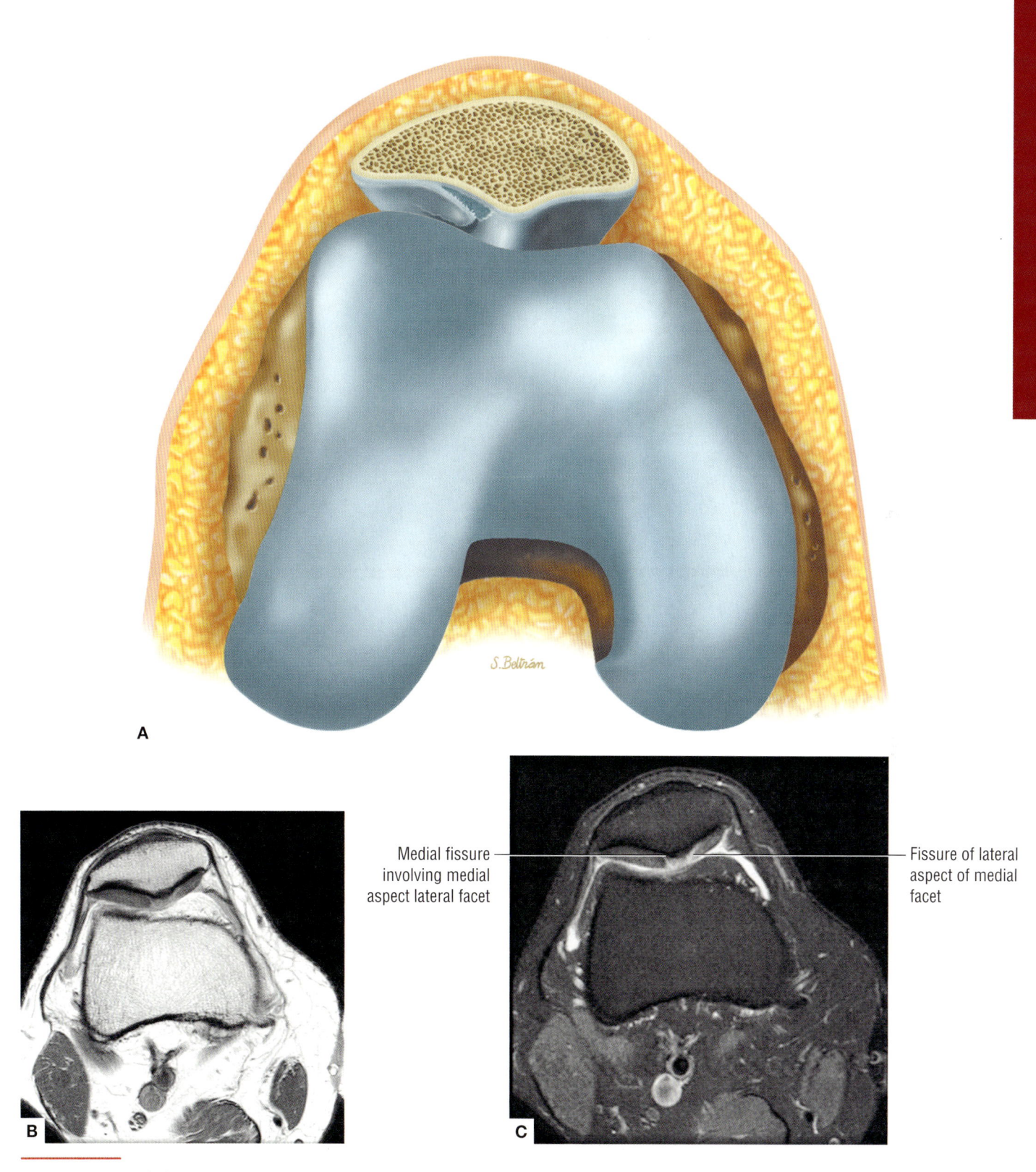

FIGURE 7.23 **(A)** Deep lateral patellar facet fissure on transverse color illustration. **(B, C)** Deep fissuring of the medial aspects of the lateral facets and lateral aspects of the medial facet. In its most frequent location, chondromalacia traverses the central area (ridge) of the patella with sparing of the superior and inferior thirds of the articular surface. Deep fissures extending to subchondral bone can be seen in grade 2 chondromalacia in both the Outerbridge and Insall classifications. **(B)** Axial T1-weighted FSE image. **(C)** Axial FS PD FSE image.

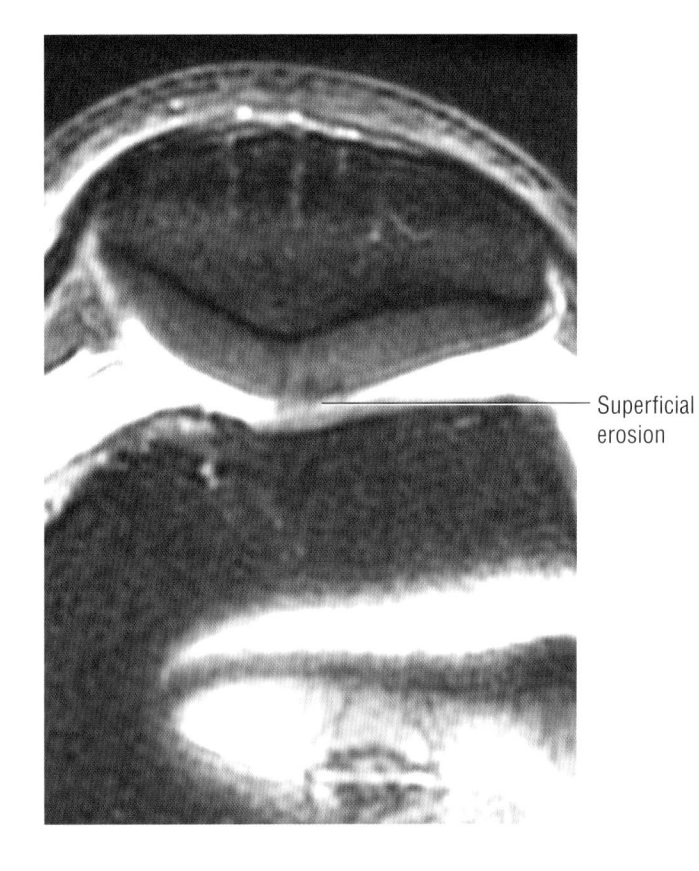

FIGURE 7.24 Superficial erosion limited to the medial aspect of the lateral patellar facet. Surface flaking can progress to fibrillation. Axial FS PD FSE image.

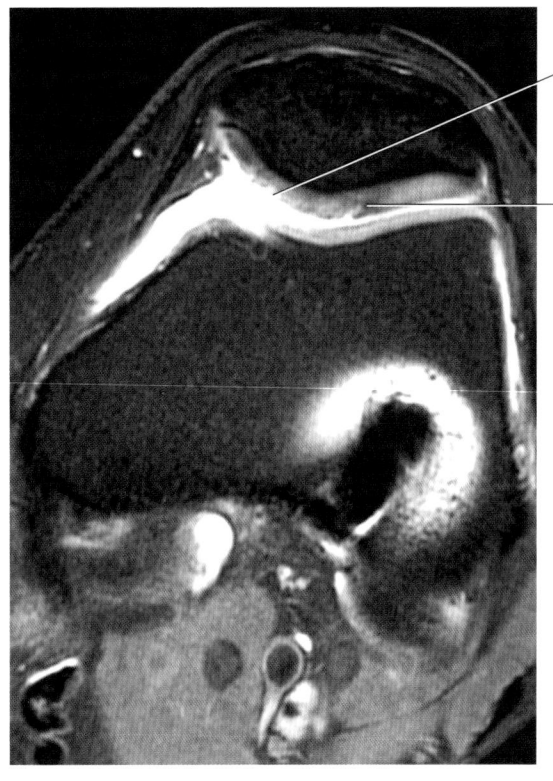

FIGURE 7.25 "Crabmeat" erosion on axial FS PD FSE image of grade 3 chondromalacia. Chondromalacia usually starts in the medial facet and progresses or extends to later involve the lateral facet.

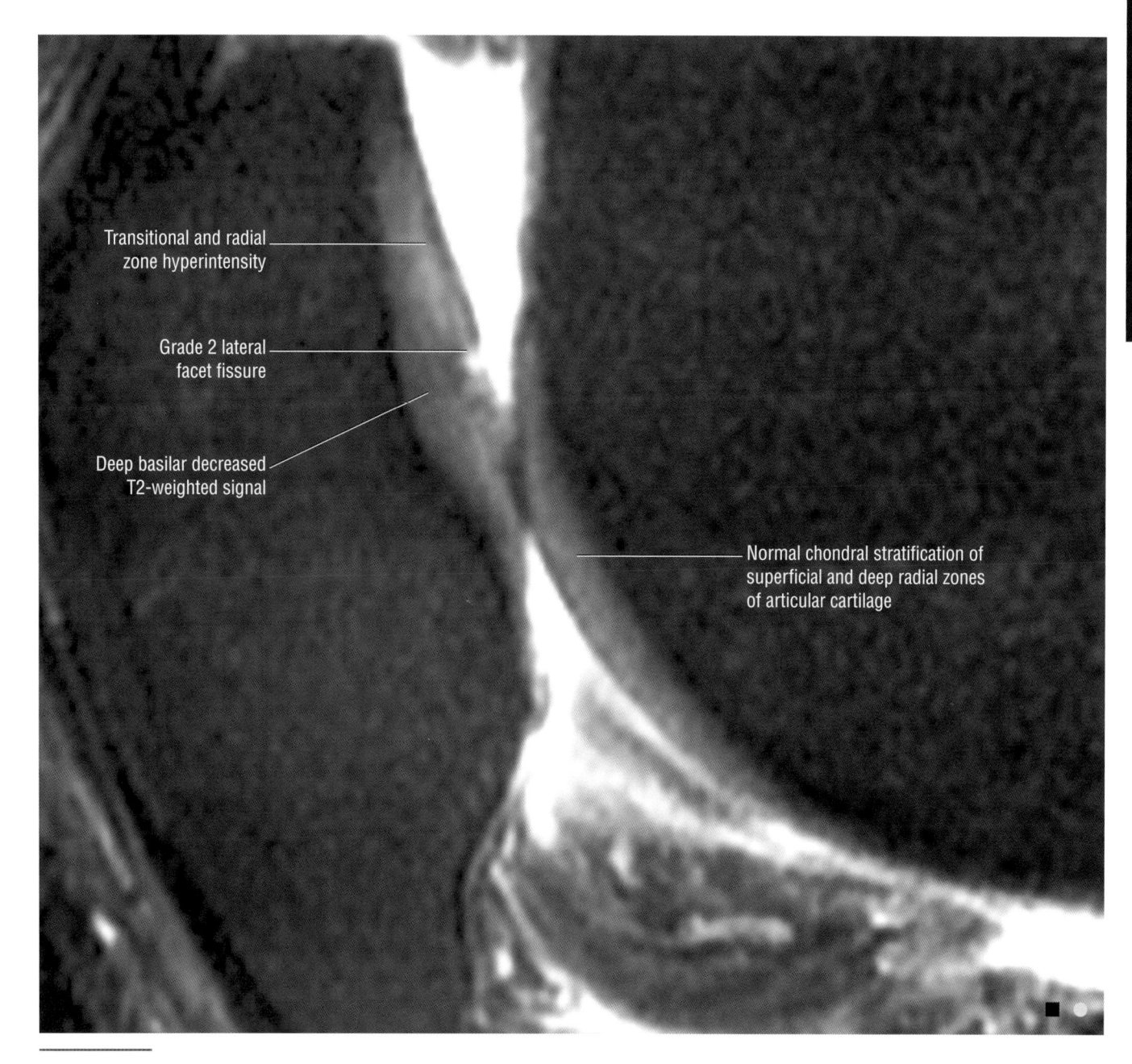

FIGURE 7.26 The normal highly anisotropic orientation of collagen type II fibrils (arranged perpendicular to the subchondral bone) produces the relative hypointense signal of the radial zone as shown in the trochlear groove. Increased T2-weighted signal superior to the grade 2 chondral fissure represents disruption of the normal chondral stratification with altered organization of the collagen matrix. Basilar hypointense T2 signal is observed deep to the grade 2 chondral fissure. Sagittal FS PD FSE image.

Chondromalacia medial aspect of lateral patellar facet with irregular crater morphology (grade 2)

Cartilage blister corresponding to area of ulcer on sagittal image

Chondrocalcinosis

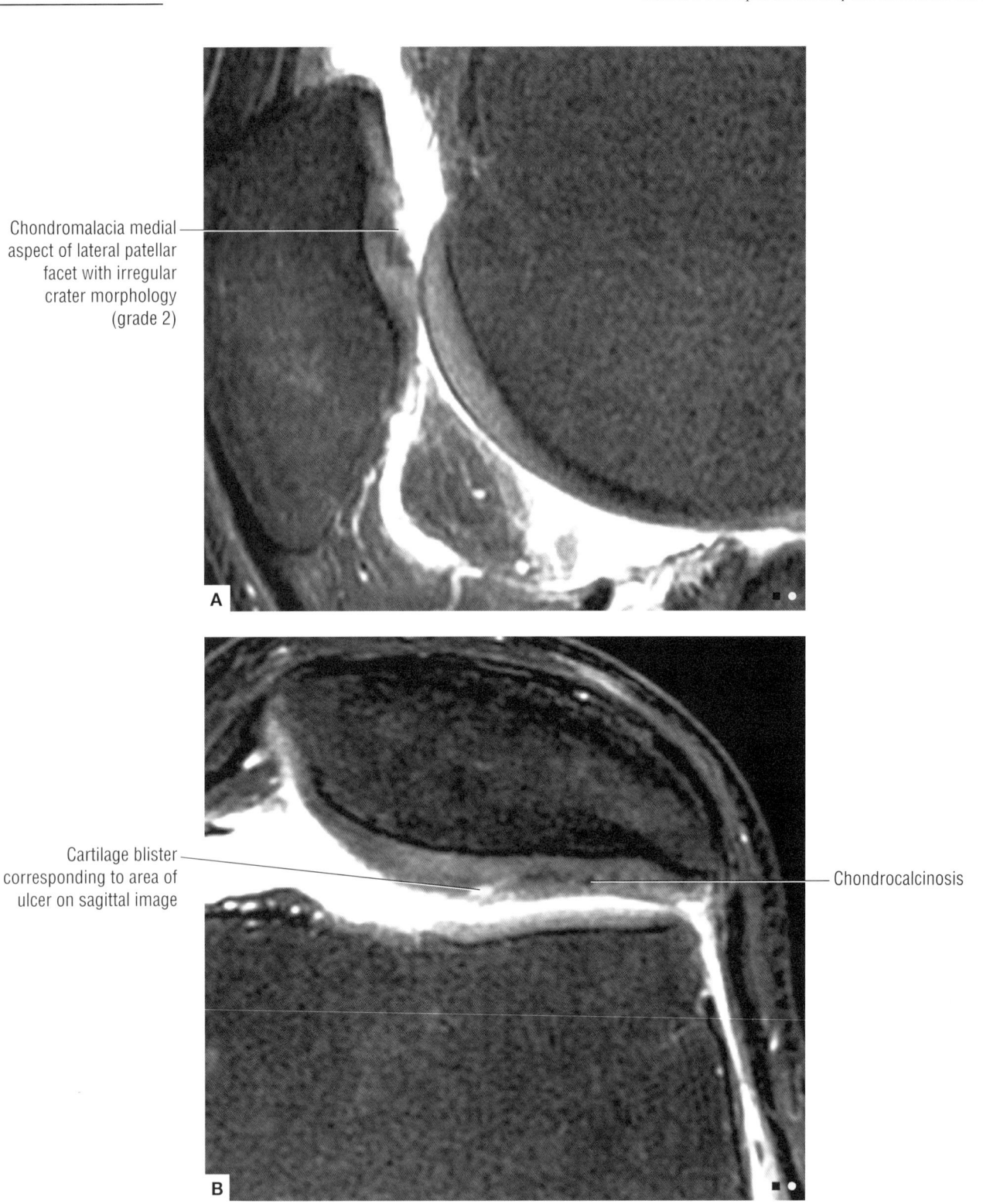

FIGURE 7.27 Chondromalacia in association with chondrocalcinosis. Chondrocalcinosis is identified with small puncture hypointense foci within the lateral facet. More generalized hypointense chondral signal is seen with collagen fragmentation. Sagittal (**A**) and axial (**B**) FS PD FSE images. When a blister ulcerates from the superficial cartilage layer, a focal crater may occur with the formation of a focal irregular crater. The term "erosion" is used to describe a more smoothly marginated area of attenuated or thinned cartilage usually seen in degenerative knees. Depth and area of chondromalacia are reported in describing the extent of chondral involvement.

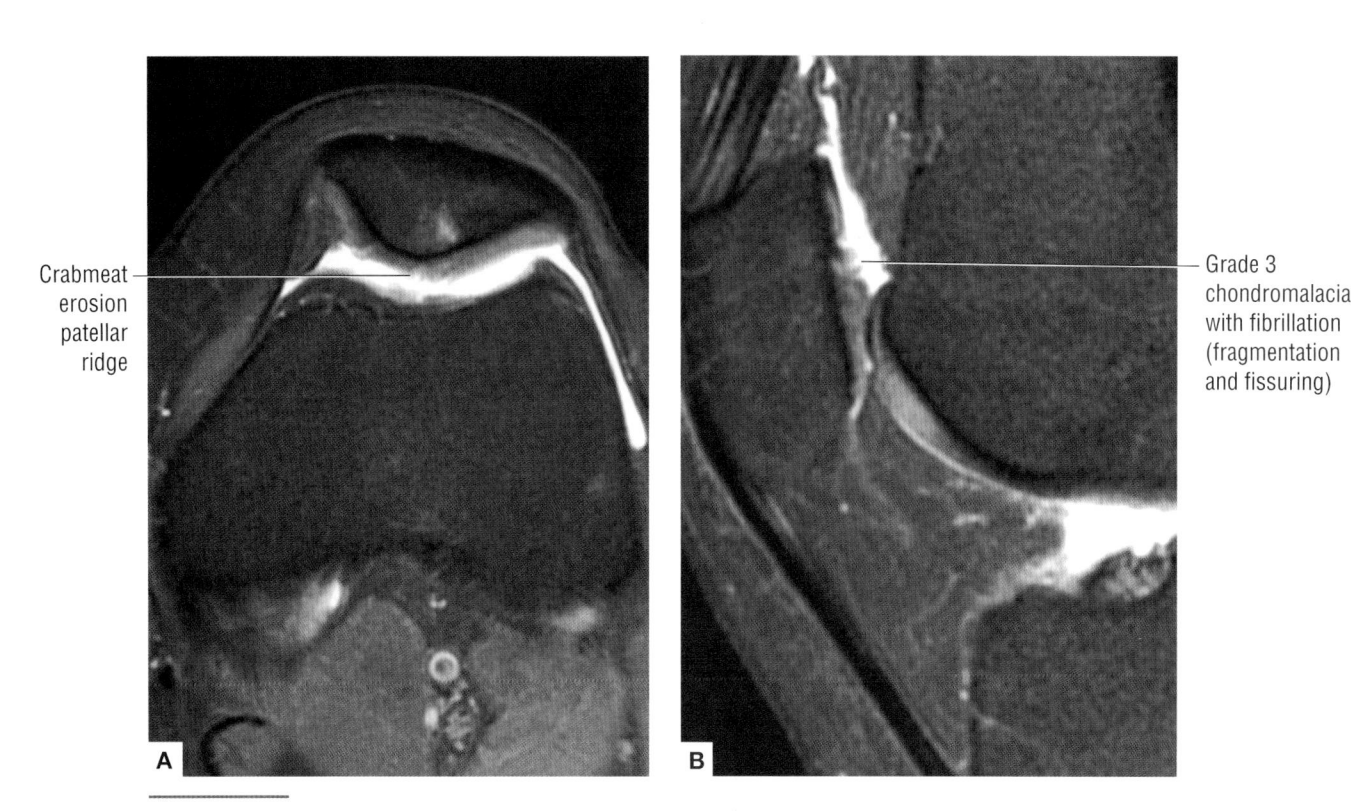

FIGURE 7.28 "Crabmeat" erosion centered on the patellar ridge. The fragmentation and fissuring in grade 3 are also referred to as fibrillation. (**A**) Axial FS PD FSE image. (**B**) Sagittal FS PD FSE image.

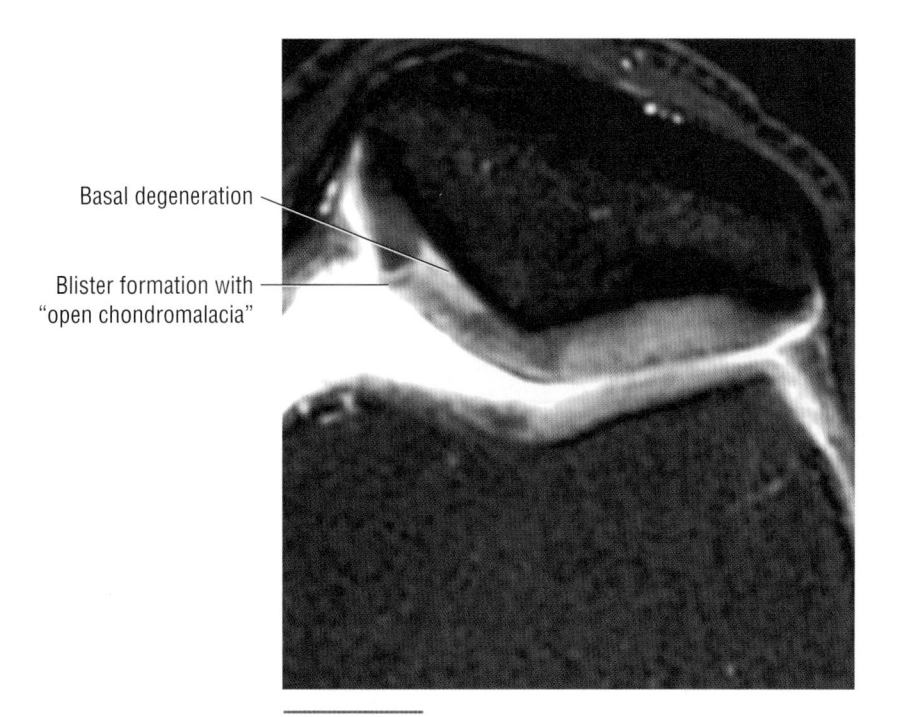

Labels (A): Crabmeat erosion patellar ridge
Labels (B): Grade 3 chondromalacia with fibrillation (fragmentation and fissuring)

FIGURE 7.29 Basal degeneration of the deep layer of the medial facet articular cartilage. Basal degeneration is associated with chondromalacia in younger patients. This degeneration erodes to form a blister, which then extends into an area of "open chondromalacia." Axial FS PD FSE image.

Labels: Basal degeneration; Blister formation with "open chondromalacia"

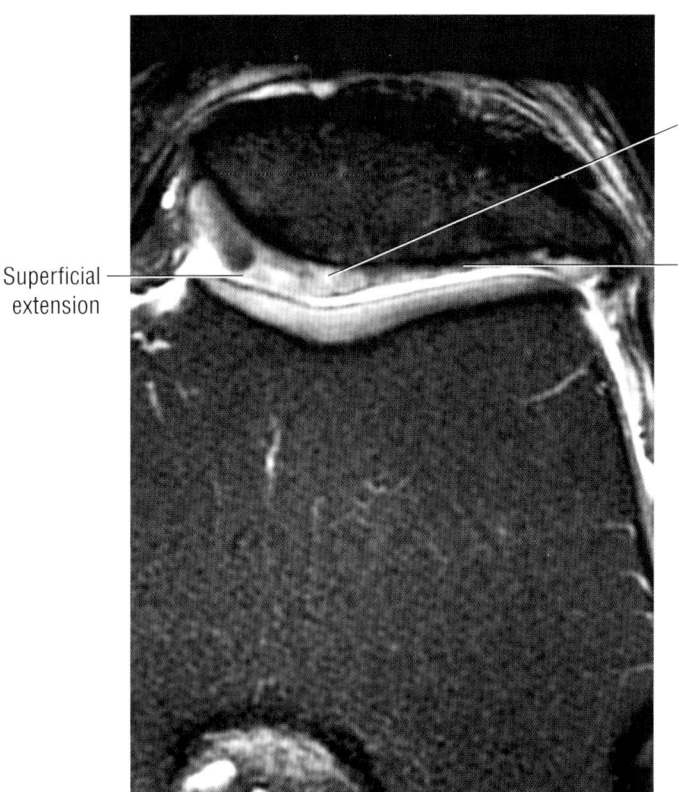

FIGURE 7.30 The inferior central ridge between the medial and lateral facets represents a preferential site for deeper basal degeneration, seen here in conjunction with superficial extension. Almost full thickness cartilage loss is shown in the lateral facet. Axial FS PD FSE image.

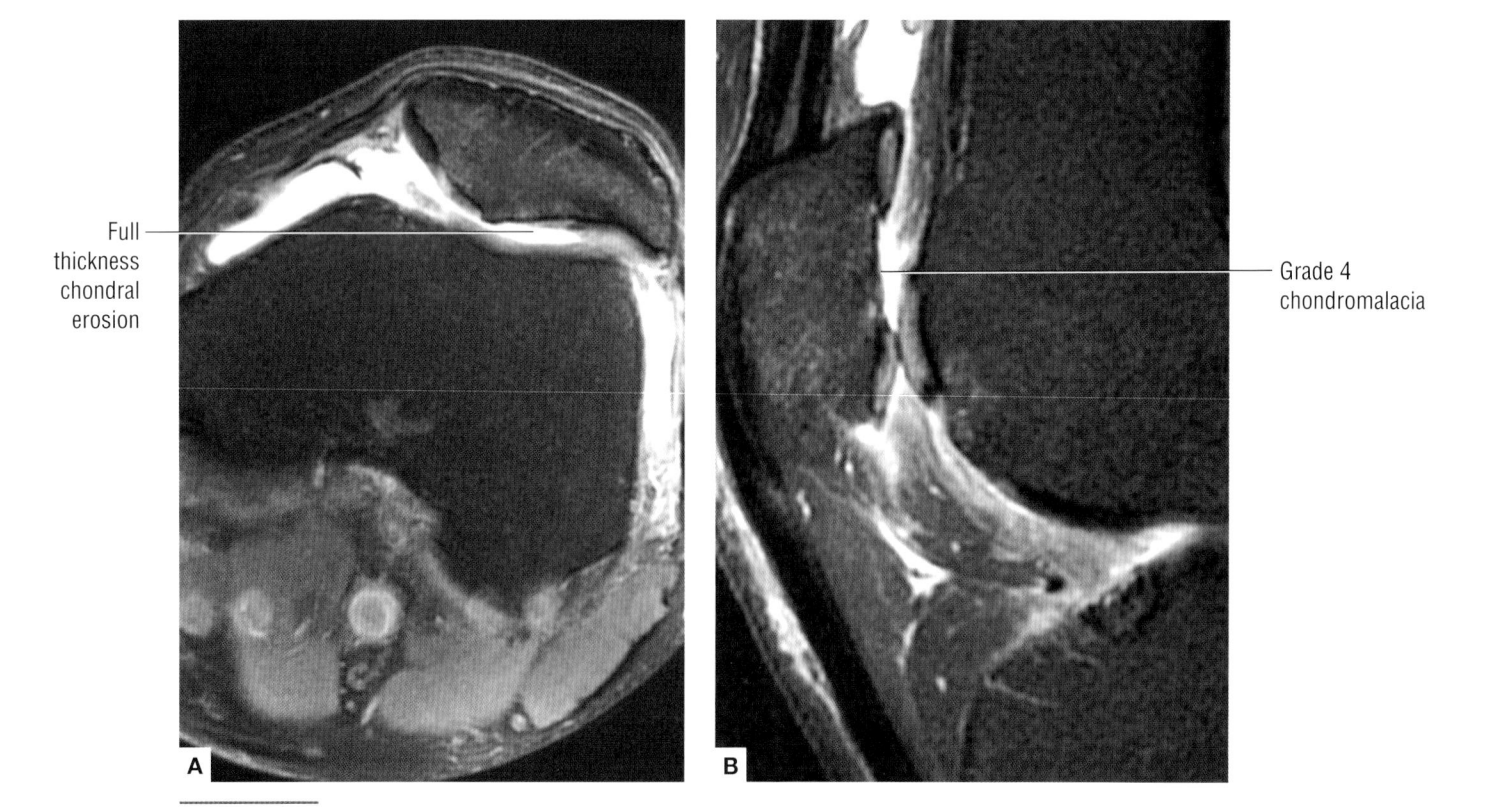

FIGURE 7.31 Lateral patellar facet full thickness chondral erosion with increasing age. Erosion to subchondral bone is more commonly seen in the lateral patellar facet. (**A**) Axial FS PD FSE image. (**B**) Sagittal FS PD FSE image.

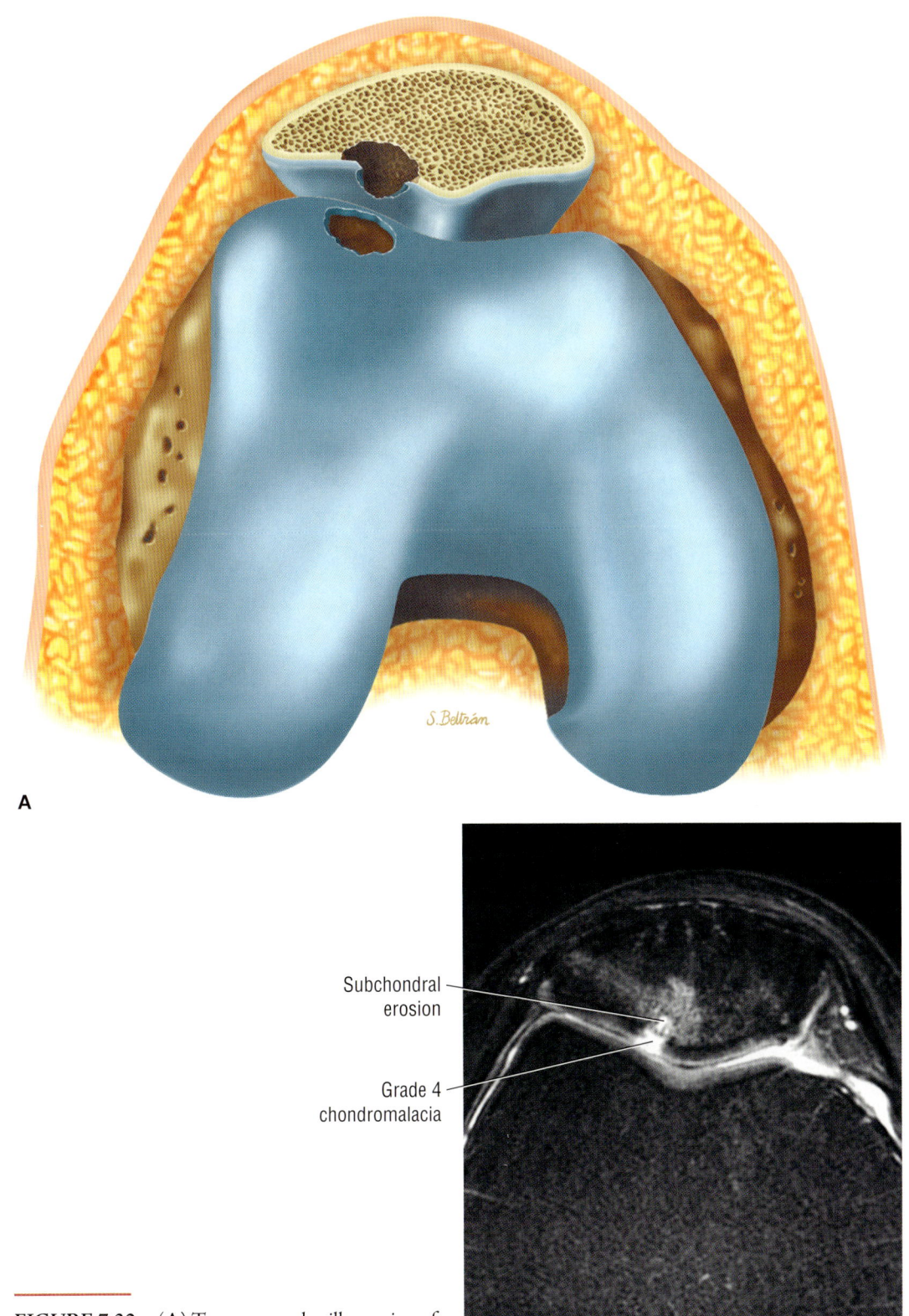

Patellofemoral Joint and the Extensor Mechanism 733

FIGURE 7.32 (**A**) Transverse color illustration of patellofemoral arthritis with lateral femoral condyle full thickness erosion and matching subchondral erosion of the lateral patellar facet. (**B**) Axial FS PD FSE image showing focal grade 4 erosion of the lateral facet with associated subchondral erosion.

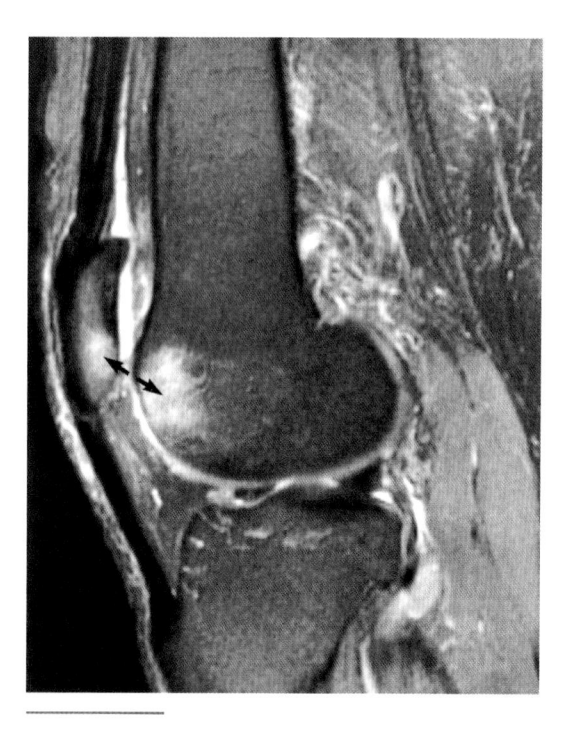

FIGURE 7.33 Subchondral kissing lesions in grade 4 chondromalacia demonstrate subchondral and cancellous hyperintensity (*arrows*) in the anterolateral femoral condyle and inferior pole of the lateral patellar facet on an FS T2-weighted FSE sagittal image. The articular cartilage surfaces are denuded in these lesions.

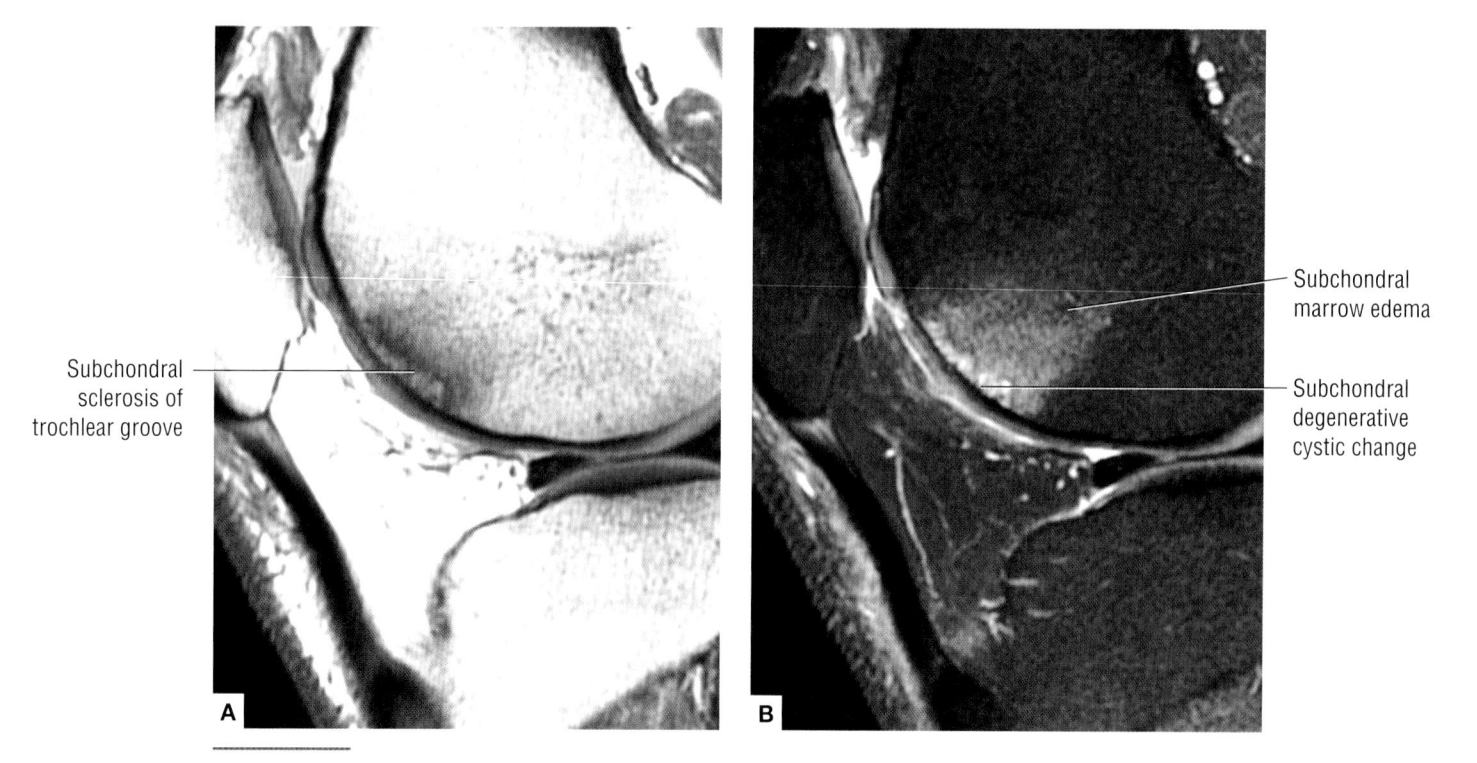

FIGURE 7.34 Subchondral sclerosis of the trochlear groove appreciated on a sagittal PD FSE image (**A**) and subchondral edema demonstrated on an FS PD FSE image (**B**).

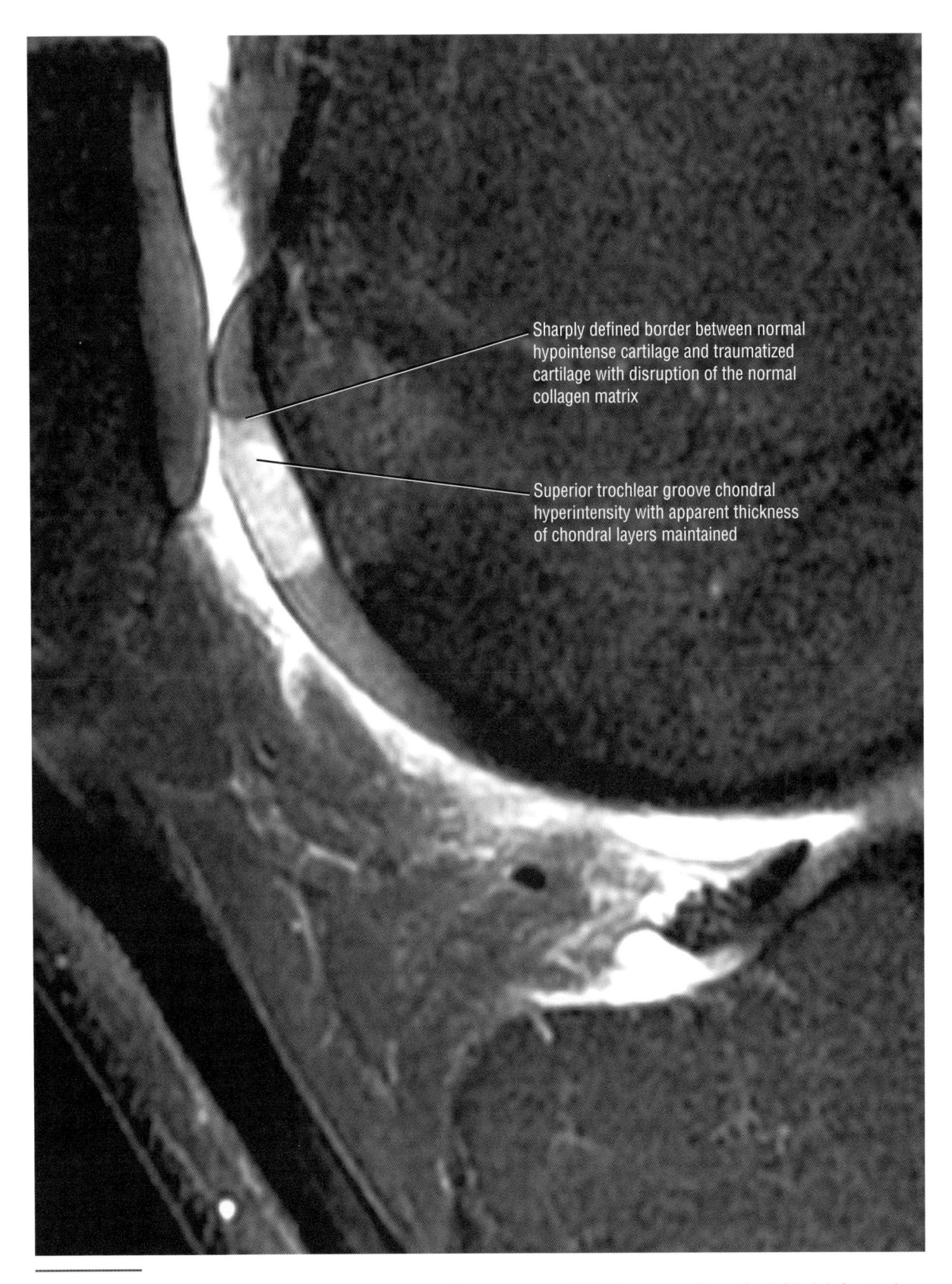

Sharply defined border between normal hypointense cartilage and traumatized cartilage with disruption of the normal collagen matrix

Superior trochlear groove chondral hyperintensity with apparent thickness of chondral layers maintained

FIGURE 7.35 Full thickness area of trochlear groove hyperintensity (T2) elevation without fluid-filled defect in the chondral contour. The sharp margination of the chondral signal hyperintensity is associated with a traumatic cartilage lesion. The hyperintense region may progress to a full thickness fluid-filled defect. Sagittal FS PD FSE image.

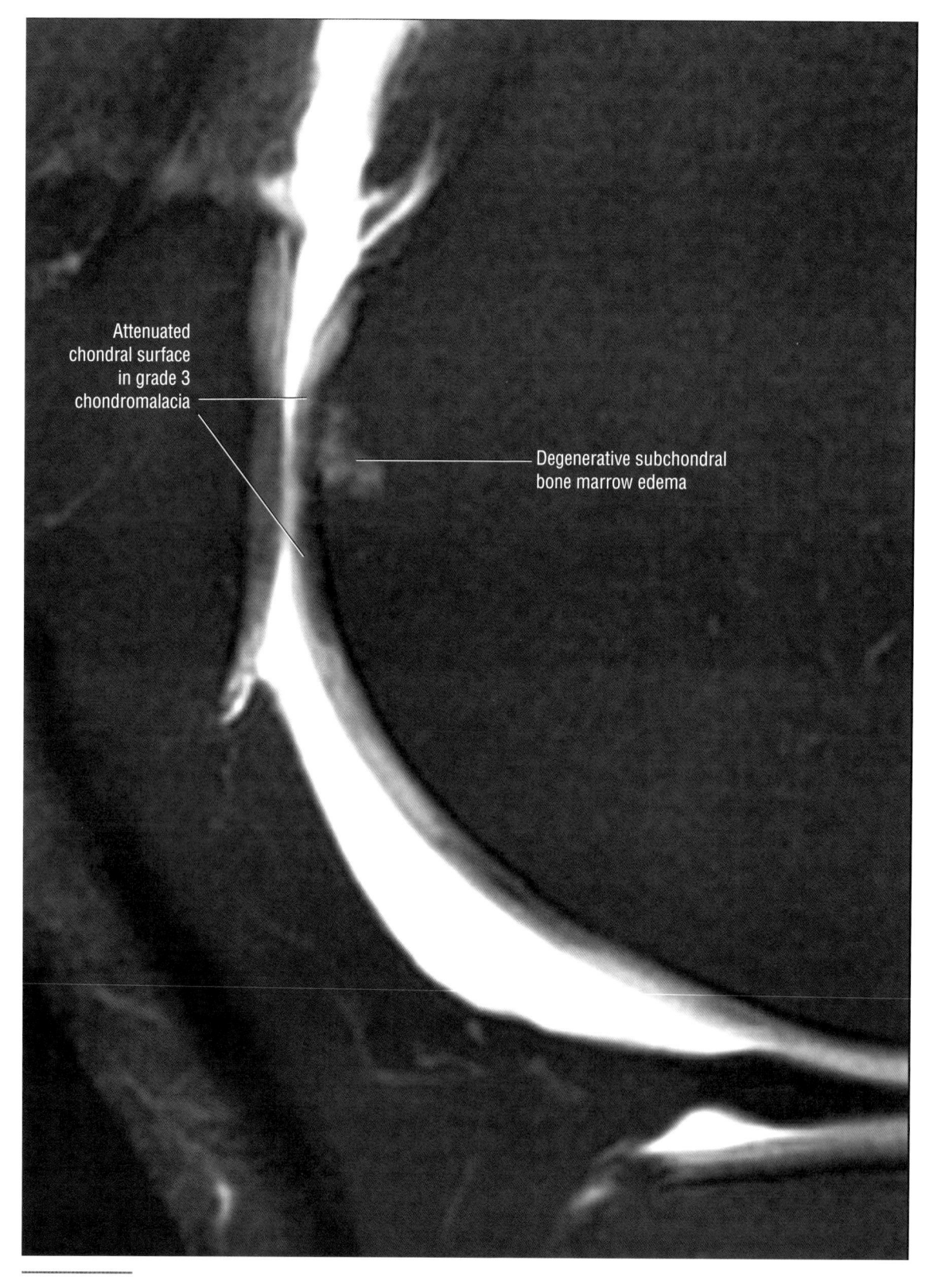

FIGURE 7.36 Larger area of trochlear groove chronic degenerative chondromalacia with attenuated articular cartilage and associated subchondral edema. The subchondral edema is related to the chronic degenerative chondromalacia and the altered patellofemoral joint biomechanics. Bone marrow edema without considering its setting is a nonspecific MR imaging finding that may also be associated with an acute traumatic or chronic osteochondral injury. Sagittal FS PD FSE image.

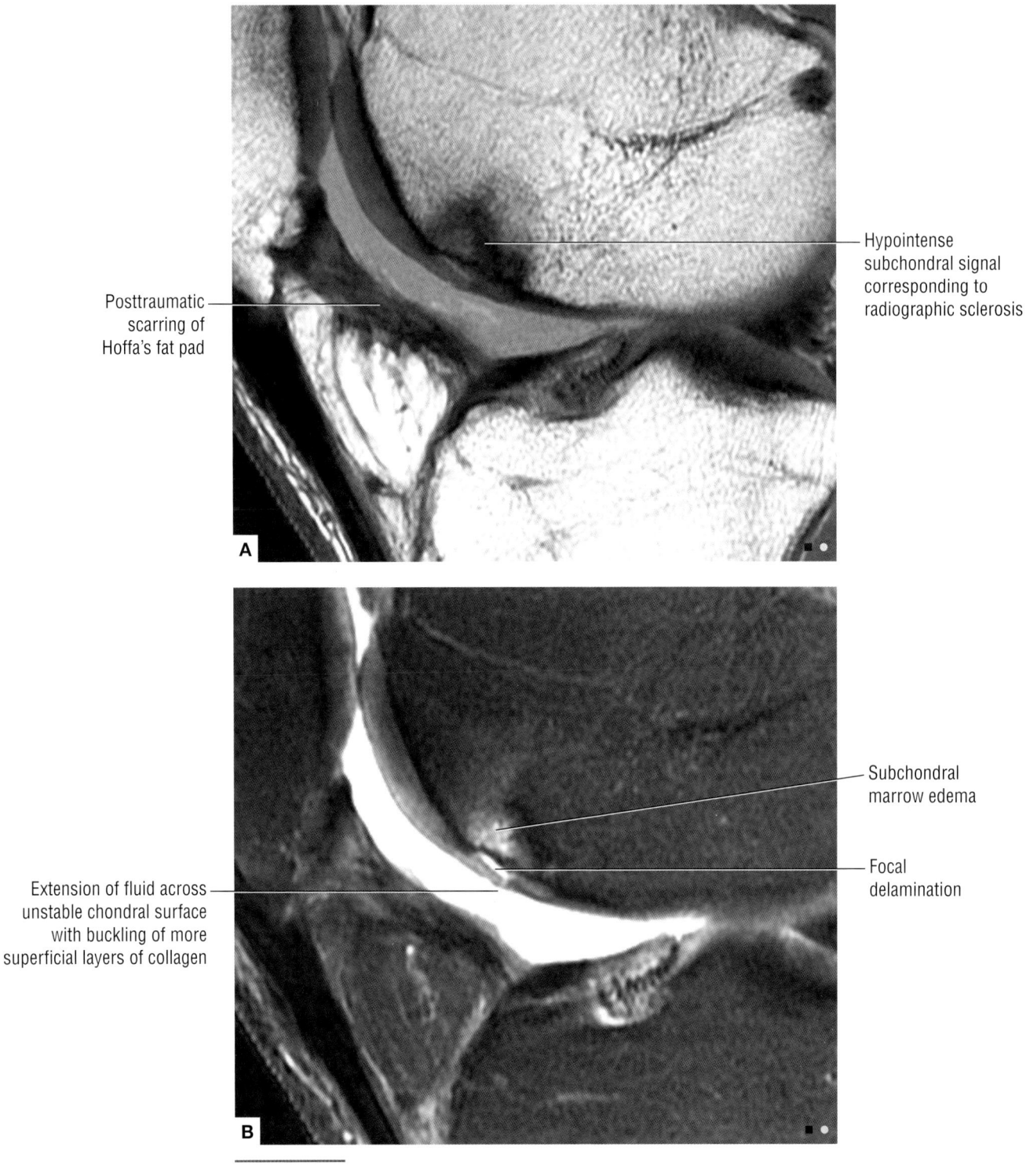

FIGURE 7.37 Delamination injury with deep radial zone focal T2 hyperintensity associated with subchondral marrow edema. Marrow edema may be seen in an acute contusion or with chronic overload and degenerative sclerosis, as in this case. Degenerative edema is more ill-defined on its borders compared to well-demonstrated acute contusions. The corresponding area of hypointense signal on T1/PD images may be associated with sclerosis and histology of necrosis, fibrosis, microcystic areas, hemorrhage, and granulation tissue. Sagittal PD (**A**) and FS PD (**B**) images.

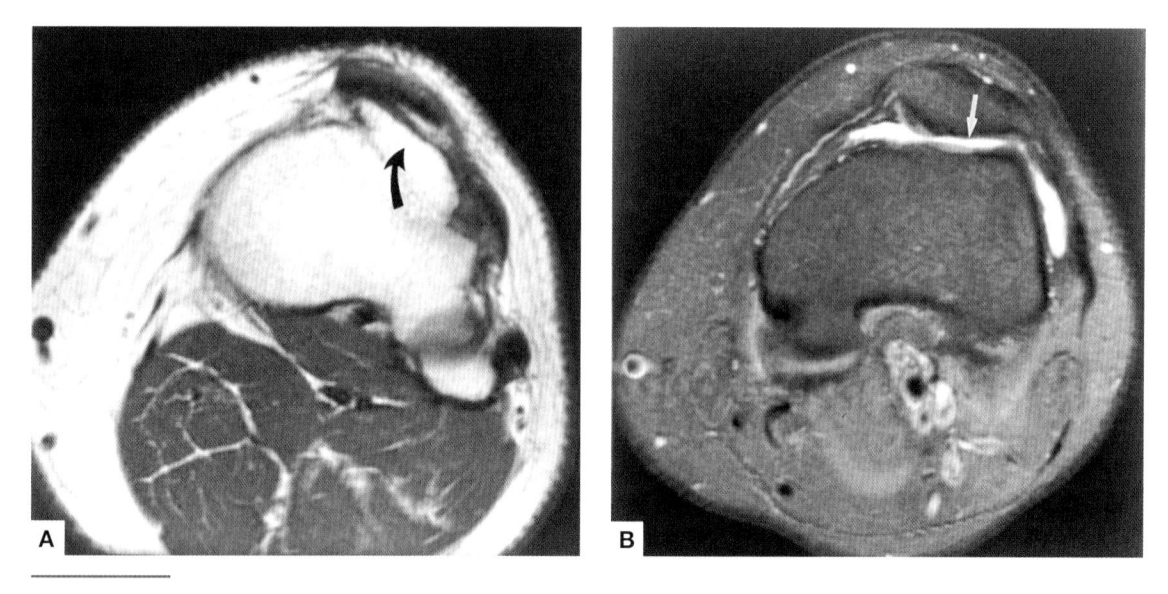

FIGURE 7.38 Fulkerson osteotomy (*curved arrow*) of the tibial tubercle on a T1-weighted axial image (**A**). This patient had denuded articular cartilage (*straight arrow*) of the lateral patellar facet, which can be seen on an FS T2-weighted FSE axial image (**B**).

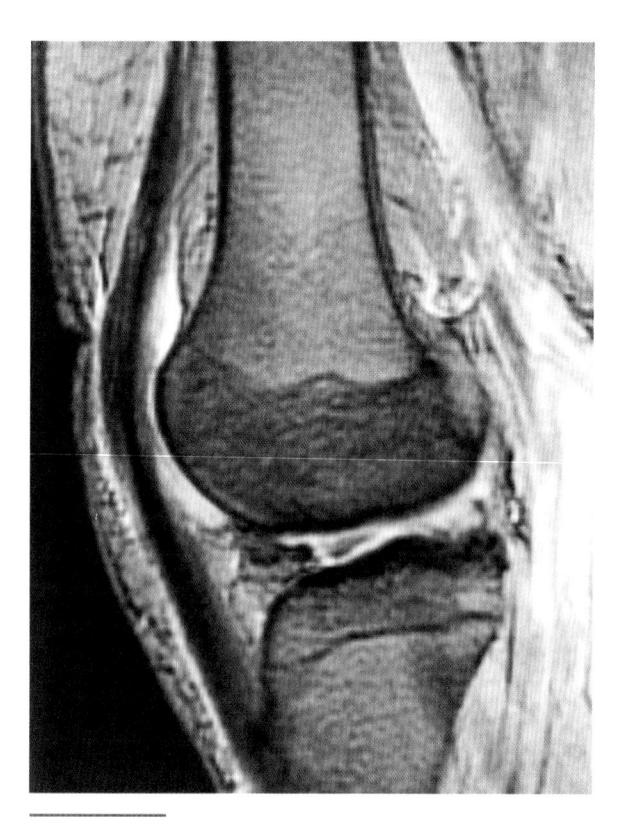

FIGURE 7.39 Patellectomy with continuity between the quadriceps and patellar tendon on a T2*-weighted sagittal image.

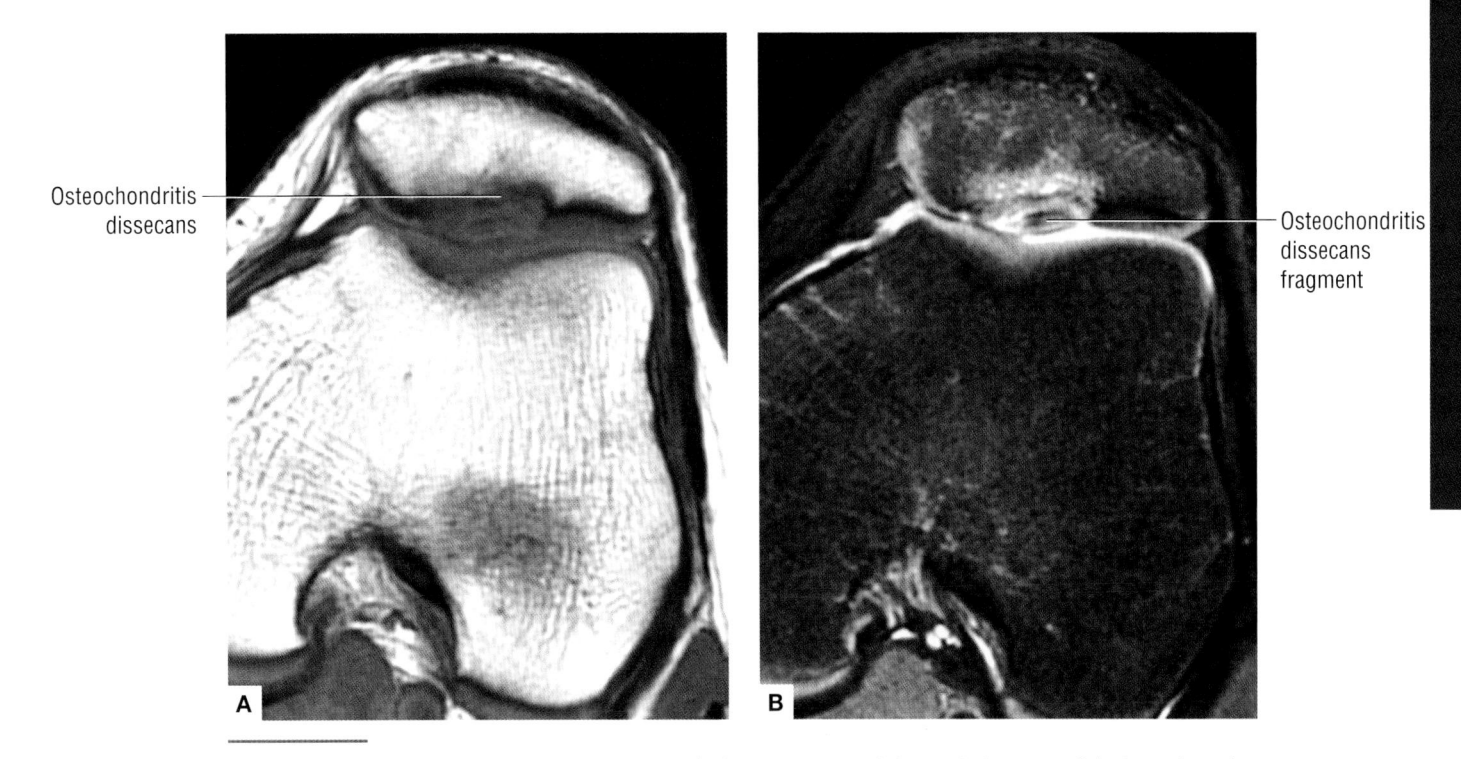

Patellofemoral Joint and the Extensor Mechanism

FIGURE 7.40 Osteochondritis dissecans with fragmentation of the medial aspect of the lateral patellar on axial PD FSE (**A**) and FS PD FSE (**B**) images.

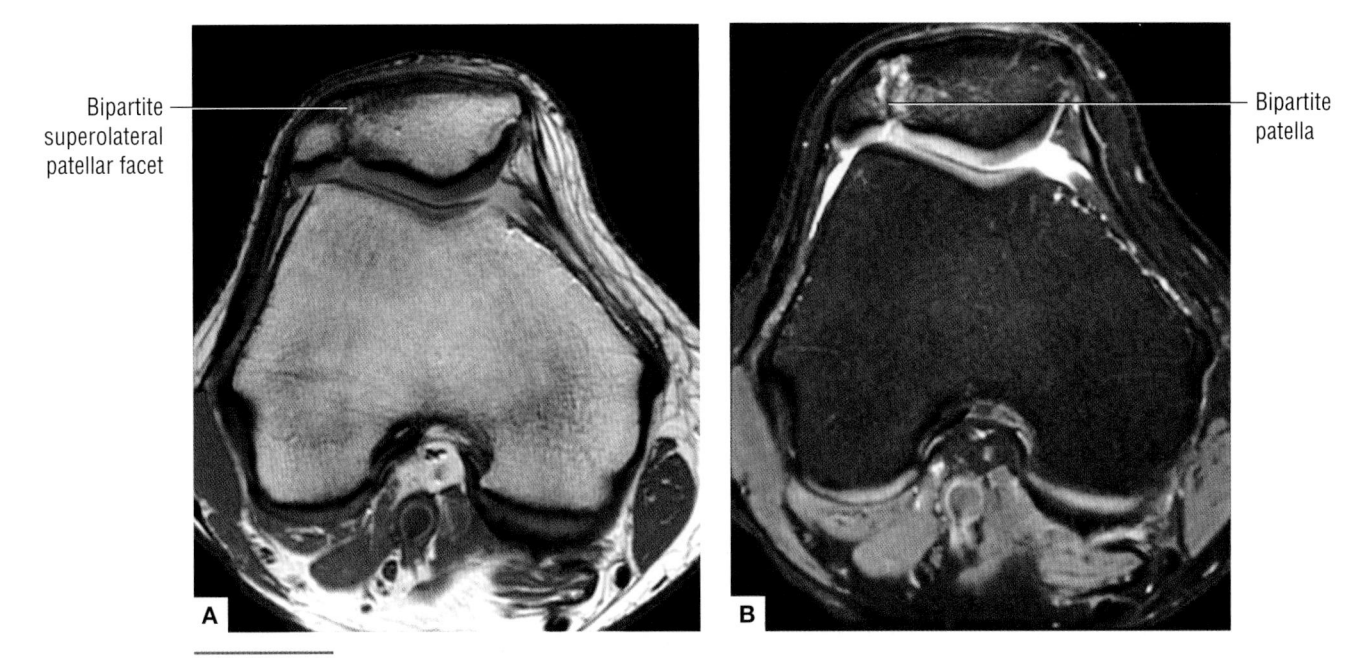

FIGURE 7.41 Bipartite lateral patellar facet involving the lateral margin of the patella on axial PD FSE (**A**) and FS PD FSE (**B**) images. Bipartite patellar dysplasia may involve the superolateral corner (most frequent) margin, apex, or superomedial pole.

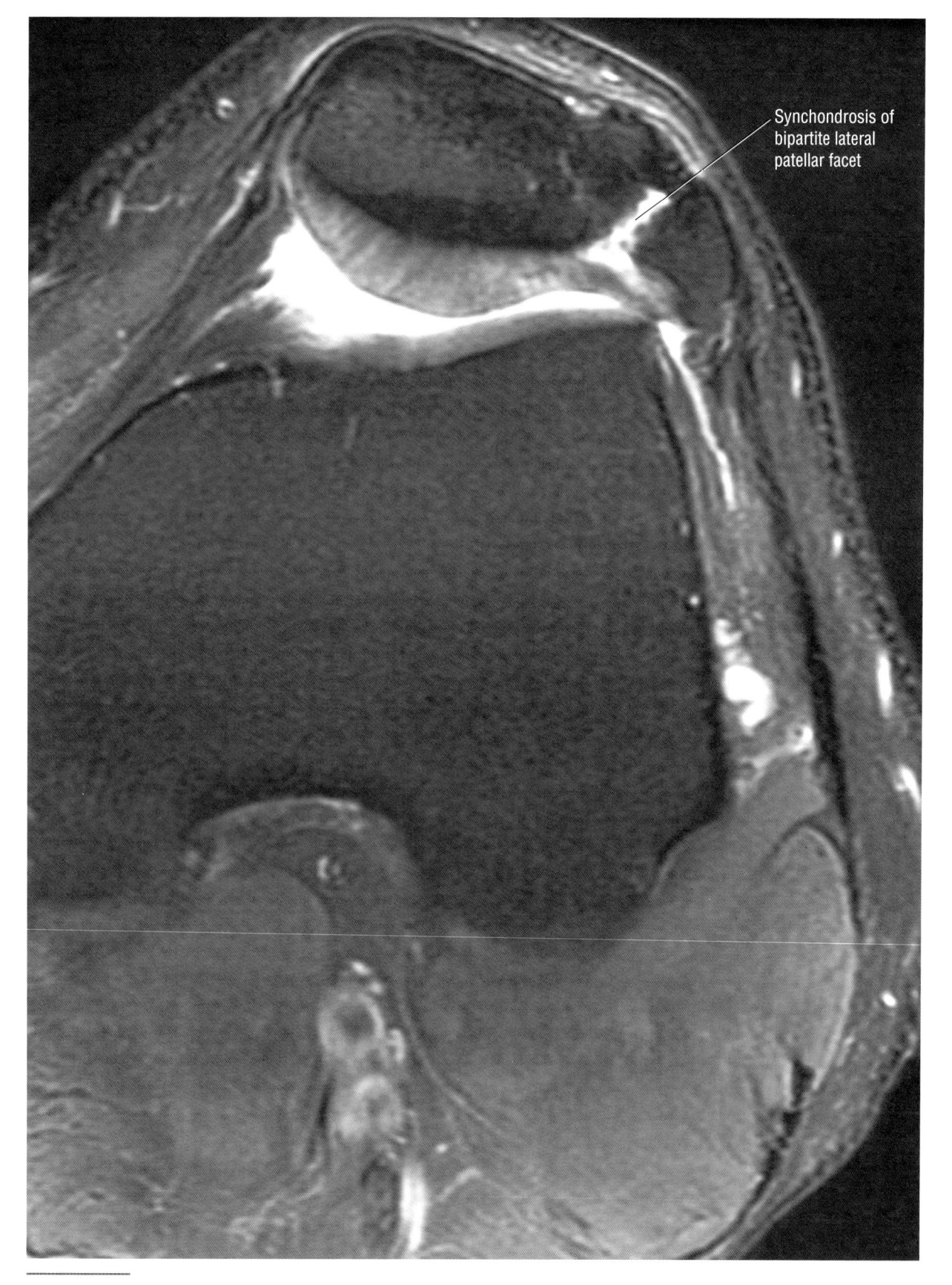

FIGURE 7.42 Bipartite patella with lateral facet cartilage undergoing chondromalacia underlying the synchondrosis of the unfused accessory ossification. Axial FS PD FSE image.

Patellofemoral Joint and the Extensor Mechanism

Bipartite superolateral patellar facet

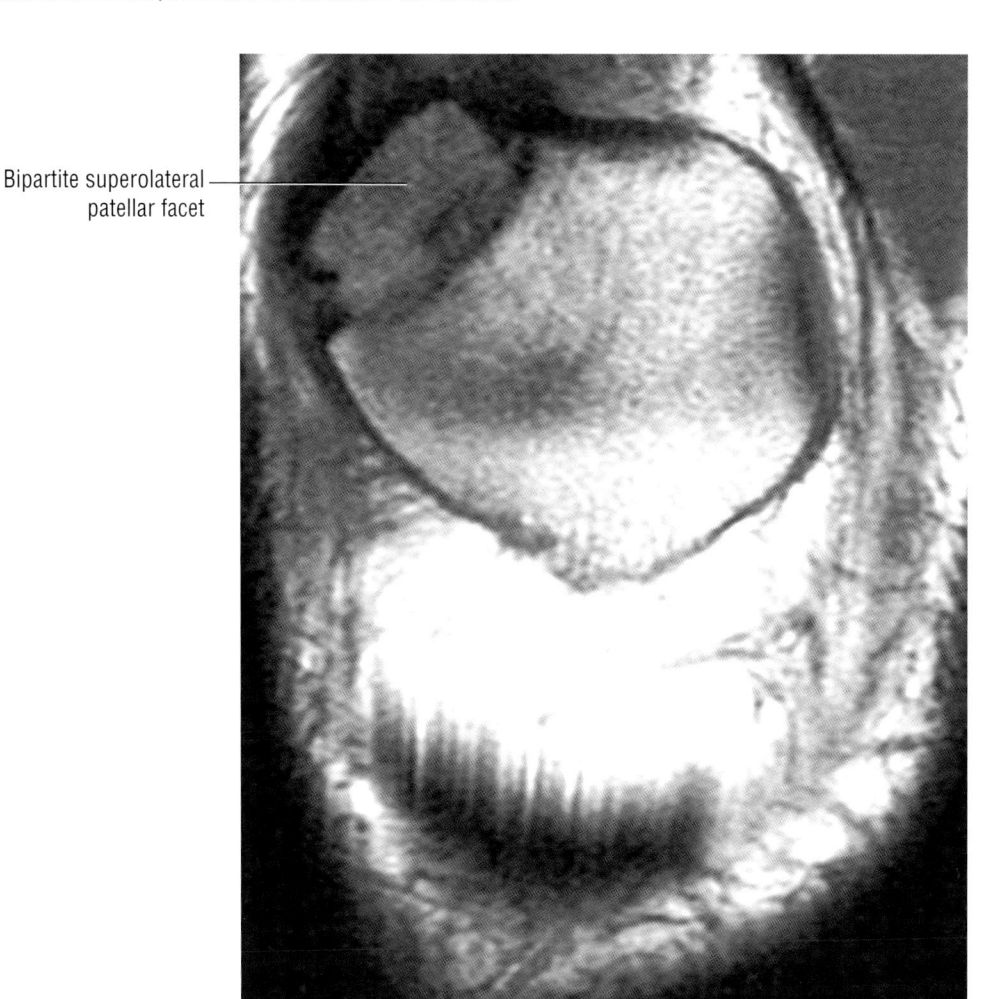

FIGURE 7.43 Characteristic superolateral location of a bipartite patella. Bipartite can be classified by location (type 1: inferior pole; type 2: lateral margin; and type 3: superolateral). Excision may be required in symptomatic superolateral bipartite patellae. Coronal PD FSE image.

Multipartite patella

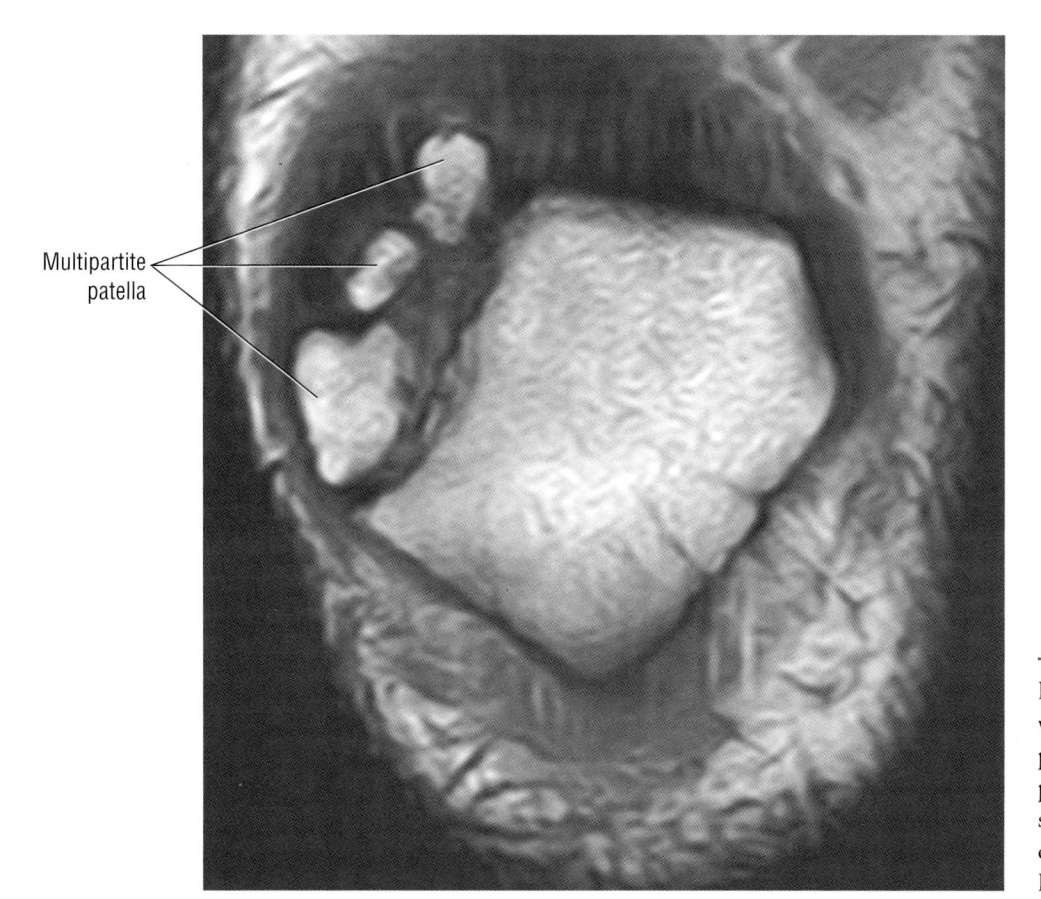

FIGURE 7.44 Multipartite patella variant of type 3 (superolateral pole). Trauma may produce a painful pseudoarticulation at the synchondrosis site in either a bipartite or multipartite patella. Coronal PD FSE image.

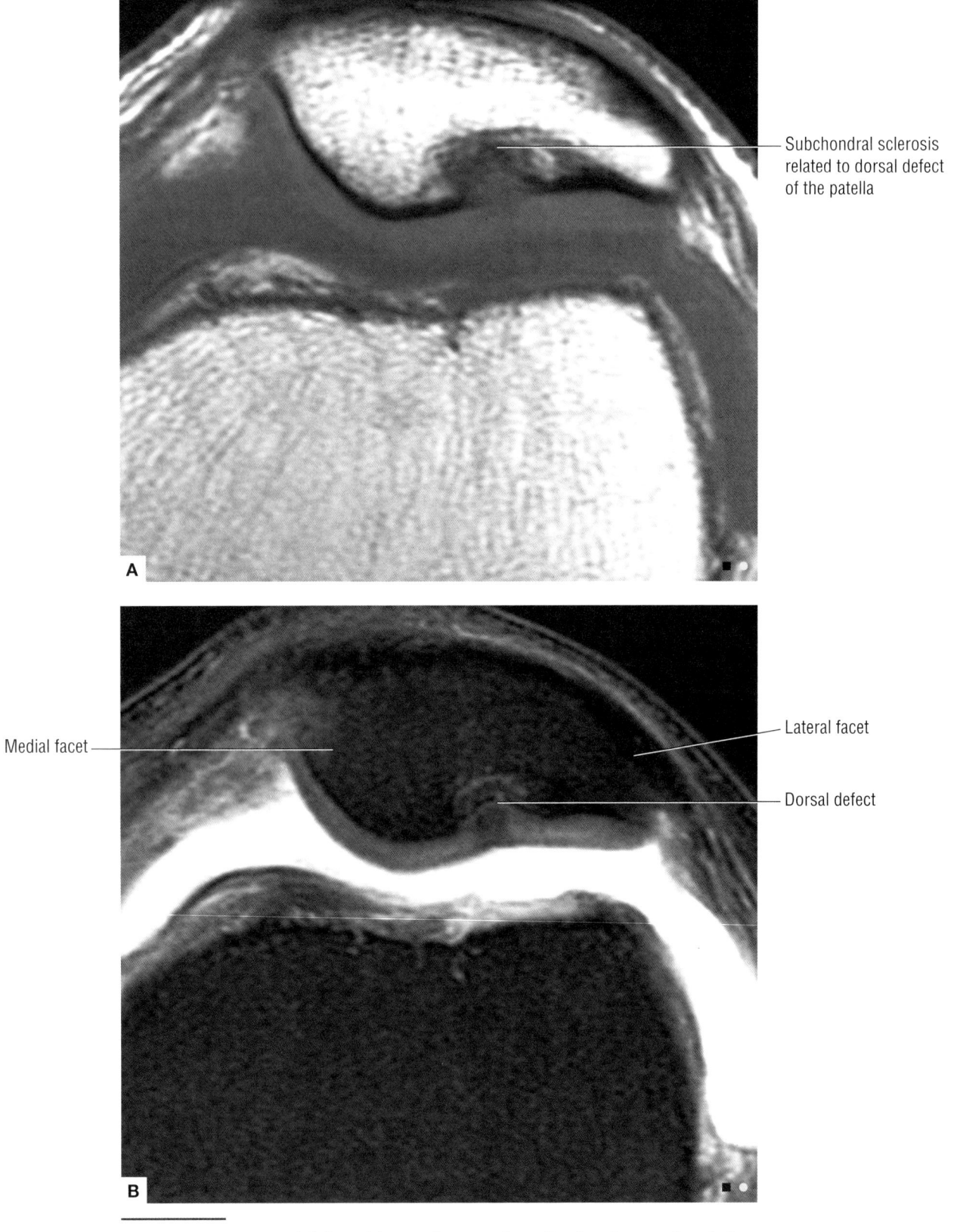

FIGURE 7.45 Dorsal defect of the patella. Lateral patellar facet benign chondral lesion (normal developmental morphology of patella) related to normal ossification of superolateral aspect involving articular surface and subchondral bone. Axial PD (**A**) and FS PD (**B**) images.

Treatment of Chondromalacia

- Initial treatment with conservative period of rehabilitation[69]
- If conservative treatment fails, instabilities or malalignment may require surgical intervention.
    - Arthroscopic shaving or removal of fibrillated and traumatized areas of articular cartilage, especially in posttraumatic chondromalacia
    - May improve patient's symptoms, although results may deteriorate over time
    - Shaving of patellar cartilage surface can be identified on MR as artificially straight articular surface with macroscopic metallic artifacts.
    - Other surgical procedures include chondroplasty with subchondral drilling, spongialization realignment procedures, tibial tubercle elevation, patellectomy, and patellar resurfacing.

Dorsal Defect of the Patella

- Superolateral aspect of the articular surface of the patella
- Well-defined benign lesion with sclerotic margins and intact overlying articular cartilage[107]
- Usually circular, about 1cm in diameter, and radiolucent on conventional radiographs
- Unclear etiology but may be related to vastus lateralis traction injury in ossification process of patella, similar to pathophysiology of bipartite patella[475]
- Asymptomatic in 50% of cases
- Histology: necrotic bone and fibrous tissue
- MR imaging: low to intermediate T1 signal intensity, central areas of increased signal intensity within the lesion
- Arthroscopy: visible cartilage surface perforations
- Differential diagnosis includes Brodie's abscess, osteochondritis dissecans, and neoplastic bony lesions.

Osteochondritis Dissecans Patellae

- Osteochondritis dissecans patellae may be associated with patellar subluxation.[89]

- Subchondral fragment usually remains in situ, causing retropatellar crepitus and pain.

- Predilection for medial facet of patella (unlike dorsal defect of the patella)

- Characterized by articular cartilage lesion (separation) with or without localized involvement of subchondral bone

Accessory Ossification of the Patella

- Classified into three types by Saupe
    - Type I: inferior pole of patella
    - Type II: lateral margin of patella
    - Type III: superolateral pole of patella

- *Bipartite patella* represents failure of fusion of secondary ossification centers
    - Symptomatic bipartite patella may be treated with surgical excision or lateral retinacular release.

- Tripartite or multipartite patella is rare.

Patellar Subluxation and Dislocation

- Lateral patellar subluxation: partial lateral displacement of patella early in process of knee flexion[6]

- Medial patellar subluxation
    - May occur secondary to overcorrection in operations for realignment of extensor mechanism, including lateral release

- Dislocations of the patella
    - Congenital and traumatic[6]

- Anatomic patellar alignment
    - Patellar groove or sulcus has median depth of 5.2mm
    - *Quadriceps angle*, or *Q angle*, defines the proximal-to-distal forces that act on and through the patella[182,475]
        - Determined by intersection of line connecting center of patella with anterior superior iliac spine (approximating line of pull of the quadriceps tendon) with a second line (in direction of the patellar tendon) that connects center of patella to tibial tubercle
        - Normal Q angle measures 14 to 15 degrees; any measurement greater than this is considered abnormal.
- Etiology
    - Ligamentous laxity
    - Abnormal iliotibial band (ITB) and vastus lateralis attachment, producing a lateral patellar pull
    - Intrinsic muscle abnormalities and soft tissue damage, including medial patellar retinaculum injuries
    - Hypoplastic femoral sulcus and lateral femoral condyle
    - Variant patellar shapes (Wiberg types), especially a patella with small and convex medial patellar facet (Wiberg type 3)
    - Patella alta, with loss of buttressing effect of lateral femoral condyle
- Radiographic measurements of patellofemoral congruence include sulcus angle, congruence angle, lateral patellofemoral angle, and patellofemoral index.[316]
    - *Sulcus angle* (depth of the trochlea)
        - Mean value of 138 degrees with standard deviation of 6 degrees
        - Increased sulcus angle indicates dysplasia and greater likelihood of malalignment and recurrent dislocation as a result of instability.
    - *Congruence angle* (degree of patellar subluxation)
        - Determined by anterior distance between articular ridge of patella and reference line that bisects the sulcus angle

- Mean congruence angle of −6 degrees with standard deviation of 6 degrees
  - *Lateral patellofemoral angle* (measures tilt and subluxation)
    - Formed by angle between intercondylar line and lateral facet
    - Should open laterally
    - Indicates tilt with subluxation if lines become parallel or open medially
  - *Patellofemoral index* (measures tilt and subluxation)
    - Closest distance of lateral facet with medial facet, expressed as a ratio
    - Normal ratio of 1:6 or less
- *Patellar tilt*
  - Malalignment that can occur with or without associated subluxation[152]
  - Chronic patellar tilt may lead to excessive lateral pressure syndrome (see discussion earlier in this chapter).
  - Subluxation or dislocation can be caused by trauma in the absence of preexisting malalignment.
- Imaging evaluation of patellar tracking
  - Especially useful for evaluation of patellofemoral mechanism during first 30 degrees of knee flexion in cases of recurrent patellar dislocations[6,271]
  - Cine-MR imaging (motion-triggered cine-MR)
    - Useful for evaluation of patellar tracking for patellar malalignment[47]
  - Kinematic MR may be used to evaluate efficacy of patellar realignment brace in counteracting patellar subluxation.[6,435]

- Treatment of recurrent patellar dislocation and patellar instability
    - Focuses on realignment and stabilization of extensor mechanism, including patella
    - Bony operations
        - Transfer of lateral tuberosity
        - Elevation of tibial tuberosity (Maquet's procedure)
        - Femoral osteotomy
        - Patellectomy
    - Soft tissue operations
        - Lateral retinacular release
        - Fascioplasty
        - Patellar ligament procedures
        - Tendon (gracilis, semitendinosus, and sartorius) and muscle transfers
        - Capsulorrhaphy[6]

Traumatic Dislocations

Key Concepts

- Medial patellofemoral ligament disruption off the adductor tubercle or medial retinaculum tear from the medial patellar facet (as defined on FS PD FSE axial images)

- Findings include osteochondral injuries of the medial patellar facet and lateral femoral condyle, strain of the vastus medialis obliquus, medial collateral ligament (MCL) sprain, and disruption of medial patellofemoral ligaments.

Traumatic Dislocations

- Occur laterally[134]

- Trauma includes both noncontact (indirect) injuries and direct injuries secondary to a blow to the knee.

- Operative findings in acute patellar dislocations
    - Medial retinacular and medial patellofemoral ligament rupture
    - Medial marginal fracture of patella
    - Intraarticular fracture of patella
    - Fracture of chondral or osseous portions of lateral femoral condyle
    - Partial patellar tendon detachment
- *Medial patellofemoral ligament* (MPFL)
    - Distinct condensation of fibers in layer 2 of the medial side of the knee[91]
    - Fibers oriented transversely and course from the superior two thirds of the medial patellar margin to an insertion point anterior to the medial epicondyle of the femur
    - Superior fibers confluent with deep fascia of distal vastus medialis
    - Functions as static restraint to lateral patellar translation (whereas distal *vastus medialis obliquus* [VMO] may play a dynamic role in this stabilization)
- *Medial retinaculum*
    - Formed by confluence of fibers from layers 1 and 2, extends from the medial patellar margin, and is continuous with the VMO fascia
    - Anteriorly confluent with fibers from layer 2, which includes the MPFL, and layer 1, accounting for its bilaminar morphology
- MR findings of patellar dislocation[124,266]
    - Injury of medial retinaculum at patellar attachments or mid-substance
    - Injury of MPFL at femoral origin (between adductor tubercle and medial epicondyle)
    - Edema with tearing of distal muscle belly of the VMO[253]
        - Rupture of the VMO muscle usually interstitial

- Lateral patellar tilt or subluxation
- Lateral femoral condyle contusion
- Osteochondral injury
    - Focal chondral defect may be associated with anterior lateral femoral condyle contusion.
    - May be overlooked on sagittal images (carefully examine coronal and axial images)
- Joint effusion
- Major ligament or meniscal injury[266]
- Adjacent superficial MCL, which is contiguous with medial retinaculum, usually demonstrates grade 1 sprain.

- Severe dislocation usually associated with complete loss of medial retinaculum and MPFL attachments

- Axial images may demonstrate the entire spectrum of findings, including:
    - Contusions in lateral aspect of lateral femoral condyle
    - Medial patellar facet contusion (with or without articular cartilage injury)
    - Medial retinacular tears/MPFL
    - Lateral patellar subluxation

- Medial retinaculum injuries
    - Range from sprains to complete disruption or avulsion
    - FS PD-weighted FSE images show areas of disruption or defect in patellar articular cartilage.
    - Pattern of contusions results from impact of medial patellar facet on the lateral aspect of the lateral femoral condyle.
        - In extension, patella spontaneously reduces back into trochlear groove.
        - Articular injury to patella usually occurs during actual dislocation but may also occur during subsequent phase of recoil of patella.

- MPFL injuries
    - Tearing in deep layer (avulsion-type tear at femoral attachment)
    - Complete rupture adjacent to femoral attachment
    - Poor visualization of medial retinaculum and MPFL with appearance of wavy fibers
        - Medial retinaculum as a whole is generally thickened because of interdigitated fluid within disrupted fibers.
        - Fibers seen in continuity may be thin or wispy.
- Nonoperative management
    - Important in treating patients with acute patellar dislocations[6]
    - Patella spontaneously reduces into trochlear groove with extension following injury.
    - Cast immobilization and rehabilitation are time-honored conservative practices.
    - Recently, importance of early return of range of motion and strength has been recognized.
    - Use of dynamic patellar brace and range-of-motion exercises with quadriceps rehabilitation reduces risk of arthrofibrosis.
- Arthroscopy
    - Diagnosis and treatment of chondral injuries and loose bodies (incidence >50%)
    - To readdress patellar tracking and intraarticular pathology
    - To perform selective lateral retinacular release (unless there is no underlying malalignment or significant patellar tilt)
- MPFL tears (especially medial femoral epicondylar tears) and defects in VMO insertion predispose patella to recurrent dislocation.
    - Redislocation treated more aggressively
    - Torn MPFL end is freed, débrided, and reattached using suture anchors.[321]
    - Intact but lax MPFL can be imbricated in pants-over-vest fashion.
    - Reattachment of MPFL to medial epicondyle may be reinforced with adductor magnus tendon.

Medial and Lateral Retinacula

- Fascicle extensions of the vastus medialis (medial) and vastus lateralis (lateral) muscle groups[87]
- Reinforce muscles and preserve normal patellar tracking
- Retinacular attachments are seen as low-signal-intensity structures converging on the medial and lateral patellar fascicles on anterior coronal images.
- Retinacula themselves are best evaluated on axial images.
- Medial retinaculum
    - Commonly torn after patellar dislocation in association with disruption of femoral attachment of MPFL
    - Free-floating retinaculum without patellar attachment or mass-like effect caused by compressed and torn retinacular fibers or chondral fragments
    - Associated edema and hemorrhage (high signal intensity on T2, FS PD-weighted FSE, or STIR images)
- Retinacular tears
    - May be associated with severe proximal patellar or distal quadriceps tendon tears
    - May involve either medial or lateral retinacular fibers
    - Valgus hyperextension stress injuries can also result in retinacular disruptions as well as MCL tears.
- Lateral retinaculum
    - Composed of two layers
        - Superficial layer (superficial oblique retinaculum): band of oblique fibers
        - Deep layer: composed of three distinct structures (epicondylopatellar band, deep transverse retinaculum, and patellotibial band)[210]
    - Tight lateral retinaculum (known as excessive lateral pressure syndrome; see discussion earlier in this chapter)
        - Tilts patella in lateral direction

- May be accompanied by patellar subluxation

- Chronic lateral patellar tilt in excessive lateral pressure syndrome generates overload, which is transmitted to the lateral patellar facet and lateral trochlea.[91]

- Chondral degeneration of lateral patellar facet and anterolateral femoral condyle

- Edema of the proximal lateral aspect of Hoffa's fat pad

- Associated patellofemoral malalignment (patellar tilt or subluxation)

- Retinacular release may be performed to minimize development of lateral facet degenerative disease.

- Site of retinacular division after release can be evaluated with MR.

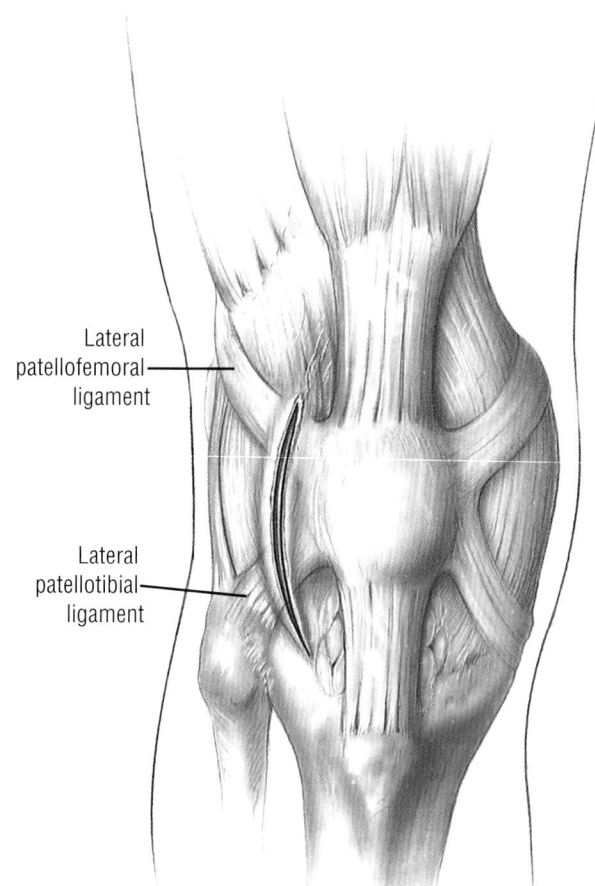

FIGURE 7.46 The lateral patellofemoral and patellotibial ligaments in relationship to a lateral release of the patella. (Reprinted from Jackson DW. *Master Techniques in Orthopaedic Surgery: Reconstructive Knee Surgery*, 3rd ed. Philadelphia, PA: Lippincott Williams & Wilkins; 2008, with permission.)

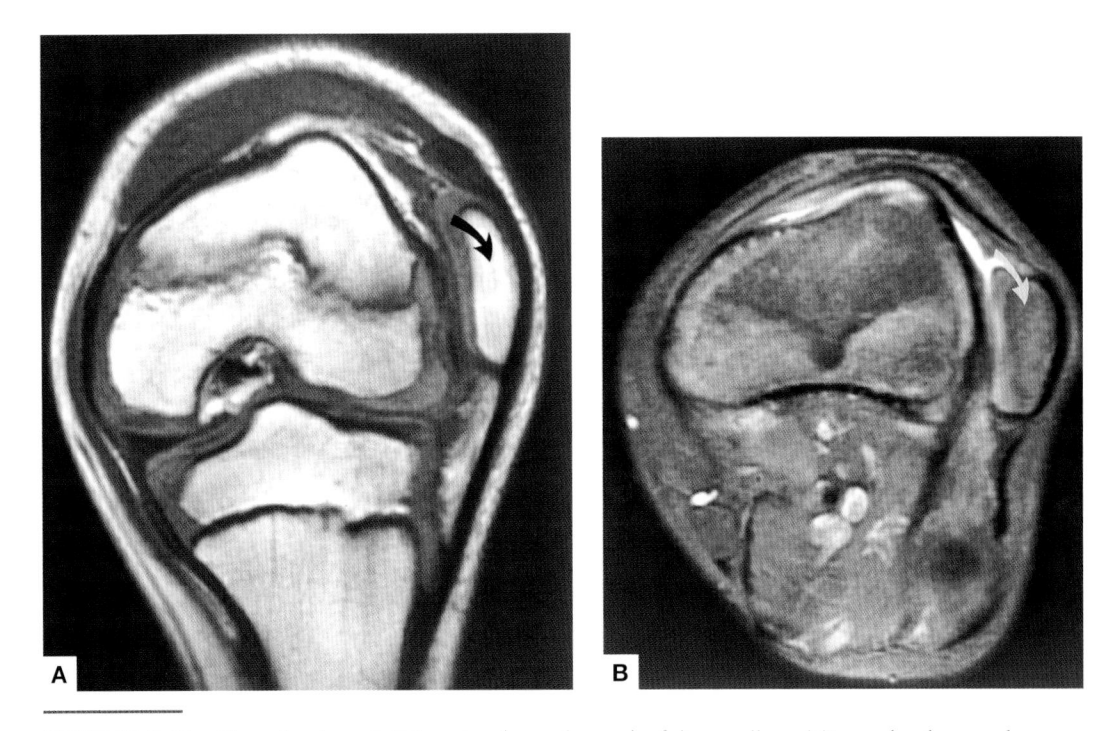

FIGURE 7.47 Complete lateral dislocation (*curved arrow*) of the patella on T1-weighted coronal (**A**) and FS PD-weighted FSE axial (**B**) images in a child with a history of recurrent dislocations. There is still relative preservation of patellar articular cartilage.

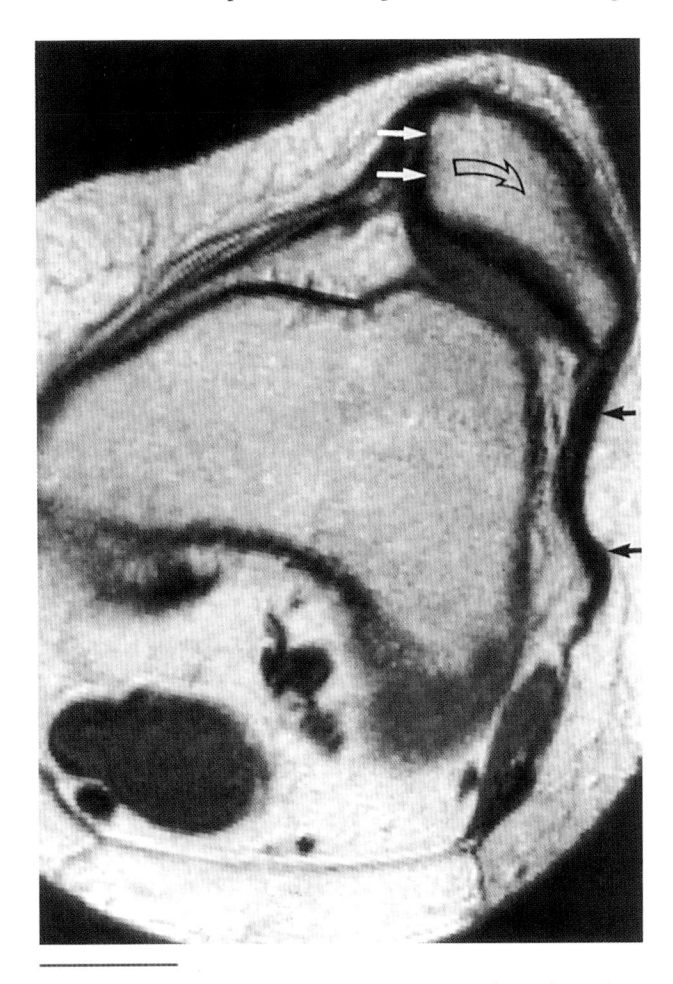

FIGURE 7.48 A T1-weighted axial image shows lateral subluxation (*curved open arrow*) of a dysplastic patella with a missing medial facet (*white straight arrows*). This defect is referred to as a Jagerhut patella. A lax lateral retinaculum is also seen (*black straight arrows*).

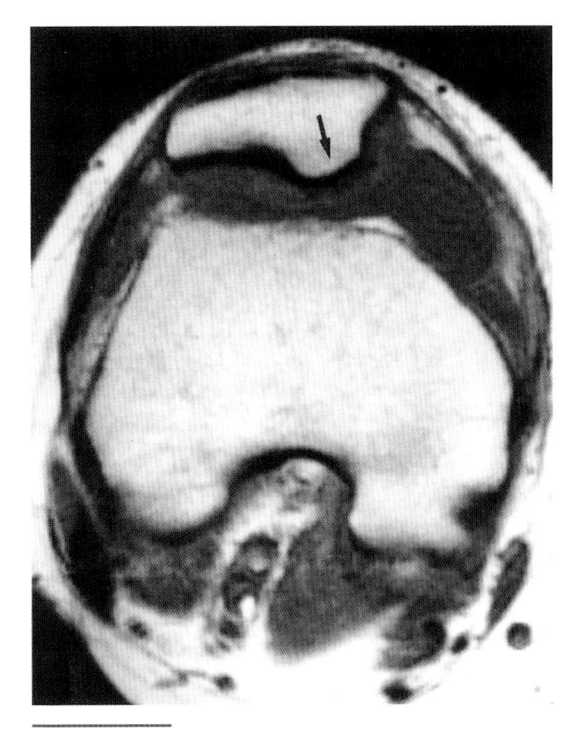

FIGURE 7.49 A Wiberg type 2 patella is indicated by concave surfaces, a smaller medial facet, and a prominent central ridge (*arrow*), as seen on a T1-weighted axial image.

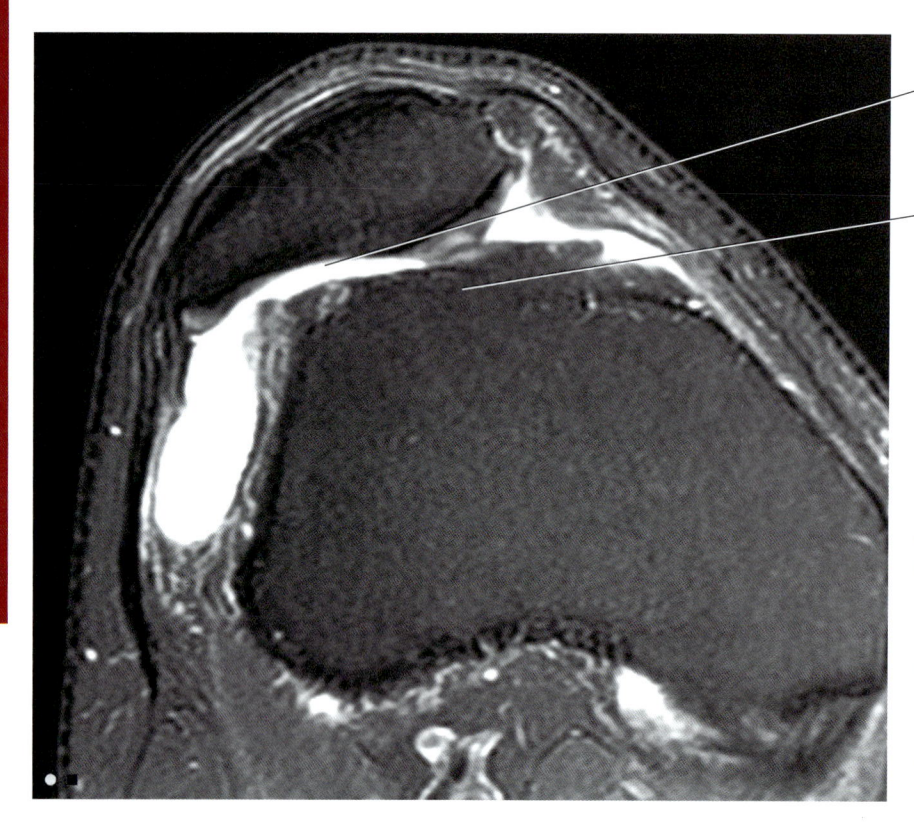

FIGURE 7.50 Trochlear dysplasia with loss of the normal trochlear groove concavity, lateral patellar subluxation, and full thickness chondral loss of the lateral facet. A shallow trochlear (3 to 5mm or less) is assessed on axial images 3cm superior to the weight-bearing femoral condylar surface. Axial FS PD FSE image.

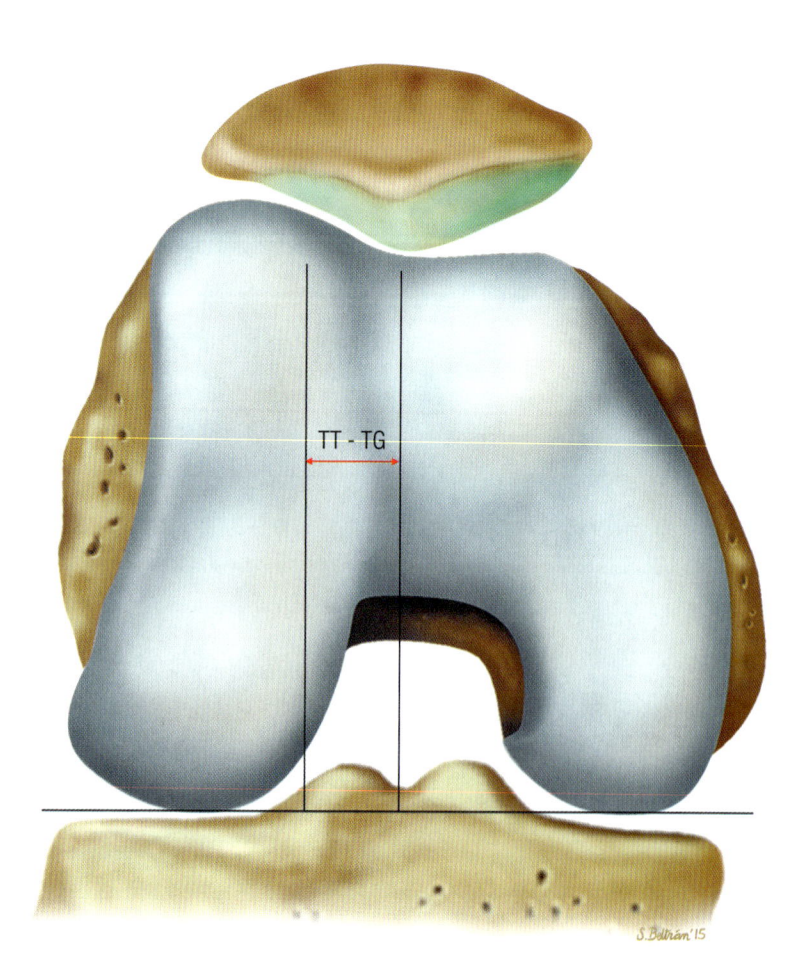

- Grade 4 chondral loss
- Trochlear dysplasia with loss of normal trochlear depth

FIGURE 7.51 Tibial tubercle (TT)–trochlear groove (TG) distance. The distance between lines drawn through the deepest point of the TG and the anterior prominence of its TT attachment of the patellar tendon is the TT-TG distance (value in millimeters). The normal TT-TG distance is in the range of 10 to 15mm. Greater than 20mm is abnormal. The TT-TG distance is a method to assess extensor mechanism valgus alignment in patellar instability.

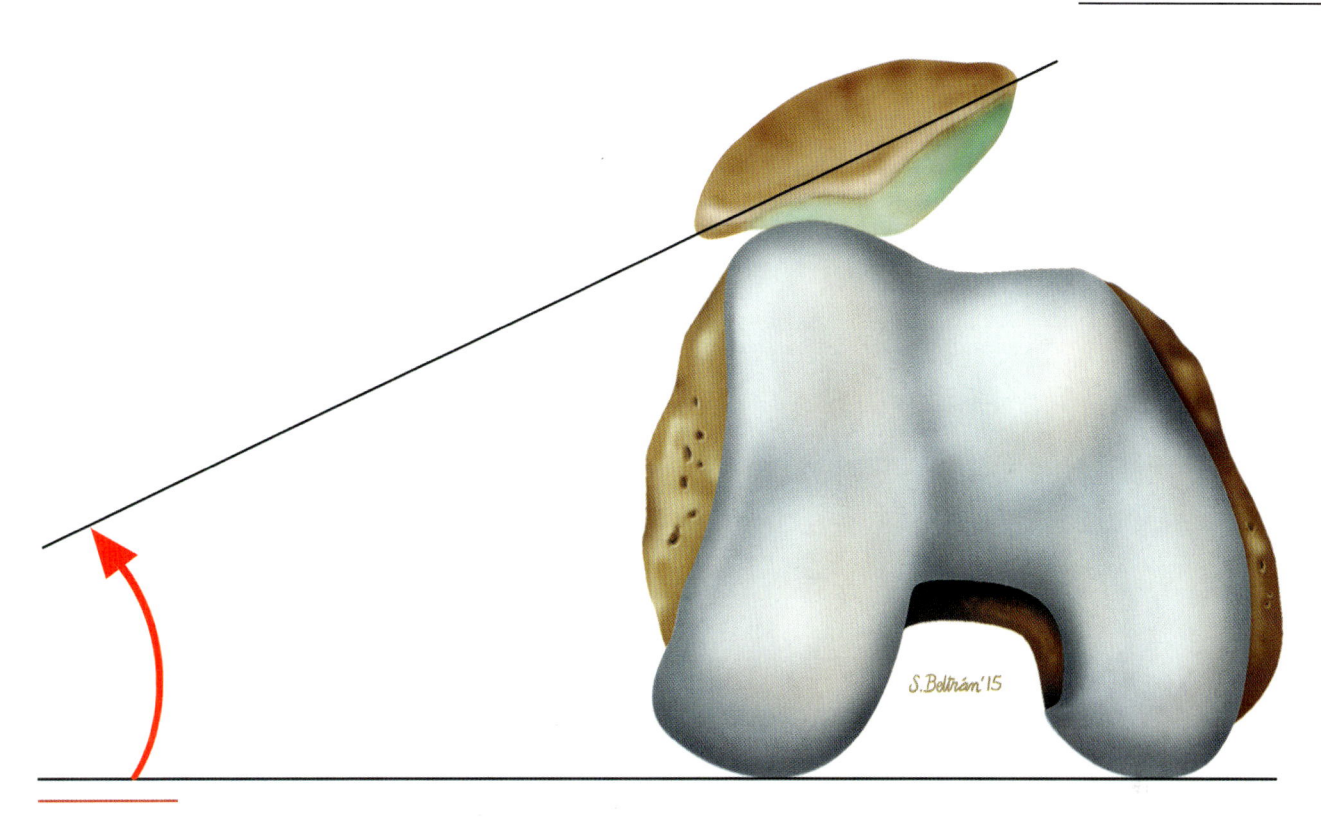

FIGURE 7.52 Patellar tilt can be assessed with CT or MR imaging. One line is parallel and tangent to the posterior femoral condyles and anterior though the long axis of the patella. Patellofemoral instability is associated with angle measurements of greater than 20 degrees.

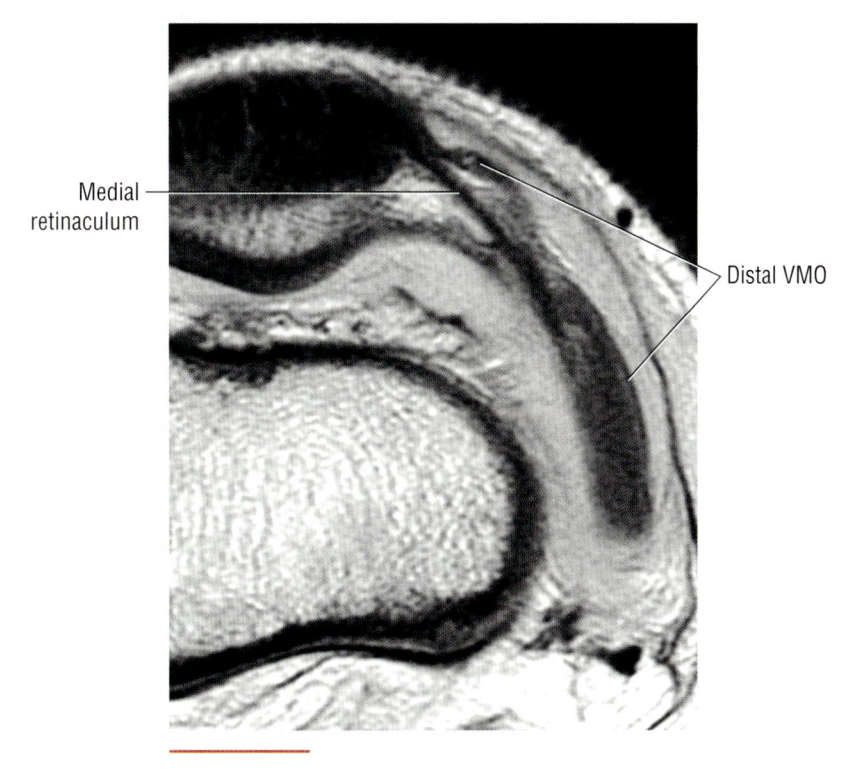

FIGURE 7.53 Axial PD FSE image showing the relationship of the distal vastus medialis obliquus (VMO) to the medial retinaculum.

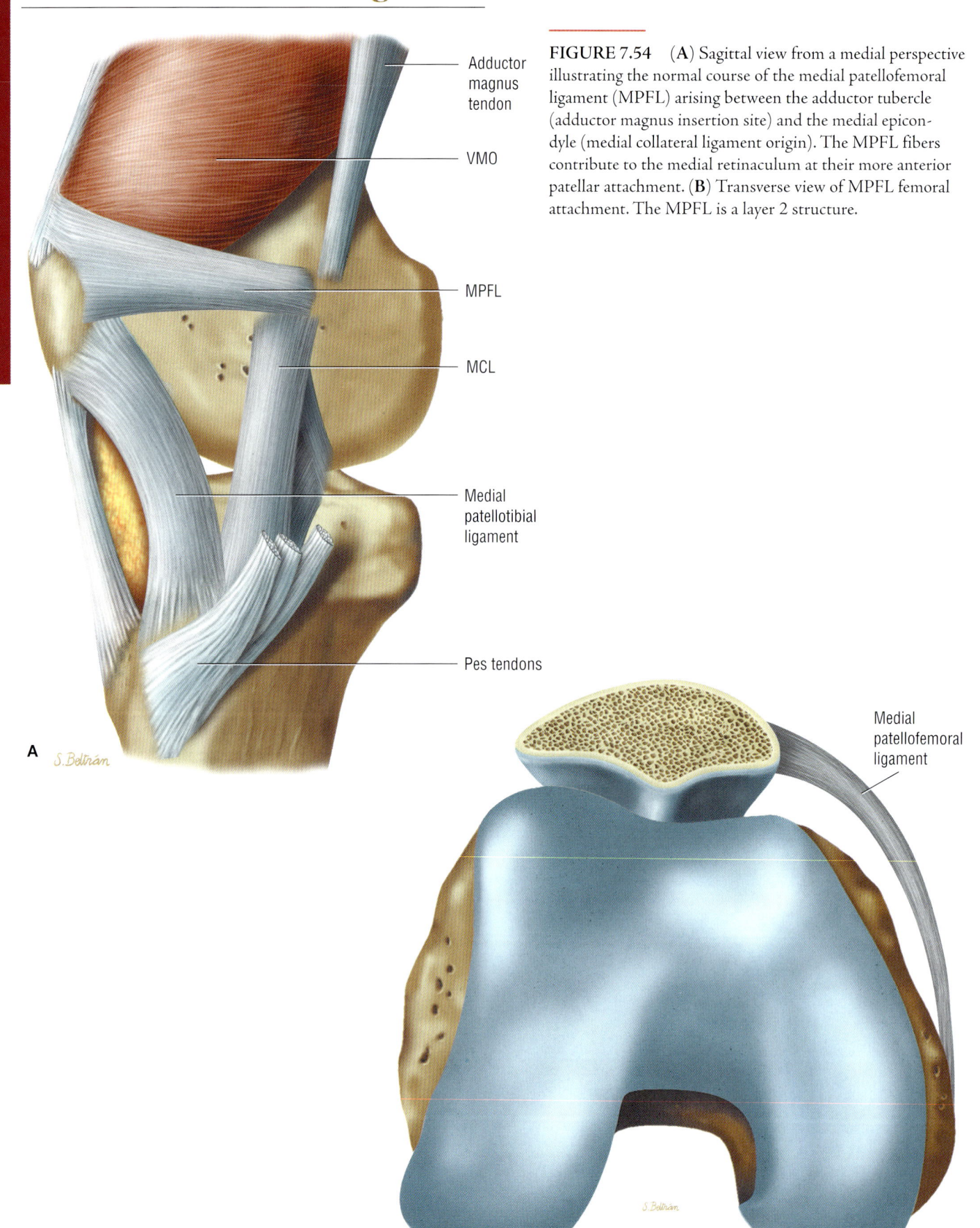

Medial Patellofemoral Ligament

FIGURE 7.54 (**A**) Sagittal view from a medial perspective illustrating the normal course of the medial patellofemoral ligament (MPFL) arising between the adductor tubercle (adductor magnus insertion site) and the medial epicondyle (medial collateral ligament origin). The MPFL fibers contribute to the medial retinaculum at their more anterior patellar attachment. (**B**) Transverse view of MPFL femoral attachment. The MPFL is a layer 2 structure.

Patellofemoral Joint and the Extensor Mechanism

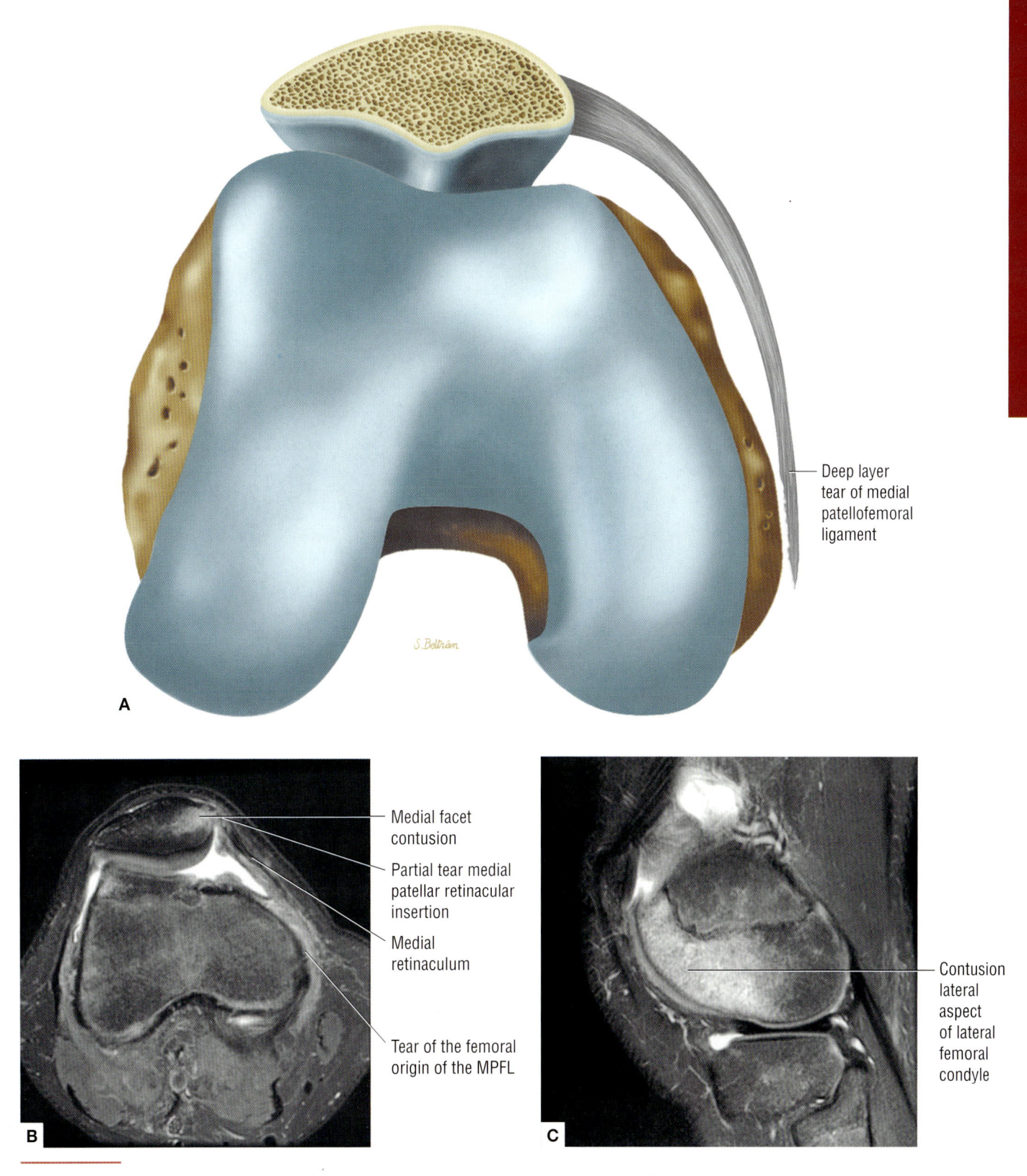

FIGURE 7.55 (**A**) Detachment or avulsion-type tear limited to the deep layer of the MPFL at its femoral attachment on a color illustration from a transverse perspective. Axial (**B**) and sagittal (**C**) FS PD FSE images showing matching contusions between the medial facet and anterolateral femoral condyle. Two common mechanisms of dislocation include noncontact, indirect injury and a direct mechanism secondary to a blow to the knee. Tearing of the deep fibers of the femoral origin of the MPFL and sprain of the medial retinacular attachment to the medial facet can be seen.

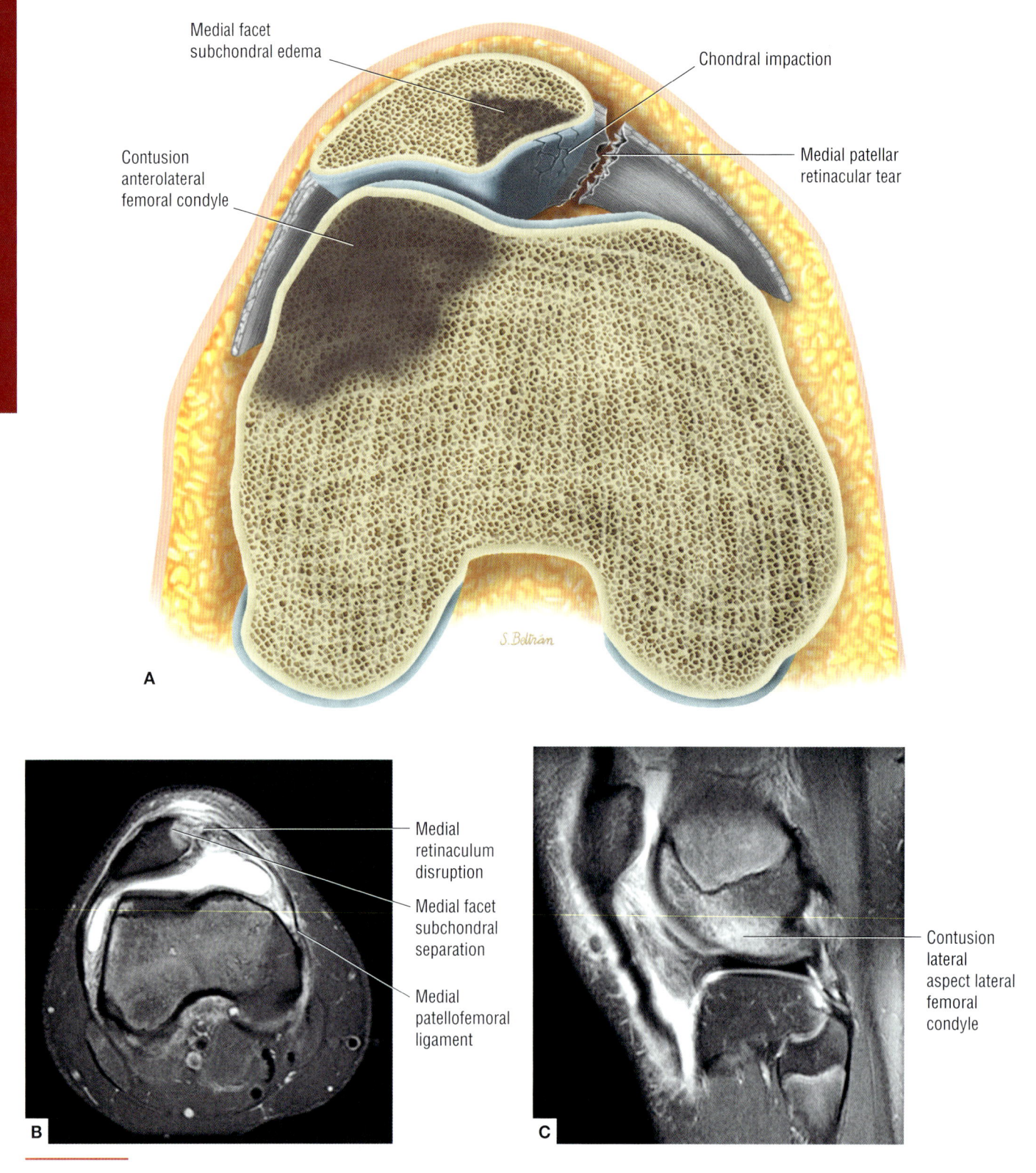

FIGURE 7.56 (**A**) Transverse plane illustration of a transient patellar dislocation with osseous contusions of the medial patellar facet (with associated chondral injury) and the anterolateral aspect of the lateral femoral condyle. Complete medial retinaculum disruption is shown. (**B**) Corresponding axial FS PD FSE image with medial retinacular disruption. There is delamination of medial patellar facet cartilage. (**C**) Sagittal FS PD FSE image with characteristic contusion of the lateral aspect of lateral femoral condyle.

Patellofemoral Joint and the Extensor Mechanism

MPFL Tear and Transient Patellar Dislocation

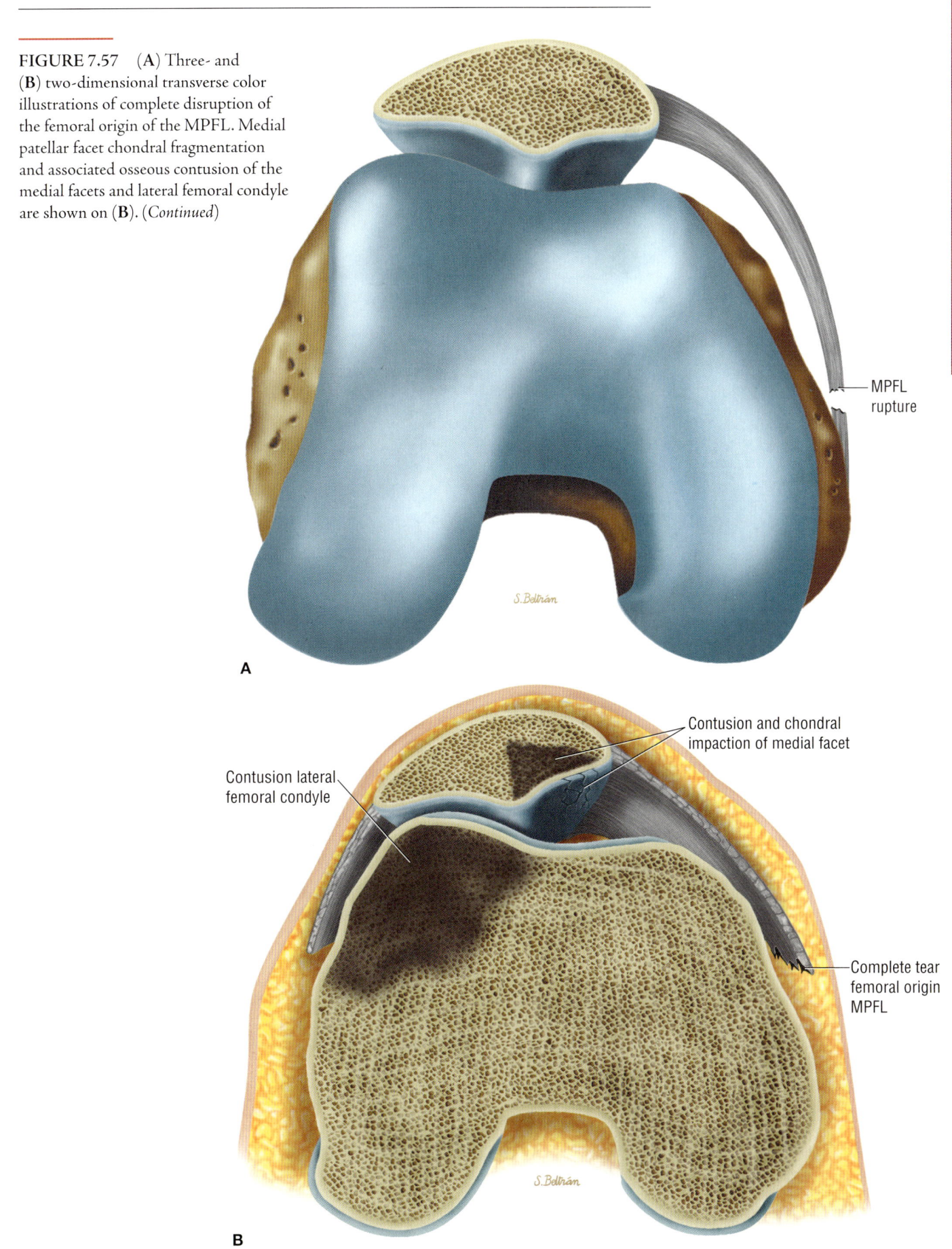

FIGURE 7.57 (**A**) Three- and (**B**) two-dimensional transverse color illustrations of complete disruption of the femoral origin of the MPFL. Medial patellar facet chondral fragmentation and associated osseous contusion of the medial facets and lateral femoral condyle are shown on (**B**). (*Continued*)

MPFL rupture

A

Contusion lateral femoral condyle

Contusion and chondral impaction of medial facet

Complete tear femoral origin MPFL

B

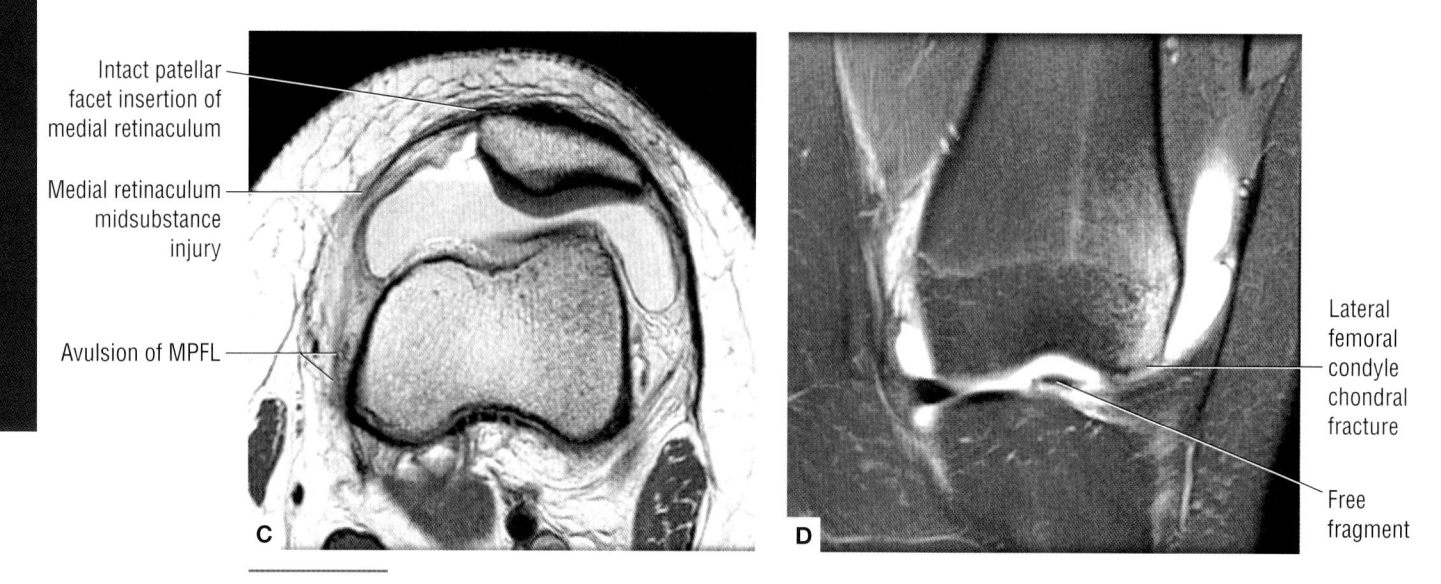

FIGURE 7.57 *(Continued)* (**C**) Discontinuity of the MPFL and mid-substance of the medial retinaculum on an axial PD FSE image. (**D**) Free fragment posterior to Hoffa's fat pad. The donor site is seen at the anterior aspect of the lateral femoral condyle. A grade 1 strain of the vastus medialis obliquus muscles is indicated.

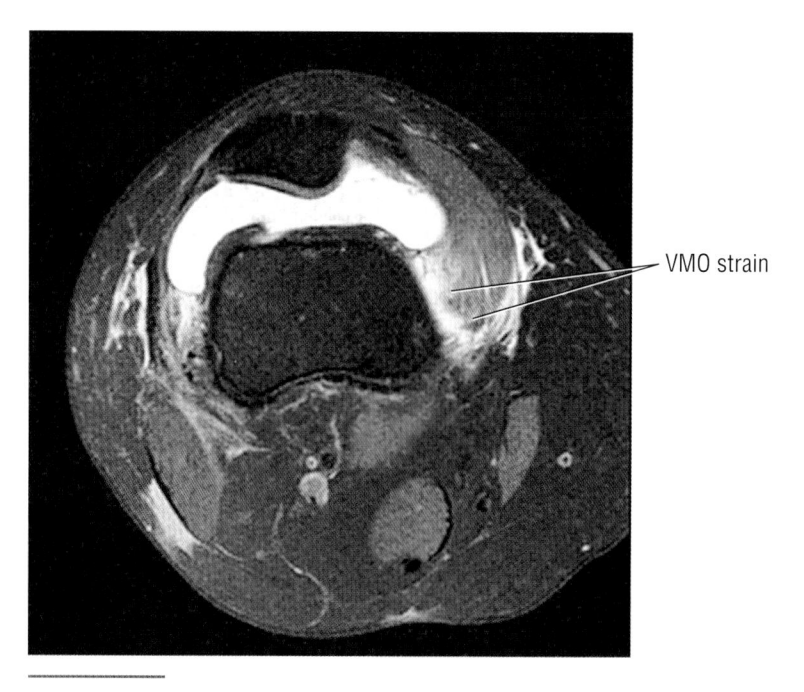

FIGURE 7.58 VMO posterior muscle strain in association with a medial retinaculum and MPFL tear.

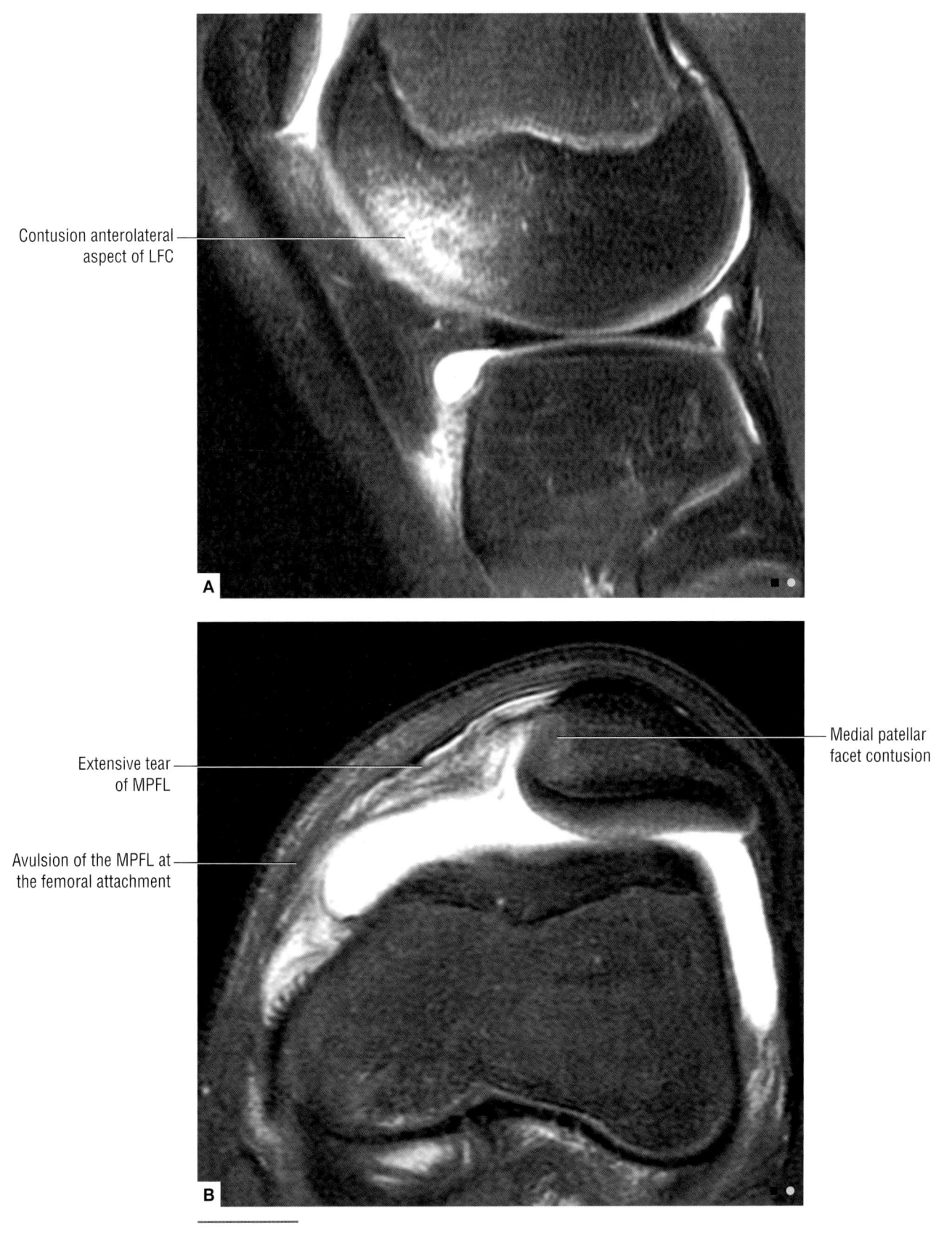

FIGURE 7.59 Transient patellar dislocation with anterolateral lateral femoral condyle (LFC) contusion and medial patellofemoral ligament (MPFL) disruption. Sagittal (**A**) and axial (**B**) FS PD FSE images.

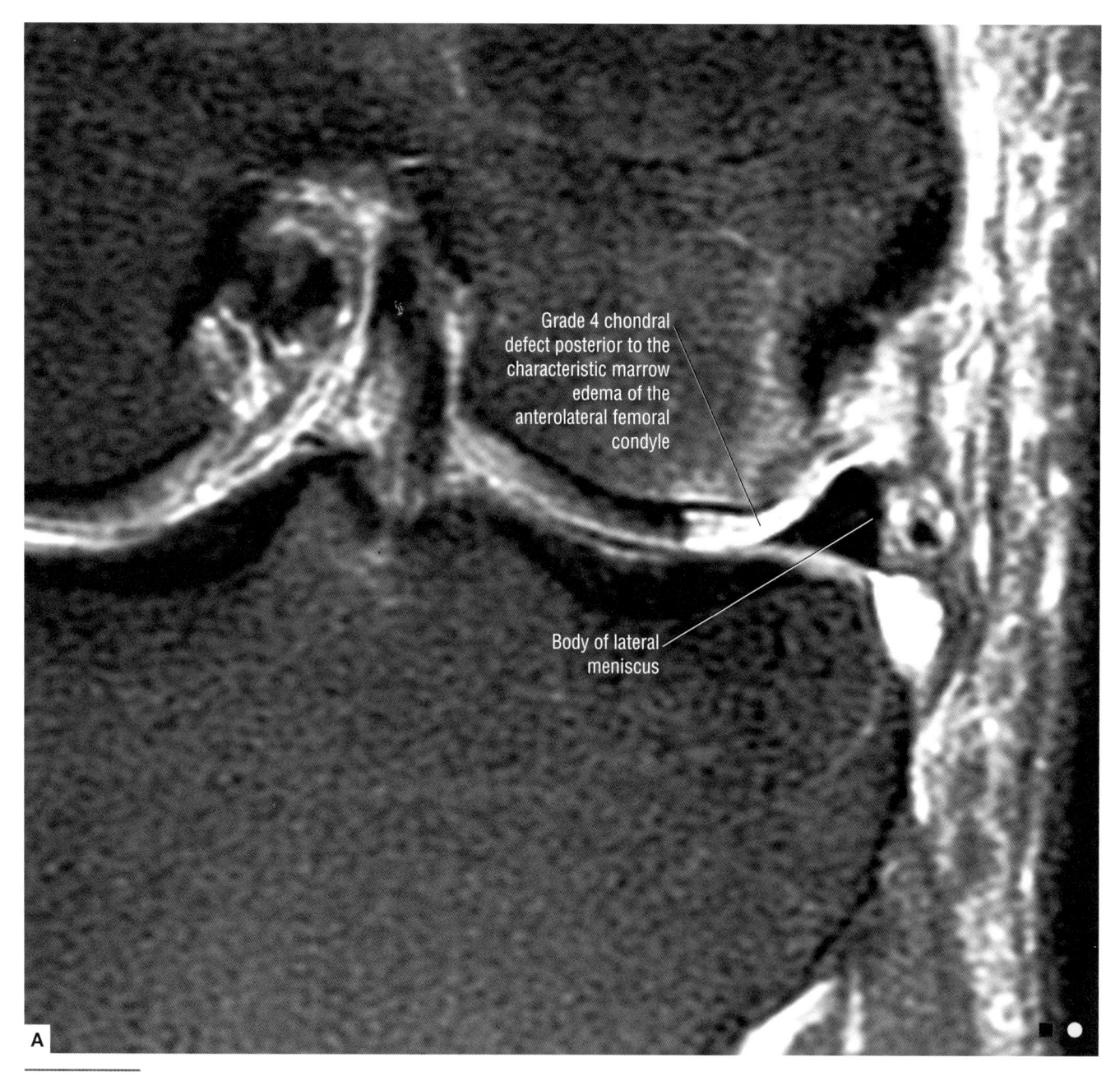

FIGURE 7.60 Full thickness lateral femoral condyle chondral lesion occurring as part of the initial sheer injury during the dislocation phase. The relocation of the patella in extension results in the non–weight-bearing anterolateral femoral condyle contusion, which would be located anterior to the grade 4 chondral injury. (**A**) Coronal FS PD FSE image.

Delamination of medial patellar facet chondral surface

Avulsion of medial patellofemoral ligament (MPFL)

Grade 4 chondral lesion of weight-bearing LFC

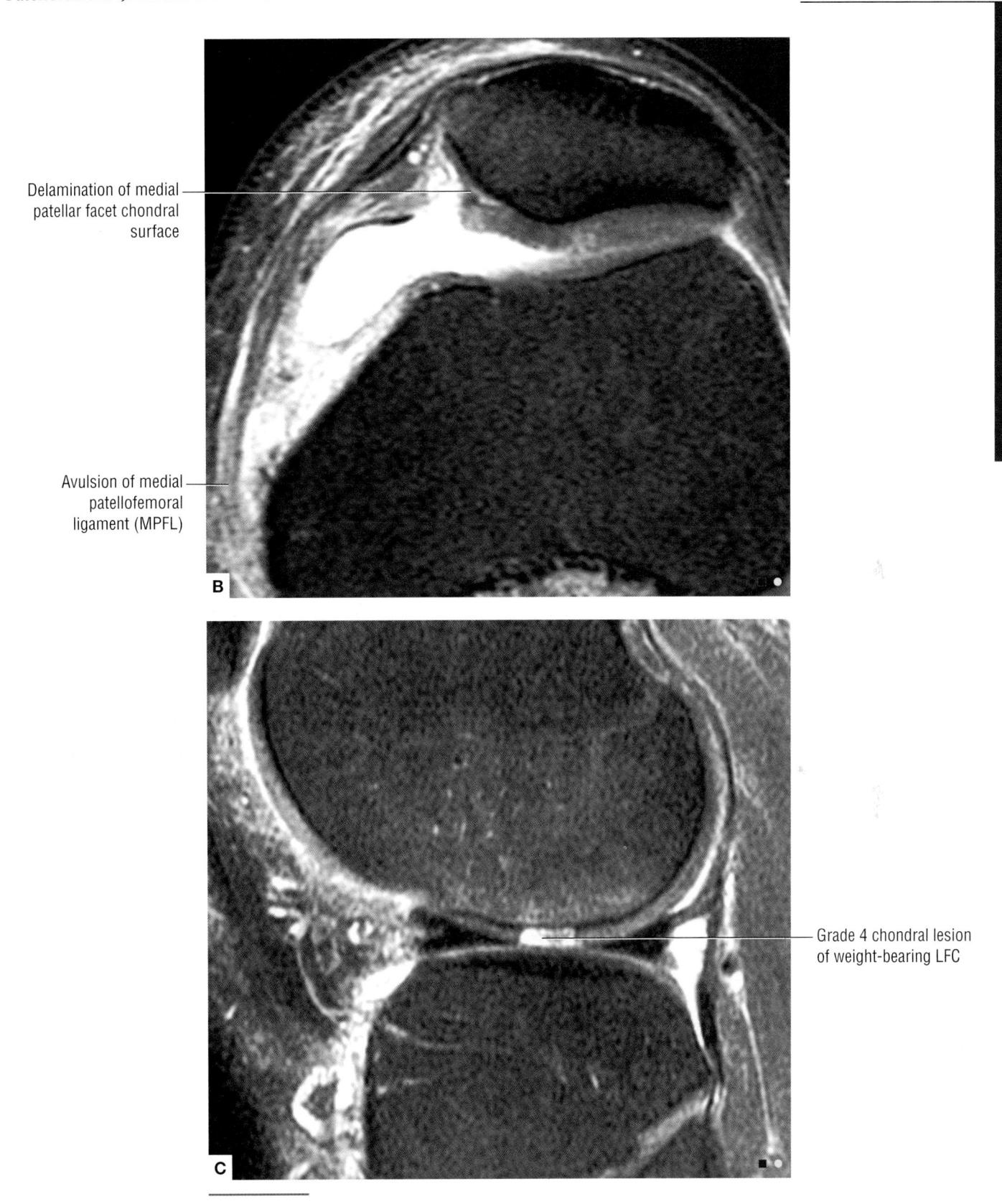

FIGURE 7.60 *(Continued)* **(B)** Shearing force of transient lateral patellar dislocation results in delamination of the medial patellar facet articular cartilage. The mechanism twisting is a valgus-flexion-external rotation (twisting motion with partial knee flexion and the femur rotating internally on a fixed foot). **(C)** Associated grade 4 chondral defect of the lateral femoral condyle occurring during the dislocation phase of transient patellar dislocation. Axial **(B)** and sagittal **(C)** PD FSE images.

Avulsed medial retinaculum

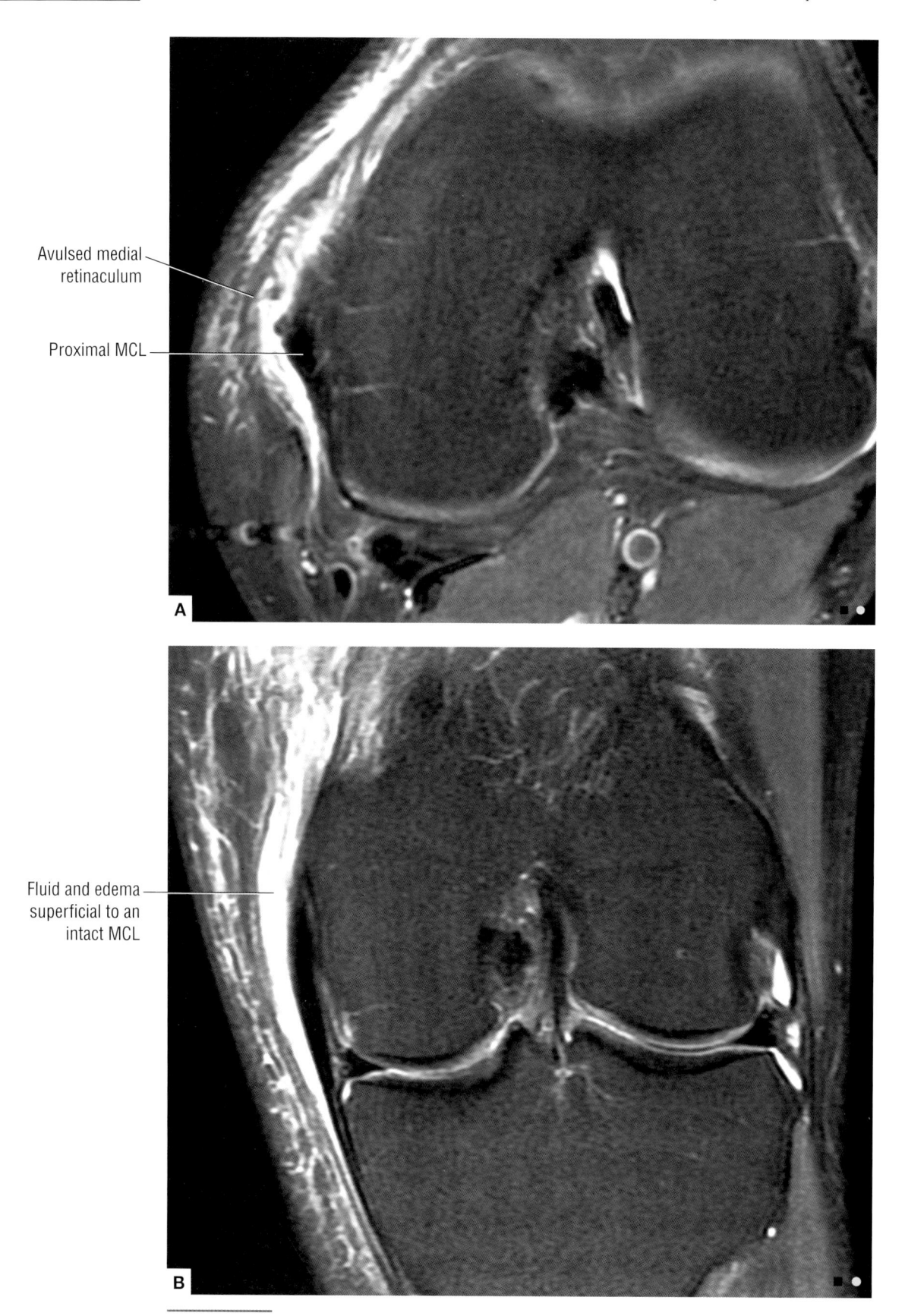

Proximal MCL

Fluid and edema superficial to an intact MCL

FIGURE 7.61 The superficial edema and fluid are the result of the medial retinaculum and medial patellofemoral ligament tear and not a sprain of the MCL. Axial (**A**) and coronal (**B**) FS PD FSE images.

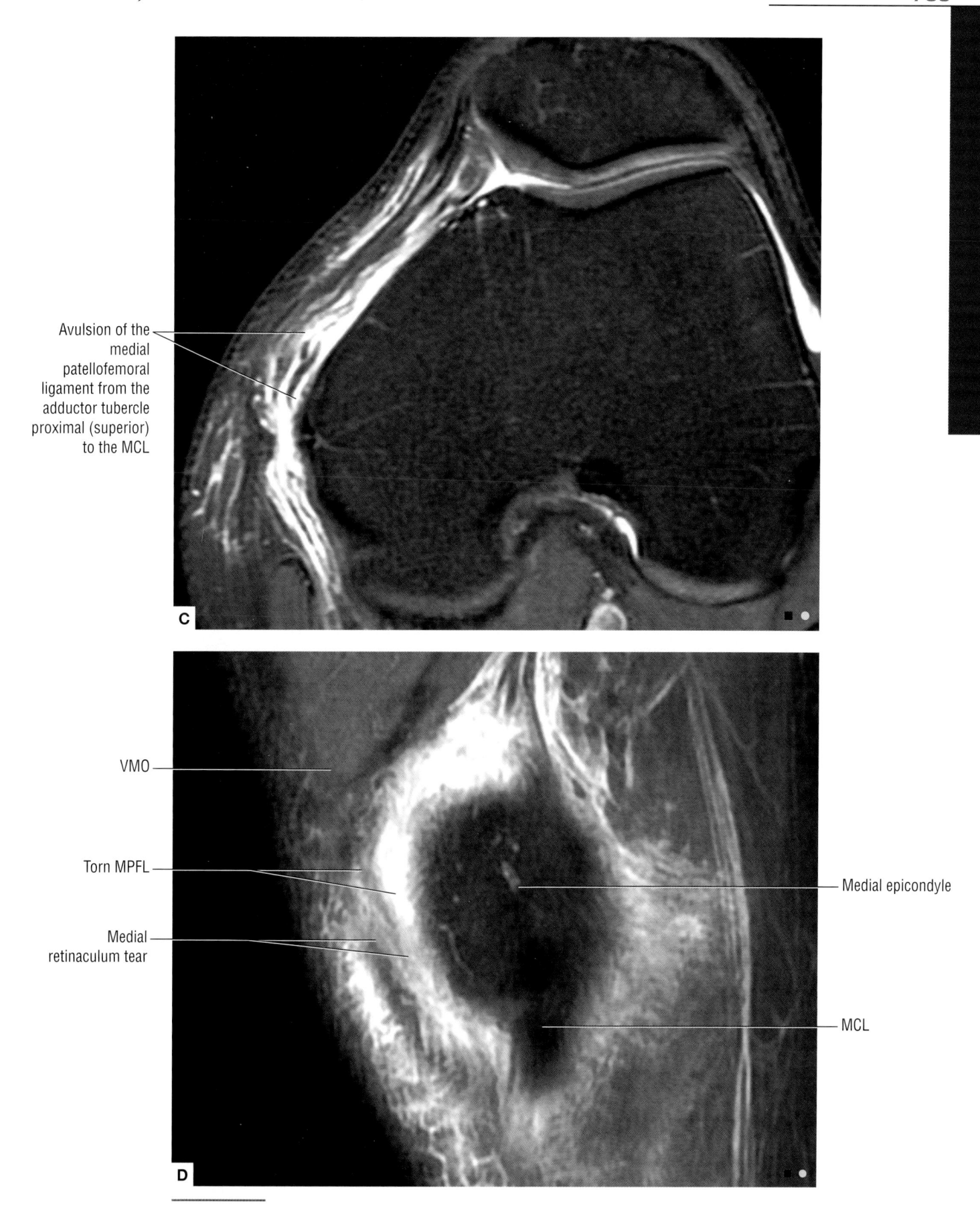

Patellofemoral Joint and the Extensor Mechanism 765

FIGURE 7.61 *(Continued)* Axial (**C**) and sagittal (**D**) FS PD FSE images.

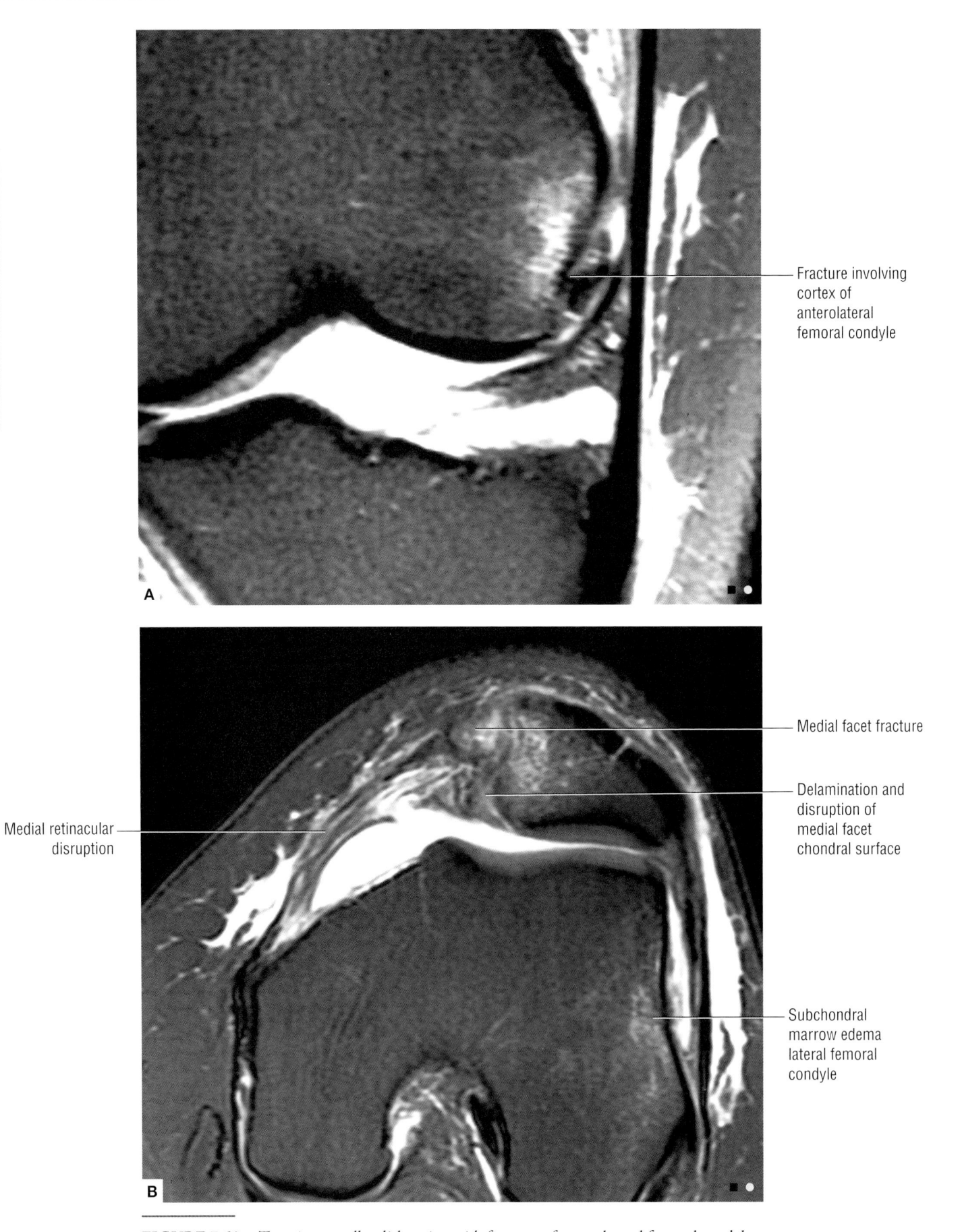

FIGURE 7.62 Transient patellar dislocation with fracture of anterolateral femoral condyle, medial retinaculum tear (middle third), and medial facet fracture fragment and shearing injury to the overlying facet articular cartilage. Coronal (**A**) and axial (**B**) FS PD FSE images.

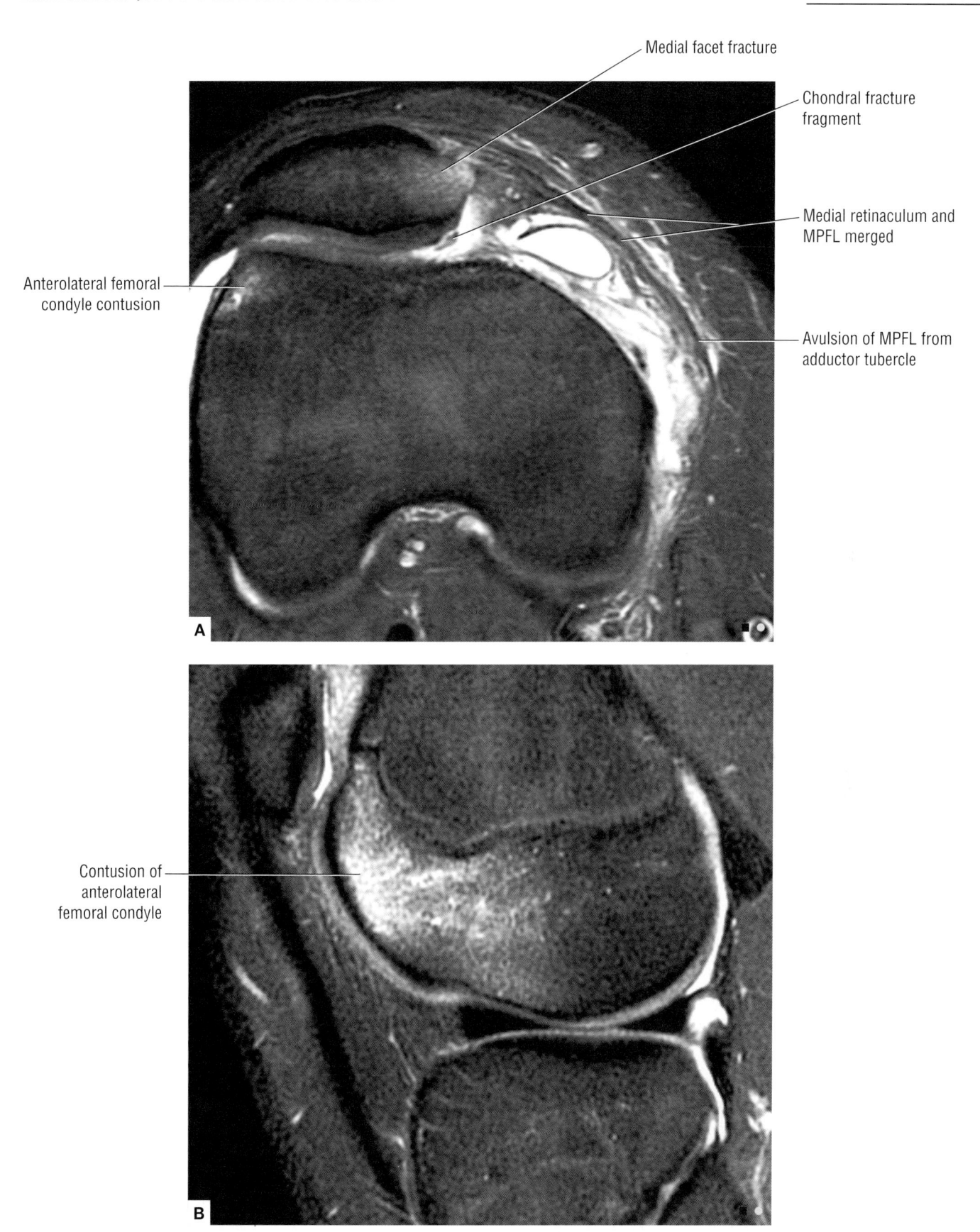

Patellofemoral Joint and the Extensor Mechanism

FIGURE 7.63 Disruption of the medial patellofemoral ligament in transient dislocation of the patella. The normal MPFL is the primary stabilizer against lateral patellar displacement. Note the MPFL, ligament, adductor magnus tendon, and the medial collateral ligament attach to the adductor tubercle. The MPFL can be located deep to the vastus medialis obliquus muscle as a landmark. Axial (**A**) and sagittal (**B**) FS PD FSE images.

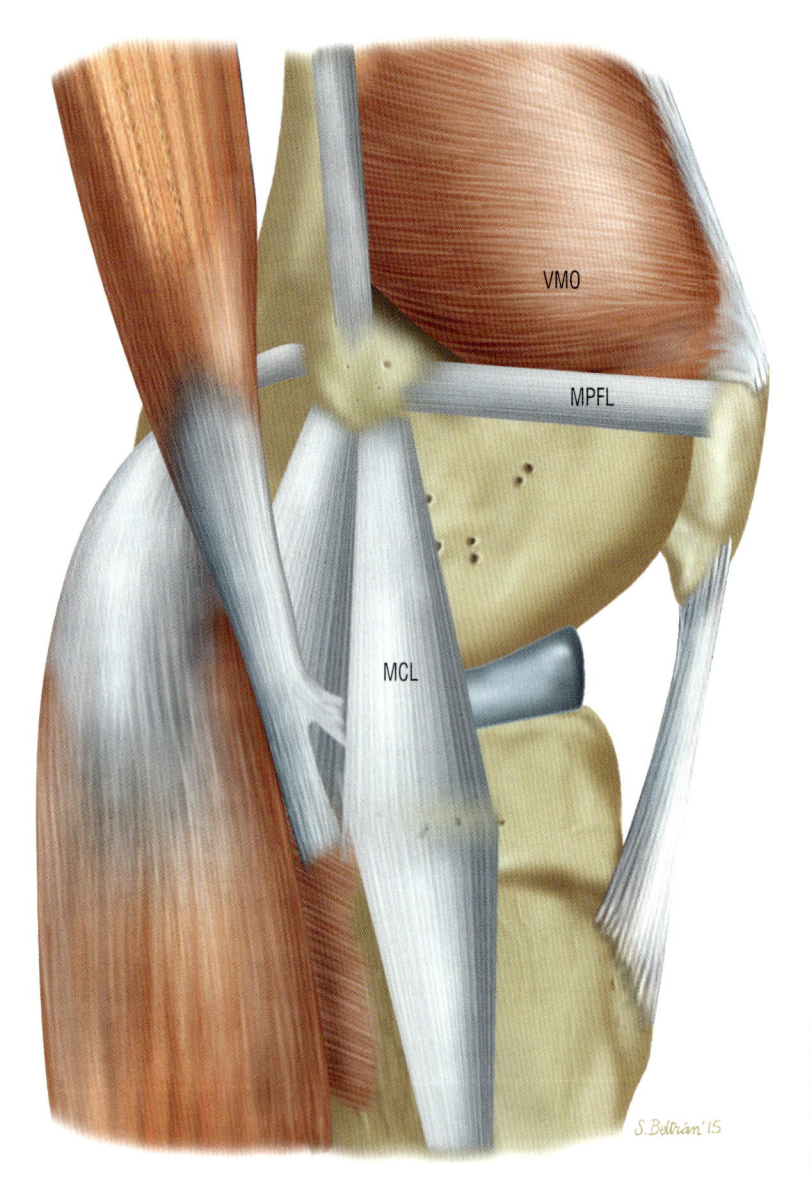

FIGURE 7.64 The normal MPFL is engaged between 0 degrees and 30 degrees of knee flexion. The trochlear is the primary restraint with flexion greater than 30 degrees.

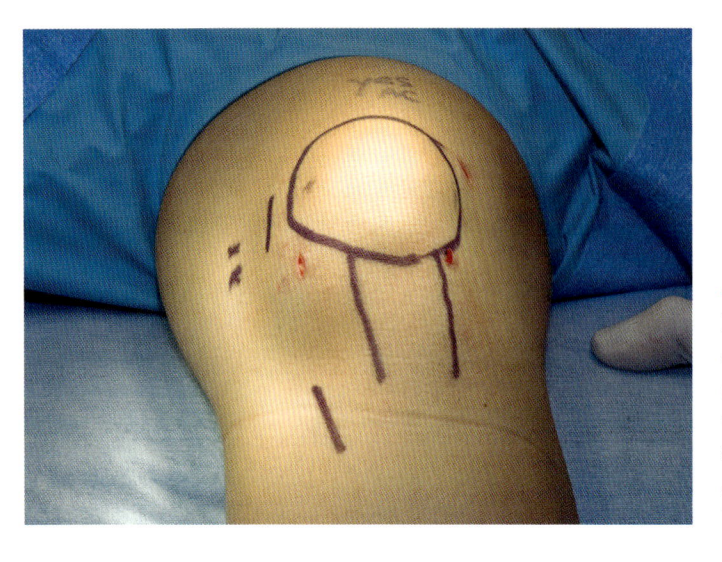

FIGURE 7.65 The patella, the edges of the patellar tendon, the adductor tubercle (proximal "X"), and the medial epicondyle (distal "X"), as well as the incision over the pes tendons and the MPFL, are marked on the skin. (Reprinted from Fu FH. *Master Techniques in Orthopaedic Surgery: Sports Medicine*. Philadelphia, PA: Lippincott Williams & Wilkins; 2010, with permission.)

Vastus Medialis Obliquus (VMO) Injury

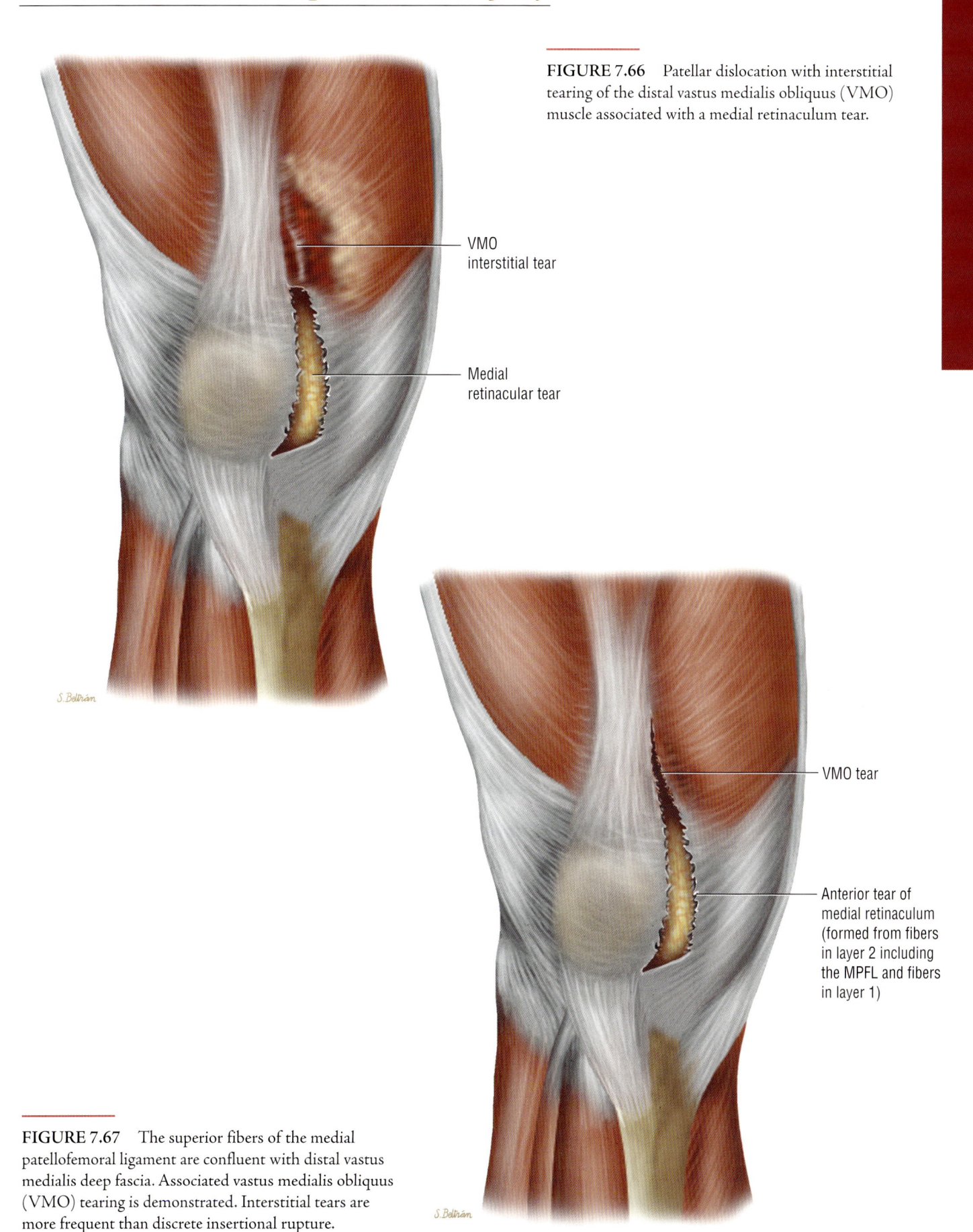

FIGURE 7.66 Patellar dislocation with interstitial tearing of the distal vastus medialis obliquus (VMO) muscle associated with a medial retinaculum tear.

- VMO interstitial tear
- Medial retinacular tear

- VMO tear
- Anterior tear of medial retinaculum (formed from fibers in layer 2 including the MPFL and fibers in layer 1)

FIGURE 7.67 The superior fibers of the medial patellofemoral ligament are confluent with distal vastus medialis deep fascia. Associated vastus medialis obliquus (VMO) tearing is demonstrated. Interstitial tears are more frequent than discrete insertional rupture.

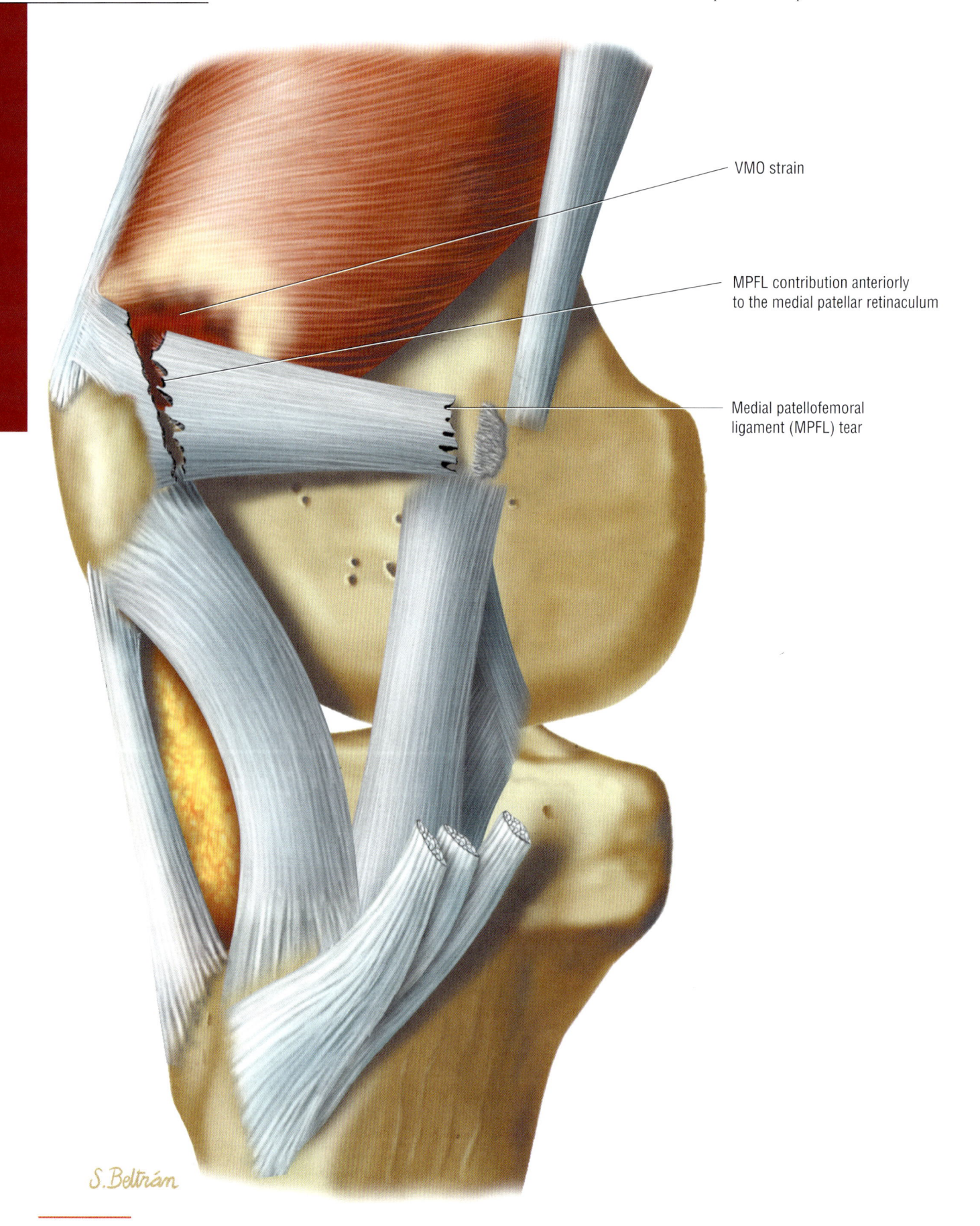

FIGURE 7.68 Sagittal view color illustration from the medial perspective of complete discontinuity of the medial patellofemoral ligament from both its femoral attachment and patellar insertion through its contribution to the medial retinaculum. Static subluxation and patellar instability result with unopposed action of the lateral retinaculum.

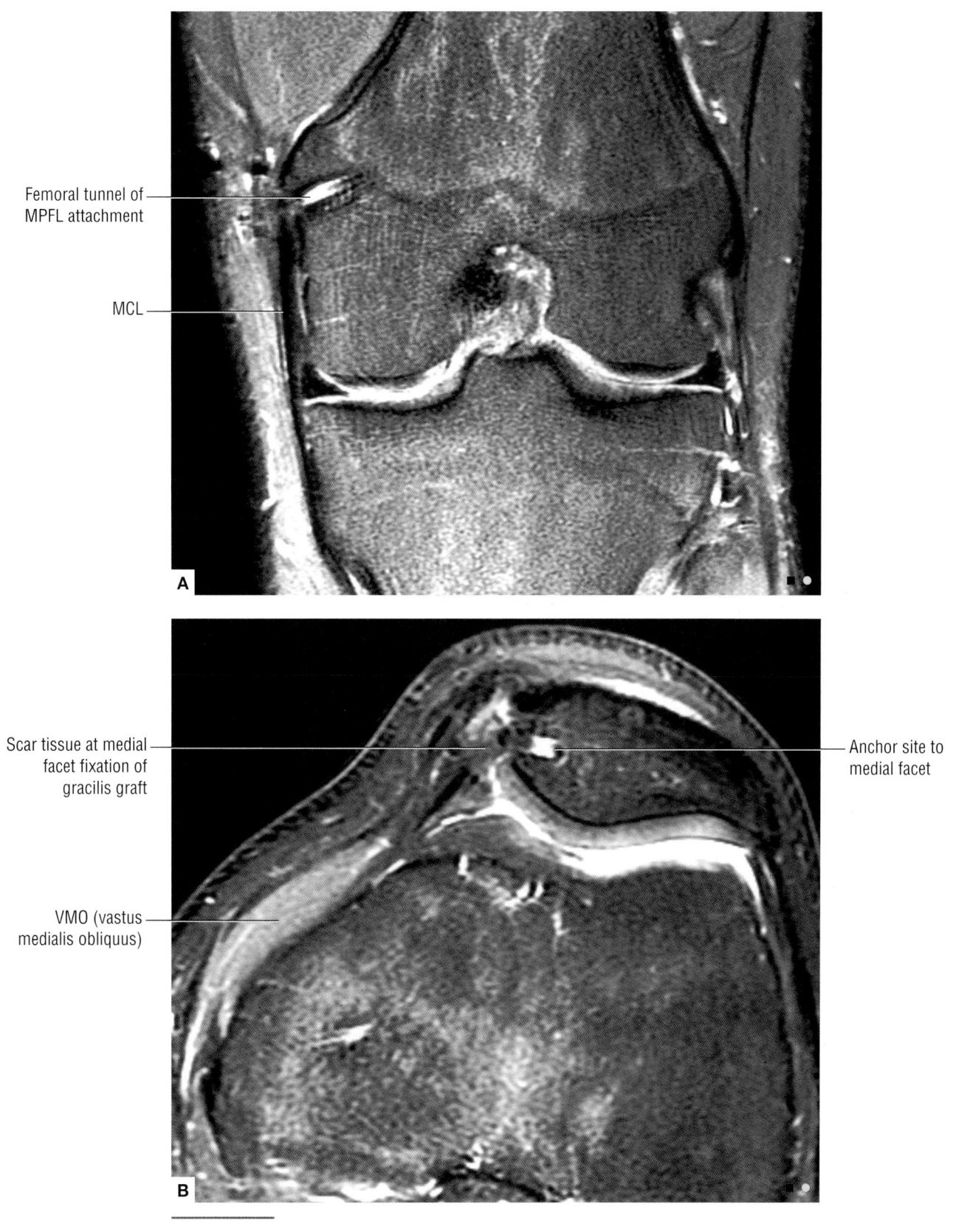

FIGURE 7.69 Reconstruction of the medial patellofemoral ligament (MPFL) using a double-stranded gracilis autograft. The MPFL insertion point is just distal to the adductor tubercle. It is important not to place the femoral tunnel too proximal or too anterior because this will increase the applied force and loading applied to the articular cartilage of the medial facet. Bone anchors were used to attach the graft to the medial facet and femoral site. Coronal (**A**) and axial (**B**) FS PD FSE images. (*Continued*)

Gracilis autograft

Femoral tunnel

Medial facet subchondral edema

Medial facet chondral wear from meniscal pressure from patellofemoral contact post MPFL reconstruction

Double stranded gracilis 4 grafts

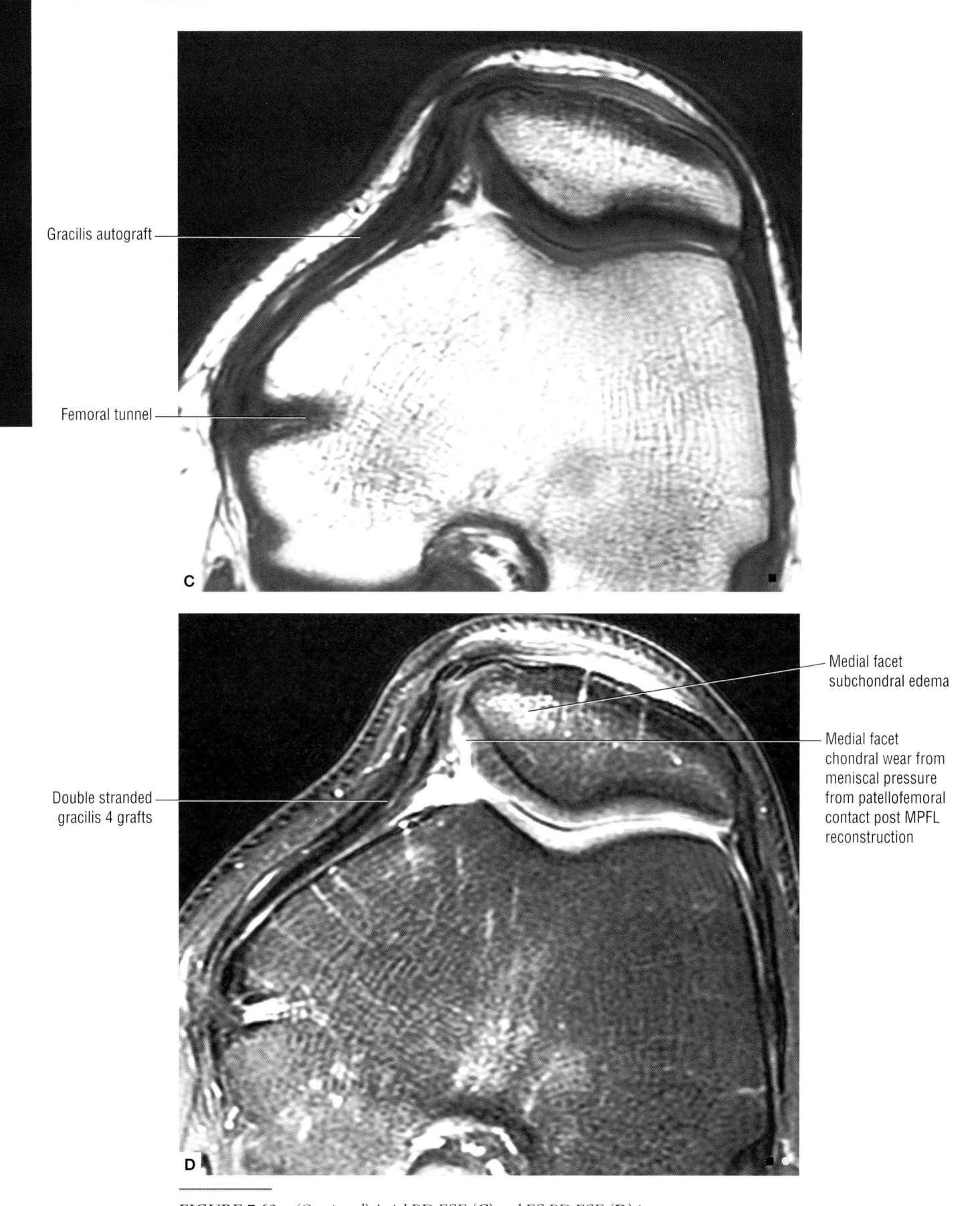

FIGURE 7.69 *(Continued)* Axial PD FSE (**C**) and FS PD FSE (**D**) images.

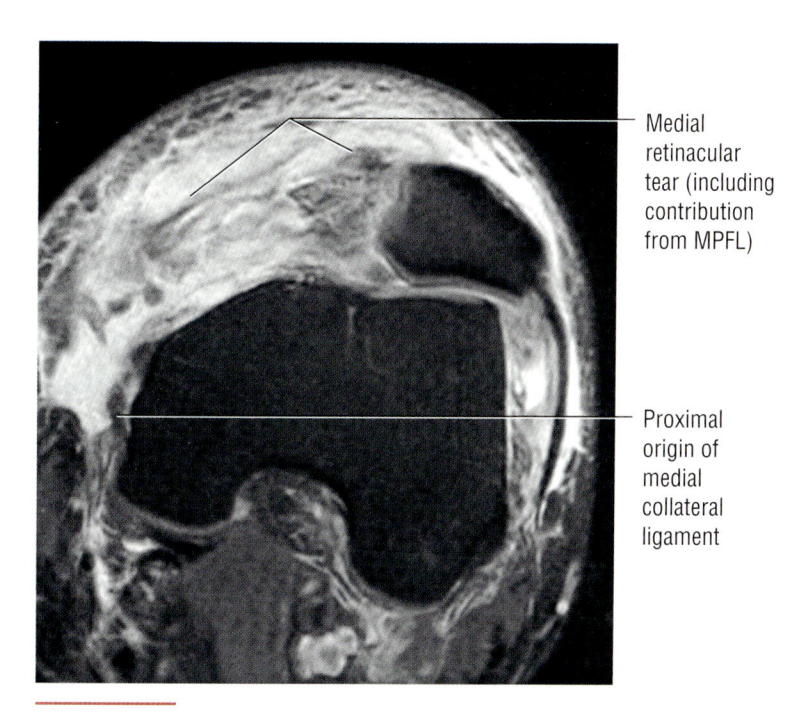

FIGURE 7.70 Complete disruption of both the femoral origin of the MPFL and its anterior continuation as the medial retinaculum on an axial FS PD FSE image. This image was obtained inferior to the adductor tubercle at the level of the proximal origin of the medial collateral ligament.

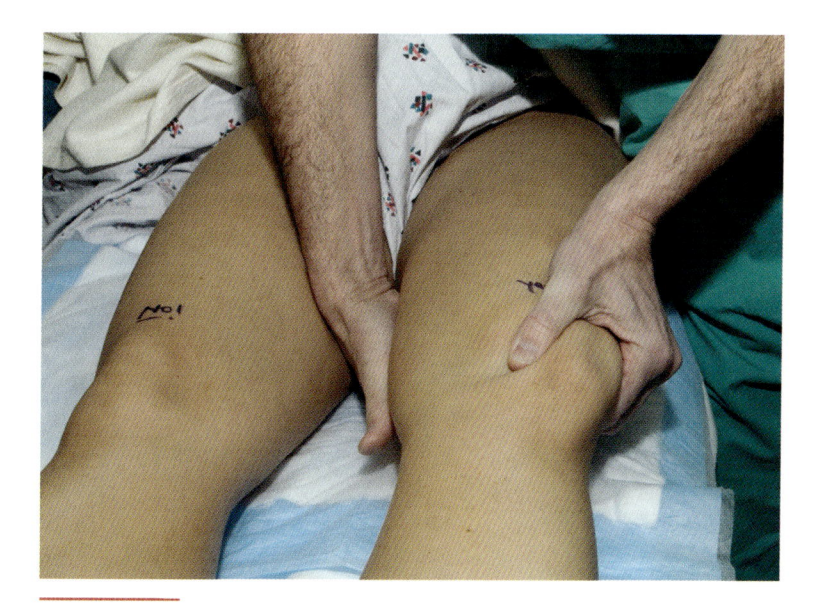

FIGURE 7.71 The glide test. In this patient, the patella can be easily dislocated laterally. (Reprinted from Fu FH. *Master Techniques in Orthopaedic Surgery: Sports Medicine.* Philadelphia, PA: Lippincott Williams & Wilkins; 2010, with permission.)

Transient Patellar Dislocation

Anterolateral femoral condyle chondral defect

Lateral femoral condyle contusion (anterior and lateral)

Chondral and subchondral impaction

Medial retinaculum tear

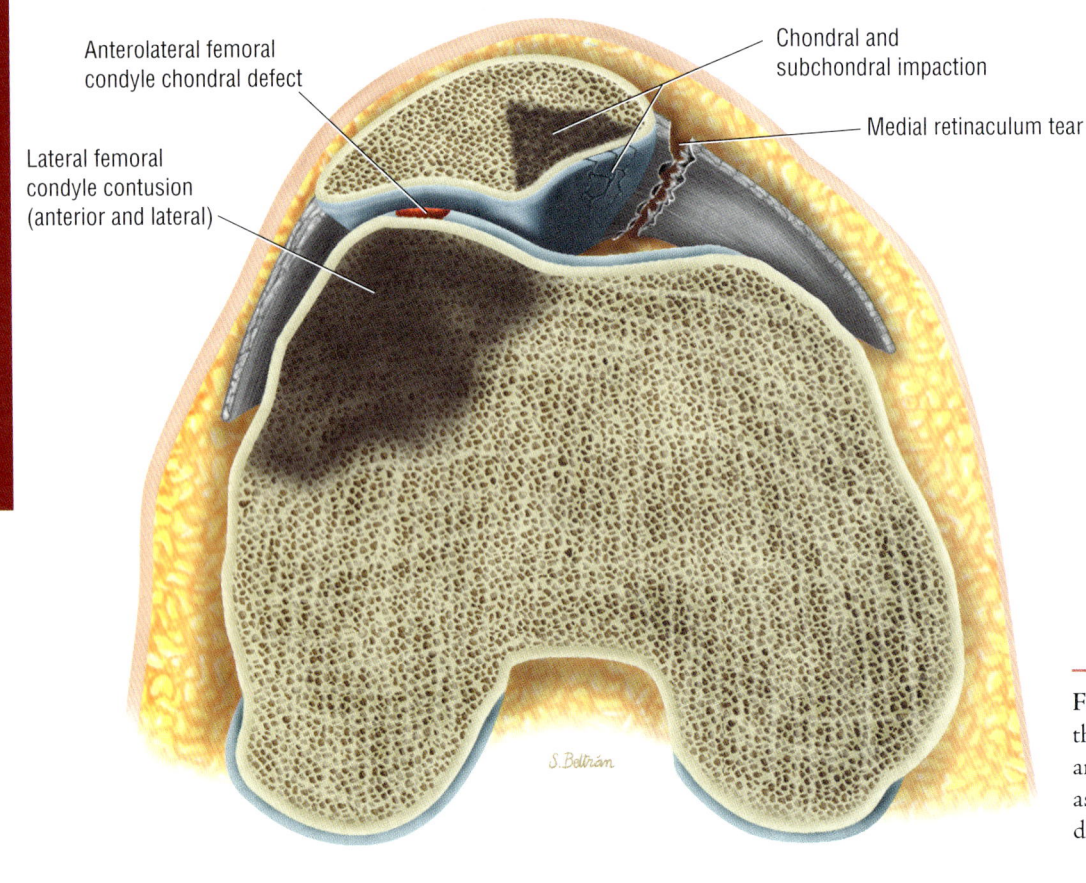

FIGURE 7.72 Focal full thickness chondral defect of the anterolateral femoral condyle associated with transient patellar dislocation.

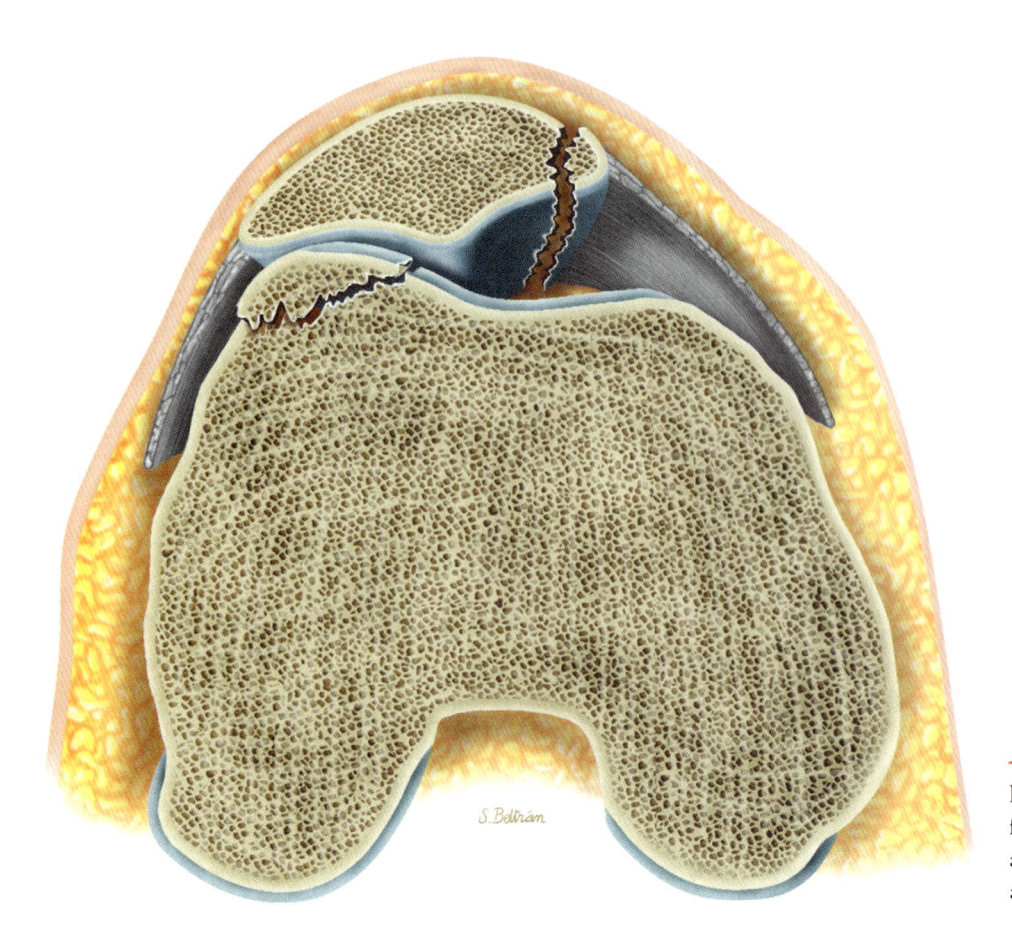

FIGURE 7.73 An osteochondral fracture of the lateral femoral condyle and the medial patellar facet is seen in association with patellar dislocation.

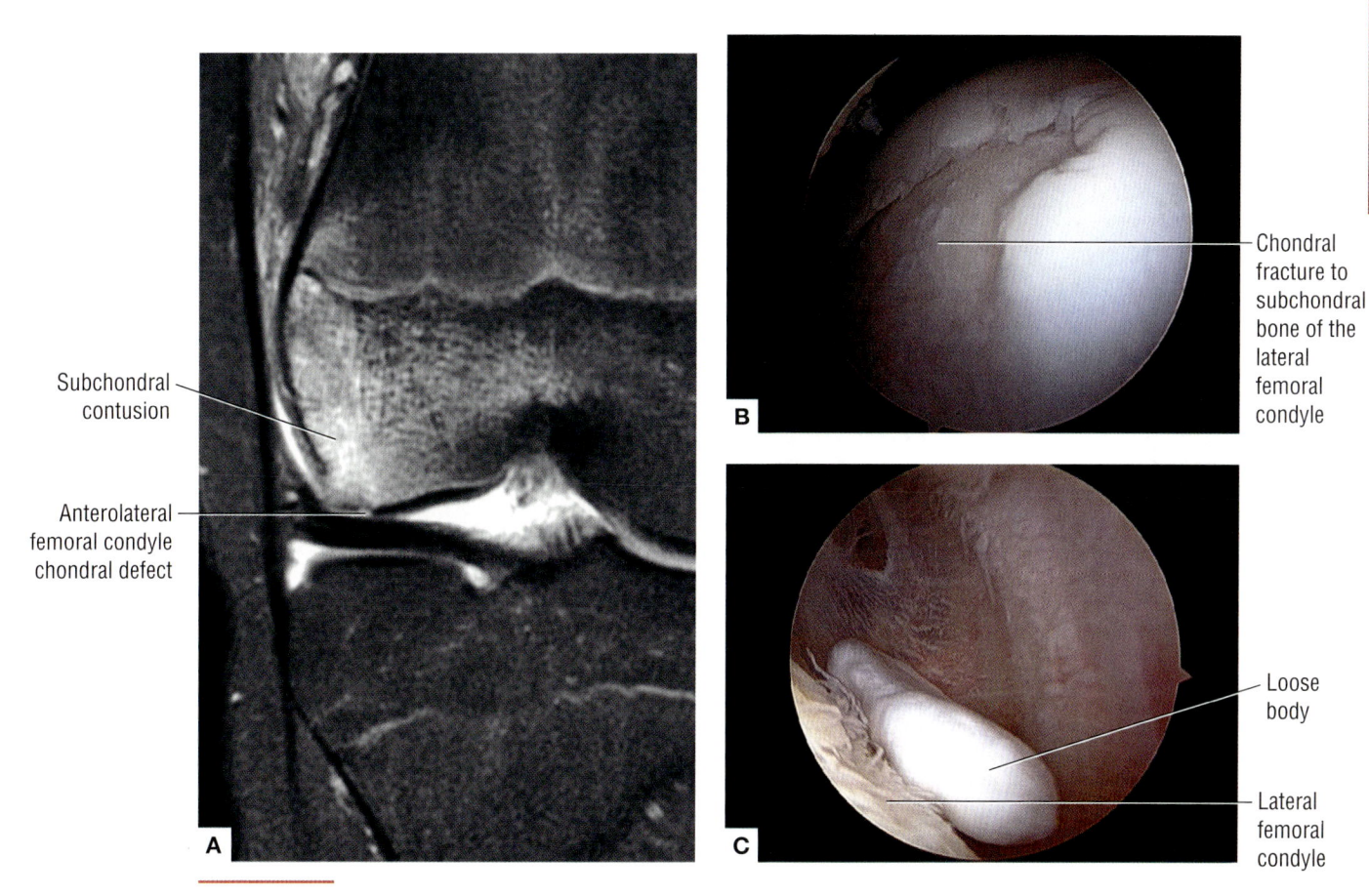

Patellofemoral Joint and the Extensor Mechanism

FIGURE 7.74 (**A**) Coronal FS PD FSE image showing a focal full thickness chondral defect of the lateral aspect of the anterolateral femoral condyle. (**B**) An arthroscopic view after transient patellar dislocation shows an anterior lateral femoral condyle full thickness chondral fracture with defect. (**C**) A corresponding chondral loose body can be seen between the lateral femoral condyle and capsule.

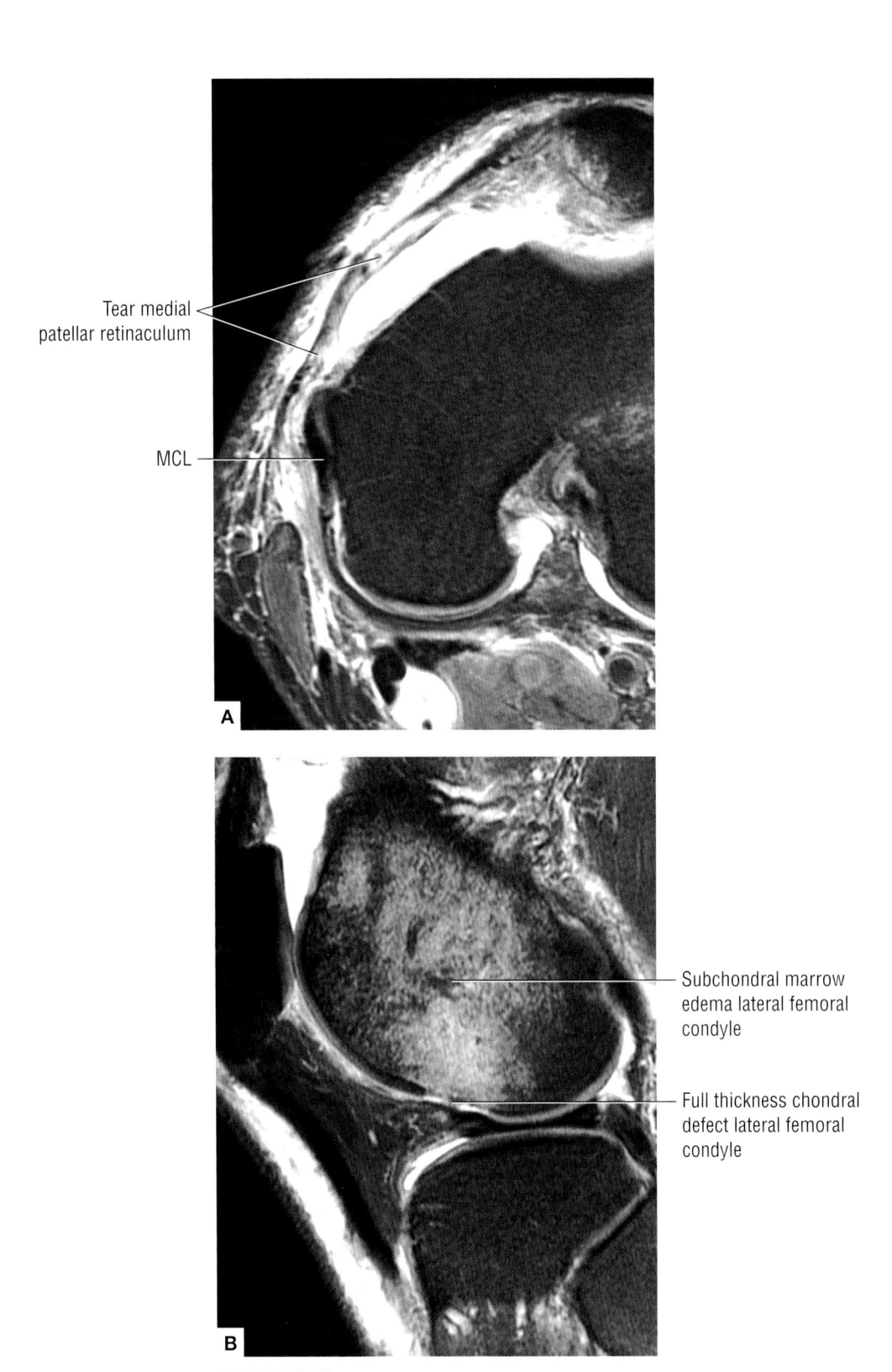

FIGURE 7.75 (**A**) A grade 1 MCL associated with a medial retinaculum tear at the level of the proximal MCL. This axial image is inferior to the origin of the MPFL. (**B**) A full thickness chondral erosion is shown on sagittal FS PD FSE image.

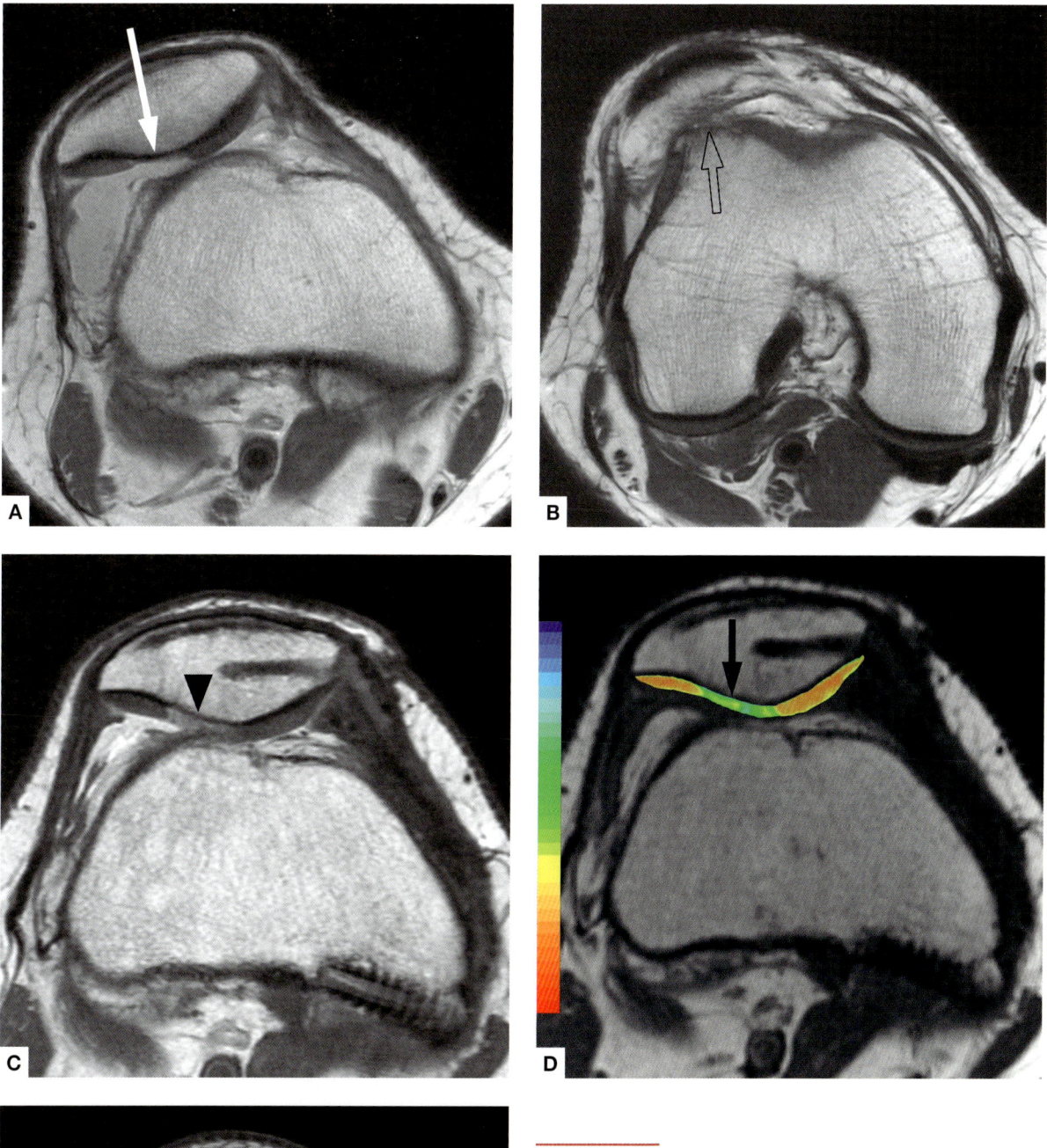

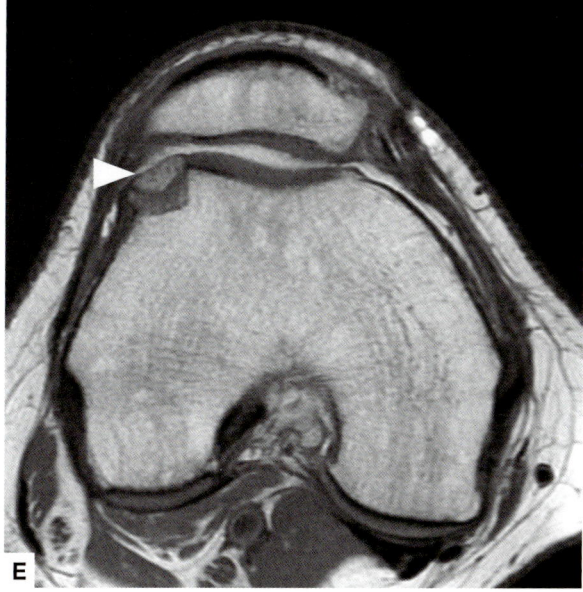

FIGURE 7.76 Cartilage repair for chronic patellofemoral instability in a 26-year-old woman. **(A, B)** Axial fast spin-echo MR images of the knee demonstrate full thickness chondral loss over the lateral patella facet extending to the median ridge (*white arrow*) and over the lateral margin of the trochlea (*open arrow*). **(C)** Axial fast spin-echo MR image 6 months following medial patellofemoral ligament reconstruction, tibial transfer, cell-based cartilage repair in the patella, and trochlea repair using a synthetic biphasic acellular copolymer scaffold. There has been progressive fill of the cartilage repair within the lateral patellar facet (*black arrowhead*). **(D)** Corresponding quantitative T2 relaxation map shows prolongation of T2 values (*black arrow*), with no matrix stratification typical of hyaline like repair. **(E)** Grayscale image of the trochlea demonstrates the biphasic nature of the scaffold (*white arrowhead*). (*Continued*)

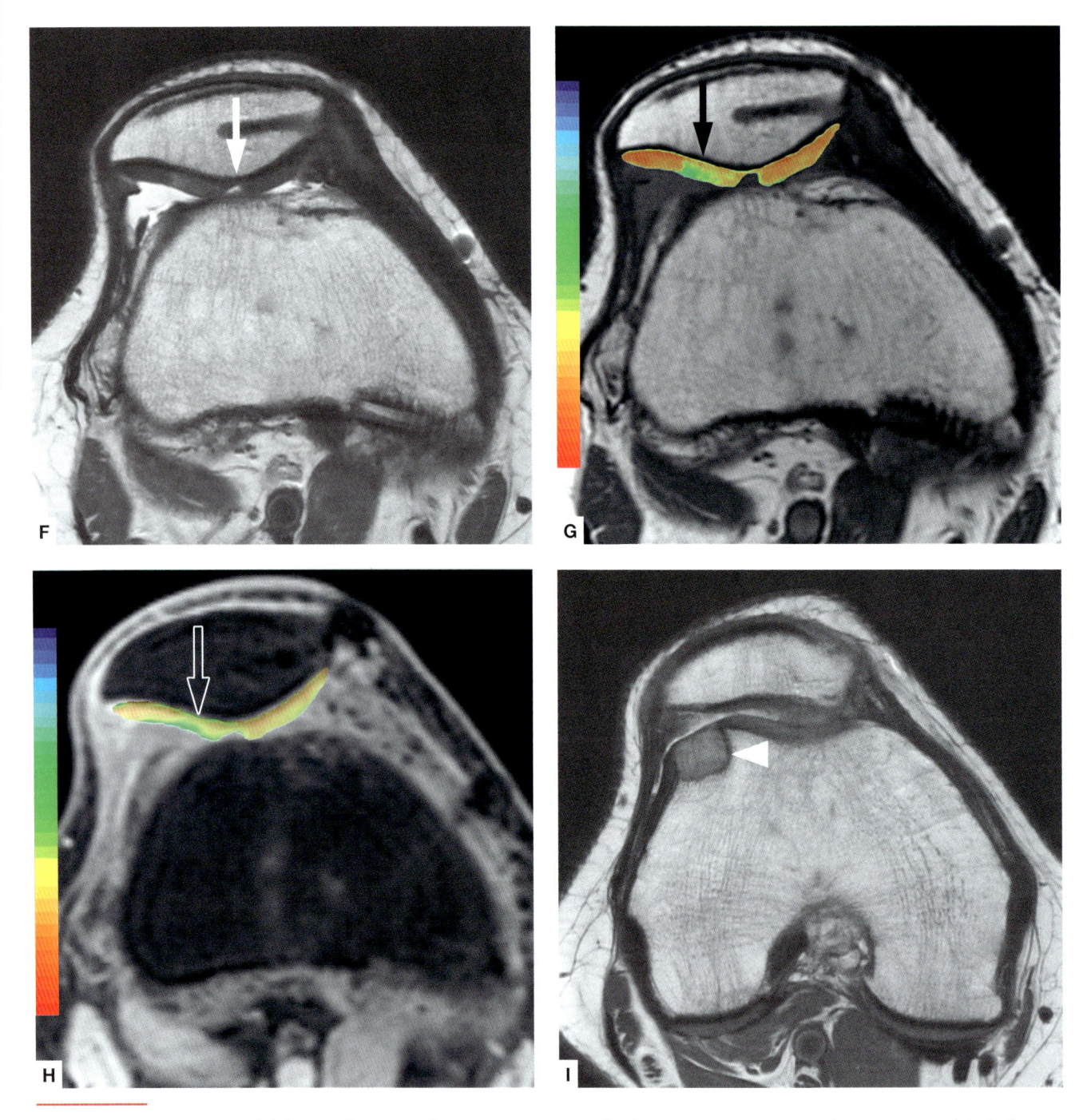

FIGURE 7.76 *(Continued)* **(F)** Axial fast spin-echo MR image 12 months following chondral repair demonstrates a full thickness chondral defect at the patellar apex (*white arrow*). **(G)** Corresponding T2 relaxation map demonstrates prolongation (*black arrow*) of T2 relaxation times. There is persistent lack of stratification on the T2 map indicative of disorganized immature repair tissue. **(H)** T1rho map shows prolonged T1rho relaxation times (*open arrow*). **(I)** The grayscale image of the synthetic plug demonstrates progressive bone ingrowth in the bone phase (*white arrowhead*) but no stratification of the cartilage repair phase. (Courtesy of Hollis G. Potter, M.D., Hospital for Special Surgery, New York, NY.)

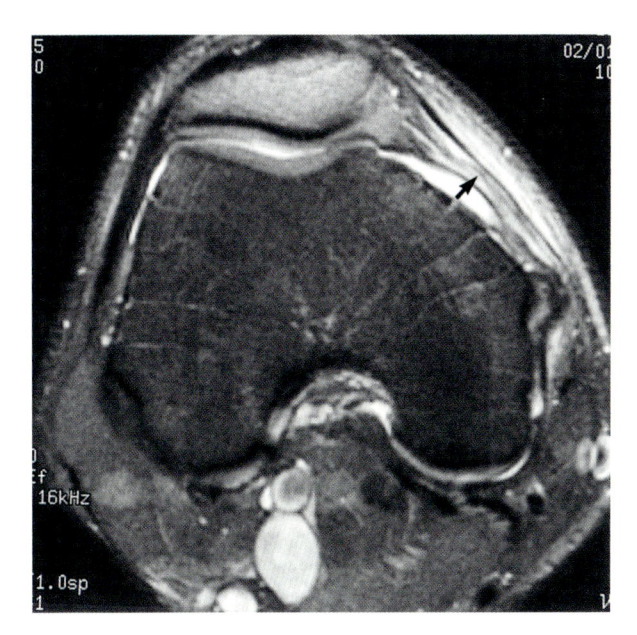

Patellofemoral Joint and the Extensor Mechanism

FIGURE 7.77 A partially torn medial retinaculum (*arrow*) displays thickening and hyperintensity on an FS T2-weighted FSE axial image. Continuity of the retinacular fibers, however, is maintained. The bilaminar morphology of the medial retinaculum is a result of its receiving contributions from both layer 1 and layer 2 fibers.

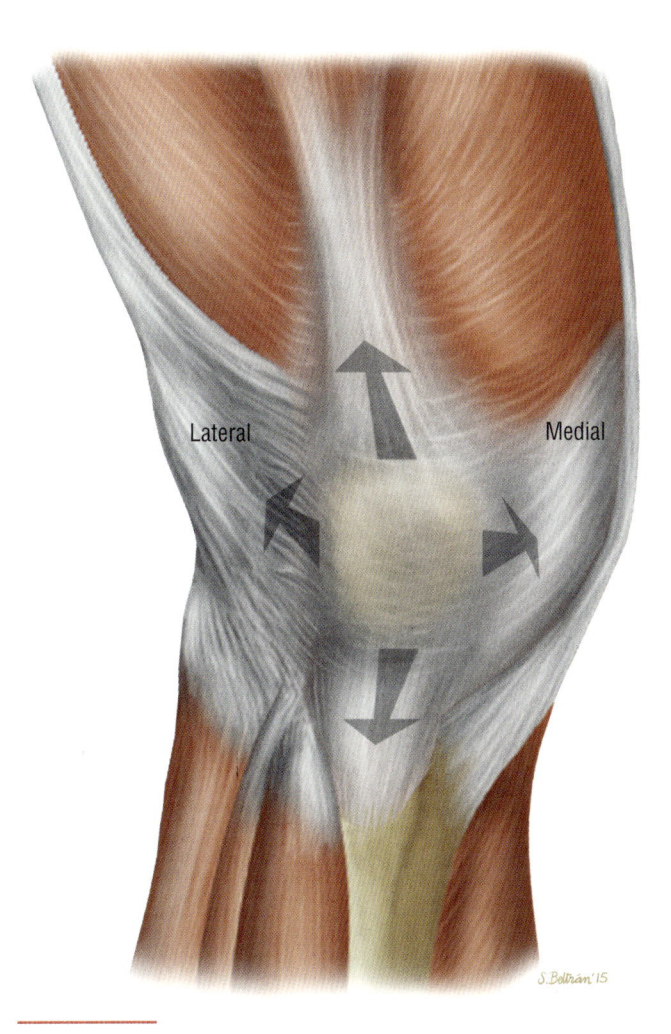

FIGURE 7.78 Stabilization of patella by the opposing forces of the patellar and quadriceps tendon and the medial/lateral retinacular attachments.

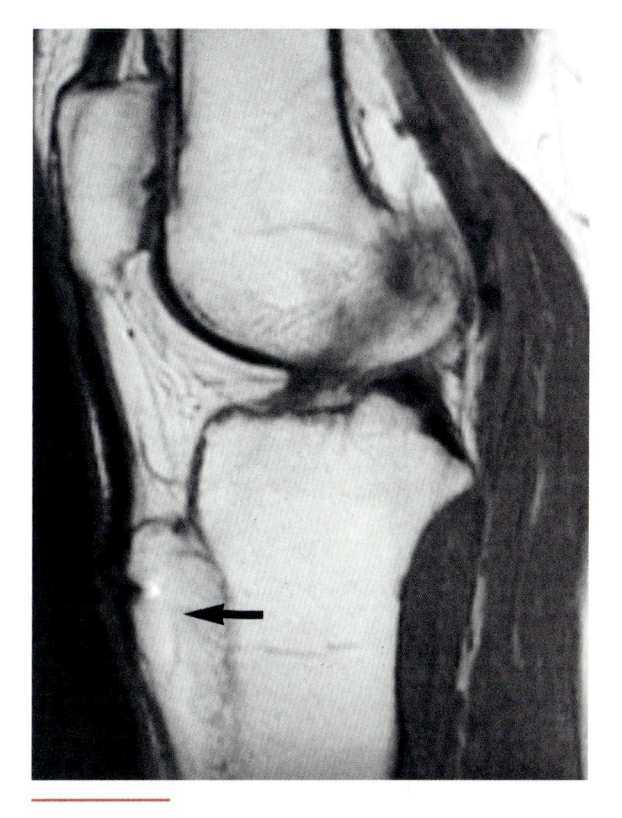

FIGURE 7.79 Maquet's procedure with advancement of the tibial tuberosity by elevation of the tibial crest, as seen on a T1-weighted sagittal image (*arrow*). Distal realignment is performed for patellar instability.

Miserable Malalignment Syndrome

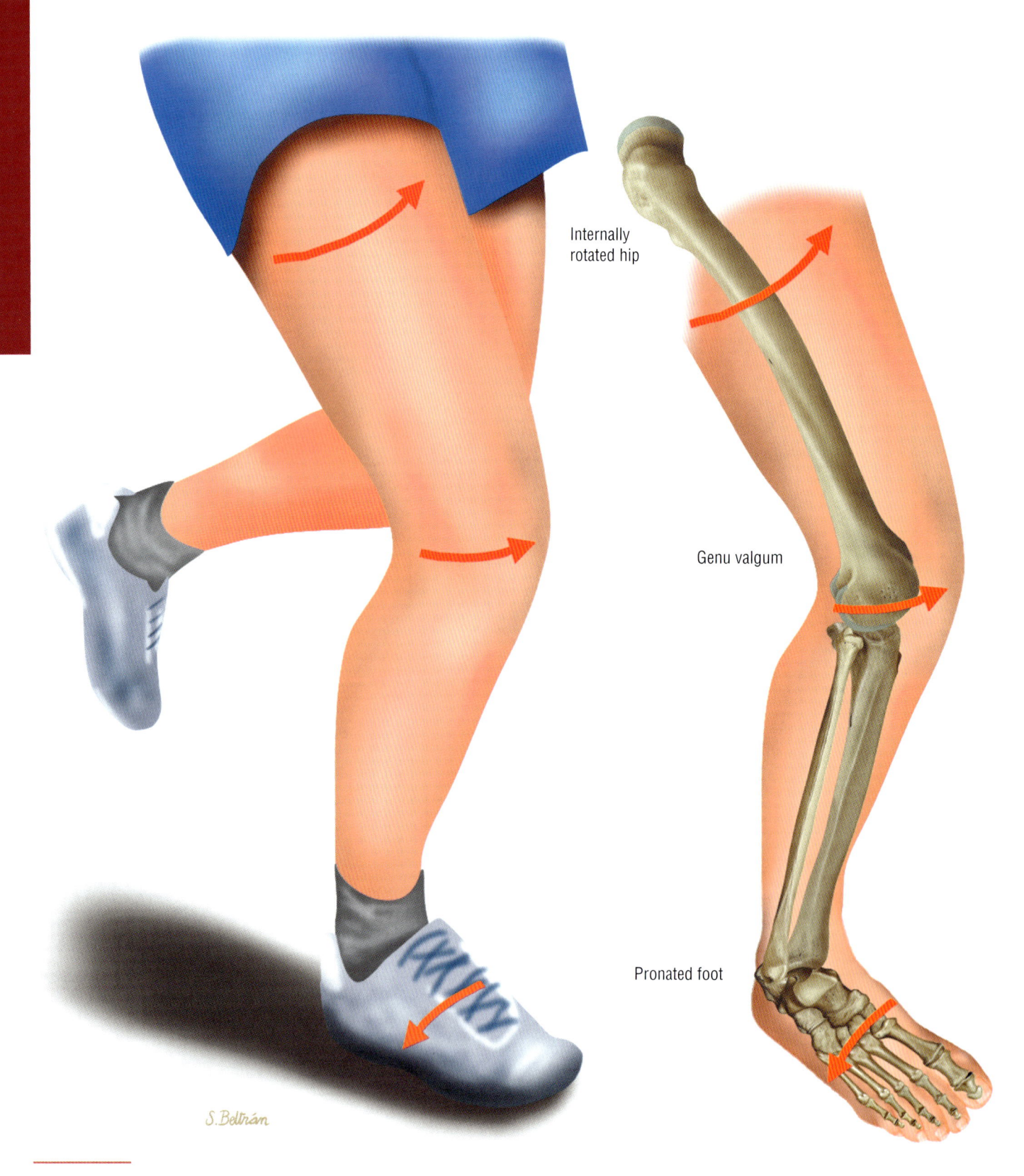

FIGURE 7.80 Miserable malalignment as a cause of anterior knee pain is associated with internal femoral rotation, a valgus knee, and hyperpronation. A hypermobile patella and hypoplastic vastus medialis obliquus (VMO) muscle may also be demonstrated features.

Tibiofibular Joint Dislocation

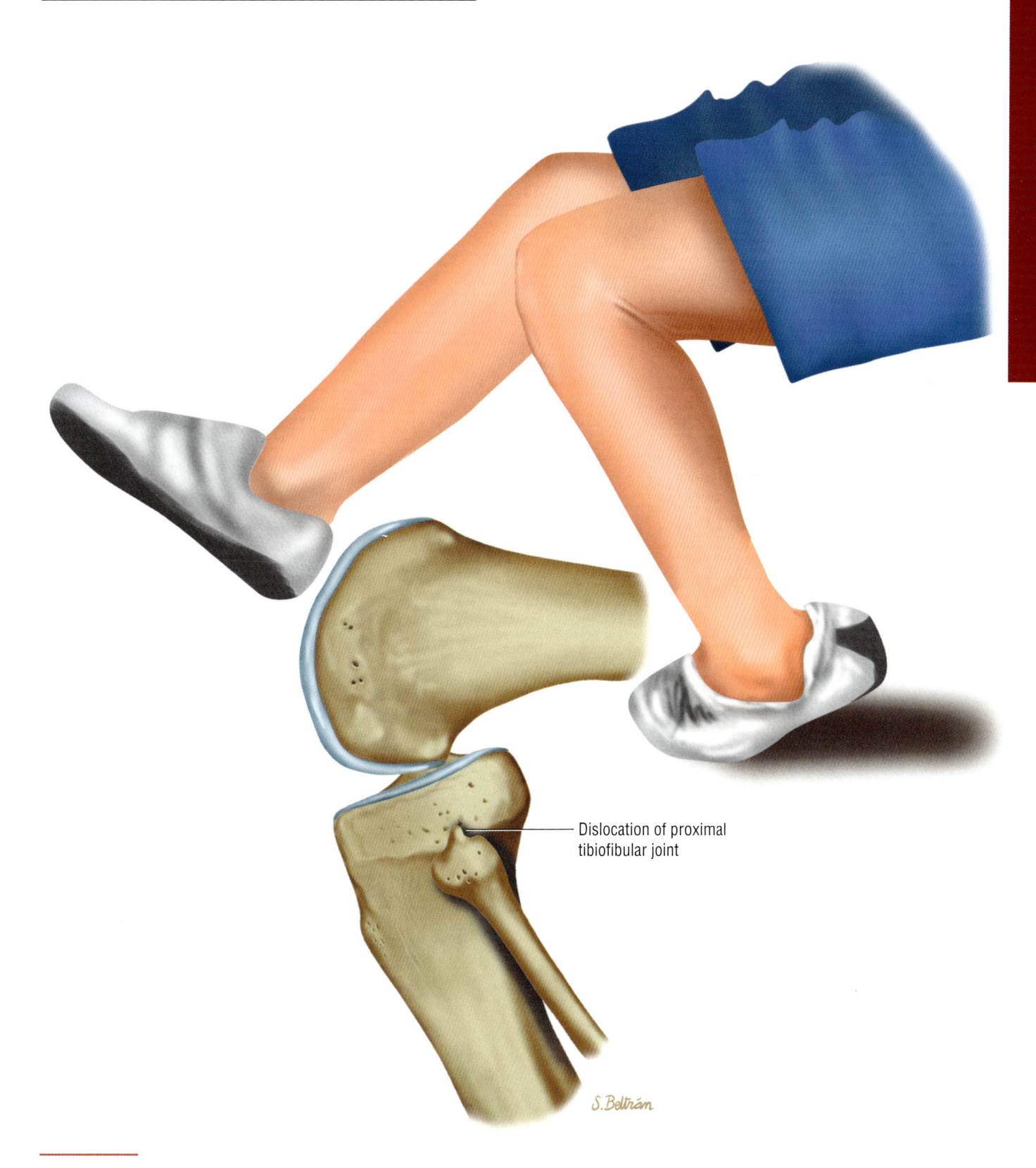

FIGURE 7.81 Dislocation of the proximal tibiofibular joint associated with adduction of the leg with the knee in flexion and a plantarflexed and inverted foot (e.g., soccer-type injury).

Patellofemoral Mechanics

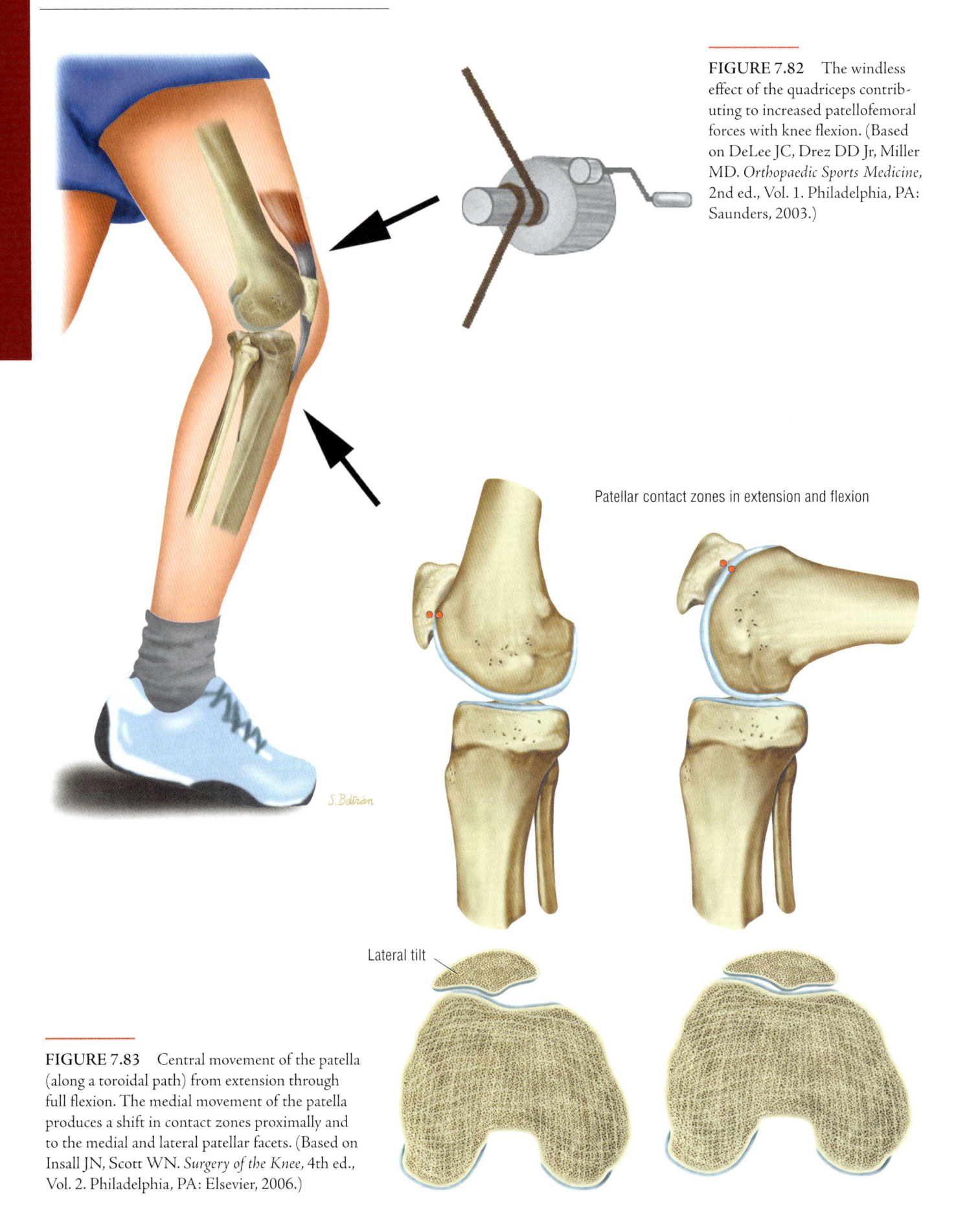

FIGURE 7.82 The windless effect of the quadriceps contributing to increased patellofemoral forces with knee flexion. (Based on DeLee JC, Drez DD Jr, Miller MD. *Orthopaedic Sports Medicine*, 2nd ed., Vol. 1. Philadelphia, PA: Saunders, 2003.)

Patellar contact zones in extension and flexion

Lateral tilt

FIGURE 7.83 Central movement of the patella (along a toroidal path) from extension through full flexion. The medial movement of the patella produces a shift in contact zones proximally and to the medial and lateral patellar facets. (Based on Insall JN, Scott WN. *Surgery of the Knee*, 4th ed., Vol. 2. Philadelphia, PA: Elsevier, 2006.)

Patellofemoral Joint and the Extensor Mechanism 783

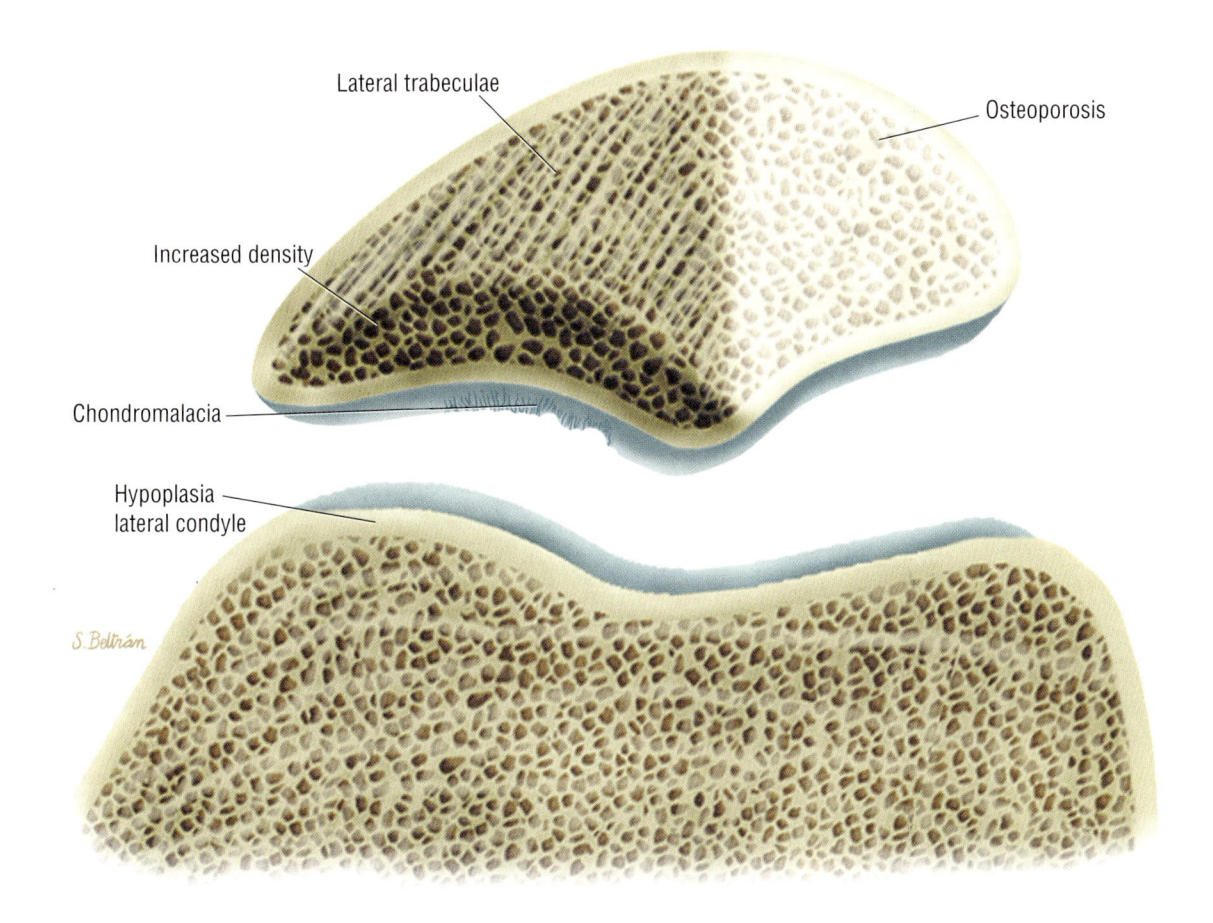

FIGURE 7.84 Excessive lateral pressure findings on radiographs are associated with MR findings of lateral facet subchondral edema and chondromalacia along with edema of the proximal lateral aspect of Hoffa's fat pad. (Based on DeLee JC, Drez DD Jr, Miller MD. *Orthopaedic Sports Medicine*, 2nd ed., Vol. 1. Philadelphia, PA: Saunders, 2003.)

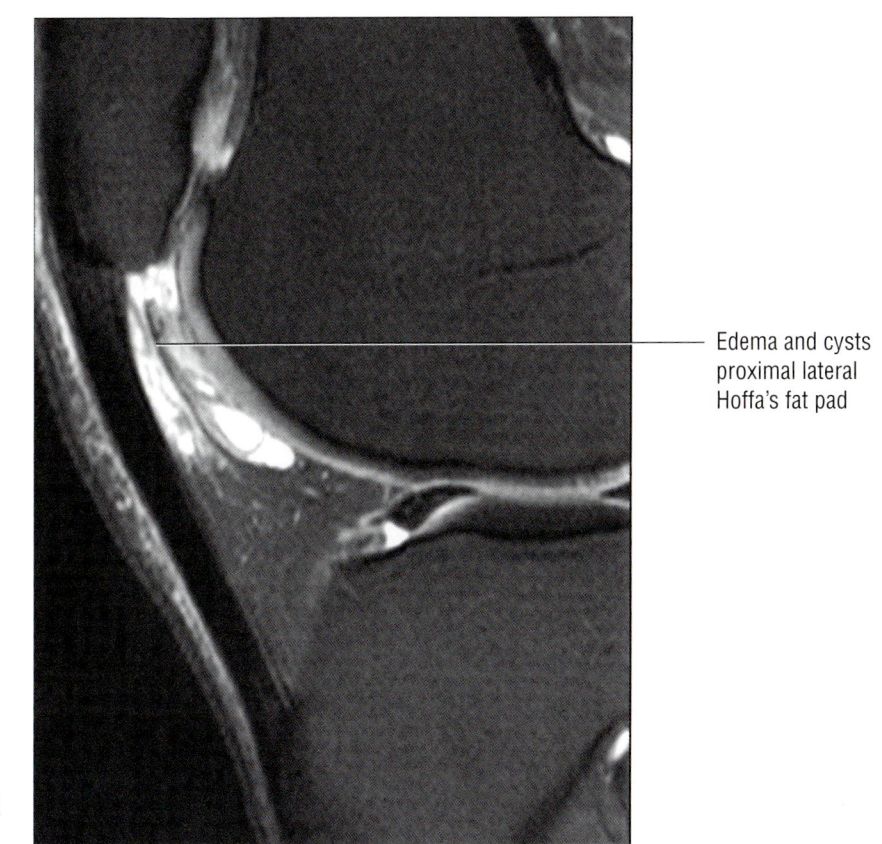

FIGURE 7.85 Edema of the superolateral aspect of Hoffa's fat pad is an indicator of potential maltracking and is associated with excessive lateral pressure. Sagittal FS PD FSE image.

Lateral Retinaculum and Illiotibial Band

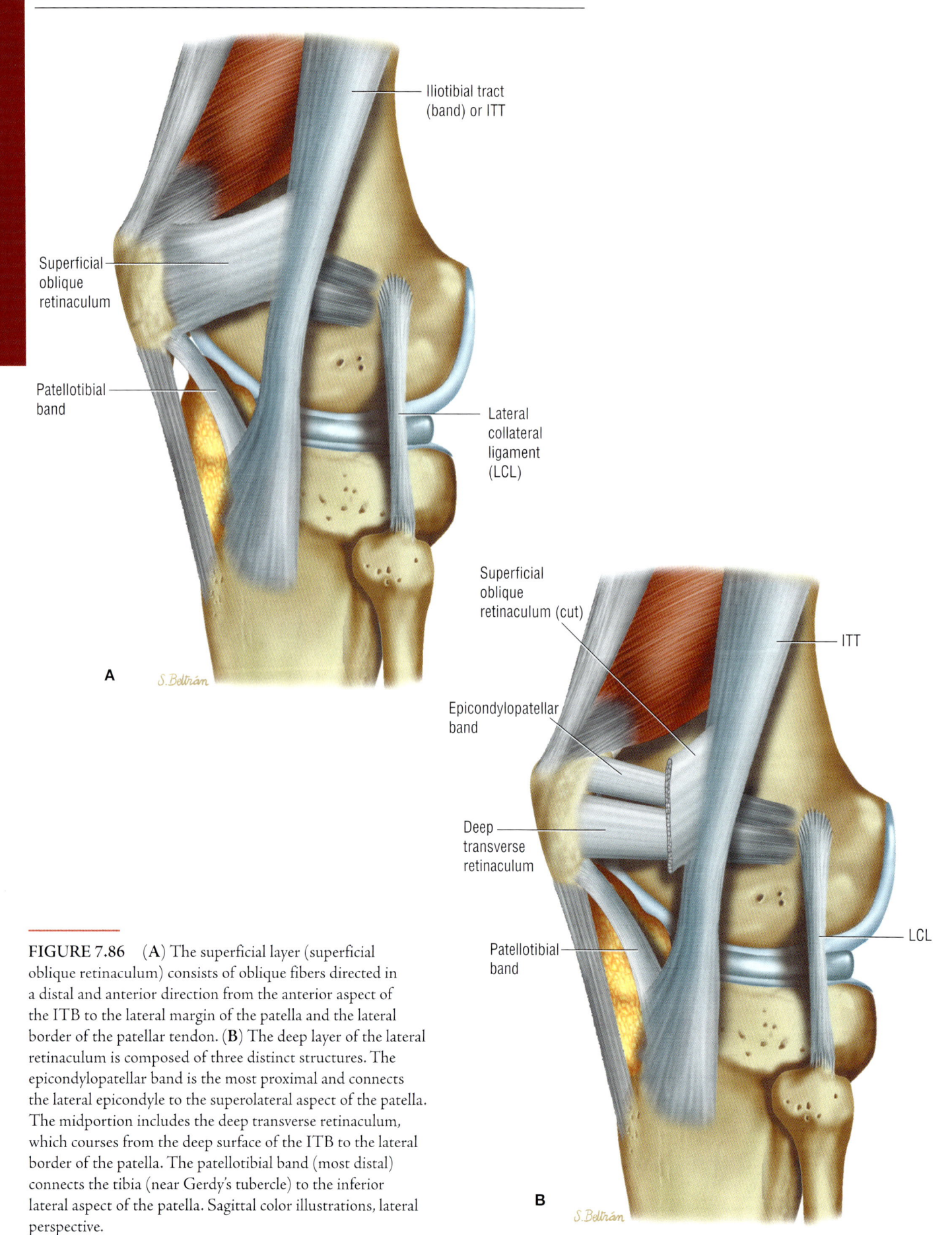

FIGURE 7.86 (A) The superficial layer (superficial oblique retinaculum) consists of oblique fibers directed in a distal and anterior direction from the anterior aspect of the ITB to the lateral margin of the patella and the lateral border of the patellar tendon. (B) The deep layer of the lateral retinaculum is composed of three distinct structures. The epicondylopatellar band is the most proximal and connects the lateral epicondyle to the superolateral aspect of the patella. The midportion includes the deep transverse retinaculum, which courses from the deep surface of the ITB to the lateral border of the patella. The patellotibial band (most distal) connects the tibia (near Gerdy's tubercle) to the inferior lateral aspect of the patella. Sagittal color illustrations, lateral perspective.

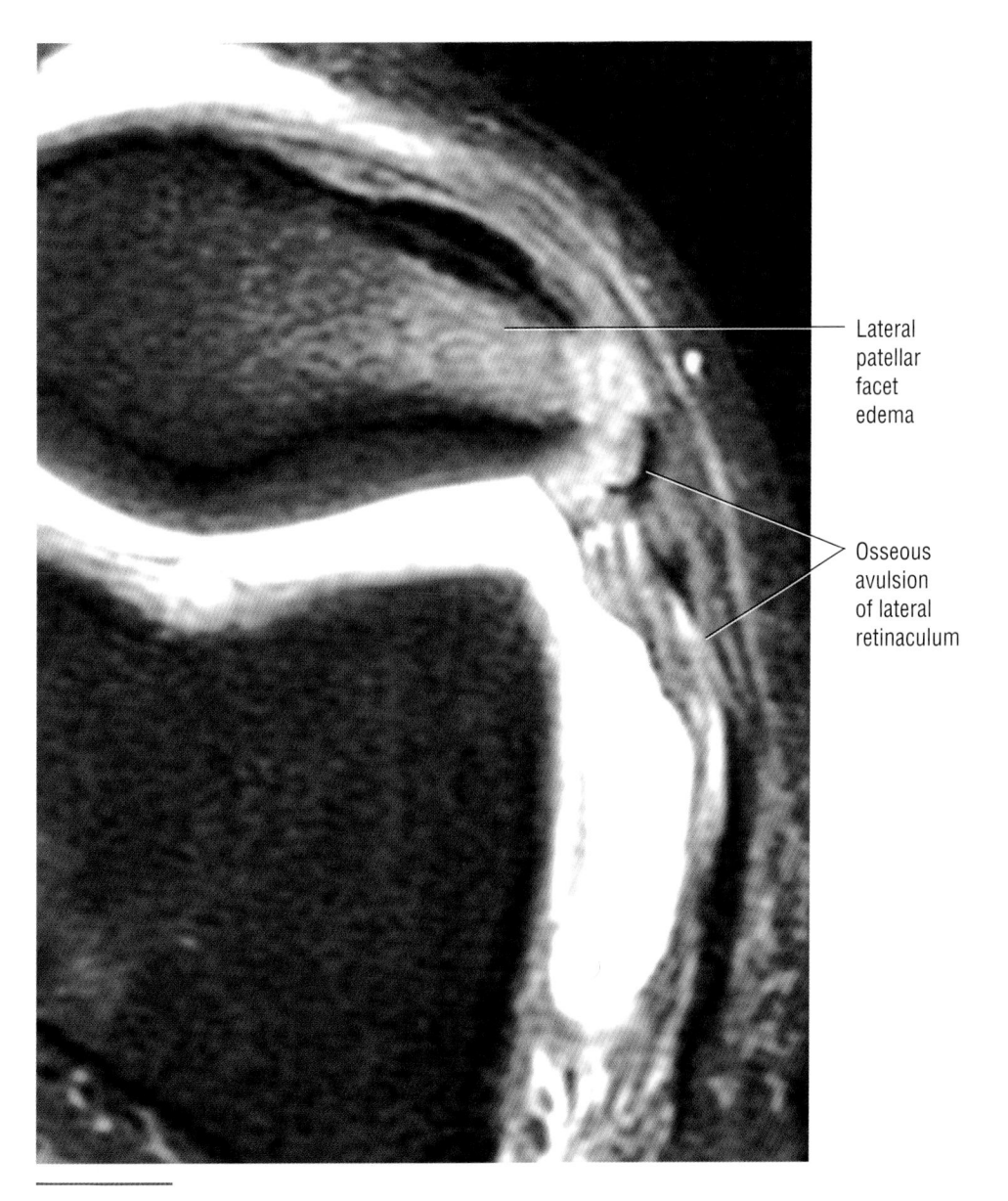

FIGURE 7.87 Osseous avulsion of the lateral retinacular attachment to the lateral patellar facet, which occurred in association with ACL trauma.

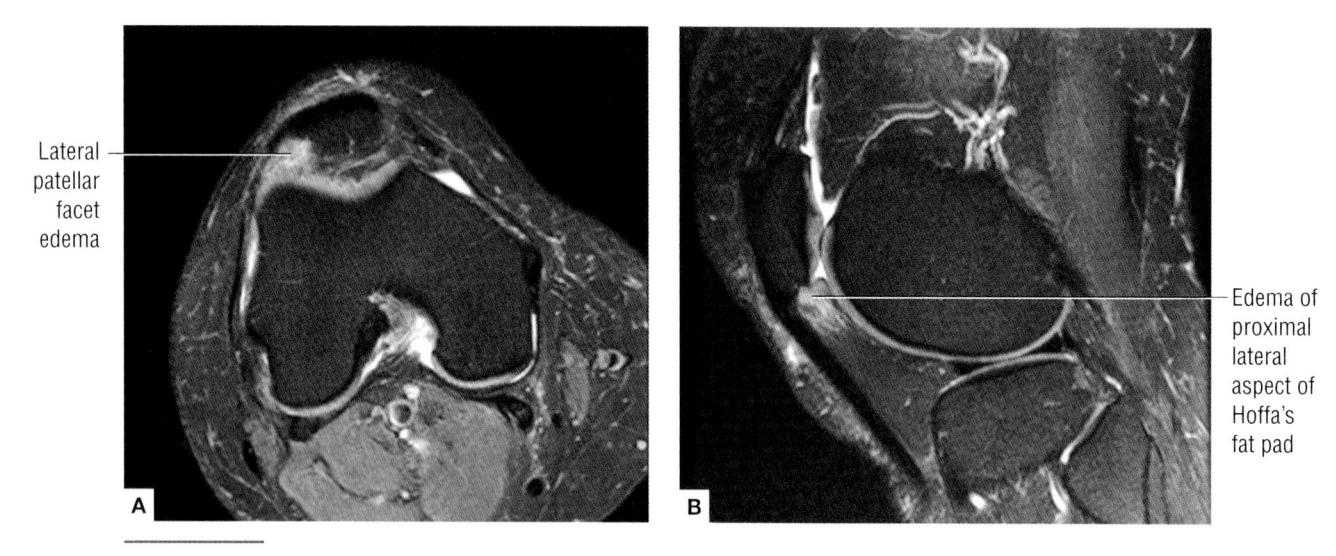

FIGURE 7.88 (**A**) Axial and (**B**) sagittal FS PD FSE images showing the excessive lateral pressure syndrome (ELPS) with articular cartilage breakdown involving the lateral facet (**A**) and edema of the proximal portion of Hoffa's fat pad (**B**).

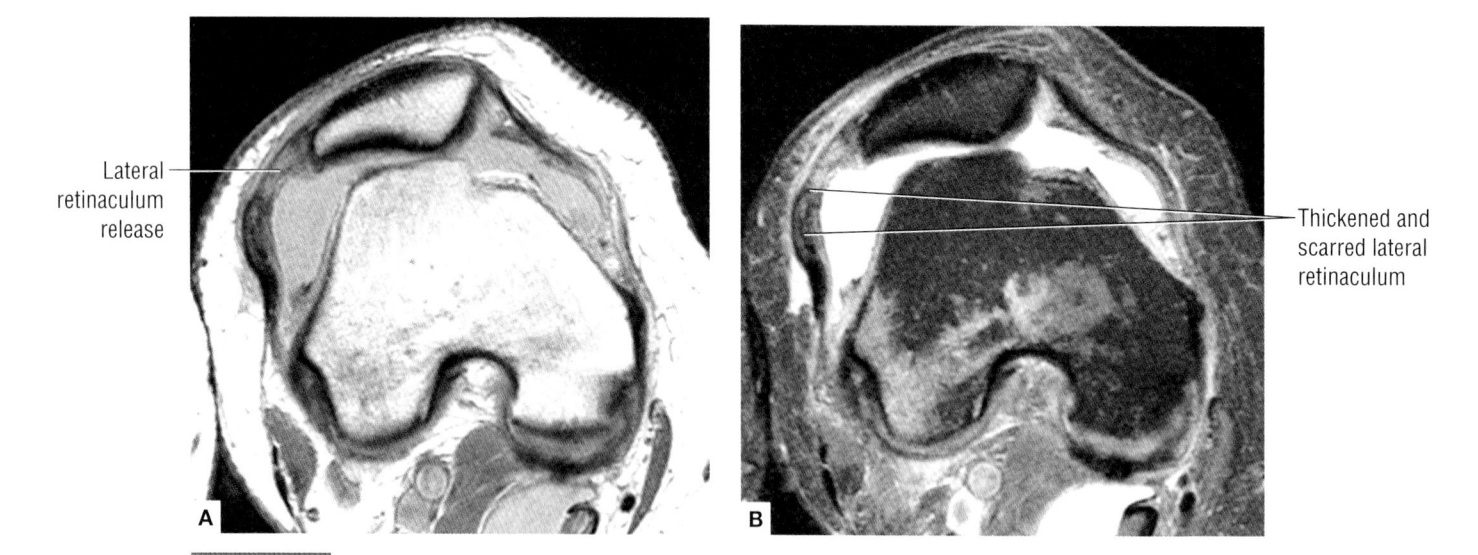

FIGURE 7.89 (**A**) Axial PD FSE and (**B**) axial FS PD FSE images showing lateral release with thickened and scarred lateral retinaculum. Note residual lateral subluxation and attenuated lateral patellar facet articular cartilage. A lateral retinacular release spares the main tendon of the vastus lateralis and sections the lateral retinaculum and the tendon of the vastus lateralis obliquus.

Iliotibial Band Syndrome

Key Concepts

- Chronic functional trauma from ITB rubbing on outer aspect of lateral femoral condyle
- FS PD FSE used to identify thickened synovium with variable degrees of inflammation within lateral synovial recess
- Thickening and signal heterogeneity of ITB visualized on anterior coronal images

Iliotibial Band Syndrome

- *Iliotibial tract* (ITT) or *band* (ITB)
    - Distal tendon of the tensor fascia lata
    - Separate from lateral retinaculum
    - Anterior to femoral epicondyle in full extension
    - Rides over lateral epicondyle in flexion
- *ITB friction syndrome*
    - Chronic inflammation proximal to insertion of ITB onto the anterolateral tibia (Gerdy's tubercle)
    - Usually seen in long-distance runners, cyclists, football players, and weight lifters
    - Causes can be either extrinsic (related to training technique) or intrinsic (related to patient's anatomic alignment).
    - Basis of syndrome is friction and inflammation between ITB and anterolateral femoral condyle.[345]
    - FS PD FSE images show high signal intensity deep to ITB and lateral to lateral femoral condyle.
    - Superficial soft tissue edema may also be seen.
    - ITB may become thickened and demonstrate internal signal heterogeneity.
    - Less frequently, distal ITB may demonstrate thickening and reactive adjacent soft tissue and osseous inflammation.
    - Circumscribed or cystic fluid collections are less common than poorly defined signal changes of the fatty tissue deep to the ITB.[338]

- *Lateral synovial recess*
    - Adventitial bursal extension from synovial capsule deep to ITB and superficial to lateral femoral condyle
    - Can be visualized arthroscopically
    - Only demonstrates inflammation or distention with fluid in the presence of ITB syndrome
- Newer theories attribute cause of inflammation in ITB syndrome to dynamic changes in knee flexion, and *not* primary inflammation of a bursa.
    - These theories account for more common presentation of edema with poorly defined margins deep to the ITB.

Clinical Presentation and Assessment

- Point tenderness or pain 3cm proximal to lateral joint line (superficial to lateral femoral epicondyle)
- Symptoms usually progressive, occurring after 2 to 3 miles of running
- Often asymptomatic at rest
- *Ober's test*
    - Used to assess ITB tightness
    - Affected knee is flexed to 90 degrees with ipsilateral hip abduction and hyperextension.
    - If tightness present, leg remains elevated secondary to shortening of ITB
- *Noble's test*
    - Performed with patient lying supine with knee flexed 90 degrees
    - Pain at 30 to 40 degrees of flexion with applied pressure to ITB during knee extension is considered a positive test.

Treatment

- Conservative therapy with resolution of symptoms associated with cessation of the inciting activity
- Steroid injection into painful site and use of orthotics often eliminate frictional trauma.

Patellofemoral Joint and the Extensor Mechanism

Illiotibial Band

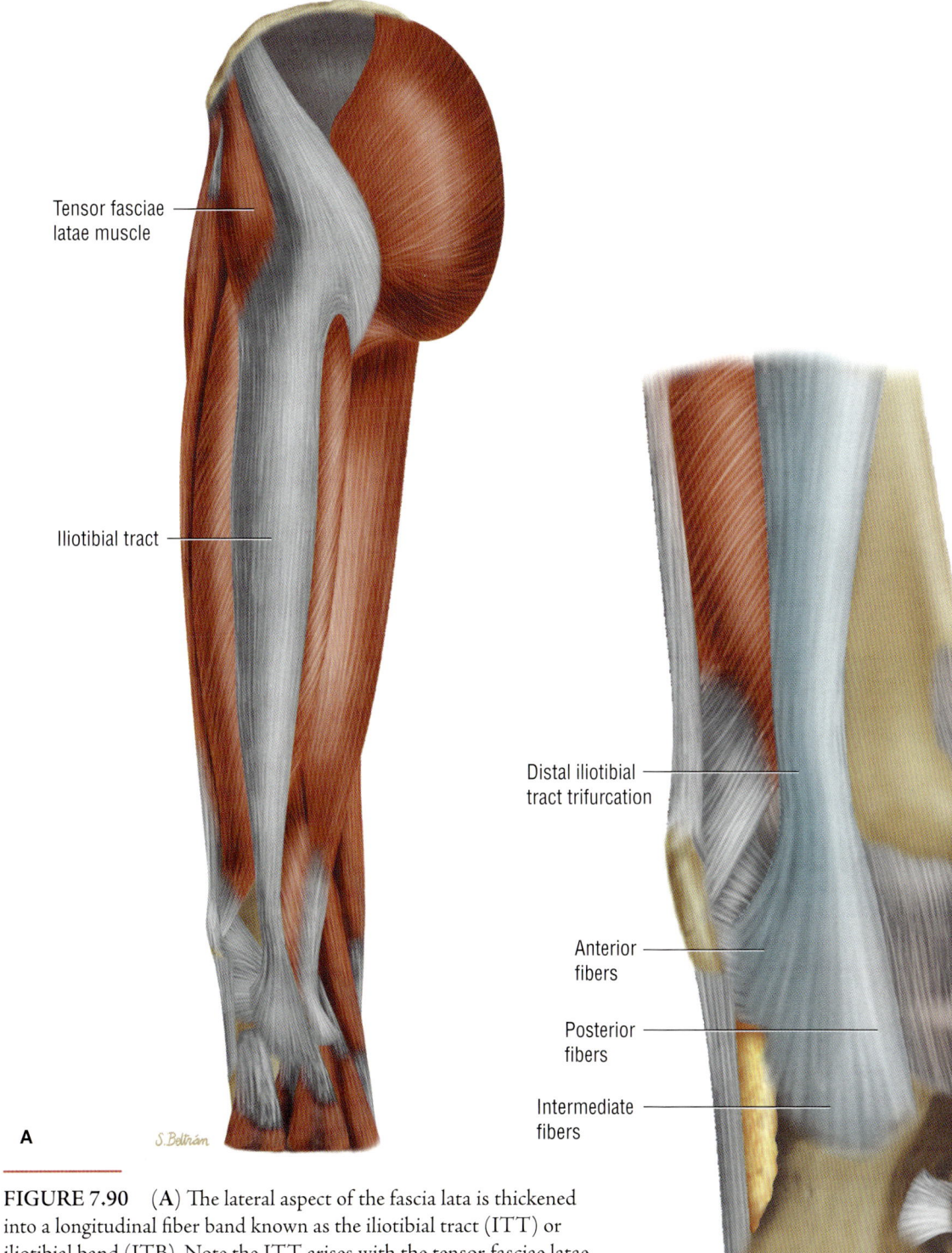

FIGURE 7.90 (A) The lateral aspect of the fascia lata is thickened into a longitudinal fiber band known as the iliotibial tract (ITT) or iliotibial band (ITB). Note the ITT arises with the tensor fasciae latae from the anterior superior iliac spine. Chronic inflammation deep to the ITT may result from the formation of a secondary or adventitious bursa instead of inflammation of a primary bursa. (B) The distal fibers of the ITT divide into anterior intermediate and posterior portions. The anterior fibers blend with the lateral retinaculum, and the posterior fibers join with distal biceps femoris expansions into crural fascia. The midportion, corresponding to the intermediate fibers of the distal ITT trifurcation, extends distally to insert anterolaterally on Gerdy's tubercle.

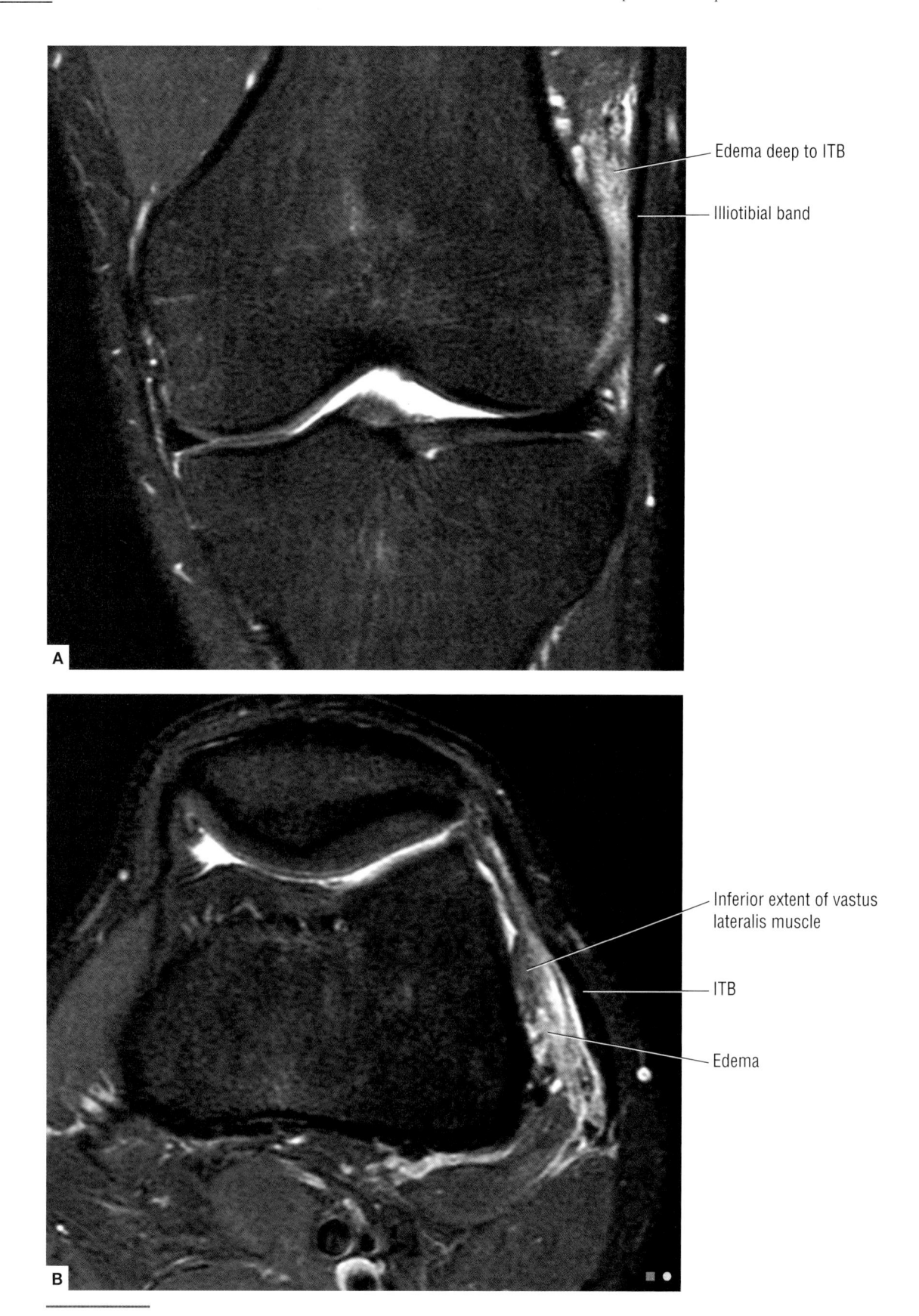

FIGURE 7.91 ITB friction syndrome may be related to compression of the highly innervated and vascularized fat between the ITB and the epicondyle and not just direct friction of the ITB over the epicondyle. Coronal (**A**) and axial (**B**) FS PD FSE images.

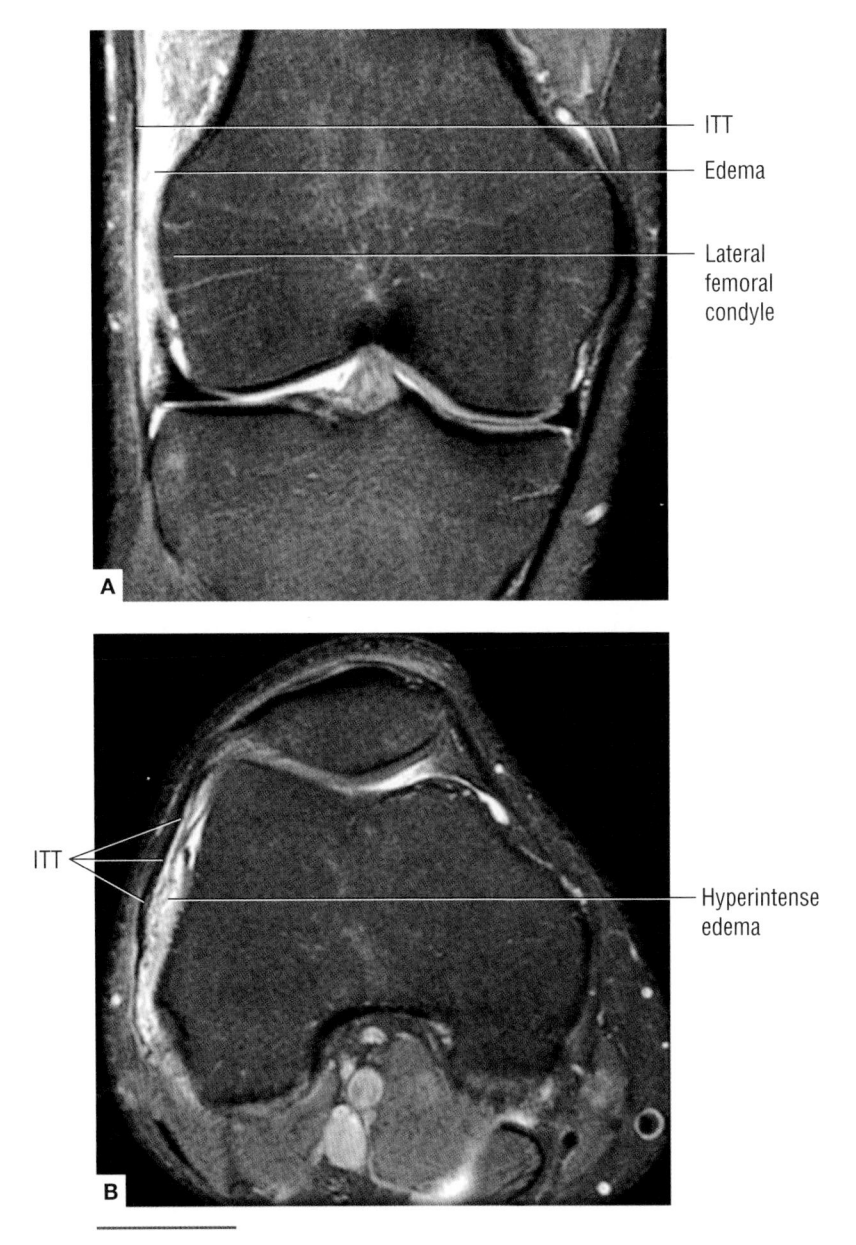

FIGURE 7.92 (**A**) Coronal FS PD FSE. (**B**) Axial FS PD FSE. There is compartmentalization of the soft tissue edema between the ITT, the meniscocapsular junction of the lateral meniscus, the lateral collateral ligament, the lateral femoral epicondyle, the fatty soft tissue distal to the vastus lateralis muscle, and the biceps femoris muscle posterolaterally.

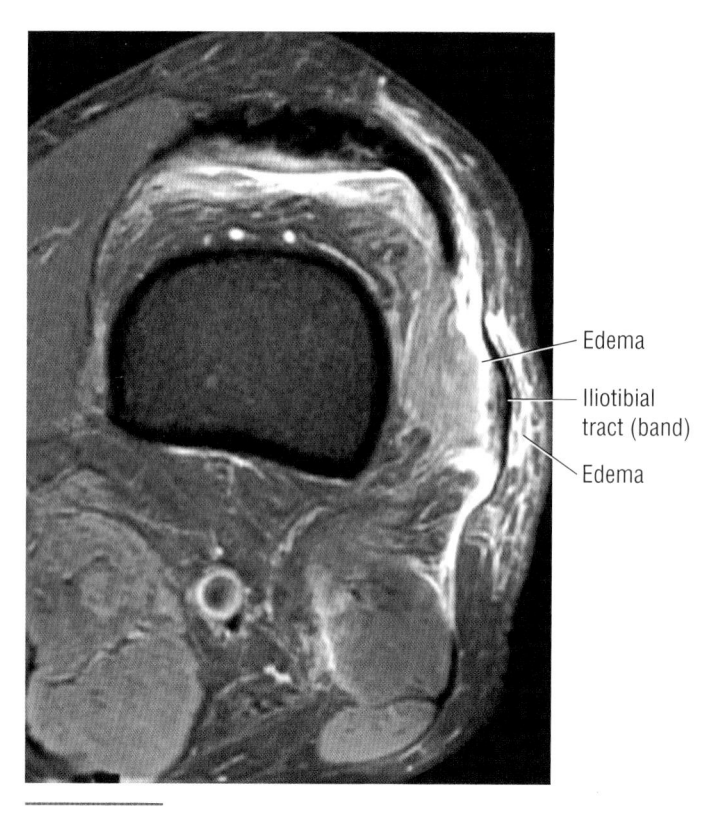

FIGURE 7.93 Extension of edema both superficial and deep to the ITT can be seen on this axial FS PD FSE image.

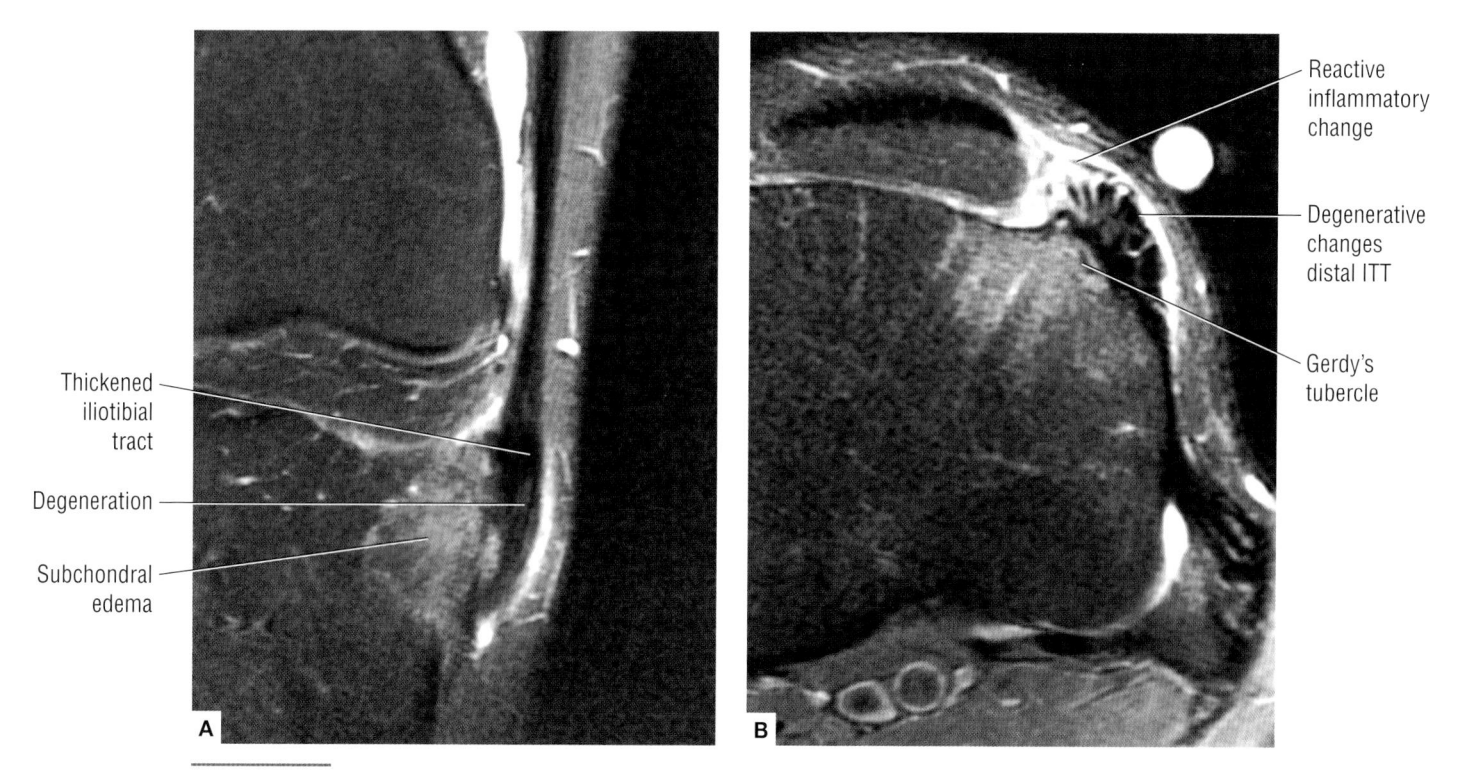

FIGURE 7.94 (**A**) Coronal and (**B**) axial FS PD FSE images displaying a thickened distal ITT with associated superficial edema and reactive proximal tibial edema at Gerdy's tubercle. Hyperintensity superficial to the ITT (ITB) is less common. Thickening of the ITT demonstrates superimposed chronic changes of ITB syndrome in addition to the more acute inflammatory changes.

Patellofemoral Joint and the Extensor Mechanism

Illiotibial Band Syndrome

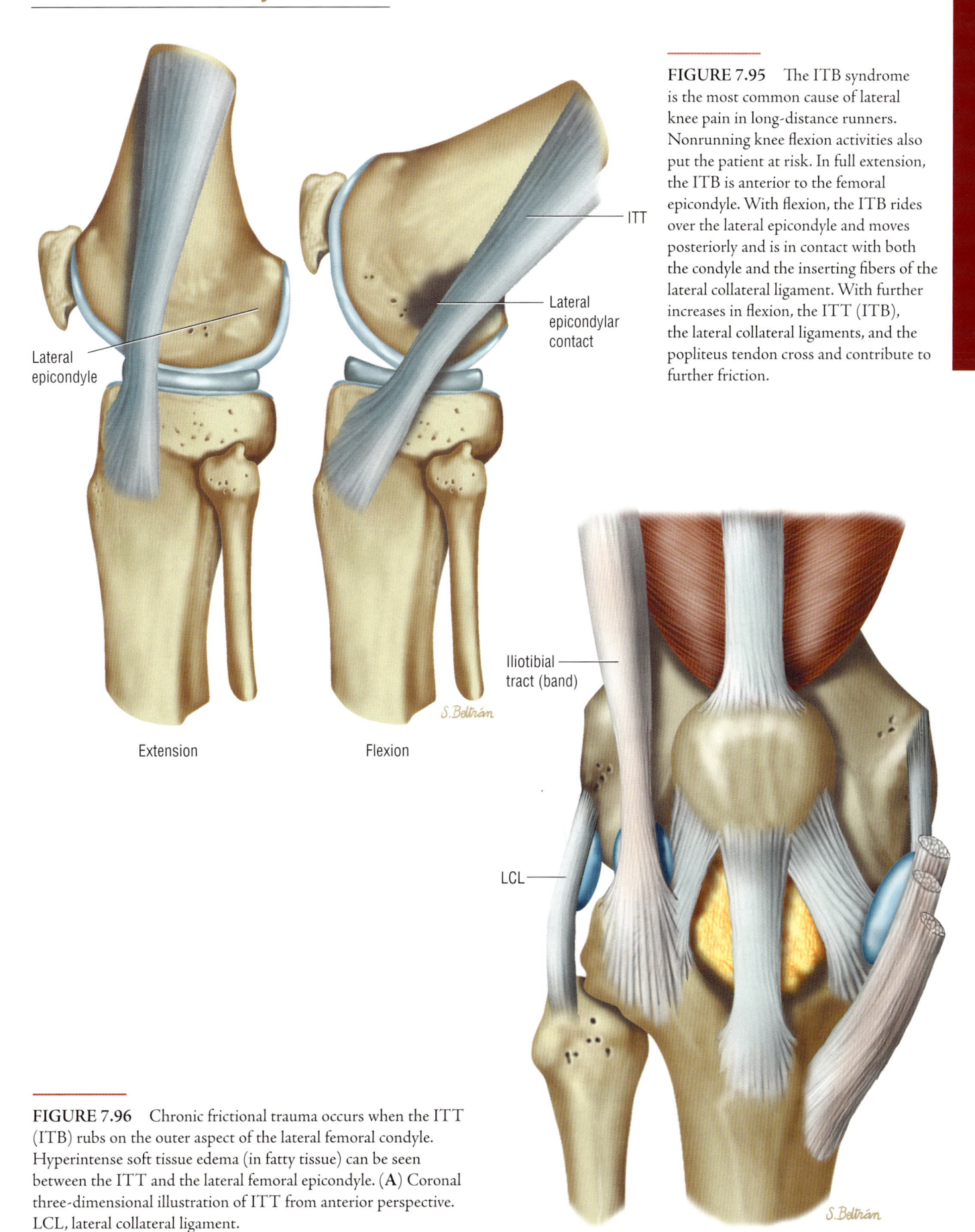

Extension

Flexion

FIGURE 7.95 The ITB syndrome is the most common cause of lateral knee pain in long-distance runners. Nonrunning knee flexion activities also put the patient at risk. In full extension, the ITB is anterior to the femoral epicondyle. With flexion, the ITB rides over the lateral epicondyle and moves posteriorly and is in contact with both the condyle and the inserting fibers of the lateral collateral ligament. With further increases in flexion, the ITT (ITB), the lateral collateral ligaments, and the popliteus tendon cross and contribute to further friction.

FIGURE 7.96 Chronic frictional trauma occurs when the ITT (ITB) rubs on the outer aspect of the lateral femoral condyle. Hyperintense soft tissue edema (in fatty tissue) can be seen between the ITT and the lateral femoral epicondyle. (**A**) Coronal three-dimensional illustration of ITT from anterior perspective. LCL, lateral collateral ligament.

Illiotibial Band Syndrome

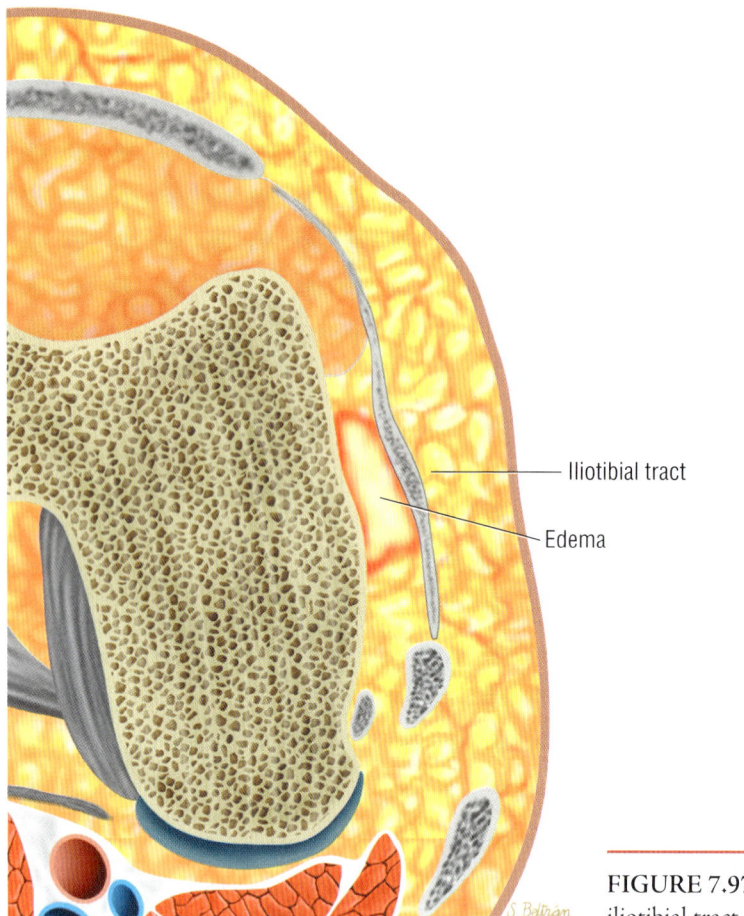

FIGURE 7.97 Localized soft tissue edema deep to the iliotibial tract.

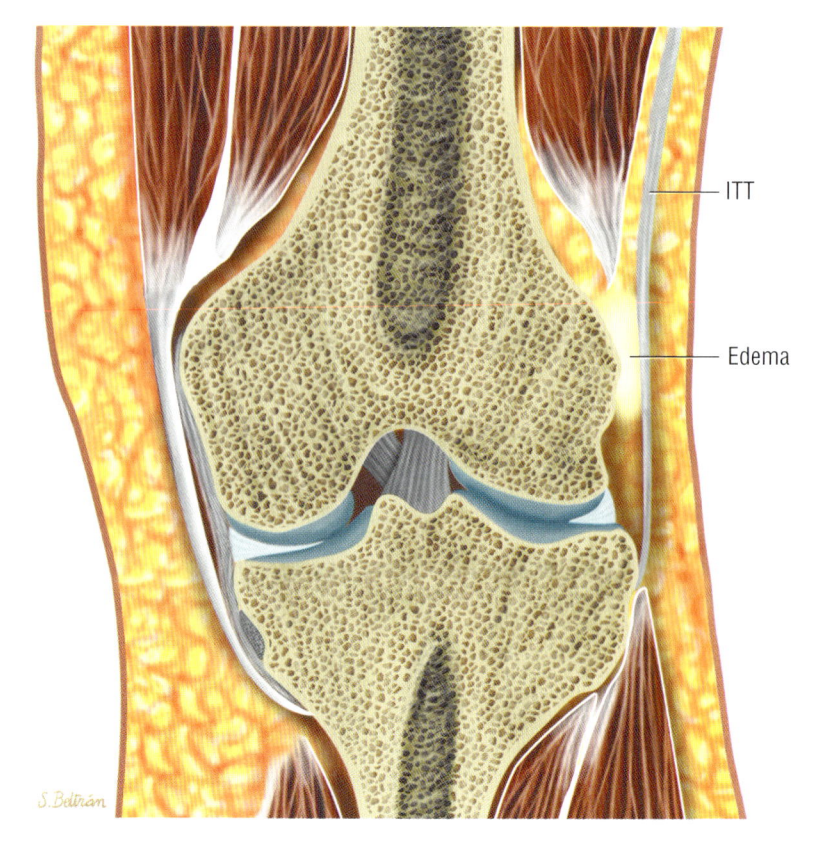

FIGURE 7.98 Edema shown deep to the ITT. Newer theories of the cause of inflammation in the ITB syndrome hold that it is not invagination of the lateral recess of the knee or inflammation of a primary bursa but rather inflammation occurring as a result of dynamic changes during knee flexion. Edema deep to the ITT (ITB) on a color coronal section.

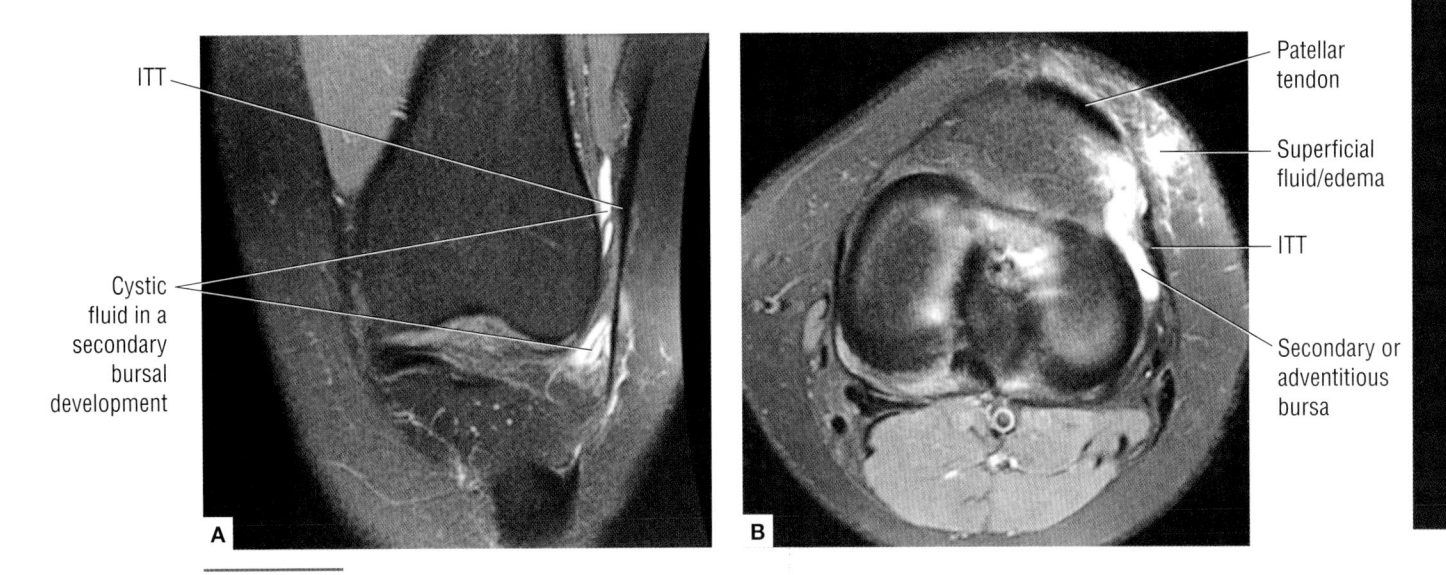

Patellofemoral Joint and the Extensor Mechanism

FIGURE 7.99 Well-defined cystic fluid collections primarily deep to the ITT (ITB) on coronal (**A**) and axial (**B**) FS PD FSE images. These fluid collections do not correspond to a primary bursa but represent formation of a secondary or adventitious bursa.

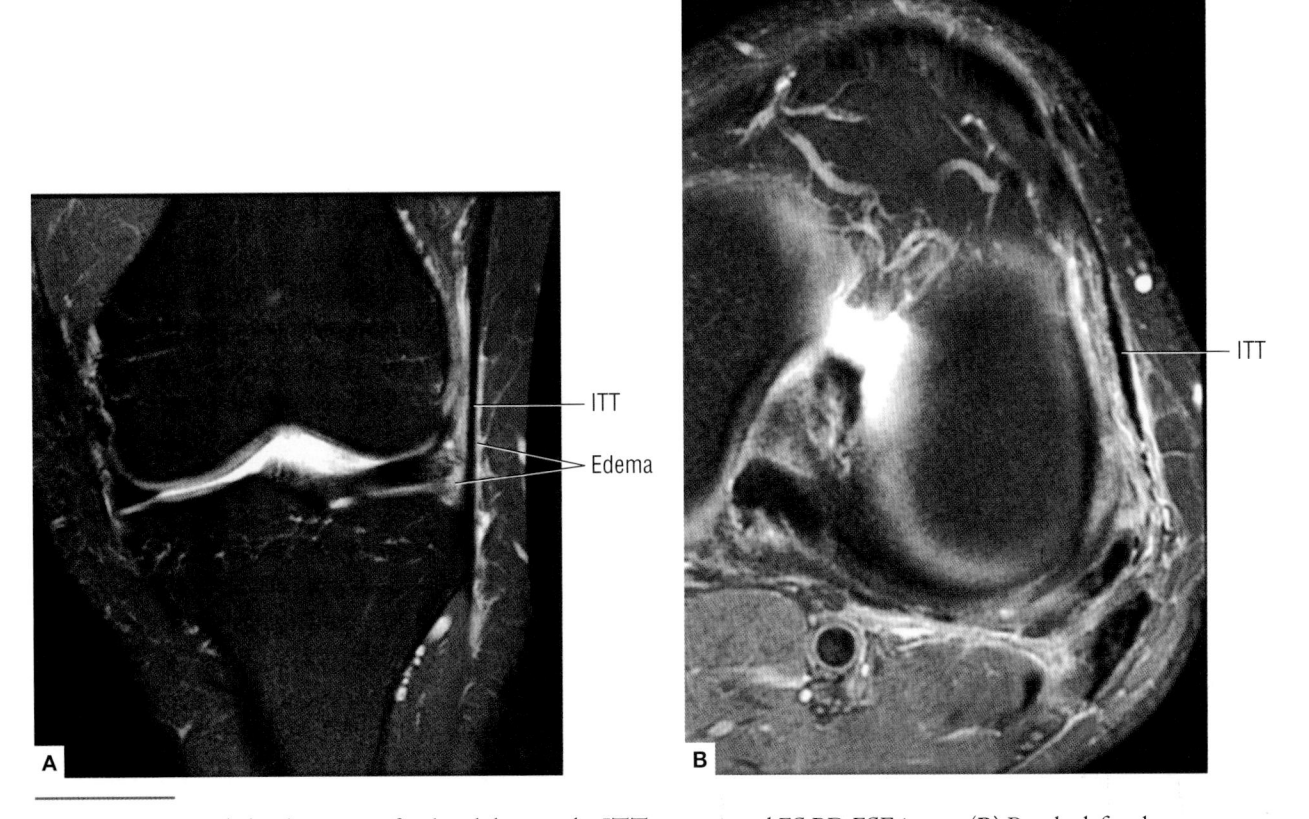

FIGURE 7.100 (**A**) Edema superficial and deep to the ITT on a coronal FS PD FSE image. (**B**) Poorly defined edema associated with ITT fibers and anterior to the biceps tendon on an axial FS PD FSE.

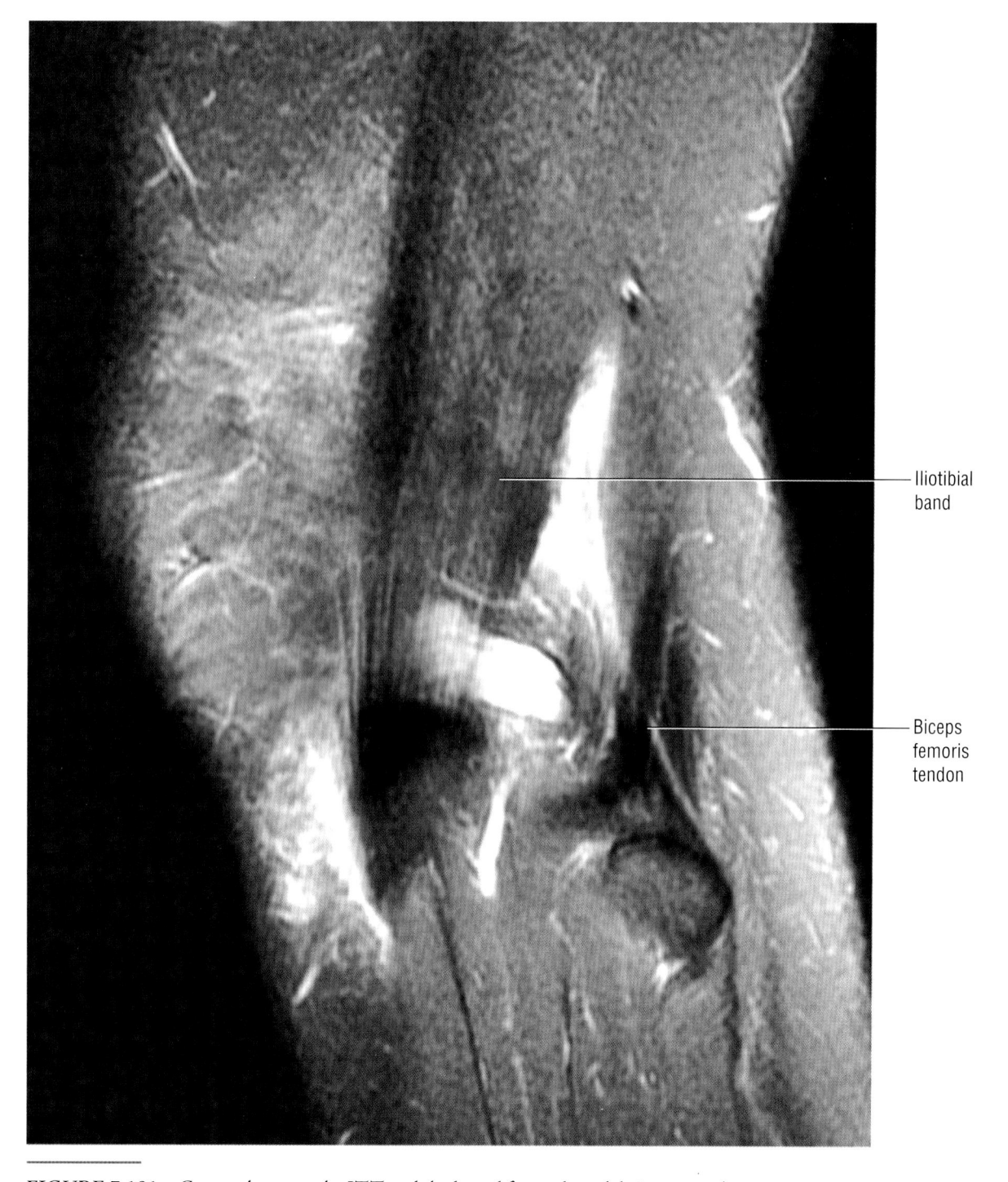

FIGURE 7.101 Contact between the ITT and the lateral femoral condyle is greatest between 20 degrees and 30 degrees. A hypointense band of longitudinal fibers can be seen converging toward the tubercle of Gerdy on this sagittal FS PD FSE image.

Patellofemoral Joint and the Extensor Mechanism

Patellar Tendinosis

Degeneration of proximal posterior fibers

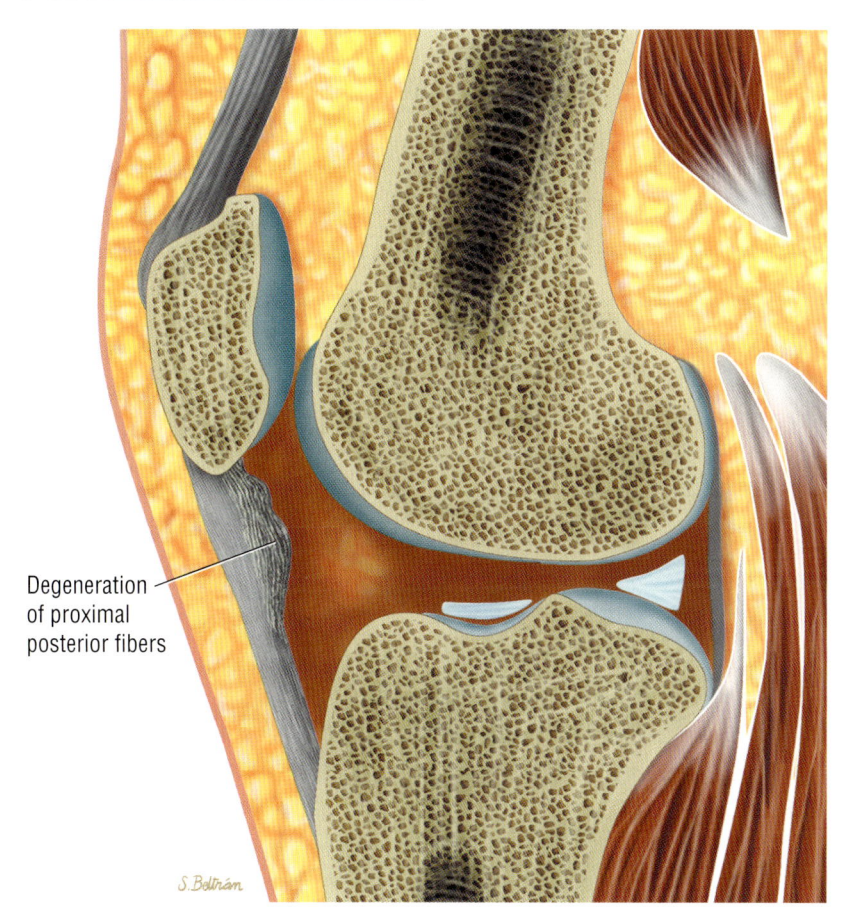

FIGURE 7.102 Patellar tendinosis involving thickening of the proximal posterior fibers. The earliest changes manifest as edema in the peritenon with normal tendon morphology. The tendinitis is a tendinopathy with tendon degeneration and collagen breakdown.

Inferior pole edema

Edema proximal Hoffa's fat pad

Patellar tendon thickening and edema

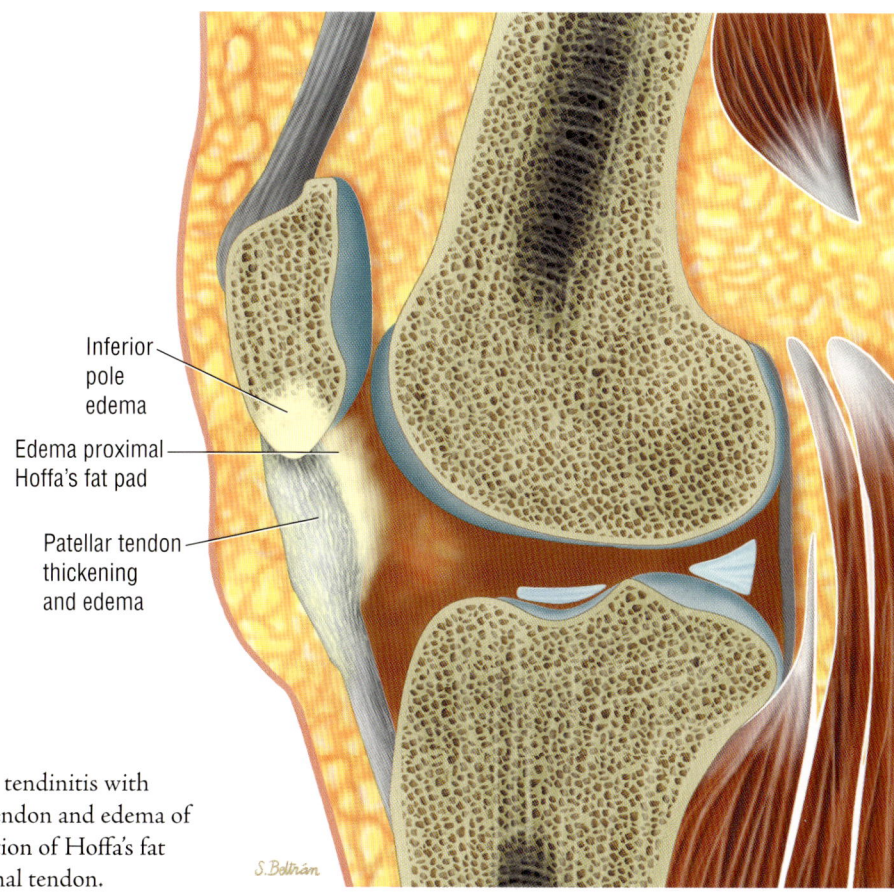

FIGURE 7.103 Advanced changes of patellar tendinitis with edema and thickening of the proximal patellar tendon and edema of the inferior pole of the patella and proximal portion of Hoffa's fat pad adjacent to the posterior fibers of the proximal tendon.

Extensor Mechanism and Patellar Tendon Abnormalities

Patellar Tendinosis

- Most commonly affects proximal posterior (deep) fibers of patellar tendon

- MR imaging findings include thickening or expansion of medial to central tendon fibers and signal hyperintensity of the tendon, adjacent proximal infrapatellar fat pad, and inferior pole of the patella.

- T2* GRE sagittal images are sensitive and specific for identifying patellar tendon collagen degeneration.

- Chronic patellar tendinitis (jumper's knee)

- Causes of inflammatory damage
    - Malalignment, instability, or overuse

- Microtear devitalization and degeneration adjacent to bone–tendon insertion.[483]

- Histologic findings:
    - Collagen degeneration without influx of inflammatory cells (tendinosis)
    - Angiogenesis with endothelial hypoplasia and loss of normal collagen architecture
    - Microtears are associated with collagen fiber separation.
    - Articular and interstitial partial tears are more common than bursal-sided pathology.
    - Affected tendon tissue develops increased levels of cyclooxygenase 2 (COX-2), which affects production of postinflammatory prostaglandins (prostaglandin E2).

MR Findings of Patellar Tendinosis

- Earliest changes are peritenon edema with normal tendon fibers.
- Later, focal thickening in the proximal third of the patellar tendon
- Medial to central portion of tendon most frequently involved[534]
    - Best appreciated on axial images, which demonstrate convexity associated with localized tendon thickening
- More diffuse tendon thickening or enlargement in severe subacute and chronic cases
- Increased signal intensity on T2, FS PD FSE, T2*, and STIR images
- T2*-weighted and STIR sequences tend to show greater tendon hyperintensity than do comparable FSE images before development of chronic tears associated with inflammation and necrosis.
- Posterior tendon margin poorly defined at level of thickening, while low-signal-intensity anterior border may be preserved
- Areas of increased signal intensity correspond to tenocyte hyperplasia, angiogenesis with endothelial hypoplasia, loss of longitudinal collagen architecture, and microtears with collagen fiber separation.[534]
- More advanced or chronic stages of patellar tendinitis have the following constellation of findings:
    - Hyperintensity in a proximal tendon partial tear
    - Hyperintense edema involving the inferior pole of the patella
    - Reactive edema and fluid associated with the adjacent proximal fat pad[314]
- In the absence of Osgood-Schlatter disease, the pathophysiology and clinical presentation of distal jumper's knee are similar to those of more proximal lesions.[363]
- Subacute versus chronic patellar tendinitis
- Acute patellar tendinitis (symptoms for <2 weeks)
    - Signal abnormalities in peritenon region without significant intrasubstance tendon changes

- Chronic patellar tendinitis (symptoms for >6 weeks)
    - Before development of associated chronic tears, changes include area of low signal intensity with enlargement within the tendon.[107]
    - If complicated by development of chronic tears, inflammation, and necrosis, the high-signal-intensity MR appearance may be similar to acute partial intrasubstance patellar tendon tears on T2-weighted sequences.

Patellar Tendon Tears

Key Concepts

- Less common than quadriceps tendon rupture
- Although degeneration of tendon fibers is a predisposing factor to rupture, the tensile and viscoelastic properties of the patellar tendon are relatively stable between younger and older age groups.
- Edema and hemorrhage are best visualized on FS PD FSE images, whereas underlying collagen degeneration is best seen on T2* GRE images.

Patellar Tendon Tears

- Result in a loss of extension and a high-riding patella
- Can occur with avulsion injuries from the tibial tubercle or the inferior pole of the patella[398]
- Most tendon ruptures occur in proximal patellar tendon at inferior patellar pole junction.
- Mid-substance ruptures are unusual and related to severe trauma with forced knee flexion against a contracted quadriceps muscle.
- Distal tears near lower pole are seen in younger patients.
- Predisposing factors for tendon rupture
    - Preexisting disease, including rheumatoid arthritis and diabetes

MR Findings of Patellar Tendon Tears

- Disruption and loss of continuity of normal low-signal-intensity tendon
- Superior retraction or patella alta is associated with complete tears.
- Lax or wavy contour of patellar tendon as a function of degree of tendon retraction
- Entire tendon may appear thickened, especially if there is an underlying or predisposing tendinitis.
- Bony fragments, with or without the signal intensity of marrow, may be identified on sagittal MR images.
- Partial tears
    - Typically involve proximal fibers and are associated with tendon thickening
    - Typically involve proximal posterior fibers of patellar tendon
    - Patellar tendon may also appear thickened after arthroscopy.

Treatment of Patellar Tendon Rupture

- Direct tendon repair
- Reconstruction with semitendinosus tendon
- Bony reattachment[69]

Patella Alta and Patella Baja

- Abnormal patellar tendon–to–patella ratio when unequal or exceeds 1:2[398]
- Patella alta (high position of the patella)
    - Associated with subluxation, chondromalacia, Sinding-Larsen-Johansson syndrome, cerebral palsy, and quadriceps atrophy[517]
- Patella baja (low position of the patella)
    - Most commonly seen as postoperative complication of anterior cruciate ligament (ACL) surgery or lateral retinacular release
    - May also be associated with polio, achondroplasia, and juvenile chronic arthritis

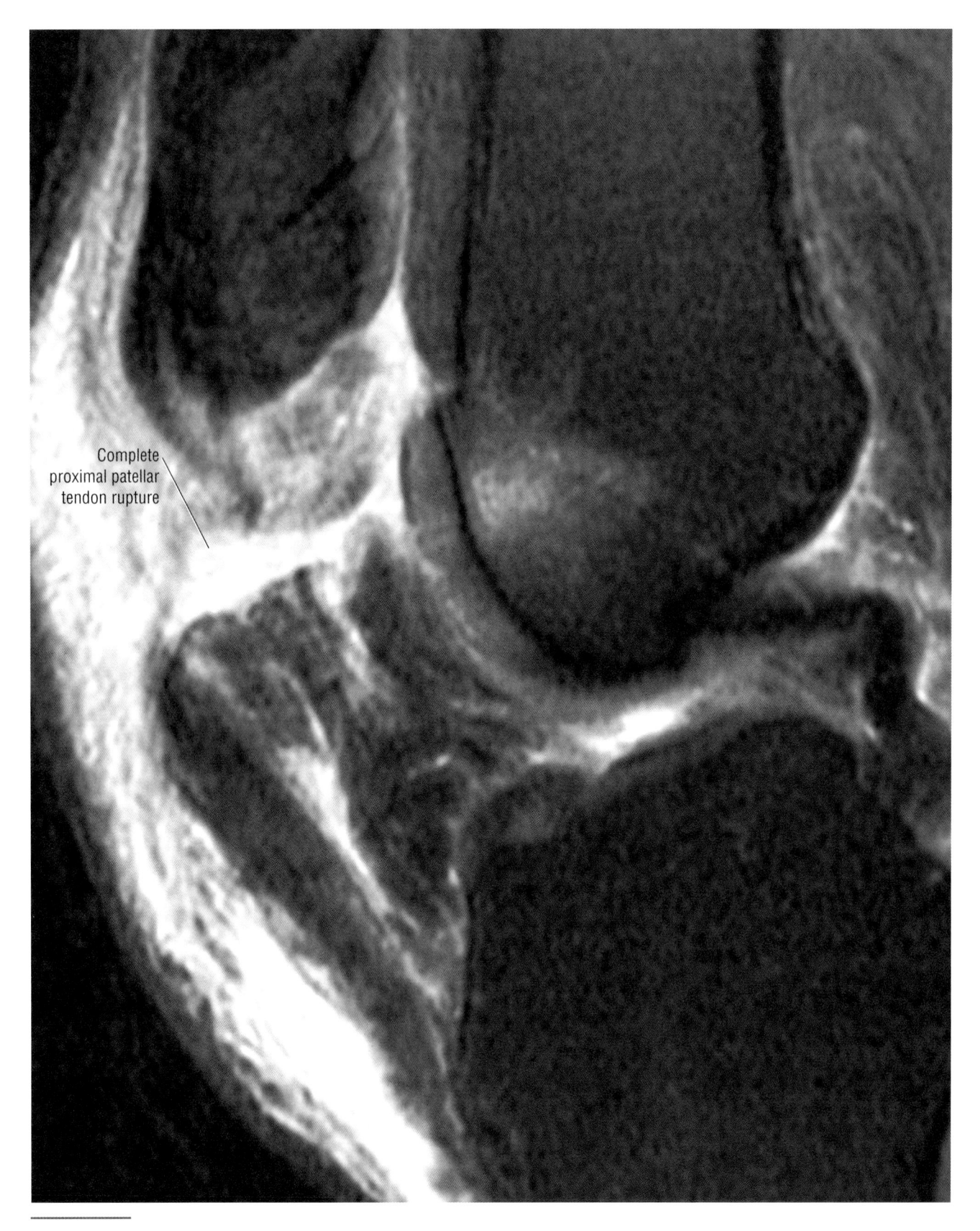

FIGURE 7.104 Complete proximal patellar tendon with tendon fiber discontinuity and hemorrhage at the tear site. Associated patella alta and anterior reactive soft tissue edema. Sagittal FS PD FSE image.

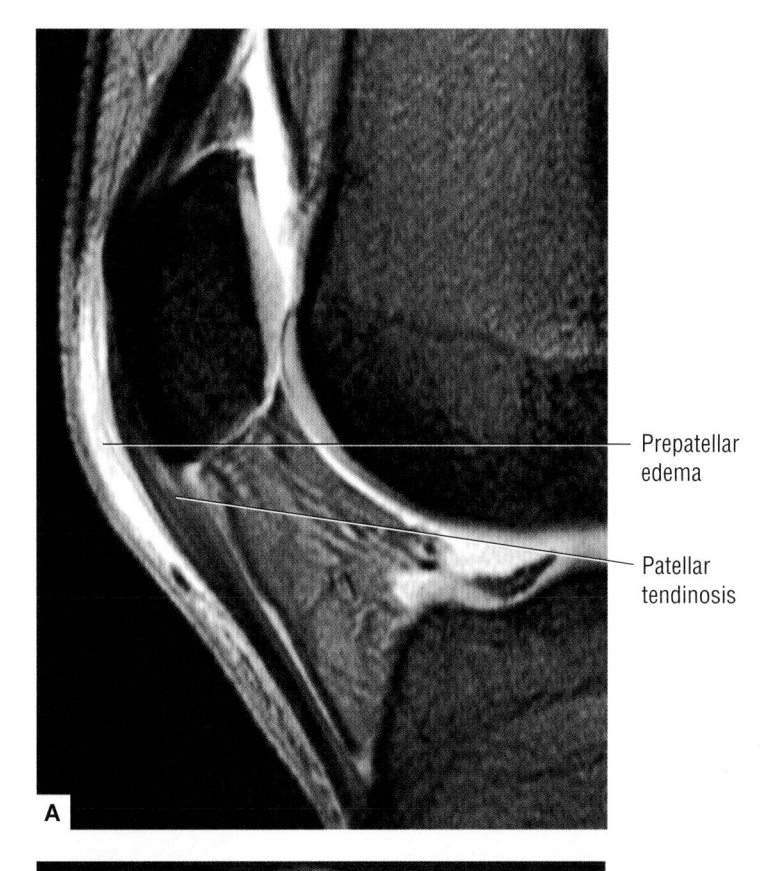

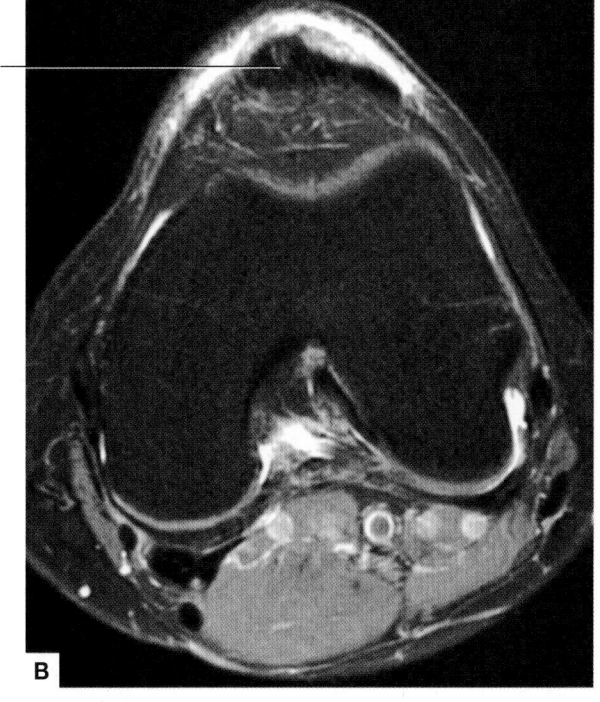

FIGURE 7.105 (**A**) Sagittal T2* GRE and (**B**) axial FS PD FSE images demonstrating proximal patellar tendon thickening with preferential degeneration of proximal posterior fibers and associated prepatellar edema. Medial involvement of the proximal patellar tendon is best seen on the axial image (**B**).

Proximal patellar tendinosis with anterior to posterior tendon thickening

Tendinosis with mucoid degeneration

Hyperintense interstitial tear

FIGURE 7.106 Severe thickening of the proximal half of the patellar tendon associated with interstitial tearing of the middle third fibers on (**A**) sagittal T2* GRE image, (**B**) sagittal PD FSE image, and (**C**) sagittal FS PD FSE image. Tendon degeneration is best visualized on the GRE image (**A**), and linear interstitial tearing is most conspicuous with FS PD FSE contrast (**C**).

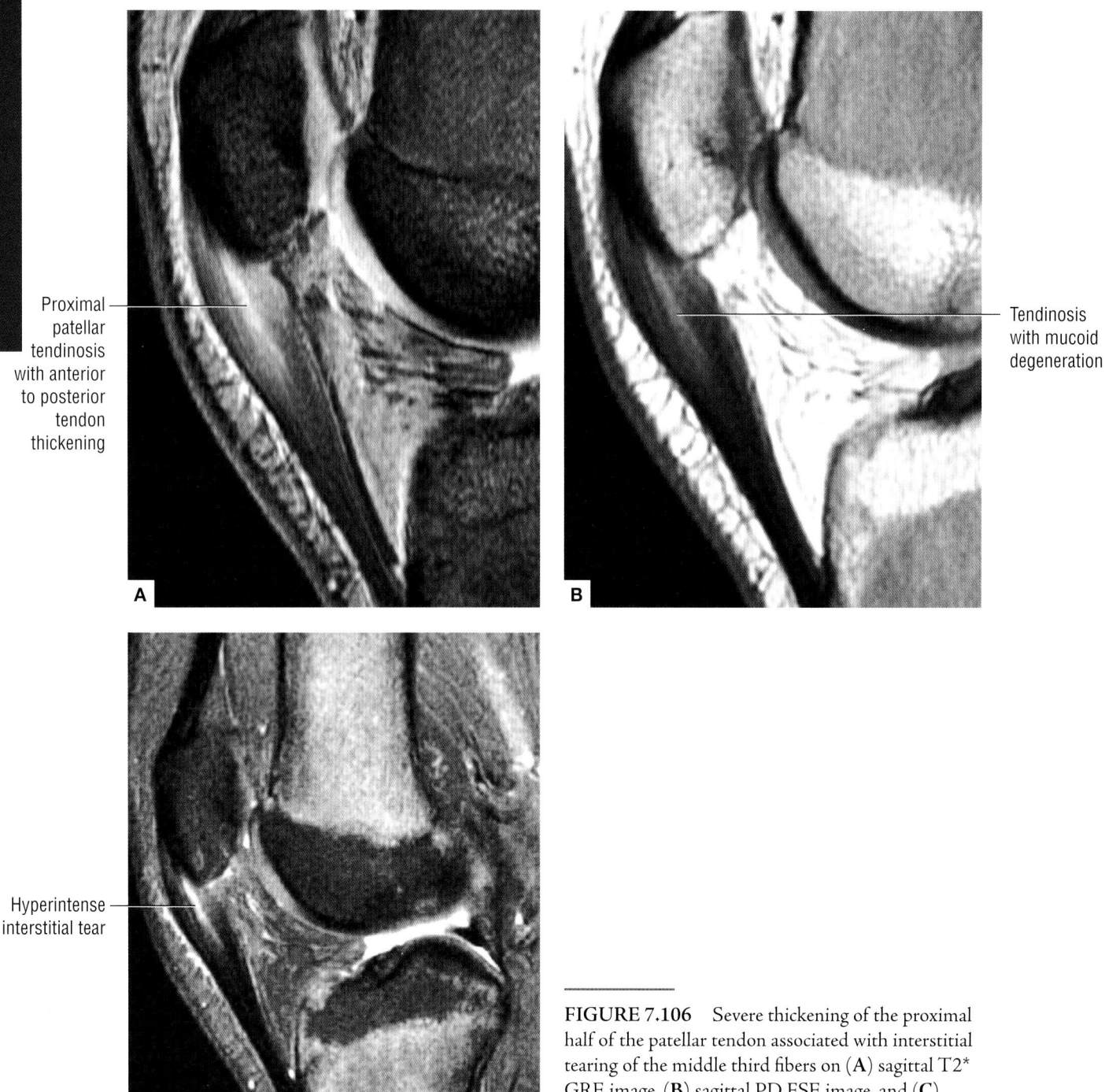

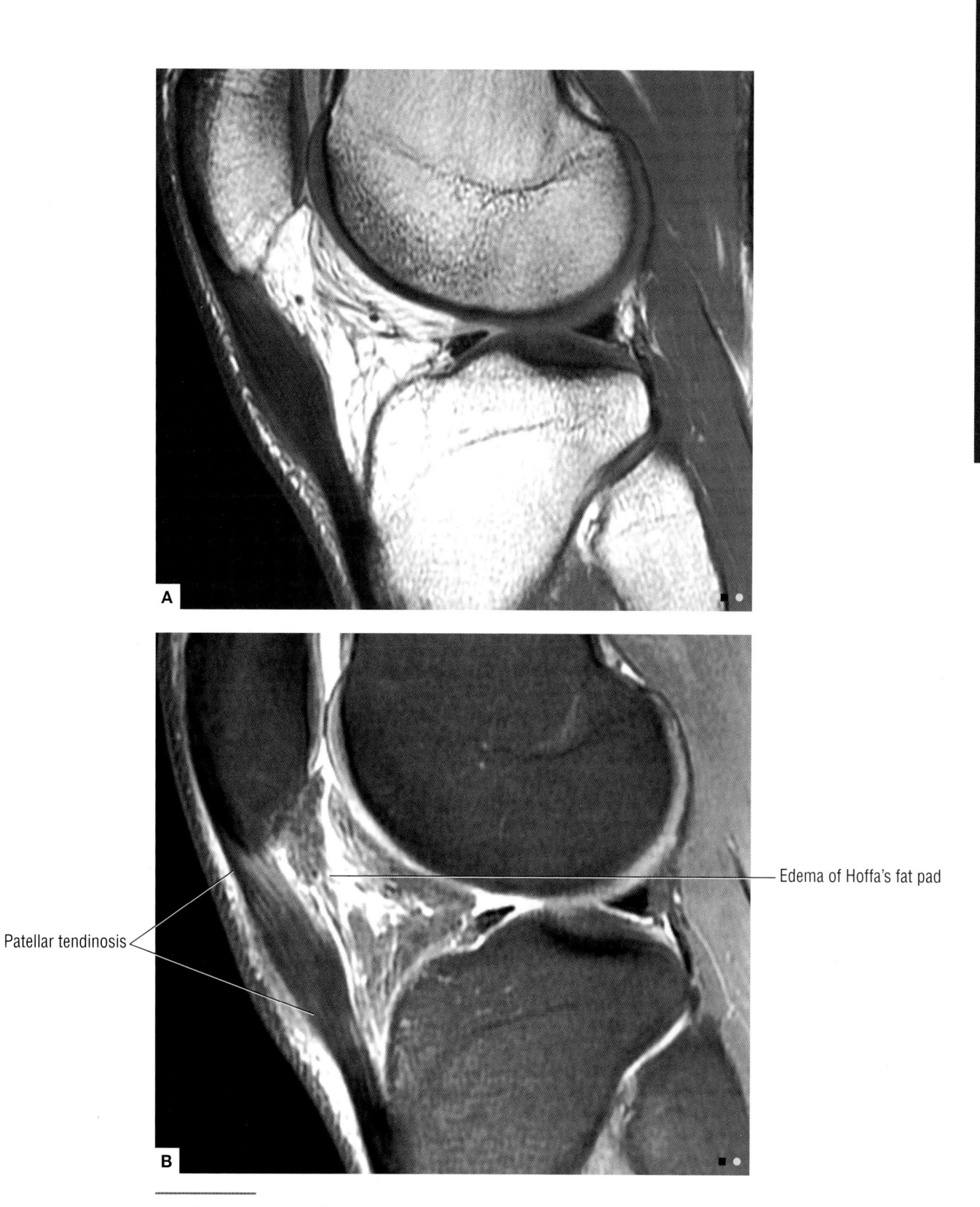

FIGURE 7.107 Patellar tendinosis with mucoid degeneration. Thickened linear striations of intermediate signal are identified in association with edema of the adjacent fat pad. Histology involves hypercellularity including atypical fibroblast and endothelial cellular proliferation and neurovascularization in an attempt at tendon healing. Sagittal PD (**A**) and FS PD (**B**) images.

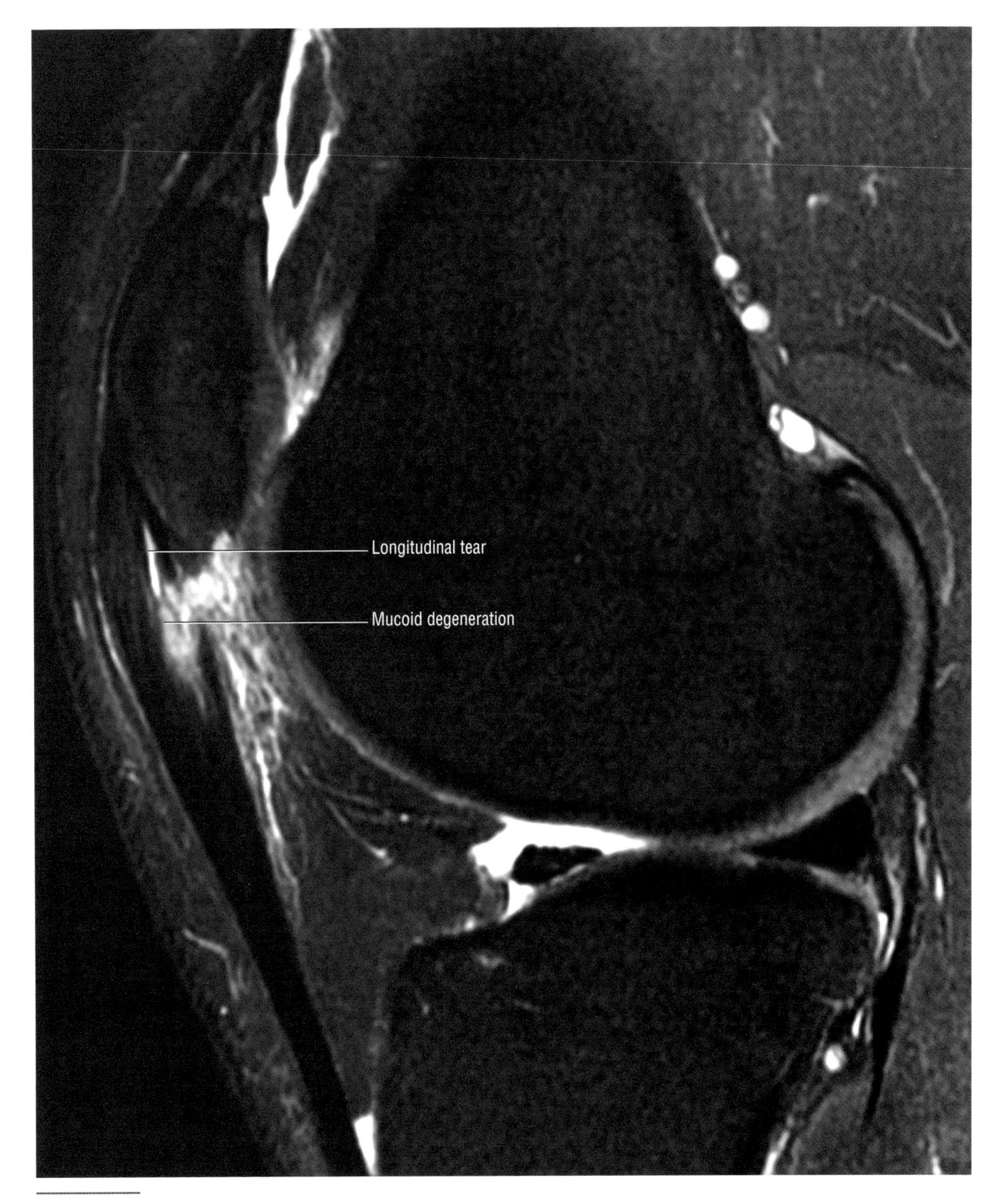

FIGURE 7.108 Intratendinous hyperintense tear (microtear) with adjacent, more ill-defined mucoid tendon degeneration. Sagittal FS PD FSE image.

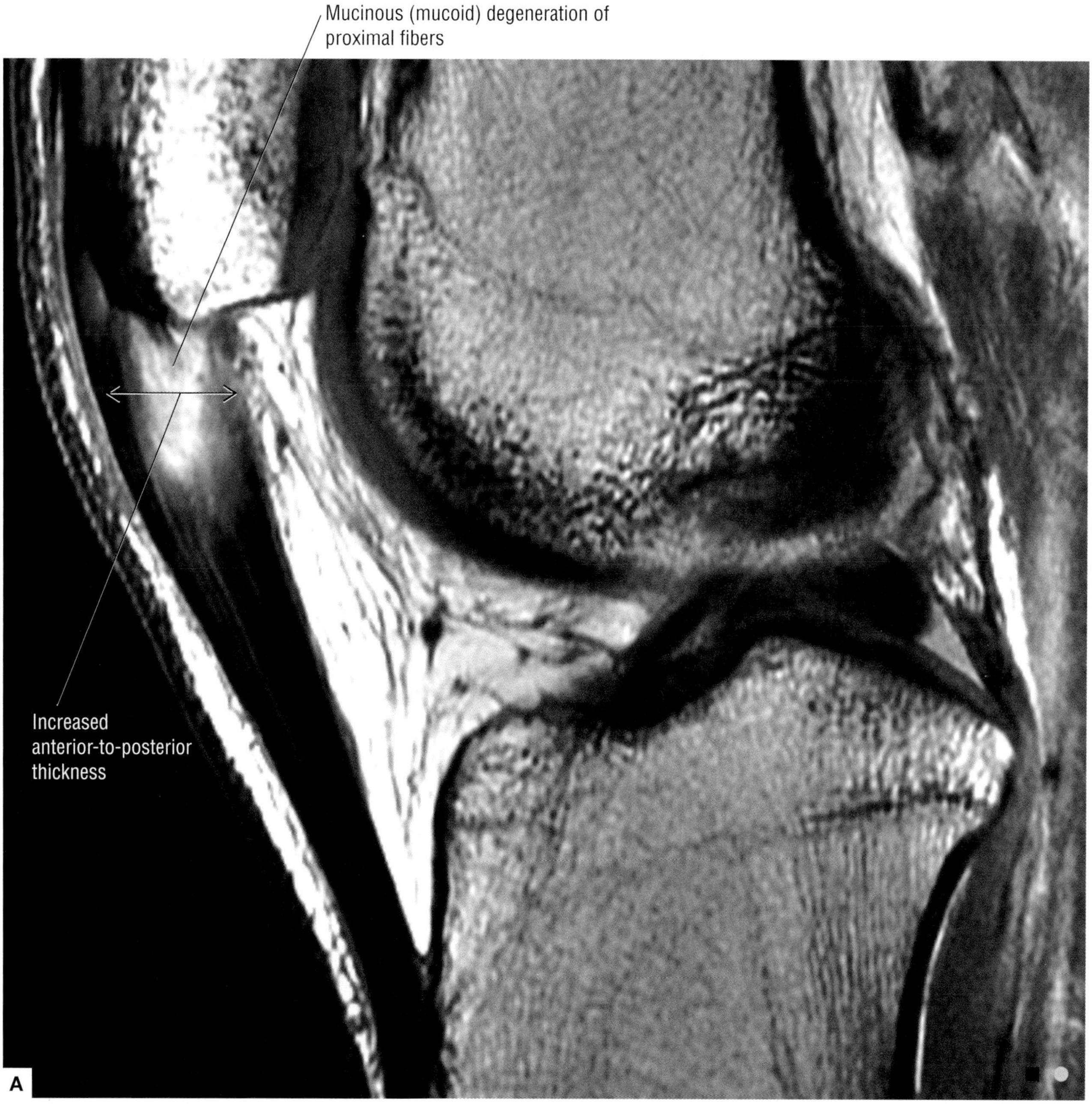

FIGURE 7.109 Proximal patellar tendinosis with involvement of proximal medial fibers. Histology correlates with loss of demarcation of collagen bundles, mucoid degeneration, intratendinous calcification, and fibrinoid necrosis without inflammatory cells. Elevated high-molecular-weight proteoglycans and type III collagen may correlate with compressive loads and adaptive changes. (**A**) Sagittal PD FSE image. (*Continued*)

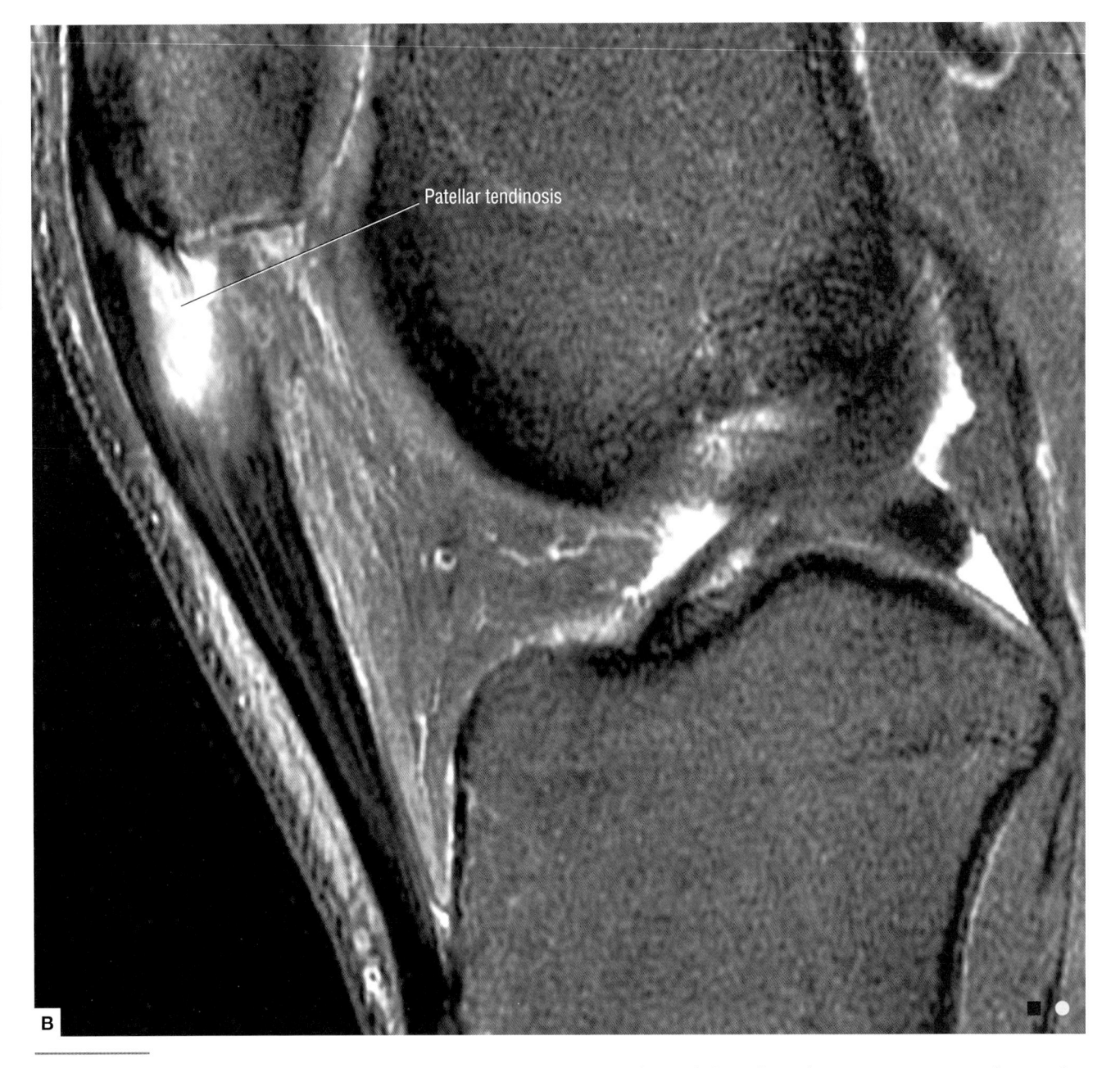

FIGURE 7.109 *(Continued)* Although the term "patellar tendinopathy" can be used clinically to characterize overuse conditions of the patellar tendon, MR can assess tendon degeneration, and thus the term "tendinosis" is more specific. (**B**) Sagittal FS PD FSE image.

Patellofemoral Joint and the Extensor Mechanism 809

Tendinosis proximal posterior fibers of patellar tendon

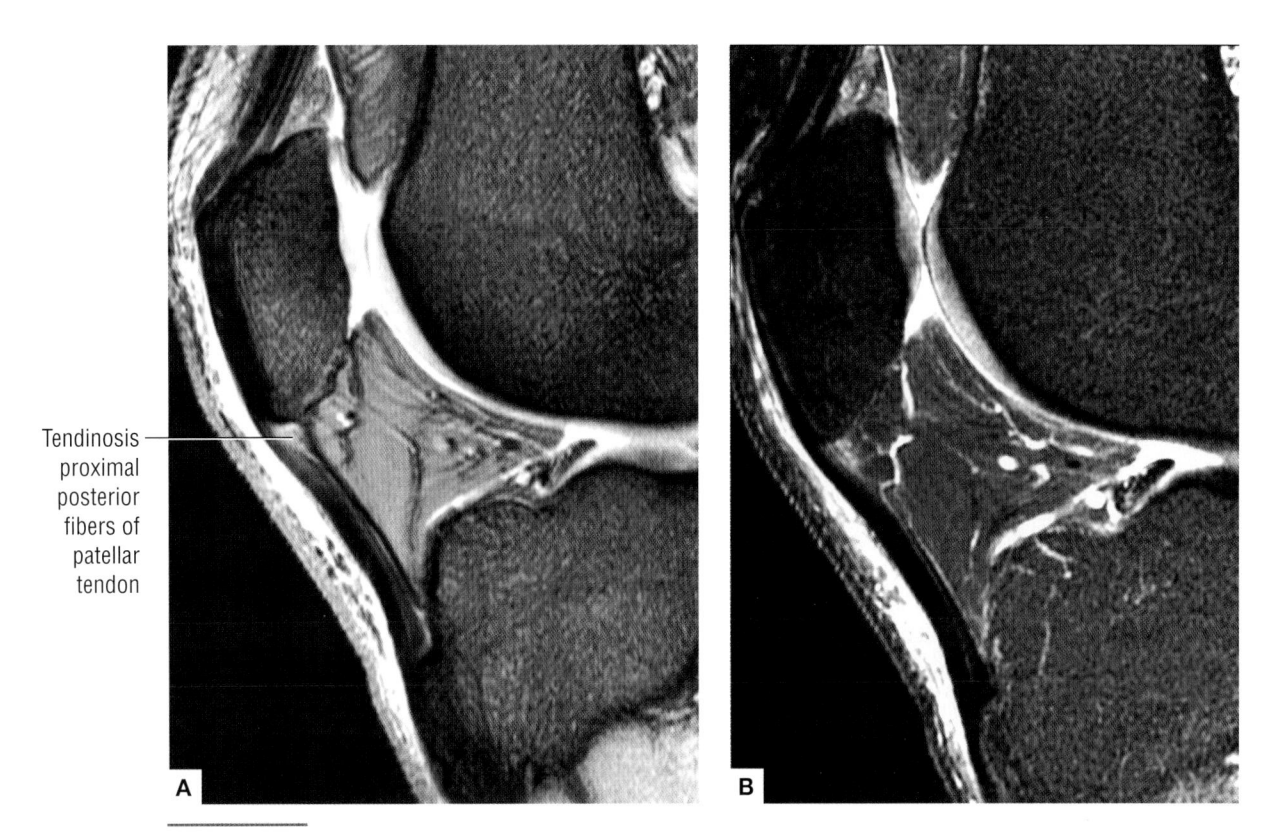

FIGURE 7.110 Comparison of proximal patellar tendinosis on a sagittal T2* GRE image (**A**) and a sagittal FS PD FSE image (**B**). Intratendinous proximal degeneration shown with hyperintense signal on the GRE image (**A**) is grossly underestimated on the corresponding sagittal FS PD FSE image (**B**).

Proximal tendon thickening

Inferior patellar pole edema
Tendon degeneration
Fluid

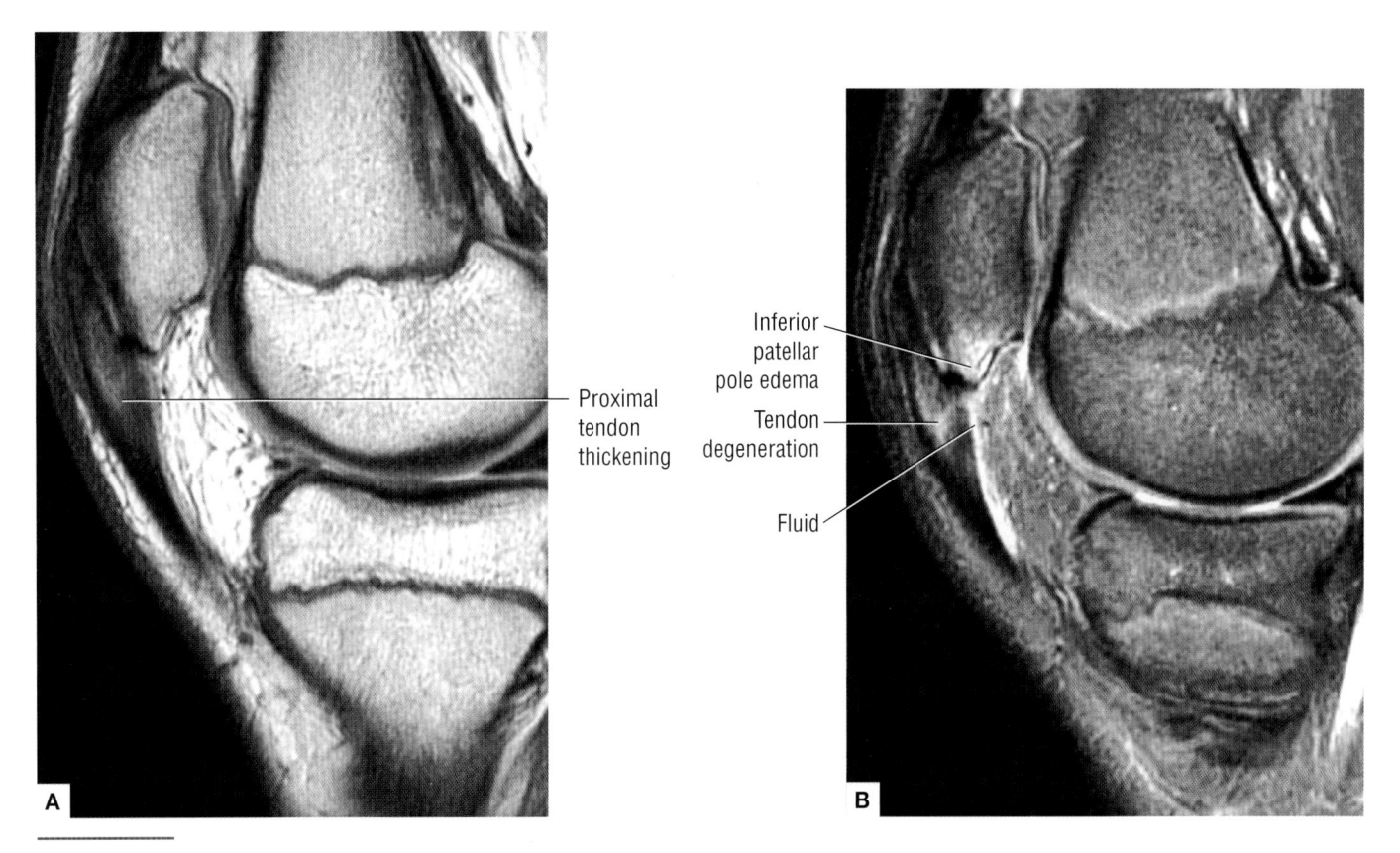

FIGURE 7.111 (**A**) Sagittal PD FSE and (**B**) sagittal FS PD FSE images show characteristic proximal patellar tendon and inferior patellar pole hyperintensity. Fluid is also seen tracking adjacent to the posterior margin of the patellar tendon. Patellar tendinosis is a degenerative condition with an absence of inflammatory cells. Repeated tensile overload may lead to microtearing and fraying followed by focal (collagen) degeneration and partial macrotearing.

Degeneration distal patellar tendon

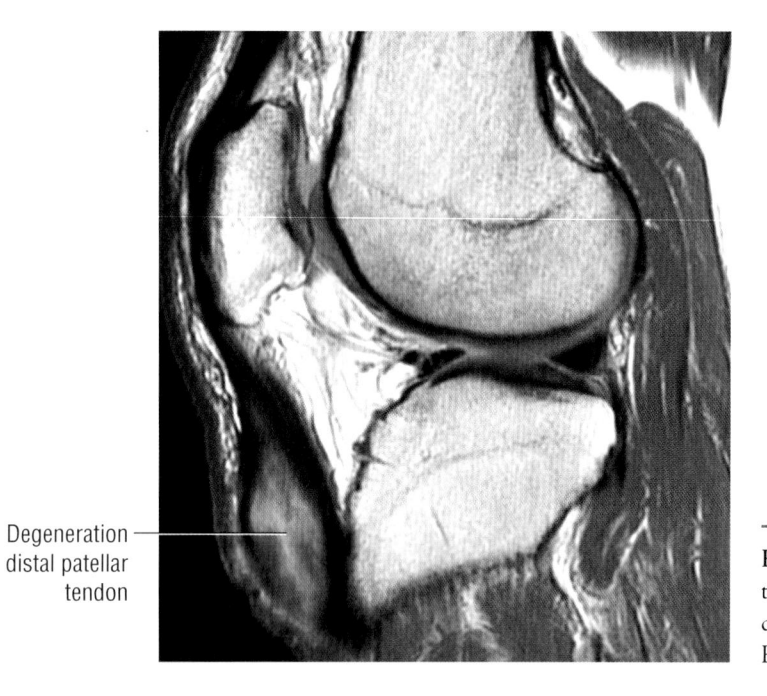

FIGURE 7.112 Distal jumper's knee with thickening, degeneration, and partial tearing of the distal third of the patellar tendon on a sagittal PD FSE image.

Interstitial tear

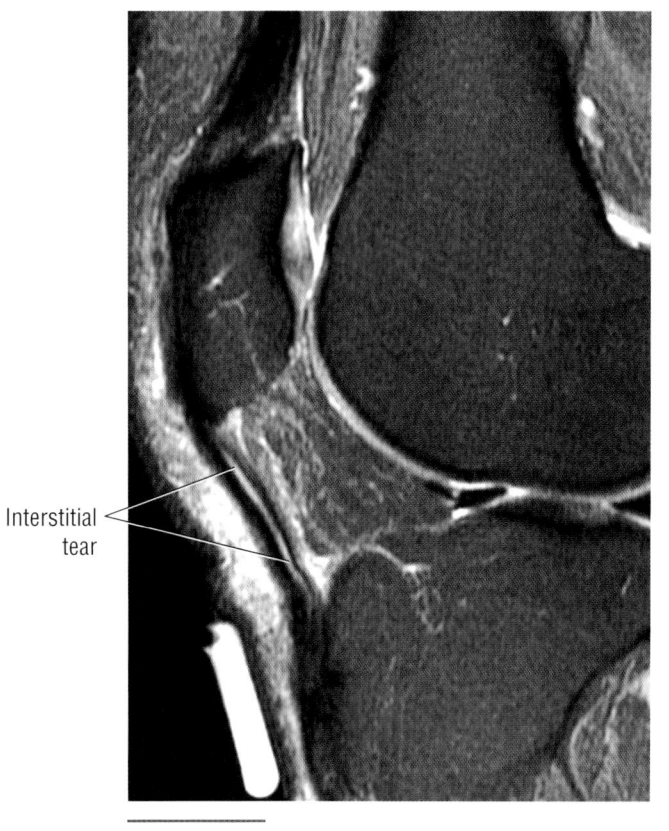

FIGURE 7.113 Acute patellar tendinitis with an atypical long-segment interstitial tear and anterior subcutaneous edema on a sagittal FS PD FSE image.

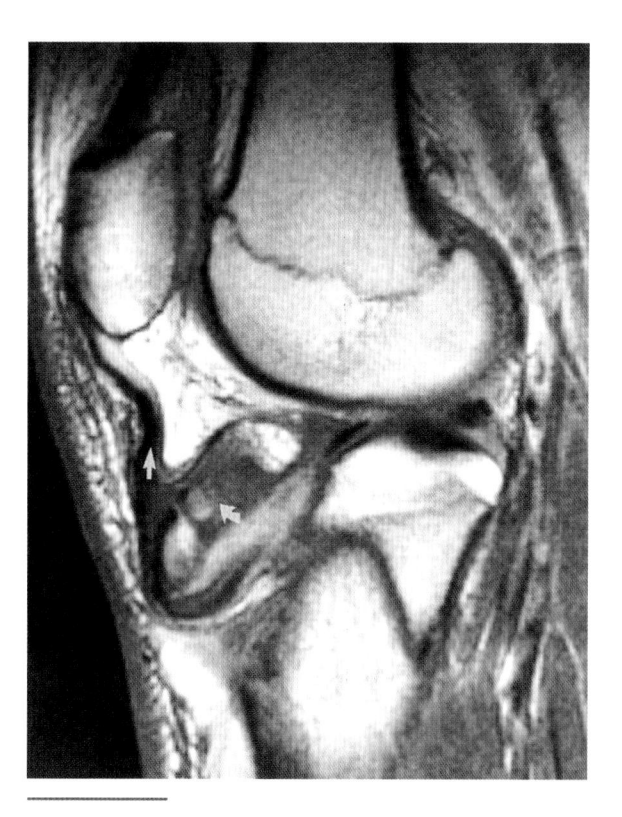

FIGURE 7.114 A T1-weighted sagittal image of a displaced anterior tibial fracture with an attached patellar tendon. Note proximal retraction of the tendon (*straight arrow*) and osseous fragment (*curved arrow*).

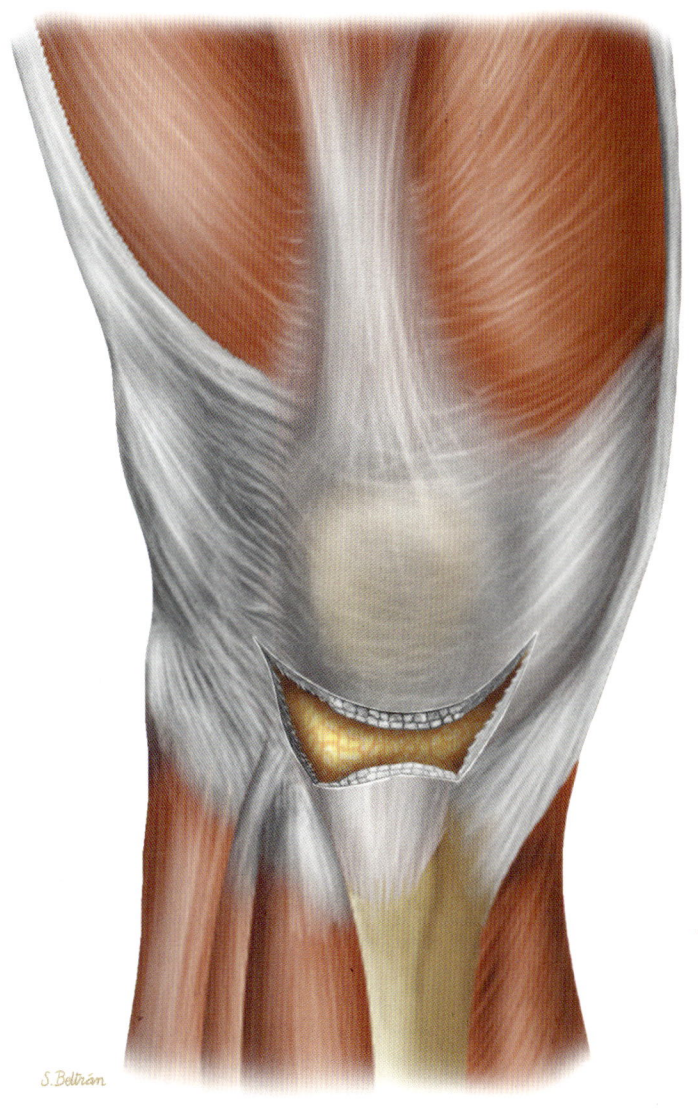

FIGURE 7.115 Rupture of the proximal patellar tendon at the inferior pole of the patella. Clinical examination may show a displaced patella, hemarthrosis, and an inability to extend the knee.

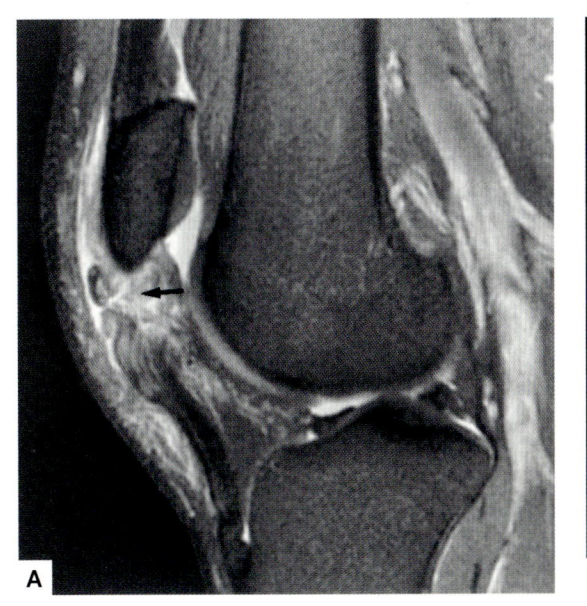

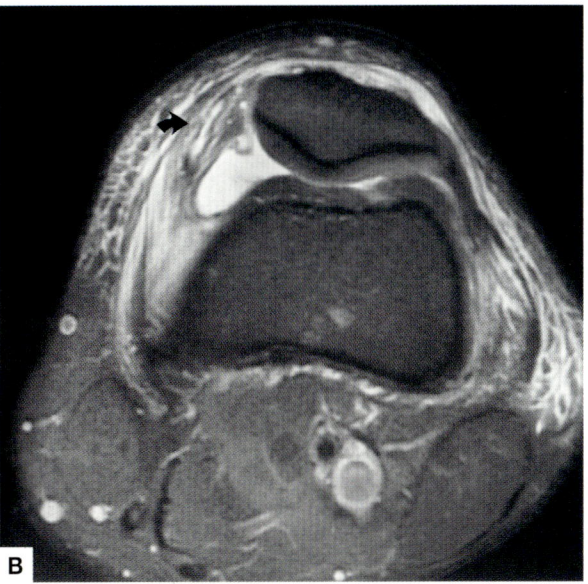

FIGURE 7.116 Acute proximal patellar tendon rupture (*straight arrow*) associated with a medial retinacular tear (*curved arrow*) on FS PD-weighted FSE sagittal (**A**) and axial (**B**) images. The proximal displacement of the patella is associated with both retinacular and capsular disruption secondary to the forceful pull of the quadriceps mechanism.

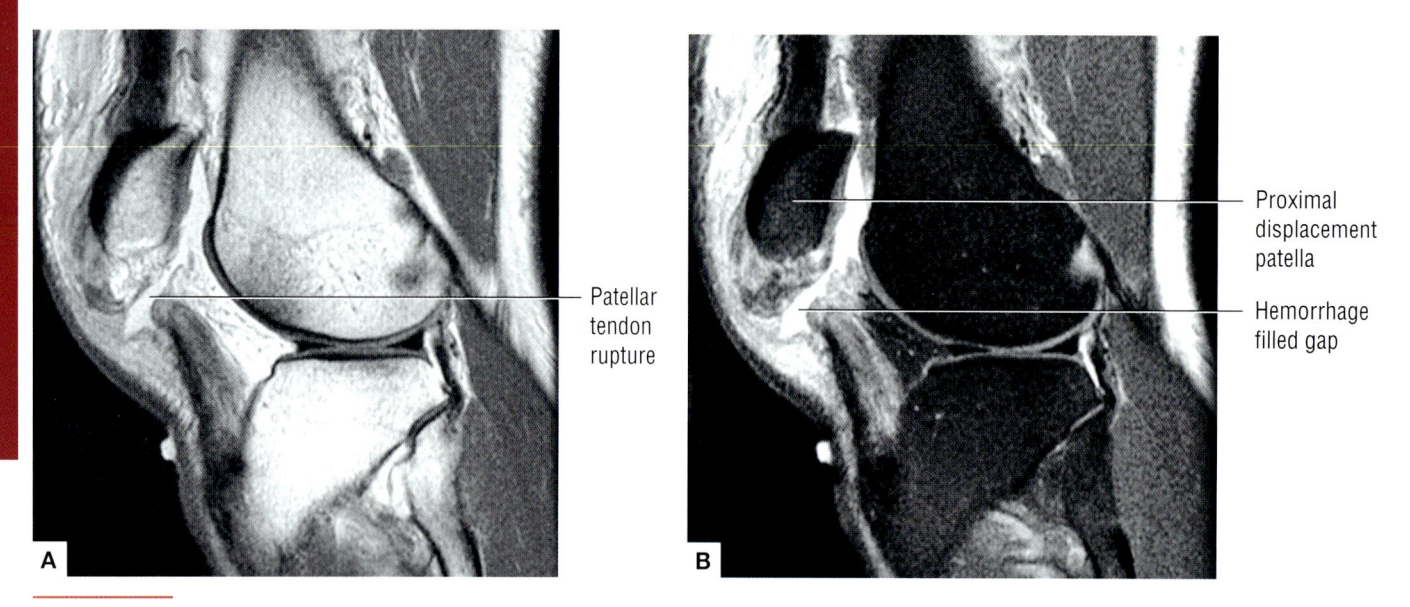

FIGURE 7.117 (A) Sagittal PD FSE and (B) sagittal FS PD FSE images show complete proximal rupture of the patellar tendon associated with proximal patellar displacement and localized hemorrhage.

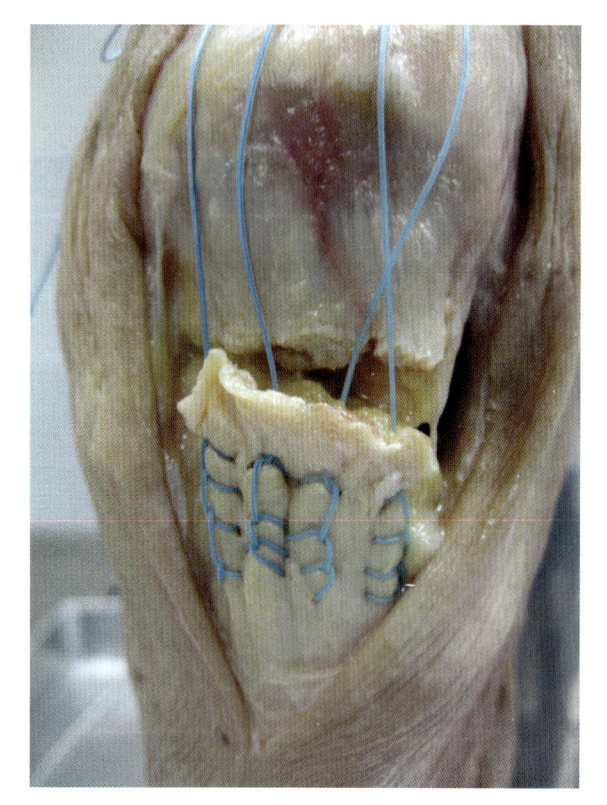

FIGURE 7.118 Cadaver specimen demonstrating medial and lateral Krackow locking stitches for patellar tendon rupture. (Reprinted from Fu FH. *Master Techniques in Orthopaedic Surgery: Sports Medicine.* Philadelphia, PA: Lippincott Williams & Wilkins; 2010, with permission.)

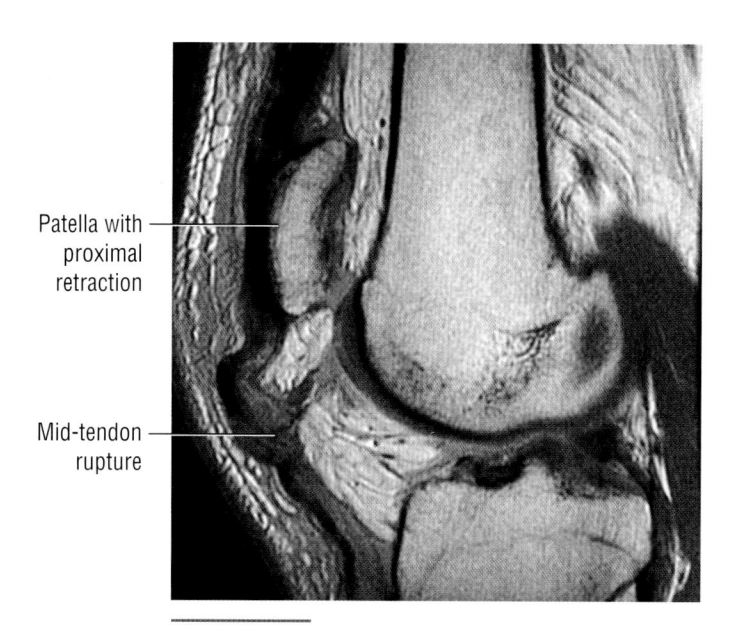

Patellofemoral Joint and the Extensor Mechanism 813

FIGURE 7.119 Sagittal PD FSE image showing mid-substance rupture of the patellar tendon. This injury is usually associated with trauma or laceration but can occur spontaneously.

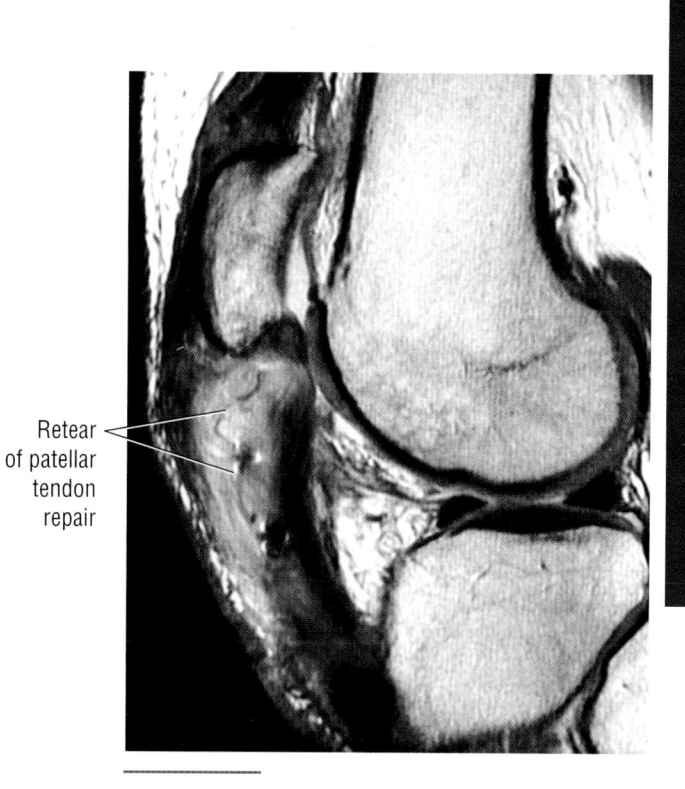

FIGURE 7.120 Sagittal PD FSE image of rerupture after a pants-over-vest patellar tendon repair. Hemorrhage and granulation tissues fill the tear site.

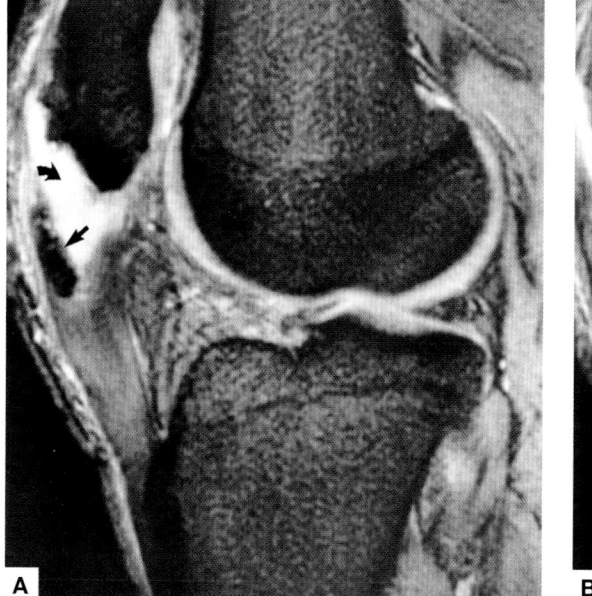

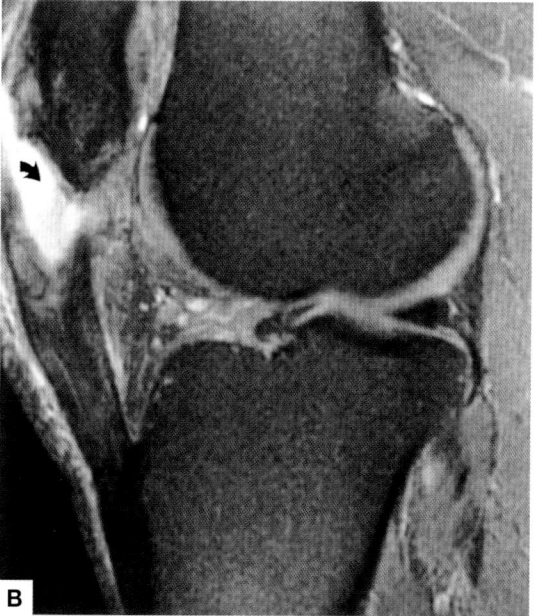

FIGURE 7.121 (**A**) Sagittal T2* and (**B**) FS PD-weighted FSE images of a proximal patellar tendon rupture (*curved arrows*) associated with diffuse tendon thickening. The avulsed inferior pole osseous fragment (*straight arrow*) is best visualized on the T2*-weighted sequence (**A**) because of the bone susceptibility effect. The greater degree of diffuse tendon hyperintensity is also shown on the T2*-weighted sequence.

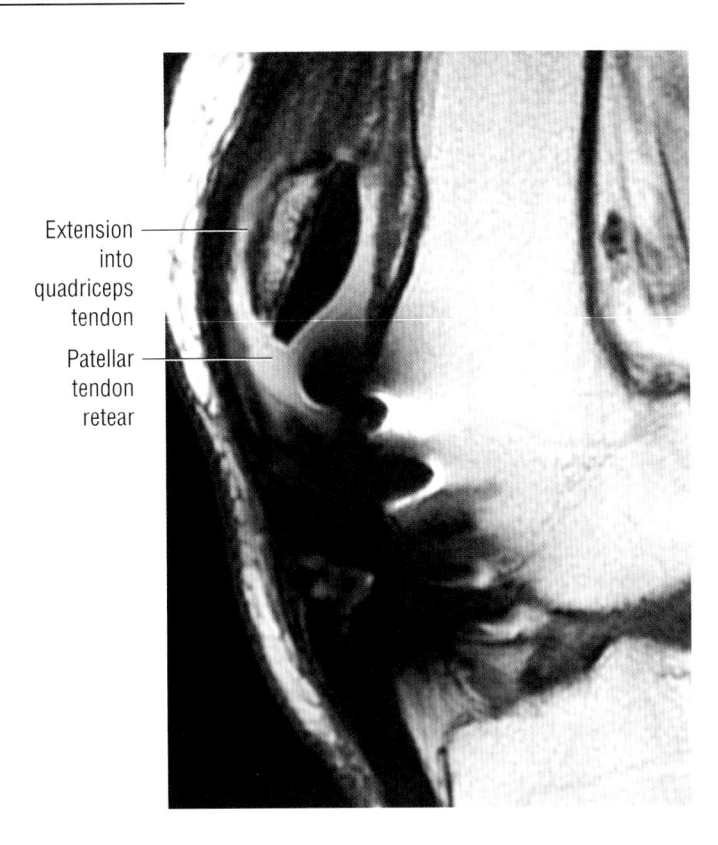

FIGURE 7.122 Sagittal PD FSE image of proximal patella tendon rerupture with extension of the tear superiorly into the distal quadriceps tendon. Patellar resurfacing is hypointense at the site of the patellar component.

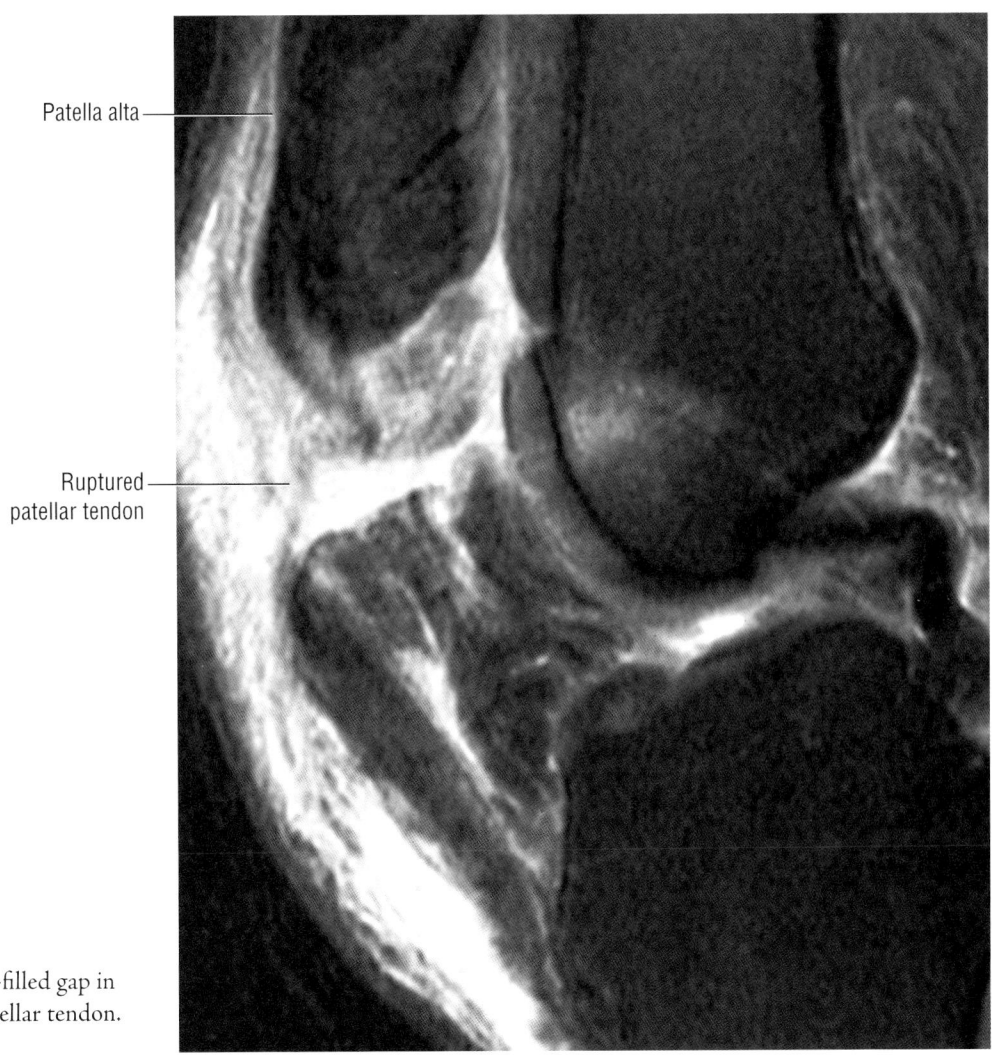

FIGURE 7.123 Hyperintense fluid-filled gap in a complete rupture of the proximal patellar tendon. Sagittal FS PD FSE image.

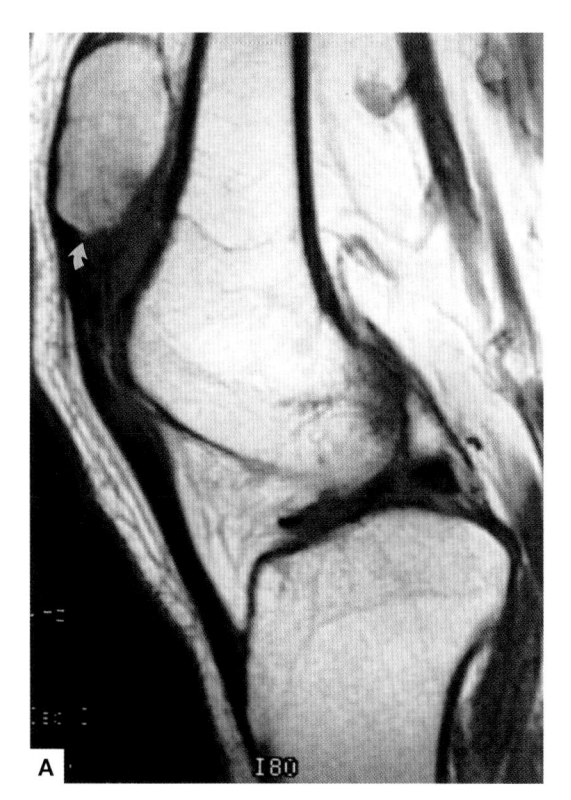

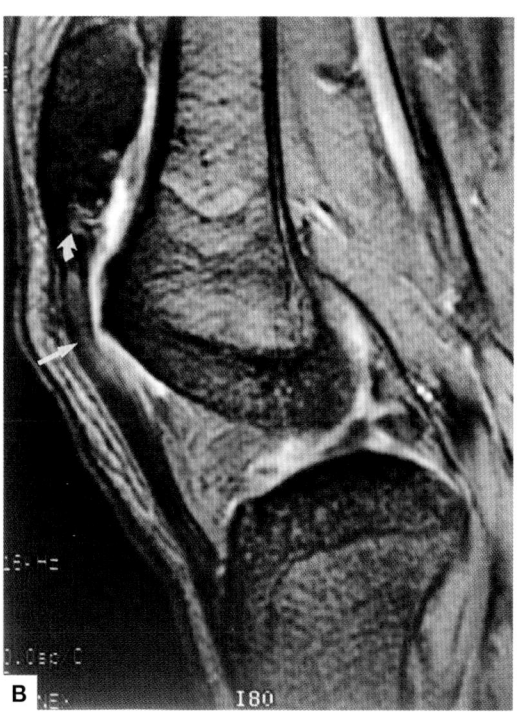

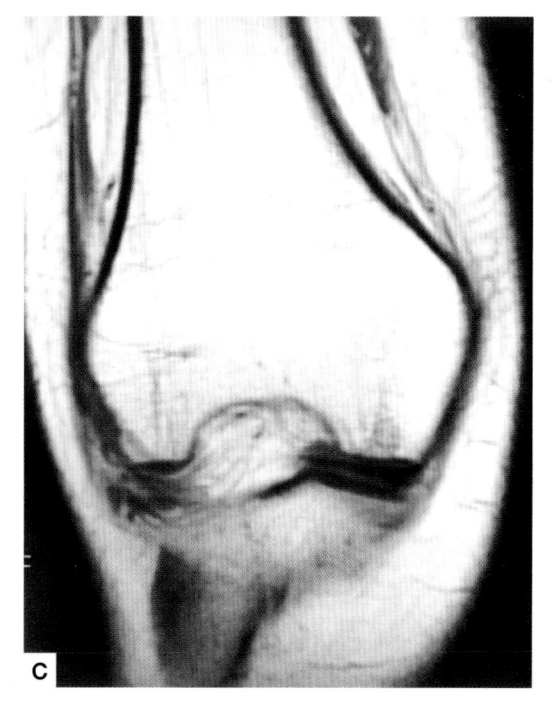

FIGURE 7.124 Patella alta (*curved arrows*) in a patient with polio. Symptomatic tendinosis (*straight arrow*) of the proximal patellar tendon is seen on (**A**) T1- and (**B**) T2*-weighted sagittal images. Trochlear groove deformity is demonstrated on T1-weighted coronal image (**C**).

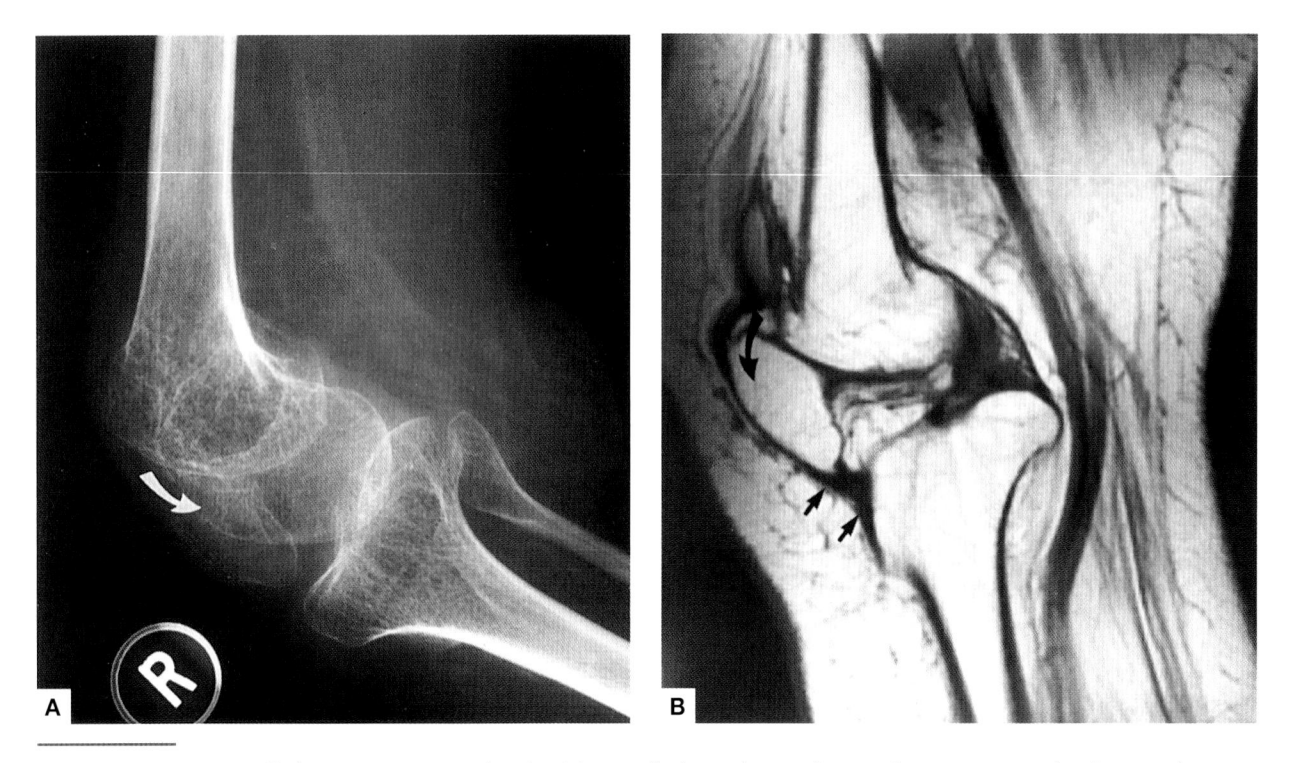

FIGURE 7.125 Patella baja in a patient with polio. The patella (*curved arrows*) is in a low position, and a shortened patellar tendon (*straight arrows*) is seen on (**A**) a lateral radiograph and (**B**) a T1-weighted sagittal image.

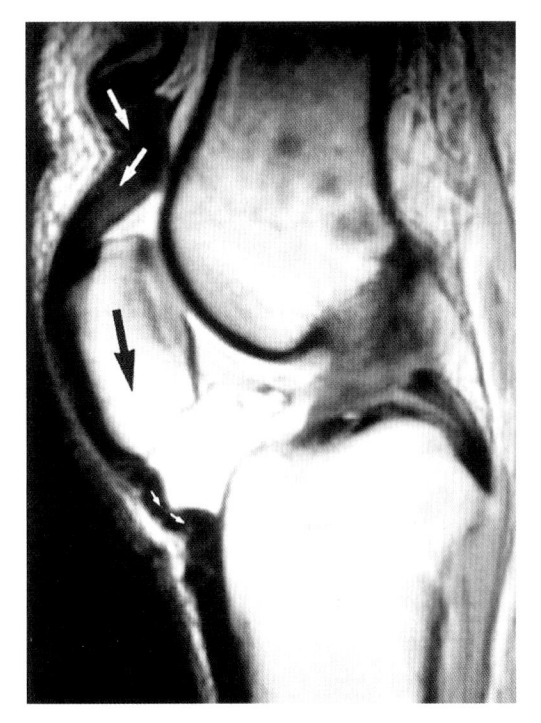

FIGURE 7.126 A proximal quadriceps tendon rupture results in patella baja (*black arrow*), lax quadriceps tendon (*white arrows*), and a foreshortened patellar tendon.

Osgood-Schlatter Disease

- Normal tibial tubercle demonstrates distinct histologic stages of development: cartilaginous, apophyseal, epiphyseal, and lastly bony incorporation into the tibia.[211]

- Clinical findings
    - Osteochondrosis of developing tibial tuberosity (apophysis)
    - Thought to be secondary to repetitive microtears during adolescent growth
    - Present with activity-related pain and/or swelling about the tibial tubercle[460]
    - Swelling and tenderness of patellar tendon and peripatellar soft tissues

- Histologic features
    - Focal tendon collagen degeneration
    - Tendon microtears
    - Influx of inflammatory cells in surrounding soft tissues
    - Bursal and synovial hypertrophy
    - Inflammatory infiltrate
    - Heterotopic bone formation and/or fragmentation

- MR findings
    - Irregularity of distal patellar tendon with thickening and localized hyperintensity on T2, FS PD-weighted FSE, STIR, and GRE images
    - May be adjacent edema within Hoffa's fat pad or fluid interposed between patellar tendon, tibial tubercle, and inferior aspect of Hoffa's fat pad
    - Multiple small ossicles or single bony fragment anterior to tibial tuberosity
    - Proximal patellar tendinosis may coexist with Osgood-Schlatter disease.

Sinding-Larsen-Johansson Syndrome

- Osteochondrosis involving distal patellar pole at insertion of patellar tendon

- Thought to be caused by persistent traction at cartilaginous junction of inferior pole of patella (traumatic origin)

- Usually occurs in the preteen or teenage years, similar to Osgood-Schlatter disease, with a greater incidence in boys.

- Differential diagnosis includes stress fracture of the patella, patellar sleeve fracture (through the cartilaginous bone junction), and a type 1 bipartite patella.

- MR findings

    - Sagittal images display area of low signal intensity on T1-weighted sequences and hyperintensity on GRE or FS PD-weighted FSE images.

    - Fragmentation of inferior pole of the patella may be associated with areas of signal alteration in adjacent proximal fat pad or proximal patellar tendon.

    - Frank displacement of distal patellar pole fragment is uncommon.

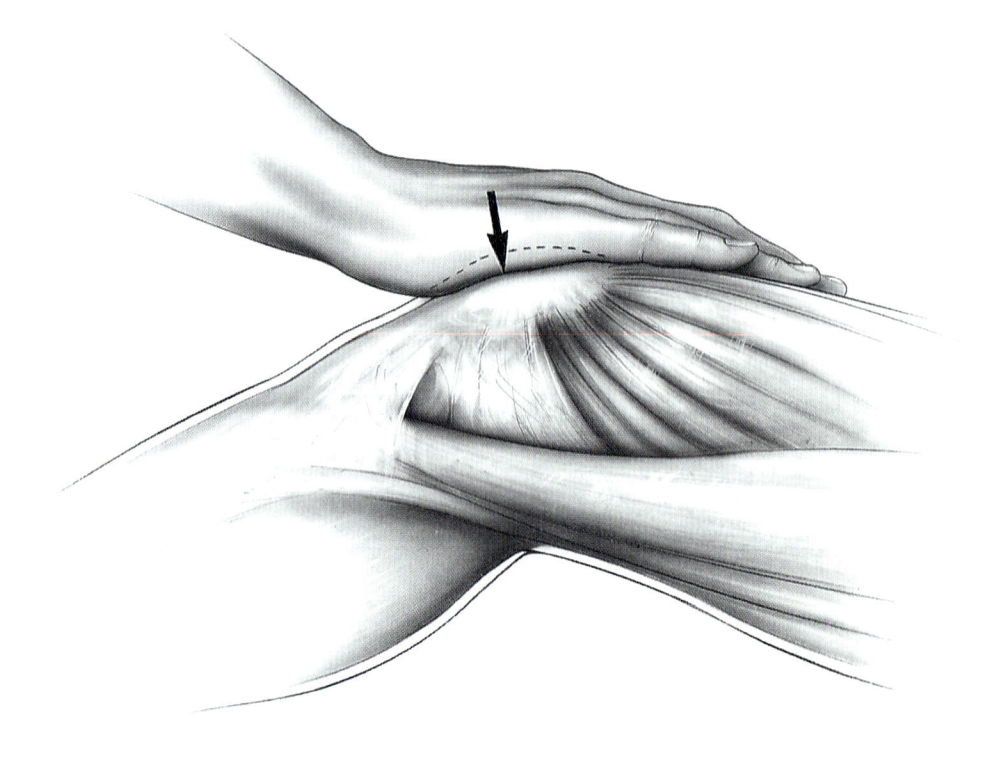

FIGURE 7.127 Compression of the patella while passing the knee through a range of motion will give an impression of the extent of articular cartilage damage and pain emanating from the articular surfaces of the patellofemoral joint. In Sinding-Larsen-Johansson syndrome, pain will be located to the inferior pole of the patella and proximal patellar tendon and not initially evident on straight anterior compression. (Reprinted from Jackson DW. *Master Techniques in Orthopaedic Surgery: Reconstructive Knee Surgery*, 3rd ed. Philadelphia, PA: Lippincott Williams & Wilkins; 2008, with permission.)

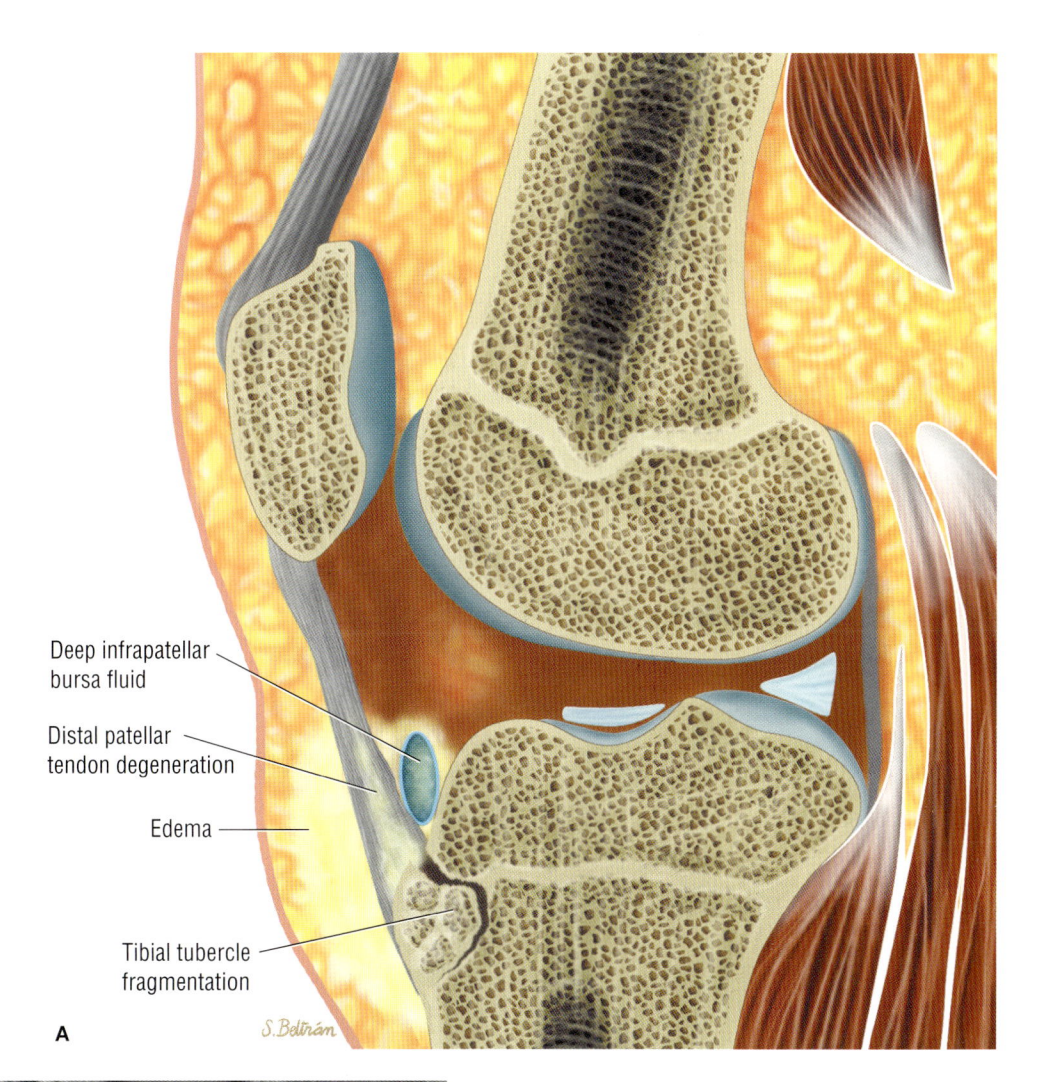

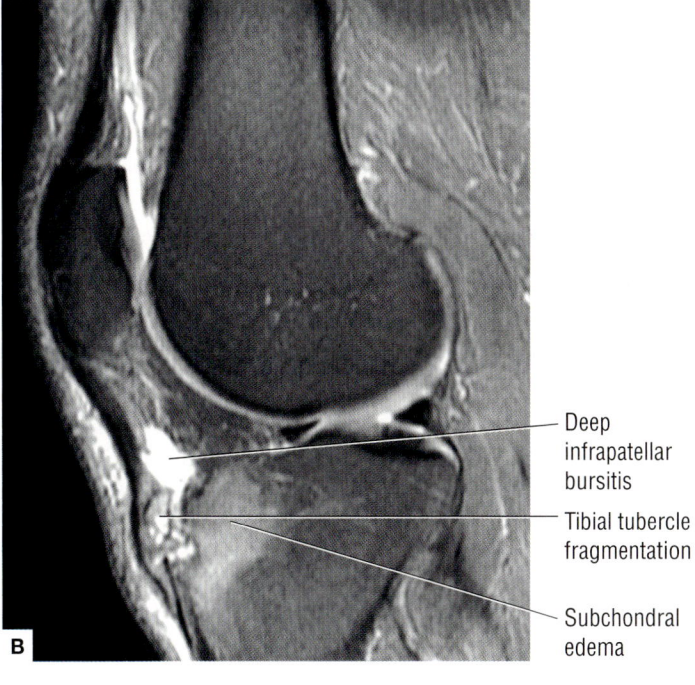

FIGURE 7.128 (**A**) Sagittal color illustration of Osgood-Schlatter disease. Tibial osteochondrosis (apophysitis) is seen at the patellar tendon insertion on the tibial tubercle. (**B**) MR findings, as seen on this sagittal FS PD FSE scan, include hyperintensity within, superficial to, and deep to the distal patellar tendon at its insertion. Variable amounts of fluid may be seen in the infrapatellar bursae, and there may be subchondral edema involving the fragmented apophysis and adjacent anterior tibia.

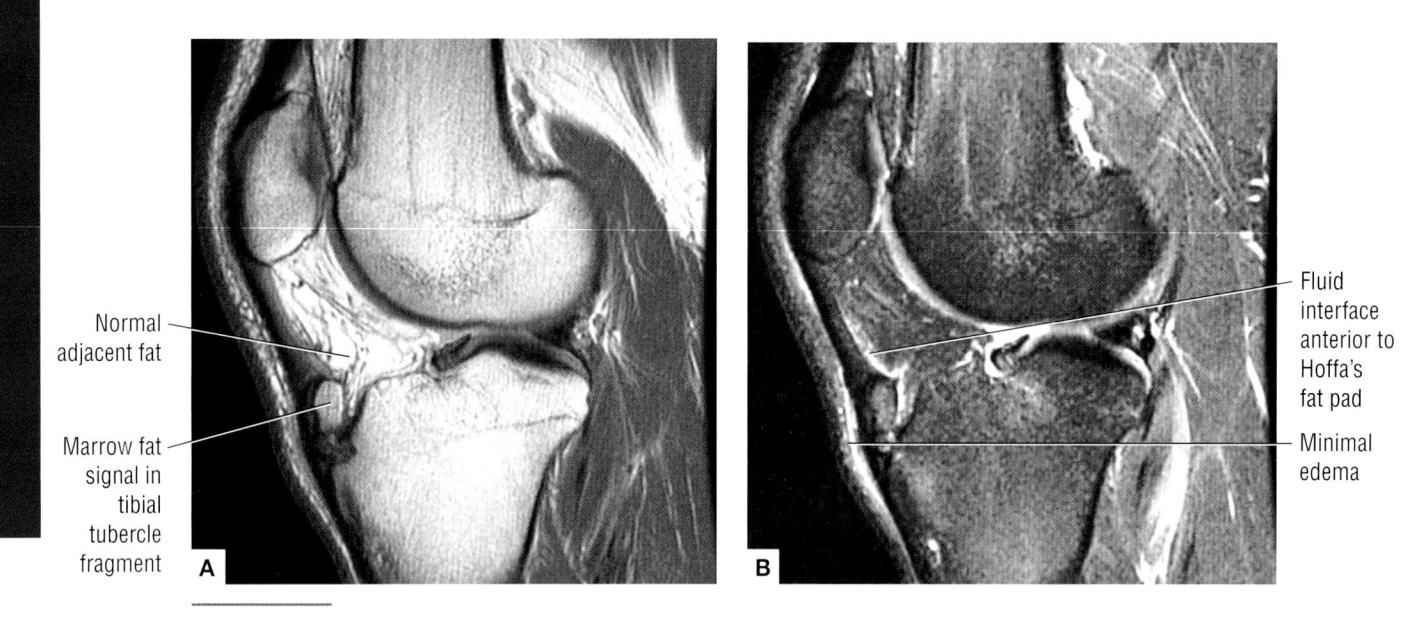

FIGURE 7.129 Chronic phase of Osgood-Schlatter disease with a marrow fat–containing fragment and minimal adjacent reactive soft tissue changes, as seen on these sagittal PD FSE (**A**) and FS PD FSE (**B**) images. Mild distal patellar tendon thickening can also be seen. Repetitive traction microtrauma that occurs during eccentric contractions of a strong extensor mechanism is common in jumping sports.

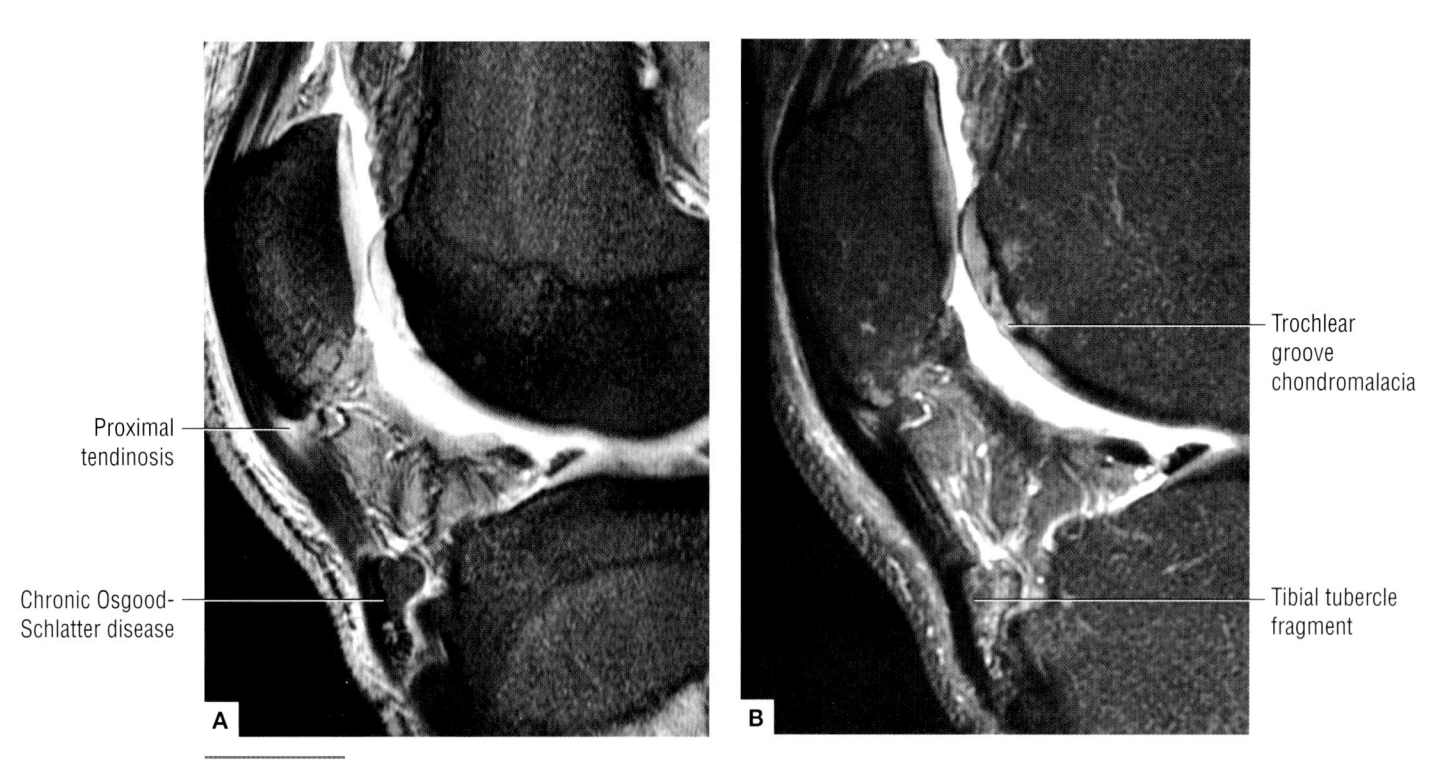

FIGURE 7.130 Chronic Osgood-Schlatter disease. Sagittal PD FSE (**A**) and FS PD FSE (**B**) images show proximal patellar tendinosis involving posterior tendon fibers with multiple submaximal avulsion fractures of the patellar tendon insertion caused by traction microtrauma.

Sinding-Larsen-Johansson Syndrome

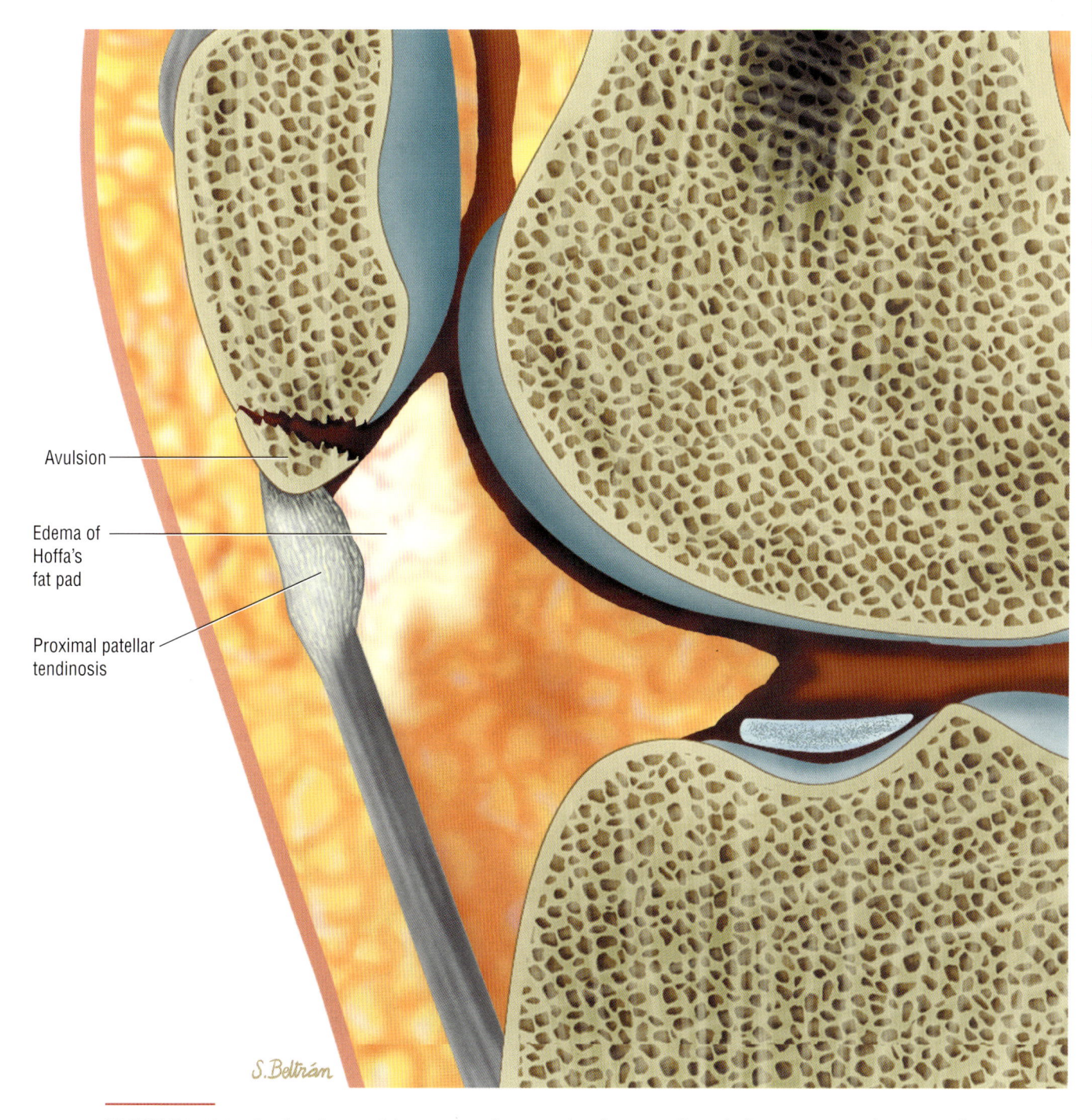

FIGURE 7.131 Sinding-Larsen-Johansson syndrome with inferior patellar pole fragmentation, adjacent patellar tendinosis, and edema of the anterior proximal aspect of Hoffa's fat pad.

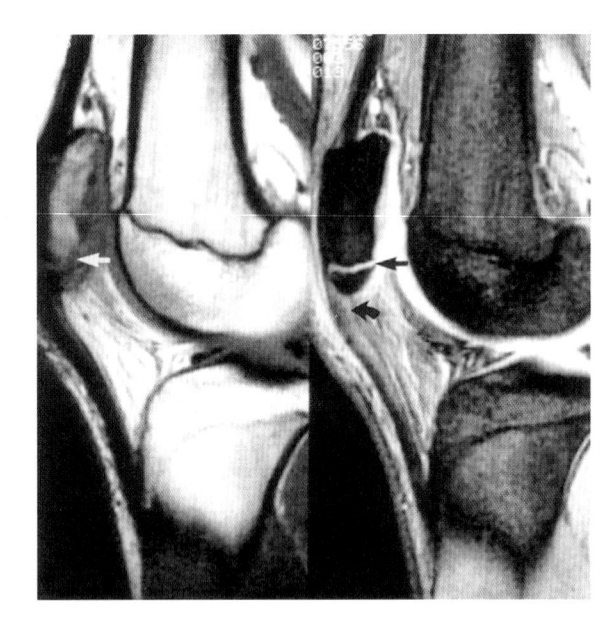

FIGURE 7.132 Accessory ossification of the inferior pole occurs in 5% of bipartite patellae and may be mistaken for Sinding-Larsen-Johansson syndrome.

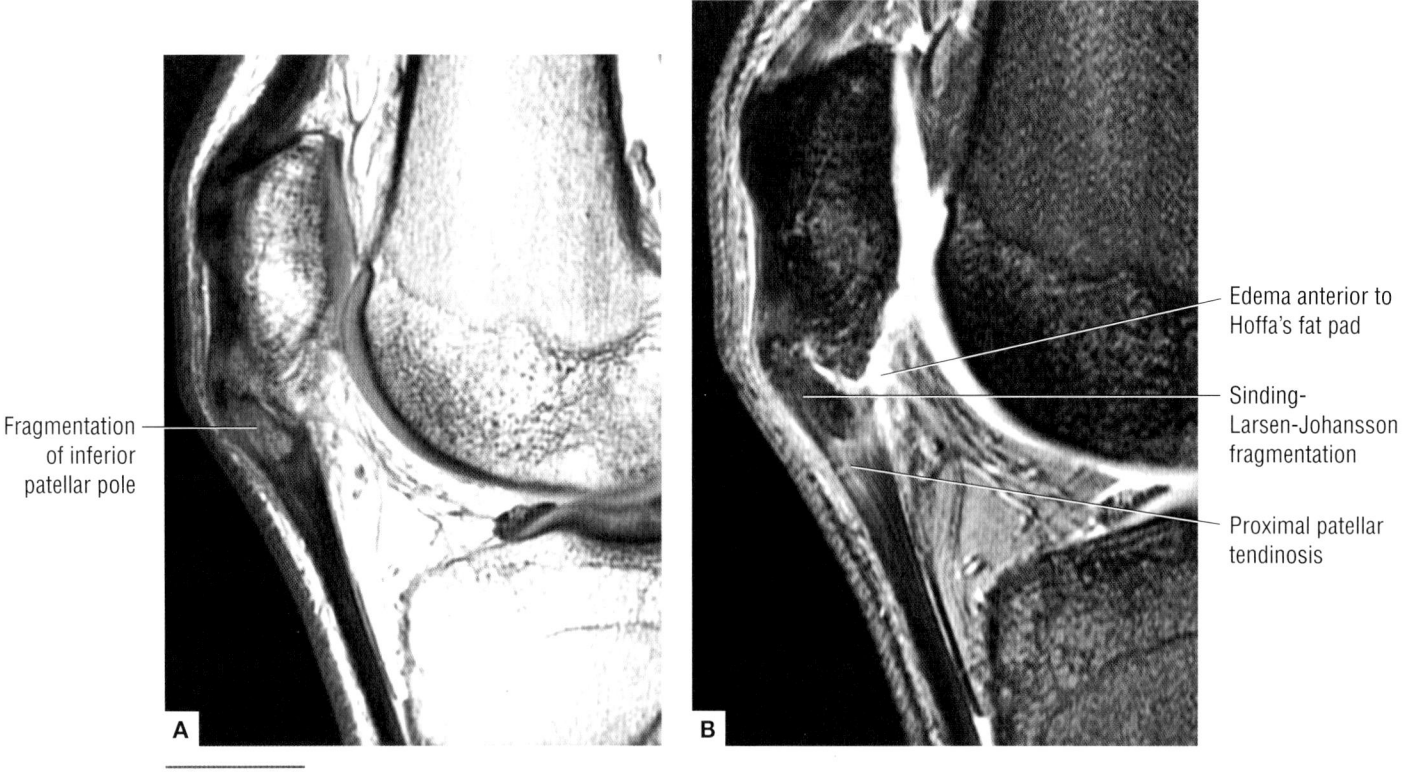

FIGURE 7.133 Sagittal PD FSE (**A**) and FS PD FSE (**B**) images in Sinding-Larsen-Johansson syndrome show patellar fragmentation from an osseous avulsion. The syndrome may also result in elongation of the distal patellar pole or a small avulsion ossicle. A patellar sleeve fracture may also produce distal pole fragmentation.

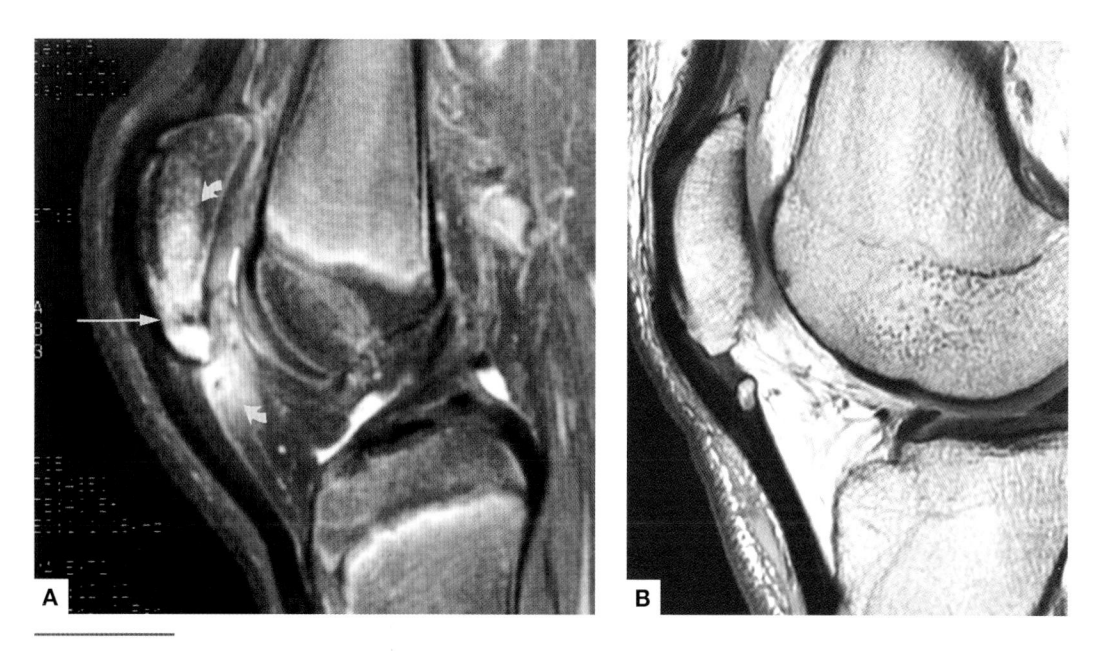

Patellofemoral Joint and the Extensor Mechanism

FIGURE 7.134 (**A**) An FS PD-weighted FSE sagittal image in a case of Sinding-Larsen-Johansson syndrome. The cause is identified as trauma with reactive marrow edema (*curved arrows*) of the inferior pole of the patella and Hoffa's fat pad adjacent to the patellar fracture (*straight arrow*). This represents overuse traction apophysitis or avulsion associated with microtrauma and dynamic stress at the proximal patellar tendon attachment site to the inferior pole of the patella. (**B**) Sagittal PD FSE image.

Inferior pole fragment in Sinding-Larsen-Johansson syndrome

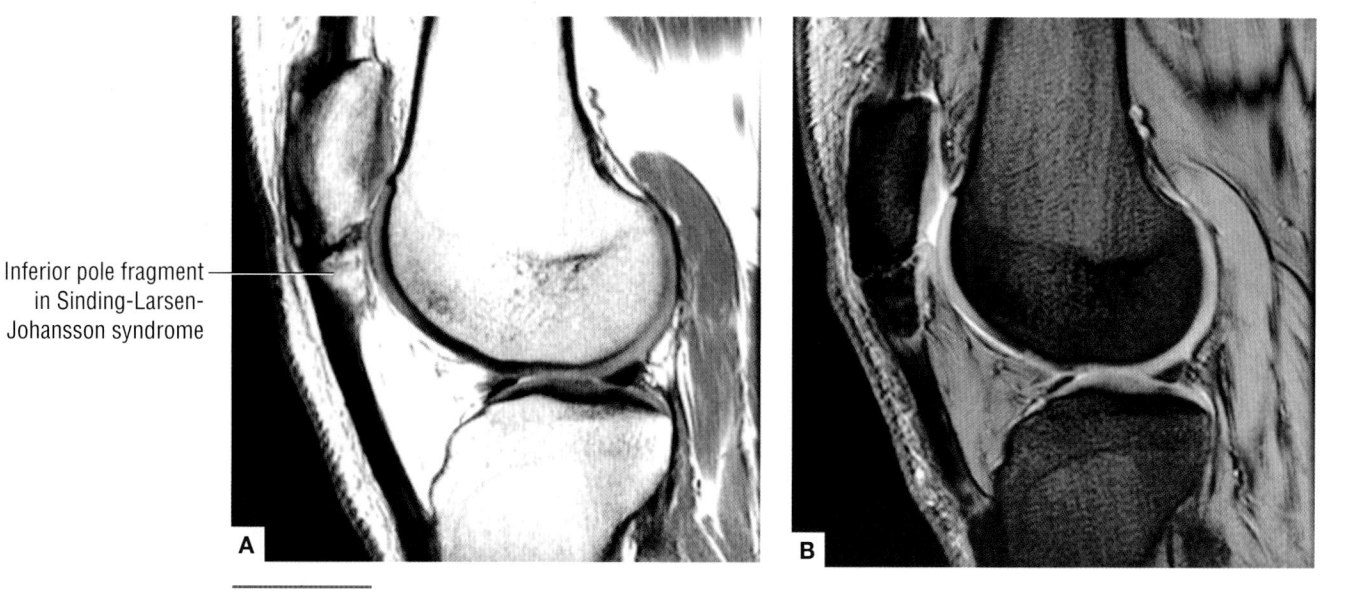

FIGURE 7.135 Chronic residual changes in Sinding-Larsen-Johansson syndrome with a large nondisplaced inferior pole fragment on sagittal PD FSE (**A**) and FS PD FSE (**B**) images.

Prepatellar and Superficial Infrapatellar Bursa

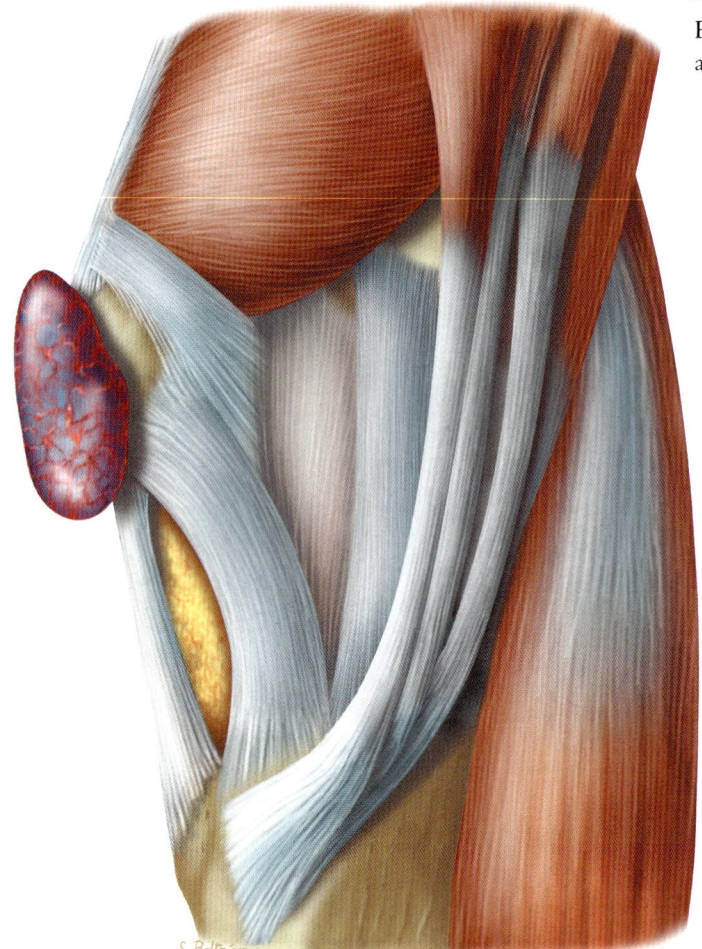

FIGURE 7.136 Subcutaneous prepatellar bursa anterior to the patella.

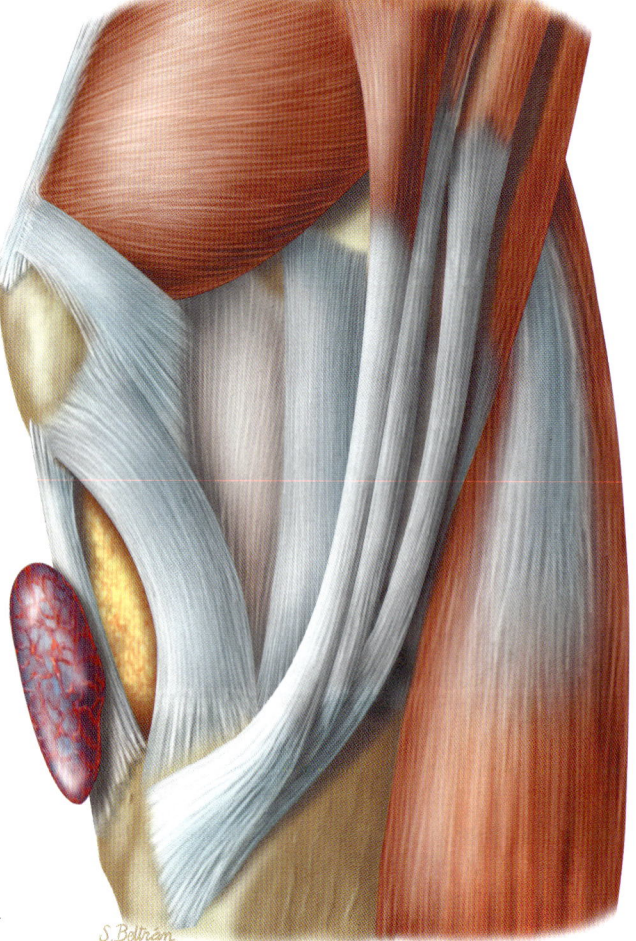

FIGURE 7.137 The superficial infrapatellar bursa between the skin and the tibial tuberosity.

Patellar Bursae

Key Concepts

- Prepatellar bursa represents one of three potential bursal spaces anterior to patella.

- Small amounts of fluid may be found normally in deep infrapatellar bursa.

- Bursae are usually not visualized on MR unless distended with fluid.

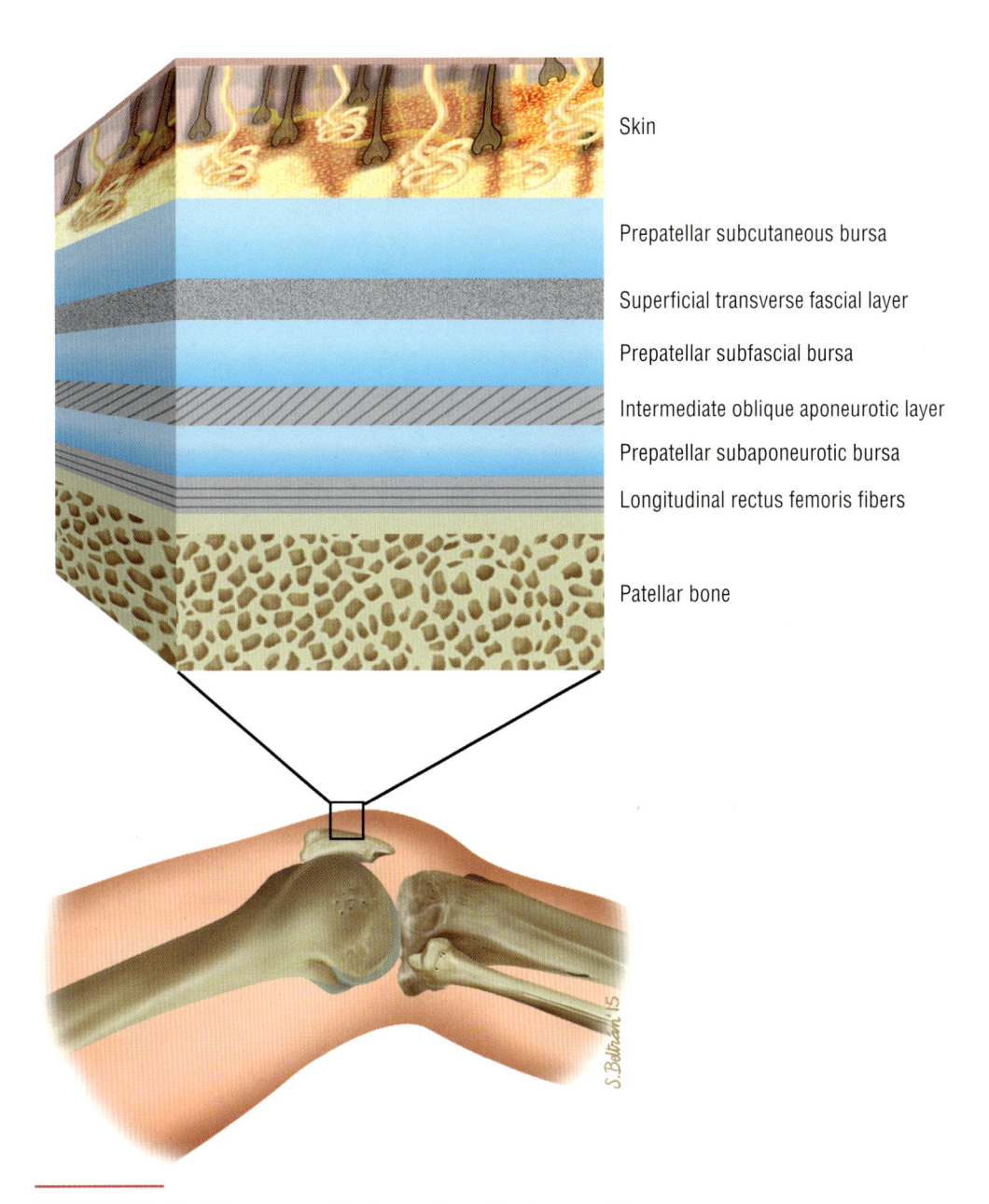

FIGURE 7.138 Three prepatellar bursae in a trilaminar model.

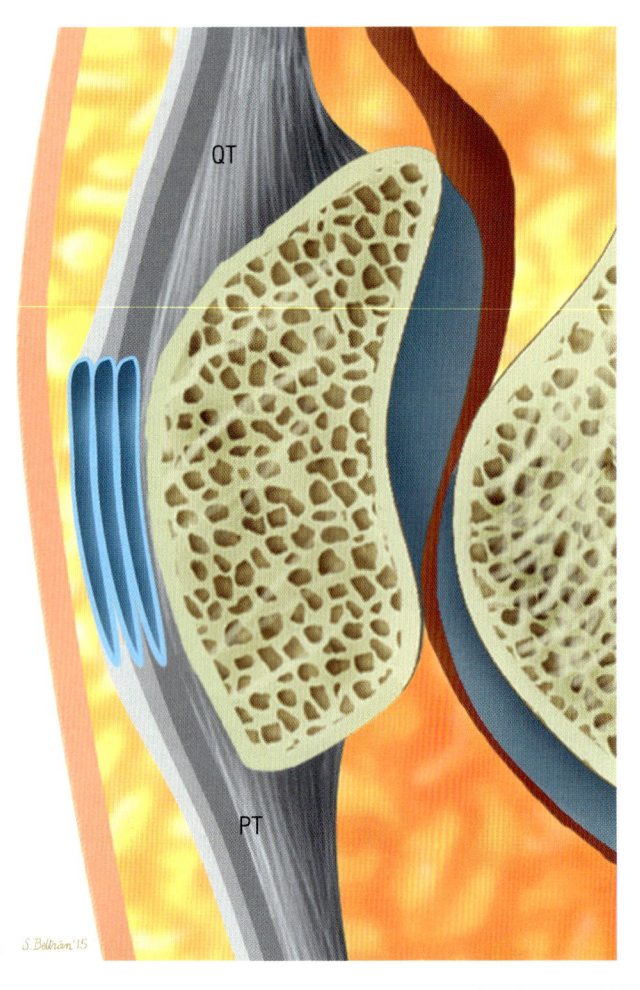

FIGURE 7.139 (**A**) Prepatellar subcutaneous (1), subfascial (2), and subaponeurosis (3) bursae. (**B**) Soft tissue anatomy anterior to the patella. Three potential prepatellar bursae as a trilaminar structure from superficial to deep includes a transversely oriented fascia, an obliquely oriented aponeurosis, and the longitudinally oriented rectus femoris fibers. Between these layers exists a prepatellar subcutaneous bursa, a prepatellar subfascial bursa, and a prepatellar subcutaneous bursa. Sagittal FS PD FSE image. PT, patellar tendon; QT, quadriceps tendon.

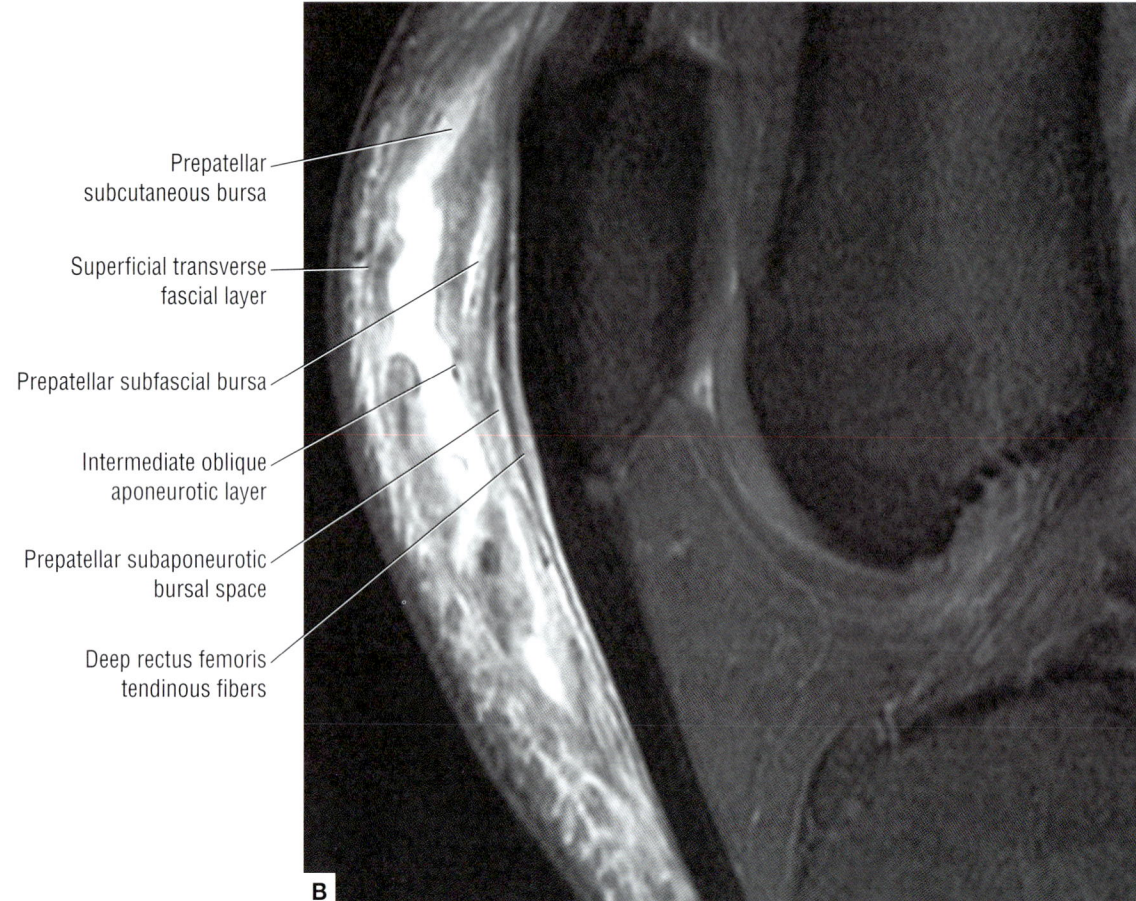

Prepatellar bursa

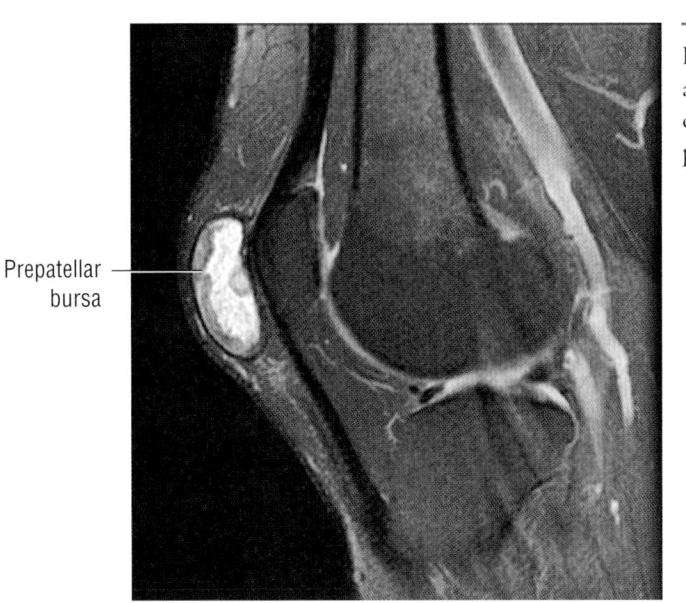

FIGURE 7.140 Sagittal FS PD FSE image showing a well-defined inhomogeneous prepatellar bursa fluid collection. Hemorrhage or synovial hypertrophy may produce signal heterogeneity.

Prepatellar bursa between arciform fascia and intermediate oblique layer

Prepatellar bursa between skin and arciform fascia

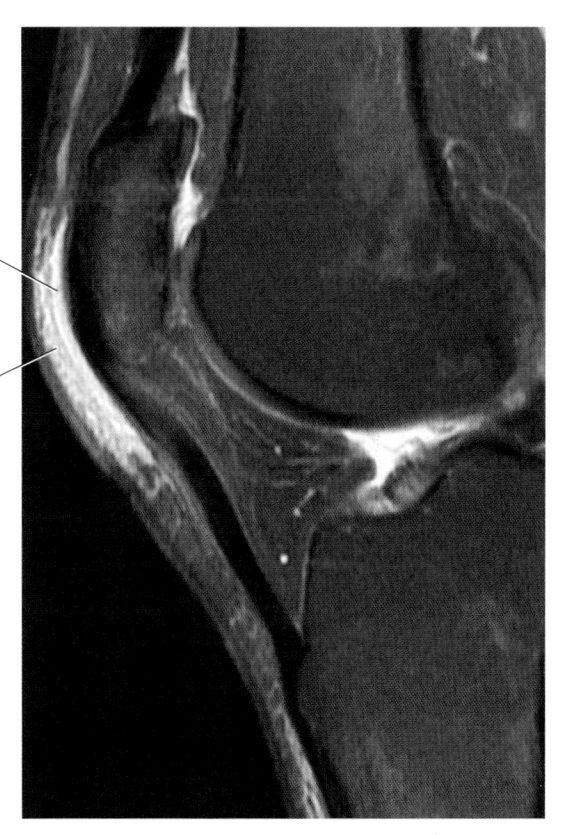

FIGURE 7.141 On this sagittal FS PD FSE image, two of the three potential bursal spaces anterior to the patella are visualized between the skin and the arciform fascia and the arciform fascia and the intermediate oblique layer.

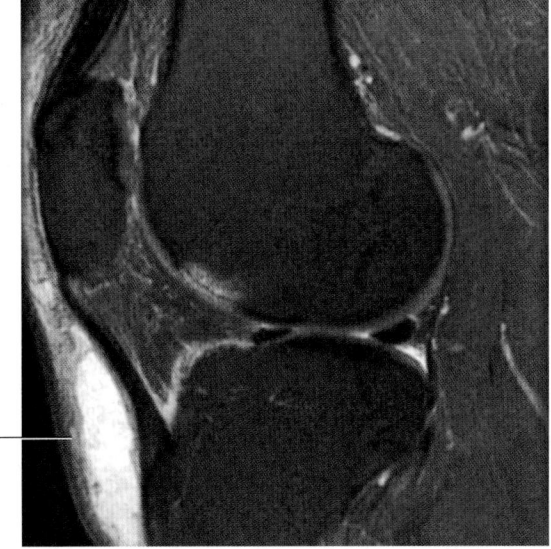

Superficial infrapatellar bursa

FIGURE 7.142 A hyperintense localized deep infrapatellar bursa fluid collection is seen on this sagittal FS PD FSE image.

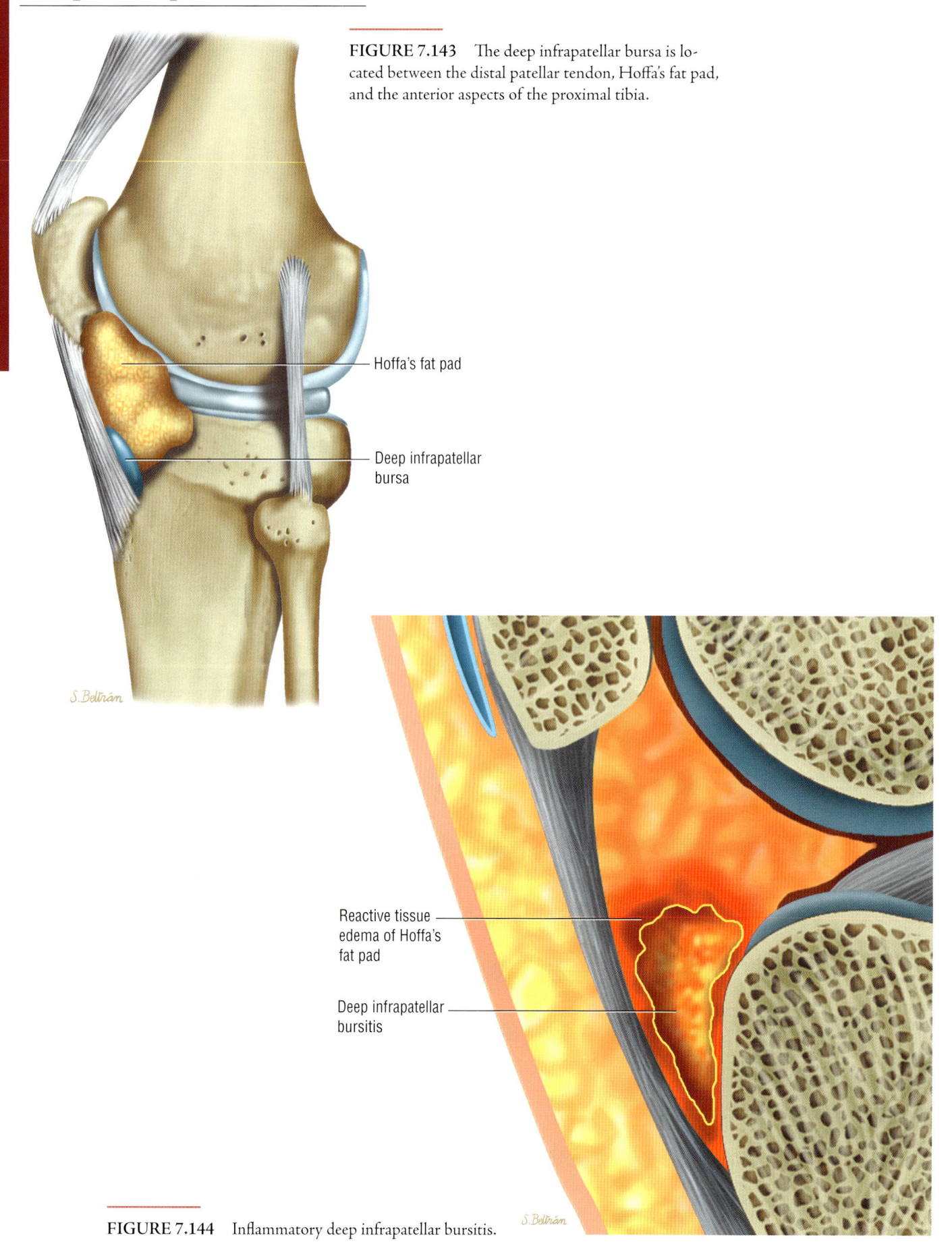

Deep Infrapatellar Bursa

FIGURE 7.143 The deep infrapatellar bursa is located between the distal patellar tendon, Hoffa's fat pad, and the anterior aspects of the proximal tibia.

- Hoffa's fat pad
- Deep infrapatellar bursa

- Reactive tissue edema of Hoffa's fat pad
- Deep infrapatellar bursitis

FIGURE 7.144 Inflammatory deep infrapatellar bursitis.

Patellar Bursae

- *Prepatellar bursitis* ("*housemaid's knee*") may involve one of the anterior subcutaneous bursa over the patella and anterior to the patellar tendon.
- Three potential bursal spaces anterior to patella
    - Prepatellar bursa: most superficial, located between skin and arciform fascia
    - Bursal space between the arciform and intermediate oblique layer
    - Bursal space between the intermediate oblique layer and deep fibers of the rectus femoris
- Soft tissue anatomy anterior to patella
    - Arciform fascia consists of transverse fibers, which partially originate from the iliotibial tract and extend over the patellar tendon.
    - Intermediate oblique layer lies between the arciform layer and the deeper longitudinal fibers of the rectus femoris.
    - Distally, the intermediate oblique layer attenuates.
    - Longitudinal fibers of rectus femoris continue over top of patella and become the patellar tendon.
- Bursitis characterized by a range of appearances
    - Edema, simple fluid or complex collection
    - More complex, septated fluid-filled collection that may contain areas of hemorrhage and proteinaceous condensations
- *Infrapatellar bursitis (clergyman's knee)*
    - Involves superficial or subcutaneous infrapatellar bursa
    - Located between skin and tibial tuberosity
- *Deep infrapatellar bursitis*
    - Bordered by distal patellar tendon, tibial tuberosity, and inferior extent of Hoffa's fat pad[87]
    - Scarring to patellar tendon associated with trochlear groove chondral abnormalities
    - Deep infrapatellar bursa, Hoffa's fat pad, and tibial tuberosity function to prevent impingement between patellar tendon and tibia in full knee flexion.

Selected Patellofemoral Surgical Procedures

Patellectomy

- May be required to treat unmanageable chondromalacia with severe pain and comminuted fracture of the patella[69]
- Usually reserved for patients who are not candidates for patellofemoral replacement or Maquet's procedure (described below)[168]

Patella Realignment Procedures

- *Lateral release*
    - Indications include pain, tight lateral retinaculum, lateral tenderness, and lateral tracking in the absence of patellar subluxation.
- *Proximal realignment*
    - Lateral release plus medial imbrications of the VMO
    - Indicated for painful lateral subluxation with a normal Q angle
- *Tibial tubercle transfers* (distal realignment)
    - Indicated for symptomatic lateral subluxation, recurrent dislocation, abnormal Q angle, abnormal flexion Q angle, and increased congruence angle
- *Maquet's procedure* (anterior tibial tubercle elevation)
    - Performed to decrease loading forces across the patellofemoral joint by raising the insertion of the patellar tendon
    - Salvage procedure for advanced patellofemoral arthrosis
- *Elmslie-Trillat procedure* (medialization of the tibial tubercle)[168]
    - Commonly performed procedure for lateral subluxations or recurrent patellar dislocations
- *Fulkerson osteotomy* (oblique osteotomy)
    - Medializes tibial tubercle and provides elevation with osteotomy

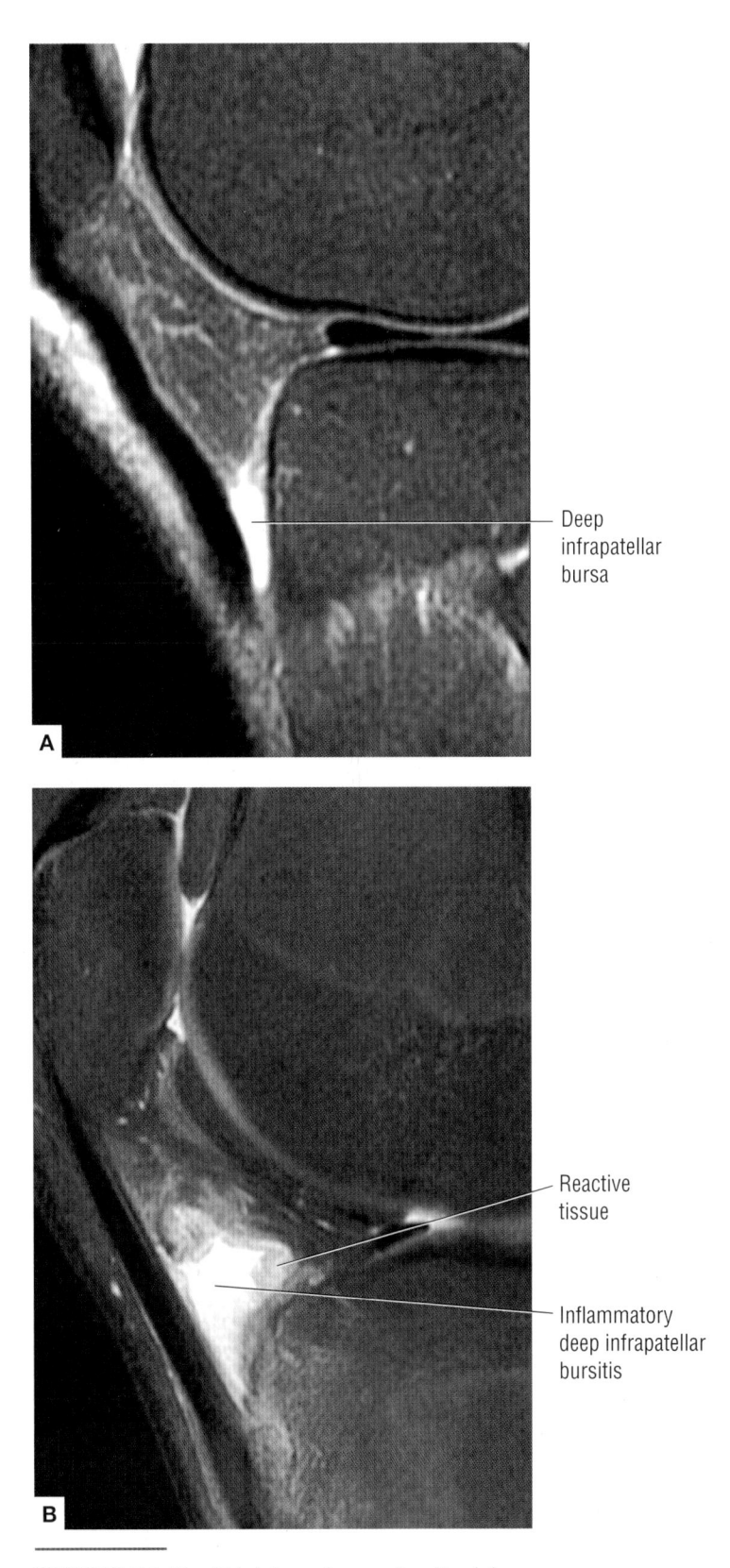

FIGURE 7.145 (**A**) A hyperintense localized deep infrapatellar bursa fluid collection is seen on this sagittal FS PD FSE image. (**B**) Large deep infrapatellar bursitis with intermediate-signal synovial thickening lining the periphery of the bursa is seen on this sagittal FS PD FSE image.

Quadriceps Tendinosis and Tear

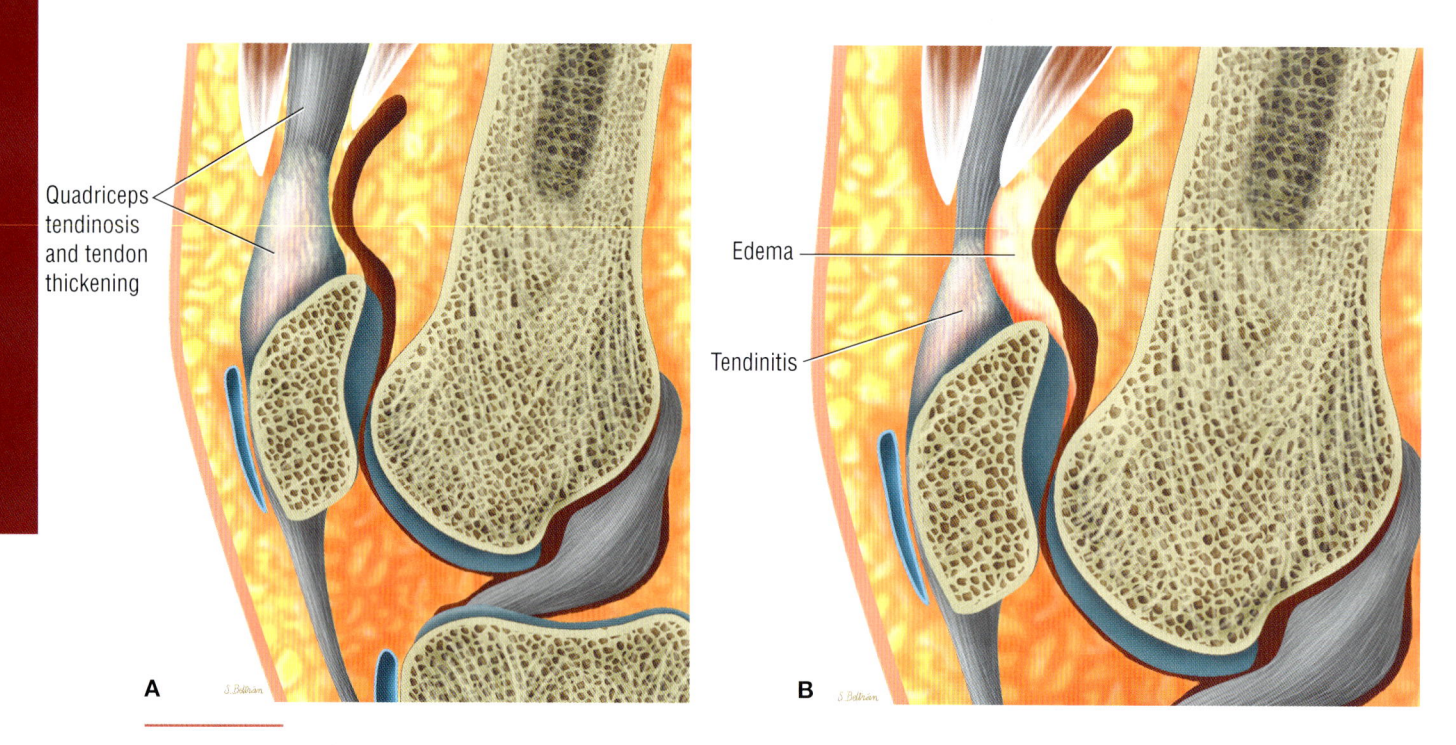

FIGURE 7.146 (**A**) Distal quadriceps tendinosis with diffuse tendon thickening. (**B**) Edema of the quadriceps fat pad associated with distal quadriceps tendinosis.

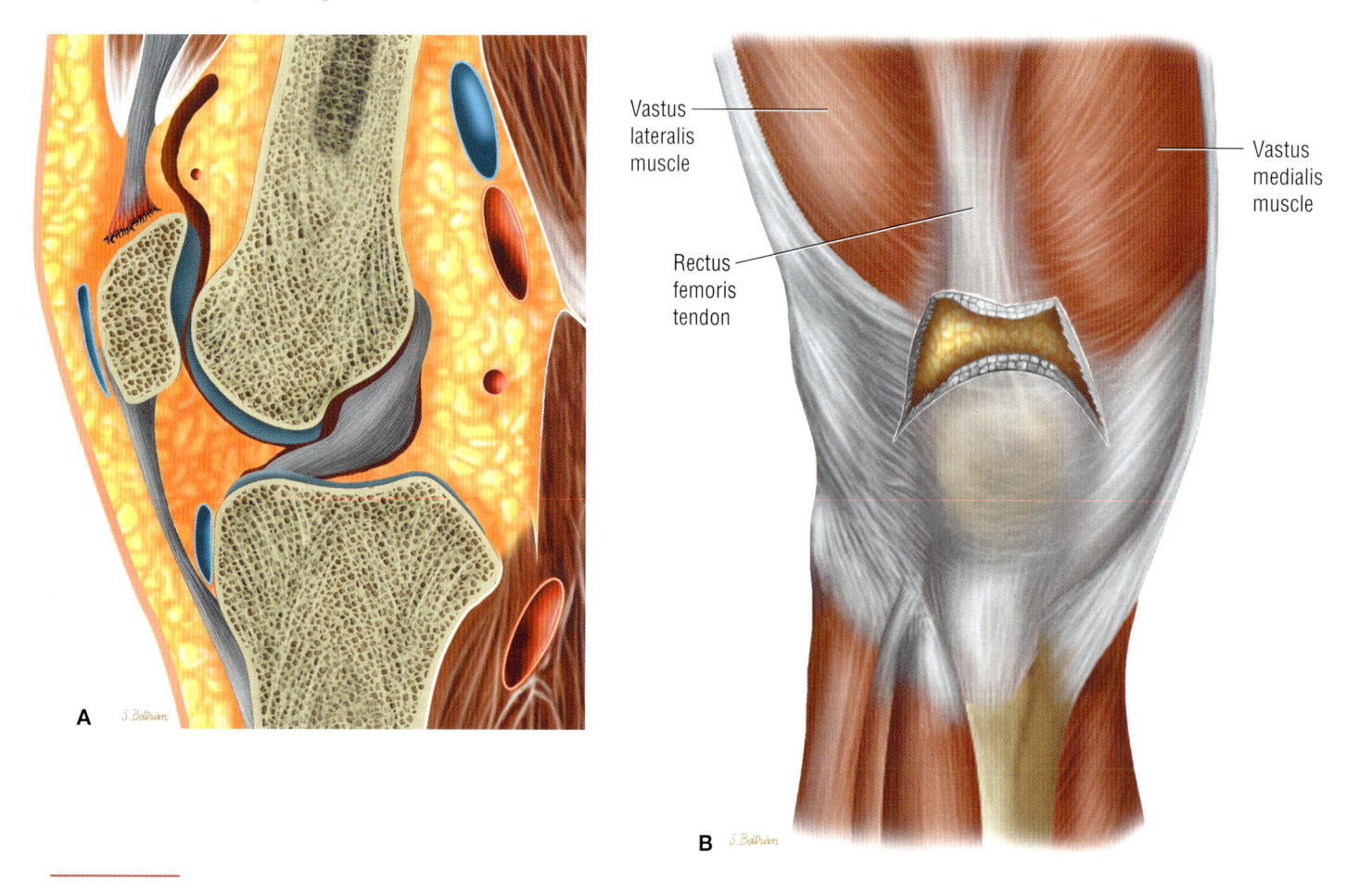

FIGURE 7.147 Grade 3 tendon strain with disruption of the tendon unit. A large hemarthrosis with a freely mobile patella, loss of extensor function, and a palpable defect occur with full thickness tears. Partial tears present with an extensor lag. (**A**) Sagittal view. (**B**) Anterior view.

Quadriceps Tendon and Muscle Tears

Key Concepts

- Quadriceps tendinosis or tears are best identified on superior aspects of sagittal images through the extensor mechanism.

- Tears usually occur proximal to the patellar insertion or expansion of the quadriceps tendon and may extend through the vastus intermedius tendon.

- Inferior migration of the patella and tendon discontinuity with interposed hemorrhage at the tendon gap are common findings in complete tendon rupture.

Quadriceps Tendon and Muscle Tears

- Quadriceps muscle group: rectus femoris and vastus intermedius muscles, which insert on the base of the patella, and the vastus lateralis and medialis muscles, which insert on the lateral and medial aspects of the patella, respectively

- Quadriceps tendon tears
    - Begin centrally and progress peripherally
    - Superficial and deep tears rarely involve the trilaminar tendon at the same level.

- Mechanism of injury
    - Repetitive microtrauma secondary to forces of explosive extension, acceleration, deceleration, jumping, and landing
    - Result in degeneration adjacent to or involving the distal quadriceps tendon insertion to the superior pole of the patella[91]
    - Chronic tendinopathy may progress to frank rupture.
    - Result from either forced muscle contraction or direct trauma
    - Usually occur in the young athlete, although in an older age group than patellar tendon ruptures
    - Acute flexion of the extended knee associated with preexisting tendinosis, chronic repetitive microtrauma, or eccentric muscle contraction can lead to tendon failure.

- Histologic findings
    - Absence of inflammatory cells in quadriceps tendinosis and partial tears
    - Microscopic features in healing include neovascularization and angioblastic hyperplasia associated with tendinosis.
    - *Myositis ossificans* can be a sequela to injury, especially when the vastus medialis is involved.
- MR evaluation of extensor muscle injuries and tears of the quadriceps tendon
    - Initial set of coronal or sagittal images display the longitudinal extent of muscle involvement.
    - Axial images identify both precise muscle group involved and adjacent anatomic relations.
    - Axial images useful in differentiating complete muscle tears with diastasis from partial tears with associated atrophy
    - Atrophy best displayed on T1-weighted images
    - Areas of edema and hemorrhage best shown on either FS T2-weighted FSE or STIR images
    - GRE images useful in showing susceptibility in hemosiderin deposits in chronic hematomas
    - MR imaging is sensitive to both acute and chronic hemorrhage in extensor muscle tears.
    - Subacute hematomas may demonstrate areas of increased signal intensity on T1-weighted images secondary to paramagnetic effect of methemoglobin.
    - Areas of chronic hemorrhage demonstrate low signal intensity, especially on GRE images.
    - Differences in signal characteristics may be important in distinguishing between areas of suspected hemorrhage and other soft tissue masses, such as synovial sarcoma.
        - Intravenous gadolinium can help clarify a differential diagnosis if an area of hemorrhage cannot be clearly characterized.
        - Hemorrhage demonstrates peripheral enhancement without central hyperintensity.
        - Malignant neoplasm, such as a synovial sarcoma, demonstrates increased intake of gadolinium centrally within the lesion.

Quadriceps tendinosis —

Partial tear — quadriceps tendon with tendinosis

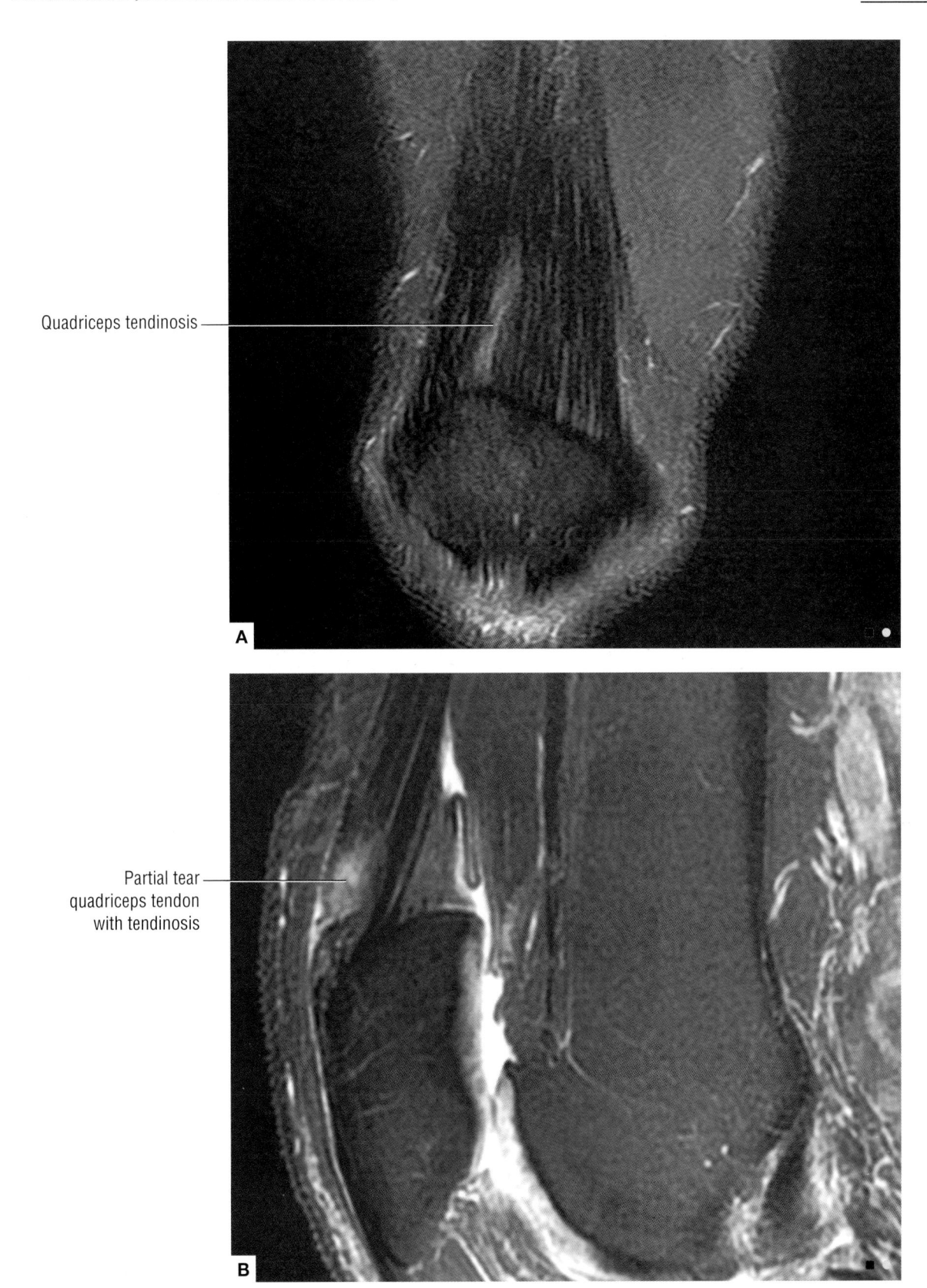

FIGURE 7.148 Quadriceps tendinosis with partial loss of anterior distal tendon contour. Tendinosis is characterized by intermediate signal in thickened distal tendon fibers. Repetitive microtrauma may be associated interstitial tears or contour abnormalities of anterior rectus femoris fibers prior to tear and retraction of intermediate and deep quadriceps tendon fibers. Coronal (**A**) and sagittal (**B**) FS PD FSE images.

Retracted anterior rectus femoris fibers

Partial tear (interstitial tear of vastus layer)

Intact deep intermedius fibers

Anterior rectus femoris tear

Interstitial tear of intermediate layer

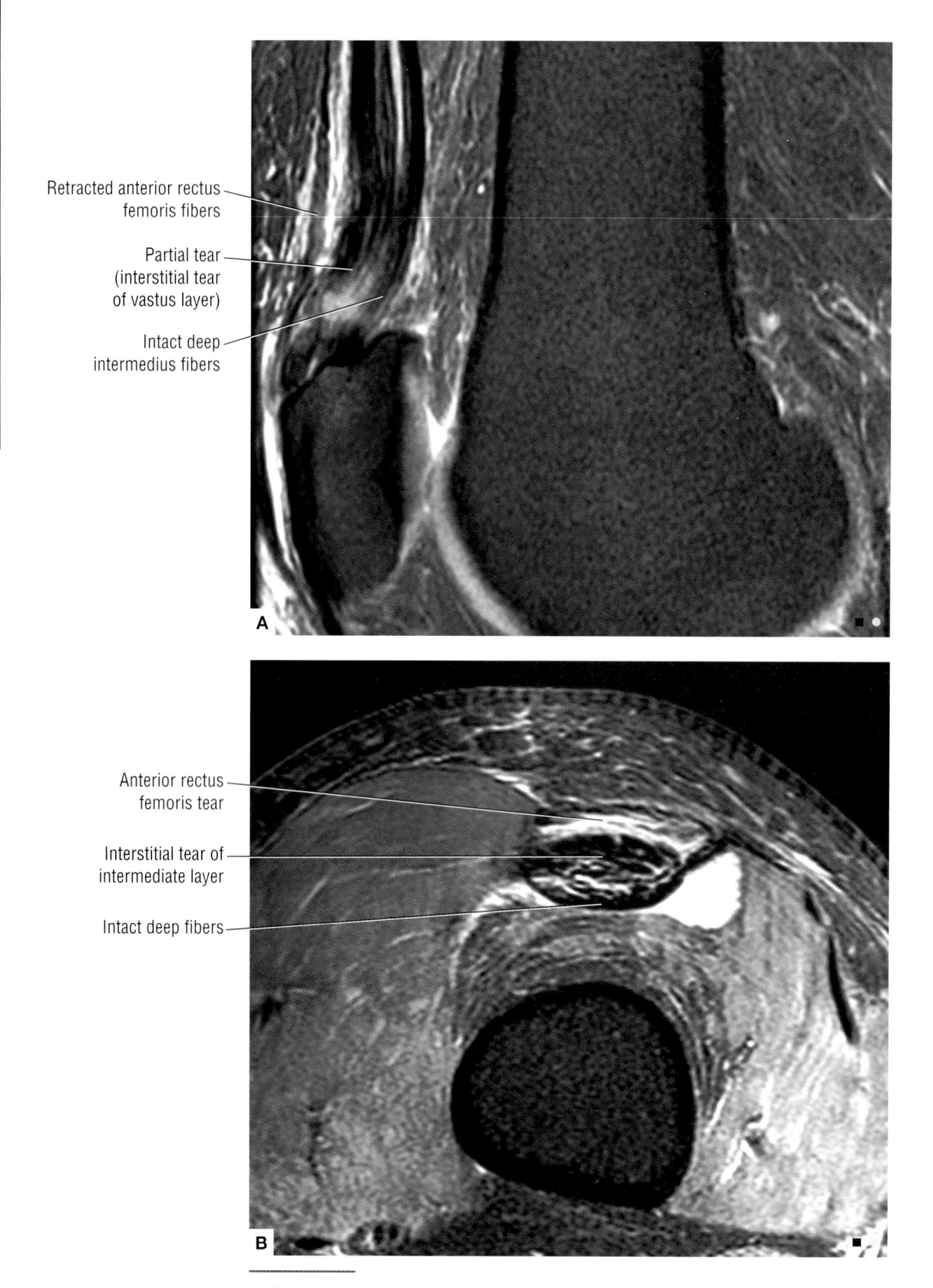

Intact deep fibers

FIGURE 7.149 Lax torn anterior rectus femoris fibers that should be oriented in line with the anterior patellar surface. Intact quadriceps tendon bulk of intermediate and deep fibers. Sagittal (**A**) and axial (**B**) FS PD FSE image.

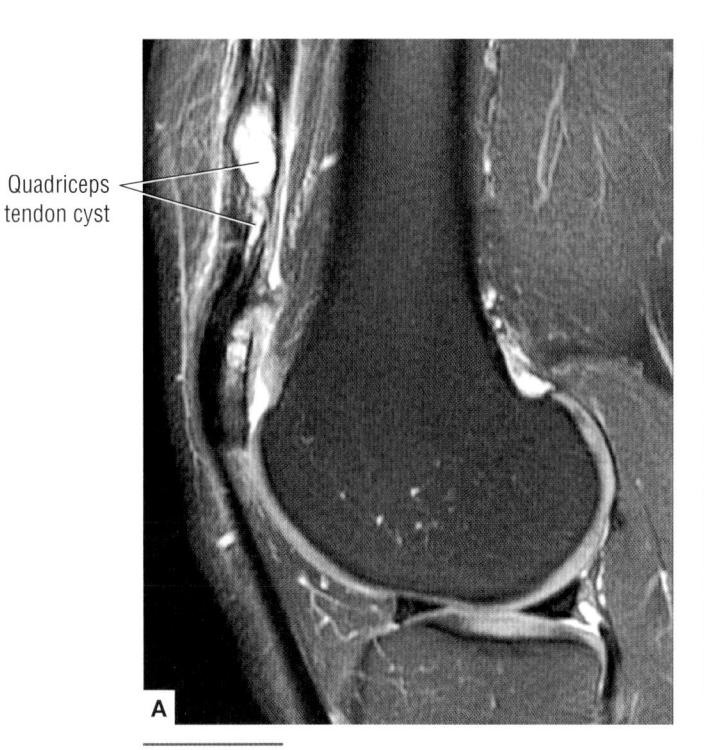

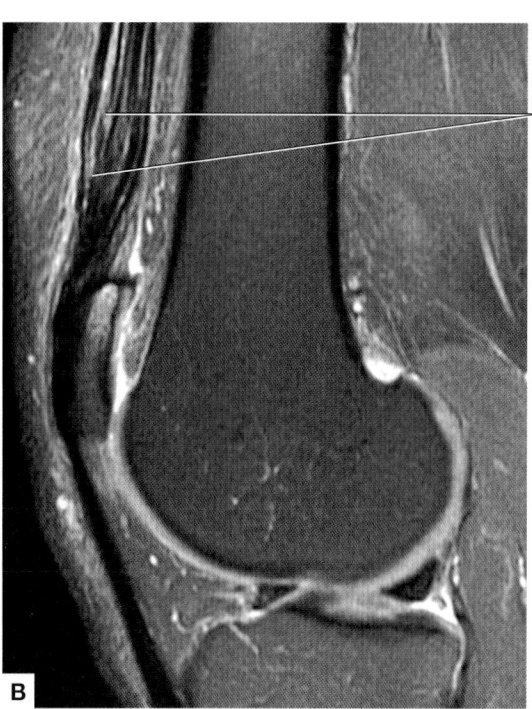

Patellofemoral Joint and the Extensor Mechanism

FIGURE 7.150 Sagittal FS PD FSE images showing quadriceps cyst (**A**) and tendinosis (**B**) with tendon thickening and linear hyperintensity. Chronic degenerative tendon areas are more common in an older population. Direct steroid injection and systemic disease can also weaken the quadriceps tendon.

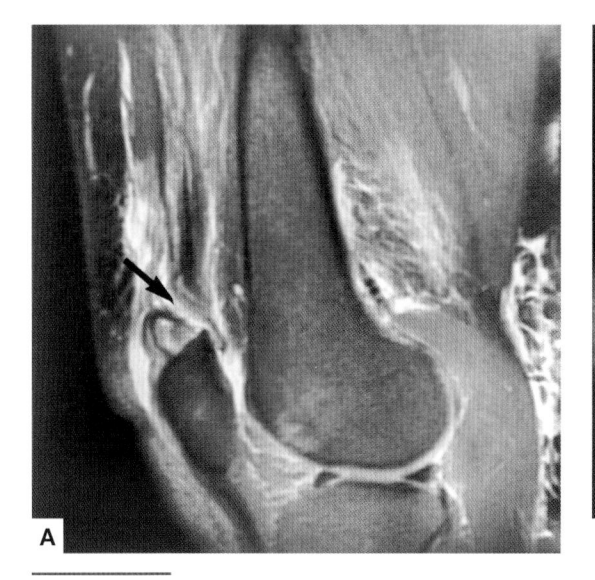

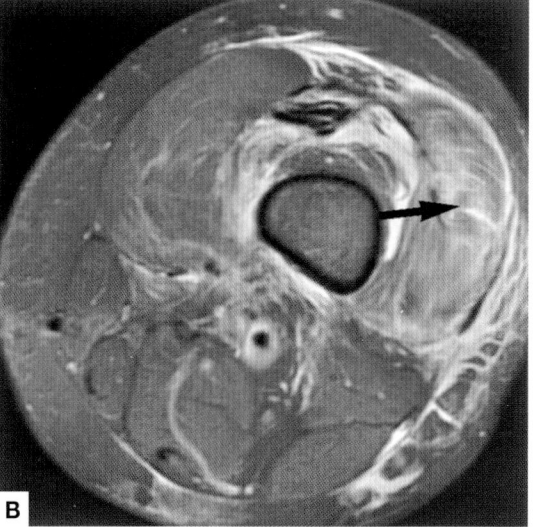

FIGURE 7.151 (**A**) An FS T2-weighted FSE sagittal image shows acute rupture of the quadriceps tendon with high-signal-intensity fluid filling the tendon gap (*arrow*). There is associated patella baja secondary to the distal pull from the patellar tendon. (**B**) An FS T2-weighted FSE axial image shows diffuse vastus lateralis muscle edema (*arrow*).

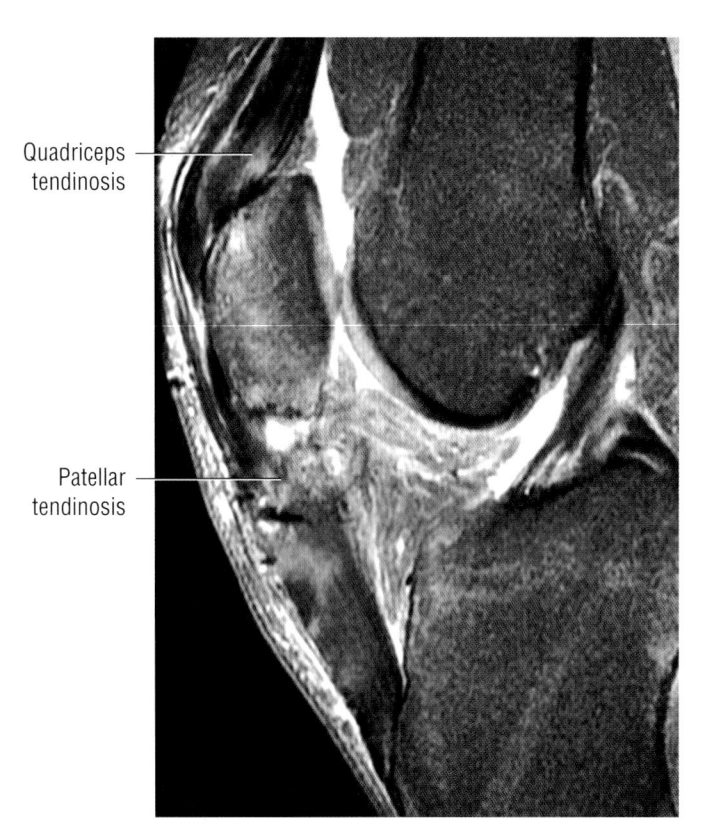

FIGURE 7.152 Distal quadriceps and patellar tendinosis. Degenerative areas of the tendon, associated with the adjacent site of rupture, are seen on this sagittal FS PD FSE image.

FIGURE 7.153 (**A**) Complete discontinuity of the distal quadriceps on a coronal PD FSE image. Eccentric contraction leads to tendon failure. The majority of ruptures occur transversely and are located within 2cm of the superior pole of the patella. (**B**) Corresponding axial FS PD FSE image showing extension of the rupture through the vastus intermedius and vastus medialis with vastus lateralis muscle strain.

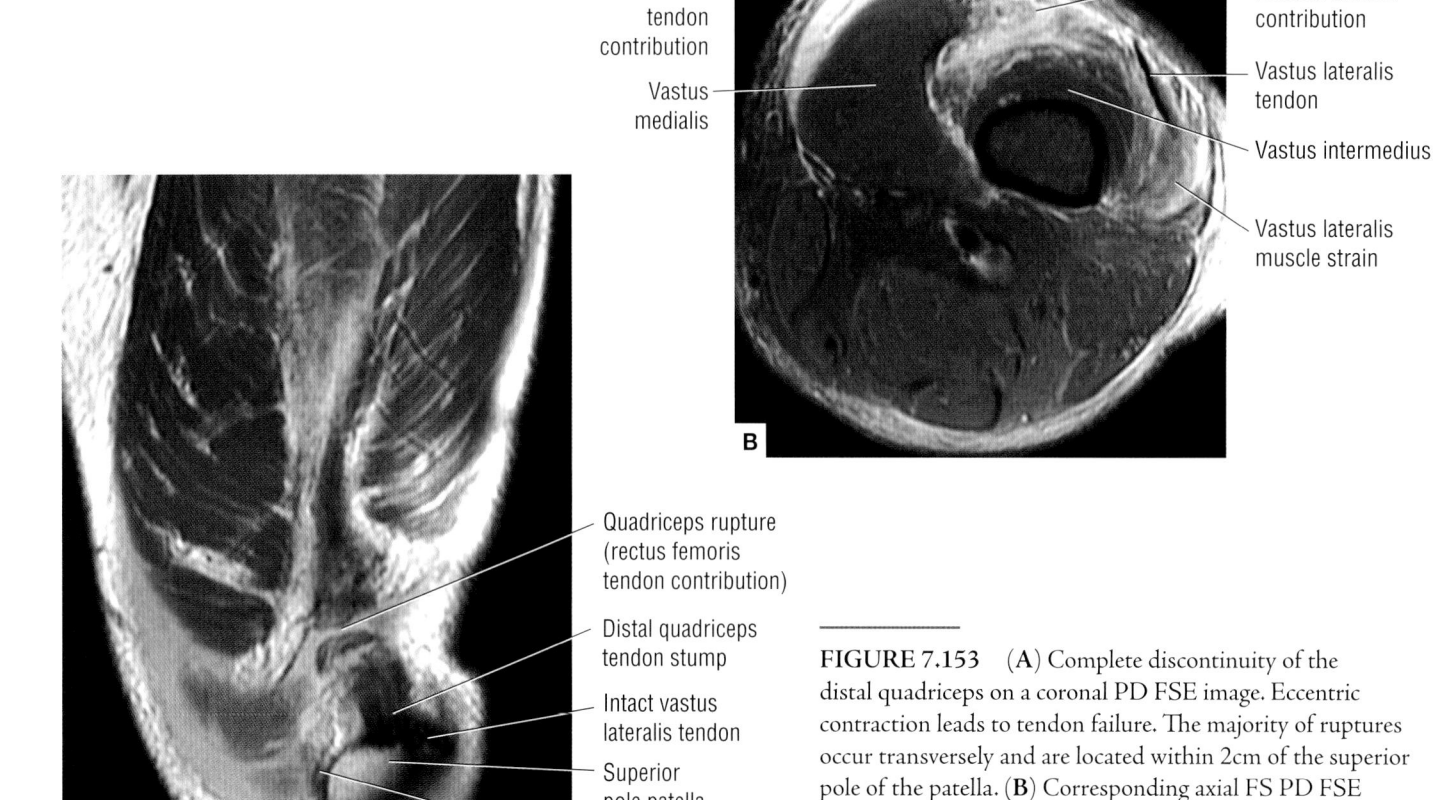

MR Findings of Quadriceps Tendon and Muscle Tears

- Edema and areas of fraying in affected muscle demonstrate intermediate signal intensity on T1-weighted images and increased signal intensity on T2, STIR, and FS PD-weighted FSE images.

- Muscle atrophy and fatty infiltration show regions of increased signal intensity on T1-weighted images.

- Retracted proximal or distal muscle bundle identified as soft tissue mass with higher signal intensity than native muscle

- Any increase in signal intensity within quadriceps tendon is abnormal.

- Increases range from intrasubstance signal in degeneration or tendinitis to high-signal-intensity hemorrhage or edema in partial or complete avulsions or ruptures of the tendon.

- Individual muscle groups should be identified in cases of partial tendon ruptures.

- MR imaging used to document an intact quadriceps tendon in superficial injuries associated with subcutaneous edema or hemorrhage

- Enlargement or increased signal intensity of the quadriceps fat pad is also within the differential of anterior knee pain.[518]

- Secondary signs of quadriceps insufficiency
    - Patellar tilting
    - Redundancy, laxity, or retraction of patellar tendon

Treatment of Quadriceps Tendon and Muscle Tears

- Acute quadriceps tendon rupture treated with direct surgical repair, with or without reinforcement of the tendon

- May include transverse drill holes across the patella for suture fixation

- Krackow and Bunnell technique together adds strength to the repair. The combined suture techniques alleviate potential shortening.

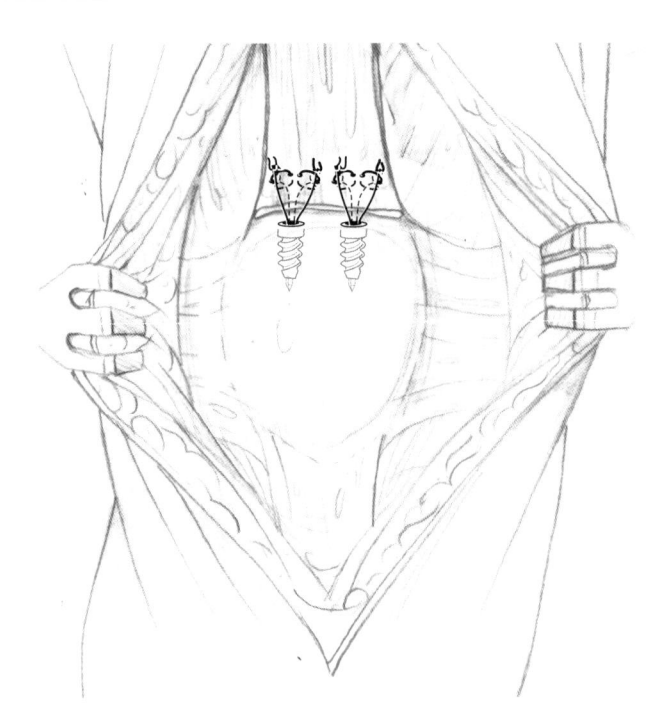

FIGURE 7.154 The final appearance of the Krackow-Bunnell weave technique before the sutures are tied. (Reprinted from Fu FH. *Master Techniques in Orthopaedic Surgery: Sports Medicine*. Philadelphia, PA: Lippincott Williams & Wilkins; 2010, with permission.)

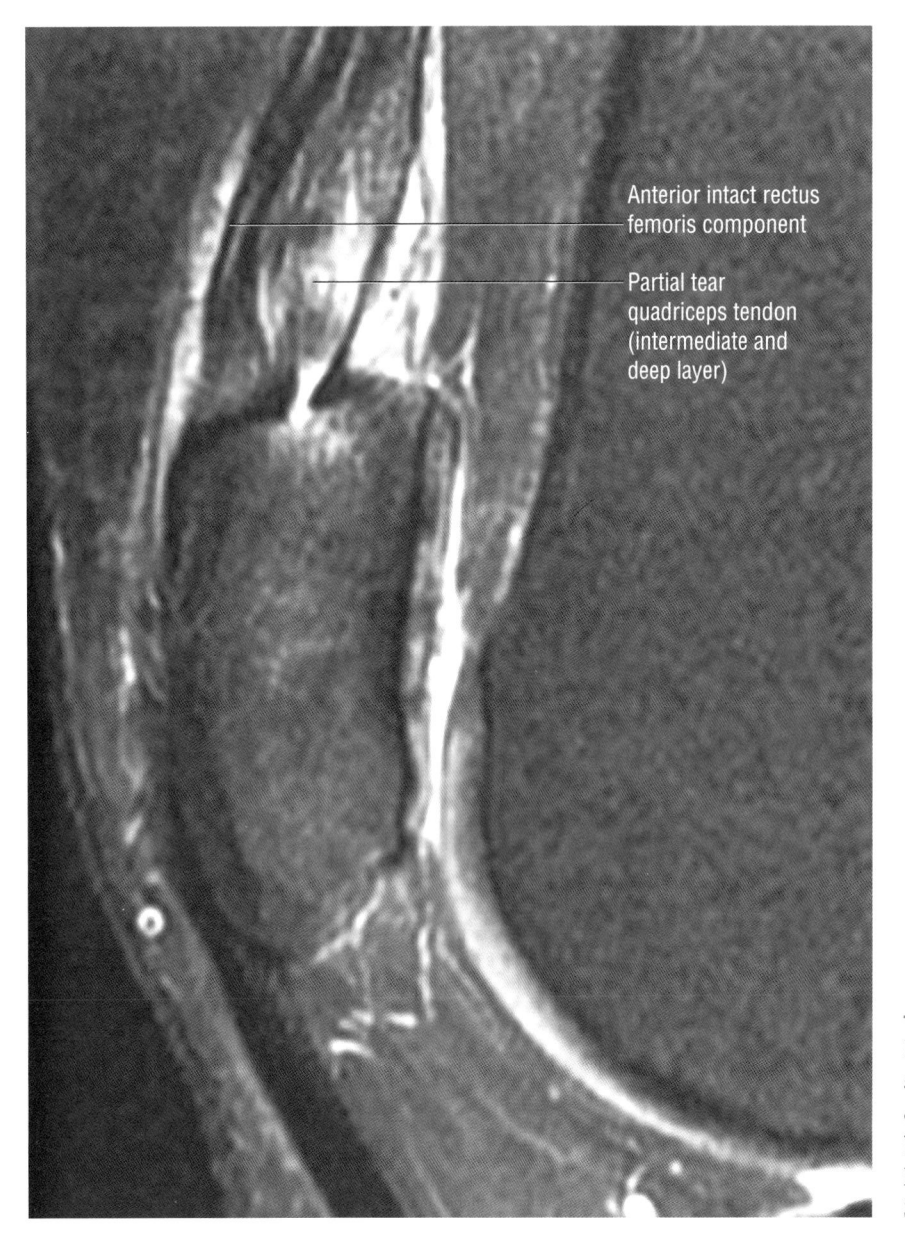

FIGURE 7.155 Partial tear of intermediate and deep quadriceps tendon layers. The normal quadriceps has a trilaminar configuration with fat between the layers of the rectus femoris, vastus lateralis, and medialis and the vastus intermedius. Sagittal FS PD FSE image.

Patellofemoral Joint and the Extensor Mechanism

Selective tear of rectus femoris tendon

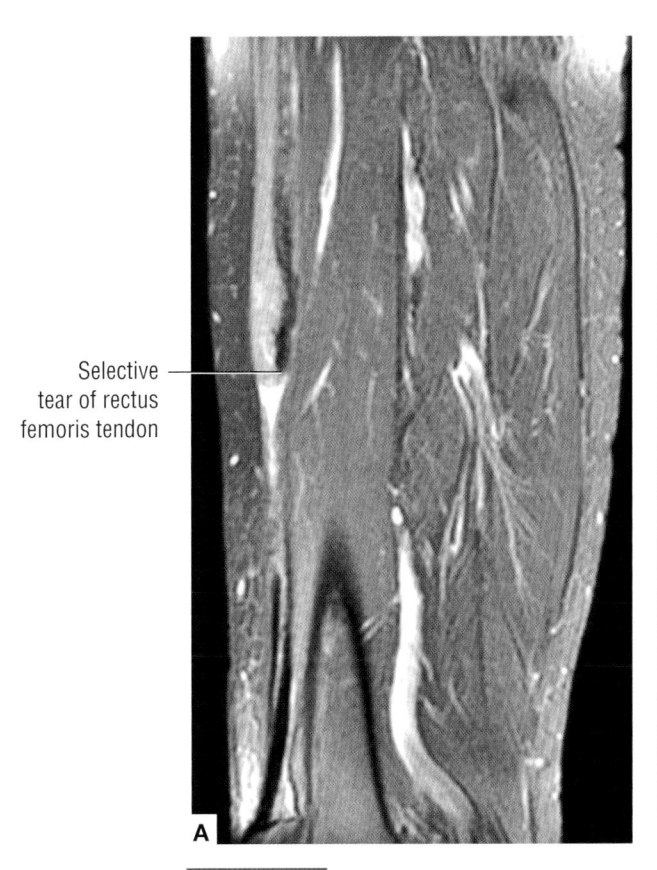

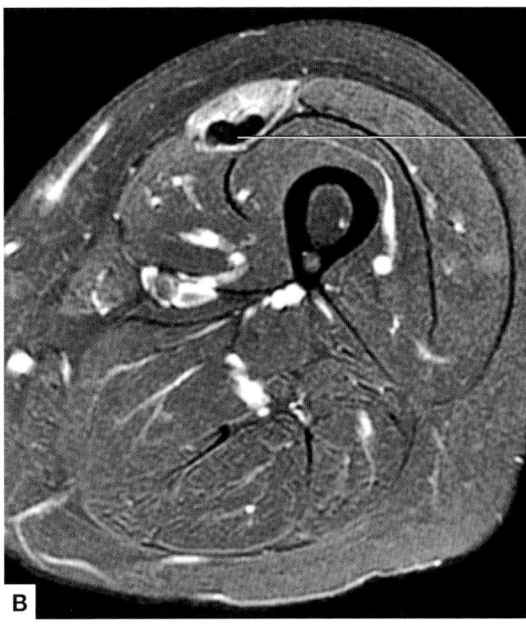

Isolated rectus femoris tear with tendon thickening secondary to proximal retraction

FIGURE 7.156 Isolated tear of the rectus femoris component of the quadriceps on sagittal (**A**) and axial (**B**) FS PD FSE images.

Quadriceps fat pad edema

Quadriceps tendinosis

Complete quadriceps tendon rupture

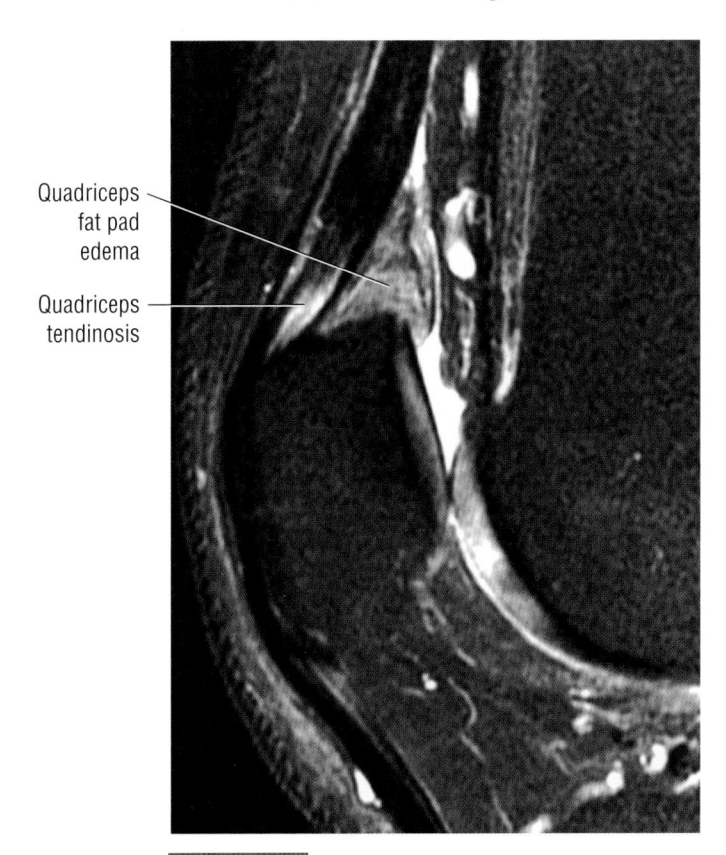

FIGURE 7.157 Diffuse edema of the quadriceps fat pad proximal to the superior pole of the patella. Hyperintense signal of the distal quadriceps tendon is also shown on this sagittal FS PD FSE image.

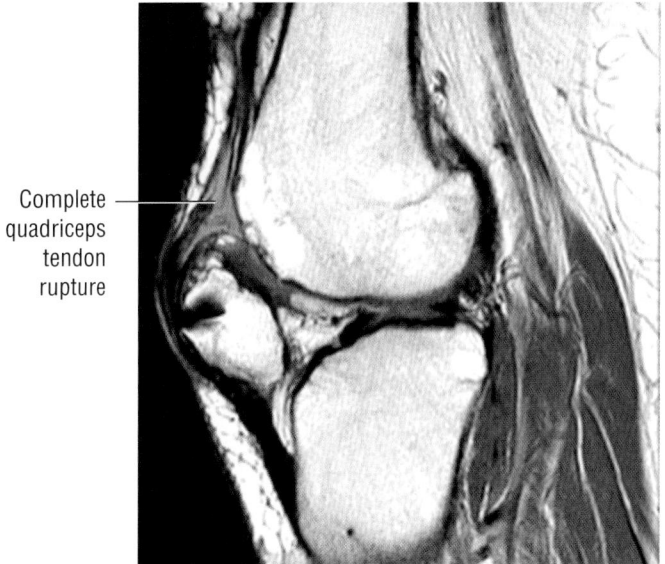

FIGURE 7.158 Sagittal PD FSE image showing patella baja with a retracted patellar tendon and diastasis at the site of quadriceps tendon rupture.

8
General Pathologic Conditions Affecting the Knee

Introduction (page 845)

Cartilage Evaluation (pages 845–856)

Evaluation of Synovium and the Irregular Hoffa's Infrapatellar Fat-Pad Sign (pages 854–864)

Arthritis (pages 865–906)

Tibiofibular Joint Arthrosis and Ganglia (page 907)

Lipoma Arborescens (pages 908–910)

Joint Effusions, Popliteal Cysts, Plicae (pages 911–932)

Osteonecrosis and Subchondral Fracture, Bone Infarcts, Osteochondritis Dissecans (pages 933–970)

Chondral and Osteochondral Lesions, Fractures, Infection (pages 971–1028)

General Pathologic Conditions Affecting the Knee

Introduction

- Magnetic resonance (MR) imaging enhances assessment of extent and progression of arthritis, as well as therapeutic response, in both adults and pediatric arthritic disorders.[398]

- MR can show joint effusions, synovial reactions, popliteal cysts, and osteonecrosis, which may not be evident on conventional radiographs.

Cartilage Evaluation

Key Concepts

- Articular cartilage extracellular matrix composed primarily of type II collagen, the proteoglycan aggrecan, noncollagenous matrix proteins, and water
    - Type II collagen has greatest concentration in upper or superficial zone where chondral ultrastructure demonstrates parallel arrangement of collagen fibers.
    - Glycosaminoglycans, especially chondroitin and keratan sulfate, are associated with swelling and water-imbibing properties of proteoglycan aggregates and have increased distribution in deeper zones.

- Early changes of osteoarthritis-related chondral degeneration may be initiated in deeper layers rather than the superficial zone.

- FS PD FSE and PD FSE routinely used as morphologic imaging techniques

- T2* gradient echo (GRE) not sensitive for chondral imaging

- Physiologic imaging techniques such as T2 mapping or contrast-enhanced imaging do not replace standard morphologic cartilage imaging techniques.

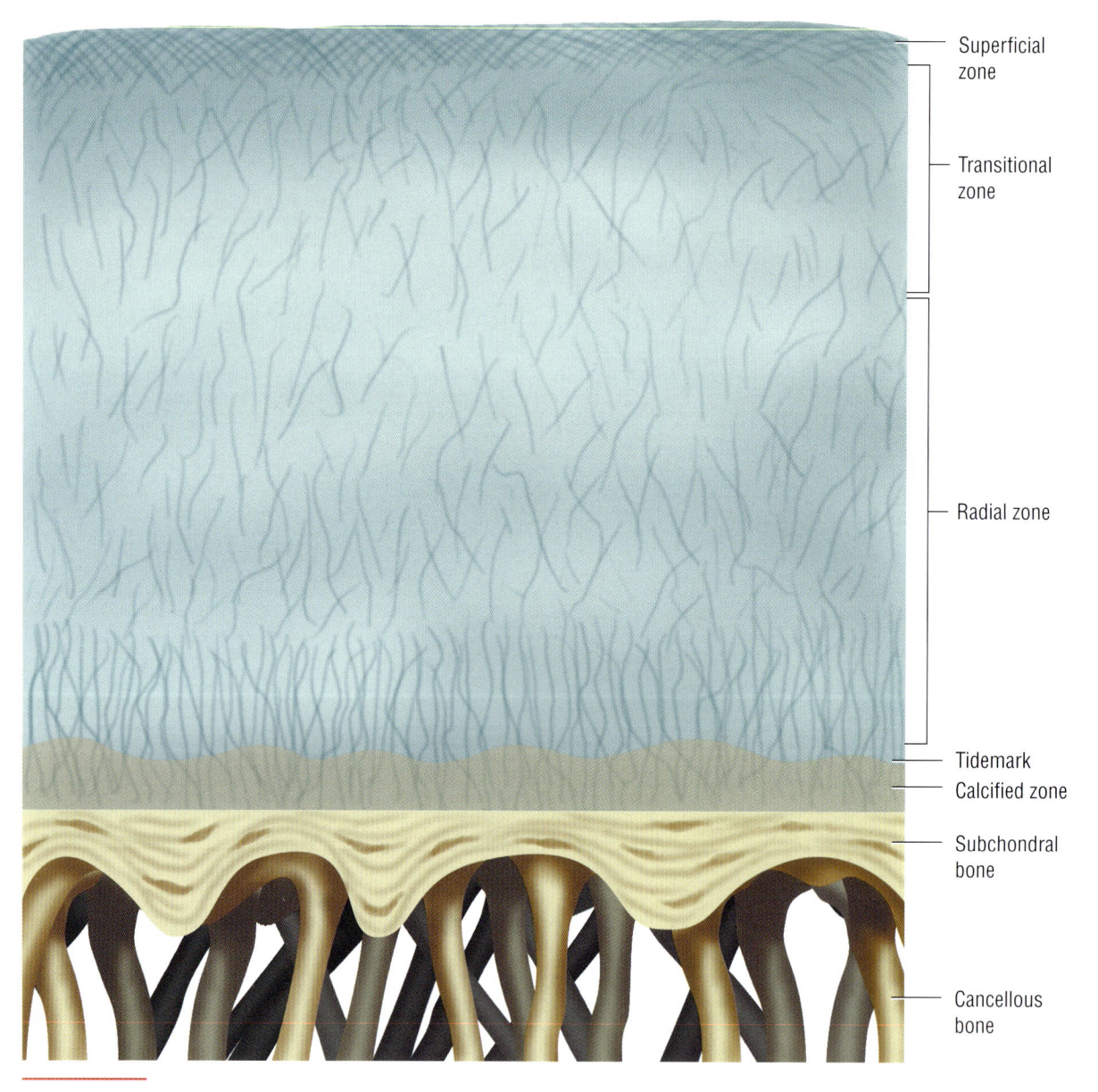

FIGURE 8.1 The collagen fibers of the radial zone are oriented perpendicular to the subchondral plate and anchor articular cartilage to bone. Collagen fibers form arcades in the transitional zone and are directed parallel to the surface in the superficial zone.

Cartilage Evaluation

- Function of articular cartilage is to assist in distribution of loads and decrease stress in subchondral bone.
- Composed of chondrocytes and extracellular matrix
    - No nerve cells or blood vessels within articular cartilage[49]
    - Chondrocytes nourished by diffusion of nutrients and metabolites through matrix, which consists of macromolecules containing water
- Structural macromolecules include collagen, proteoglycans, and noncollagenous proteins.
    - Proteoglycan aggregates are formed from hyaluronan, link protein, and aggrecan components, and exist as functional structures in extracellular matrix.
    - Collagens in fibrillar meshwork provide tensile strength and form.
    - Articular cartilage collagen is primarily type II collagen (90% to 95%).
    - Type IX (surface binding) and type XI (internal core formation) collagens help organize and stabilize type II collagen fibers.
- Lamellar organization of articular cartilage with four zones based on proximity of chondrocytes in the composition of matrix
    - *Gliding or superficial zone*
        - Most superficial; forms articular surface of joint
        - Flattened or ellipsoid chondrocytes and collagen fibers parallel to articular surface
        - Deep to thin cell-free layer of overlying matrix
    - *Transitional zone*
        - Deep to superficial zone
        - Larger with more random distribution of collagen fibers
    - *Radial or deep zone*
        - Deep to transitional zone
        - Largest zone with cells arranged or aligned into short columns
        - Has largest collagen fibers, highest proteoglycan content, and lowest water content
        - *Tidemark,* or *calcification line,* demarcates transition from radial zone to calcified zone of cartilage.

Proteoglycan Complex and Collagen Fibers

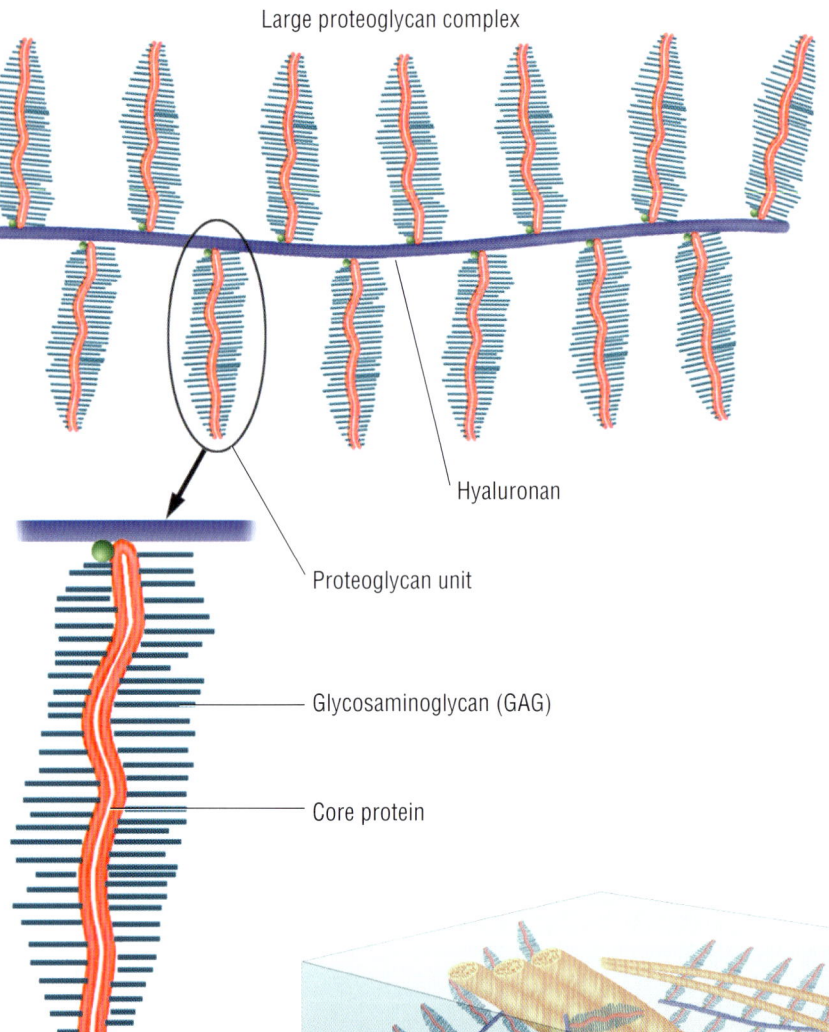

FIGURE 8.2 Proteoglycan complex with proteoglycan side units. The relationship of the core protein and the glycosaminoglycan (GAG) chains is shown relative to the hyaluronan backbone. The large aggregating proteoglycan is known as an aggrecan. The high density of negatively charged GAG side chains contributes to the mechanical stiffness of cartilage by creating an osmotic swelling pressure. Repulsive forces generated by compression of negatively charged aggrecan molecules also function to stiffen the extracellular matrix.

FIGURE 8.3 The organization and relationship of large proteoglycan complexes to both large- and small-diameter type II collagen fibers. The proteoglycan complexes or aggrecan molecules bind to the surface of the collagen fibers and link them together. (Based on "Functional anatomy of the musculoskeletal system." In: Standring S, ed. *Gray's Anatomy*. New York: Churchill Livingstone, 2005. Chapter 6, pp. 83–136.)

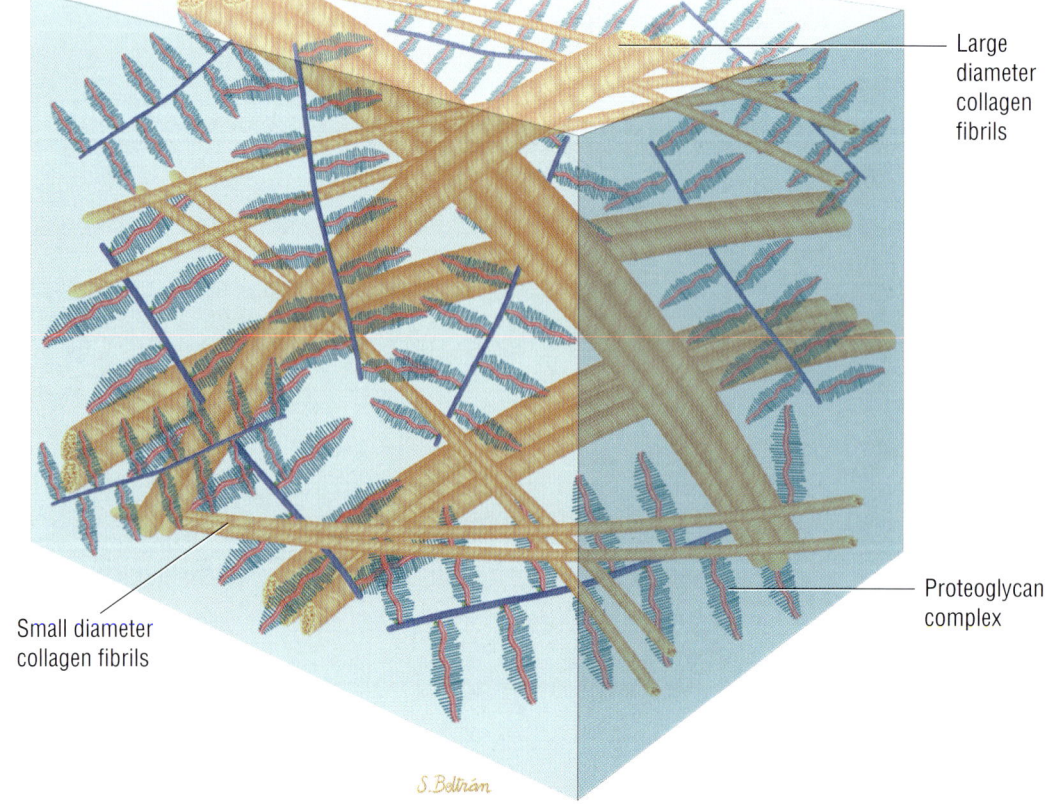

- **Calcified zone**
    - Deepest zone, dividing articular cartilage from underlying subchondral bone (including subchondral plate and deeper cancellous bone)
    - Thin layer
- Normal age-related increases in T2 values may be seen from deep radial zone to outer transitional zone in asymptomatic patients.
    - These changes are different from the focally increased T2 values seen in chondral erosions.[335]

Pathology

- Early changes of localized fibrillation, which represents disruption of superficial articular cartilage layers[49,334]
- When extensive, fibrillation may have deep projections that reach subchondral bone.
- Disruption of molecular framework of the matrix leads to increased water content and decreased proteoglycan content.[49]
- Consequent increased permeability and decreased stiffness of matrix, which may make articular cartilage more susceptible to further damage
- Fissures develop, leading to tears of the tips of fibrillated cartilage.
- Release of cartilage fragments and enzymatic degradation of matrix contribute to decrease in overall cartilage thickness and volume.
- Simultaneously, anabolic cytokines stimulate production of matrix macromolecules and proliferation of chondrocytes (attempt to repair).
- Unsuccessful repair response leads eventually to end-stage changes with exposed subchondral bone, sclerosis, subchondral cysts, joint space narrowing, and osteophytes.

Imaging of Articular Cartilage

- Patellar, femoral, and tibial articular surfaces routinely observed on MR imaging[385]
- Normal hyaline cartilage demonstrates intermediate signal intensity on T1, PD, and FS PD FSE images because of its hydropic composition (as compared with low signal intensity of cortex and fibrocartilaginous menisci).
    - Changes in signal intensity of cartilage are believed to be caused by loss of water-binding proteoglycan molecules.

- Hyaline cartilage displays intermediate signal intensity on conventional T2-weighted images.
    - If a joint effusion is present, FS PD FSE and T2-weighted images create arthrogram-like effect with hyperintense synovial fluid improving delineation of thinner cartilage surfaces (e.g., medial and lateral compartments).
    - Compared with FS PD FSE images, there is less contrast between articular cartilage and subchondral bone on conventional T2-weighted images.
    - In the absence of a joint effusion, surface or contour irregularities may not be resolved.[393]
- With GRE, chemical-shift, and fast low-angle–shot techniques, hyaline cartilage demonstrates high signal intensity.
    - Although articular cartilage defects smaller than 3mm have been identified with T2*-weighted images, degeneration is generally underestimated with these technique.
    - It may be difficult to distinguish high-signal-intensity fluid from high-signal-intensity articular cartilage with accuracy.
    - Surface articular cartilage fissures and early articular cartilage softening may be missed on T2*-weighted images.
    - This sequence is not recommended as a routine cartilage imaging protocol.
    - T2*-weighted echo technique shows delineation of the fluid–cartilage interface because effusions generate higher signal intensity than adjacent cartilage surfaces; however, the technique is not sensitive to spectrum of chondral degeneration.
- Overall approach includes incorporation of morphologic imaging technique, fast T2 mapping sequence, and rapid version of delayed gadolinium-enhanced imaging.
- Three-dimensional (3D) sequences for thin-section capability with multiplanar reformatting
    - FS 3D spoiled gradient recalled (SPGR) technique has 95% accuracy rate (with 96% sensitivity and 95% specificity) in evaluating patellofemoral articular cartilage defects in cadavers with use of intraarticular saline.[113,114,370,383,393]

- **Spin-echo and GRE sequences**
    - Bilaminar or trilaminar appearance[385]
    - Trilaminar appearance on FS SPGR images[383] consists of superficial region of high signal intensity, middle area of low signal intensity, and deep area of high signal intensity.[114,383]
    - Isotropic arrangement of collagen and position relative to magnetic field thought to influence MR imaging characteristics of the three layers
    - Outer area of high signal intensity thought to represent superficial gliding zone
    - Middle layer may represent transitional zone.
    - Deep layer corresponds to combination of the radial (deep) zone, calcified zone, and subchondral bone.[393]
- FS PD-weighted FSE techniques more successful in separating cartilage–fluid interface and identifying early changes[45,480]
    - FSE images may suffer from loss of spatial resolution along phase-encoded axis (increased blurring with short echo times [TEs]).
    - Blurring effect can be minimized and resolution increased by using 256 or 512 matrix and sequences with lower echo train lengths (ETLs; ≤4) and higher TEs.
    - Without FS techniques, FSE images limited by higher signal intensity from fat-containing tissues relative to conventional T2 spin-echo sequences
    - Requires use of longer repetition time (TR; >4000ms) and TE (>100ms) sequences to produce T2 effect.
    - Chondral surfaces can also be evaluated with high-resolution PD FSE images by using matrix of 512 × 384, increasing bandwidth, and modifying field of view (FOV) to optimize signal-to-noise ratio (SNR).
- With short tau inversion recovery (STIR) image contrast, it is possible to differentiate brighter signal intensity of fluid from intermediate to high signal intensity of articular cartilage.[385]
    - Also effective for demonstrating early changes in subchondral bone in areas of overlying articular cartilage damage

- Intraarticular MR arthrography with conventional T1 spin-echo sequences, FS, and gadolinium contrast
    - May allow identification of smaller chondral lesions than intraarticular studies performed with saline[176]
    - Compared with FS PD-weighted FSE sequences, MR arthrography not as useful for detection of internal articular cartilage alterations or deep/basal layer changes
    - More sensitive to superficial articular cartilage changes
    - Do not accurately reflect internal changes of water composition within degenerating cartilage
- Magnetization transfer contrast is sensitive to interaction between water molecules.
    - Improves contrast on GRE sequences (e.g., SPGR)[527]
    - Not yet been shown to be superior to FS T2-weighted FSE contrast in routine articular cartilage visualization[3,385,527]
- Morphologic cartilage imaging techniques include driven equilibrium Fourier transform (DEFT) imaging and steady-state free precession (SSFP).[165]
    - DEFT imaging uses a tip-up pulse (90 degrees) following a spin-echo train to return magnetization to the Z axis.
        - Tissues with long T1 values, including synovial fluid, demonstrate enhanced signal (improved cartilage–fluid interface) at short echo and repetition times.
        - DEFT contrast is dependent on the ratio of T1 to T2 tissue contrast, in comparison to conventional T1- or T2-weighted imaging.
    - SSFP imaging generates high SNR 3D images.
        - In fluctuating equilibrium MR (FEMR), a variant of SSFP, each phase-encoding step is repeated twice with reconstructed fat and water images.
        - Both FEMR and SSFP techniques are limited by sensitivity to off-resonance artifacts.
        - Dixon SSFP imaging is used for FS at high resolution as a replacement for FS 3D spoiled GRE imaging.
- Novel methods that sample K-space in a radial fashion have also shown potential in producing 3D high-resolution images with FS PD FSE-like contrast obtained with relatively short imaging times.

- Physiologic imaging techniques
    - T2 mapping: as a function of water content in damaged cartilage
    - Sodium MR imaging: identifying regions of glycosaminoglycan depletion
    - Diffusion-weighted imaging: diffusion of water as a function of cartilage degradation
    - Contrast-enhanced imaging: cartilage matrix evaluation with delayed contrast-enhanced MR to map the distribution of glycosaminoglycans or GAG depletion

Articular Cartilage in Children

- Thicker cartilage, allowing increased sensitivity in detection of focal erosions and cartilage thinning

- In infants, articular cartilage seen before appearance of distal femoral and proximal tibial ossific nuclei; demonstrates higher signal intensity than adjacent marrow

- Before any radiographic evidence of joint space narrowing is found, focal erosions and uniform attenuation of articular cartilage can be observed in MR studies of patients with juvenile chronic arthritis, hemophilia, or degenerative joint disease.

- Loss of subchondral signal intensity has also been observed in association with initial cartilage loss in patients with sclerosis.

- Areas of suspected subchondral sclerosis may show regions of high signal intensity on FS PD-weighted FSE or STIR images.

- Interosseous cysts and hemorrhage (high signal intensity on T2-weighted images) may develop at sites of denuded hyaline cartilage.

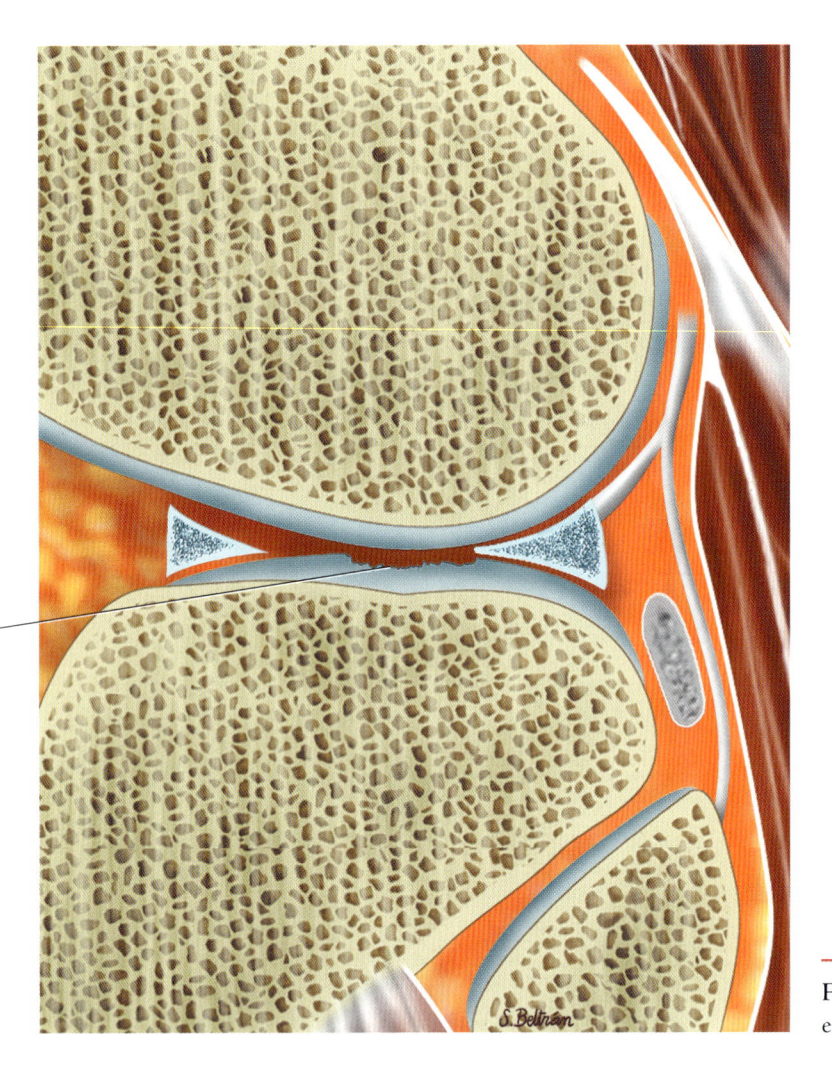

Lateral tibial plateau chondral erosion

FIGURE 8.4 Lateral tibial chondral erosion.

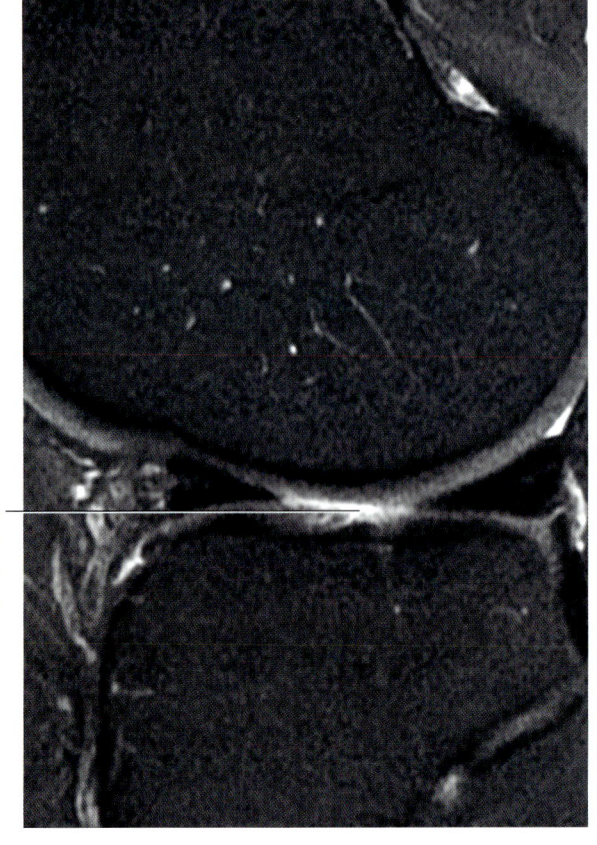

Lateral tibial plateau chondral erosion

FIGURE 8.5 Sagittal FS PD FSE contrast with arthrogram-like effect allowing visualization of mid-lateral tibial plateau chondral erosion.

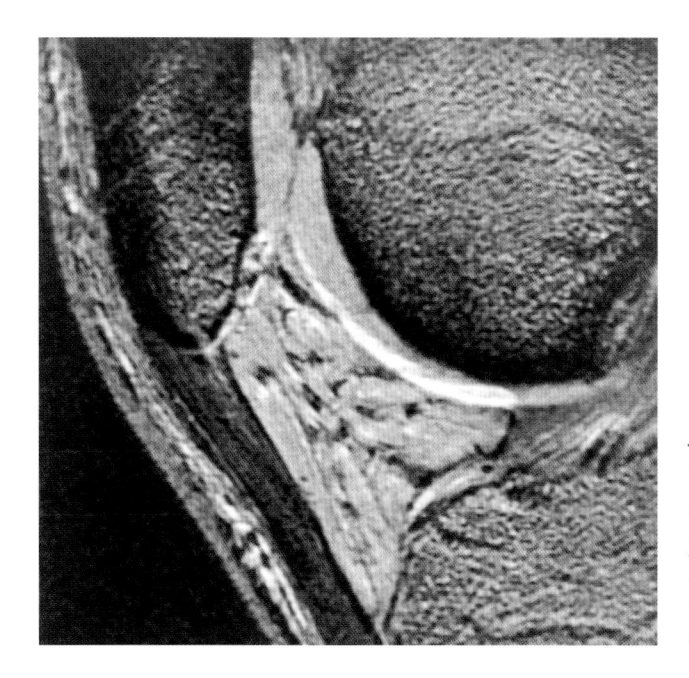

General Pathologic Conditions Affecting the Knee

FIGURE 8.6 A sagittal 3D SPGR image obtained without fat suppression shows the patellofemoral articular cartilage in excellent anatomic detail. However, the sensitivity of this technique for surface and intrasubstance degeneration is limited.

Subchondral erosions

Basal degeneration

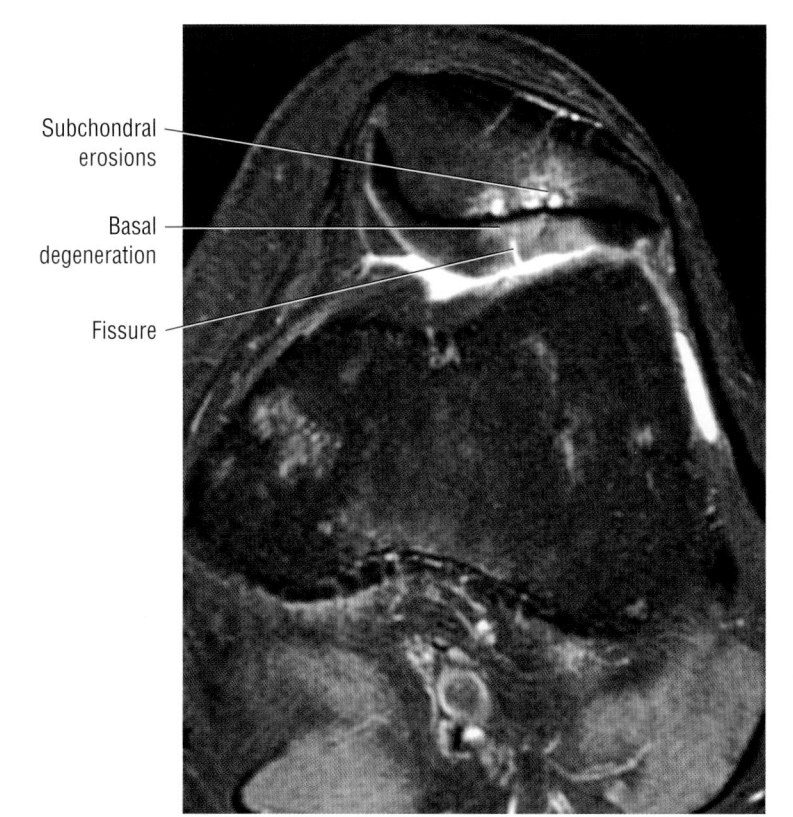

Fissure

FIGURE 8.7 Various stages of chondromalacia, including fissures, fibrillation, basal degeneration, and subchondral erosion, on an axial FS PD FSE image.

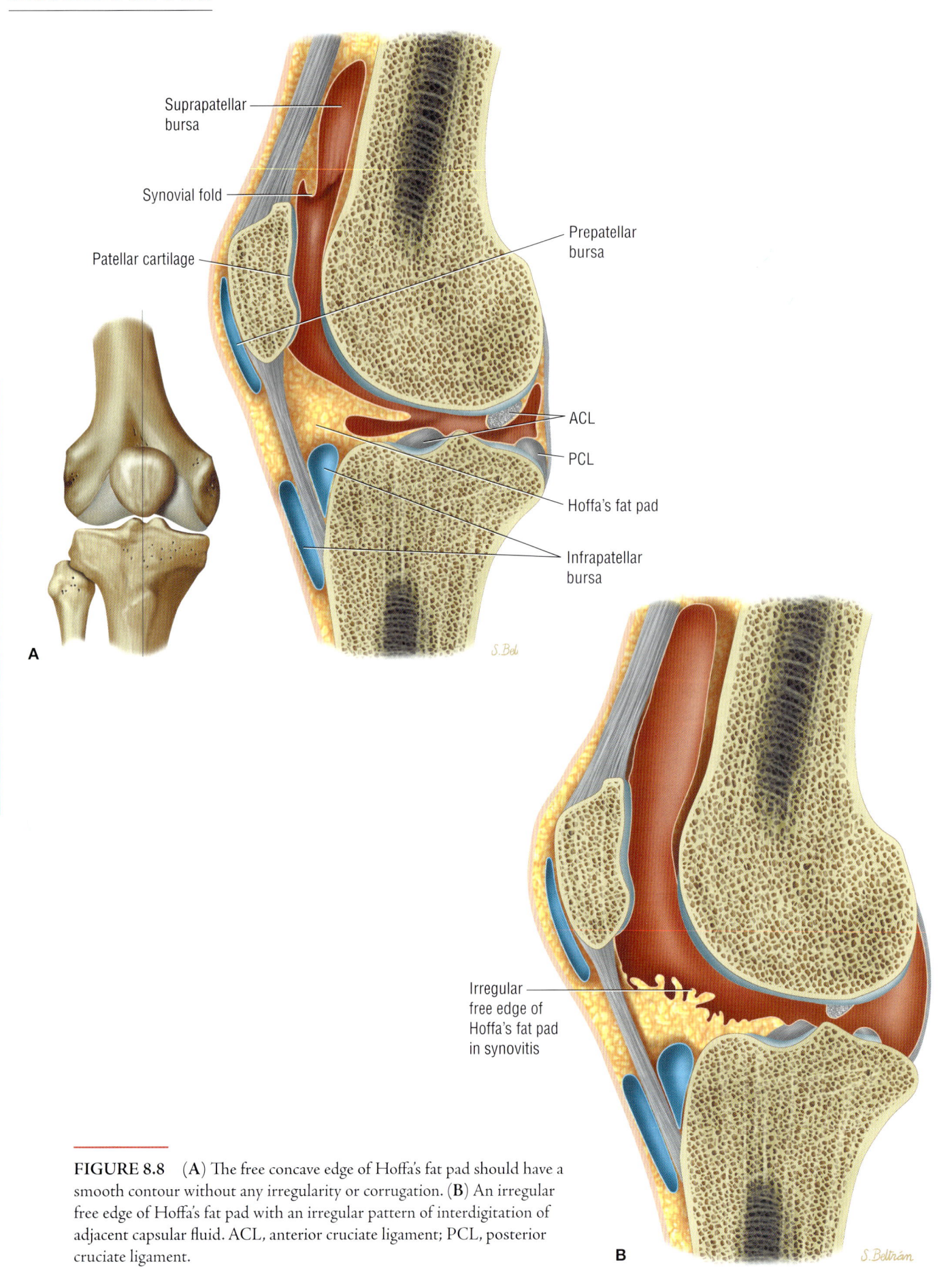

Hoffa's Fat Pad

FIGURE 8.8 (**A**) The free concave edge of Hoffa's fat pad should have a smooth contour without any irregularity or corrugation. (**B**) An irregular free edge of Hoffa's fat pad with an irregular pattern of interdigitation of adjacent capsular fluid. ACL, anterior cruciate ligament; PCL, posterior cruciate ligament.

Evaluation of Synovium and the Irregular Hoffa's Infrapatellar Fat-Pad Sign

Key Concepts

- Irregular free edge of Hoffa's infrapatellar fat pad associated with synovitis

- Inflammation of synovial lining and reflection is seen in:
    - Trauma (hemorrhagic effusions with anterior cruciate ligament [ACL] tears and fractures)
    - Inflammatory arthritis
    - Pigmented villonodular synovitis
    - Hemophilia
    - Fluid associated with synovial masses generates increased signal intensity on T2-weighted images.

- *Hoffa's disease*
    - Should be distinguished from irregular infrapatellar fat-pad sign
    - Represents impingement of fat pad characterized by both inflammation and subsequent fibrosis
    - May be secondary to trauma
    - Areas of signal alterations with hyperintensity on T2, FS PD-weighted FSE, STIR, and GRE images
    - Areas of scarring and fibrosis with low signal intensity on T1- and T2-weighted images
    - Hypertrophy of the fat pad occurs after trauma when the fat pad enlarges beyond the margins of the patellar tendon.
    - Resultant impingement produces pain and inflammation.
    - Infection (septic arthritis)

- Synovial hypertrophy (hypertrophic villous fronds) in thickened synovium typically located between periarticular fat and joint fluid and visualized as intermediate signal intensity on PD or FS PD FSE images

Evaluation of Synovium and the Irregular Hoffa's Infrapatellar Fat-Pad Sign

- Synovial reaction and proliferation characterized on MR by changes in contour of synovial reflections

    - *Irregular infrapatellar fat-pad sign*: irregularity with loss of smooth posterior concave free border of Hoffa's infrapatellar fat pad

    - Although synovium cannot be imaged directly in early synovitis, a corrugated surface along Hoffa's infrapatellar fat pad is evident in the early stages of synovial irritation.

    - When present, hypertrophied synovium is intermediate in signal intensity on PD or FS PD FSE images.

    - Irregular infrapatellar fat-pad sign may be seen in hemophilia, rheumatoid arthritis, pigmented villonodular synovitis, Lyme arthritis, inflammatory osteoarthritis, and hemorrhagic effusions (caused by arthritis or trauma) with reactive synovium

    - Swelling of retropatellar fat pad may occur in chronic patellofemoral chondromalacia and instability.[69]

    - Postoperative scarring of Hoffa's fat pad may also be associated with reactive synovial thickening.

- Gadolinium–diethylene triamine pentaacetic acid (DTPA) contrast-enhanced T1-weighted images (with FS)

    - Useful in accurate identification of pannus tissue, seen as areas of increased signal intensity adjacent to low-signal-intensity joint fluid[33]

    - Improve contrast differentiation between bright-signal-intensity pannus and low-signal-intensity joint fluid

    - On T1, T2, FS PD-weighted FSE, and T2*-weighted protocols, synovial hypertrophy and pannus demonstrate low to intermediate signal intensity and are more difficult to identify.

Synovitis and Hoffa's Disease

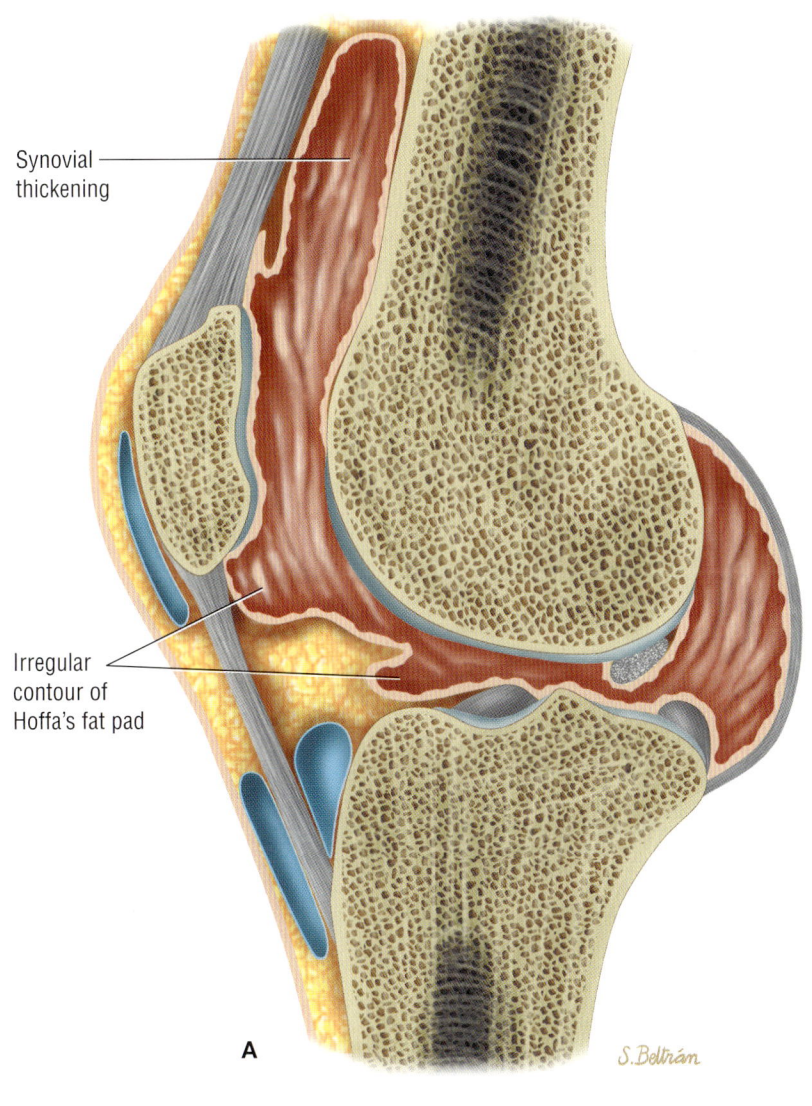

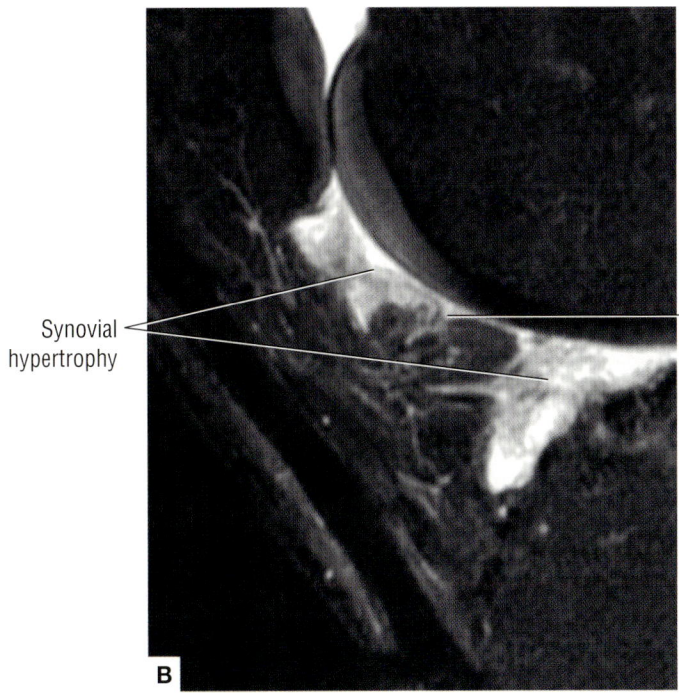

FIGURE 8.9 (**A**) Synovitis with thickened synovium and irregular contour of Hoffa's fat pad. (**B**) Intermediate-signal-intensity hypertrophied synovium in synovitis associated with an irregular contour of Hoffa's fat pad.

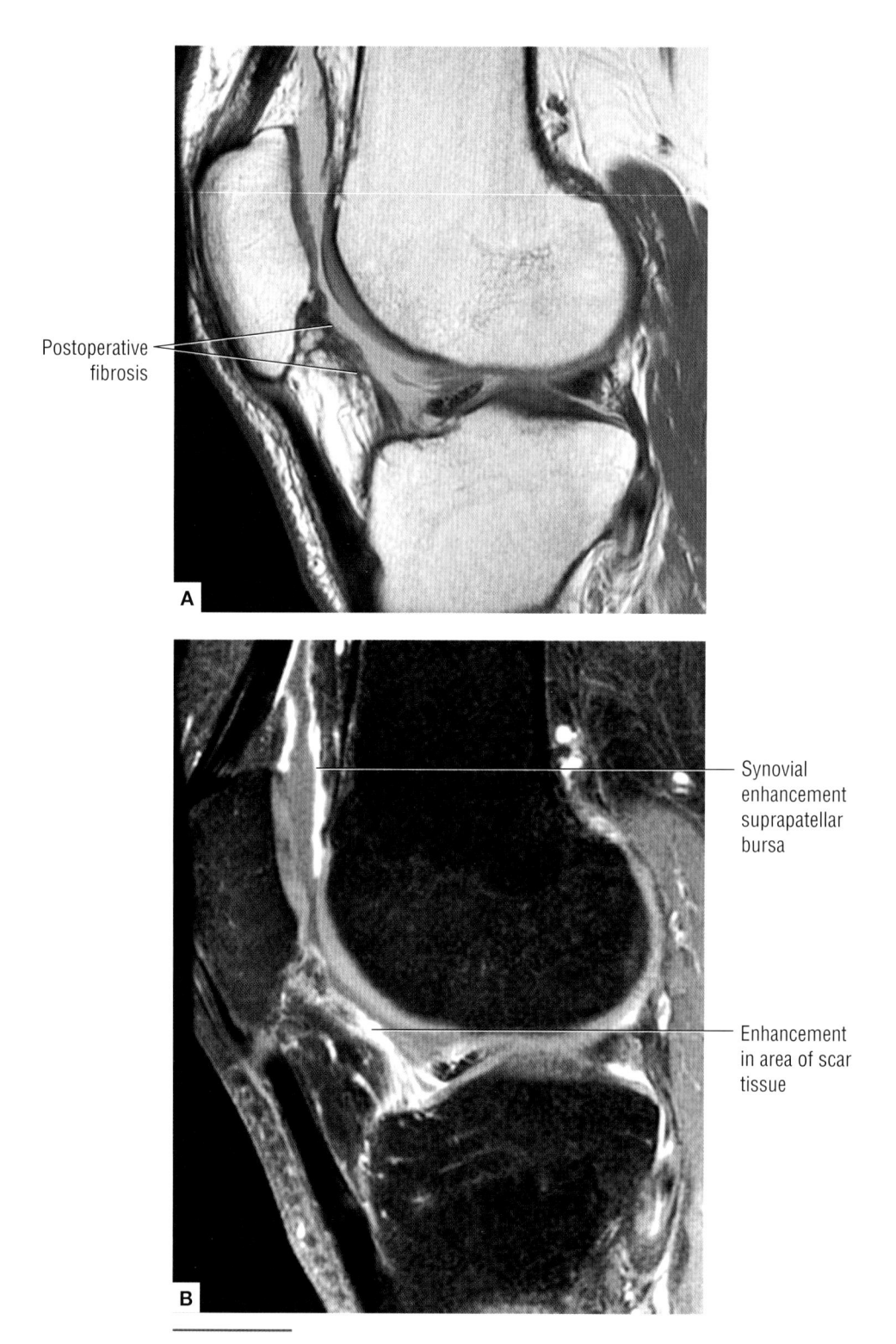

FIGURE 8.10 Postoperative fibrosis of Hoffa's fat pad with hyperintense synovial enhancement on sagittal (**A**) PD FSE and (**B**) FS T1-weighted FSE postintravenous contrast images.

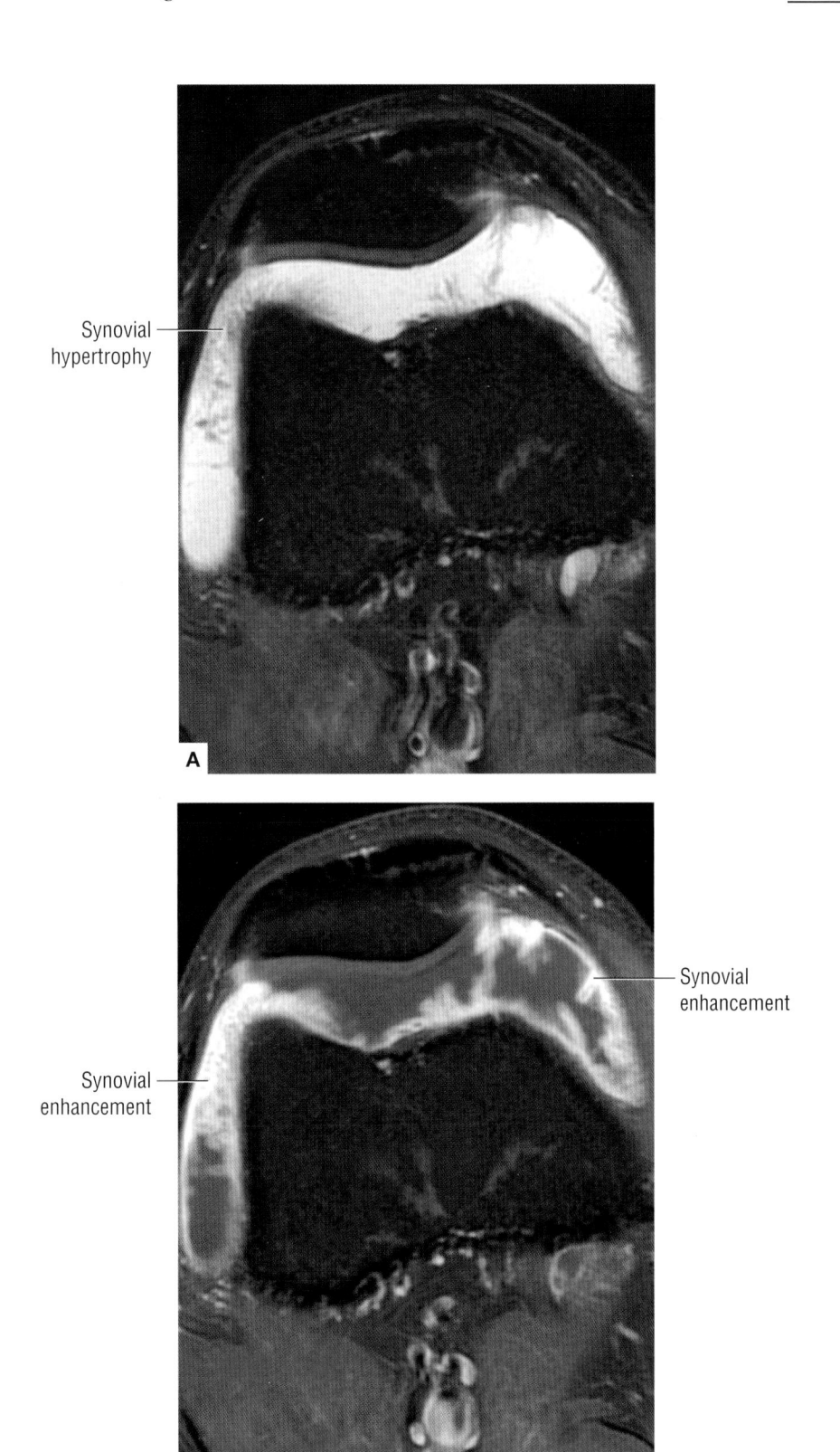

FIGURE 8.11 (**A**) Intermediate-signal-intensity fronds of synovial hypertrophy on an axial FS PD FSE image. (**B**) Corresponding axial FS T1-weighted contrast-enhanced (intravenous) image identifying thickened synovium.

862　Stoller's Orthopaedics and Sports Medicine: The Knee

Edema, hemorrhage, fibrosis, and calcification in Hoffa's infrapatellar fat pad

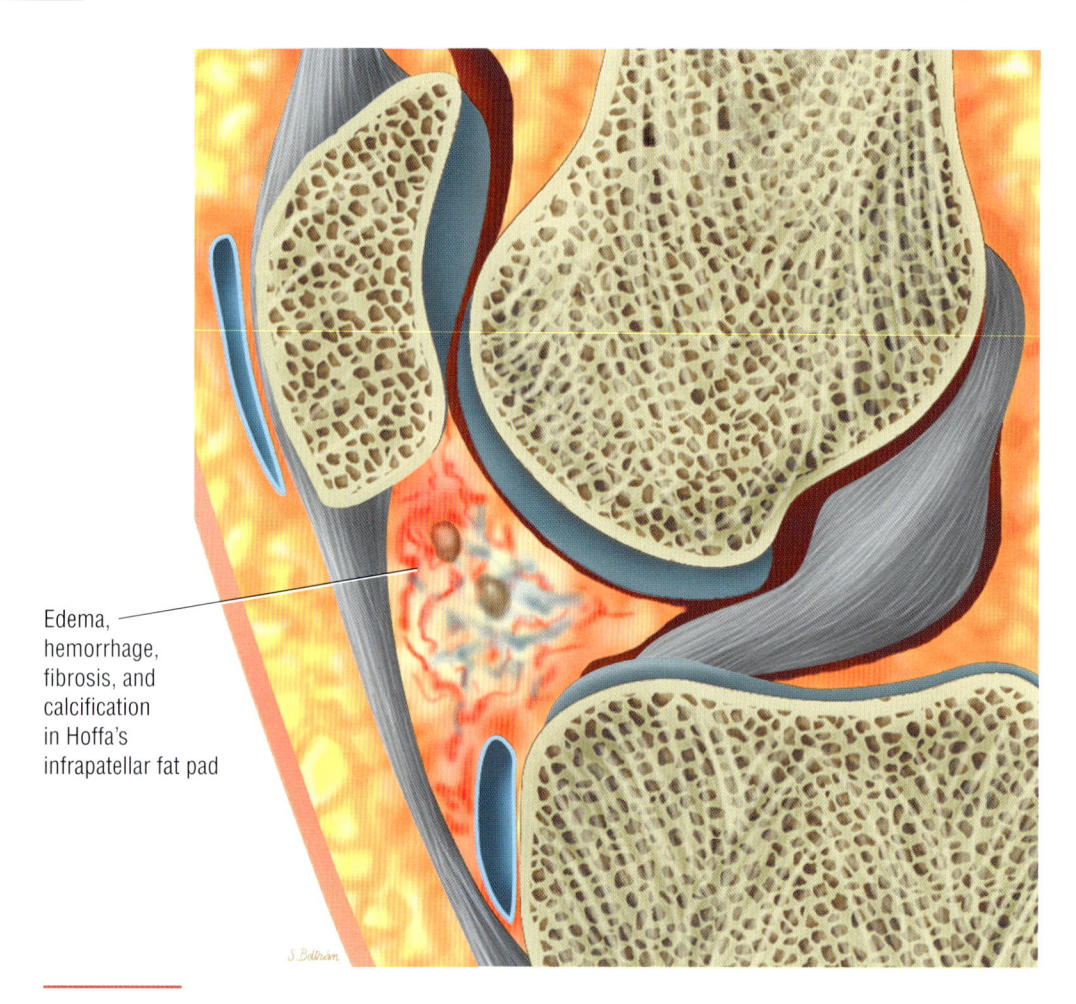

FIGURE 8.12 Hoffa's disease with enlargement of the infrapatellar fat pad associated with edema, hemorrhage, or chronic changes, including fibrosis and calcifications.

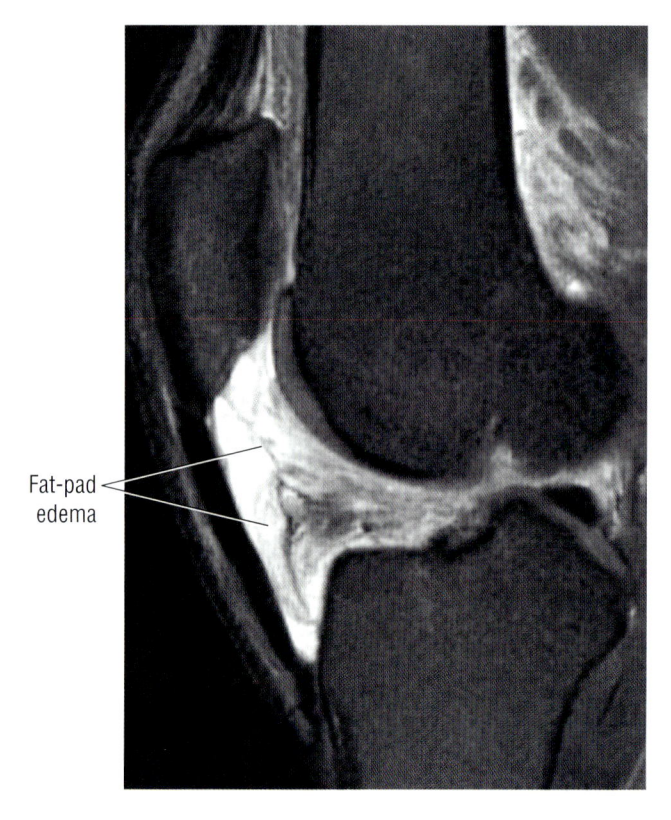

Fat-pad edema

FIGURE 8.13 Hyperintense edema of Hoffa's fat pad on a sagittal FS PD FSE image. In Hoffa's disease, there is enlargement of the infrapatellar fat pad associated with edema, hemorrhage, or chronic changes including fibrosis and calcifications.

General Pathologic Conditions Affecting the Knee

Synovial enhancement in juvenile chronic arthritis

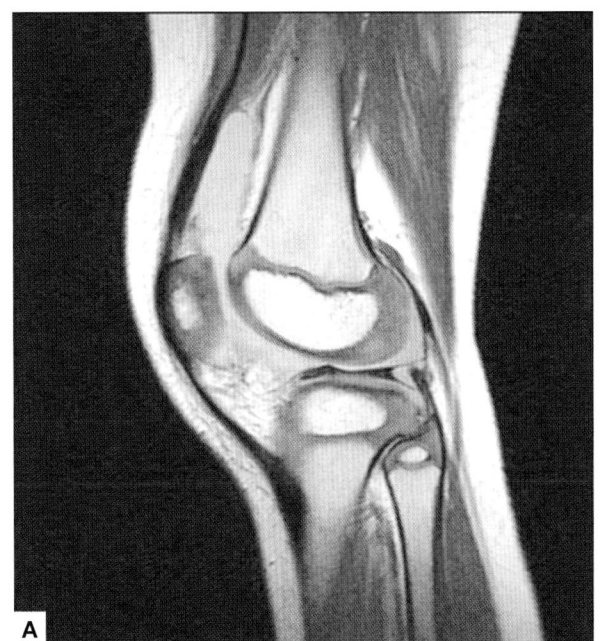

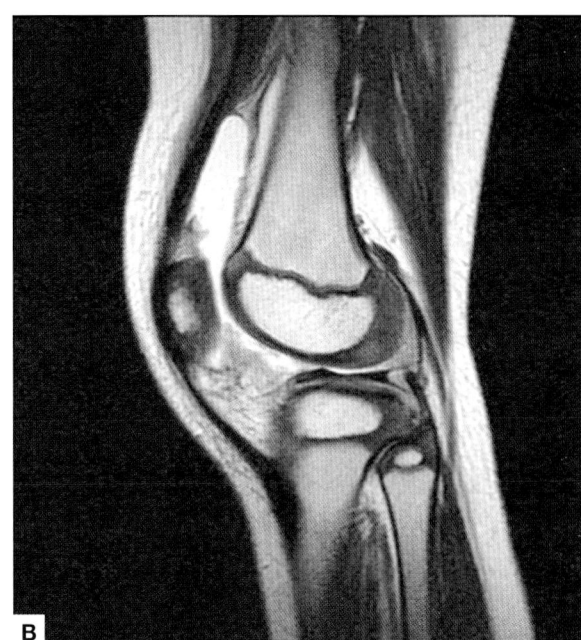

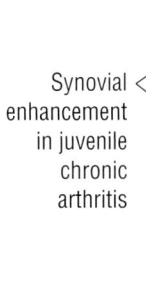

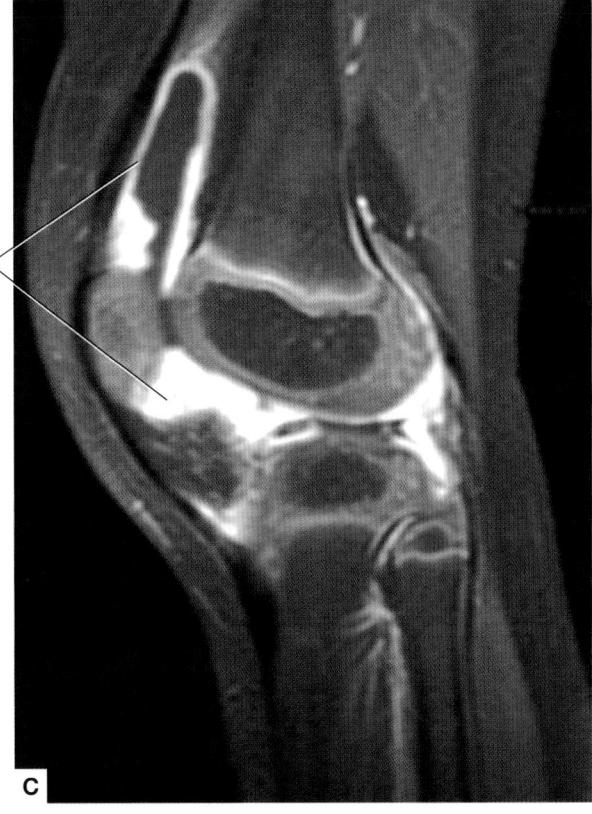

FIGURE 8.14 Initial presentation of juvenile chronic arthritis with joint effusion, synovitis, and hyperintense thickened synovium on sagittal (**A**) PD FSE, (**B**) T2-weighted FSE, and (**C**) FS T1-weighted FSE with intravenous contrast enhancement.

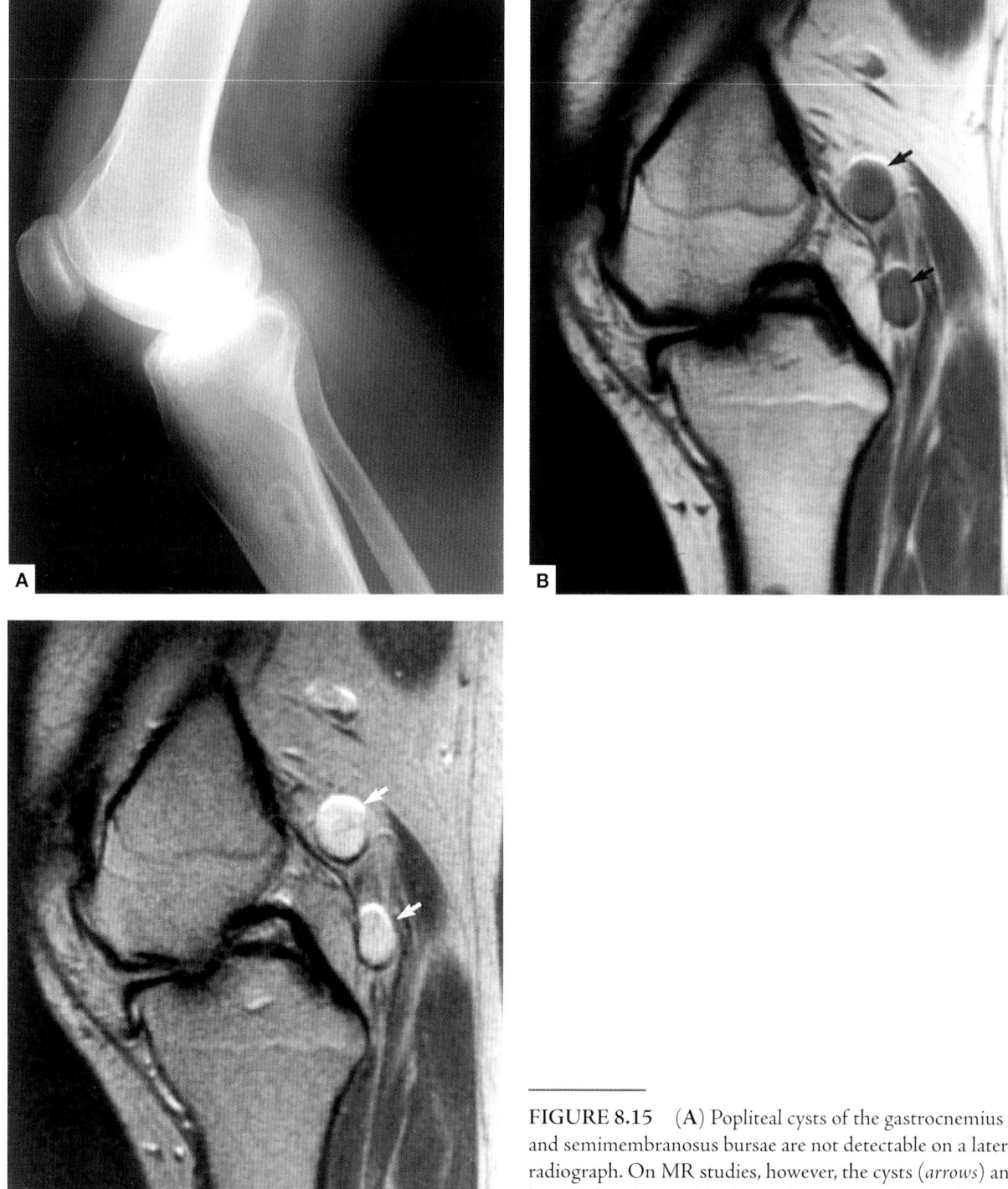

FIGURE 8.15 (**A**) Popliteal cysts of the gastrocnemius and semimembranosus bursae are not detectable on a lateral radiograph. On MR studies, however, the cysts (*arrows*) and bursae show low and high signal intensity, respectively, on (**B**) T1-weighted and (**C**) T2-weighted sagittal images.

Juvenile Chronic Arthritis

Key Concepts

- Juvenile chronic arthritis is divided into pauciarticular, polyarticular, and systemic-onset patterns.

- Joint effusions, synovitis (irregular fat-pad sign), and synovial thickening are seen in early disease.

Juvenile Chronic Arthritis

- Formerly known as juvenile rheumatoid arthritis
- Subdivided into three types, depending on type of onset[399]
    - *Pauciarticular juvenile chronic arthritis*
        - Most common subtype in absence of other rheumatic disorders
        - Typically a female toddler presenting with a limp or decreased range of motion at the knee
        - Hip or shoulder involvement is rare.
        - Up to 20% of children have chronic uveitis (iridocyclitis).
            - Asymptomatic or may result in permanent visual impairment
    - *Polyarticular juvenile chronic arthritis*
        - Less common
        - Slightly older age group
        - Symmetric arthritis targets knees, wrists, and elbows.
        - Five or more joints involved within the first 6 months of disease
    - *Still's disease (systemic-onset juvenile arthritis)*
        - Least common form of juvenile chronic arthritis
        - High-spiking fever, erythematous macular rash, and visceral involvement, including hepatosplenomegaly, lymphadenopathy, and pericarditis

- Other pediatric rheumatic diseases
    - Seronegative spondyloarthropathies, including juvenile forms of ankylosing spondylosis, psoriatic arthritis, arthritis associated with inflammatory bowel disease, and collagen vascular disease (systemic lupus erythematosus)
    - Transient synovitis may produce joint swelling secondary to inflammation but is self-limiting and does not represent a chronic arthritis.
- MR studies in the initial stages of juvenile chronic arthritis demonstrate synovitis with irregularity of Hoffa's infrapatellar fat pad.[175]
    - Articular cartilage erosions and synovial hypertrophy (identified before joint space narrowing evident on plain-film radiography)
    - Popliteal cysts of gastrocnemius and semimembranosus bursae.
    - Thickening of synovium of suprapatellar bursa
    - Enhancing synovium on contrast-enhanced studies
    - Marrow signal abnormalities reflect bone marrow edema or hyperemia prior to development of epiphyseal overgrowth.
    - In more advanced disease → subarticular cysts, subchondral cysts, and osteonecrosis of femoral and tibial surfaces
    - Hypoplastic menisci
        - Alteration in synovial fluid composition may impair normal fibrocartilage development
        - Also correlated with increased synovial volume
    - Enlarged epiphysis, widening of the intercondylar notch, and squaring of the inferior margin of the patella (seen on conventional radiographs and MR)
- MR evaluation of signs of disease progression
    - Increasing use of more aggressive treatment protocols
    - Can demonstrate pannus tissue changes
    - May be a cost-effective way of monitoring the effectiveness of therapy

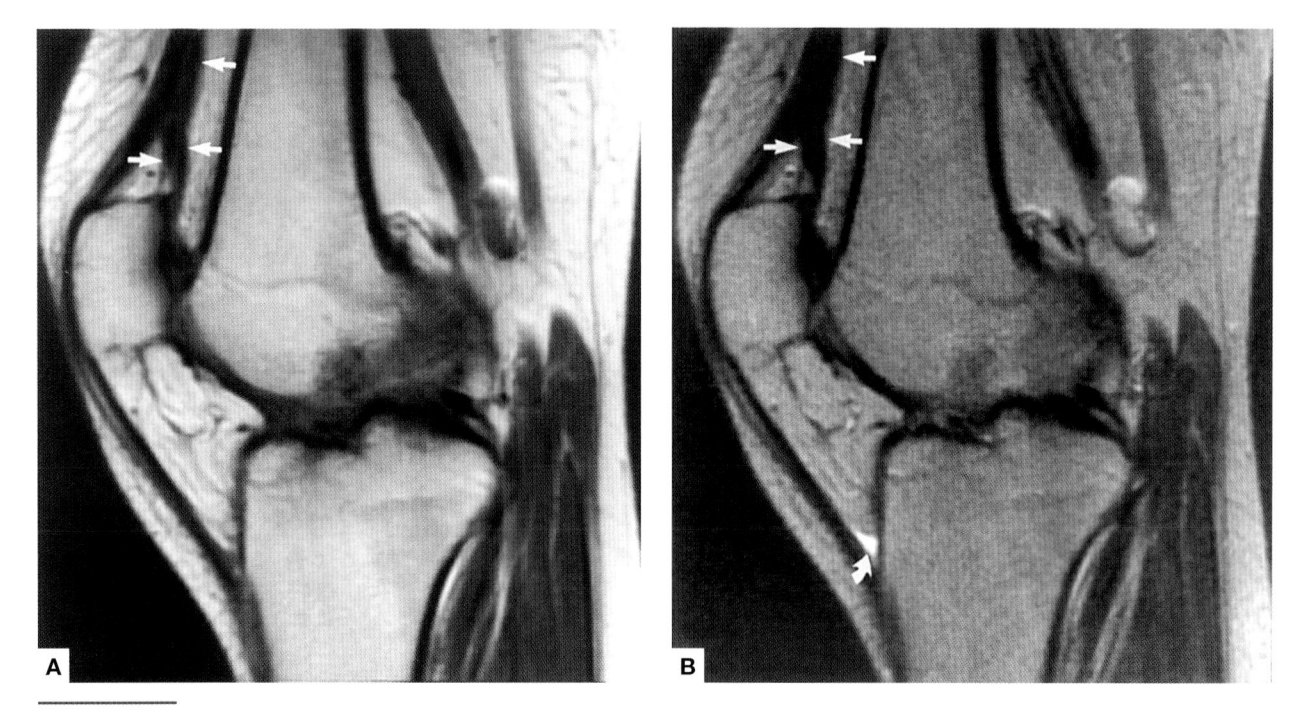

General Pathologic Conditions Affecting the Knee

FIGURE 8.16 Juvenile chronic arthritis causes suprapatellar synovial hypertrophy (*straight arrows*), seen as low signal intensity on both (**A**) T1-weighted and (**B**) T2-weighted sagittal images. In contrast, a focus of fluid demonstrates bright signal intensity (*curved arrow*) on the T2-weighted image.

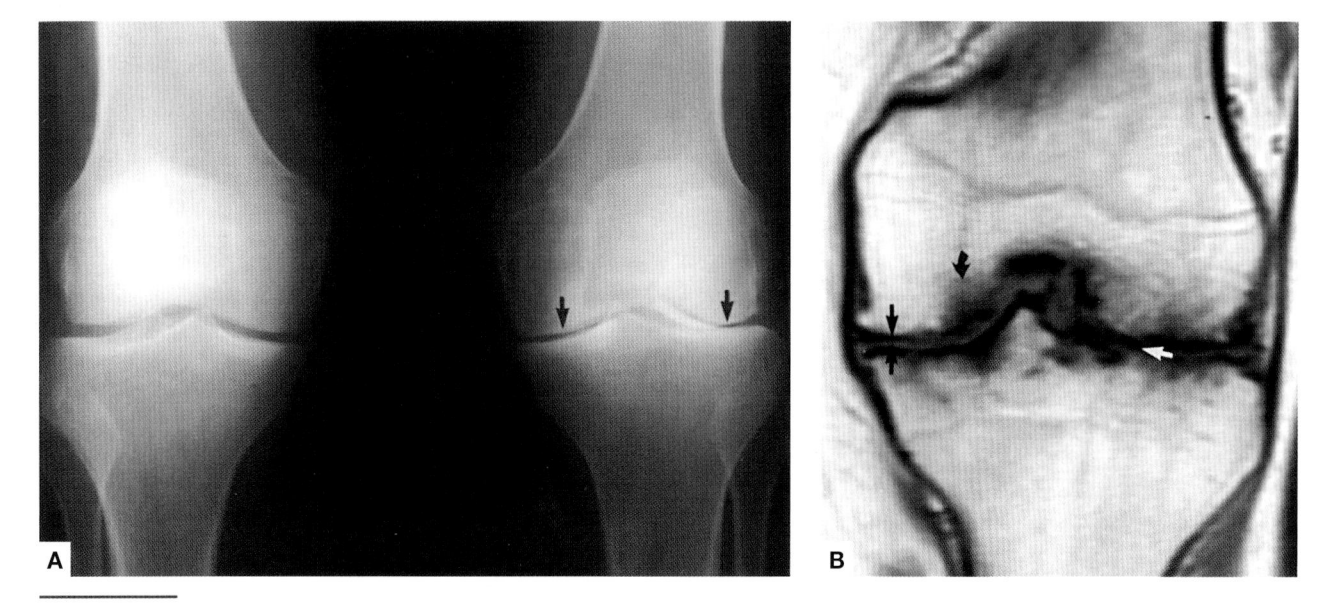

FIGURE 8.17 Advanced juvenile chronic arthritis with marked joint space narrowing (*black arrows*) is seen on (**A**) an anteroposterior radiograph and (**B**) a T1-weighted coronal image. Articular cartilage erosion (*white arrow*) and subchondral sclerosis (*curved arrow*) are best seen on MR images.

Pannus in Rheumatoid Arthritis

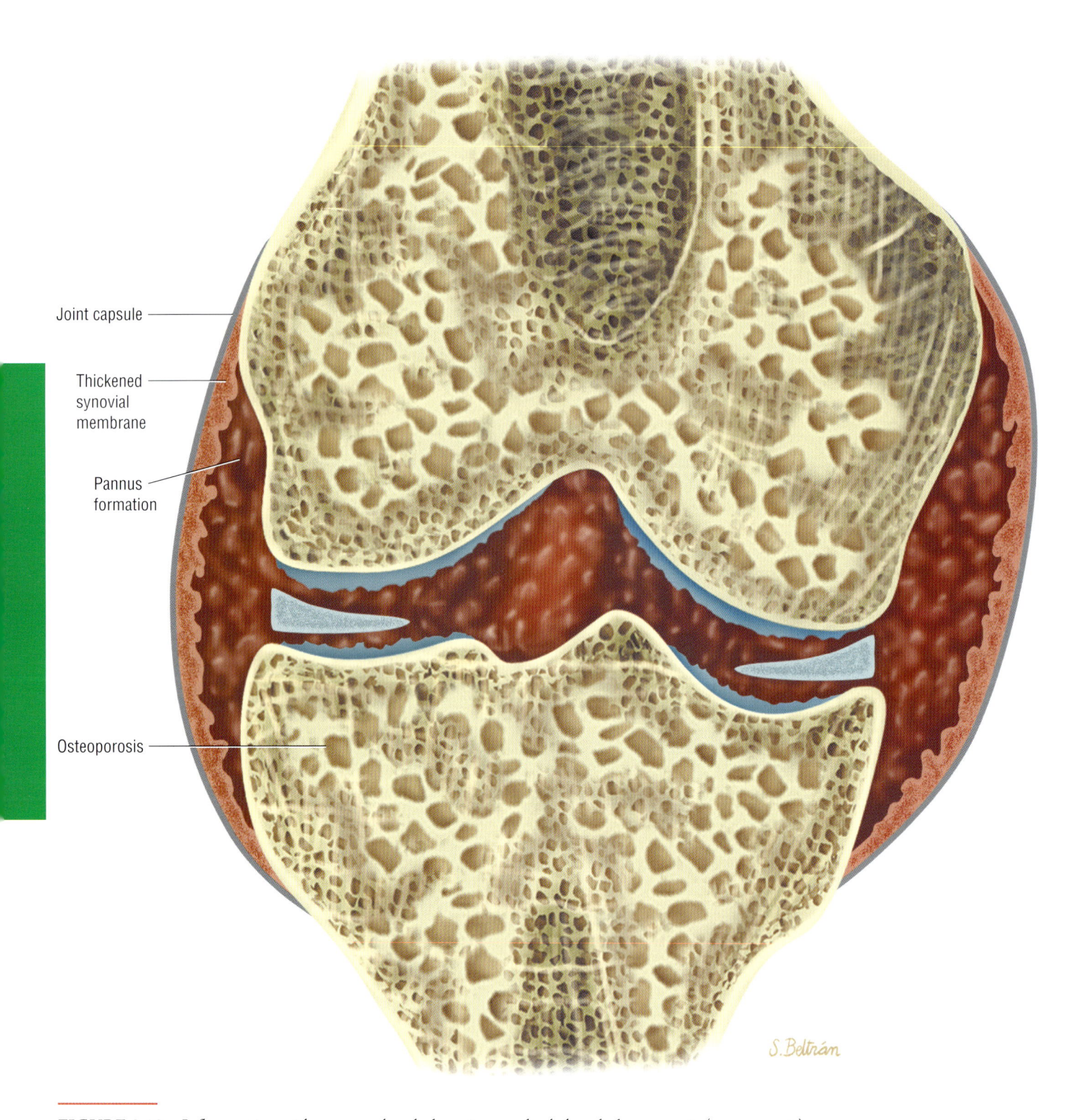

FIGURE 8.18 Inflammation with pannus, chondral erosions, and subchondral osteopenia (osteoporosis).

Rheumatoid Arthritis

Key Concepts

- MR imaging signs
    - Soft tissue swelling with synovial thickening
    - Direct visualization of intermediate-signal-intensity pannus tissue
    - Juxtaarticular osteoporosis (marrow inhomogeneity)
    - Loss of subchondral plate
    - Erosion
    - Subchondral cysts
    - Joint space narrowing
- FS PD FSE images demonstrate subchondral marrow edema.
- IV contrast enhances thickened synovium.

Rheumatoid Arthritis

- Systemic inflammatory arthritis
- Four of seven criteria must be present for more than 6 weeks:
    - Morning stiffness
    - Oligo- or polyarthritis in three or more joints or several joint groups
    - Arthritis of wrist, metacarpophalangeal joint, or proximal interphalangeal joint
    - Symmetric arthritis
    - Rheumatoid nodules (juxtaarticular or over bony prominences or extensor surfaces)
    - Serum positive for rheumatoid factor
    - Radiographic changes including erosions and juxtaarticular demineralization
- First involves synovium, then cartilage and bone (MR detects early disease and can be used to monitor the effects of disease-modifying drugs)

MR Findings of Rheumatoid Arthritis

- Bicompartmental and tricompartmental disease in the knee
- Marginal and subchondral erosions with diffuse loss of hyaline articular cartilage on both medial and lateral femoral articular surfaces
- Large joint effusions with popliteal cysts with uniform high signal intensity on T2, FS PD-weighted FSE, and T2*-weighted images
- Subchondral marrow edema associated with erosions and marrow heterogeneity in osteopenia on FS PD FSE images
- Less frequently, signs of degenerative arthritis with osteophytosis and subchondral sclerosis (low signal intensity)
- Irregular fat pad in more active stages of the disease
- Hypertrophied synovial masses with intermediate signal intensity on T1- and T2-weighted contrast image
- Thickened synovium may line joint capsule or present as more diffuse and irregular villous hypertrophy.
- In chronic stages, there is subsidence of inflammation and progression from fibrous to bony ankylosis.
- Osteonecrosis and infarcts can be identified before corresponding radiographic changes are evident.
- Gadolinium-DPTA contrast-enhanced images
    - Useful in identifying pannus or granulation tissue that grows over cartilage surfaces[4,255,361]
    - Pannus or exuberant inflammatory synovium can extend to margins of joints and may be associated with tendon sheath involvement (tendinomuscular).
    - Pannus tissue erodes both cartilage and bone.
    - Contrast-enhanced images more effective than non–contrast-enhanced T1, T2, FS PD-weighted FSE, T2*, or STIR images for separating fluid from adjacent pannus
    - Pannus tissue may be underestimated without IV gadolinium enhancement.
    - Ability to map out pannus useful in examining patients with severe inflammatory arthritis when synovectomy is considered before total joint arthroplasty

General Pathologic Conditions Affecting the Knee

Synovial Hypertrophy

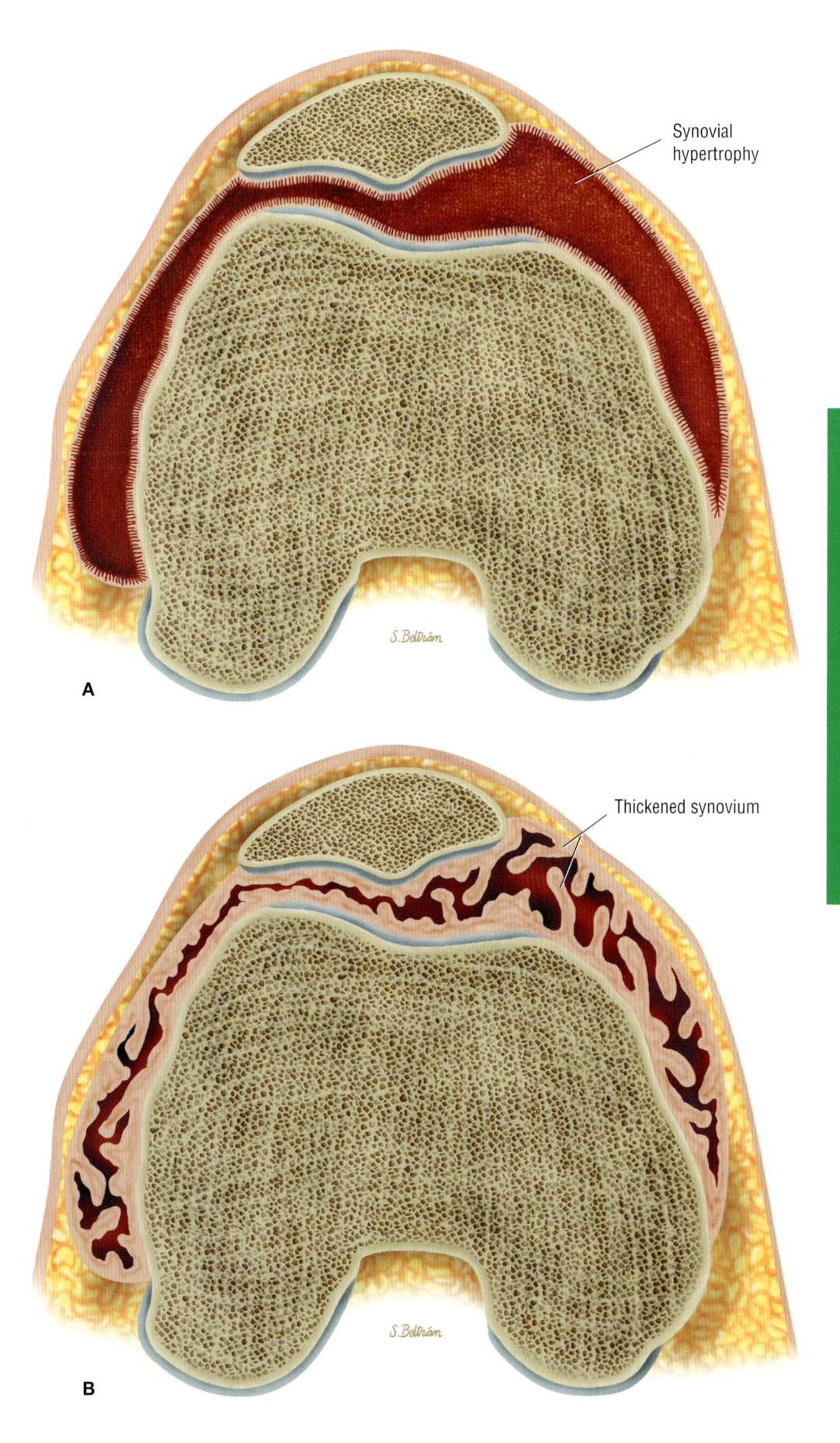

FIGURE 8.19 (**A**) Synovial hypertrophy. (**B**) Characteristic thickened synovium that is demonstrated on contrast-enhanced MR images.

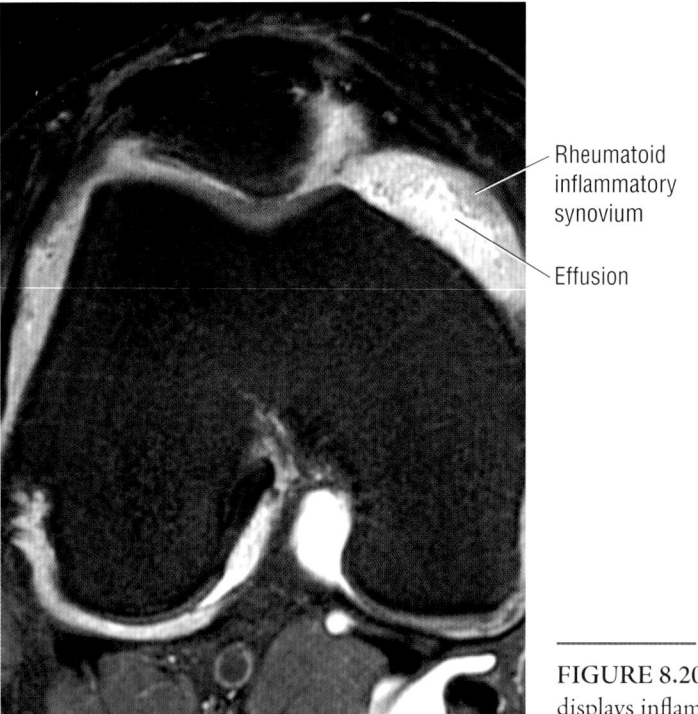

FIGURE 8.20 Axial FS PD FSE image displays inflammatory synovium of intermediate signal intensity.

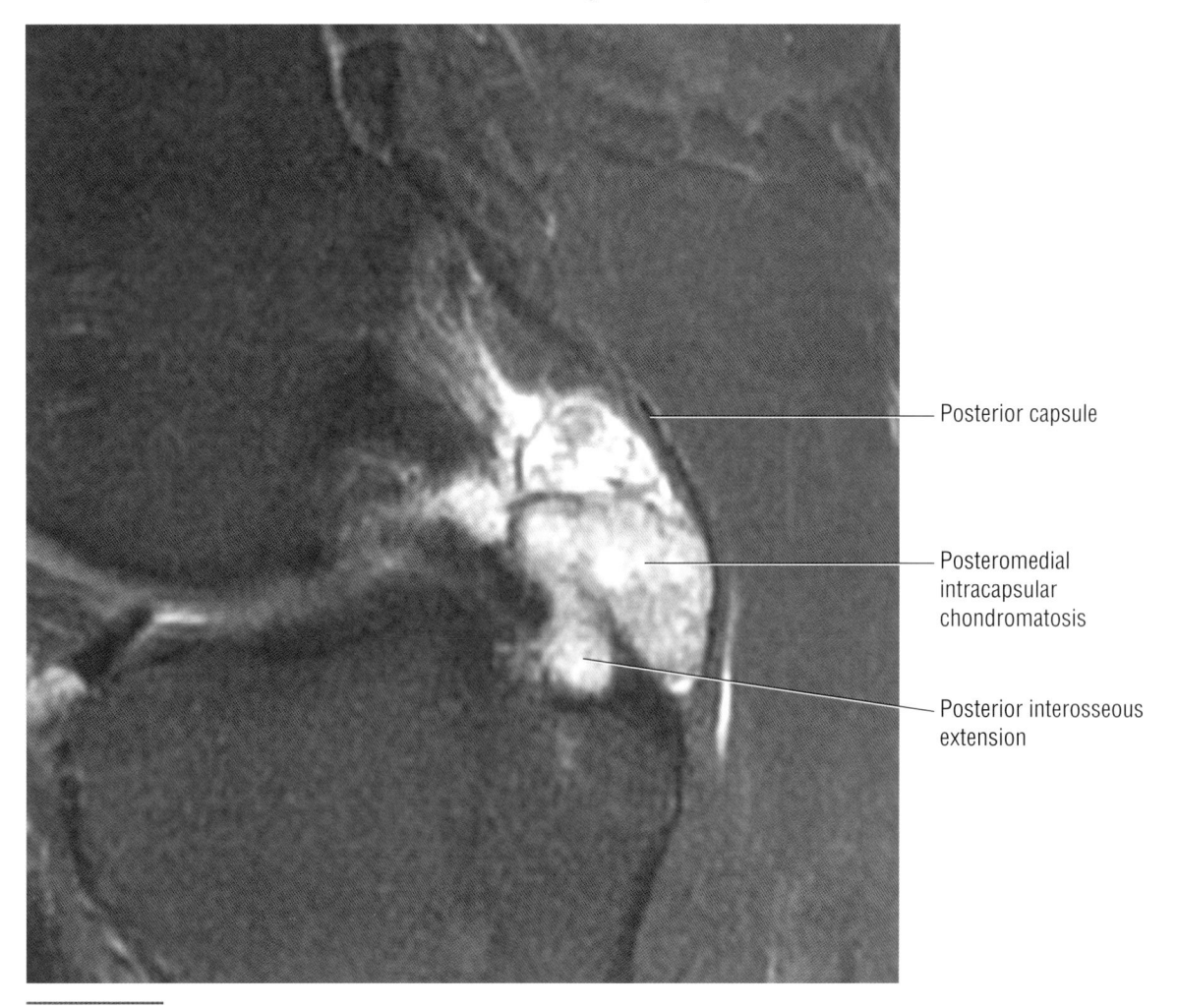

FIGURE 8.21 Extrusion of the posterior tibia with chondromatosis. Note that the cartilage intermediate signal could be mistaken for synovial thickening. This lesion was focal in contrast to rheumatoid inflammatory synovium. Sagittal FS PD FSE image.

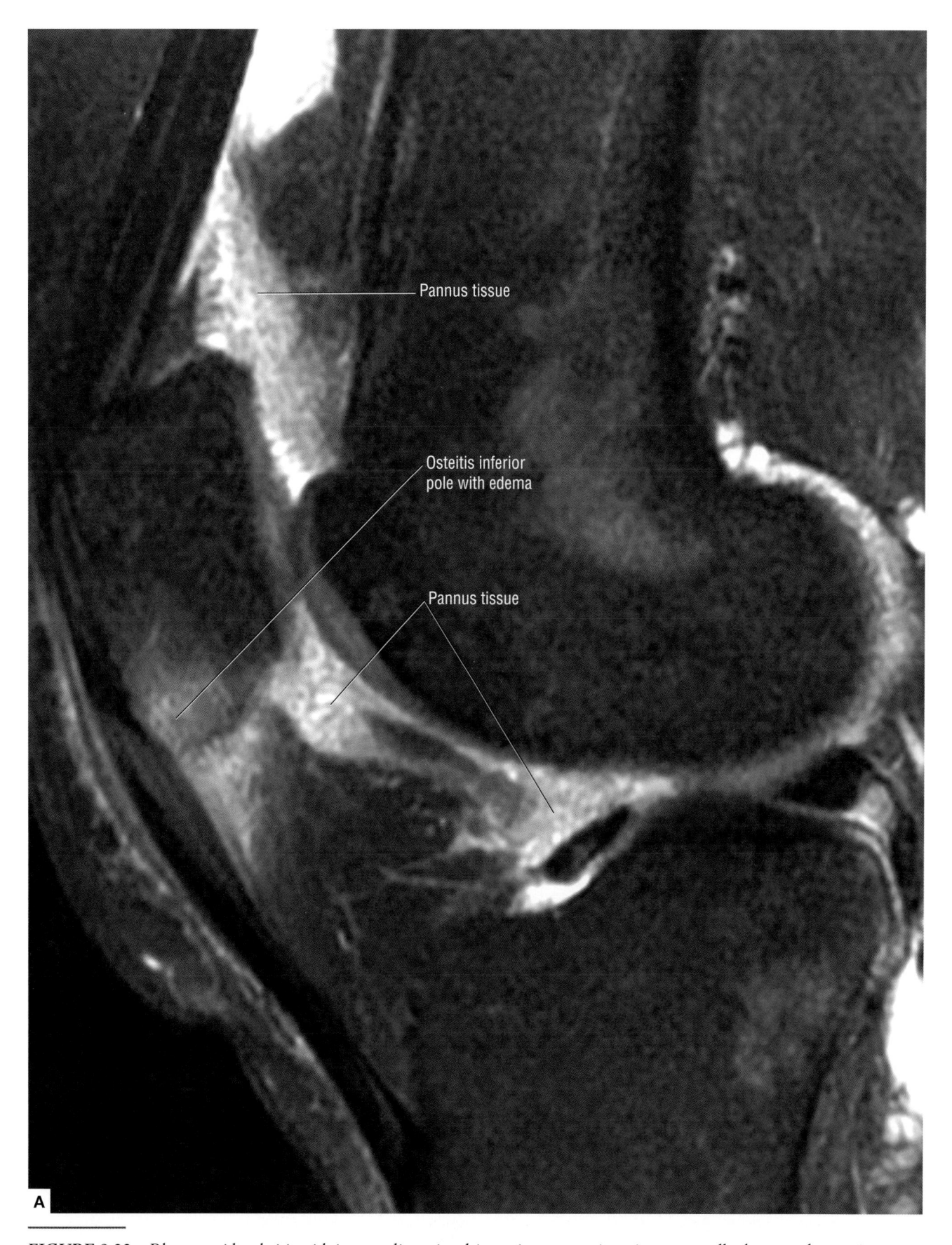

FIGURE 8.22 Rheumatoid arthritis with intermediate-signal-intensity pannus tissue in suprapatellar bursa and posterior to Hoffa's fat pad. Identification of joint fluid and synovial hypertrophy is useful in earlier stages of inflammation especially since the advent of disease-modifying antirheumatic drugs. Thickened synovium and pannus tissue can be identified prior to osteitis to affect treatment prior to the development of erosions. (**A**) Sagittal FS PD FSE image. *(Continued)*

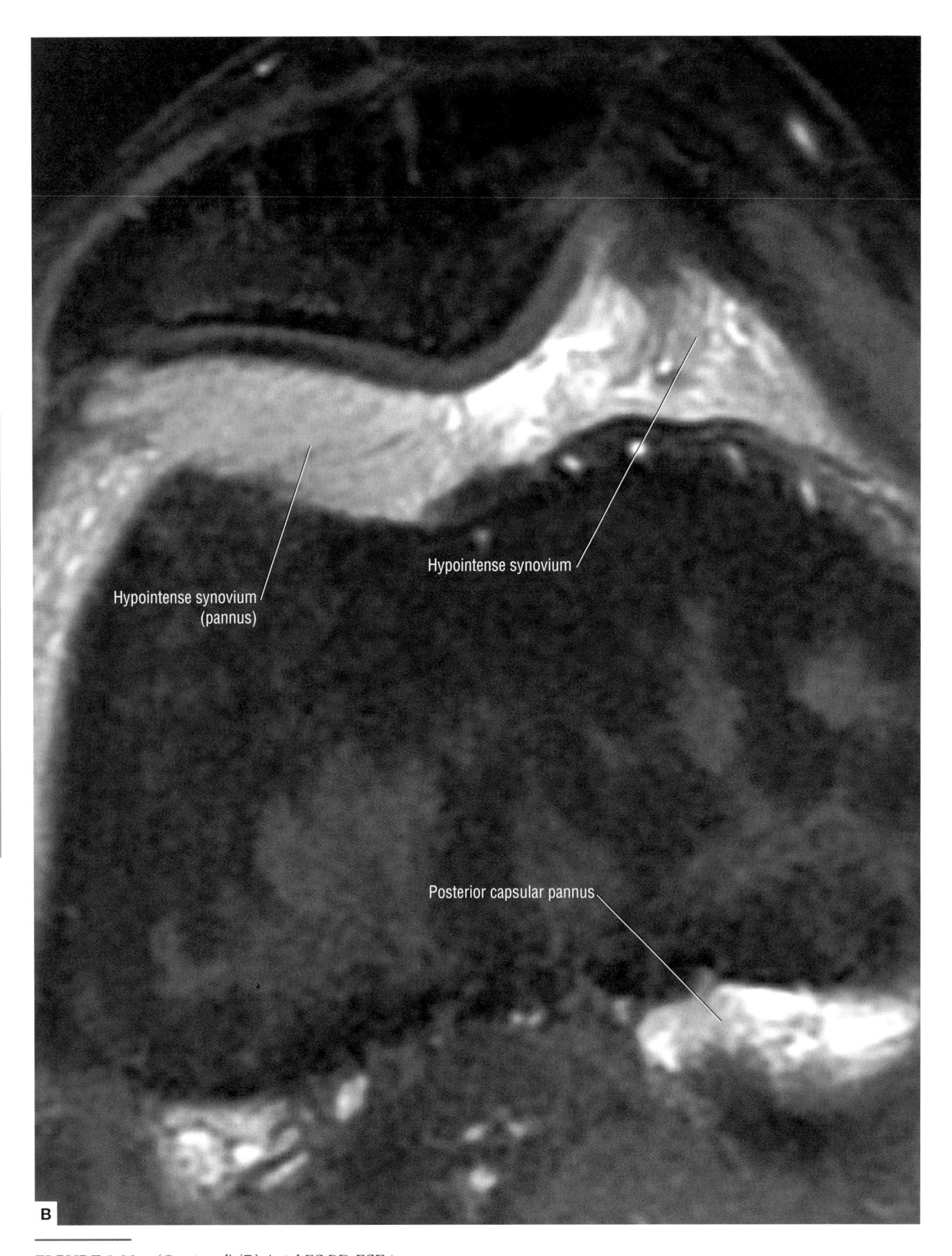

FIGURE 8.22 *(Continued)* **(B)** Axial FS PD FSE image.

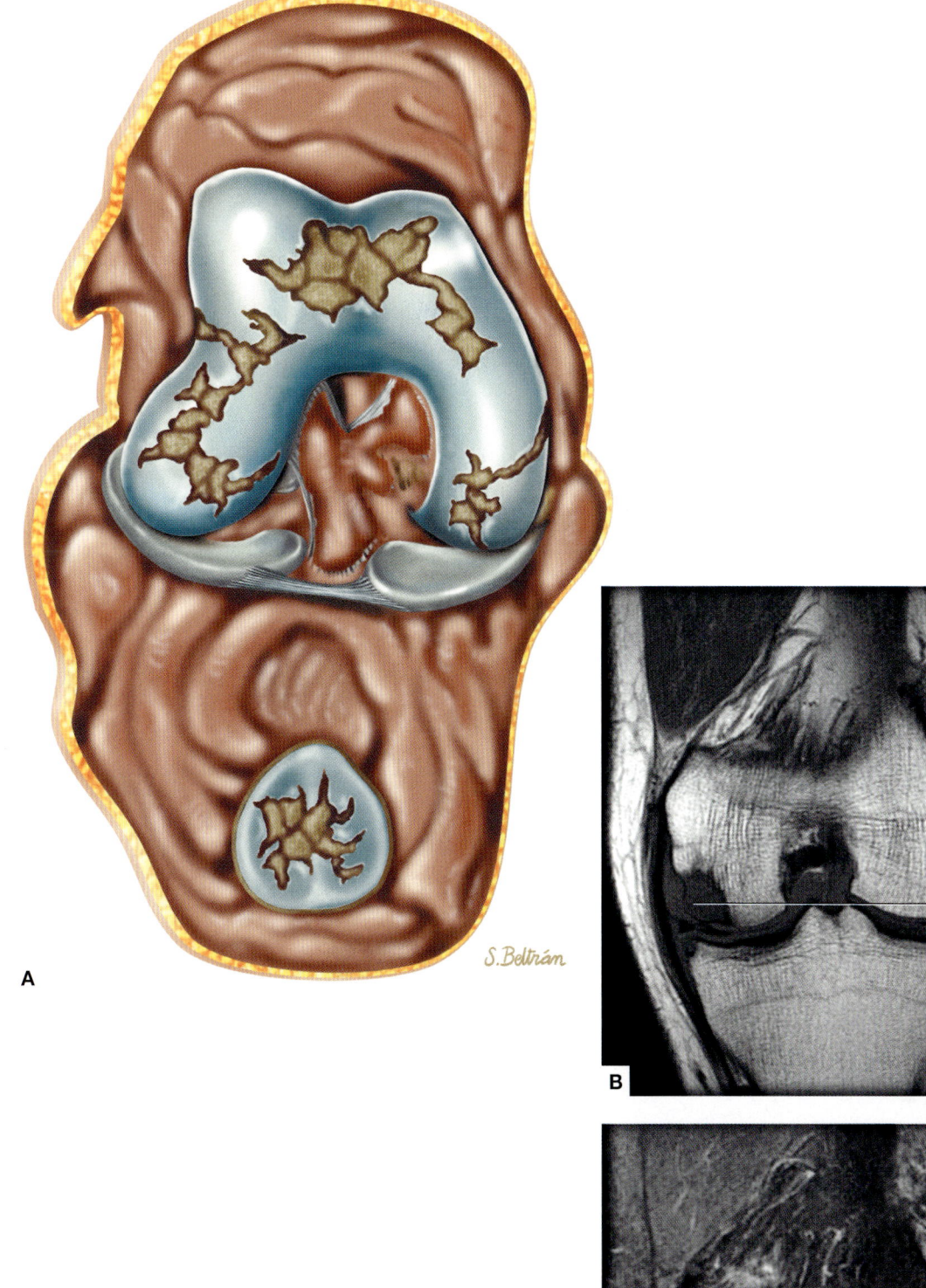

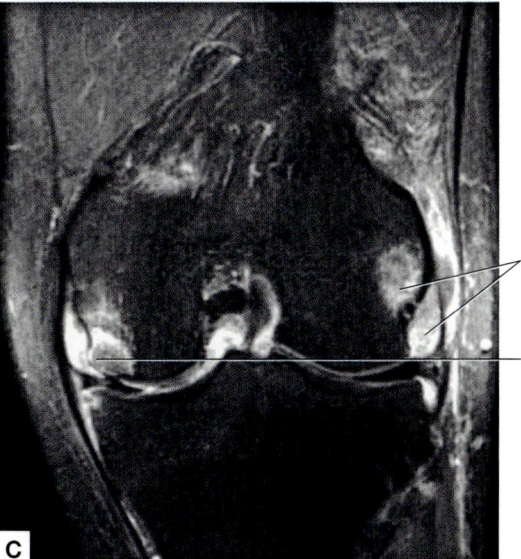

General Pathologic Conditions Affecting the Knee

Erosion lateral femoral condyle
Erosion medial femoral condyle

Pannus tissue with adjacent erosion
Pressure erosion with pannus tissue

FIGURE 8.23 (**A**) Chondral erosions of the distal femur and patella associated with synovial thickening on an anterior view color (coronal perspective) illustration with the patella retracted inferiorly. There is direct extension of pannus to the margins of the joint. Tendinomuscular involvement of pannus and popliteal fossa synovial cysts are frequently seen. Pannus tissue resulting in marginal erosions is seen on coronal PD FSE (**B**) and FS PD FSE (**C**) images.

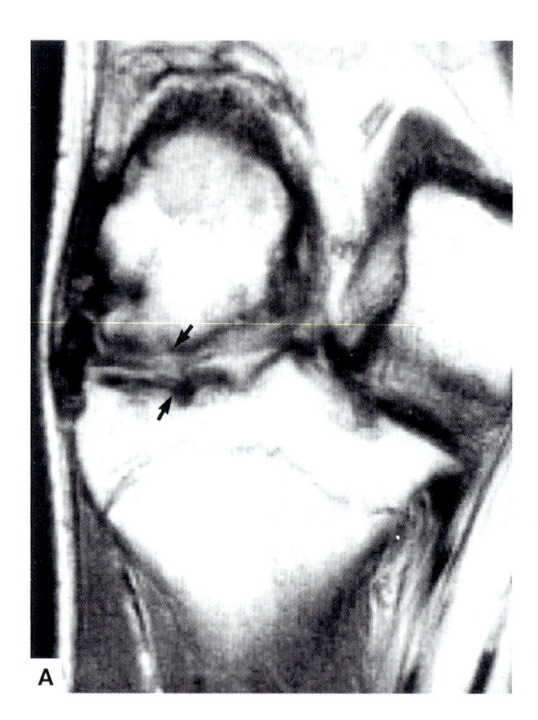

FIGURE 8.24 (**A**) Coronal T1-weighted image in the more chronic phase of rheumatoid arthritis with joint space narrowing, sclerosis (arrows), and decreased inflammatory response. (**B**) More advanced stage of rheumatoid arthritis with fibrous ankylosis and less prominent inflammatory component.

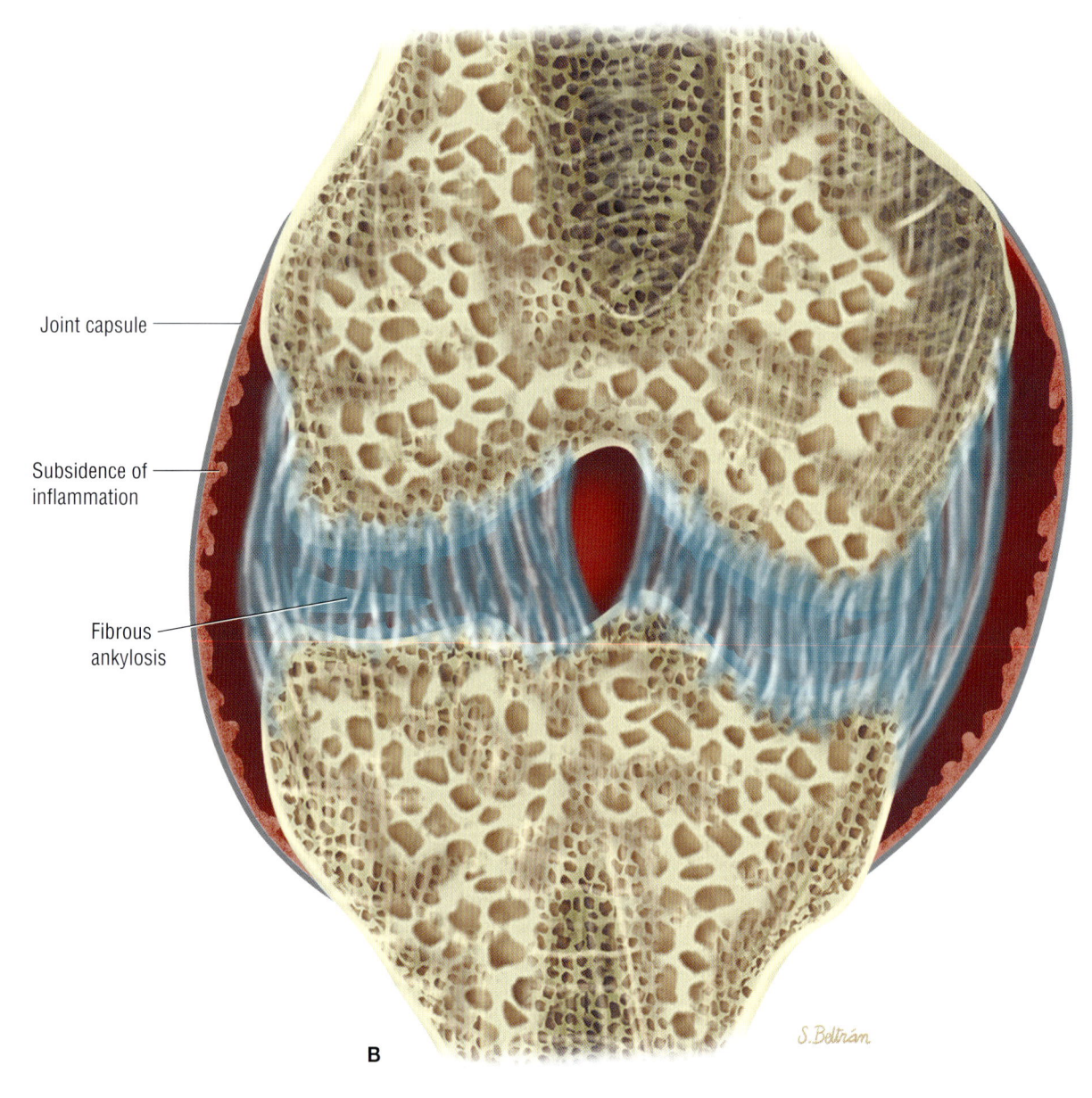

- Joint capsule
- Subsidence of inflammation
- Fibrous ankylosis

Pigmented Villonodular Synovitis (PVNS)

Key Concepts

- Presents as either localized or nodular type of mass posterior to Hoffa's fat pad or diffuse type with distribution through joint recesses

- Localized or nodular PVNS is also known as localized nodular synovitis, emphasizing its common location involving the infrapatellar fat pad, lack of diffuse frond-like projections of synovium, and decreased hemosiderin deposition compared to diffuse PVNS.

- T2* GRE images demonstrate greater susceptibility to increased hemosiderin content in diffuse PVNS than in localized or nodular PVNS.

Pigmented Villonodular Synovitis

- Monoarticular synovial proliferative disorder[288]

- Occurs in diffuse and nodular forms

- Usually presents as nonpainful soft tissue mass

- Most common site of involvement is the knee, especially in the diffuse form of the disease.

- Localized or nodular PVNS is also known as *localized nodular synovitis*.[200]

    - Lacks diffuse frond-like synovial projections and abundance of hemosiderin found in diffuse PVNS

    - Well circumscribed, lobular, and usually less than 4cm in diameter

    - Combination of fat and hemosiderin contributes to white, yellow, gray, and brown areas on gross cut surface examination

    - Corresponding histologic findings include dense collagenous capsule, fibrous scarring, multinucleated giant cells, mononuclear cells, xanthoma cells, histofibroblastic hyperplasia, and hemosiderin deposits (although less than in the diffuse type of PVNS)

- *Diffuse* PVNS

    - Hemosiderin-laden macrophages frequently deposited in hyperplastic synovial masses

    - May be associated sclerotic bone lesions

- On gross examination, characterized by multiple soft spongy lesions; brown, yellow, or rust-like tissue (based on hemosiderin content); and absence of a well-defined collagenous capsule

- Microscopic features include hemosiderin within histiocytes, villous hyperplasia of synovial membrane, capillary hyperplasia, sheets of polymorphic rounded cells, and hyalinized appearance of stromal collagen.

- Fewer multinucleated giant cells are present compared with localized PVNS.

MR Findings of Pigmented Villonodular Synovitis

- Hemosiderin-infiltrated synovial masses demonstrate low signal intensity on T1-, T2-, FS PD-weighted FSE, and T2*-weighted images because of the paramagnetic effect of iron.[257,347,374,466]

- Condylar erosions may be associated with a synovial mass and fibrous tissue.

- Localized nodular PVNS
    - Well-circumscribed mass within or posterior to Hoffa's infrapatellar fat pad
    - Less commonly within the posterior capsule of the knee joint

- Diffuse PVNS
    - Visualized in any recess in communication with the joint, including popliteus tendon sheath, coronary (meniscotibial) and meniscofemoral recesses, suprapatellar bursa, popliteal cyst, and the intercondylar notch

- Intermediate-signal-intensity soft tissue–like mass associated directly with patellar tendon is seen in chronic tophaceous gout and may be confused with PVNS.
    - Gouty tophi tend to be deposited about extensor tendons such as the quadriceps and patellar tendons.[288]

General Pathologic Conditions Affecting the Knee

Pigmented Villonodular Synovitis (PVNS)

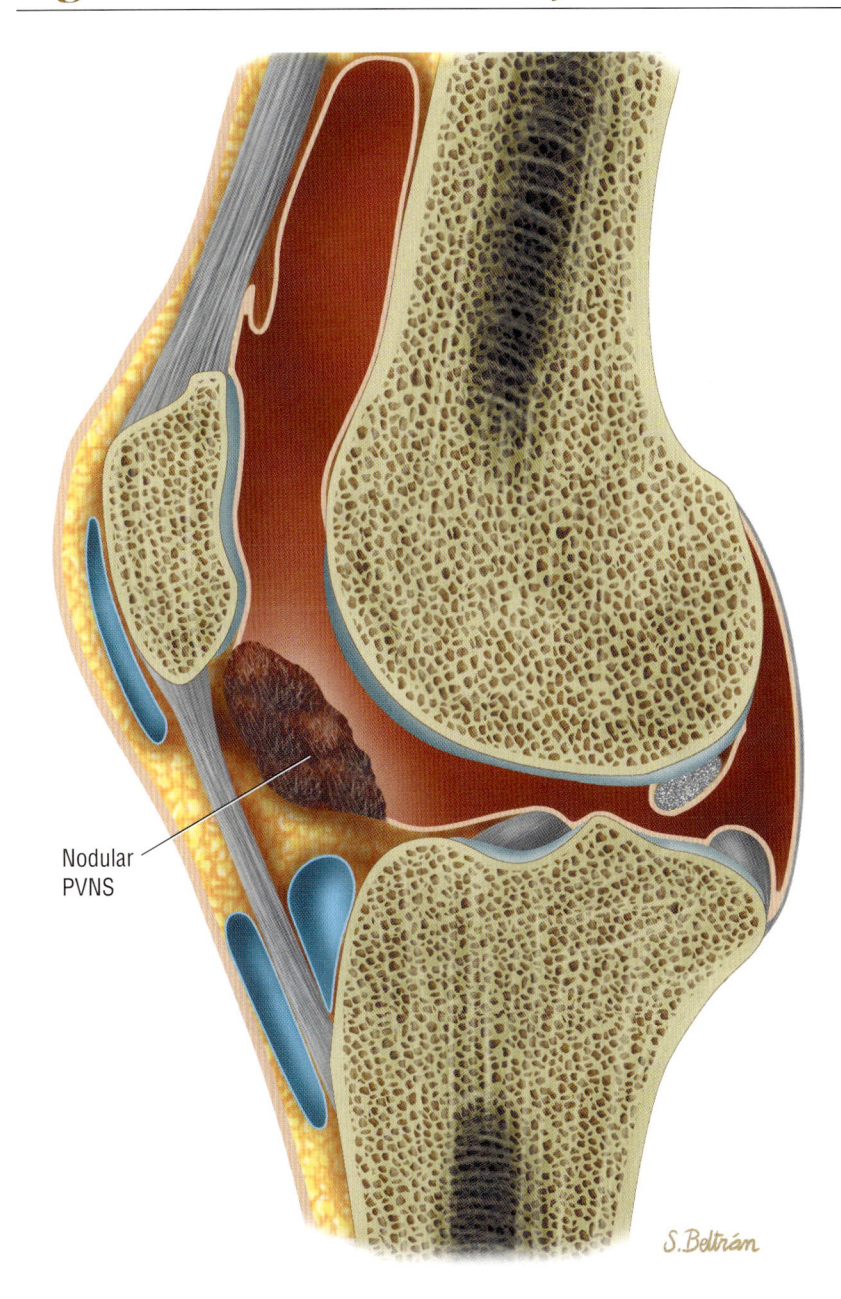

FIGURE 8.25 Characteristic location of focal nodular PVNS deforming the posterior margin of Hoffa's fat pad.

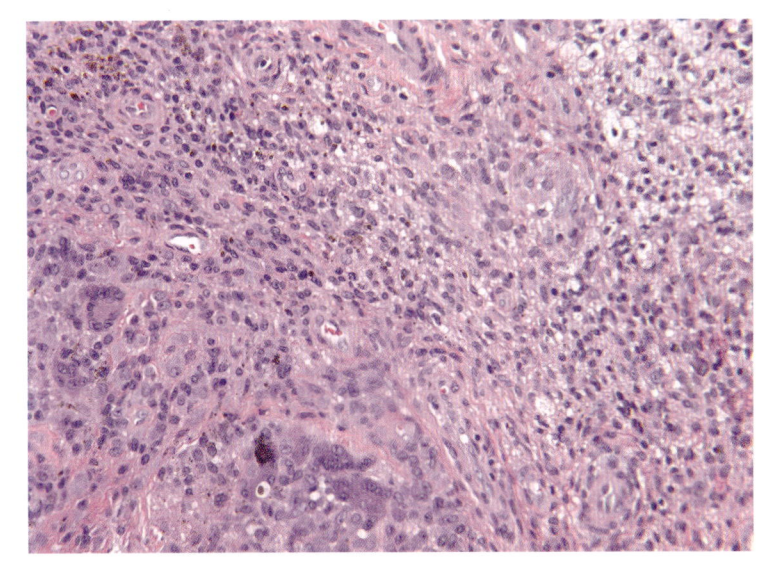

FIGURE 8.26 Histologic photomicrograph (20× power) of PVNS. (Reprinted from Jackson DW. *Master Techniques in Orthopaedic Surgery: Reconstructive Knee Surgery*, 3rd ed. Philadelphia, PA: Lippincott Williams & Wilkins; 2008, with permission.)

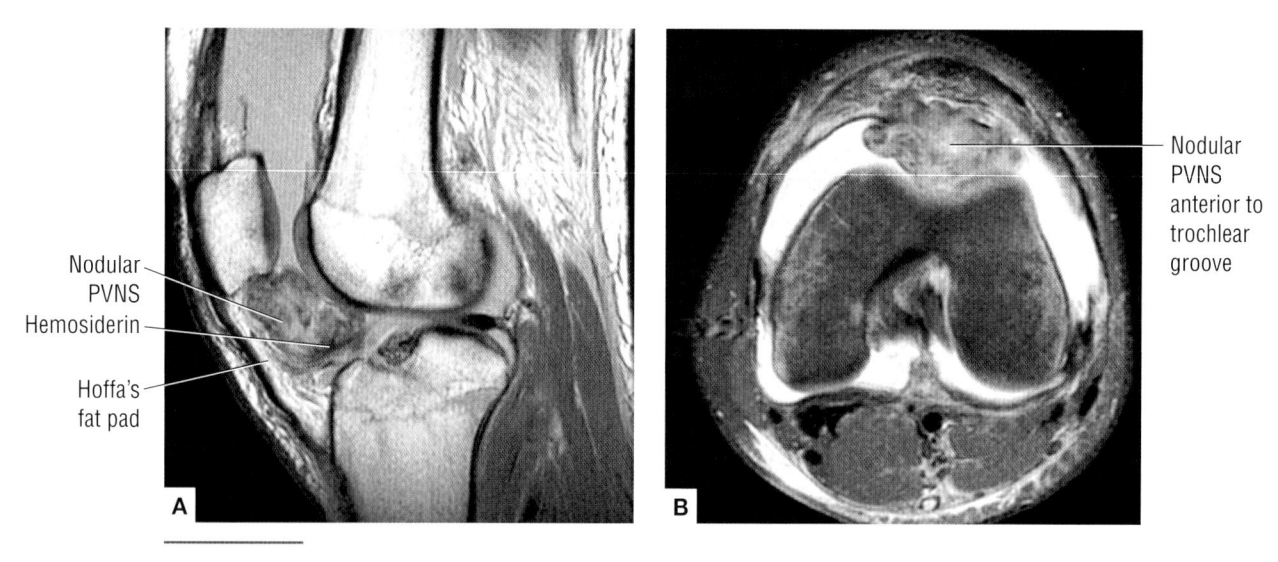

FIGURE 8.27 Sagittal PD (**A**) and axial FS PD FSE (**B**) images showing localized or nodular PVNS hypointense to intermediate in signal intensity.

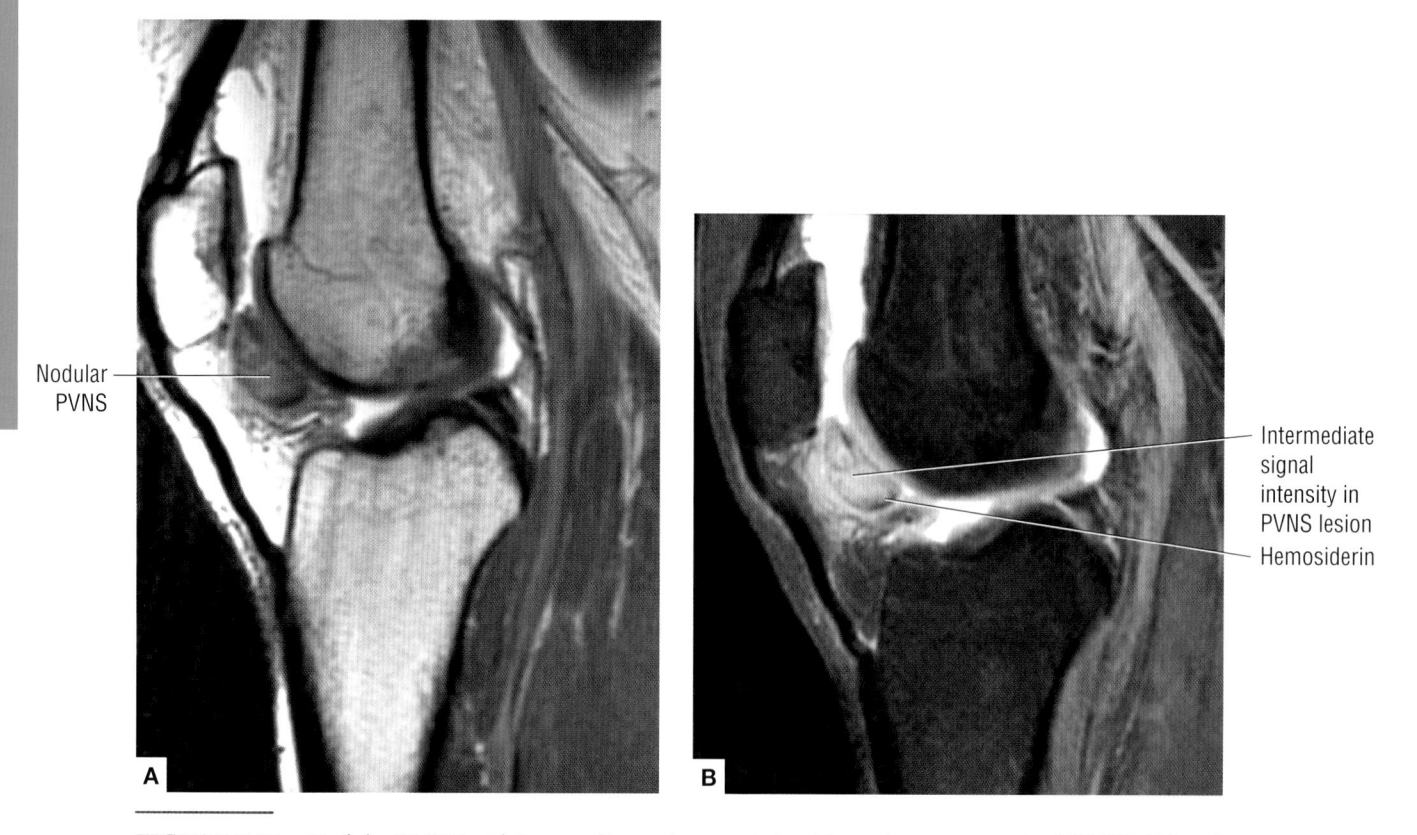

FIGURE 8.28 Nodular PVNS with intermediate to increased signal intensity seen on sagittal FS PD (**A**) and FS PD FSE (**B**) images. The localized form of PVNS has less hemosiderin content than the diffuse form.

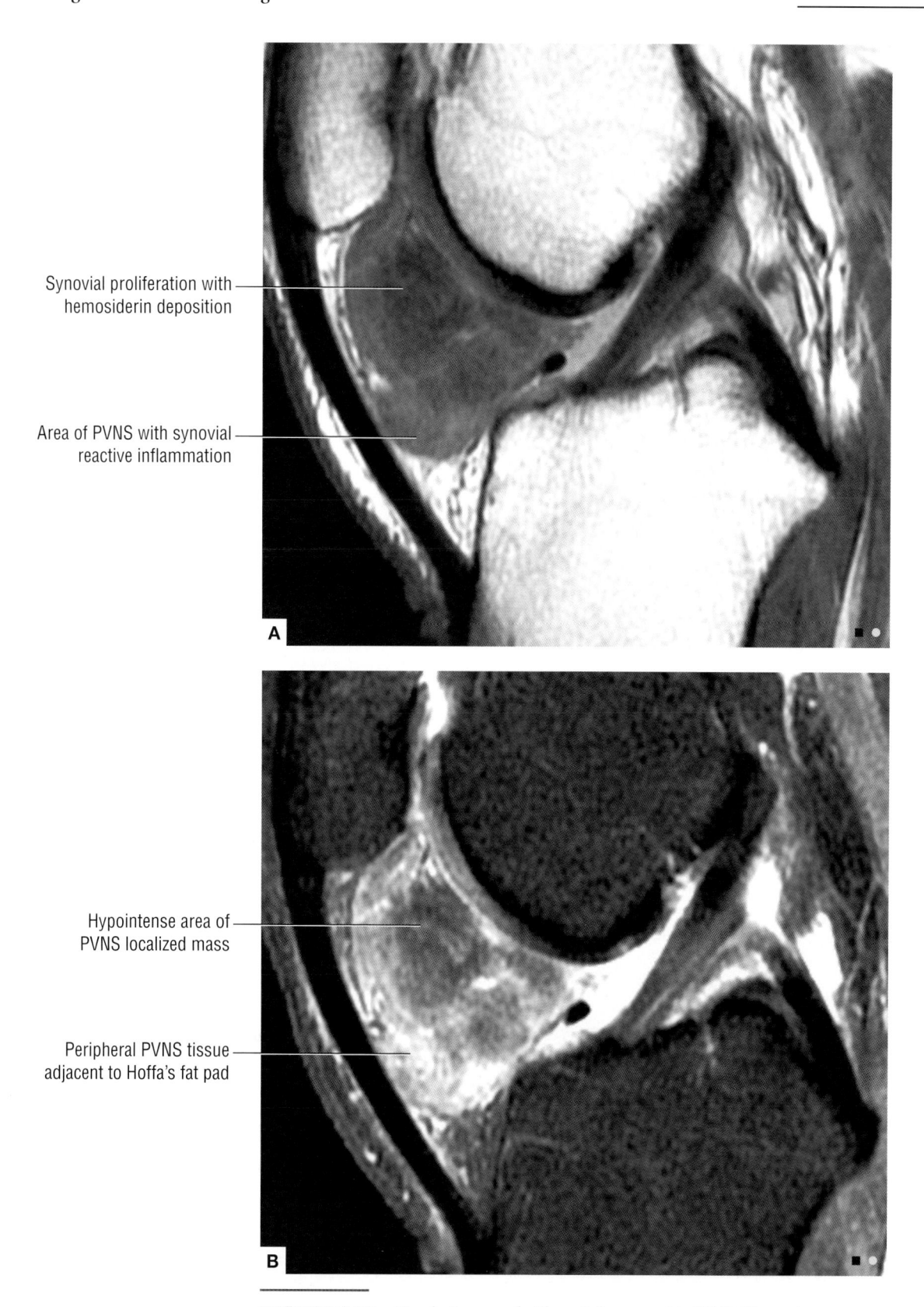

FIGURE 8.29 Focal pigmented villonodular synovitis (PVNS) as a heterogenous mass posterior to Hoffa's fat pad. Lobulated margin with areas of hypointense or intermediate signal intensity may exist adjacent to regions of relative hyperintensity. Distinct contrast between hypointense area with greater hemosiderin content and intermediate/hypointense thickened synovium. Inflammation with multinucleated giant cells, repeated hemorrhage with hemosiderin deposition, and xanthoma cells from altered lipid metabolism are included in the pathophysiologic mechanisms. Sagittal PD (**A**) and FS PD (**B**) images.

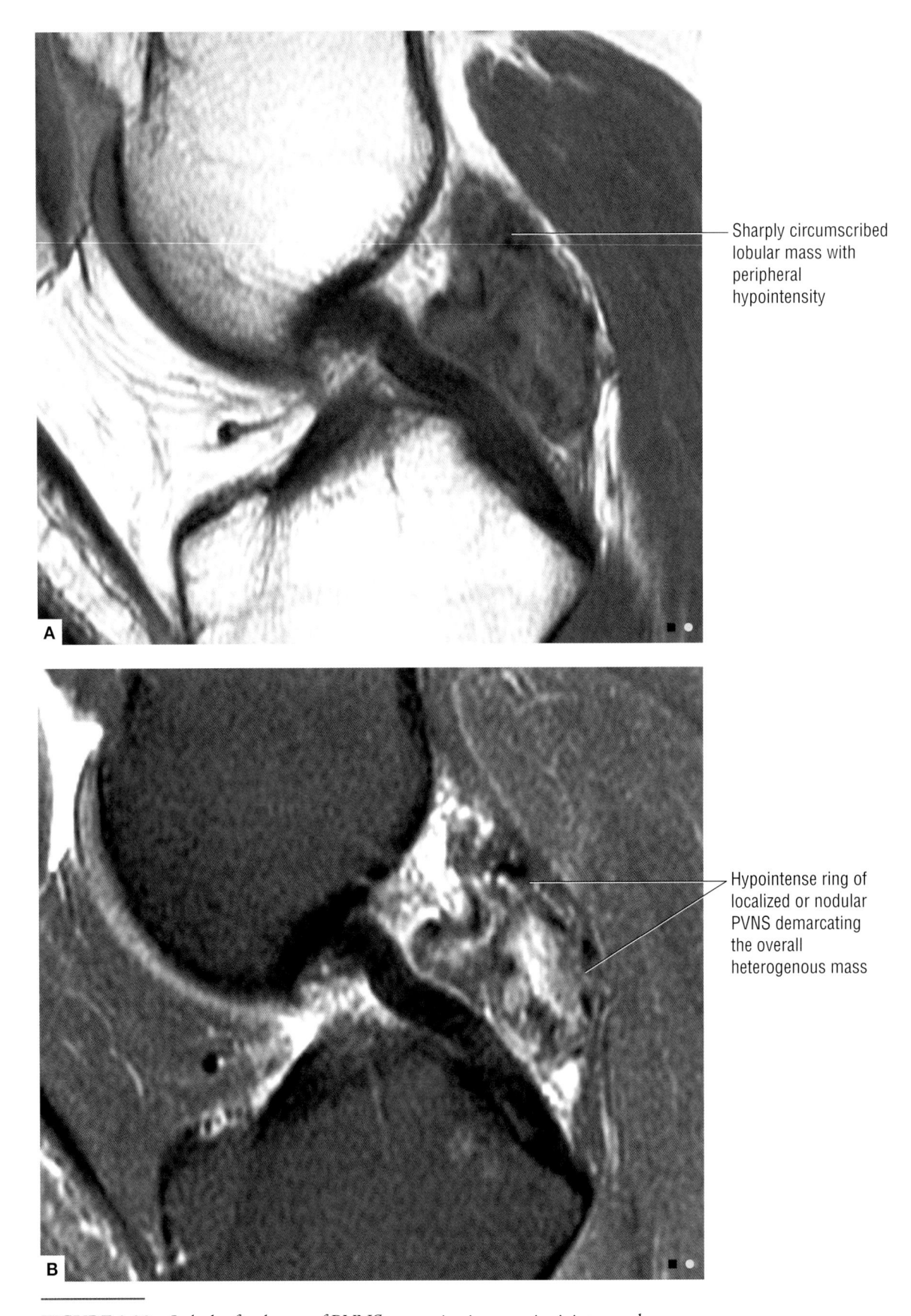

FIGURE 8.30 Lobular focal mass of PVNS presenting in posterior joint capsule instead of the more common location posterior to Hoffa's fat pad in the anterior compartment. The hypointense peripheral border reflects the higher content of hemosiderin. PD (**A**) and FS PD (**B**) sagittal images.

Hypointense nodular localized PVNS

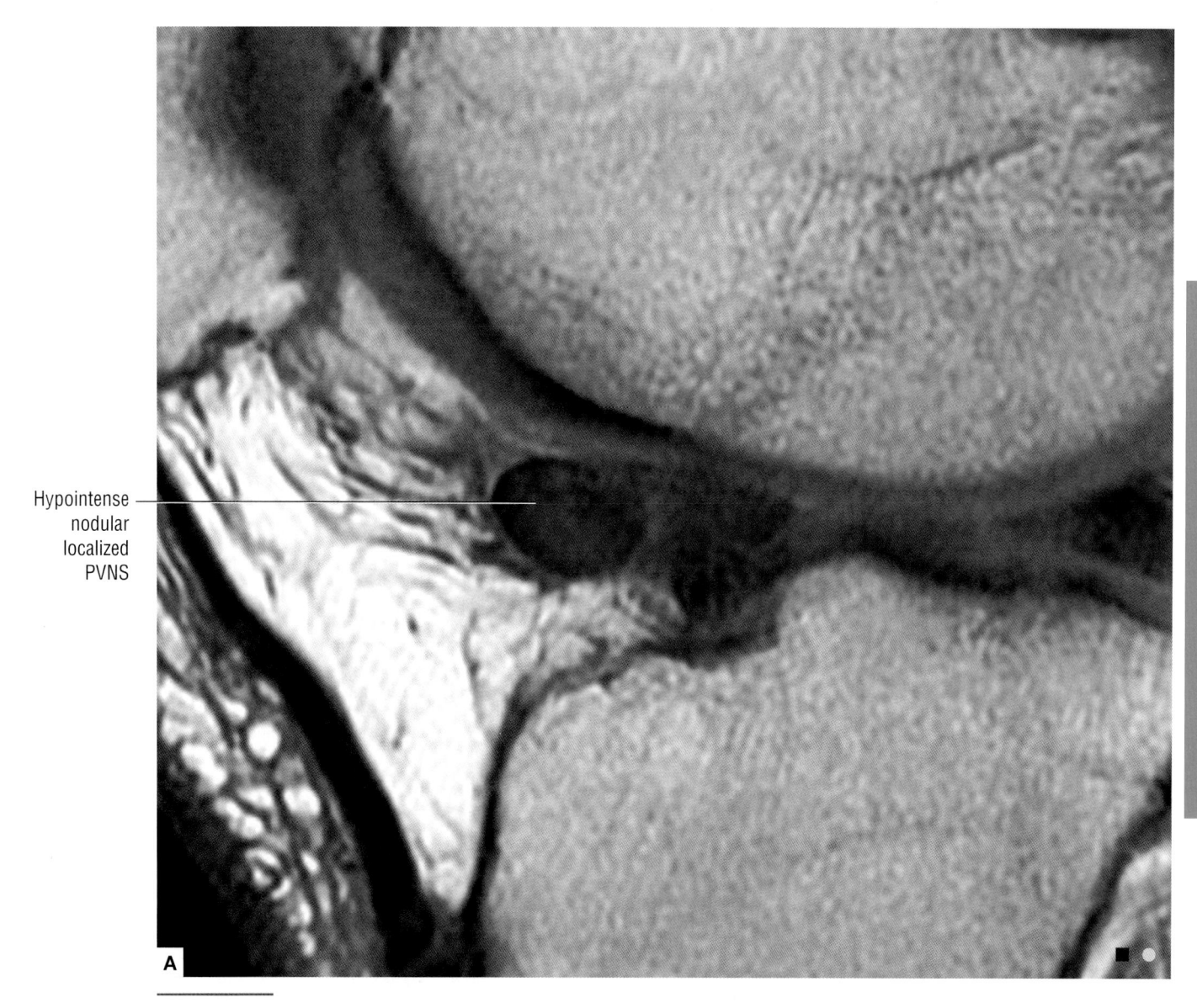

FIGURE 8.31 Localized PVNS is low to intermediate signal on T1/PD and intermediate/heterogenous centrally on fluid-sensitive sequences. The hypointense hemosiderin ring outlining the peripheral borders of the tissue is characteristic in the localized form of PVNS, which otherwise may be more difficult to diagnose compared to the significant susceptibility of hemosiderin when imaged in the diffuse form of PVNS. Sagittal PD (**A**) image. *(Continued)*

Hypointense peripheral border of localized PVNS

Hypointense periphery of hemosiderin

Intermediate heterogenous central area of nodular PVNS tissue

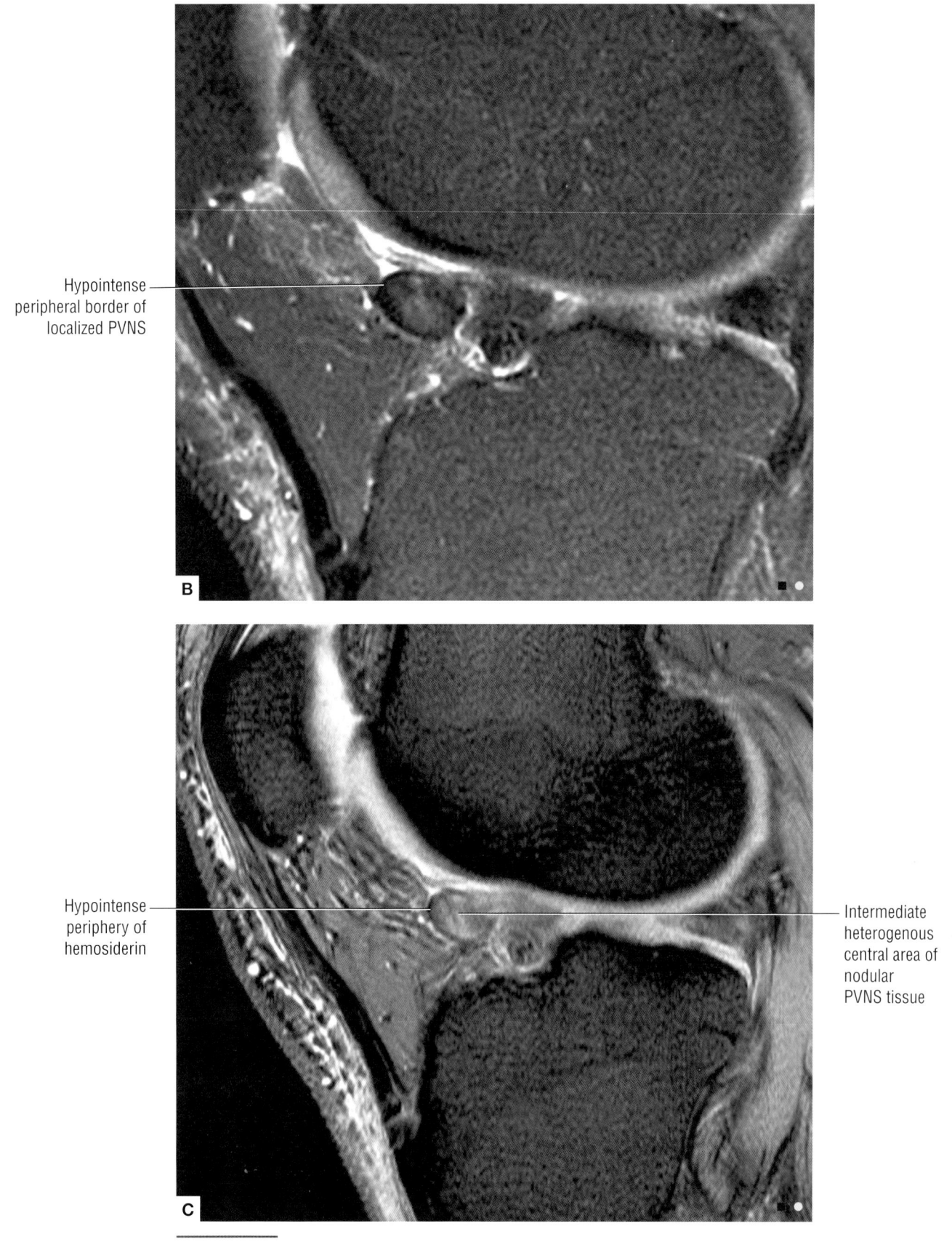

FIGURE 8.31 *(Continued)* Sagittal FS PD- (**B**) and gradient echo T2*- (**C**) weighted images.

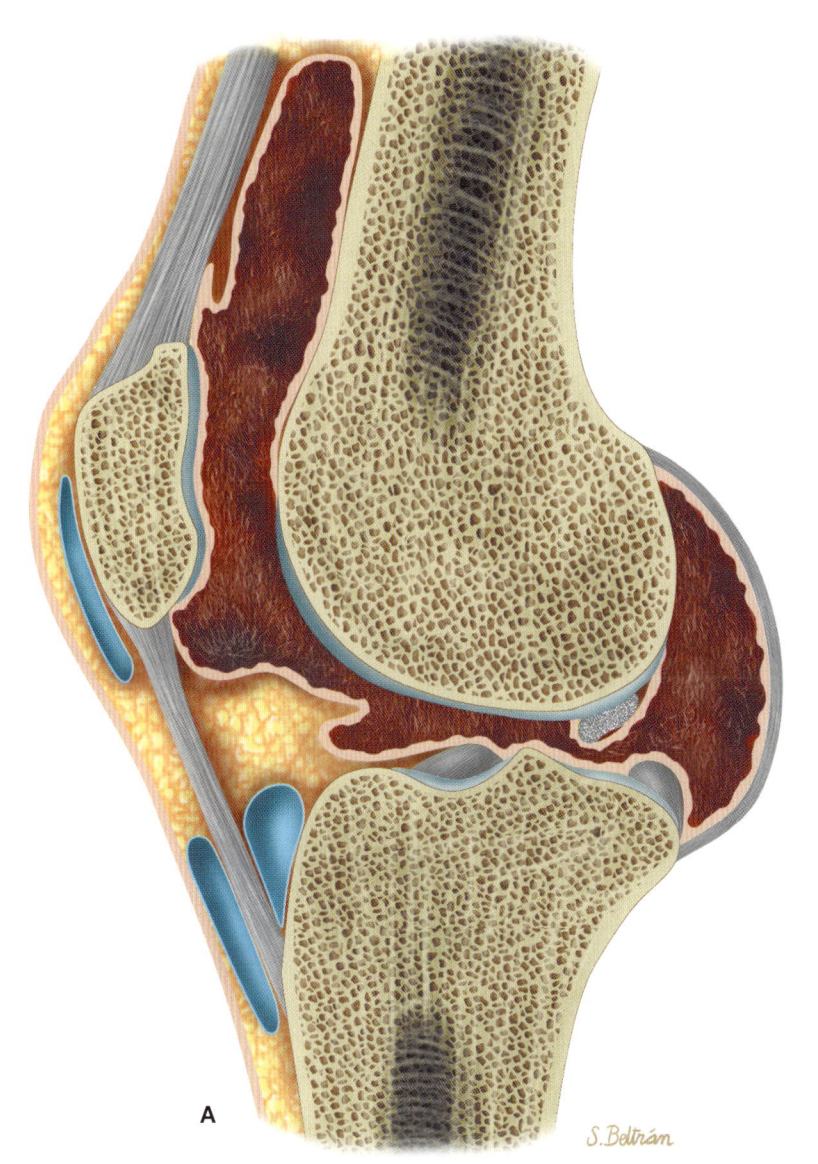

FIGURE 8.32 **(A)** The diffuse form of PVNS involving the suprapatellar bursa and posterior capsule. Progressive synovitis with pain and effusions are common. **(B)** Sagittal T2* GRE image displays hypointense hemosiderin deposits in the posterolateral capsule and along the free edge of Hoffa's fat pad.

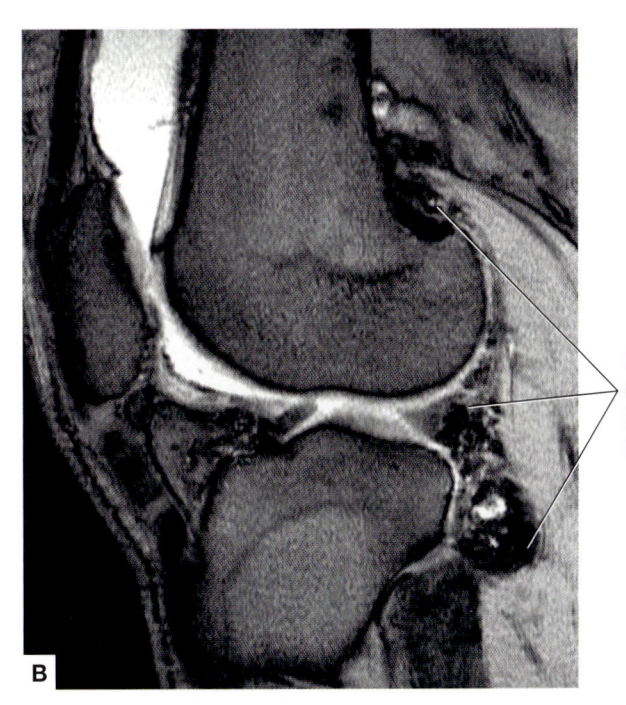

Posterolateral distribution of hemosiderin in PVNS tissue

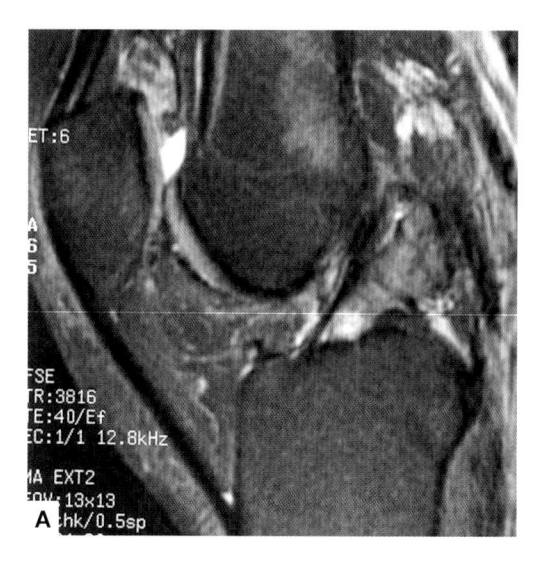

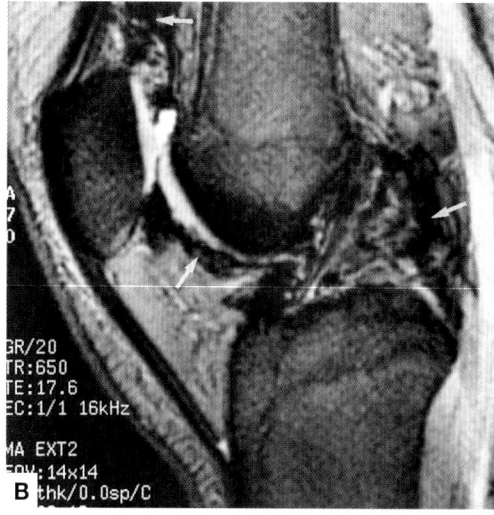

FIGURE 8.33 Comparison of FS PD-weighted FSE (**A**) and T2*-weighted (**B**) sagittal images used in the assessment of the diffuse form of PVNS. The FS PD-weighted FSE sequence (**A**) is less sensitive to hemosiderin (*arrows*) in pannus tissue and synovium than is the T2*-weighted sequence (**B**).

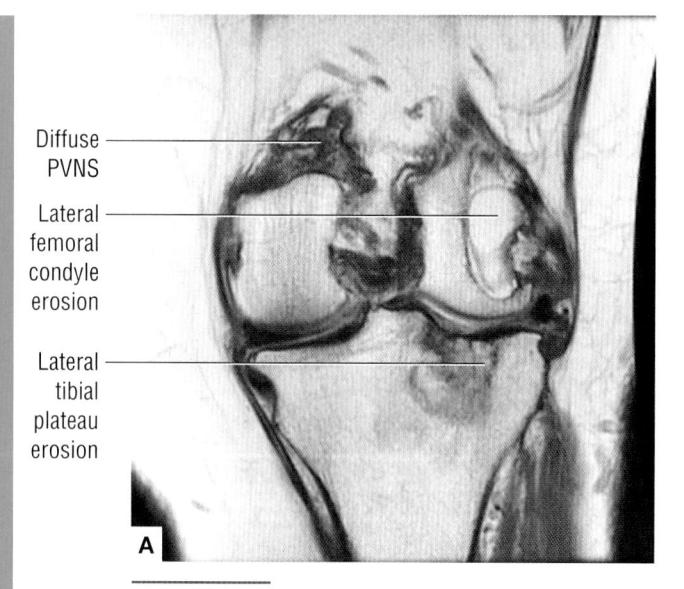

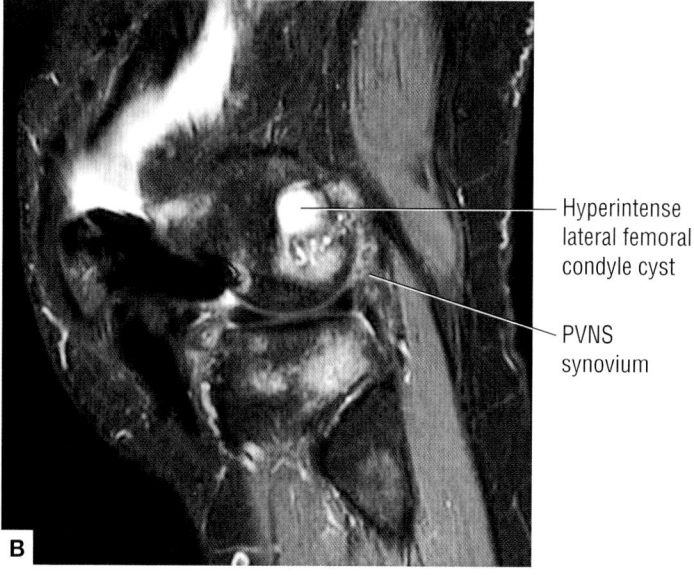

FIGURE 8.34 (**A**) Coronal PD FSE and (**B**) sagittal FS PD FSE images showing osseous cyst-like erosions involving the lateral femoral condyle and lateral tibial plateau in diffuse PVNS. No calcifications are associated with the erosion.

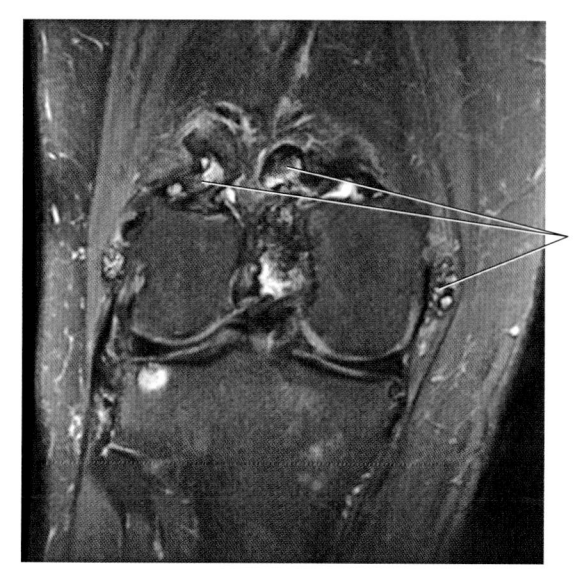

FIGURE 8.35 Posterior capsular involvement in diffuse PVNS is usually evident on posterior coronal images superior to the femoral condyles. Coronal FS PD FSE image.

General Pathologic Conditions Affecting the Knee

- Hypointense paramagnetic effect of hemosiderin
- Suprapatellar PVNS tissue
- Hoffa's fat pad free edge susceptibility

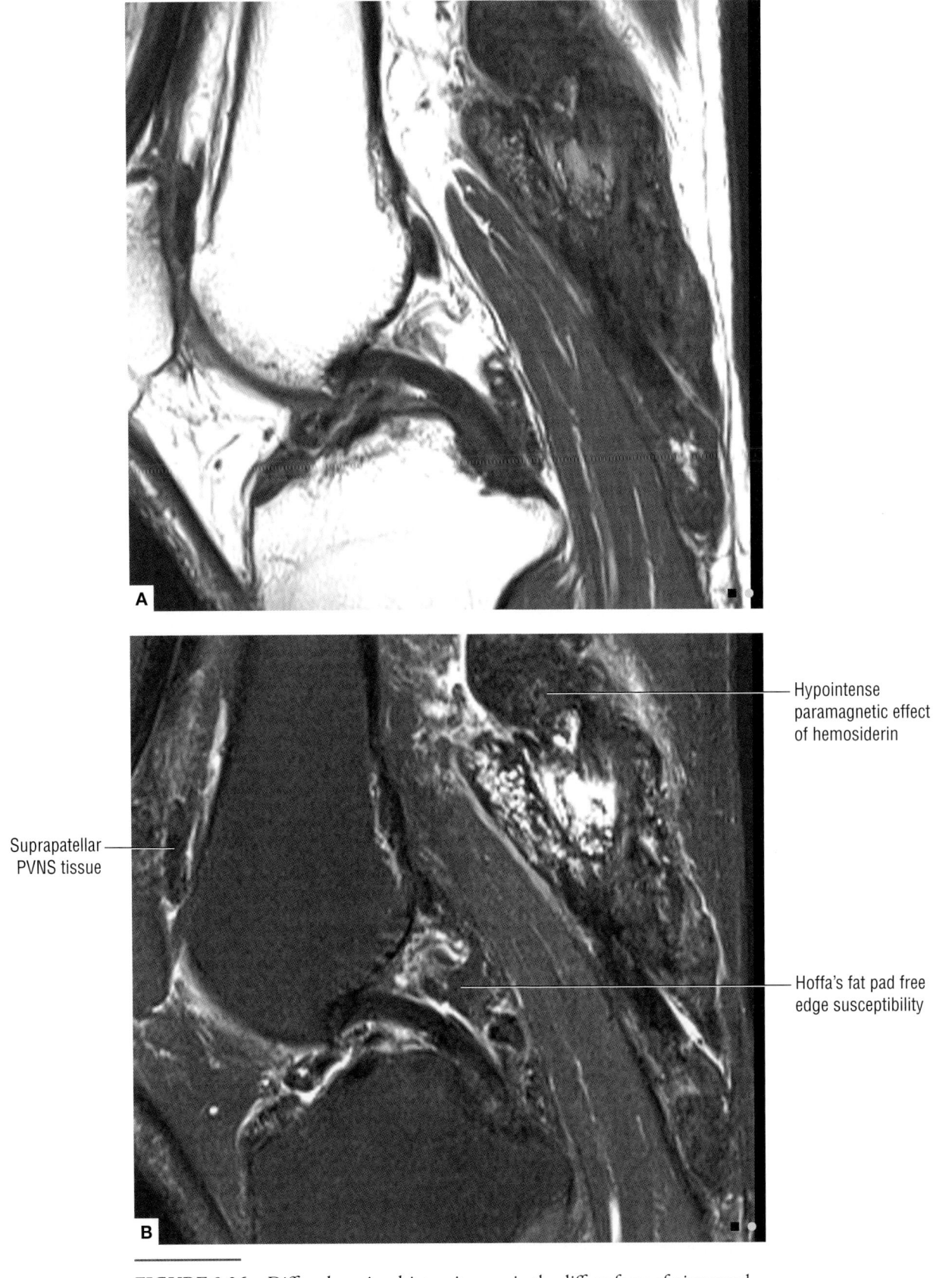

FIGURE 8.36 Diffuse low-signal-intensity area in the diffuse form of pigmented villonodular synovitis (PVNS). The paramagnetic effect of hemosiderin is detected as hypointense or dark areas throughout the joint and within the popliteal cyst. The diffuse form results in hypertrophic synovial tissue throughout the knee joint. Sagittal PD (**A**) and FS PD (**B**) images.

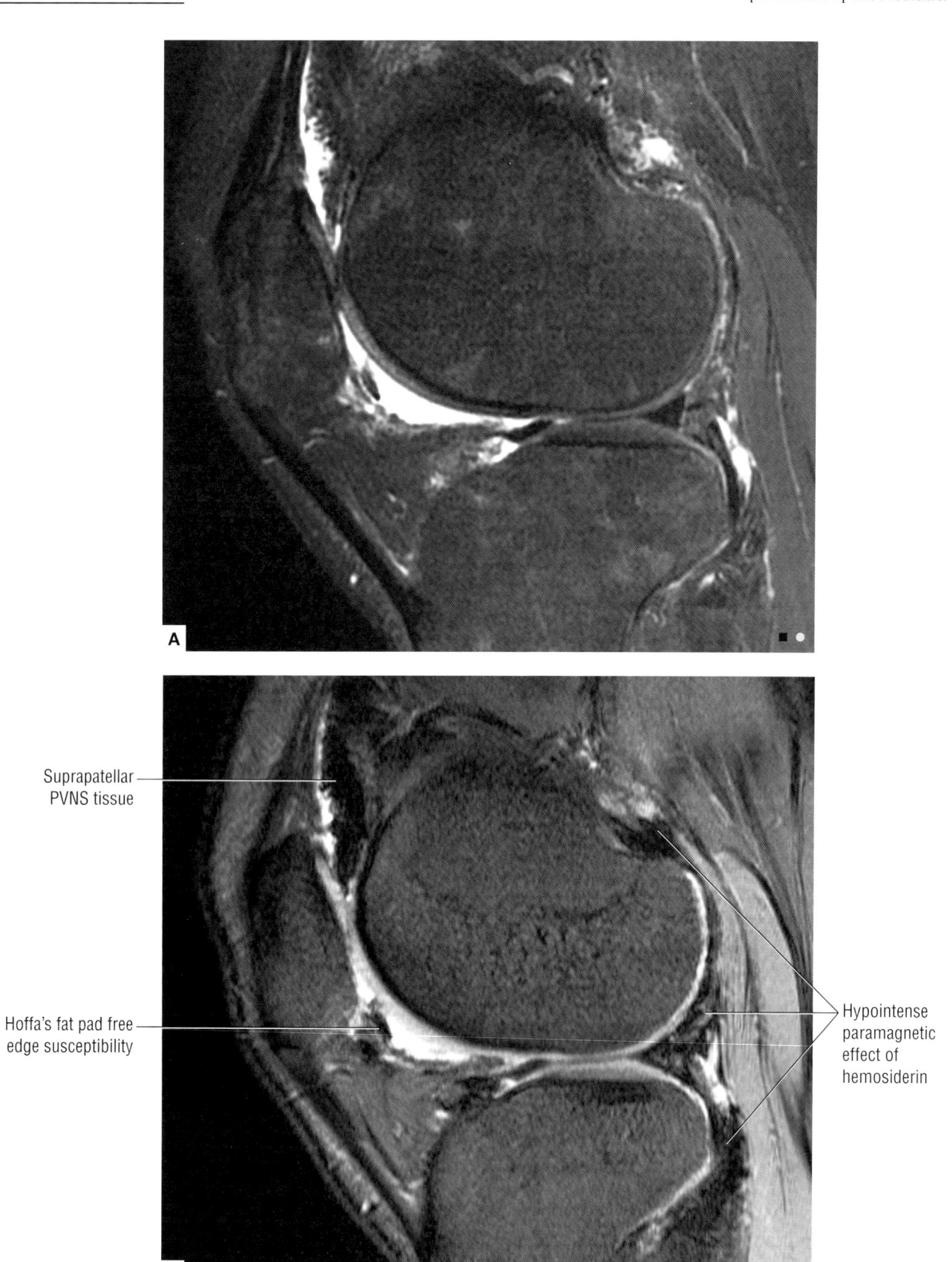

FIGURE 8.37 Diffuse PVNS with typical hypointense paramagnetic effect of hemosiderin deposits specific for diagnosis. Exaggerated susceptibility or blooming of hypointense signal occurs on gradient echo images. Sagittal FS PD (**A**) and T2* gradient echo (**B**) images.

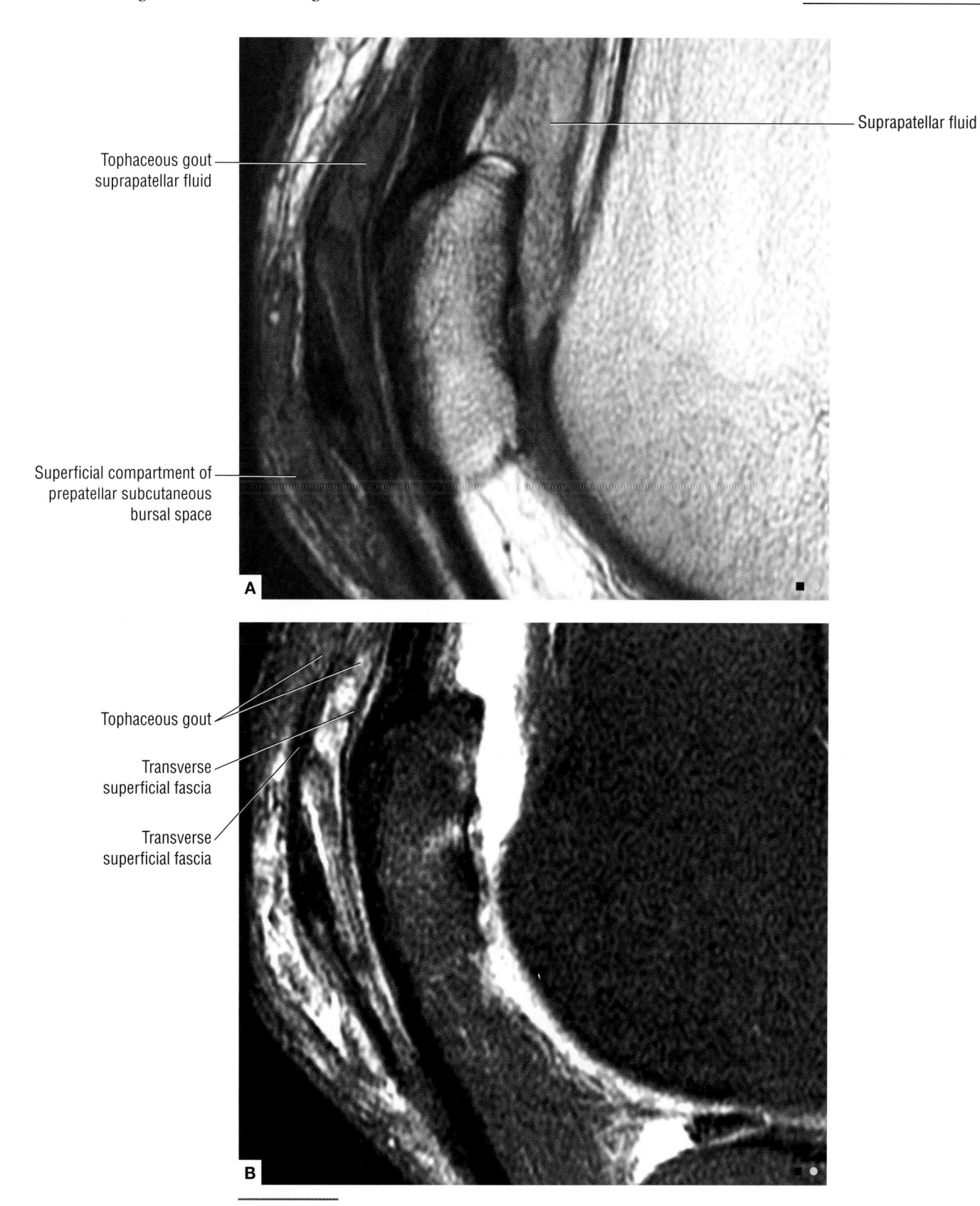

FIGURE 8.38 Low–intermediate signal intensity of tophaceous gout on PD-weighted sagittal image. Fascial thickening and compartmental soft tissue gout deposits help define the trilaminar prepatellar bursa. Tophaceous gout soft tissue masses involving the prepatellar bursae of the knee. Characteristic heterogenous signal intensity on sagittal FS PD FSE image. Common locations for soft tissue deposits of gout include the medial aspect of the infrapatellar fat pad and anterior joint recess. Gout is present as bursal distension of all three compartments of the prepatellar bursa as separated by two layers of fascia. Sagittal PD (**A**) and FS PD (**B**) images.

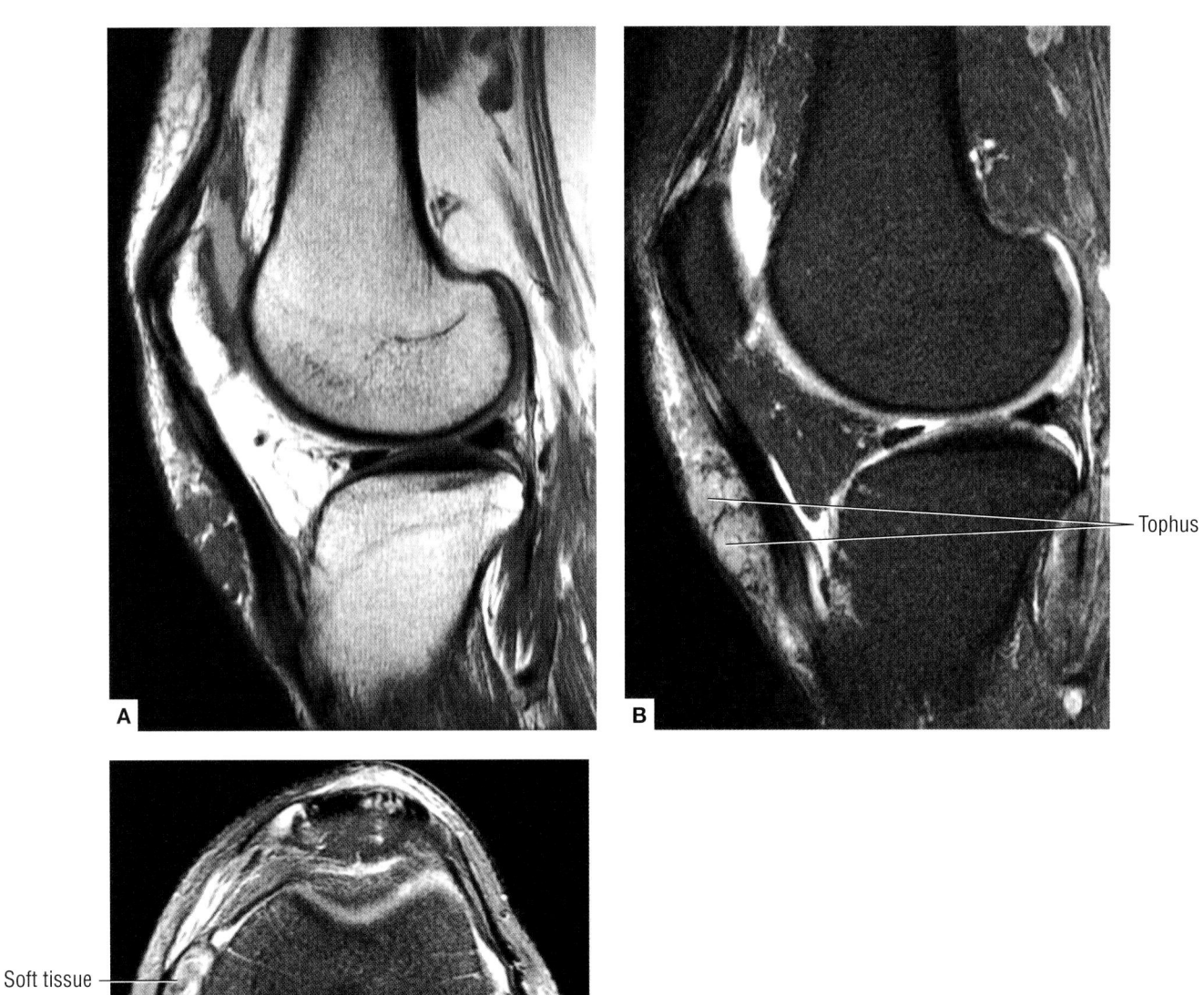

FIGURE 8.39 Sagittal (**A**) PD FSE and (**B**) FS PD FSE and (**C**) axial FS PD FSE images display gouty soft tissue tophi anterior to the distal patellar tendon and deep to the medial retinaculum. Synovial fluid, tendon sheath bursae, and subcutaneous tissue have low pH values, allowing precipitation of uric acid and crystal deposition. Tophi result when this precipitation induces chronic local inflammatory reactions.

Hemophilia

Key Concepts

- Recurrent hemorrhage into knee joint is typical in hemophilic arthropathy.

- Irregular infrapatellar fat-pad sign with hypointense hemosiderin deposited in a thickened synovial reflection is characteristic.

Hemophilia Pathology

- Initial synovial reaction to intraarticular hemorrhage is associated with synovial hypertrophy, hemosiderin deposition in phagocytic cells, perivascular infiltrates of inflammatory cells, and fibrosis of subsynovial layer.

- Vascular hyperplasia of the synovium contributes to further hemorrhage.

- Pannus formation, unlike in rheumatoid disease, is limited.

- Articular cartilage destruction in hemophilia is attributed to toxic or chemical factors, including hydrolytic enzymes.

MR Findings of Hemophilic Arthropathy

- Hemosiderin and fibrous tissue, formed from repeated episodes of joint hemorrhage, demonstrate low signal intensity on T1- and T2-weighted images.[261,536]

- Irregular contours of Hoffa's fat pad and markedly thickened, hemosiderin-laden synovial reflections of low signal intensity are common findings.

- Articular cartilage irregularities and erosions detected on MR scans (when conventional radiographs are normal in early stages of disease)

- Subchondral and intraosseous cysts or hemorrhage identified on coronal and sagittal MR images

- Fluid-filled cysts generate high signal intensity on T2-weighted images.

- Articular and subchondral abnormalities of the femoral condylar and tibial surfaces are relatively common, seen in 75% to 85% of cases.

Lyme Arthritis

Key Concepts

- Identified on MR by irregular fat pad within the affected knee without pannus formation

Lyme Arthritis

- Lyme disease and resultant arthritis caused by spirochete *Borrelia burgdorferi*, which is transmitted by *Ixodes* ticks
- Characterized by delayed appearance of oligo- or polyarticular inflammatory arthritis[226]
- Knee most commonly affected
    - Inflammatory synovial effusions
    - Synovial hypertrophy
    - Infrapatellar fat-pad edema
    - Cartilage erosions (in severe chronic cases)
- Pain, warmth, and swelling of knee associated with circular erythematous migratory rash, headaches, and malaise after exposure to carrier deer tick
- MR is sensitive to the joint changes in synovitis, but diagnosis requires presence of elevated titers of immunoglobulin (Ig) M and IgG antibodies against the spirochete.

MR Findings of Lyme Arthritis

- Joint effusion and irregular, corrugated Hoffa's infrapatellar fat pad.
- Enthesopathic changes may occur in tendons (quadriceps and patellar).
- New bone may form at capsular insertion sites.
- Loss of articular cartilage in 25% of patients with chronic Lyme arthritis[228,272]
- Requires antibiotic treatment with penicillin or tetracycline

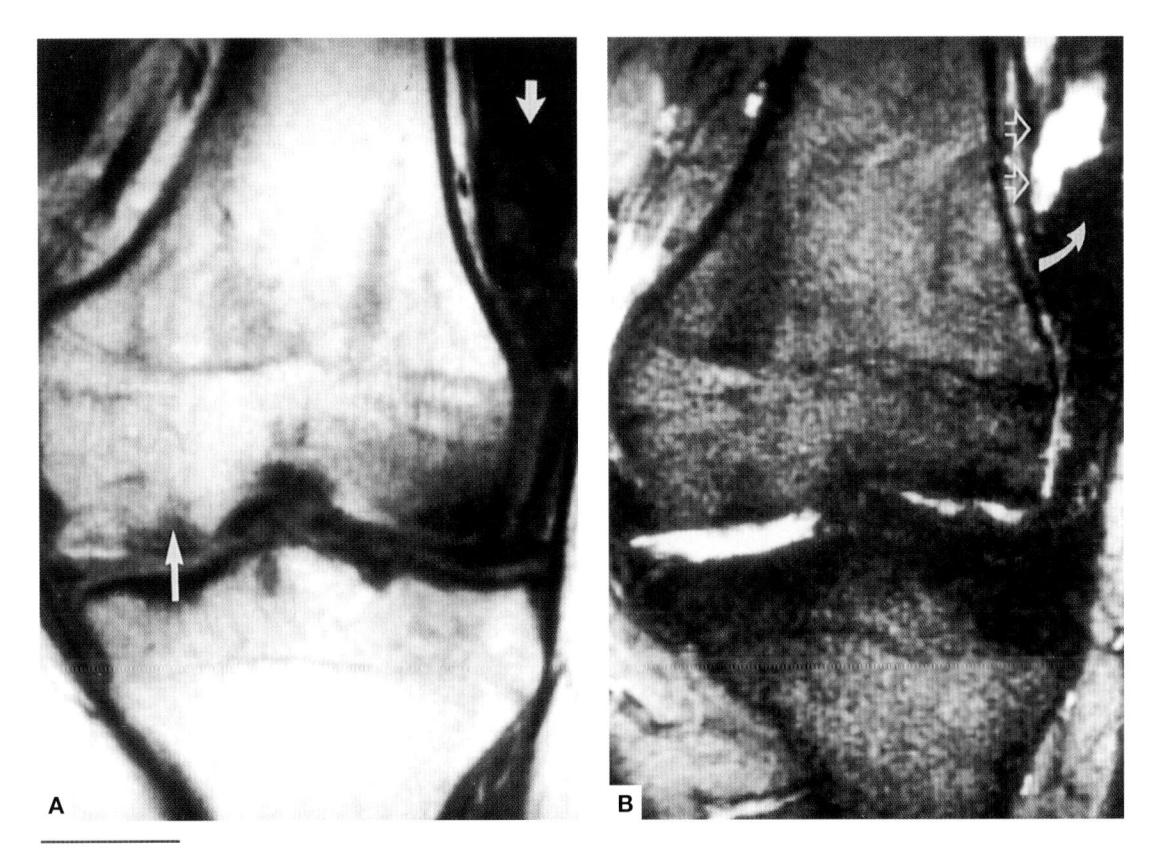

General Pathologic Conditions Affecting the Knee

FIGURE 8.40 (**A**) A T1-weighted coronal image demonstrates erosive changes (*long arrow*) and surrounding low-signal-intensity areas along the lateral femur (*short arrow*) in a patient with hemophilia. (**B**) On a T2*-weighted image, high-signal-intensity fluid or hemorrhage (*open arrows*) is distinguished from chronic hemosiderin deposition (*curved arrow*).

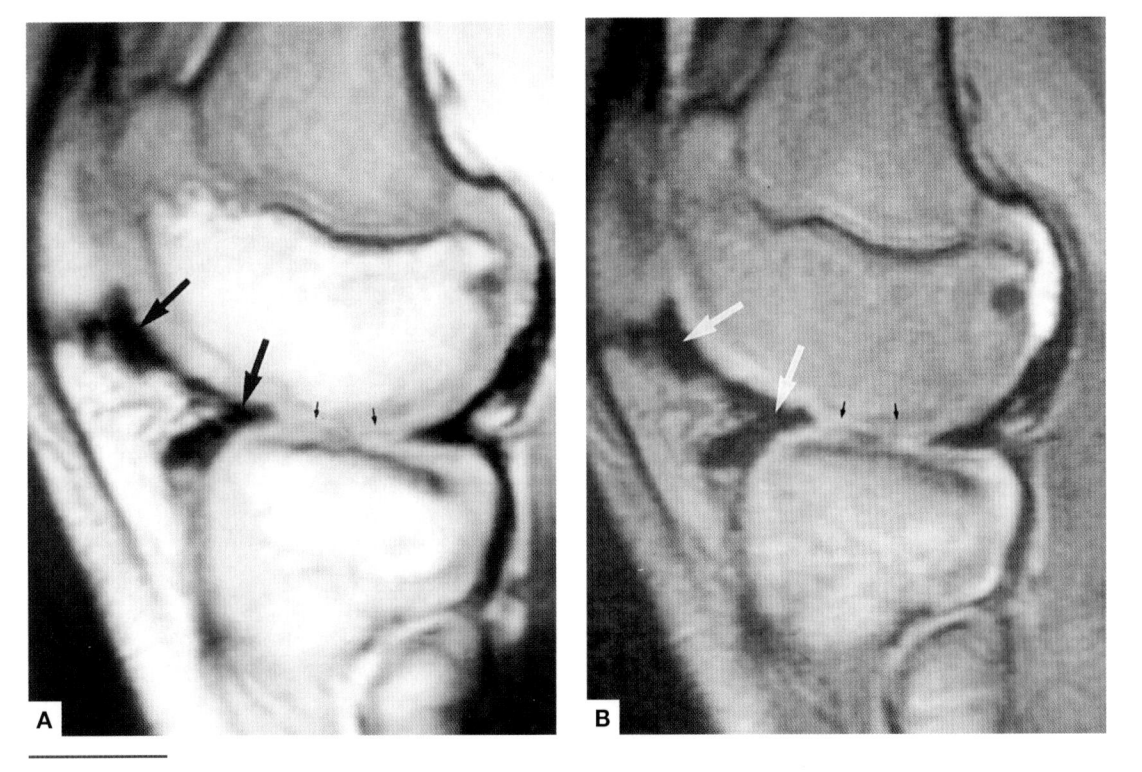

FIGURE 8.41 The knee of a patient with hemophilia showing early cartilage erosions (*small arrows*) and a thickened hemosiderin-laden synovium that demonstrates low signal intensity (*large arrows*) on (**A**) T1-weighted and (**B**) T2-weighted images. The irregularity of Hoffa's infrapatellar fat pad indicates synovial irritation. There is subchondral erosion in the posterior aspect of the lateral femoral condyle.

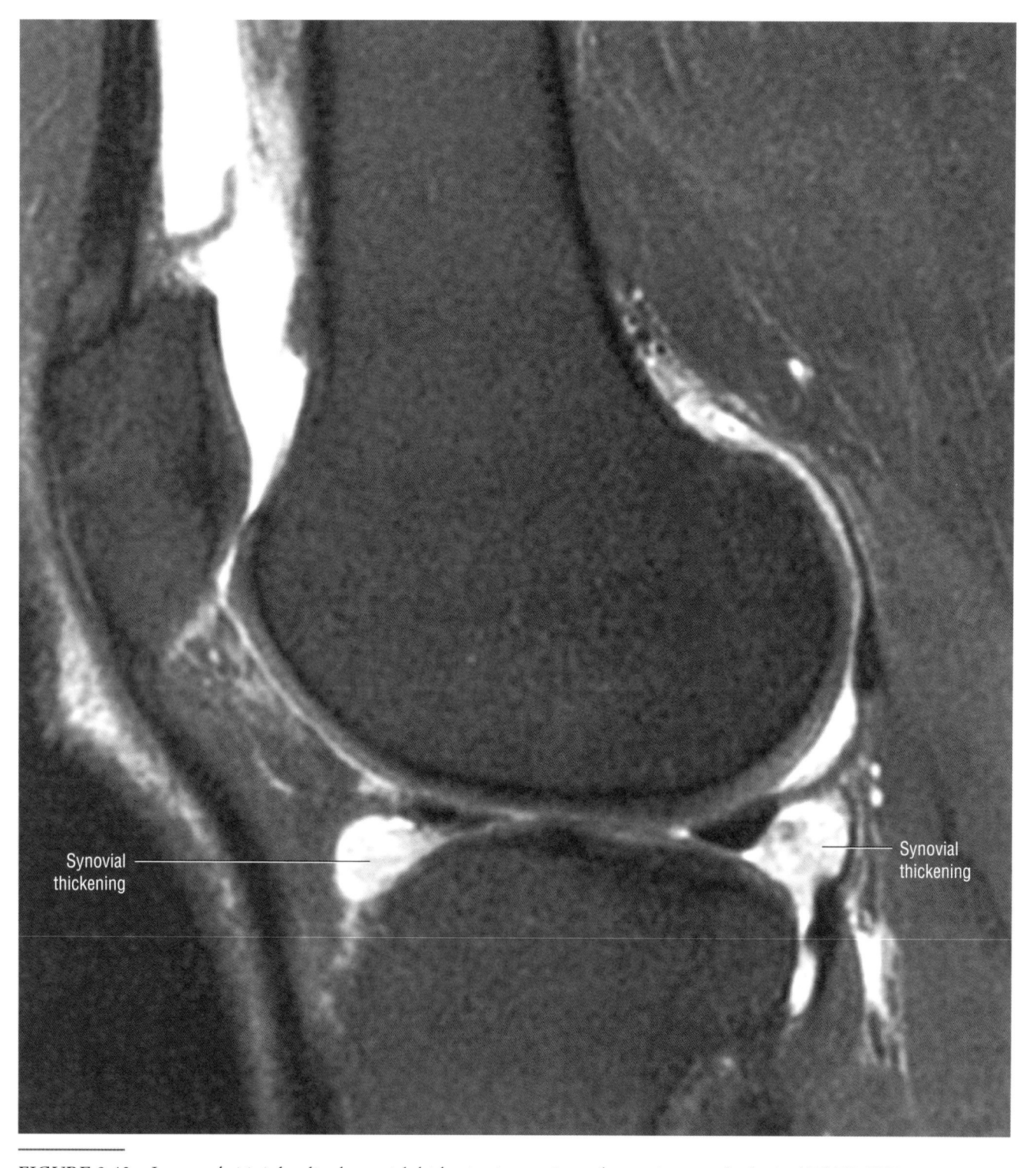

FIGURE 8.42 Lyme arthritis is localized synovial thickening in anterior and posterior capsule. Sagittal FS PD FSE image.

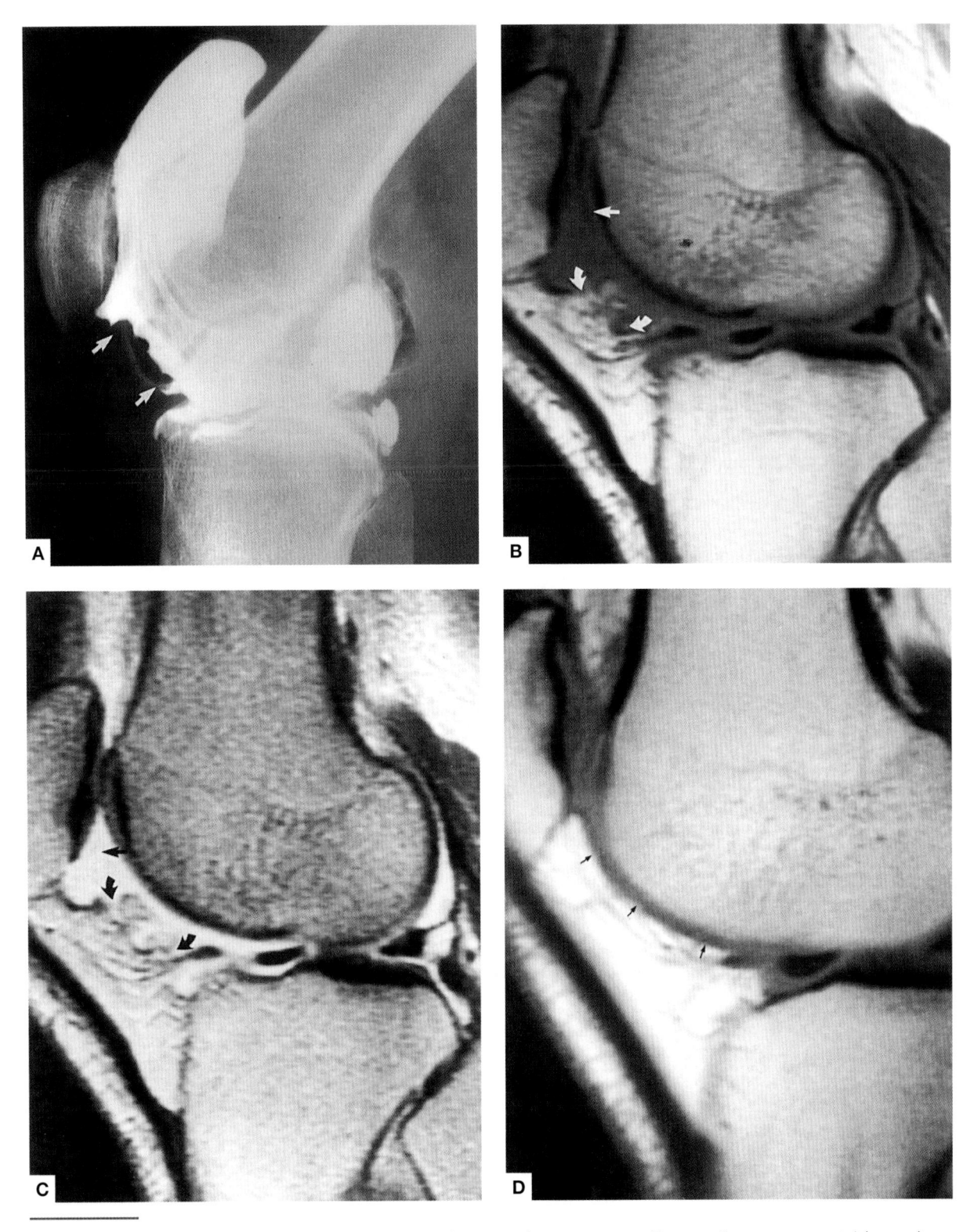

General Pathologic Conditions Affecting the Knee 895

FIGURE 8.43 Lyme arthritis. (**A**) A lateral-view arthrogram demonstrates scalloping of contrast material (*arrows*), indicating synovitis. (**B**) T1-weighted and (**C**) T2-weighted sagittal images show an irregular Hoffa's infrapatellar fat pad (*curved arrows*) with interdigitation of synovial effusion (*straight arrows*). Joint effusion is bright on the T2-weighted image. (**D**) On an intermediate-weighted sagittal image in the same patient, the asymptomatic knee displays the normal concave contour of the free edge of Hoffa's infrapatellar fat pad (*arrows*).

MCL Sprain

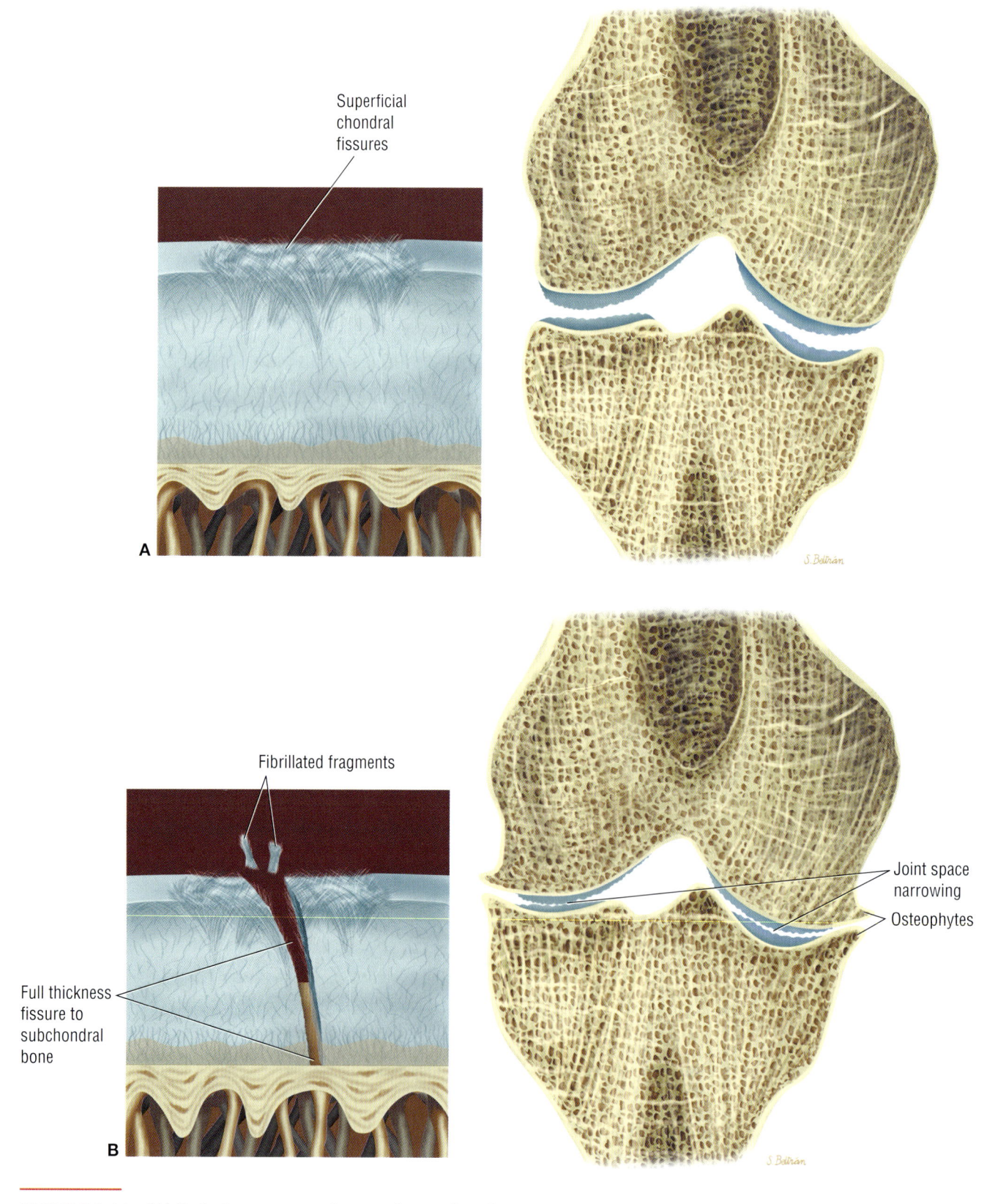

FIGURE 8.44 (**A**) Early degenerative arthritis with superficial fissures of the articular cartilage. (**B**) Progression to more advanced degenerative arthrosis. Chondral fissures extending down to the subchondral bone, release of fibrillated cartilage debris, joint space narrowing, subchondral sclerosis, and osteophyte formation are seen. (*Continued*)

Osteoarthritis

Key Concepts

- Process of osteoarthritis begins as fatigue fracture of collagen meshwork followed by increased hydration of articular cartilage, as opposed to the desiccated cartilage seen with aging.
- Irregular fat-pad sign is associated with inflammatory component to osteoarthritis process.

Osteoarthritis

- Primary osteoarthritis: gradual process of destruction and regeneration resulting from chronic microtrauma
- Secondary osteoarthritis: noninflammatory degenerative joint disease resulting from predisposing events such as trauma, congenital deformity, infection, or metabolic disorder
- Loss of articular cartilage, associated new bone formation and capsular fibrosis
- Pathology of early osteoarthritis
    - Increase in volume of the damaged cartilage as it swells
    - Related to decrease in tensile properties of collagen network, which usually resists swelling pressure generated by osmotic properties of proteoglycans
    - Marked by decreased amounts of aggrecan and release of proteoglycan fragments into synovial fluid
    - Changes in matrix macromolecules result in increased synthesis of cartilage oligomeric matrix protein (COMP) and cartilage intermediate layer protein (CILP) in deeper layers of articular cartilage.
    - Surface degradation may be result of deterioration of molecules linking collagen fibrils.
    - Mechanically impaired collagen network is susceptible to surface disruption during mechanical loading.

MR Findings of Osteoarthritis

- Vary from osteophytic spurring to compartment collapse, denuded articular cartilage, torn and degenerative meniscal fibrocartilage, and diminished marrow signal intensity in areas of subchondral sclerosis[252,285]

- Regions of bone remodeling are associated with degenerative articular cartilage and represent subchondral sclerosis, subchondral cystic cavities (with myxoid, fibrous, or cartilaginous tissue), regenerative cartilage, and new layers of bone formation.[49]

- MR can accurately assess articular cartilage[45]
    - Preoperative planning for joint replacement procedures, especially in unicondylar arthroplasties
    - Posterior-to-anterior bent-knee standing radiograph of both knees still allows accurate assessment of remaining articular cartilage in tibiofemoral compartments.[405]

- Chondral fragments (intermediate signal intensity) and loose bodies (high signal intensity of marrow fat) may be associated with more advanced degenerative disease.
    - Central knee osteophytes are associated with high-grade to full thickness chondral erosions.[311]
    - Exclusive use of FS-type sequences may result in confusion between areas of fat and marrow-containing loose bodies
    - Fatty marrow contrast of osteochondral fragments is decreased on T2*-weighted, FS PD-weighted FSE, and STIR images.

- Tibiofibular joint may also be affected by degenerative arthrosis, ganglia, or trauma.

- *Synovial chondromatosis*
    - Multiple synovium-based chondral fragments with low to intermediate signal intensity
    - Osseous fragments may be sclerotic (hypointense) with intermediate signal properties of cartilage.
    - Primary chondromatosis: fragments of similar size
    - Secondary chondromatosis: fragments vary in size

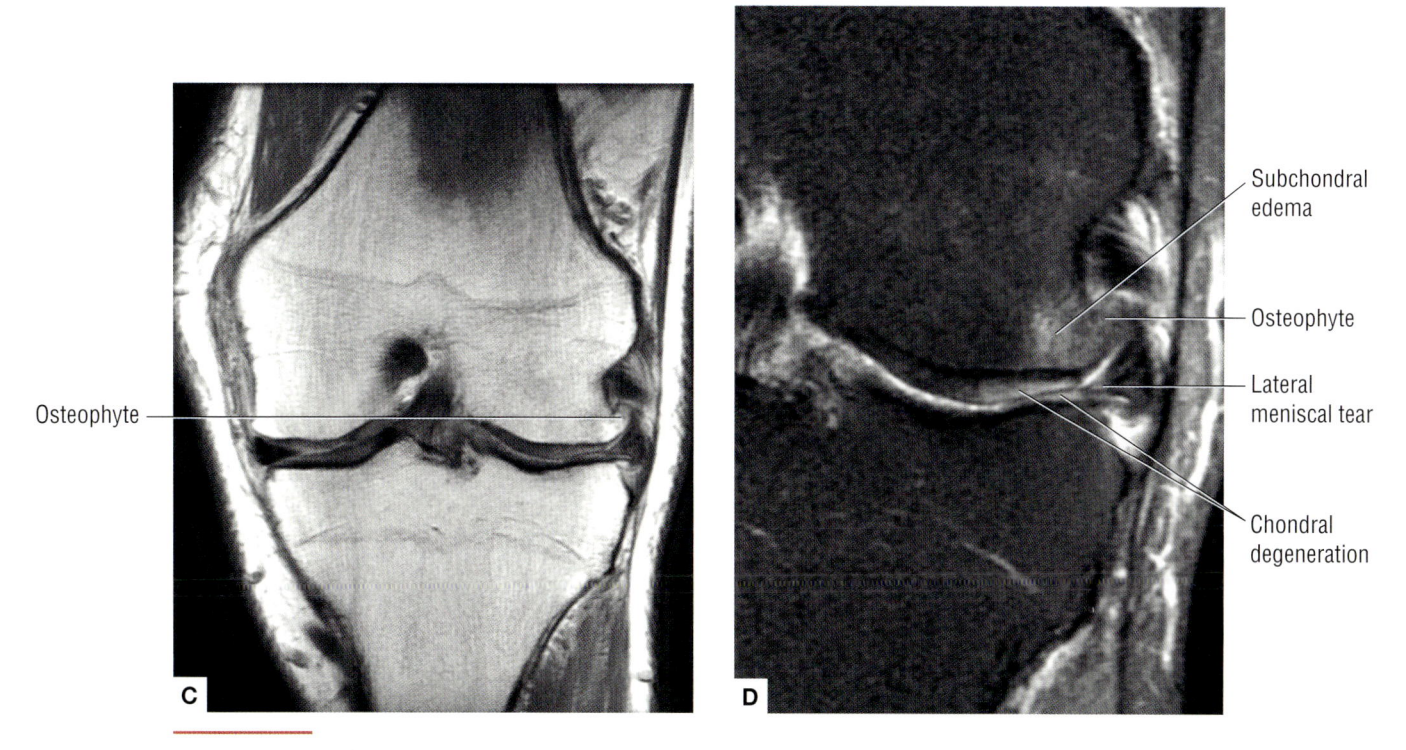

FIGURE 8.44 *(Continued)* **(C)** Coronal T1-weighted FSE image showing joint space narrowing and osteophytic spurring of the lateral compartment. **(D)** Chondral loss and degeneration are more accurately depicted on this coronal FS PD FSE image.

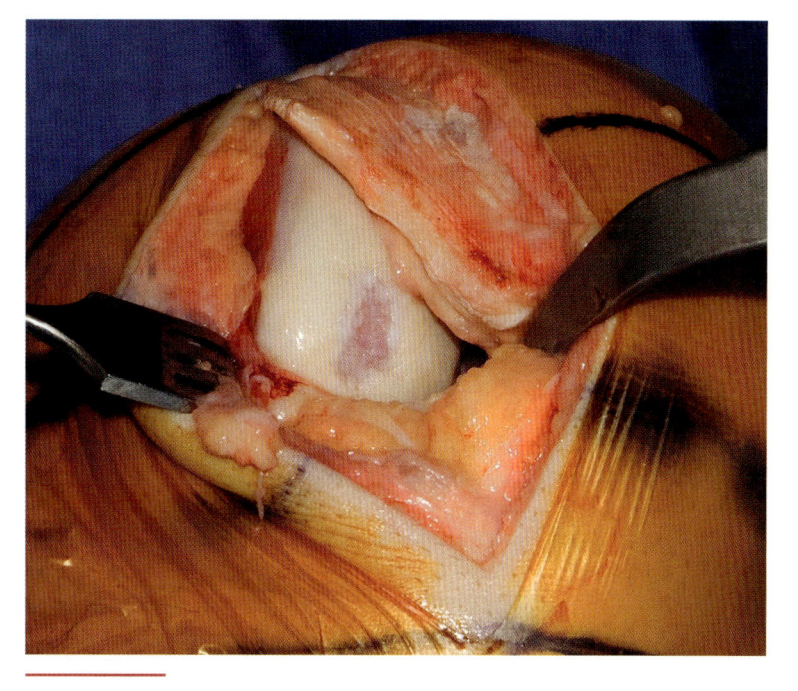

FIGURE 8.45 Lateral femoral condyle chondral degeneration exposed using a lateral peripatellar arthrotomy. (Reprinted from Fu FH. *Master Techniques in Orthopaedic Surgery: Sports Medicine.* Philadelphia, PA: Lippincott Williams & Wilkins; 2010, with permission.)

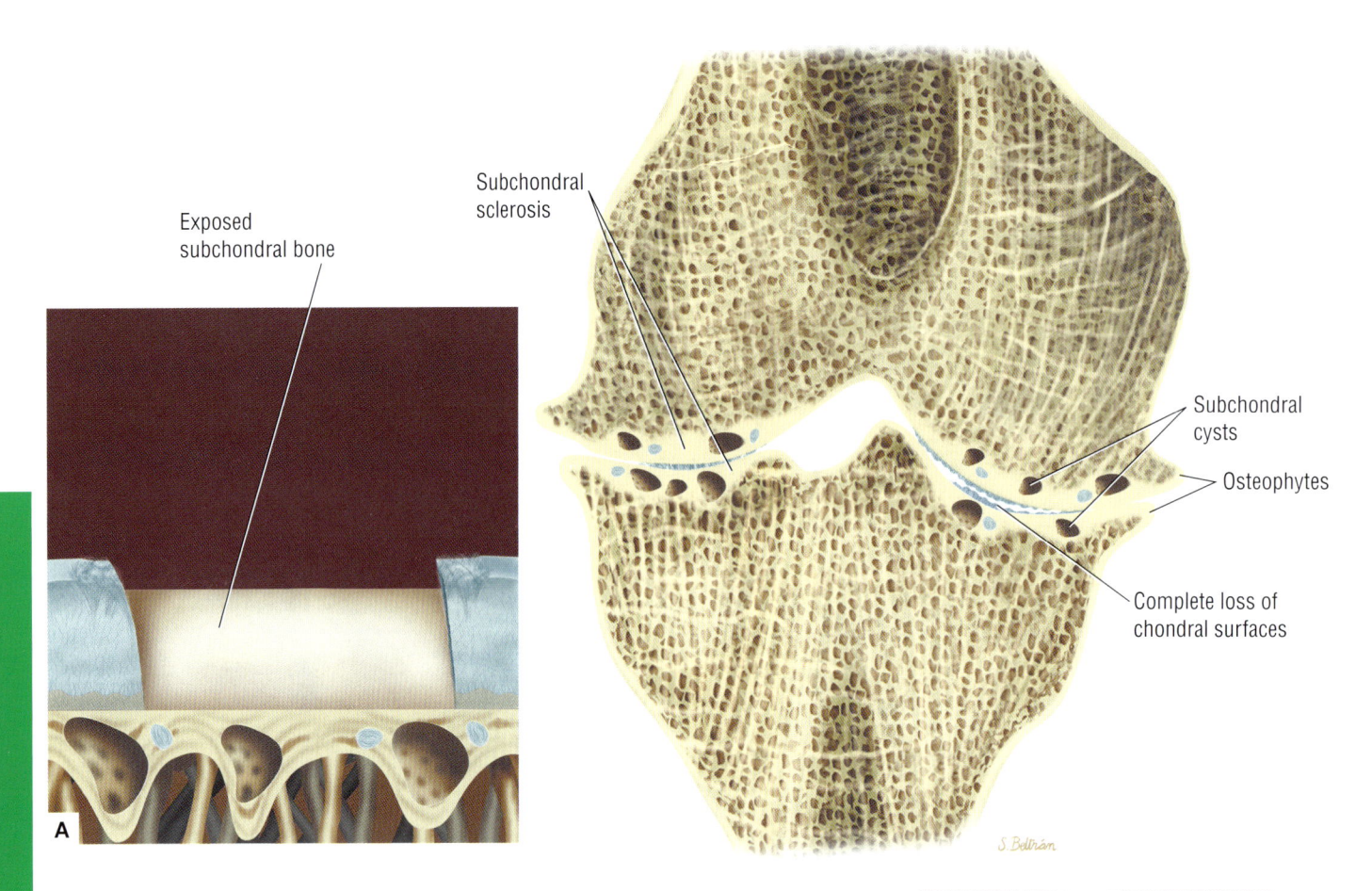

FIGURE 8.46 (**A**) End-stage degenerative arthritis (osteoarthrosis) with full thickness erosions and exposure of subchondral bone. Subchondral sclerosis, cysts, loss of joint space, and osteophytes occur at this stage. (**B**) Degenerative osteoarthritis as seen on a T1-weighted sagittal image with multiple marrow fat-containing suprapatellar loose bodies (*small straight arrows*), joint effusion, osteophytosis (*small curved arrow*), joint space narrowing, loss of lateral compartment articular cartilage, a torn lateral meniscus (*large curved arrow*), subchondral sclerosis and edema (*large straight arrow*), and patellofemoral involvement. Inflammatory osteoarthritis is seen with synovitis and an irregular fat-pad sign.

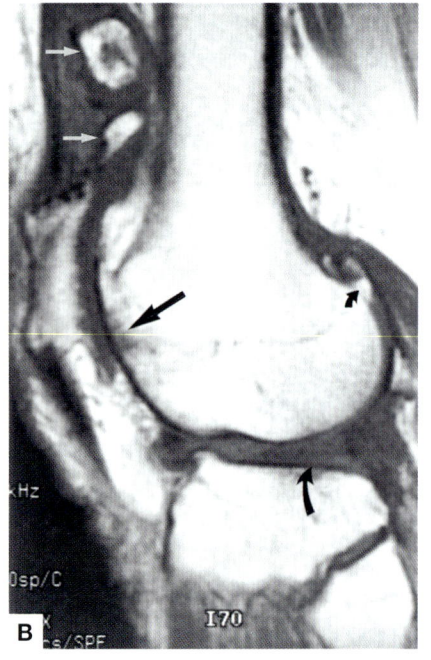

General Pathologic Conditions Affecting the Knee 901

Loose body (chondral fragment)

Chondral loose body

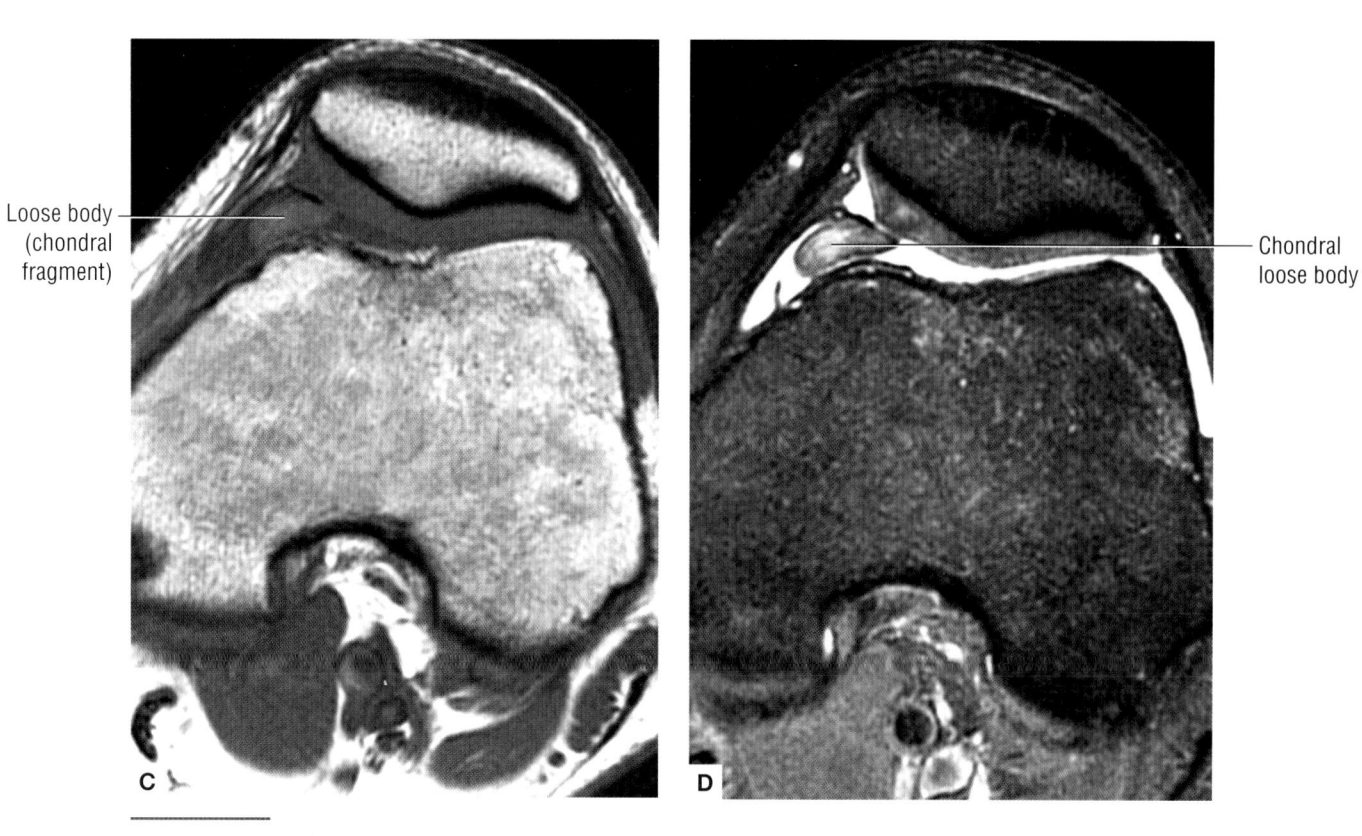

FIGURE 8.46 *(Continued)* (**C, D**) Medial suprapatellar bursa non-marrow fat-containing chondral fragment shown in a separate case. Both chondral and osteochondral loose bodies may be identified in degenerative osteoarthritis. (**C**) Axial T1-weighted FSE. (**D**) Axial FS PD FSE.

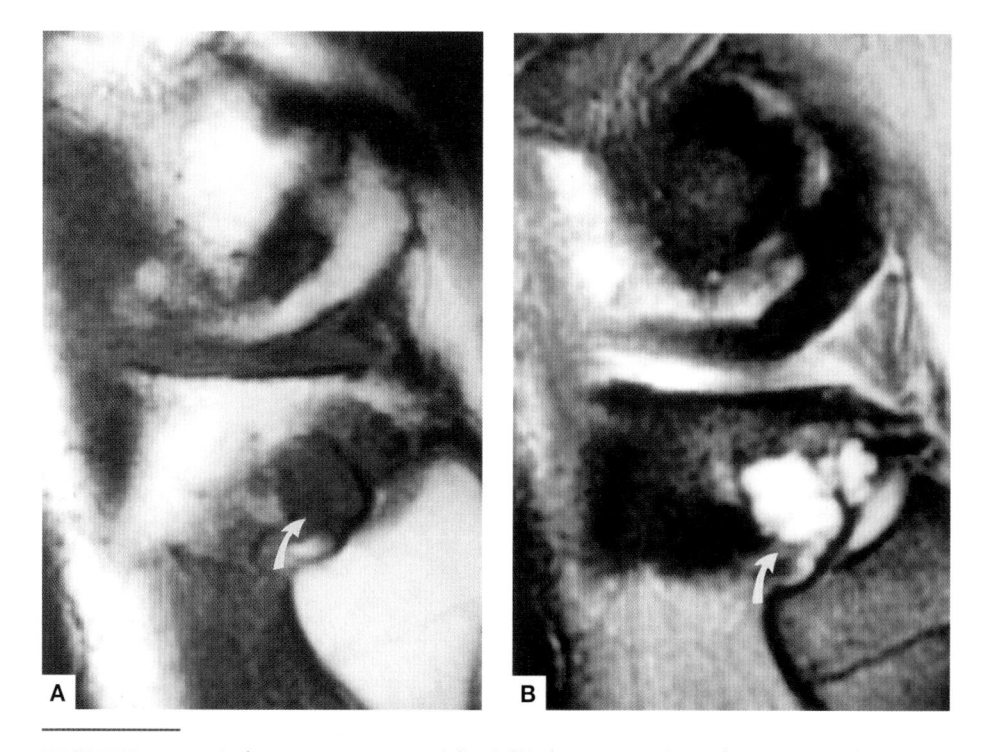

FIGURE 8.47 A degenerative synovial fluid-filled extraneural cyst (*curved arrows*) of the superior tibiofibular joint demonstrates (**A**) low signal intensity on a T1-weighted image and (**B**) high signal intensity on a T2*-weighted image. The lateral meniscus is completely absent, and there is associated joint space narrowing.

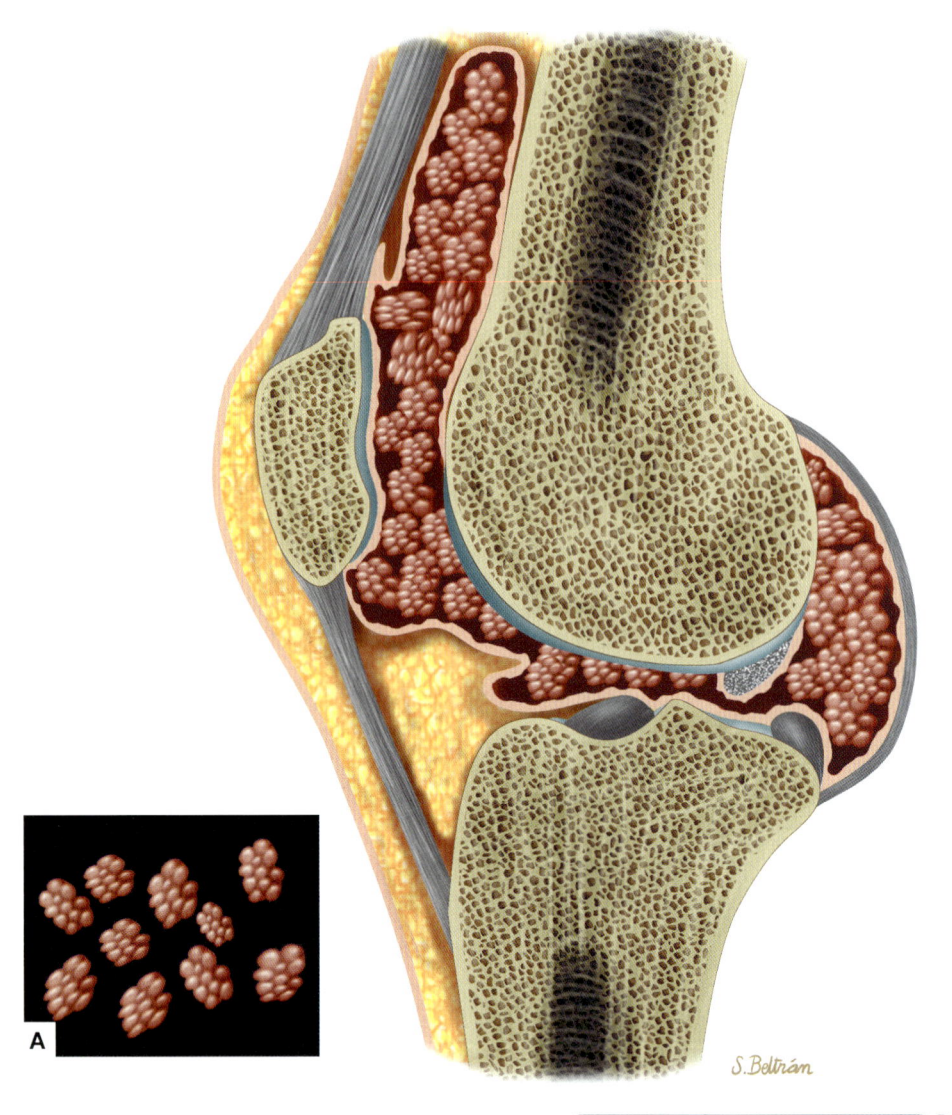

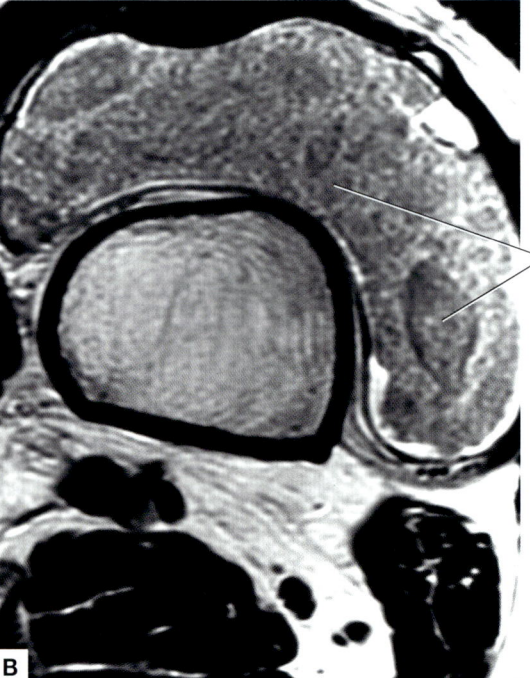

FIGURE 8.48 (**A**) Sagittal color illustration with inset of synovial chondromatosis derived from synovial metaplasia producing multiple chondromas in contact with and receiving nutrients from the joint capsule synovial lining. (**B**) Axial T2-weighted FSE image demonstrating hypertrophic synovium and multiple chondral fragments. In contrast to synovial chondromatosis, degenerative arthritis would typically present with fewer intraarticular loose bodies.

General Pathologic Conditions Affecting the Knee

FIGURE 8.49 Synovial chondromatosis may also present with numerous osseous bodies and is also referred to as osteochondromatosis. Sagittal PD FSE (**A**) and FS PD FSE (**B**) images.

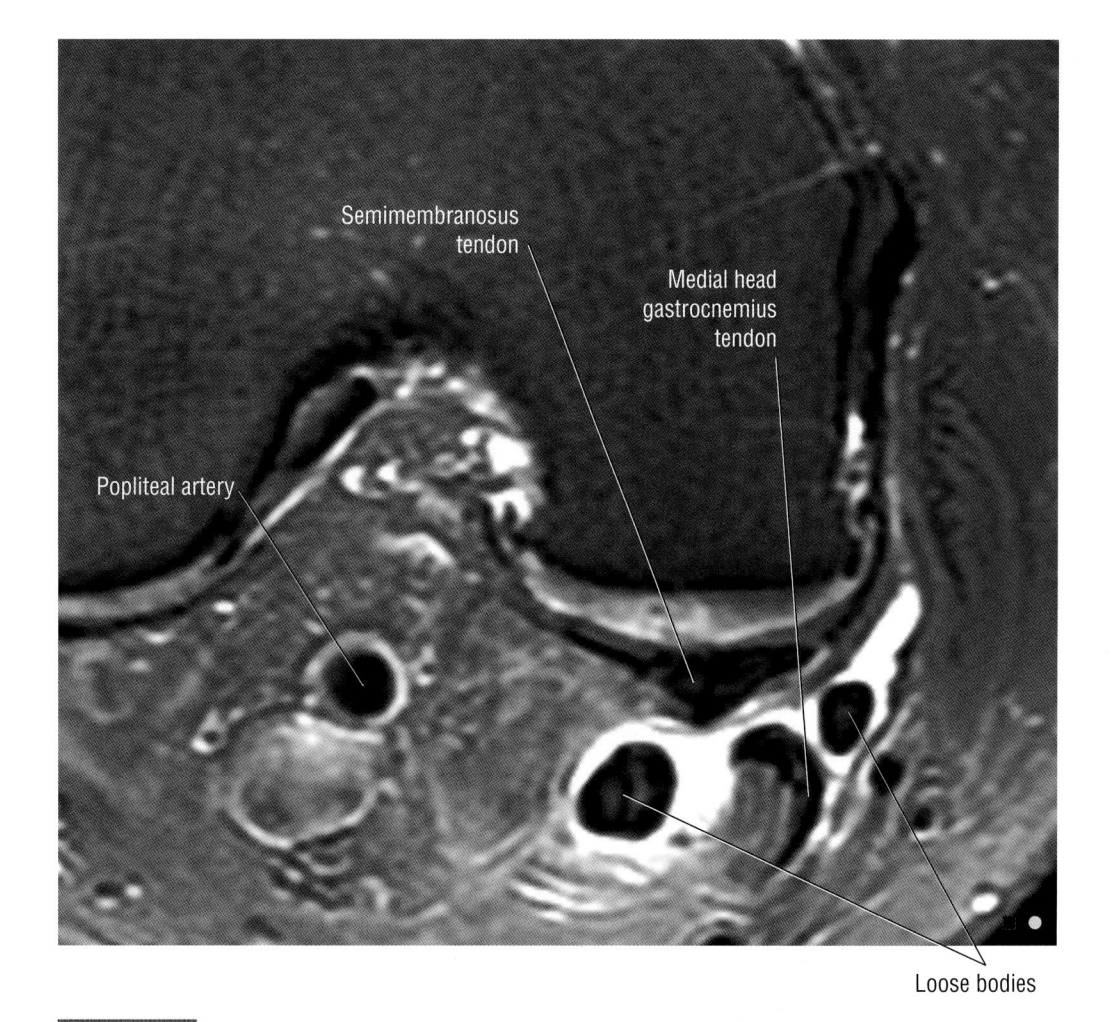

FIGURE 8.50 Loose bodies in a medial popliteal cyst. Axial FS PD FSE image.

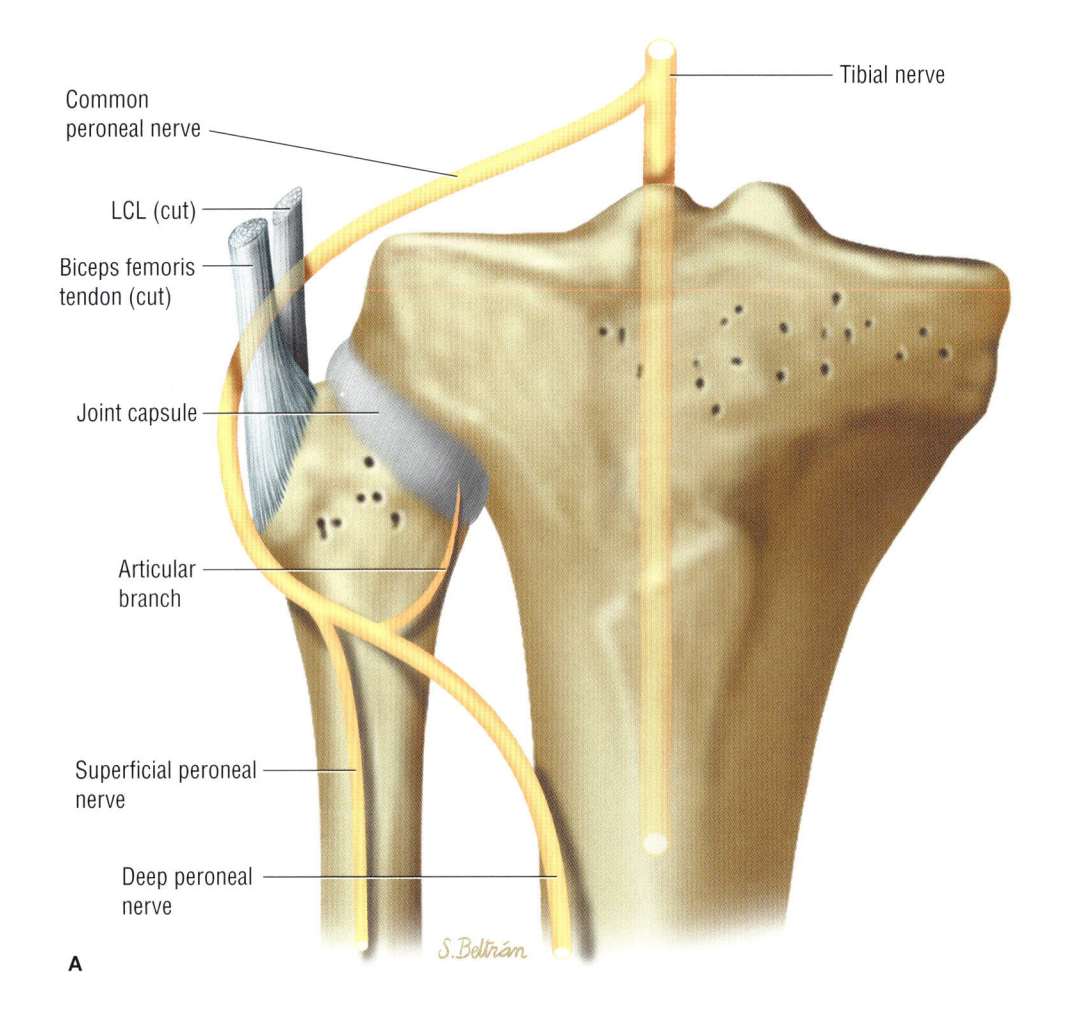

FIGURE 8.51 (**A**) Common peroneal nerve and its anterior branches, which include the articular branch (anterior to the tibiofibular joint), the superficial branch, and the deep branch. The common peroneal nerve separates from the sciatic nerve in the upper popliteal fossa. (**B**) A sagittal FS PD FSE image showing the normal anterior inferior course of the common peroneal nerve posterior to the fibular head. The articular branch of the common peroneal nerve is the conduit for the intraneural dissection (involving the epineurium) of fluid across a capsular defect into the superior tibiofibular joint. Extraneural ganglion at the anterior aspect of the tibiofibular joint does not follow the course of the common peroneal nerve. LCL, lateral collateral ligament.

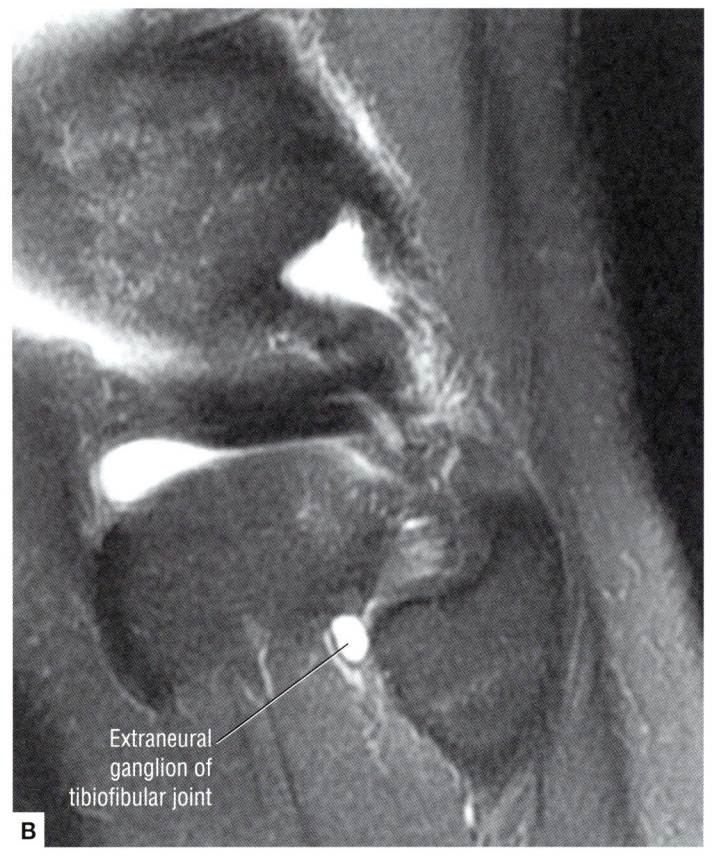

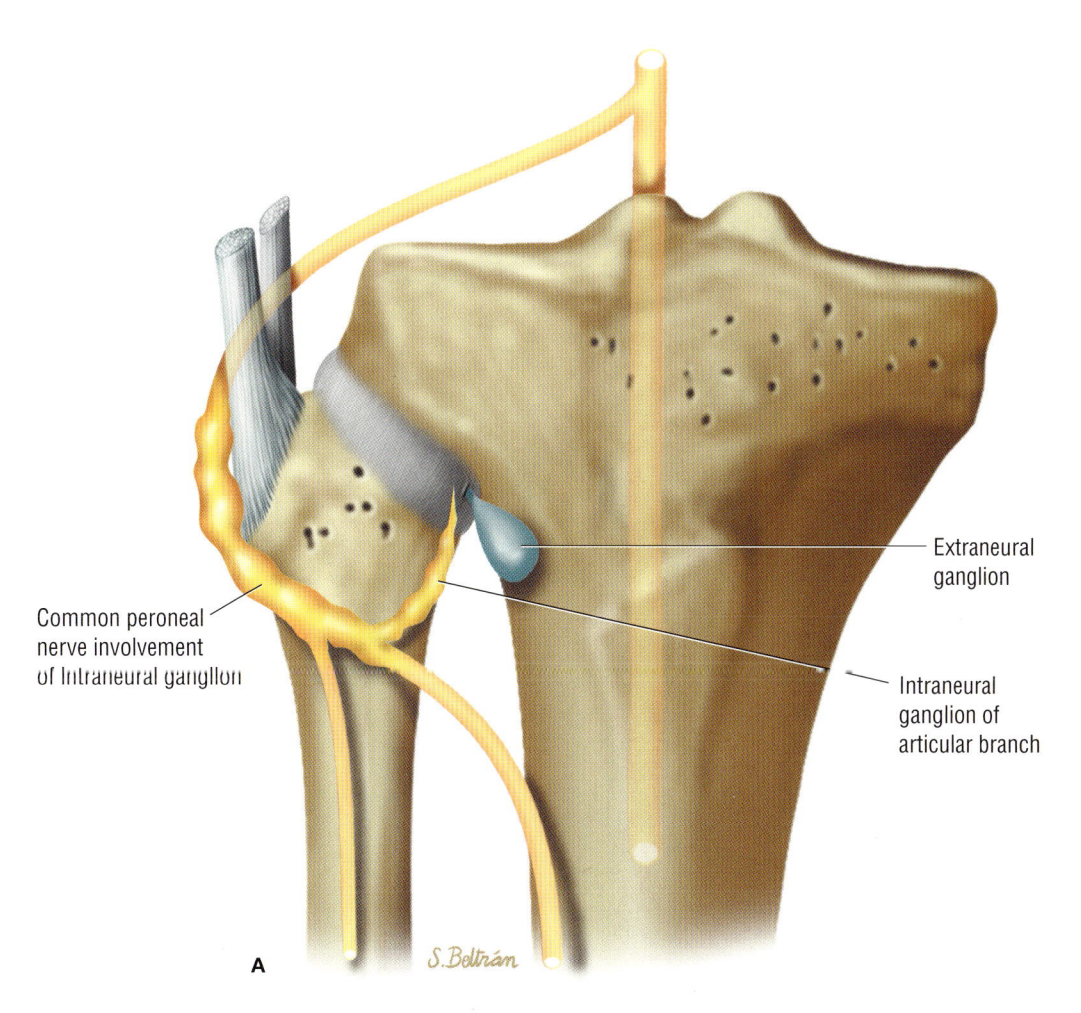

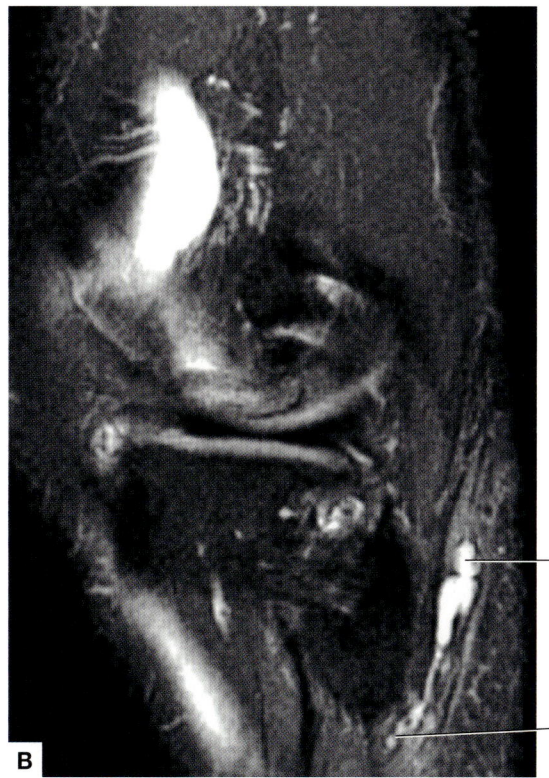

FIGURE 8.52 **(A)** Intraneural ganglion (*yellow*) involving the articular branch of the common peroneal nerve. There is associated proximal dissection of the ganglion through the epineurium to involve the deep peroneal nerve and distal common peroneal nerve proper. A separate extraneural ganglion (*blue*) shows direct superior tibiofibular joint communication without neural involvement. **(B)** Articular branch and proximal common peroneal nerve involvement from the proximal dissection of an intraneural ganglion on a sagittal FS PD FSE image.

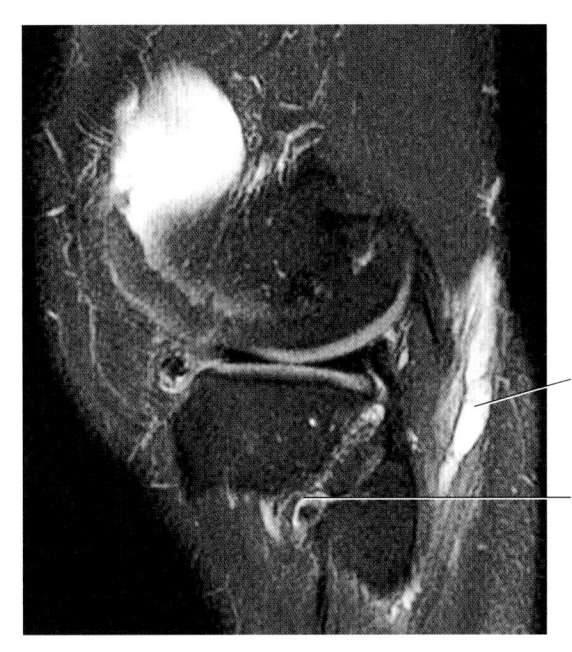

FIGURE 8.53 Sagittal FS PD FSE image of common peroneal nerve propagation of the intraneural ganglion toward the sciatic nerve.

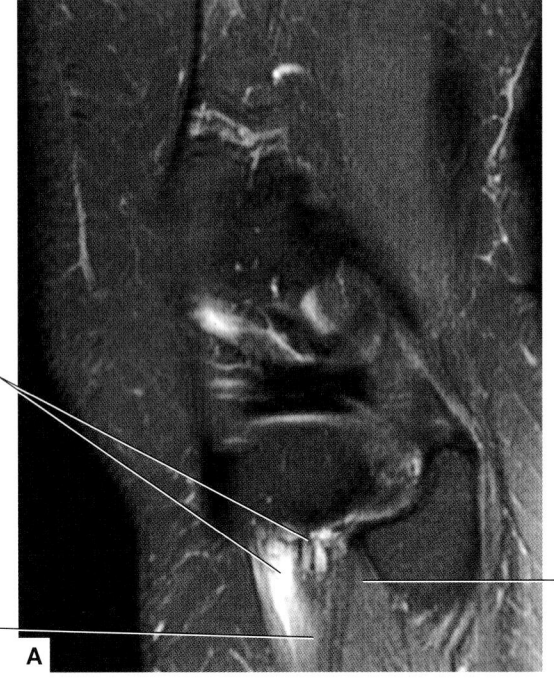

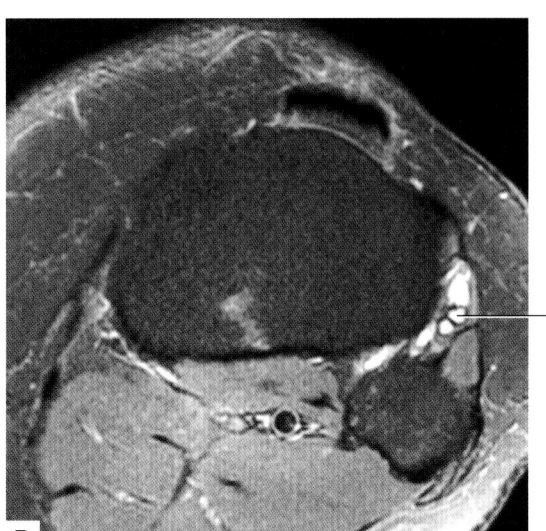

FIGURE 8.54 (**A**) Sagittal FS PD image and (**B**) axial FS PD image showing extraneural ganglion with anterior intramuscular extension. Direct communication with the superior tibiofibular joint is seen in the axial plane. The common peroneal nerve is unaffected.

Tibiofibular Joint Arthrosis and Ganglia

- Dislocation of proximal (superior) tibiofibular joint may occur with either indirect or direct trauma in athletic activities.

- Participation in sports that generate high torquing forces may result in an increased rate of degenerative change, especially in anterior third of the joint.

- Degenerative arthrosis of the tibiofibular joint is associated with hypointense subchondral sclerosis and hyperintense joint fluid.

- Spectrum of tibiofibular-related ganglia and relationship to the common peroneal nerve, described by Spinner et al.[457]

- Cysts or ganglia in proximity to proximal tibiofibular joint can be classified as intraneural, extraneural, or combined.

- Stage 0: cyst restricted to the tibiofibular joint without neural involvement; extraneural ganglia may produce symptoms secondary to extrinsic neural compression.

- Intraneural ganglia progress from the superior tibiofibular joint to:
    - Stage I: articular branch of the peroneal nerve
    - Stage II: deep peroneal nerve
    - Stage III: common peroneal nerve
    - Stage IV: sciatic nerve

- Articular branch of the peroneal nerve provides path or conduit for fluid dissection (from capsular defect) through the epineurium, producing a deep peroneal nerve deficit.

- Identify normal intermediate signal intensity of the common peroneal nerve. The nerve is posterolateral to the proximal fibula

- Classify ganglion as intraneural if the cystic area corresponds to the linear course of the common peroneal nerve through its articular branch.

- Classify the ganglion as extraneural if there is no relationship to the course of the articular branch or common peroneal nerve.

Lipoma Arborescens

Key Concepts

- Intraarticular fatty villonodular proliferation with well-vascularized fat covered by a uniform thickened cell lining
- T1-weighted sequences required to document fat signal
- FS PD FSE or STIR sequences used to demonstrate uniform fat suppression
- Fatty villonodular proliferation should not be mistaken for inflammatory synovitis.
- Rare intraarticular lesion consisting of villous lipomatous proliferation of the synovium
- Arthroscopy: numerous fatty-appearing globules and villous projections[35]

MR Findings of Lipoma Arborescens

- Large frond-like masses originating from the synovium
- Intraarticular masses with signal characteristics similar to fat in all pulse sequences[132]
- Joint effusions are common.
  - MR may demonstrate susceptibility artifact if there is recurrent hemarthrosis.
- MR useful in differentiating lipoma arborescens from other causes of chronically swollen and painful joint, including rheumatoid arthritis, PVNS, and synovial chondromatosis[35]
- Intraarticular hemangioma may be present with either local or diffuse presentation.
  - Diffuse variety may display series of vascular channels that are predominantly venous in origin.
  - Channels may result in low-signal-intensity penetrations within infrapatellar fat pad.[424]
- Compare T1 and FS PD FSE (fluid sensitive) images in the sagittal plane to document fatty villonodular composition

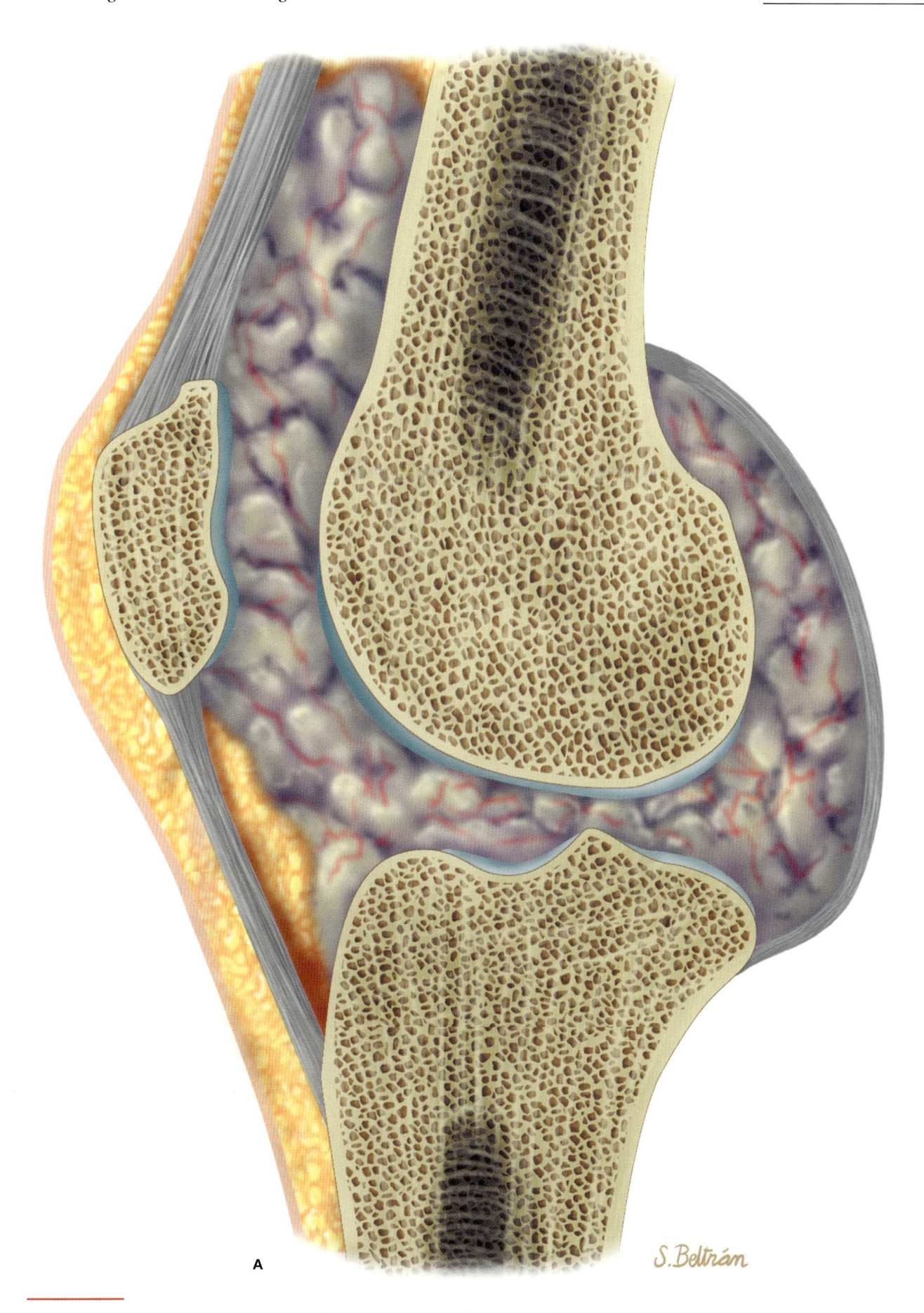

FIGURE 8.55 Lipoma arborescens or villous lipomatous proliferation of the synovium is a nonneoplastic condition. It may be associated with osteoarthritis, rheumatoid arthritis, psoriasis, or diabetes mellitus. **(A)** Color sagittal section. *(Continued)*

FIGURE 8.55 (*Continued*) (**B**) Sagittal PD FSE image. (**C**) Sagittal FS PD FSE image.

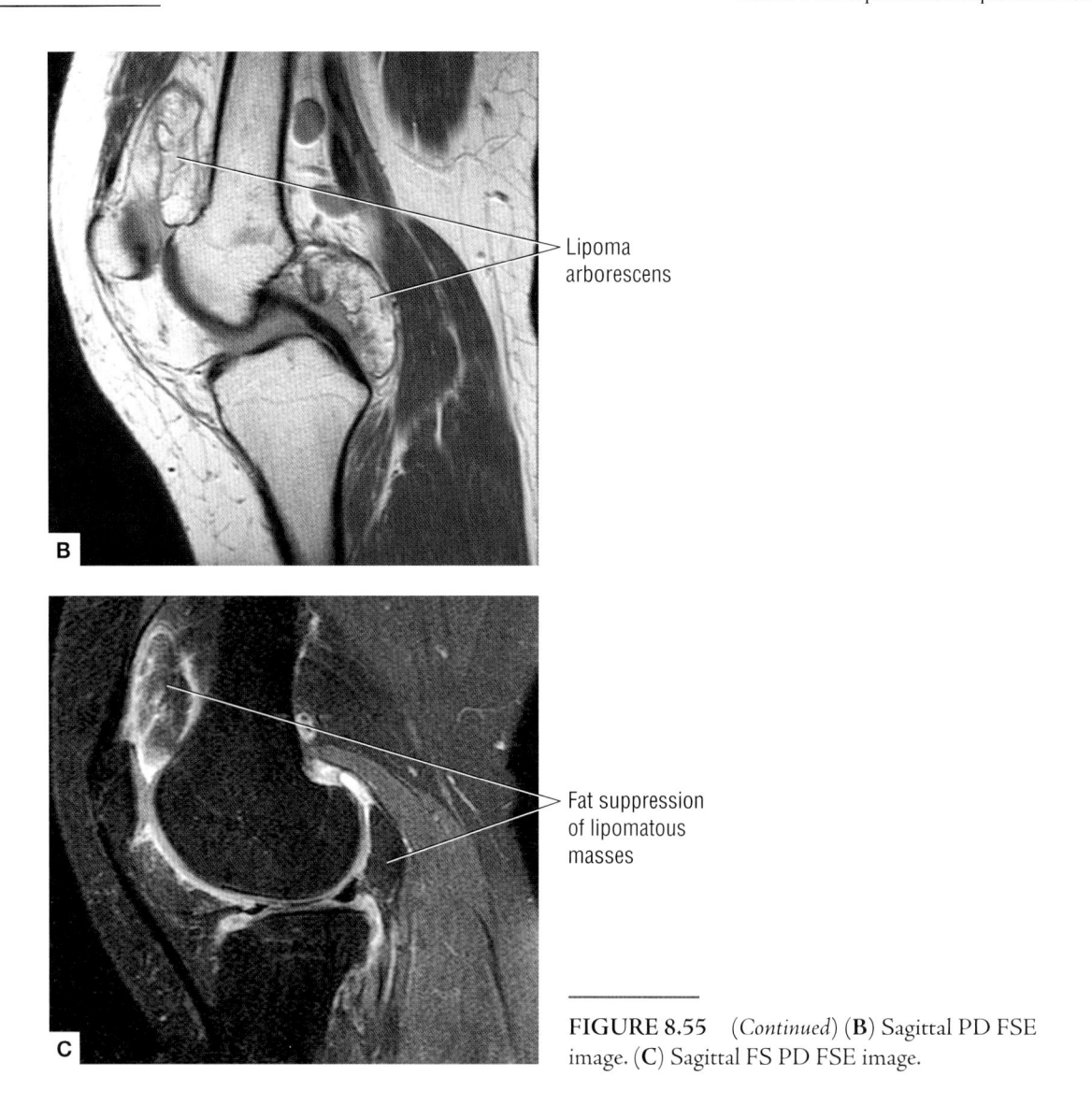

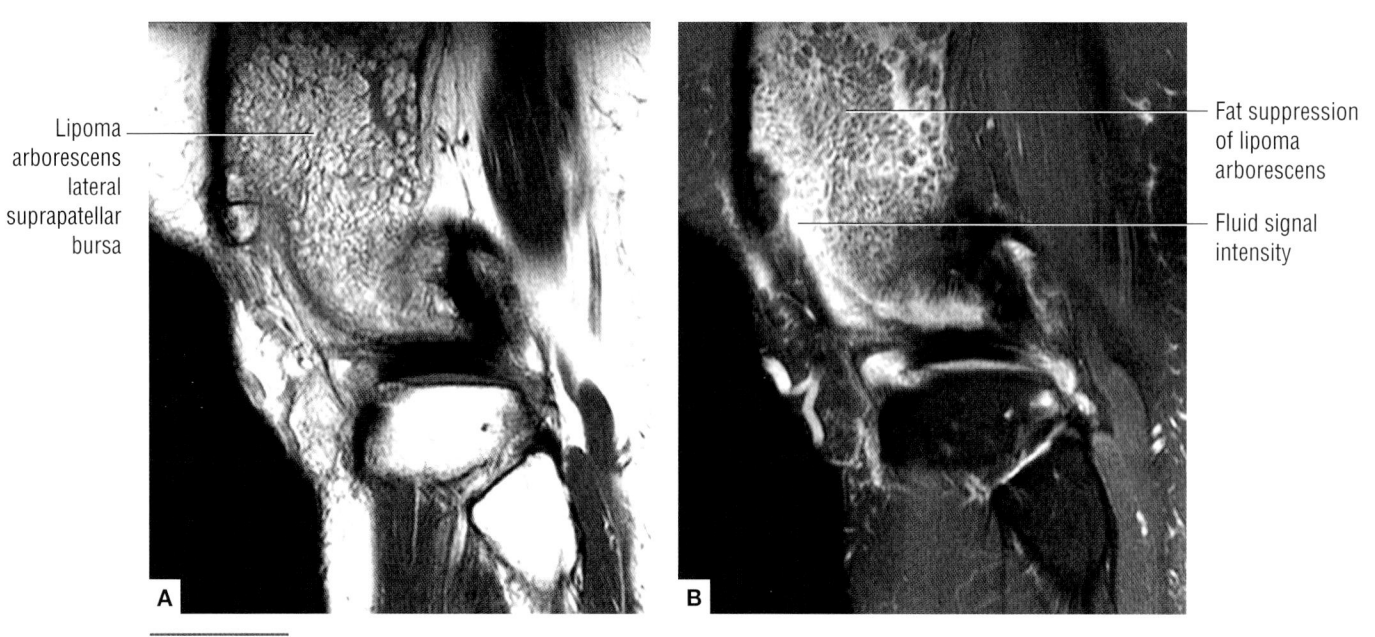

FIGURE 8.56 (**A**) Lipoma arborescens with intraarticular lipomatous tissue demonstrating high signal intensity on a PD FSE sagittal image. (**B**) The lesion is hypointense on this FS PD FSE sagittal sequence.

Joint Effusions

Key Concepts

- Modifying window level and width to the threshold of the constituents of a joint effusion increases MR sensitivity in evaluation of synovial disorders.

- Evaluate for contour irregularity of Hoffa's fat pad, indicative of synovitis.

Joint Effusions

- Characterized by low signal intensity on T1-weighted images and bright signal intensity on corresponding conventional T2, FS PD-weighted FSE, GRE T2*, and STIR images

- Fluid preferentially accumulates in suprapatellar recess and central portions of the joint in traumatized knee.[231]

- Layers of postaspiration fat–fluid, fluid–fluid, and air–fluid levels demonstrated in suprapatellar fluid collections
    - When MR is performed after arthrography, contrast can be seen coating articular cartilage and extending into the suprapatellar recess.

- On FS PD FSE images, fluid trapped between meniscal surfaces is seen with bright-signal-intensity interface (does not interfere with evaluation of the meniscal fibrocartilage)
    - As little as 1 mL of fluid can be detected within the joint on MR scans.
    - Normal knee contains 4 mL or less of synovial fluid.

MR Appearance of Joint Effusions

- Inflammation and infection usually associated with synovial thickening or hypertrophy, easily identified by modifying window level and width

- Quantitative mapping of synovial inflammation performed with IV contrast to enhance pannus

- On coronal images, distribution of fluid in the medial and lateral gutters extends into suprapatellar bursa, taking on a saddle-bag appearance.

- Hemorrhagic synovial fluid is associated with an irregular fat pad and may demonstrate a serum–sediment level in subacute hemorrhagic effusions.
- Fat–serum–sediment level in lipohemarthrosis often associated with severe bone contusion and fracture
- Low-signal-intensity artifacts may be seen after knee aspirations or secondary to MR arthrography.
- Arthrographic effect can be produced by intraarticular diffusion of gadolinium after IV injection.[119]
- Increased signal intensity can be seen within 10 minutes of contrast administration and immobilization of the knee.
- Peaks within 30 minutes
- Technique can be used to improve identification of meniscal surfaces and various tear patterns.

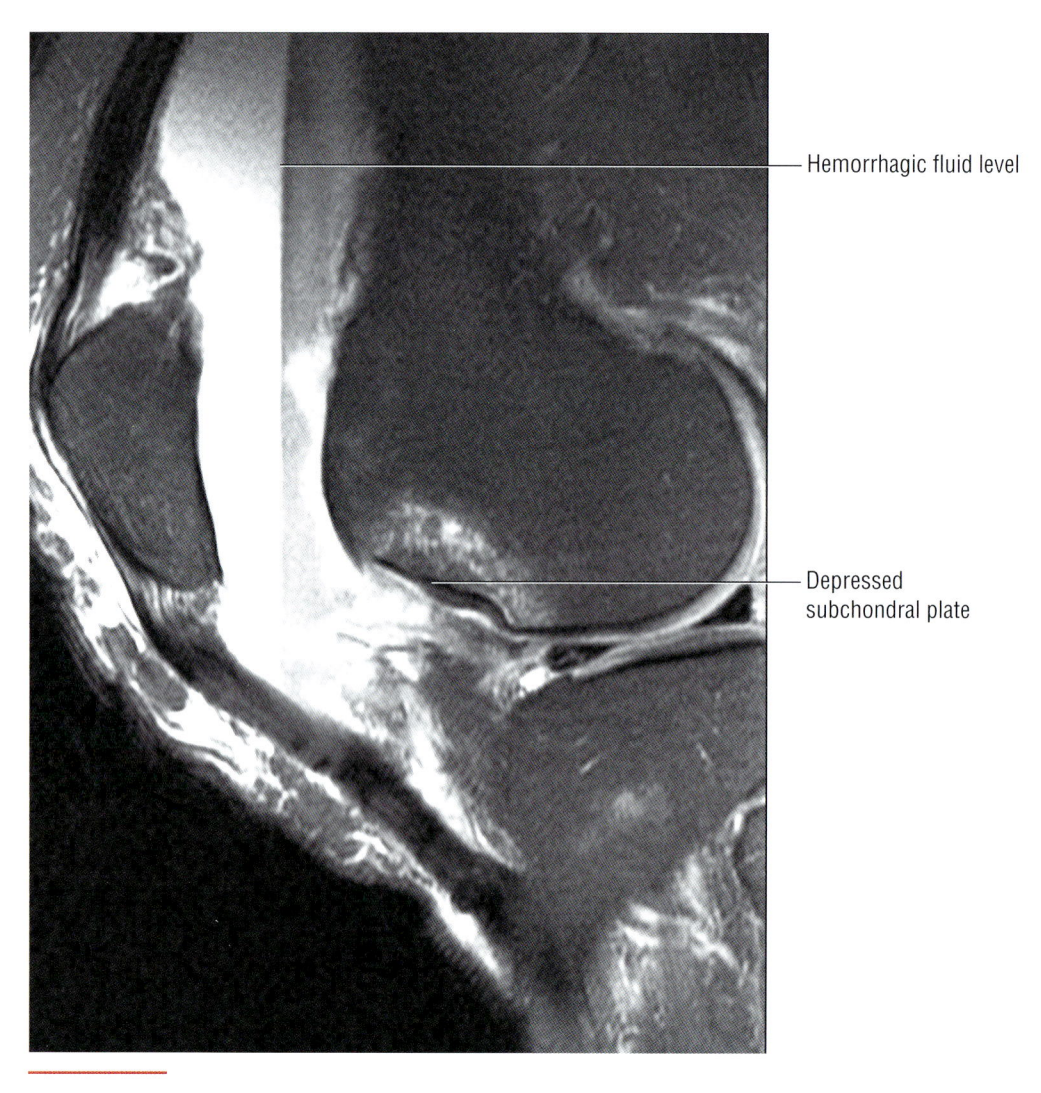

FIGURE 8.57 Layering of serum–sediment in hemarthrosis associated with impaction fracture of the lateral femoral condyle. Sagittal FS PD FSE image.

Popliteal and Atypical Cysts

Key Concepts

- Atypical popliteal cysts that are not adjacent to the semimembranosus or medial head of the gastrocnemius and cysts with nonuniform signal intensity require follow-up, including IV contrast, to exclude a soft tissue sarcoma.

- Hemorrhagic popliteal cyst demonstrates characteristic susceptibility of blood product degradation.

- It is important to appreciate that the articular branch of the common peroneal nerve serves as a conduit for superior (proximal) tibiofibular joint ganglia.

Popliteal and Atypical Cysts

- Classic popliteal cysts (also known as *Baker's cysts*)
    - Arise from the gastrocnemius–semimembranosus bursae between the medial head of the gastrocnemius muscle and the more medial semimembranosus tendon[173,284]
    - Demonstrate low signal intensity on T1-weighted images and uniformly increased signal intensity on T2-weighted images as well as FS PD-weighted FSE images[485]
    - Septations may be seen, usually in cysts that arise in atypical locations.
    - Narrow neck connecting cyst to joint usually identified on axial images, just below proximal attachment site of medial head of gastrocnemius
    - Axial images particularly useful in identifying relations of medial head of gastrocnemius muscle and semitendinosus and semimembranosus tendons
    - Popliteal cysts may arise from any condition that causes increase in synovial fluid within the joint.
        - Frequently seen in association with tears of the posterior horn of the medial meniscus
        - Intraarticular communication and associated pathology may be seen on contiguous sagittal images.
    - Hemorrhagic joint effusions with fluid–fluid level in the cyst
    - Loose bodies may collect in posterior popliteal cysts.

- Dissecting or ruptured popliteal cyst with subacute hemorrhage demonstrates increased signal intensity on T1-weighted and FS PD FSE images because of presence of blood.
    - Blood creates areas of inhomogeneity that may generate intermediate signal intensity.
    - Susceptibility artifact with areas of low signal intensity in subacute and chronic hemorrhage on GRE images
- Atypical locations for other cysts include tibiofibular joint (see discussion above) and bursa between the lateral head of gastrocnemius muscle and biceps femoris.
    - Tibiofibular cysts need to be classified as intraneural or extraneural.[457]
        - Intraneural cysts may produce a deep peroneal nerve deficit as the cyst preferentially dissects proximally within the epineurium of articular branch of deep peroneal nerve.
    - Cysts may also present as soft tissue masses proximal and distal to popliteal fossa.
- In very young children, popliteal cysts may occur as primary disorder in absence of concurrent intraarticular pathology.[122]
- Cysts are frequently seen in patients with juvenile chronic arthritis or adult rheumatoid arthritis.

MR Evaluation of Popliteal and Atypical Cysts

- MR evaluation useful for differentiating cyst from popliteal artery aneurysm and venous malformation, which may have a similar clinical appearance
    - Cystic adventitial disease of popliteal artery, which may present as popliteal fossa soft tissue mass, is well displayed on MR images.
    - Multiple cystic masses can be seen arising from wall of popliteal artery.[372]
    - Popliteal artery entrapment syndrome may be associated with anomalous structures that may be mistaken for posterior popliteal fossa masses.
    - Frequently, popliteal cysts show peripheral or wall enhancement, which is a normal finding.

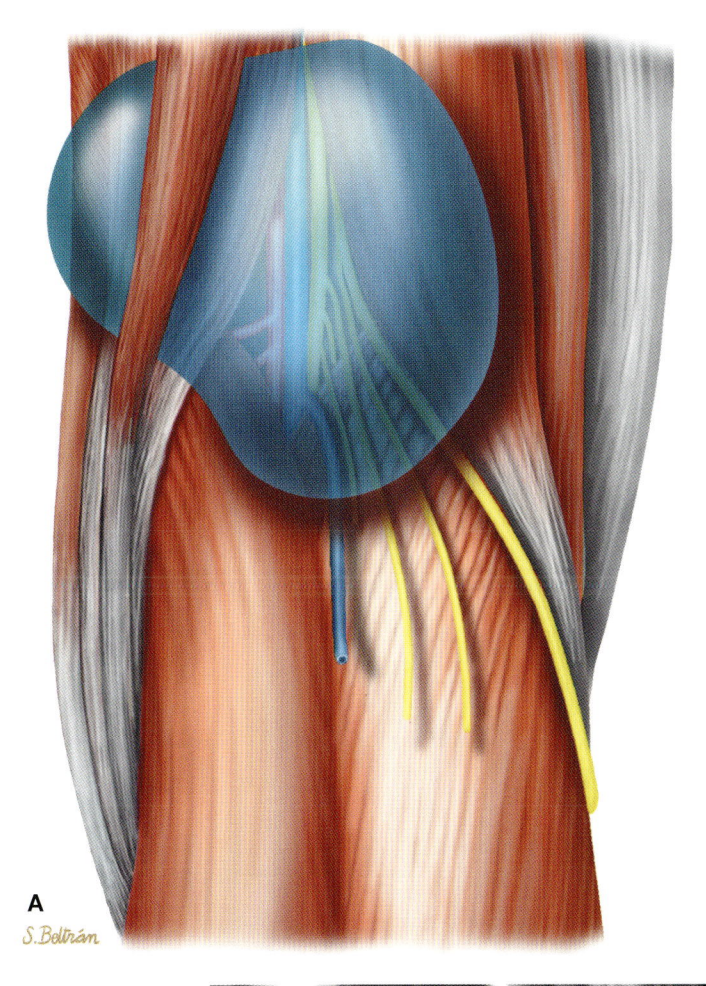

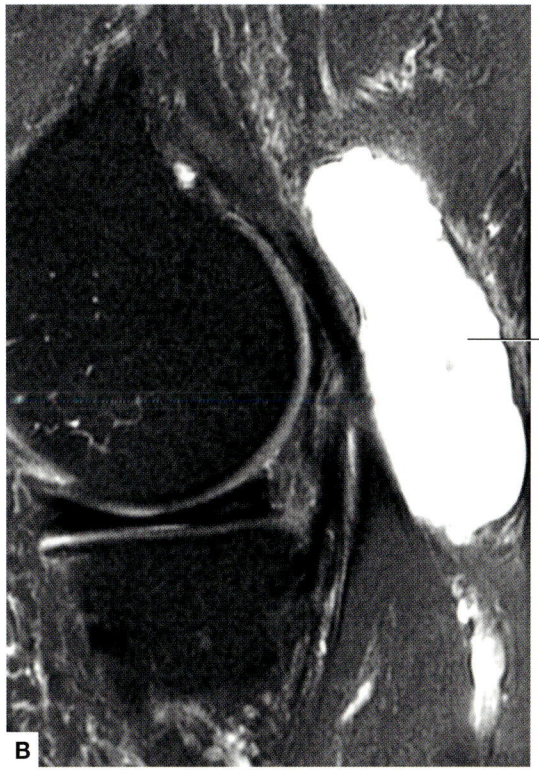

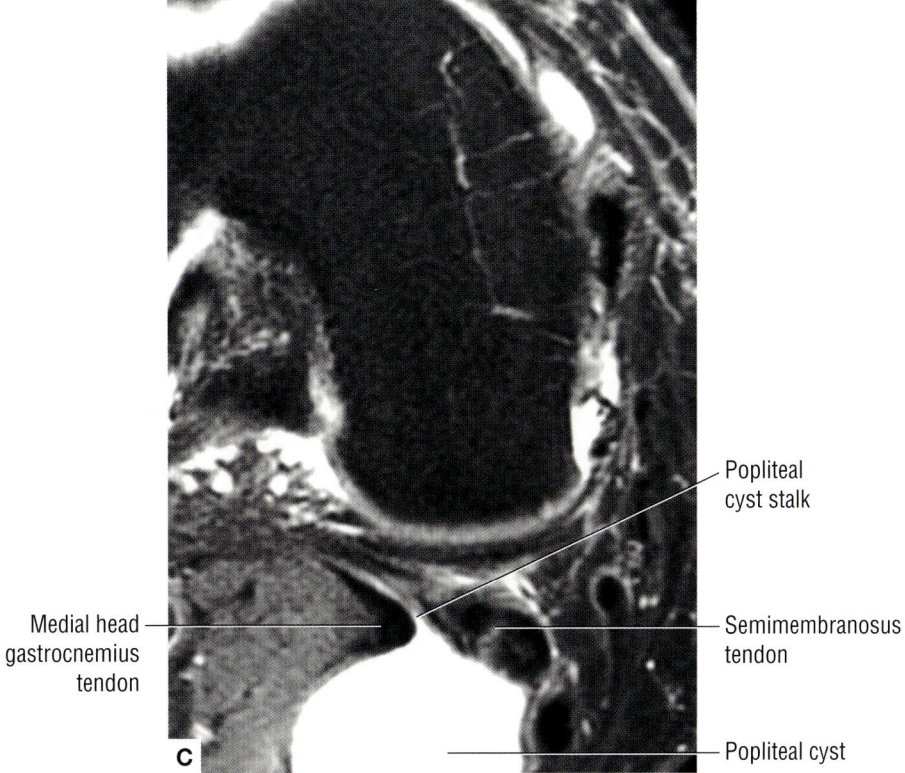

General Pathologic Conditions Affecting the Knee

FIGURE 8.58 (**A**) Popliteal cysts are either primary or secondary to intraarticular pathology. Their characteristic location is adjacent to the semimembranosus or medial head of the gastrocnemius. If the cyst is located in an atypical location or cannot be aspirated, further evaluation including intravenous contrast is recommended to exclude a soft tissue sarcoma. A typical medial popliteal cyst adjacent to the medial head of the gastrocnemius displays hyperintense signal on sagittal (**B**) and axial (**C**) FS PD FSE images. The stalk communicating with the joint and passing between the medial head of the gastrocnemius tendon and the semimembranosus tendon is appreciated on the axial image.

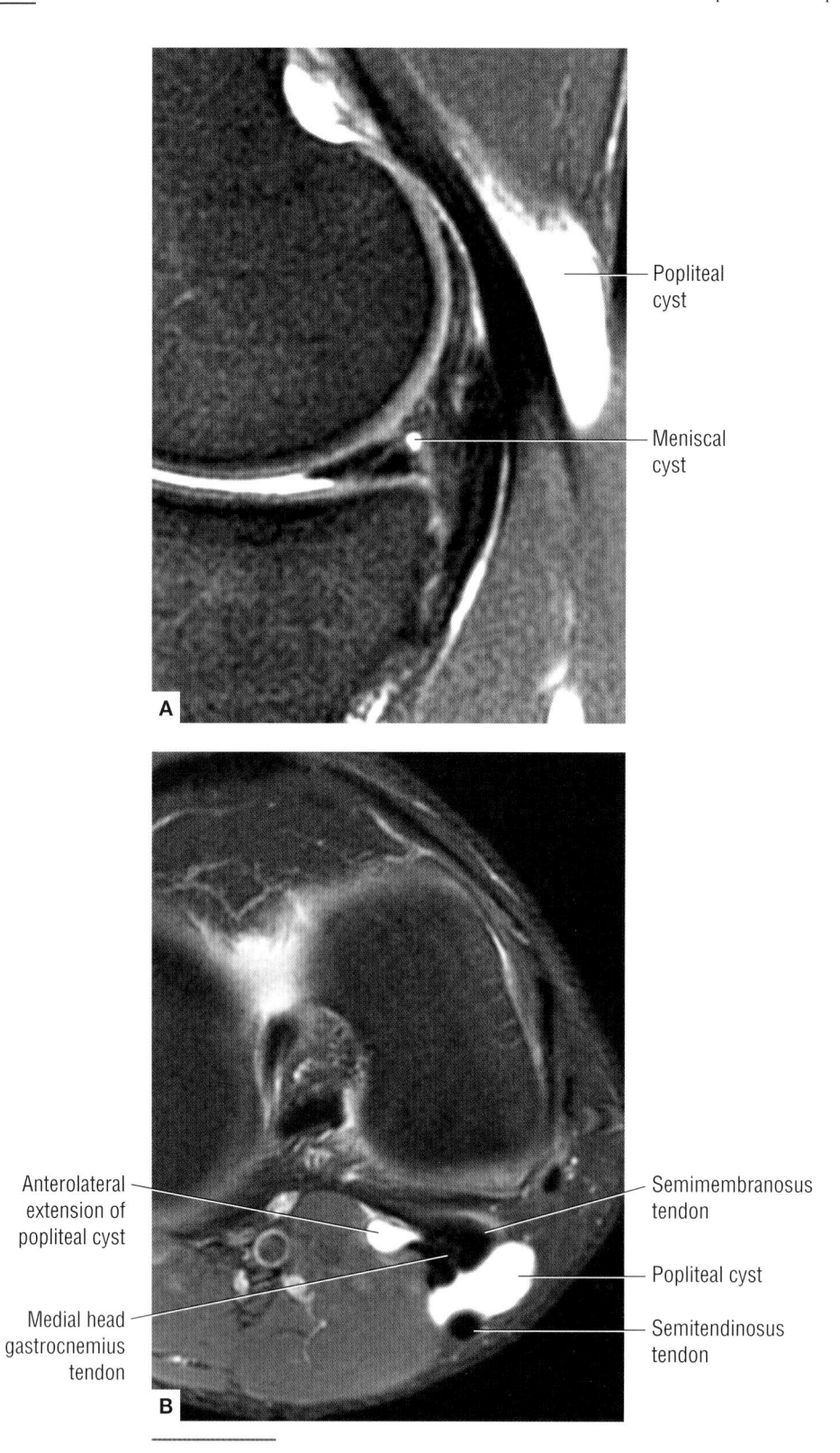

FIGURE 8.59 (**A**) Meniscal cyst and popliteal cyst shown on the same sagittal FS PD FSE image. Intraarticular abnormalities associated with popliteal cysts include meniscal tears, ACL tears, and degenerative osteoarthritis or inflammatory arthritis. The association between posterior horn medial meniscus tears and popliteal cysts is high. (**B**) Axial FS PD FSE image showing that the popliteal cyst also extends between the medial head of the gastrocnemius and semimembranosus anteriorly and the semitendinosus posteriorly.

General Pathologic Conditions Affecting the Knee

- Treating underlying joint pathology usually results in disappearance of the cyst.

- If suspected soft tissue mass shows central or irregular gadolinium enhancement, differential diagnosis must include soft tissue neoplasms (e.g., synovial sarcoma).

Ganglion Cysts

- Viscous synovium-filled masses with hyaluronic acid– and mucopolysaccharide-rich contents (unlike popliteal cysts)[387]

- May be intraarticular or extraarticular (joint capsule, pes anserinus tendons, and Hoffa's fat pad) in location

- Usually a connection or stalk traceable to the joint

- Septations common

- Unless associated with hemorrhage, ganglion cysts are low signal intensity on T1-weighted images and hyperintense on T2-weighted images.

- Deep venous thrombosis may present with hyperintense, prominent venous collaterals in the medial head of the gastrocnemius muscle in the presence of clinical calf or popliteal fossa pain.

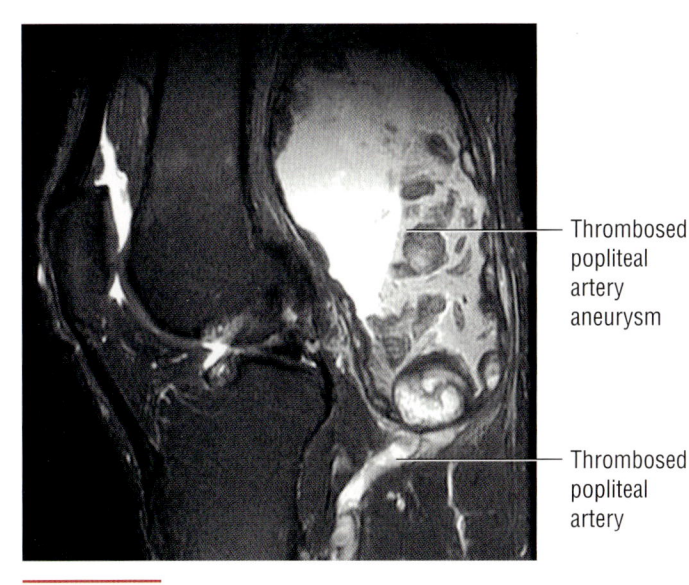

FIGURE 8.60   Sagittal FS PD FSE image showing popliteal artery aneurysm in Ehlers-Danlos syndrome. Joint hypermobility, skin bruising and elasticity, and vascular abnormalities are seen in the group of syndromes related by abnormal collagen synthesis/production.

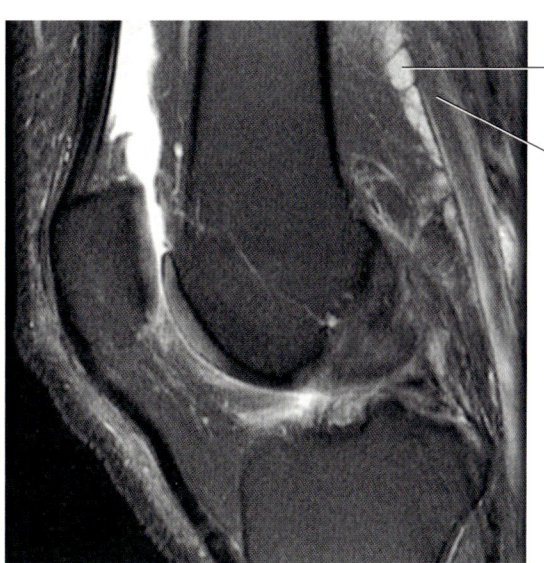

FIGURE 8.61   Cystic adventitial disease results in compression of the popliteal artery by mucoid cysts that develop within the adventitia of the popliteal artery. Men in their mid-40s present with intermittent claudication. Sagittal FS PD FSE image.

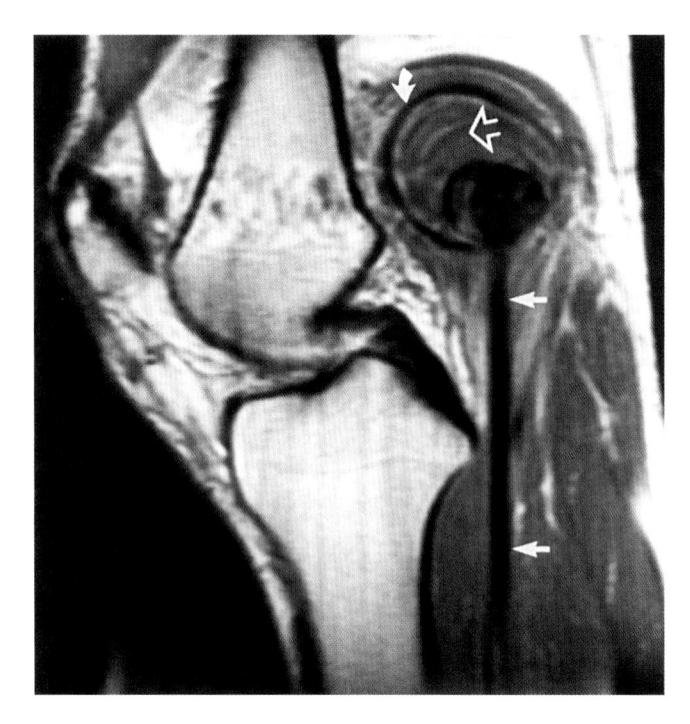

FIGURE 8.62 A T1-weighted sagittal image displays an enlarged aneurysm of the popliteal artery. The normal low-signal-intensity popliteal artery (*solid arrows*), an intermediate-signal-intensity thrombus (*open arrow*), and a low-signal-intensity peripheral rim of calcification (*curved arrow*) are identified. Popliteal artery aneurysms are associated with thrombosis, venous occlusion, peripheral embolization, and ulceration and gangrene. MR shows continuity with the popliteal artery. Thrombus formation is best evaluated in the axial plane.

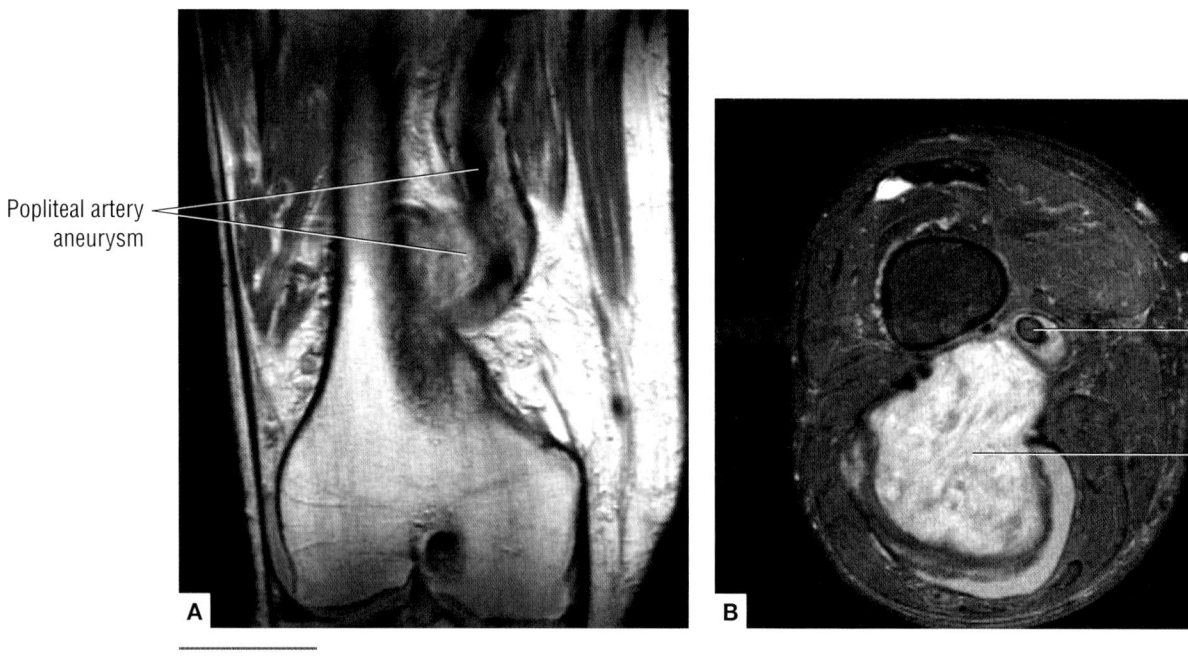

FIGURE 8.63 True aneurysms, which involve all the layers of the arterial wall, are common in the popliteal artery. MR studies are useful for identification of patients at risk for thrombotic complications since MR has the advantage of demonstrating the aneurysmal sac and mural thrombus, even if the artery is occluded. (**A**) Coronal PD FSE. (**B**) Axial FS PD FSE.

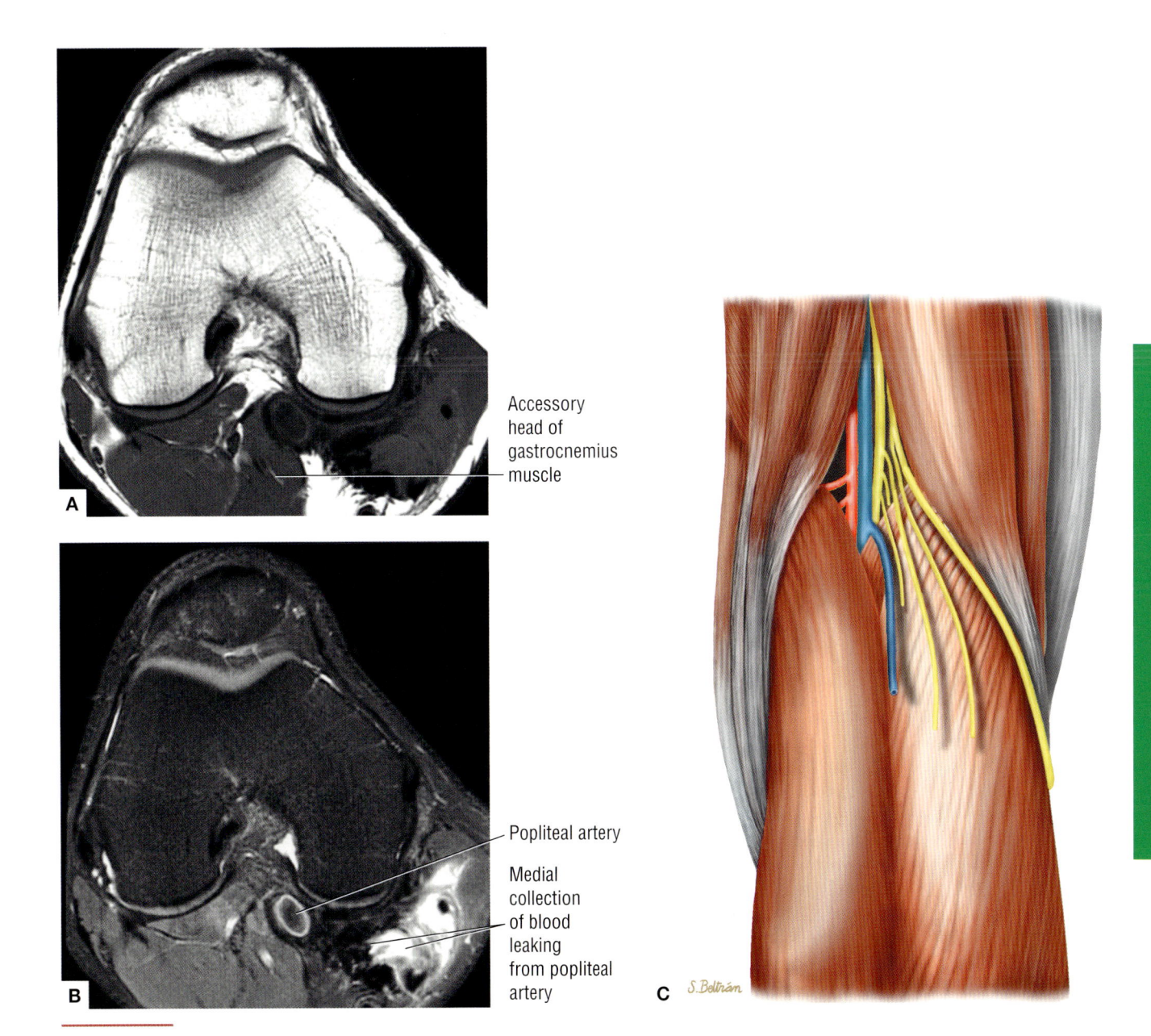

FIGURE 8.64 Postoperative popliteal artery entrapment with medial leaking of blood, which is in direct communication with the popliteal artery. Popliteal artery entrapment was the result of an accessory head of the gastrocnemius muscle. A fibrous band between the medial head gastrocnemius and lateral condyle or hypertrophy of the plantaris or semimembranosus may also cause compression of the popliteal artery. (**A**) Axial T1-weighted FSE image. (**B**) Axial FS PD FSE. (**C**) Posterior view of normal neurovascular structures for reference (color illustration).

Plicae

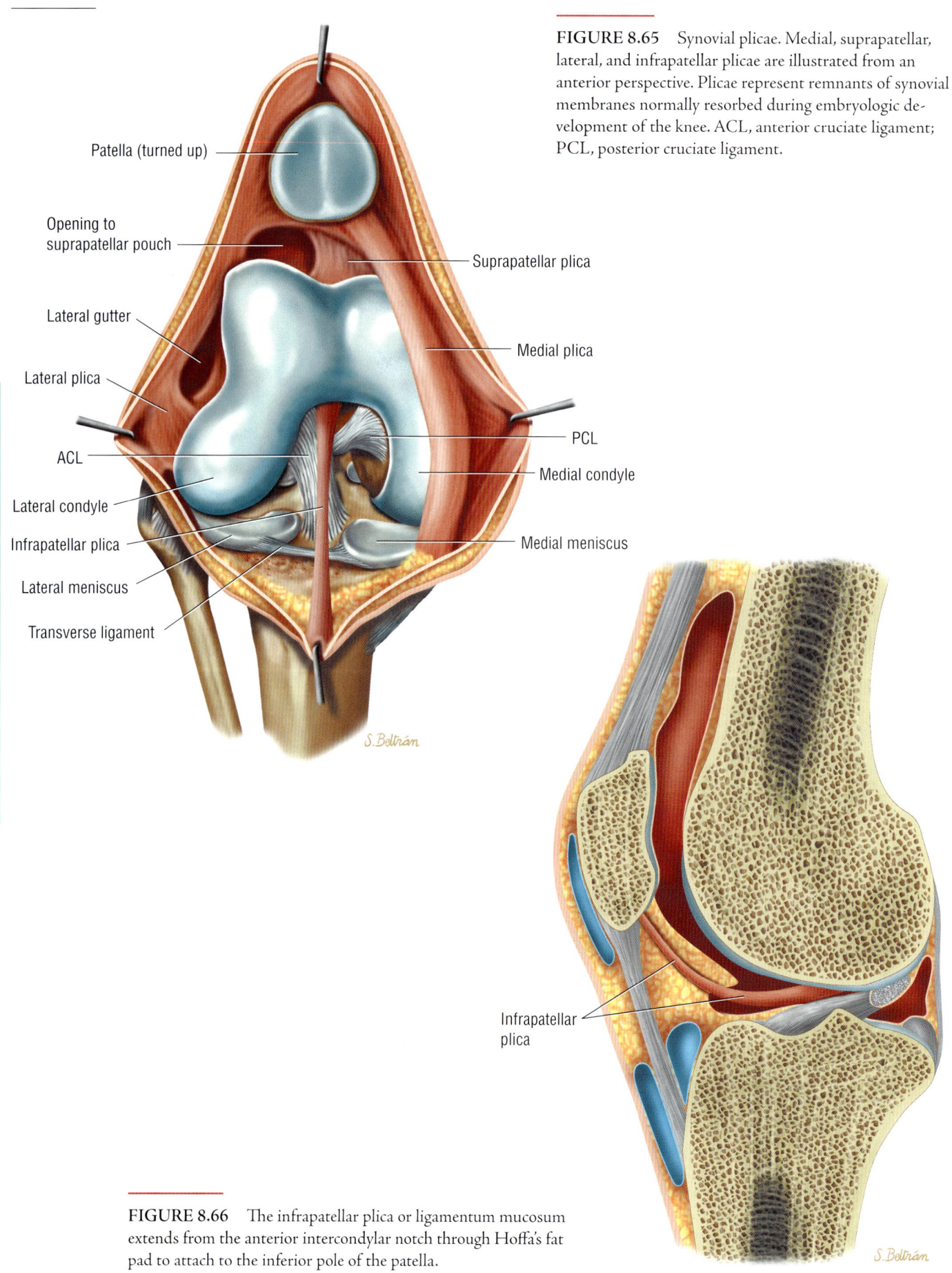

FIGURE 8.65 Synovial plicae. Medial, suprapatellar, lateral, and infrapatellar plicae are illustrated from an anterior perspective. Plicae represent remnants of synovial membranes normally resorbed during embryologic development of the knee. ACL, anterior cruciate ligament; PCL, posterior cruciate ligament.

FIGURE 8.66 The infrapatellar plica or ligamentum mucosum extends from the anterior intercondylar notch through Hoffa's fat pad to attach to the inferior pole of the patella.

Plicae

Key Concepts

- Suprapatellar plica can impinge on articular cartilage of superomedial angle of trochlea in knee flexion.
    - Suprapatellar septum or complete shelf may result in fluid build-up in suprapatellar bursa and present as a soft tissue mass.
- Infrapatellar plica, anterior to ACL, coursing through Hoffa's fat pad to inferior patellar pole attachment.
    - Anterior meniscofemoral ligament thought to attach to transverse ligament or anterior horn medial meniscus and posterior to infrapatellar plica.
- Medial or mediopatellar plica visualized on medial sagittal images and axial images through patellofemoral joint
    - Thick or shelf-like medial plica frequently associated with medial patellar facet chondromalacia

Synovial Plicae

- Represent one of several differential diagnoses for anterior knee pain[224]
    - Plica syndrome may include anterior knee pain or clicking, catching, or locking of the knee.
- Anatomy
    - Embryologic remnants of septal division of knee into three compartments[13,56,224]
    - May be present as a large shelf in slightly fewer than 20% of knees[155] (medial plicae)
- MR findings
    - Medial plicae best seen on axial images
    - Suprapatellar plicae seen on sagittal images, traversing the suprapatellar bursa
    - Infrapatellar plicae best seen on sagittal images, most likely to be found anterior and parallel to ACL
        - *Ligamentum mucosum*, an incomplete infrapatellar plica

Infrapatellar Plica

- Classified as having a vertical septum as a separate structure from the ACL, split or bipartite, or fenestrated
- Narrow femoral origin at anterior aspect of intercondylar notch
- Widens as it proceeds through the joint space
- Thickest segment is its intercondylar component
- Course of infrapatellar plica through Hoffa's fat pad to inferior pole of the patella is more delicate or attenuated in caliber.
- Should not be mistaken for the ACL
  - In axial plane, anterior location of the infrapatellar plica relative to the ACL is characteristic.
- Trochlear groove chondromalacia is associated with infrapatellar plicae.

Suprapatellar Plica

- Can be seen in patients with suprapatellar soft tissue mass
  - Persistent plica dividing suprapatellar bursa into two separate compartments containing hemorrhagic synovial fluid and debris
- Several types of suprapatellar plicae, including superomedial and superolateral types
- Can also exist as a cord or membrane (with or without a perforation)
- Zidorn classification of suprapatellar plicae (four groups based on morphology)
  - Type I, or *septum completum*: completely separates suprapatellar bursa and knee joint
  - Type II, or *septum perforatum*: has one or more openings in the septum
    - Opening or perforation (porta) permits communication of joint fluid between suprapatellar bursa and knee joint
  - Type III, or *septum residual*: remaining fold, usually in medial location
  - Type IV, or *septum extinctum*: involuted septum

Medial Patellar Plica

- Inflamed medial patellar plica thickens and may interfere with normal quadriceps function and patellofemoral articulation.

- Erosion or abrasion of femoral condylar or patellar articular cartilage can occur as plica loses flexibility and gliding motion.

- Sakakibara arthroscopic classification for medial plica:
    - Type A: cord-like elevation in the synovial wall
    - Type B: shelf-like without covering the anterior medial femoral condyle
    - Type C: large and shelf-like, covers anterior medial femoral condyle
    - Type D: central defect or fenestrated
    - Symptomatic impingement (types C and D) can occur when thick and shelf-like medial plicae interfere with articular cartilage of medial patellar facet (in flexion) or medial femoral condyle (in extension).

- MR appearance
    - Abnormal medial patellar plica seen as thickened band of low signal intensity with underlying irregularity of medial patellar facet cartilage surface (axial images)
    - Sagittal images show longitudinal orientation of medial plica extending toward Hoffa's infrapatellar fat pad, anterior to anterior horn of medial meniscus.
    - Plical thickness is not measured quantitatively.
    - Fibrotic hypertrophy secondary to chronic irritation can be identified and is considered symptomatic when impingement on medial femoral condyle in knee flexion is present.

Plicae

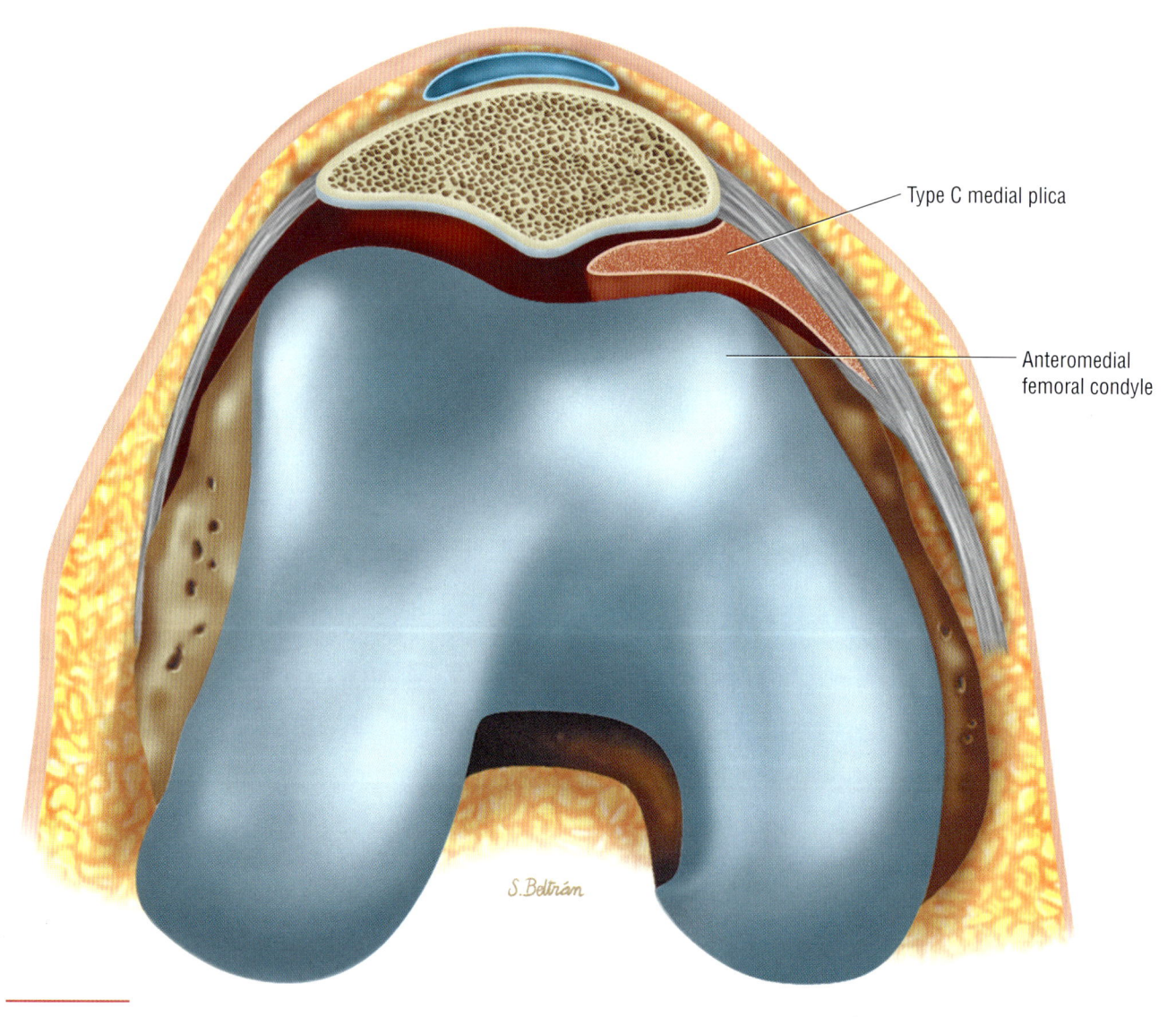

FIGURE 8.67 Type C medial patellar plica that covers the anteromedial femoral condyle. Axial color illustration.

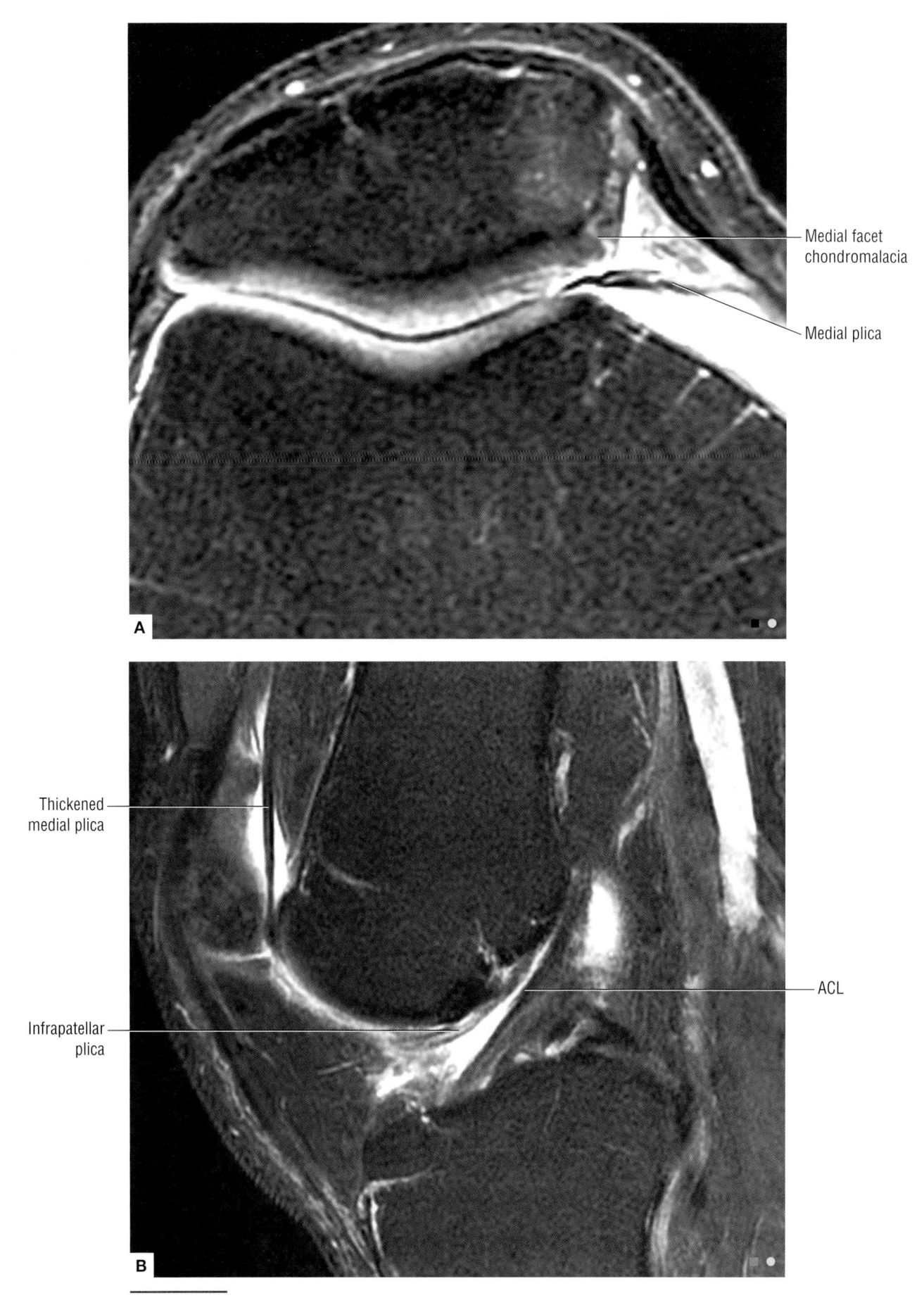

FIGURE 8.68 Thickened shelf-like medial plica intraarticular component of the infrapatellar plica on axial (**A**) and sagittal (**B**) FS PD images.

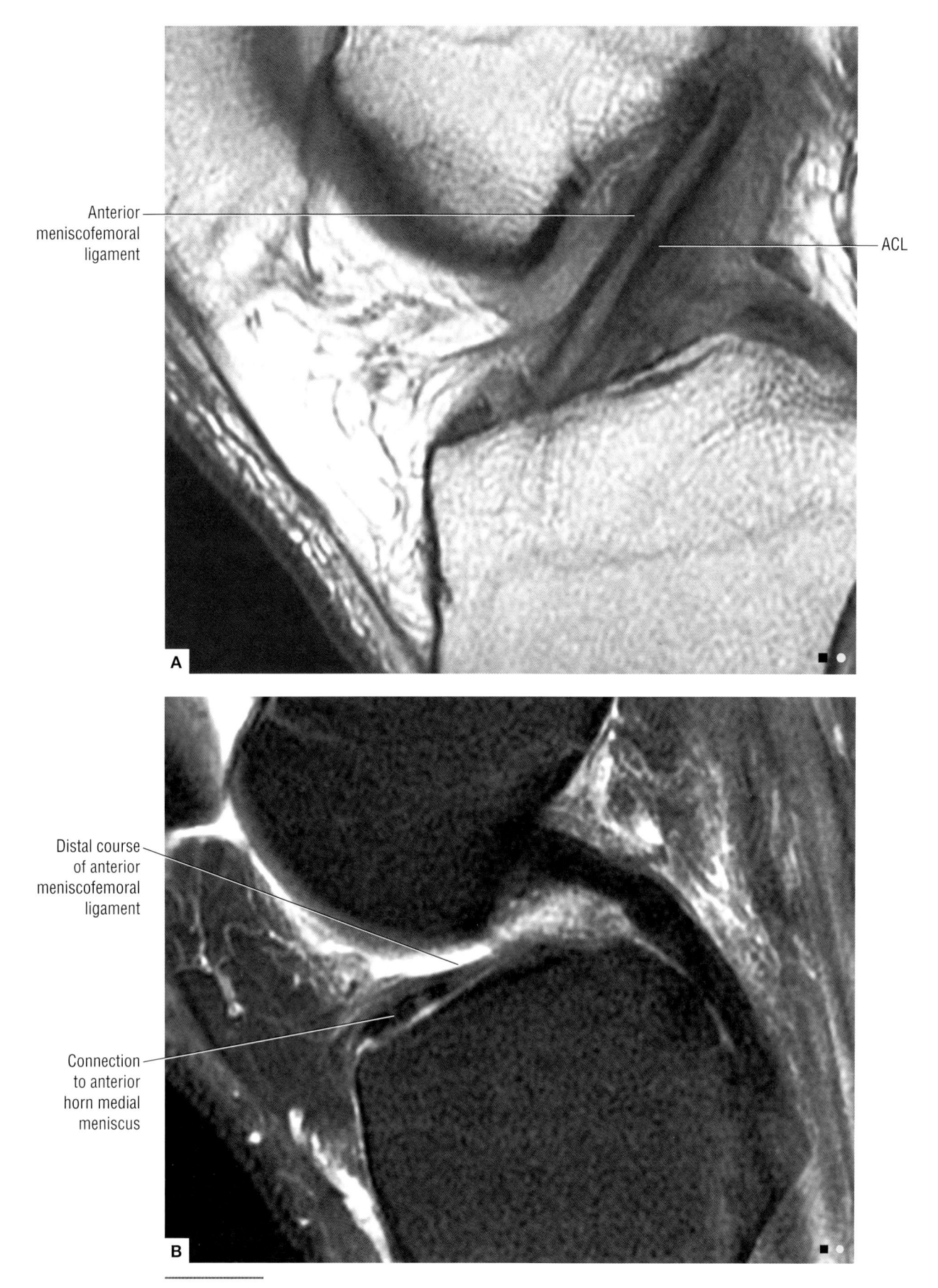

FIGURE 8.69 The anterior meniscofemoral ligament can be mistaken for an infrapatellar plica but lies posterior and parallel to the ligamentum mucosum. Sagittal PD (**A**) and FS PD (**B**) images.

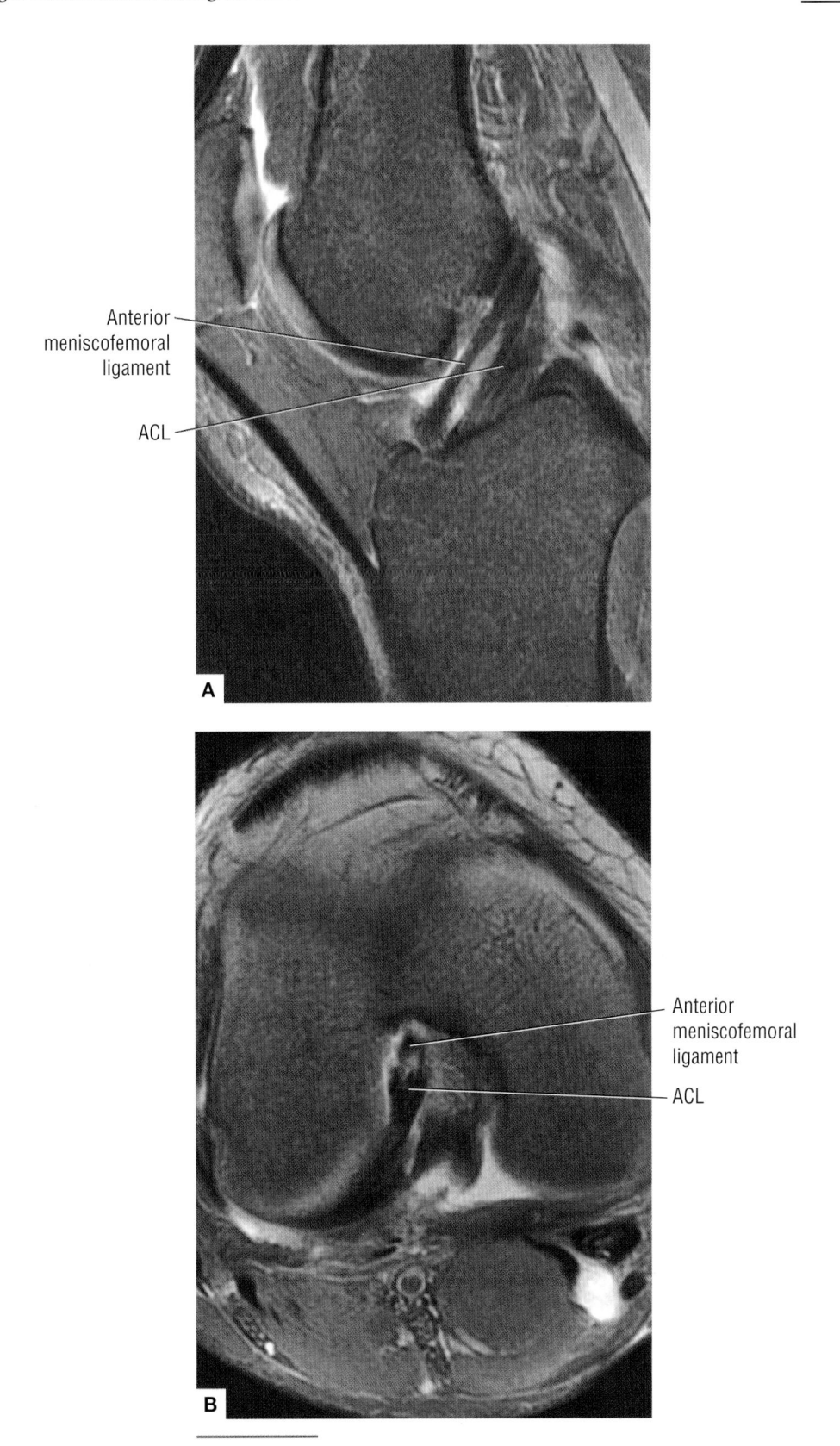

FIGURE 8.70 (**A**) Sagittal FS PD FSE image showing a large (wide and thick) anterior meniscofemoral ligament variant, which may be mistaken for the ACL or infrapatellar plica. This structure also has been referred to as a infrapatellar plica historically, even though there is no connection to the inferior pole. (**B**) On axial images, a thick anterior meniscofemoral ligament is characteristically seen as a hypointense structure anterior to the ACL. Axial FS PD FSE image.

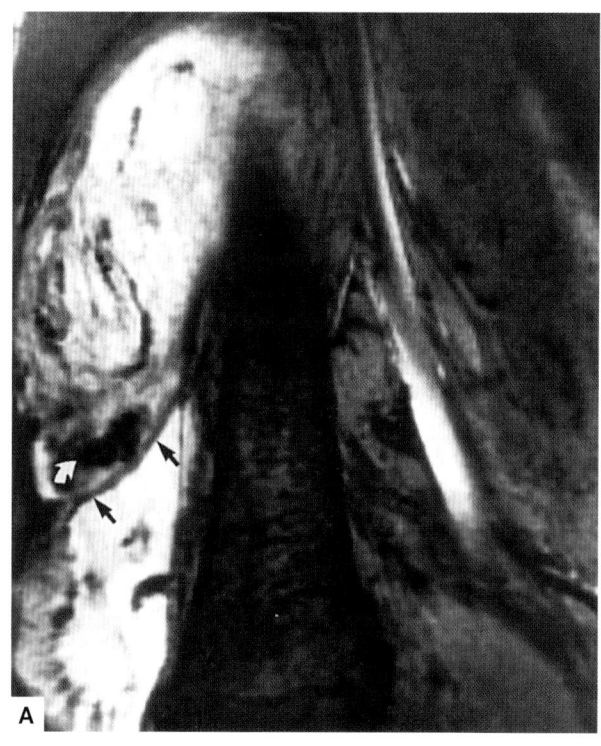

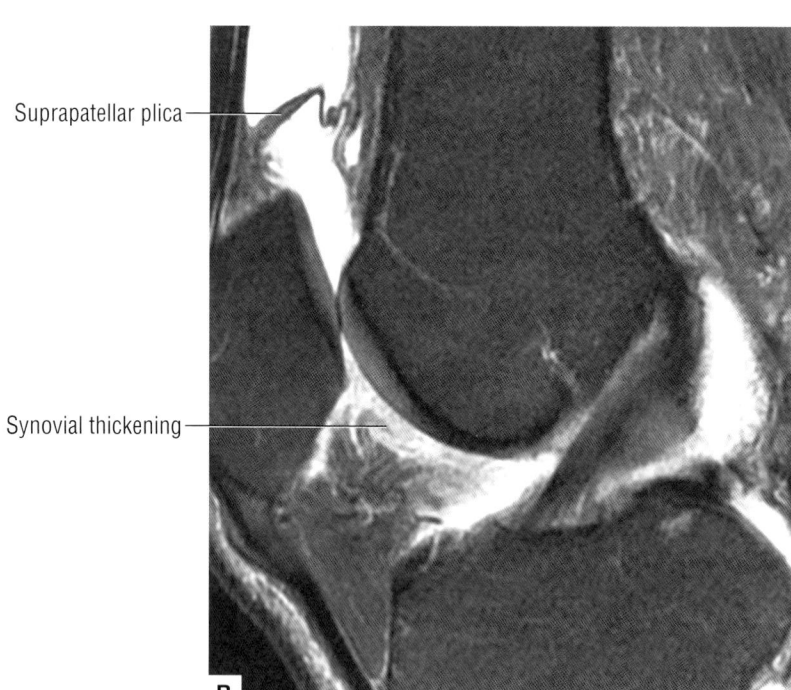

FIGURE 8.71 (**A**) Division of the suprapatellar bursa into two compartments with an intact suprapatellar plica is seen as a low-signal-intensity band (*solid arrows*) on T2*-weighted sequence. Low-signal-intensity hemosiderin deposits (*curved arrow*) contrast with the surrounding bright-signal-intensity hemorrhagic fluid. (**B**) Asymptomatic suprapatellar plica on a sagittal FS PD FSE image for comparison. An infrapatellar plica is also present.

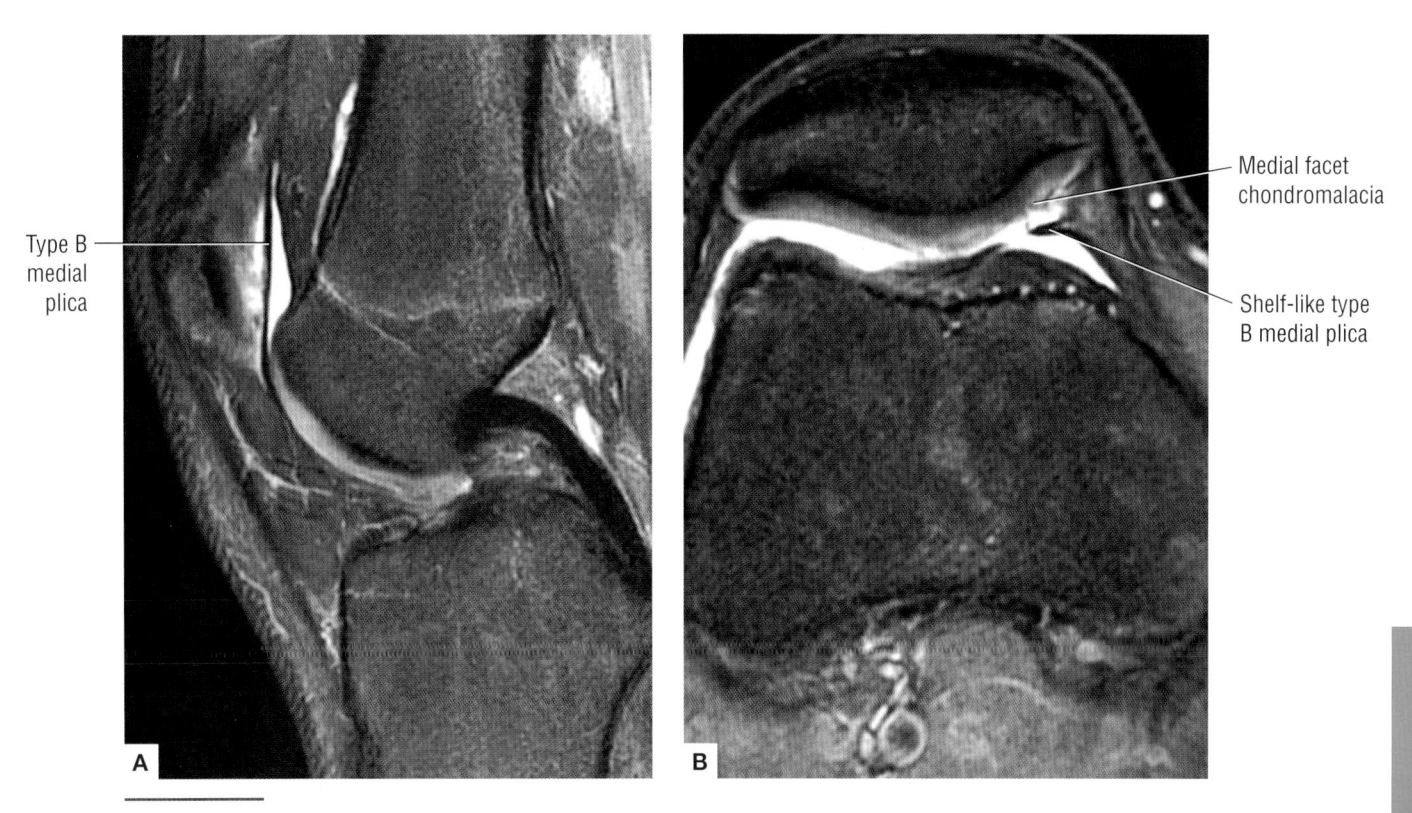

General Pathologic Conditions Affecting the Knee

FIGURE 8.72 (**A**) Sagittal FS PD FSE and (**B**) axial FS PD FSE images showing a mildly thickened type B medial plica with hypointense shelf-like morphology. The plica does not fully cover the anteromedial femoral condyle, and there is associated superficial chondromalacia of the medial patellar facet.

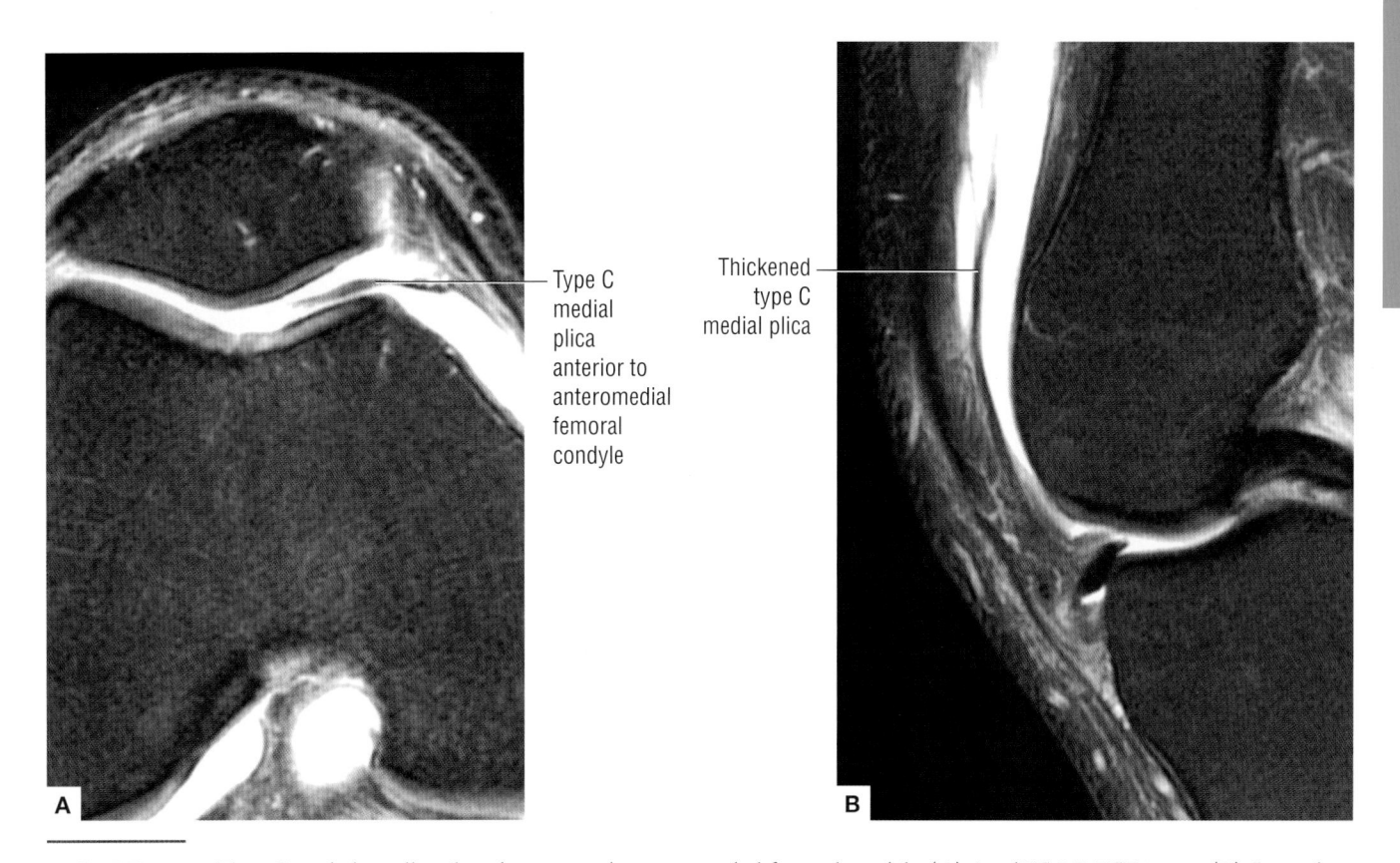

FIGURE 8.73 Type C medial patellar plica that covers the anteromedial femoral condyle. (**A**) Axial FS PD FSE image. (**B**) Sagittal FS PD FSE image.

Lateral Patellar Plica

- Thickened lateral patellar plica is uncommon.
- Visualized in lateral recess deep to lateral retinaculum[155]
- Coronal plane provides excellent perspective of course of lateral plica above popliteus hiatus and transverse ligament to infrapatellar fat-pad attachment.
- Lateral alar fold, another structure in the lateral gutter, is separate from the lateral patellar plica.

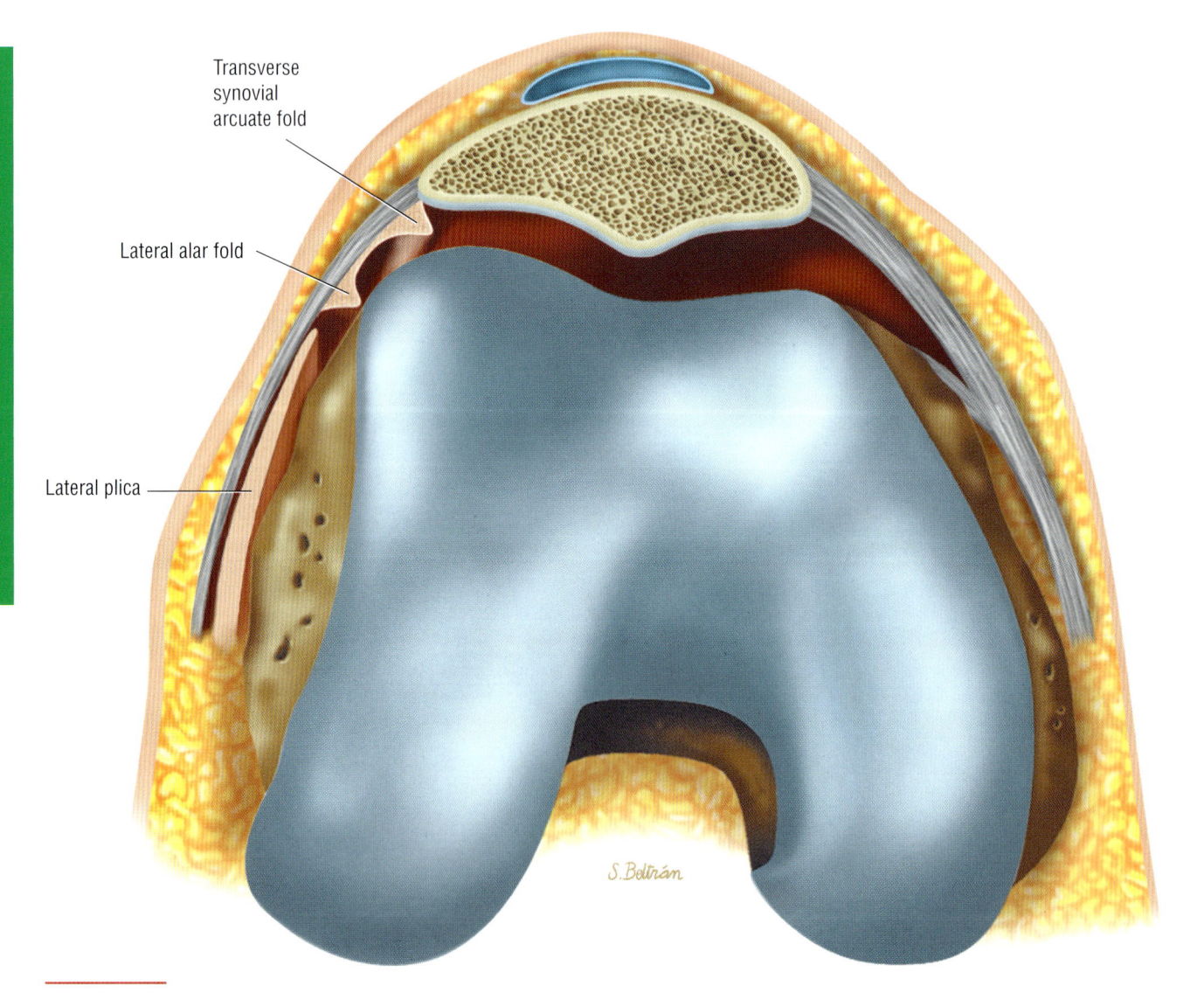

FIGURE 8.74 Longitudinal course of a lateral patellar plica demonstrated on a cross-sectional color illustration. A lateral plica may interfere with access to the anterolateral portal at arthroscopy.

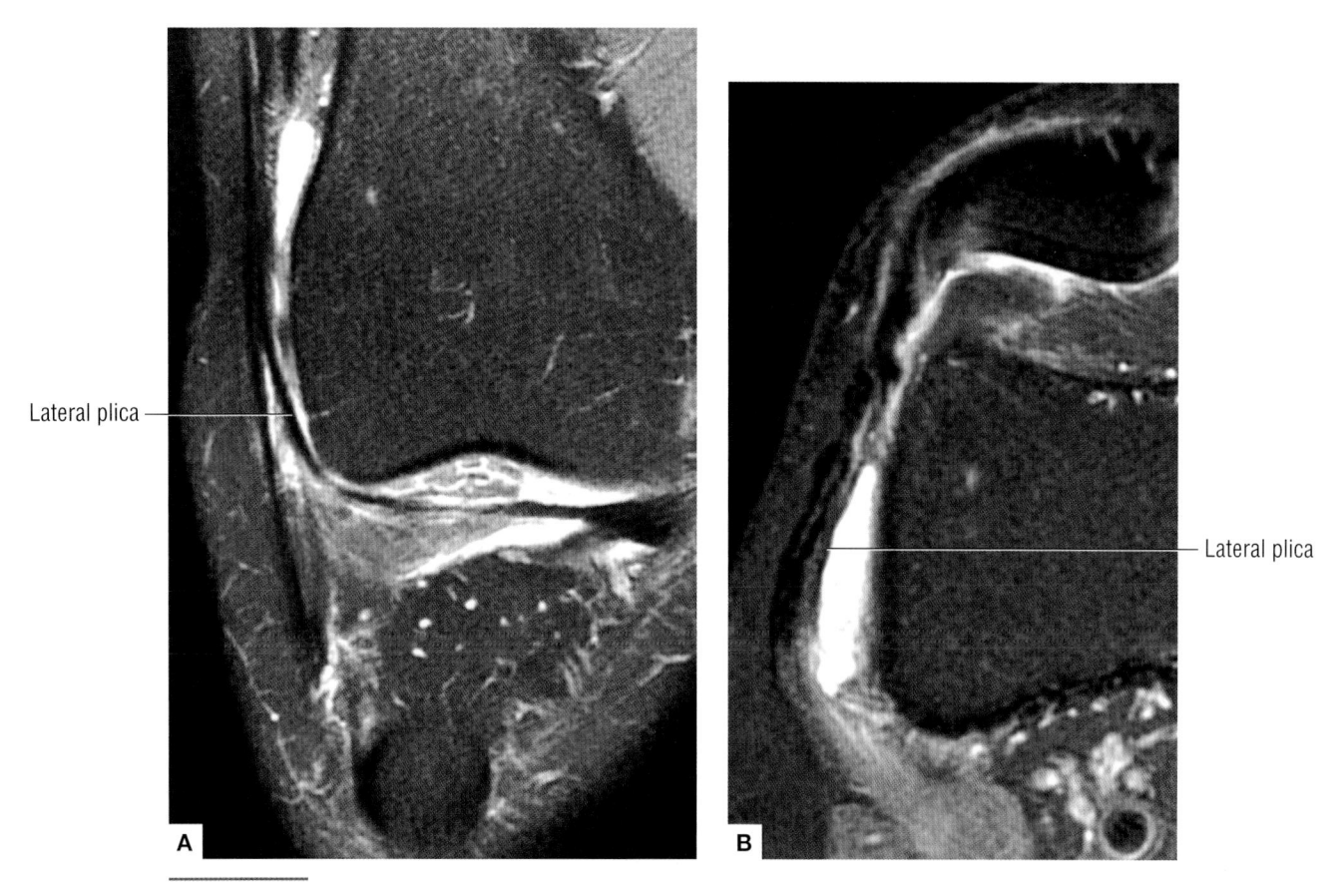

General Pathologic Conditions Affecting the Knee

FIGURE 8.75 (**A**) Distal course of the lateral plica and attachment to the infrapatellar fat pad on an anterior coronal FS PD FSE image. (**B**) Lateral patella plica on an axial FS PD image.

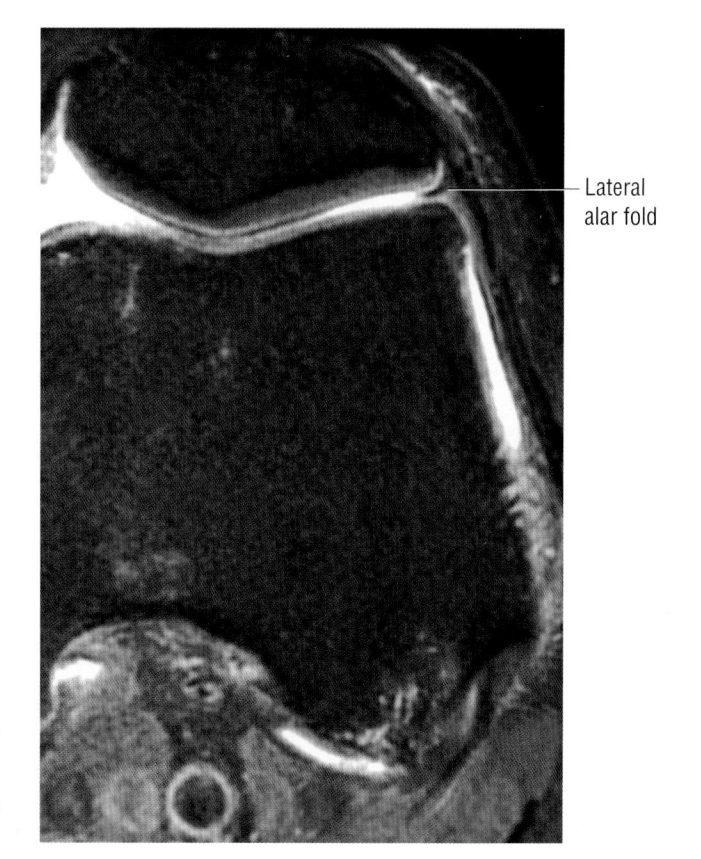

FIGURE 8.76 The normal lateral alar fold should not be confused with a lateral patellar plica and is located closer to the patella. Axial FS PD FSE image.

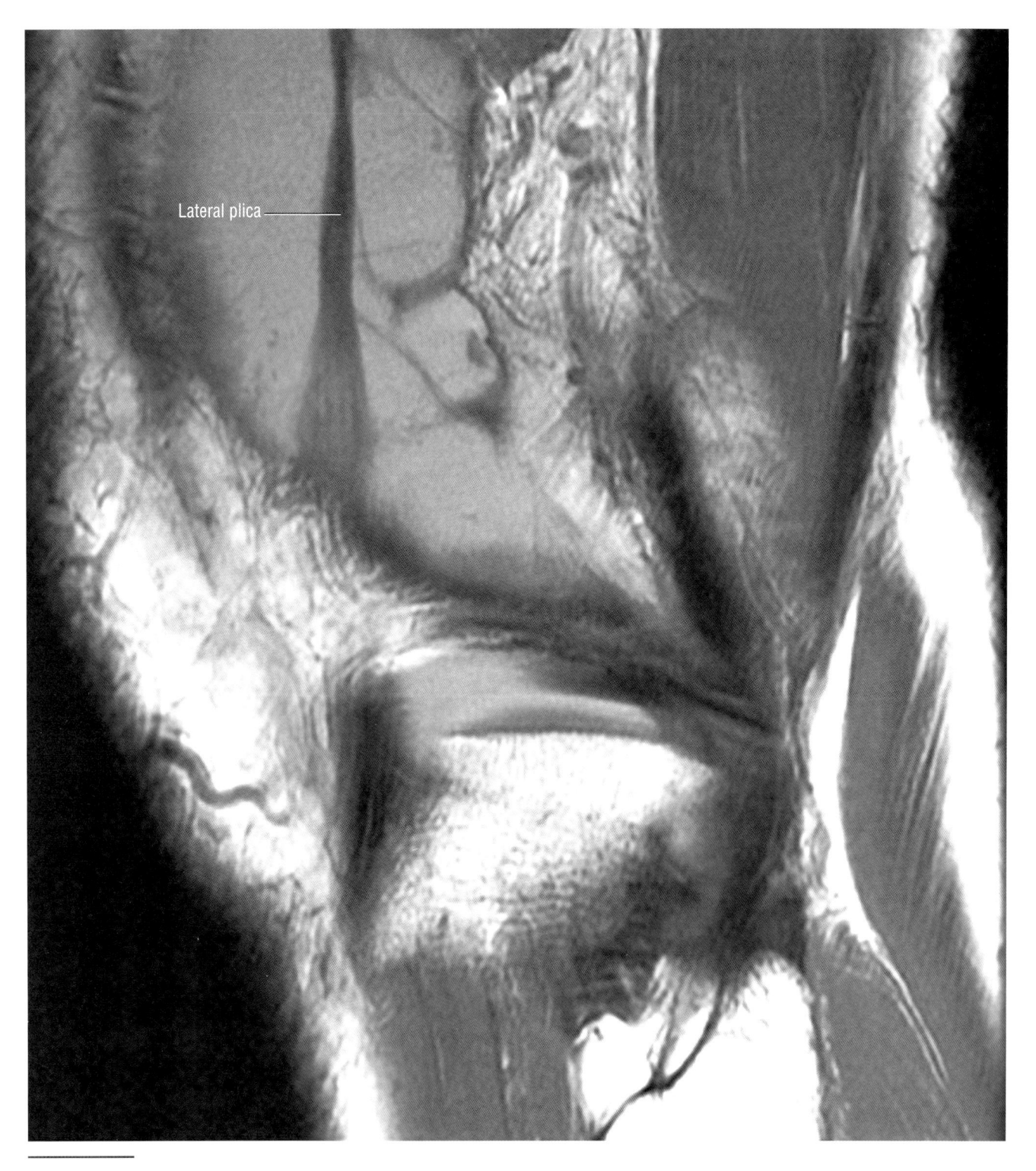

FIGURE 8.77 Prominent wide symptomatic lateral plica that usually has an oblique course in the axial plane may be visualized with a vertical or vertical oblique course on sagittal images. Sagittal PD FSE image.

Osteonecrosis and Related Osseous Disorders

Key Concepts

- Subchondral fracture of spontaneous osteonecrosis of the knee in fact represents insufficiency fracture without associated cellular necrosis.

- Healed or healing stages of osteochondritis dissecans may demonstrate return to subchondral marrow fat signal intensity with varying degrees of overlying chondral degeneration.

- Epiphyseal subchondral hypointensity with overlying chondral heterogeneity can represent normal epiphyseal maturation during ossification of immature skeleton.

Spontaneous Osteonecrosis and Insufficiency Fractures

- Osteonecrosis can occur spontaneously or in association with medical conditions, such as:
    - Steroid use
    - Renal transplantation
    - Alcoholism
    - Hemoglobinopathies
    - Gaucher's disease
    - Caisson's decompression sickness
    - Systemic lupus erythematosus[371]

- Steroid-induced osteonecrotic lesions tend to be larger than those seen in spontaneous osteonecrosis, possibly because of frequent development of related bone infarct pattern.
    - *Spontaneous (idiopathic) osteonecrosis of the knee*
    - Typically affects older, predominantly female patients who present with acute medial joint pain[25,52,523]
    - Often involves weight-bearing surface of medial femoral condyle
    - Medial and lateral tibial plateaus and lateral femoral condyle may also be affected.[293]

- Two theories of pathogenesis: vascular and traumatic[378]
- Vascular model
  - Thrombotic venous occlusion leads to interruption of microcirculation of femoral condyle, resulting in edema and increased intraosseous pressure, which in turn lead to ischemia and hypoxic death of bony tissue.
  - Revascularization with new vessel ingrowth may weaken remaining bone architecture, causing subchondral collapse and articular destruction.
  - If revascularization is successful, however, it does not lead to collapse of healing necrotic segment.
- Traumatic model
  - Insufficiency fractures occur in an osteoporotic patient following trivial trauma.
  - Subchondral bone is then at risk for necrosis.
  - Secondary reflux of synovial fluid through damaged articular cartilage contributes to increased interosseous pressure and resultant compromise of vascular supply to subchondral bone.
  - At present, traumatic theory is accepted.

- Clinical history of osteonecrosis
  - Intense pain for 2 to 3 months, dissipating by 12 to 15 months
  - Lesions with area greater than 50% of condyle and measuring 5cm or greater in diameter are classified as large and frequently progress to radiographic collapse.

- Subchondral fractures
  - Associated with significant diffuse condylar marrow edema, which is of greatest intensity in area adjacent to microtrabecular fracture
  - Insufficiency fractures tend to be located parallel and directly subjacent to subchondral plate.

General Pathologic Conditions Affecting the Knee

- Necrotic focus in primary ischemic change may occur in a deeper subchondral location, may not be directly in contact with the subchondral plate, and may demonstrate greater superior-to-inferior length and a convex or irregular and greater depth.

- Meniscal tears often associated with spontaneous osteonecrosis and insufficiency fractures

- Differential diagnosis of osteonecrosis includes osteochondritis dissecans, osteoarthritis, meniscal tears, stress fractures, and pes anserinus bursitis.

- Conventional radiographs
  - Not sensitive in evaluating an osteonecrotic focus before development of sclerosis and osseous collapse
  - Radiographic classification of necrotic lesion consists of five stages[328,378]:
    - Stage 1: normal
    - Stage 2: mild flattening of weight-bearing aspect of femoral condyle
    - Stage 3: area of radiolucency with sclerosis distal to lesion
    - Stage 4: radiolucent area surrounded by sclerotic halo; collapsed subchondral bone visible as calcified plate
    - Stage 5: secondary degenerative changes and erosions with subchondral sclerosis of both femur and tibia

MR Patterns of Osteonecrosis

- Osteonecrotic focus associated with adjacent bone marrow edema, similar to transient osteoporosis of the hip
  - Necrotic focus is low signal intensity on T1- and T2-weighted images.
  - Adjacent subchondral bone may display hyperintensity on T2, FS PD-weighted FSE, or STIR images.
  - T2*-weighted images are less sensitive to this associated marrow edema or hyperemia.
  - Subchondral sclerosis may be masked on T2*-weighted images.

- Necrotic focus involves weight-bearing surface of femoral condyle and may involve both condyles simultaneously.

- Discrete morphology of low-signal-intensity necrotic focus and localization to medial femoral condyle help distinguish this pattern of osteonecrosis from that caused by traumatic trabecular bone injuries, which show a similar medullary hyperintensity on T2, FS PD-weighted FSE, or STIR images.

- Area of marrow hyperintensity in spontaneous osteonecrosis can be much greater and deeper within subchondral bone than would be typically expected in localized trauma.

- Osteonecrotic focus without any associated marrow changes

  - In early stages, necrotic focus itself may display some degree of hyperintensity on heavily weighted T2, FS PD-weighted FSE, or STIR images.

  - Even with negative radiographs, low-signal-intensity changes detected within area of osteonecrosis on T1- and T2-weighted MR images

  - Overlying articular cartilage and status of meniscal cartilage evaluated on T1- and T2-weighted images

  - Reports of osteonecrosis occurring after arthroscopic reconstruction of cruciate ligament and after laser-assisted arthroscopic surgery[35,424]

  - Osteonecrosis also reported after arthroscopic medial meniscectomy

Treatment of Osteonecrosis

- Initially conservative, including protected weight bearing[293,378]

- Advanced stages require surgical intervention, including arthroscopic débridement, core decompression, high tibial osteotomy, drilling with or without bone grafting, osteochondral allografts, unicompartmental arthroplasty, and total knee replacement.

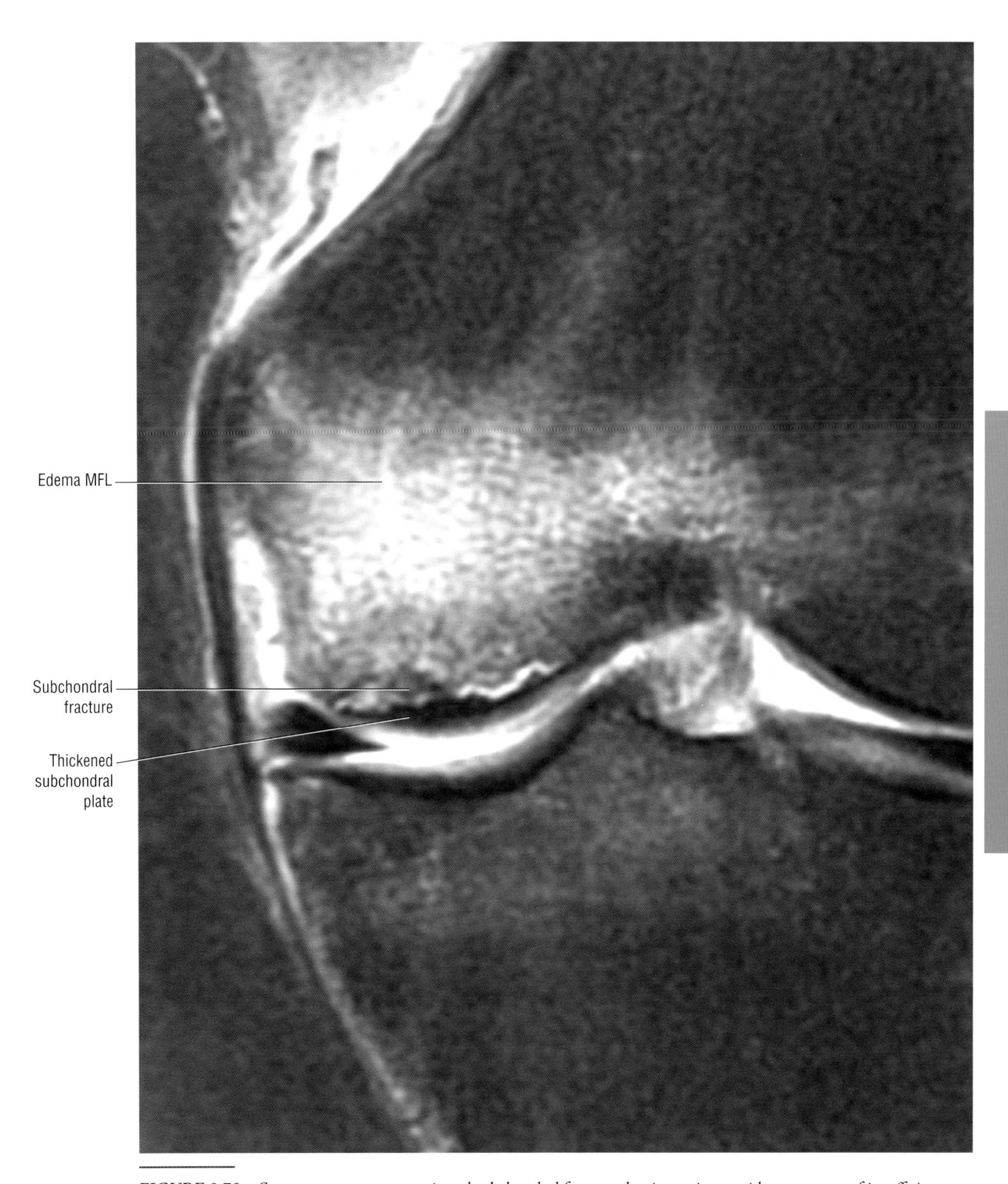

General Pathologic Conditions Affecting the Knee

FIGURE 8.78 Spontaneous osteonecrosis and subchondral fracture that is consistent with a spectrum of insufficiency fracture of the femoral condyle. The thickened subchondral plate is a more chronic response to the initial linear fracture line that is subarticular in location. Coronal FS PD FSE image.

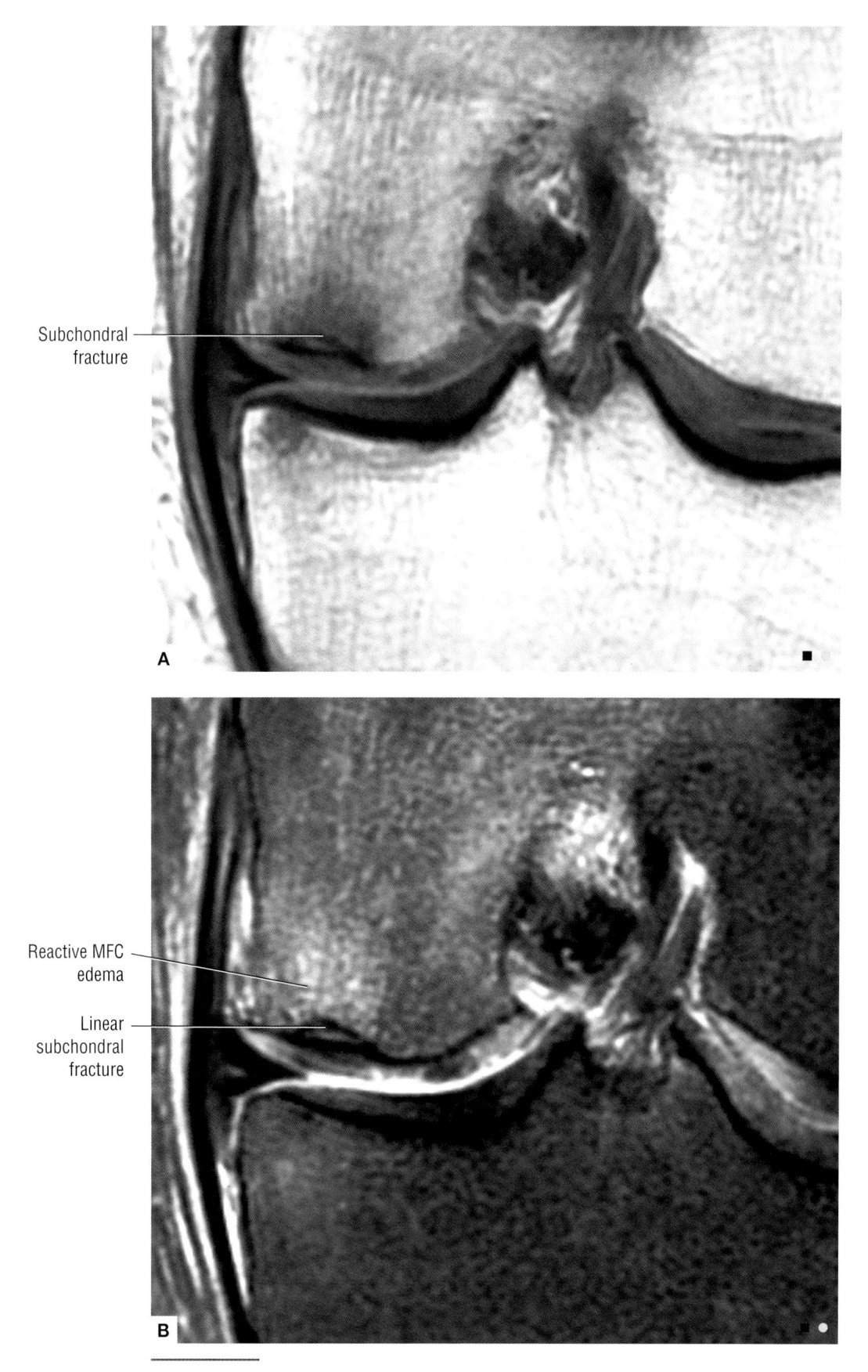

FIGURE 8.79 Discrete thin hypointense subchondral insufficiency fracture with associated edema in medial femoral condyle. Acute fractures will demonstrate hypointensity of the fracture line itself, whereas subacute fractures will develop hyperintensity in the linear subchondral fracture independent from the associated bone marrow edema of the femoral condyle. Coronal PD (**A**) and FS PD (**B**) images.

General Pathologic Conditions Affecting the Knee

Necrotic zone of medial femoral condyle

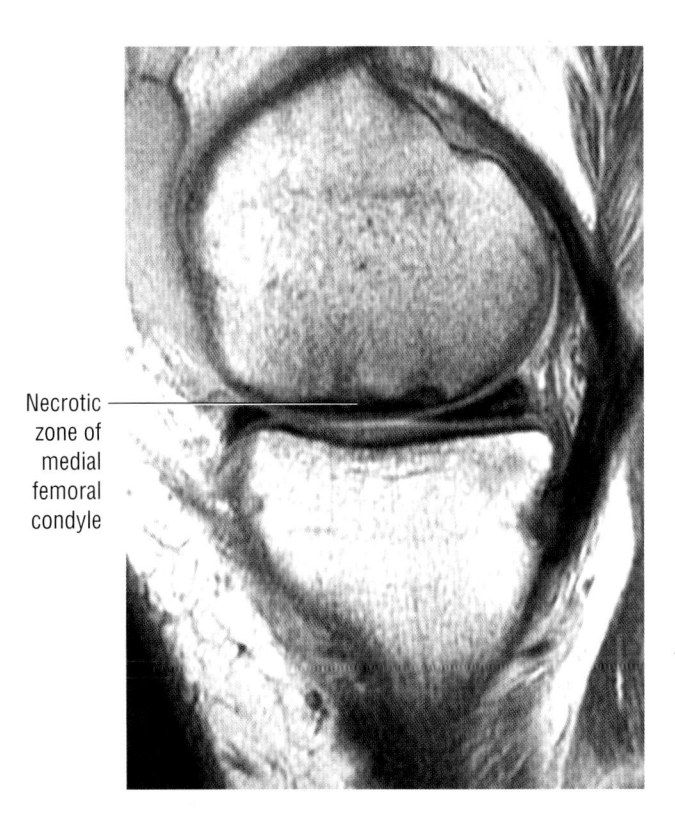

FIGURE 8.80 The shape of the lesion is relatively ovoid, and the sagittal anterior-to-posterior length is greater than the coronal medial-to-lateral measurement. Sagittal PD FSE image.

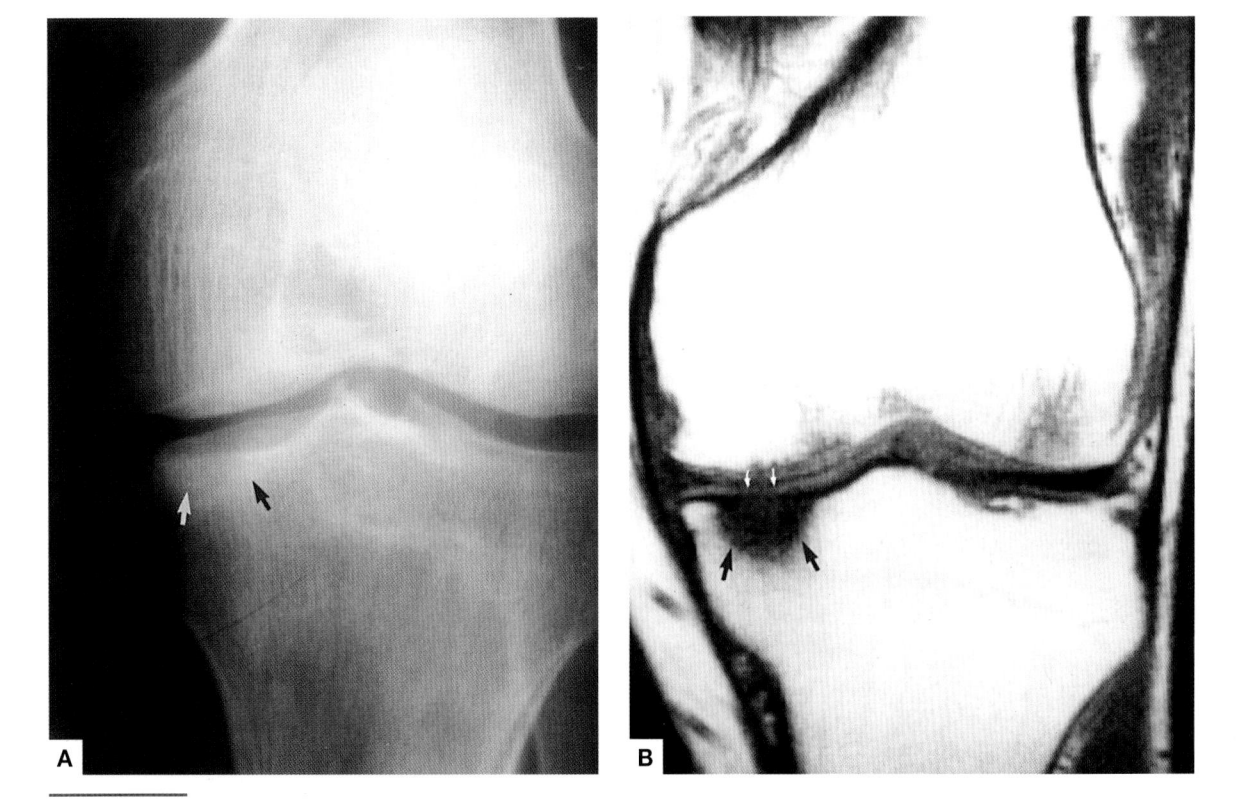

FIGURE 8.81 (**A**) On an anteroposterior radiograph, a sclerotic focus in the medial tibial plateau (*arrows*) indicates osteonecrosis. (**B**) On a T1-weighted coronal image, a well-defined region of subchondral low signal intensity is seen in the medial tibial plateau (*black arrows*). Thinning of overlying hyaline articular cartilage (*white arrows*) also is observed.

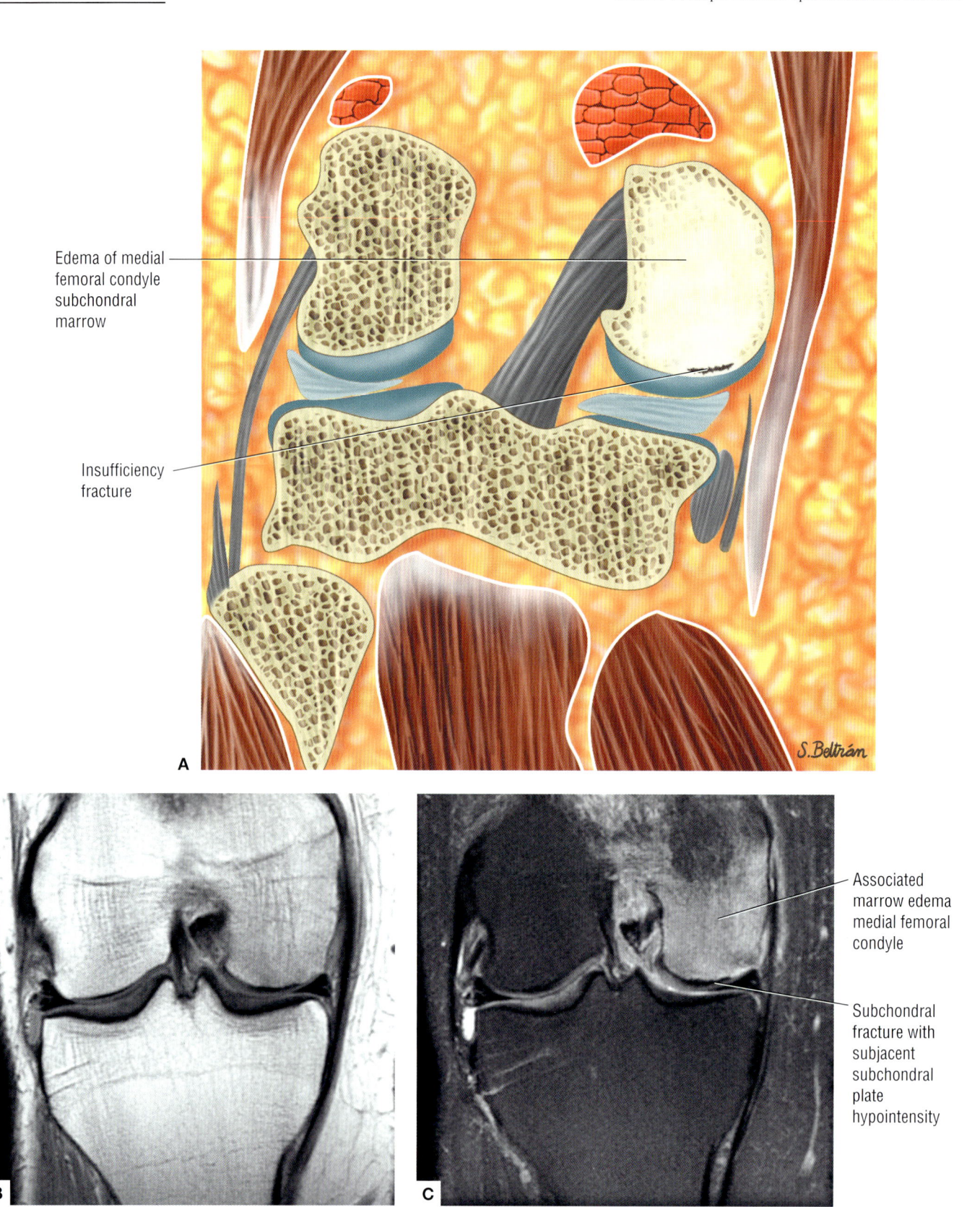

FIGURE 8.82 (**A**) Insufficiency fracture of the medial femoral condyle with discrete linear subchondral fracture. These fractures may heal or develop into osteonecrosis in marrow at risk for ischemia. Insufficiency fractures were previously attributed only to the subchondral bone of the medial tibial plateau in older osteopenic women. (**B, C**) A medial femoral condyle subchondral (subcondylar) fracture resulting in thickening of the subchondral plate. Associated edema of the medial femoral condyle is hyperintense on (**B**) coronal PD FSE and (**C**) coronal FS PD FSE images.

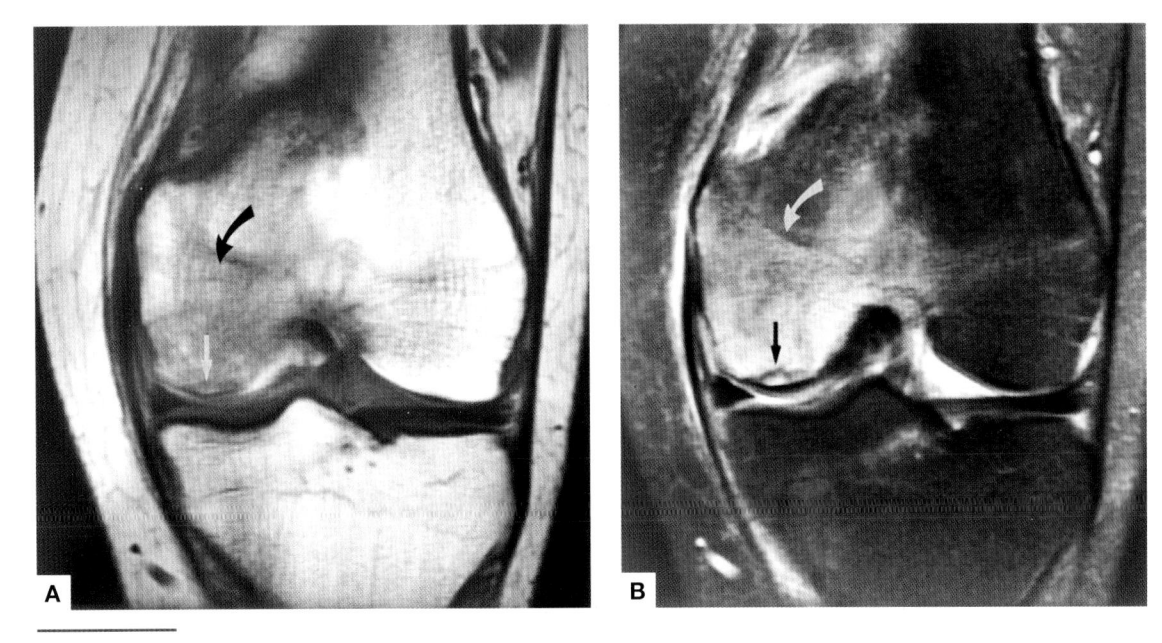

General Pathologic Conditions Affecting the Knee

FIGURE 8.83 (**A**) Coronal T1-weighted FSE image and (**B**) coronal FS PD FSE image displaying a subcondylar fracture of the medial femoral condyle with subchondral bone at risk for necrosis. Ischemia-related subchondral fractures may occur in a deeper location and may not be in direct contact with the subchondral plate. *Curved arrow*, edema; *straight arrow*, subchondral fracture.

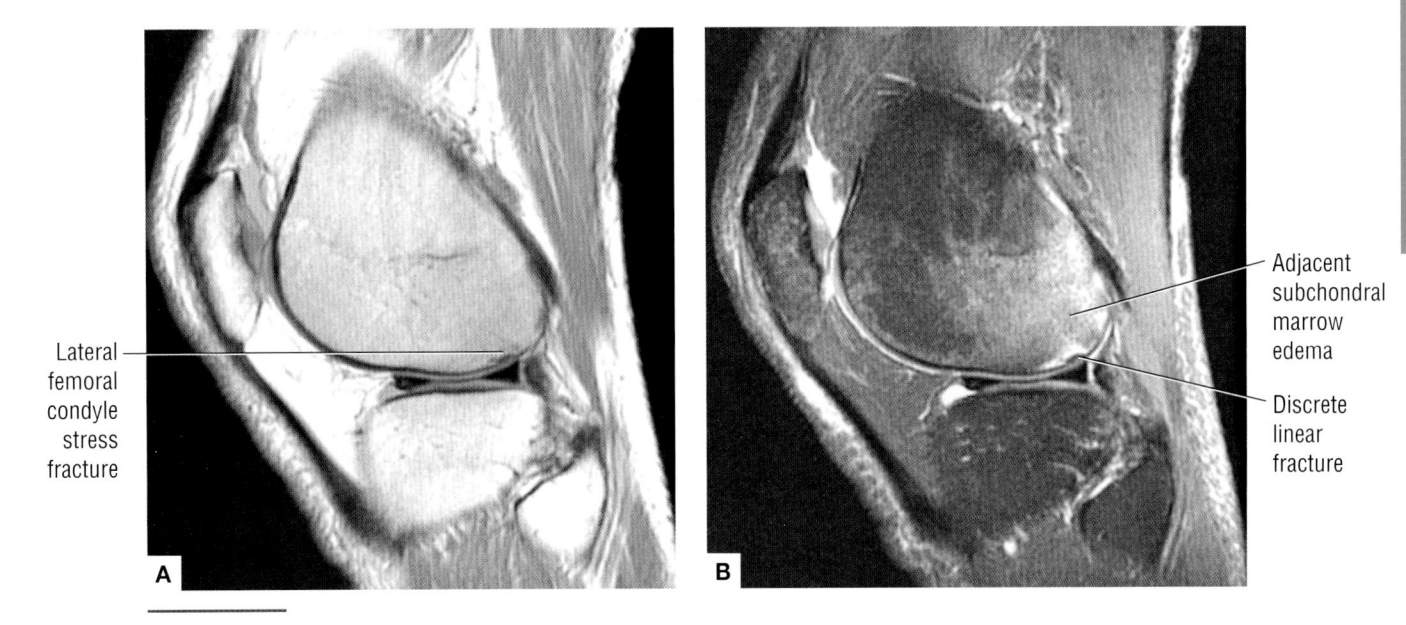

FIGURE 8.84 Discrete femoral condyle linear subcondylar stress fracture located lateral and posterior within the lateral femoral condyle. Based on its eccentric location and lack of a convex upper border, osteonecrosis can be excluded. (**A**) Sagittal PD FSE image. (**B**) Sagittal FS PD FSE image.

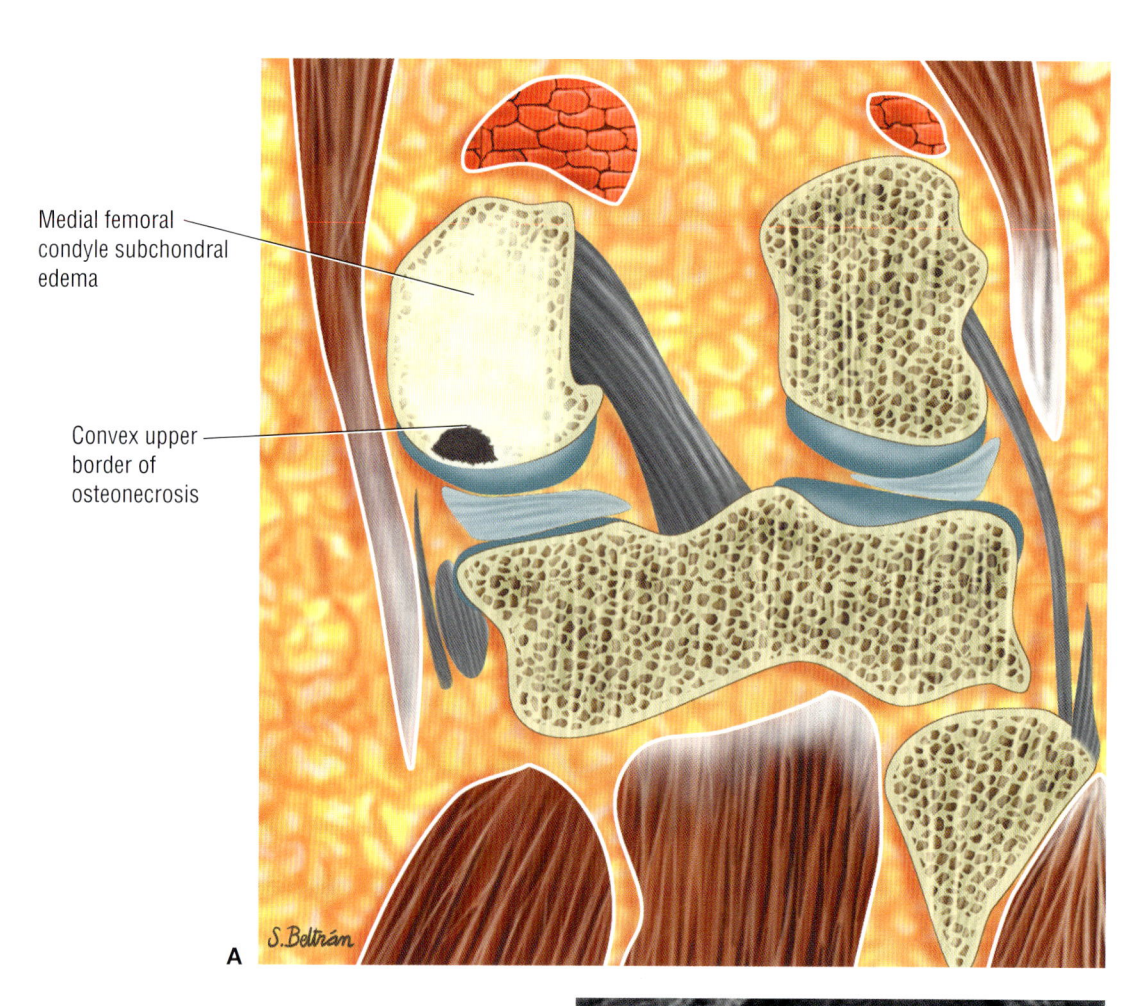

FIGURE 8.85 (**A**) The characteristic convex upper border demarcating a subchondral focus of osteonecrosis in spontaneous osteonecrosis of the knee (SONK). This morphology would be unusual in an insufficiency or stress fracture. Convex interface of hypointense necrotic defect in the medial femoral condyle on (**B**) a coronal FS PD FSE image.

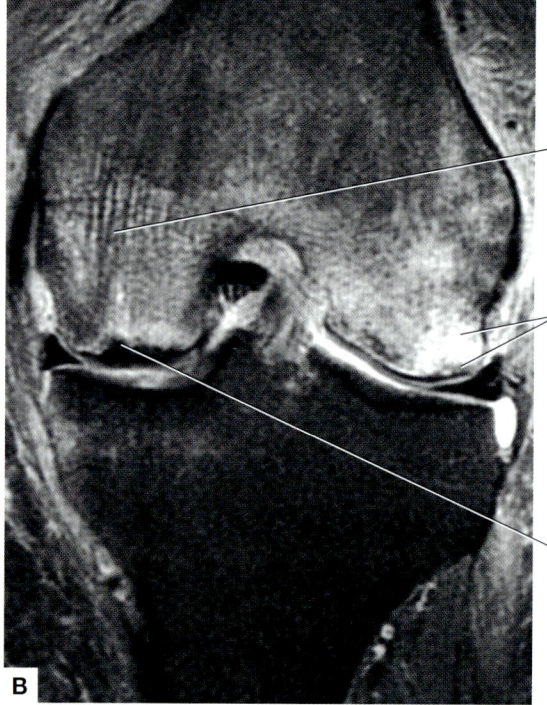

General Pathologic Conditions Affecting the Knee

Subtle subchondral fracture indicating acute on chronic

Thickened subchondral plate

Hyperintense bone marrow edema

Thickened subchondral plate

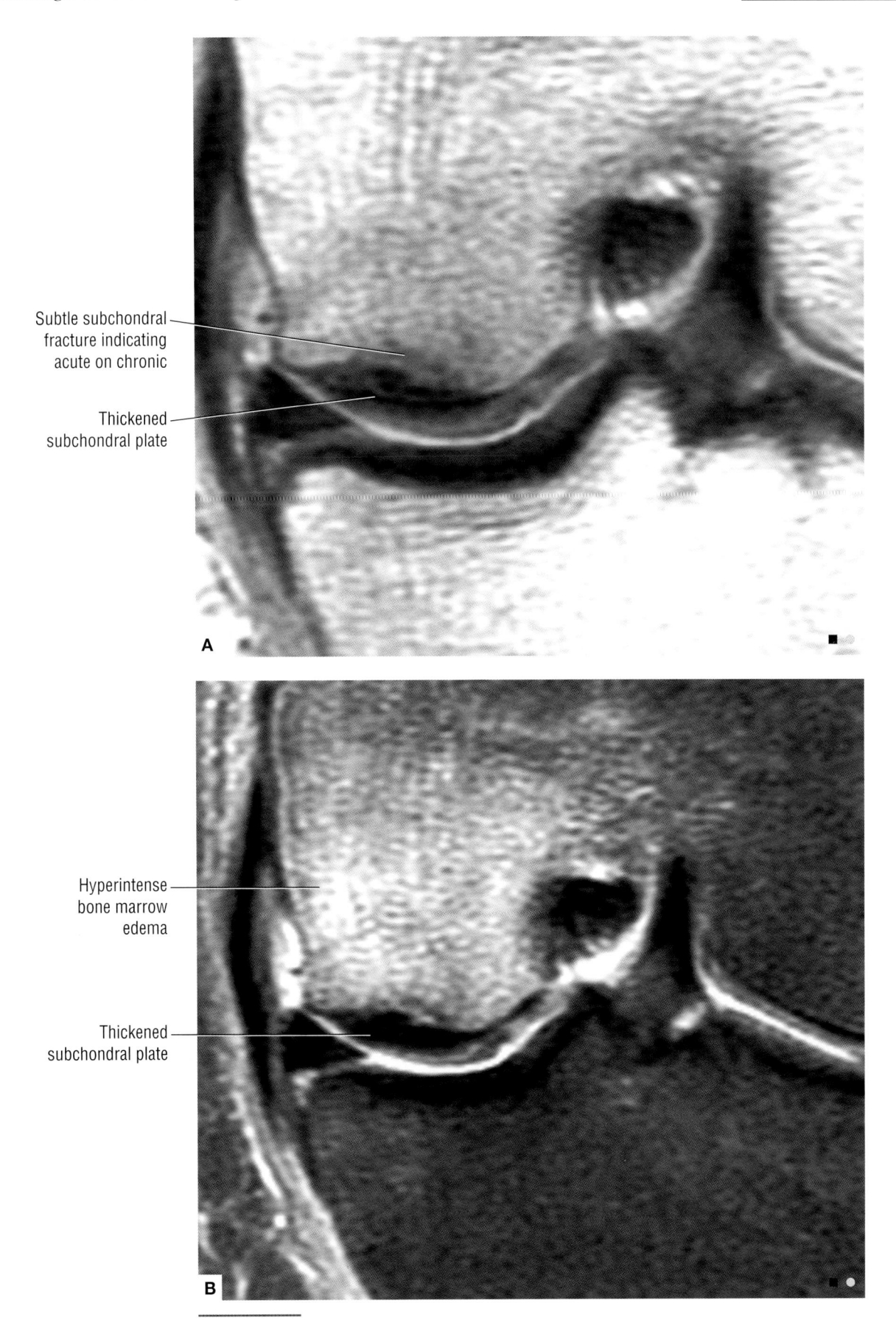

FIGURE 8.86 Acute-on-chronic changes with MR features of spontaneous osteonecrosis of the knee (SONK) with thickened head in reparative phase of a subchondral fracture with adjacent, subtle, more acute insufficiency fracture in deep subchondral bone. Coronal PD (**A**) and FS PD (**B**) images.

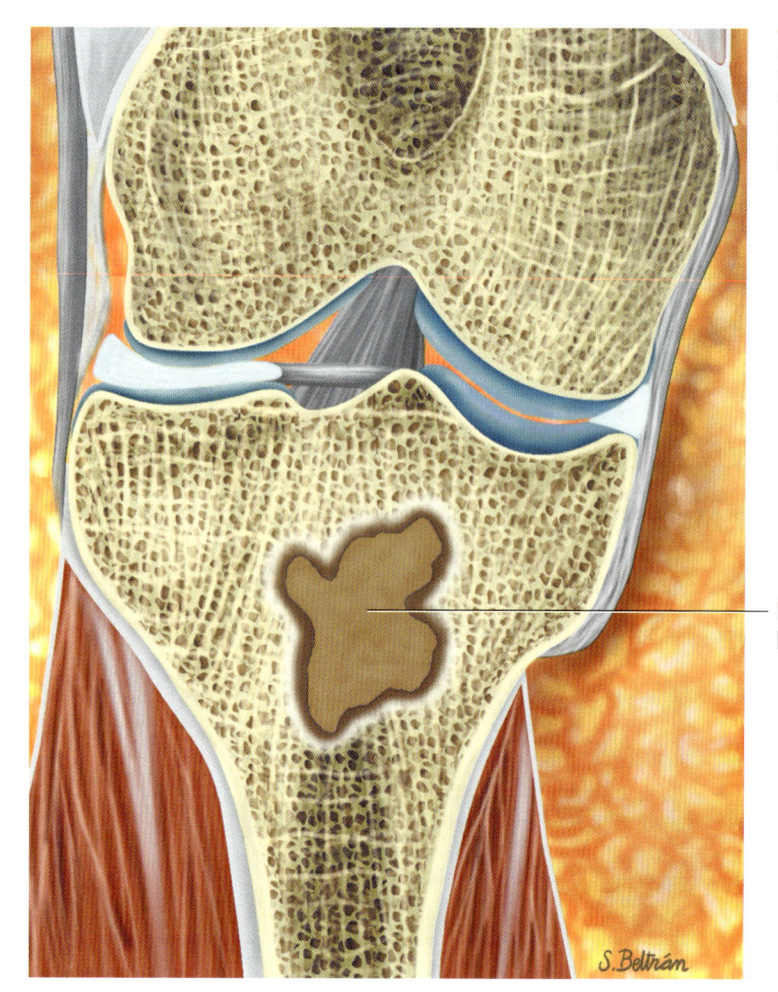

FIGURE 8.87 Serpiginous border of medullary infarct. Metaphyseal involvement is more common than epiphyseal or diaphyseal involvement.

Metaphyseal bone infarct

Bone Infarcts

- Usually metaphyseal in location, but also found in epiphyseal and diaphyseal locations

- May be seen in association with steroid therapy when part of a chemotherapy protocol

- MR appearance

    - Characteristic serpiginous low-signal-intensity border of reactive bone and central component of high-signal-intensity yellow or fat marrow

    - On T2-weighted images, chemical-shift artifact seen as high-signal-intensity line paralleling outline of infarct

    - May also demonstrate areas of mild contrast enhancement with IV gadolinium administration

    - When calcified, demonstrate low signal intensity on T1- and T2-weighted images

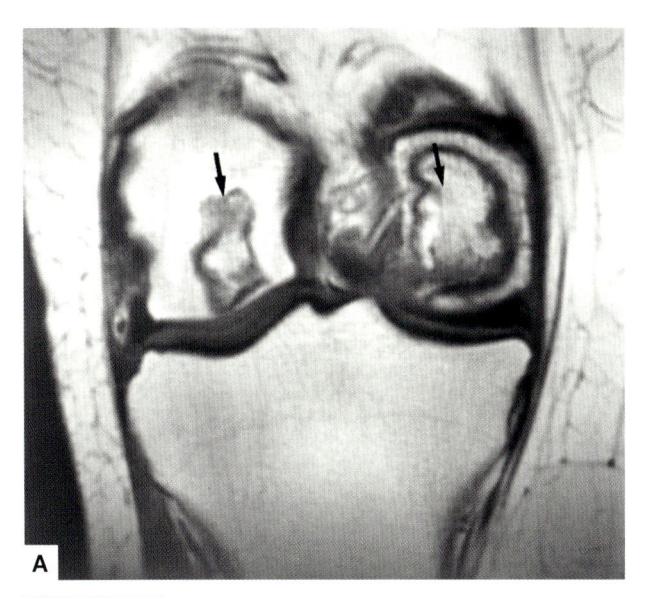

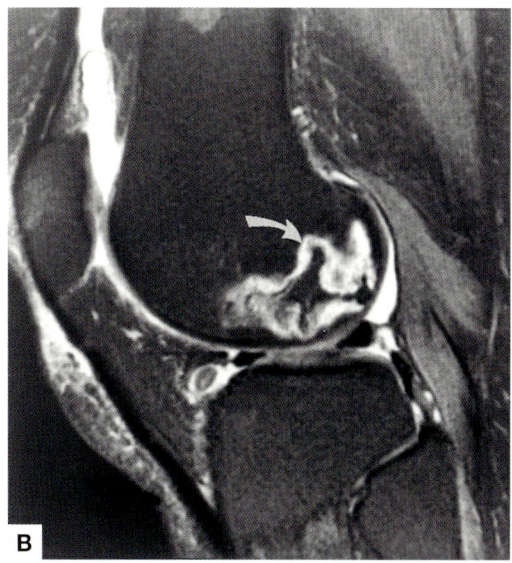

General Pathologic Conditions Affecting the Knee

FIGURE 8.88 Subchondral bone infarcts (*straight arrows*) of the medial and lateral femoral condyle on (**A**) T1-weighted coronal image and (**B**) FS PD-weighted FSE sagittal images. The infarcts display central fatty marrow signal characteristics and are associated with a peripheral rim (*curved arrow*) of reactive tissue (hypointense on T1-weighted images and hyperintense on T2-weighted images) that is involved in the process of gradual substitution. New bone is found at the circumference of the infarct.

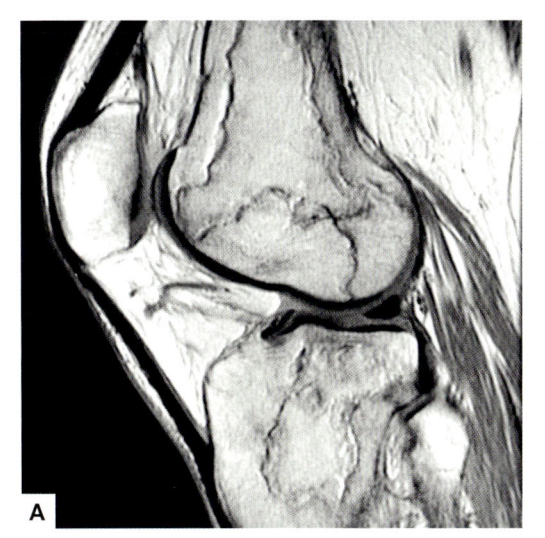

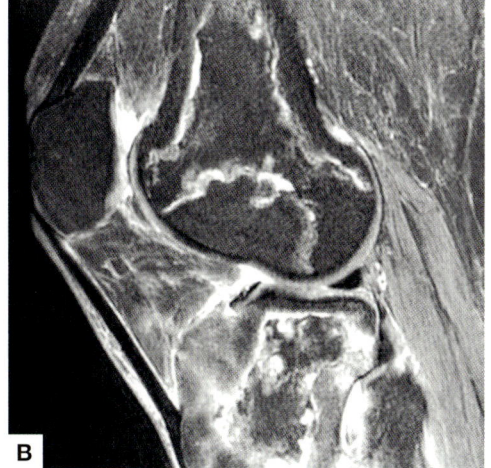

FIGURE 8.89 Sagittal PD (**A**) and FS PD FSE (**B**) images with subcondylar extension of diffuse medullary infarcts.

- Fibroblastic reactive tissue at healing interface of infarct demonstrates hyperintensity on heavily T2-weighted, FS PD-weighted FSE, and STIR images

- Epiphyseal infarcts or infarcts abutting subchondral surface may weaken subchondral plate, resulting in microfractures and articular surface collapse.

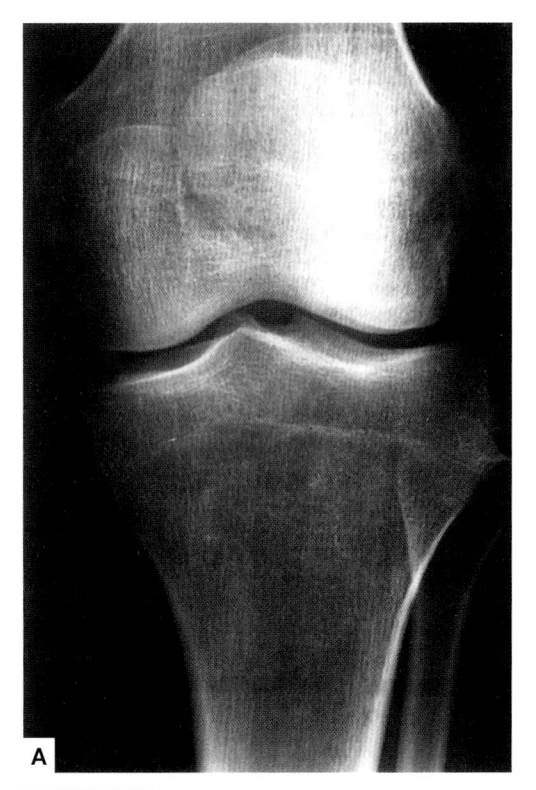

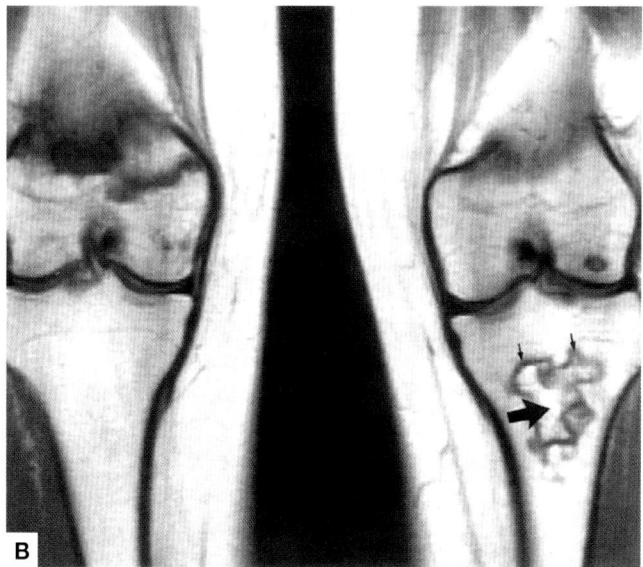

FIGURE 8.90 A bone infarct that is not seen on an anteroposterior radiograph (**A**) is revealed on a T1-weighted coronal image (**B**) with characteristic serpiginous low-signal-intensity peripheral sclerosis (*small arrows*) and a high-signal-intensity central portion (*large arrows*).

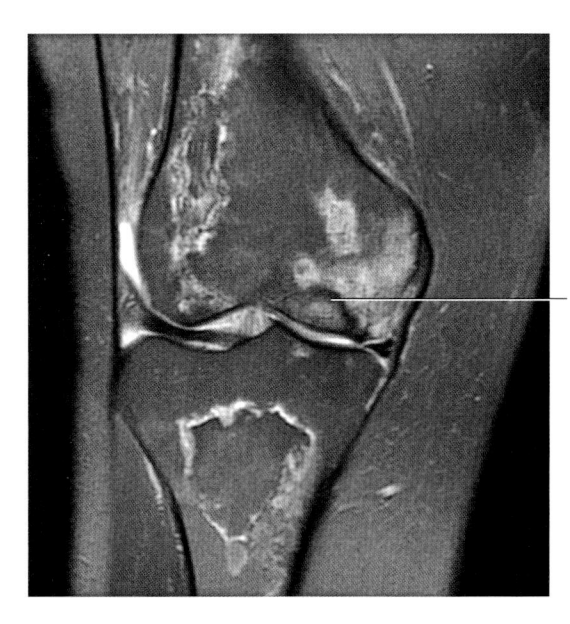

Medial femoral condyle osteonecrosis demarcated from the adjacent medullary infarcts

FIGURE 8.91 The subchondral extension of the medial femoral condylar infarct is associated with the complication of a subchondral fracture characteristic of medial femoral condyle osteonecrosis. Predisposing factors include trauma, steroids (endogenous and exogenous), and collagen vascular disease (e.g., systemic lupus erythematosus), renal transplant, pancreatitis, alcoholism, Gaucher's disease, sickle cell anemia, gout, and arteritis. Coronal FS PD FSE image.

Osteochondritis Dissecans

- Differs from spontaneous osteonecrosis of the knee in that it primarily affects male patients 10 to 20 years of age and typically involves the lateral surface of the medial femoral condyle[41,282,318,392]

- Represents an osteochondrosis characterized by necrosis of bone followed by reossification and healing[385]

- Subchondral bone changes may demonstrate areas of signal inhomogeneity and direct extension of subchondral fluid.

- Imbibed high-signal-intensity subchondral fluid implies fissuring of overlying articular cartilage.
    - Has high correlation with lesion instability, especially when fluid circles entire fragment in its circumference[99]
    - Focal cystic regions deep to lesion also associated with instability
    - IV gadolinium enhancement of granulation tissue between the necrotic fragment and parent bone also correlates with fragment loosening and instability.[122]

Osteochondritis Dissecans Pathology

- History of knee trauma found in as many as 50% of patients

- Granulation tissue advances into region between necrotic fragment and healing bone.

- Articular cartilage (the only remaining support for necrotic bone) may fail, resulting in detachment or fragmentation of articular cartilage into joint.

- Fluid in base of necrotic lesion, without direct communication with joint, usually implies abnormal overlying articular cartilage surface, which may or may not allow extension of intraarticular injected contrast or saline.

- Hyperintensity between lesion and adjacent bone on FS PD FSE images represents either fluid or granulation tissue.

- Lesion stability is related to absence of increased signal intensity at fragment interface on T2-weighted images.[114]

- Healed lesions
    - Do not demonstrate bright-signal-intensity interface between fragment and adjacent bone of femoral condyle
    - Return of marrow fat signal intensity in previously necrotic fragment
    - Intact overlying articular cartilage surface without any residual contour irregularities
- Normal subchondral epiphyseal hypointensity with overlying chondral inhomogeneity may be seen in both femoral condyles in immature skeleton.[498]
    - May represent normal pattern of ossification during epiphyseal maturation
- Classically, lesions located in lateral aspect of medial femoral condyle (55%)
    - Less commonly involve central portion of medial femoral condyle (25%)[41]
    - May also affect lateral femoral condyle (18%)
        - Association between osteochondritis dissecans of lateral femoral condyle and discoid lateral meniscus
        - May uncommonly involve anterolateral femoral condyle or lateral aspect of trochlear groove
    - May occur bilaterally (24%)
- Arthroscopic staging system for osteochondritis:
    - Stage 1: 1- to 3-cm lesion with intact articular cartilage
    - Stage 2: articular cartilage defect without loose body
    - Stage 3: partially detached osteochondral fragment, with or without fibrous tissue interposition
    - Stage 4: loose body with a crater filled with fibrous tissue[69,318]
        - Dislodged or free fragment may be seen on a different MR image than the donor site.
        - Free fragment may still contain a chondral surface.

MR Findings of Osteochondritis Dissecans

- Focus of osteochondritis demonstrates low signal intensity on T1- and T2-weighted images (before it can be detected on conventional radiographs).

- Follow-up imaging will exclude development of osteochondritis dissecans focus.

- Articular cartilage of distal femoral epiphysis becomes progressively heterogeneous with age.

- In patients 3 to 5 years of age, increased signal intensity can be seen in stippled pattern.

- With increasing age and advancing ossification, appearance progresses to ill-defined pattern and then a well-defined pattern of increased signal.

- MR particularly useful for identifying posterior condylar lesions in children

- T2 or STIR imaging techniques may reveal adjacent hyperintensity of medullary bone in unstable lesions, although it is unusual to see extensive marrow reaction (as seen in adult spontaneous osteonecrosis).

- Fragmentation or full-thickness fluid-filled fissures can be assessed on coronal and sagittal images.

- Edema of subchondral bone margin sclerosis, or anterior/posterior or medial/lateral fragment breakdown can be used to describe an unstable lesion or lesion at risk for further fragmentation.

Treatment of Osteochondritis Dissecans

- In young patients, range from nonoperative treatment to arthroscopic drilling of osteochondral fragment (stable intact lesion)

- Drilling may be used with internal fixation with screws or autogenous bone pegs in skeletally mature patients.

- Cancellous grooves used for internal fixation of fragments when healing more difficult to achieve

- Loose osteochondral fragments removed

- Partially detached fragments treated with débridement before reduction and stabilization[510]

OCD of medial femoral condyle

Subchondral edema
OCD fragment
Chondral fissure

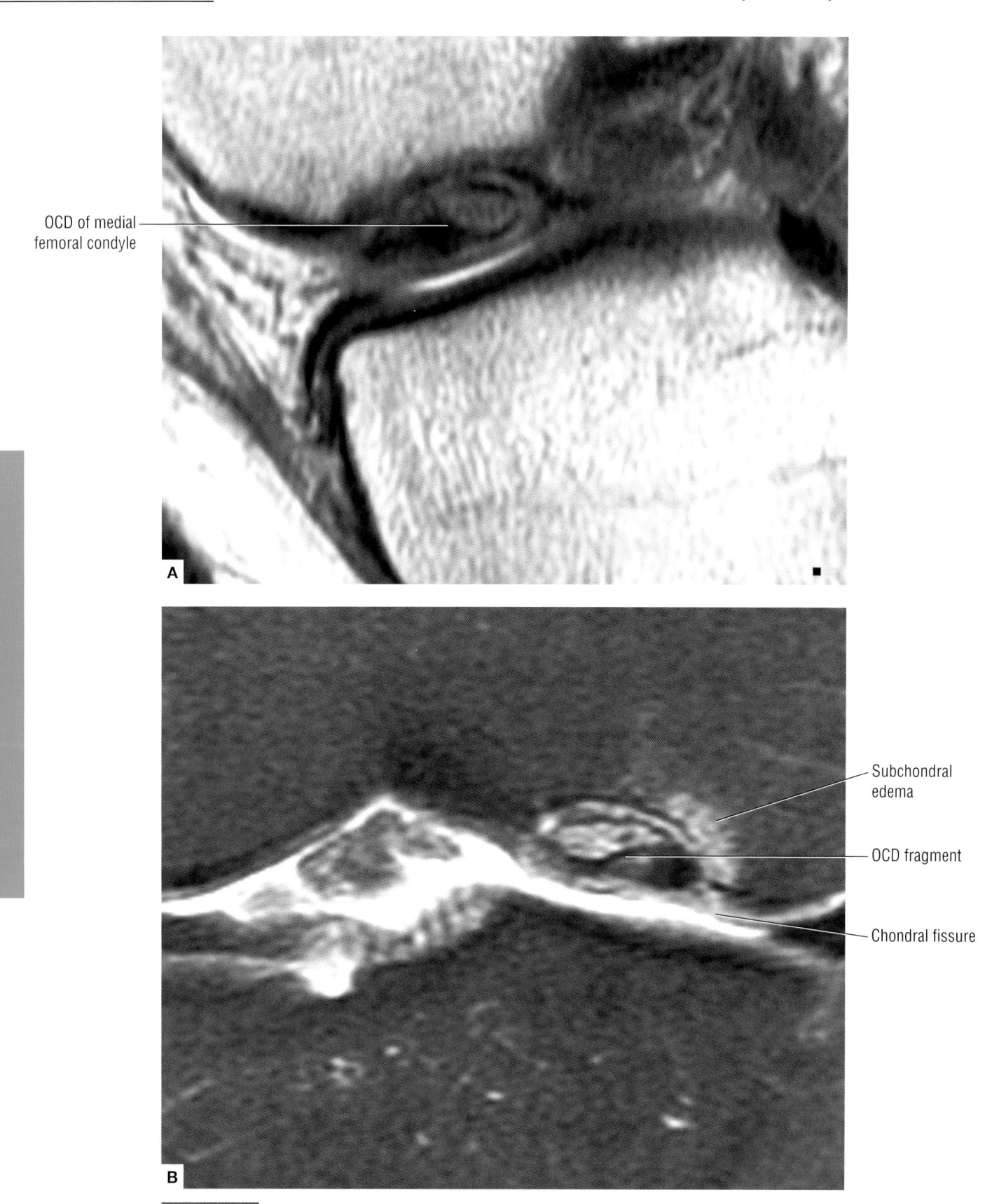

FIGURE 8.92 Osteochondritis dissecans with subchondral edema and chondral fissures placing this lesion at risk for further fragmentation. Sagittal (**A**) and coronal FS PD (**B**) images.

Osteochondritis Dissecans

FIGURE 8.93 Extended pattern of osteochondritis dissecans (OCD) of the medial femoral condyle involving a portion of the weight-bearing surface. Osteochondritis dissecans is common in adolescents and young adults. Chronic injury may result in this form of osteochondral fracture.

- OCD extended pattern involving weight bearing medial femoral condyle

- Uninvolved lateral aspect of medial femoral condyle
- Inferocentral OCD

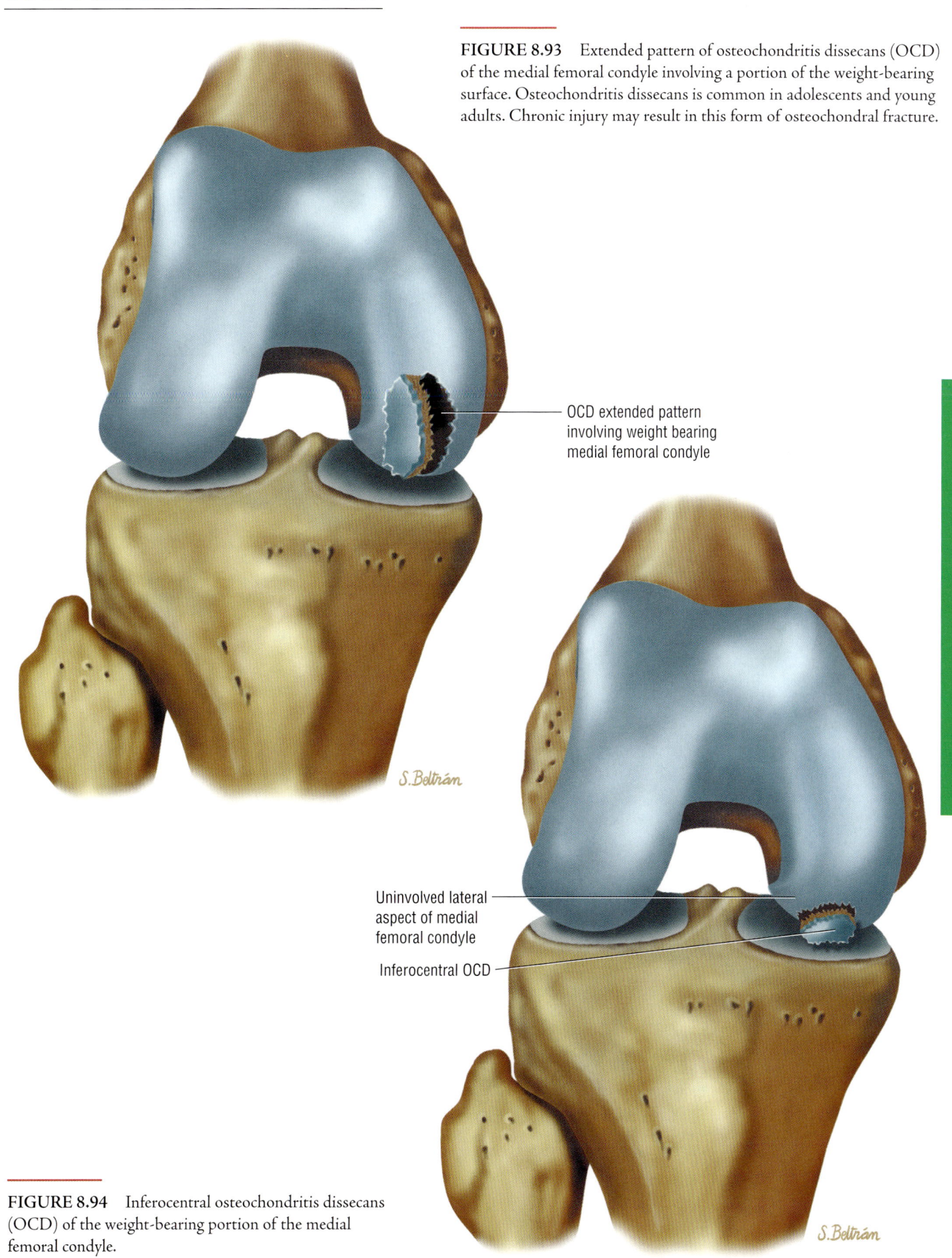

FIGURE 8.94 Inferocentral osteochondritis dissecans (OCD) of the weight-bearing portion of the medial femoral condyle.

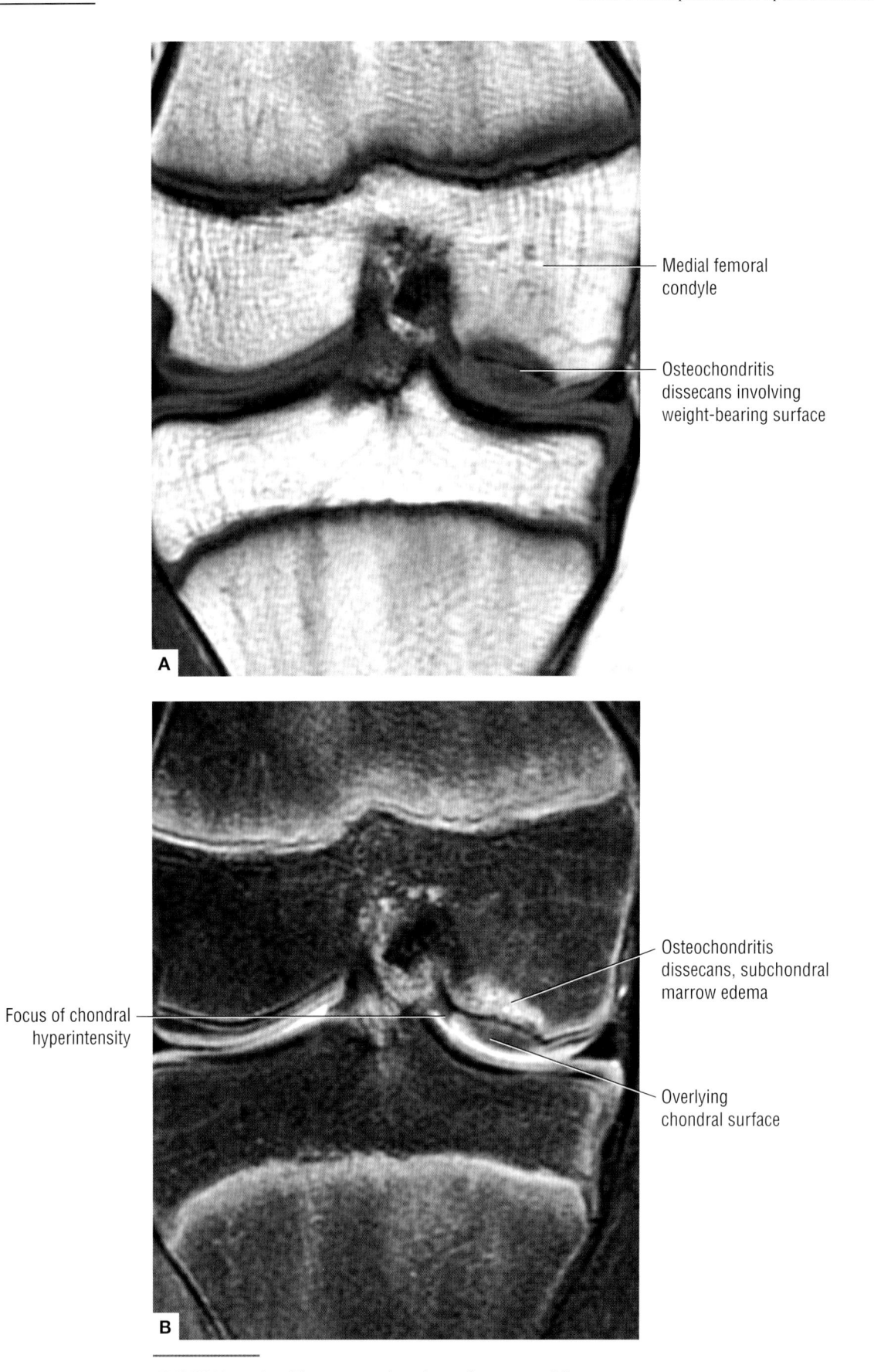

FIGURE 8.95 Classic osteochondritis dissecans of the non-weight-bearing lateral aspect of the medial femoral condyle and intercondylar notch. (**A**) Coronal T1-weighted FSE image. (**B**) Coronal FS PD FSE image.

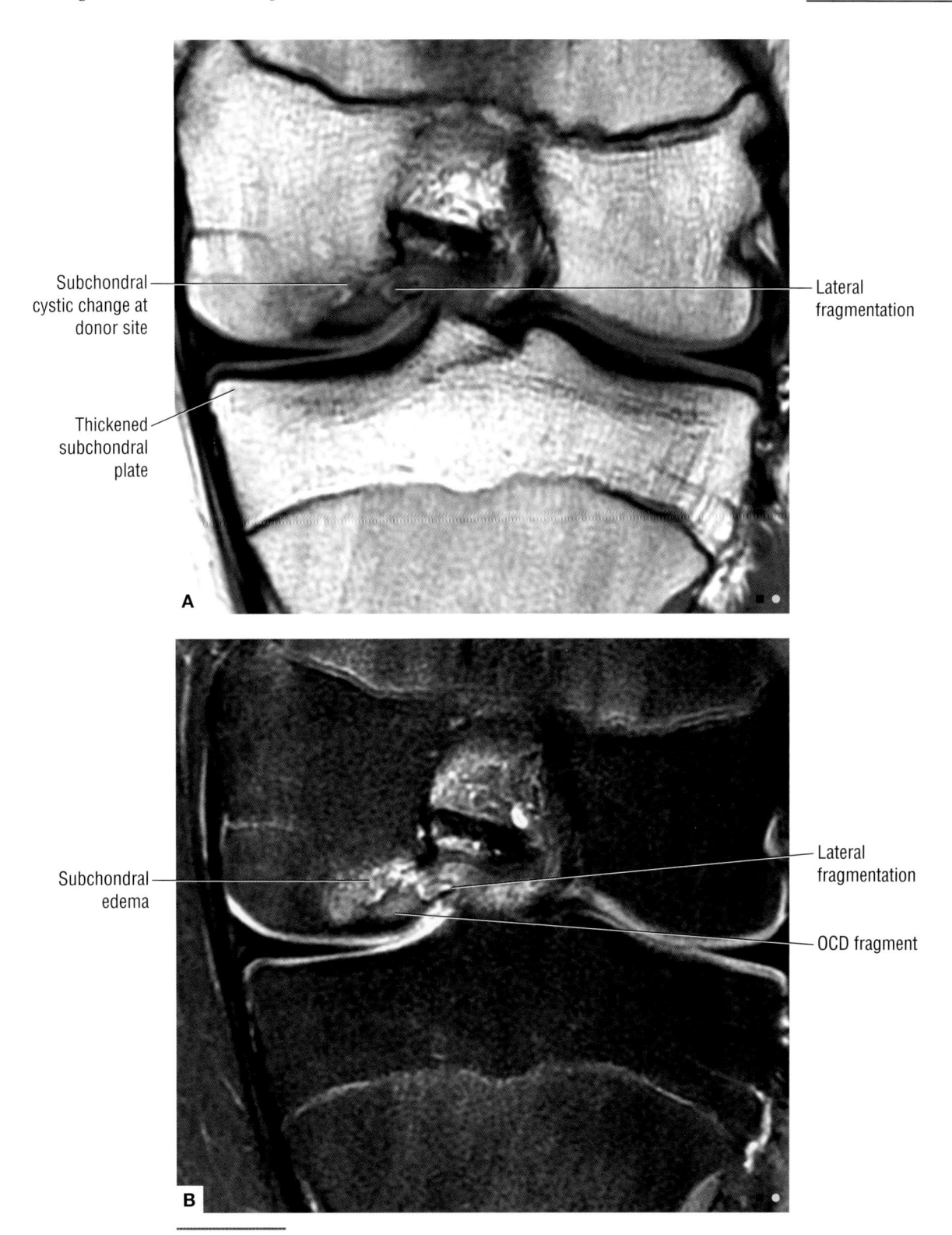

FIGURE 8.96 Unstable osteochondritis dissecans (OCD) involving the lateral aspect of the medial femoral condyle. Fragmentation of the lateral aspect of the fragment and full thickness chondral fissures at posterior region of the lesion are associated with segment instability. Although there is no hyperintense fluid circumscribing the lesion, the multiple small hyperintense cysts at the fragment interface increase specificity for an unstable lesion. The gradient echo sequence displaced more segment hyperintensity than the corresponding FS PD FSE. A T1-weighted image, however, may be more accurate in predicting vascular potential for healing than hyperintense edema on a fluid-sensitive sequence. Coronal PD (**A**) and FS PD (**B**) images. (*Continued*)

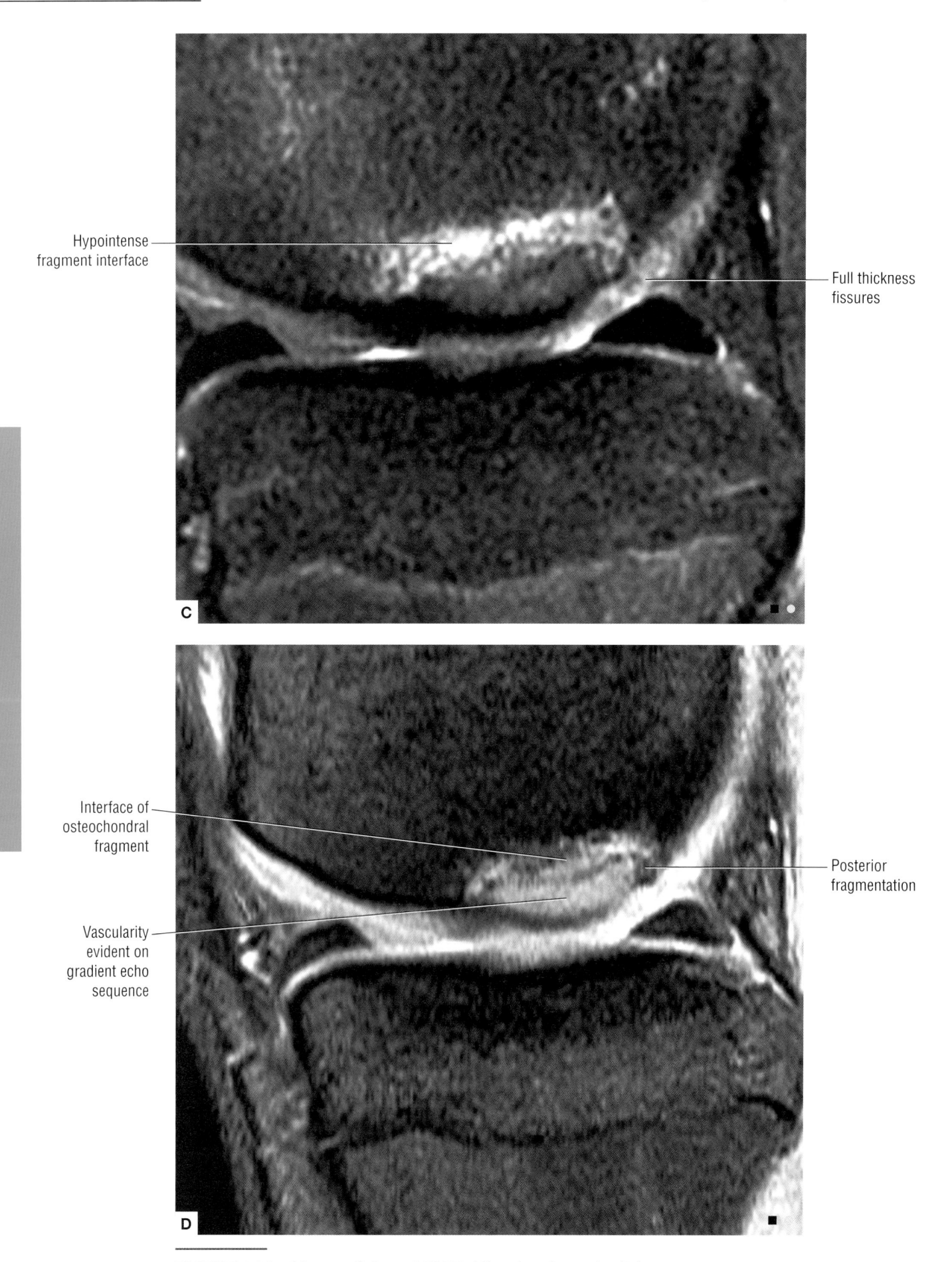

FIGURE 8.96 (*Continued*) Sagittal FS PD (**C**) and gradient echo (**D**) images.

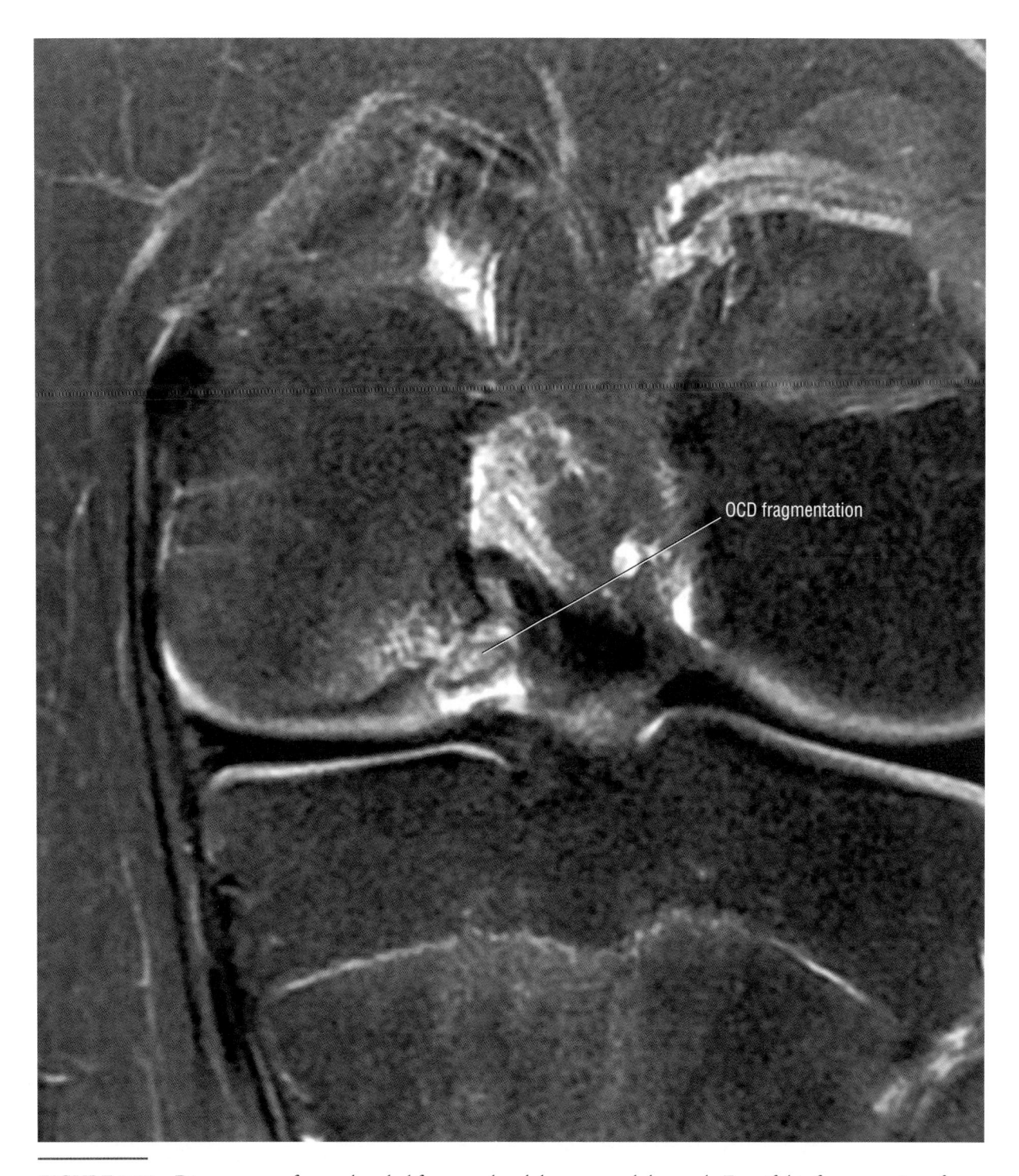

General Pathologic Conditions Affecting the Knee

FIGURE 8.97 Discrete area of osteochondral fragment breakdown toward the notch. Even if this fragmentation of the lateral aspect of the osteochondritis dissecans is attached by synovium, it is still an unstable lesion at risk for further fragmentation. Coronal FS PD FSE image.

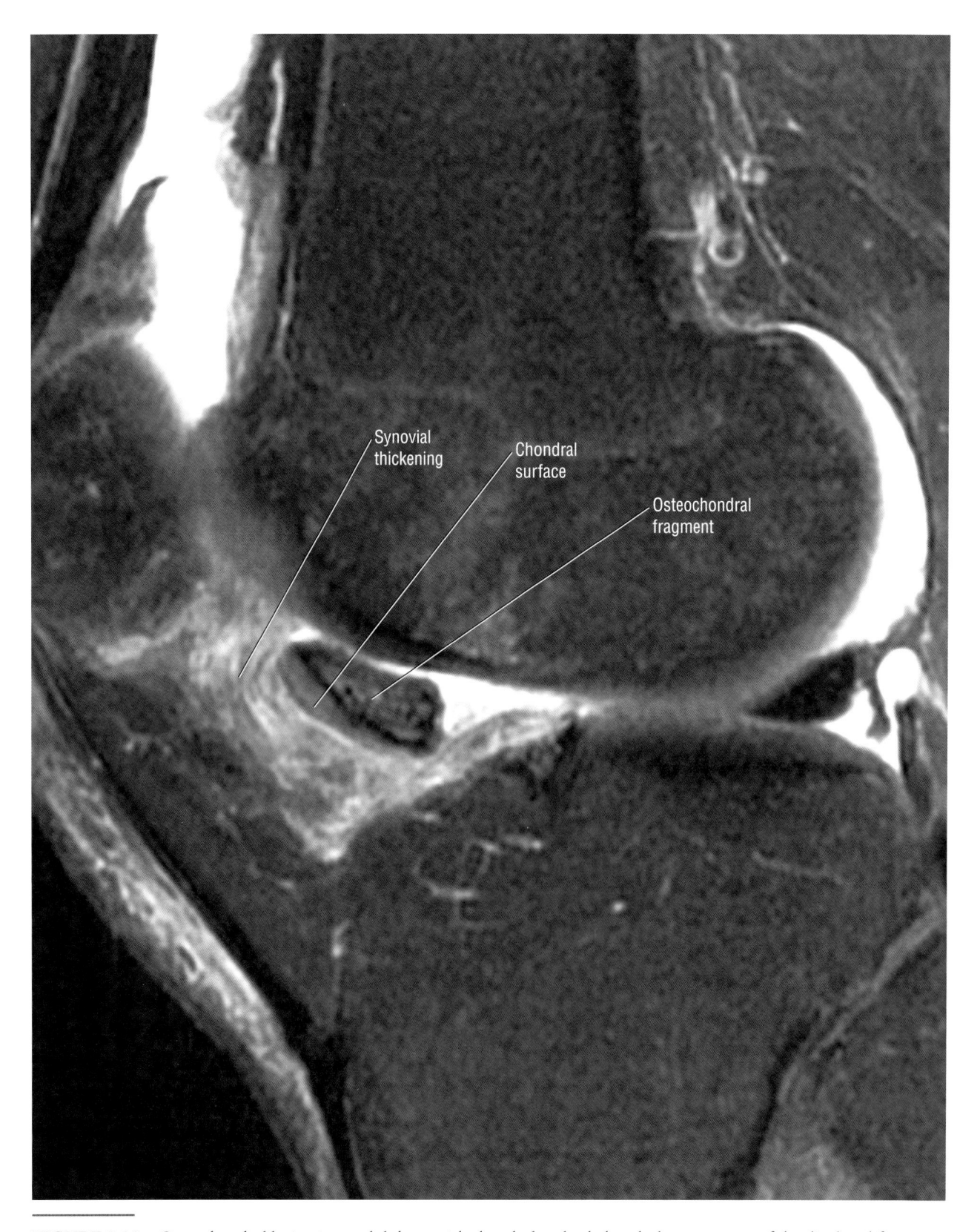

FIGURE 8.98 Osteochondral lesion in an adult knee with chondral and subchondral components of the displaced fragment visible posterior to Hoffa's fat pad. Localized inflammation and synovial thickening occur adjacent to the osteochondritis dissecans fragment. Chondral pathology is usually associated with synovitis. Sagittal FS PD FSE image.

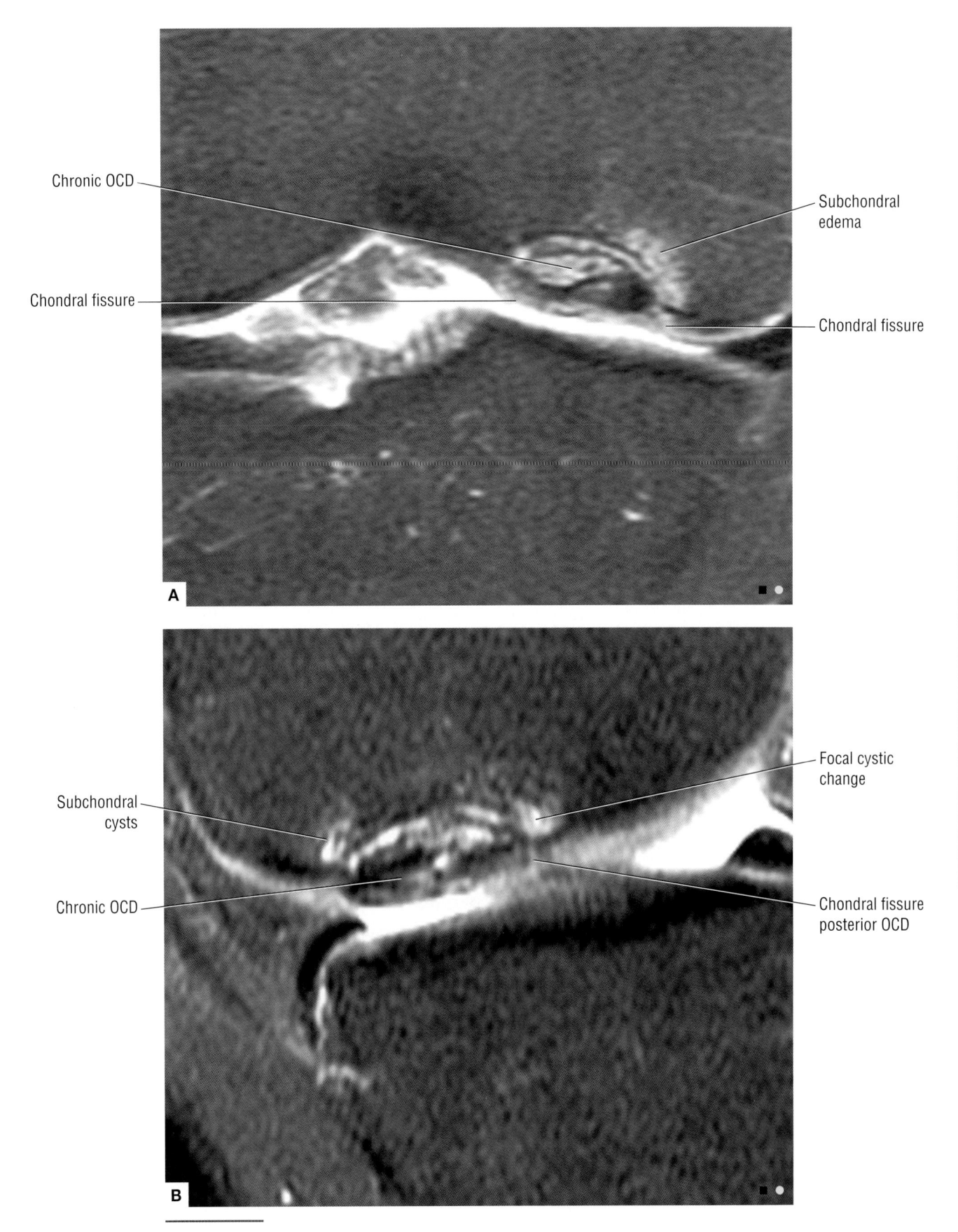

FIGURE 8.99 Young adult sequela of osteochondritis dissecans with linear hyperintense interface and development of multiple small cysts in parent bone bed of the medial femoral condyle. Fragment size is also reported in two planes. Larger fragments (>1cm) are also associated with instability. Focal subchondral cystic change is often associated with adjacent full thickness chondral fissures. Coronal (**A**) and sagittal (**B**) FS PD FSE image.

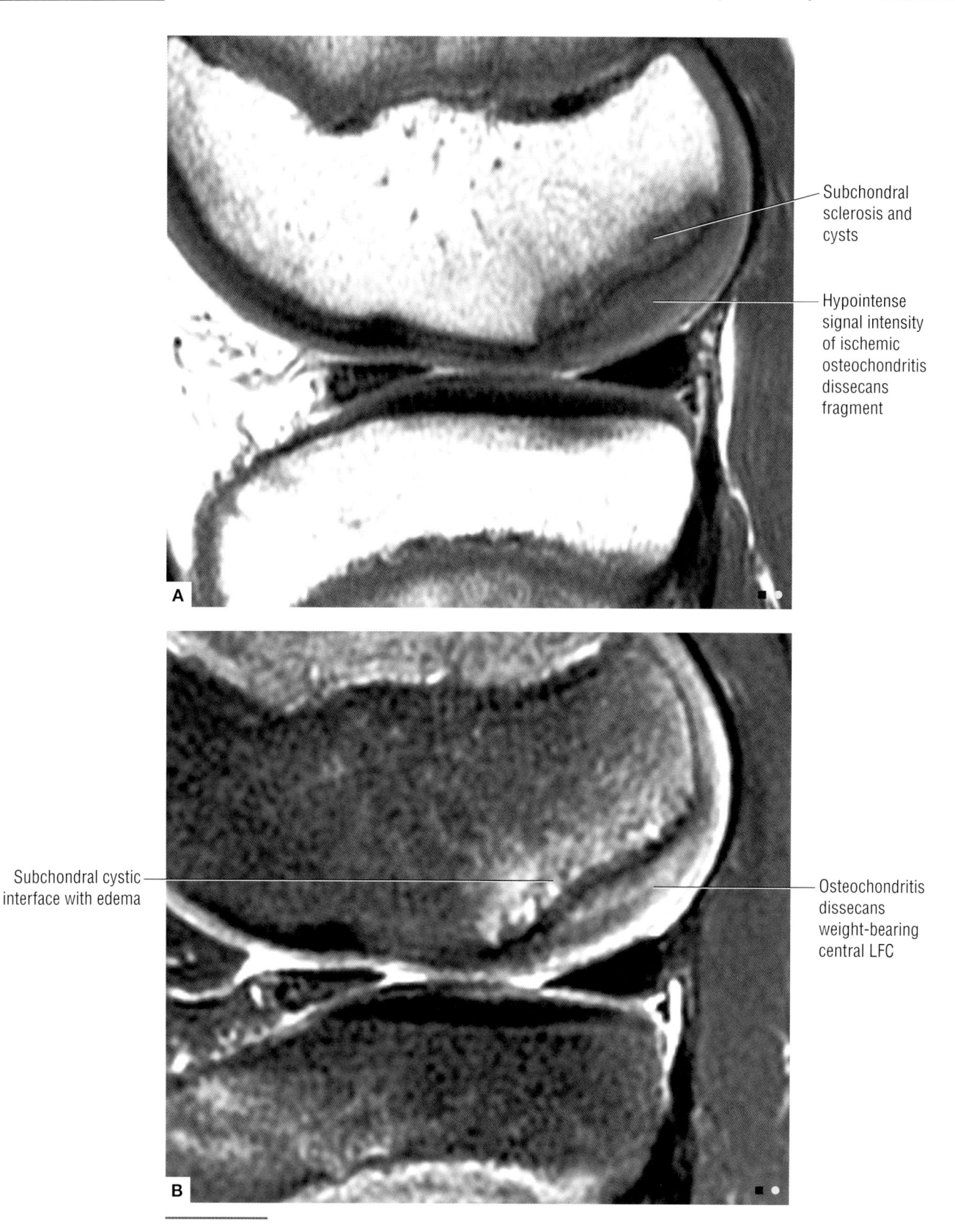

FIGURE 8.100 Osteochondritis dissecans of the lateral femoral condyle (LFC). There is continuity of overlying articular cartilage at this stage. The edema and cystic change at the junction with the deeper subchondral bone imply excessive loading of the LFC as a result of the structurally weakened subchondral ischemic bone. The lesion of osteochondritis dissecans occurs in the growing (immature) skeleton and involves trauma, ischemia, and an ossification center at risk. Disruption of the epiphyseal plate may disrupt osteogenesis and chondrogenesis, producing disordered endochondral ossification and subsequent subchondral ischemic or avascular necrosis. Sagittal PD (**A**) and FS PD (**B**) images.

General Pathologic Conditions Affecting the Knee

Osteochondritis Dissecans

FIGURE 8.101 Inferocentral osteochondritis dissecans (OCD) of the lateral femoral condyle.

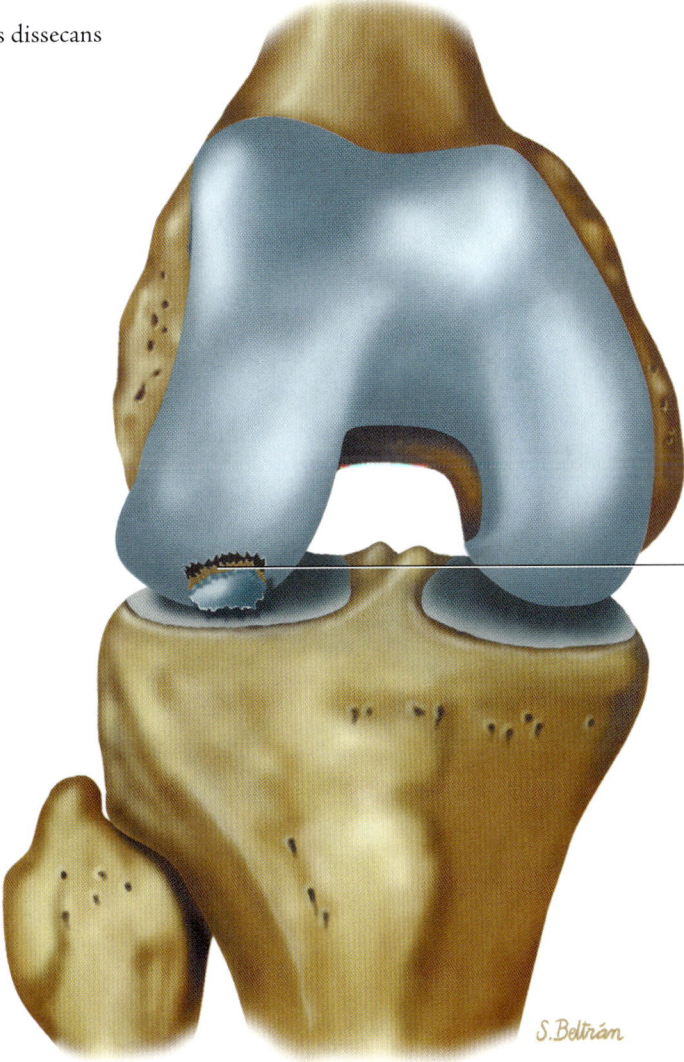

- Inferocentral OCD of the lateral femoral condyle

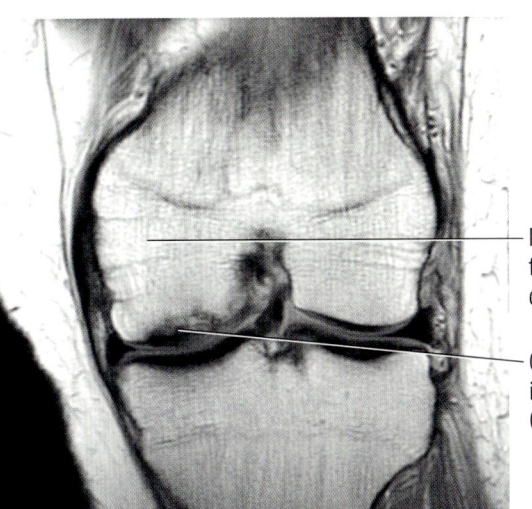

FIGURE 8.102 Inferocentral osteochondritis dissecans (OCD) of the weight-bearing portion of the medial femoral condyle. Note that the more lateral aspect of the medial femoral condyle is spared. Coronal T1 image.

- Medial femoral condyle
- Chronic inferocentral OCD

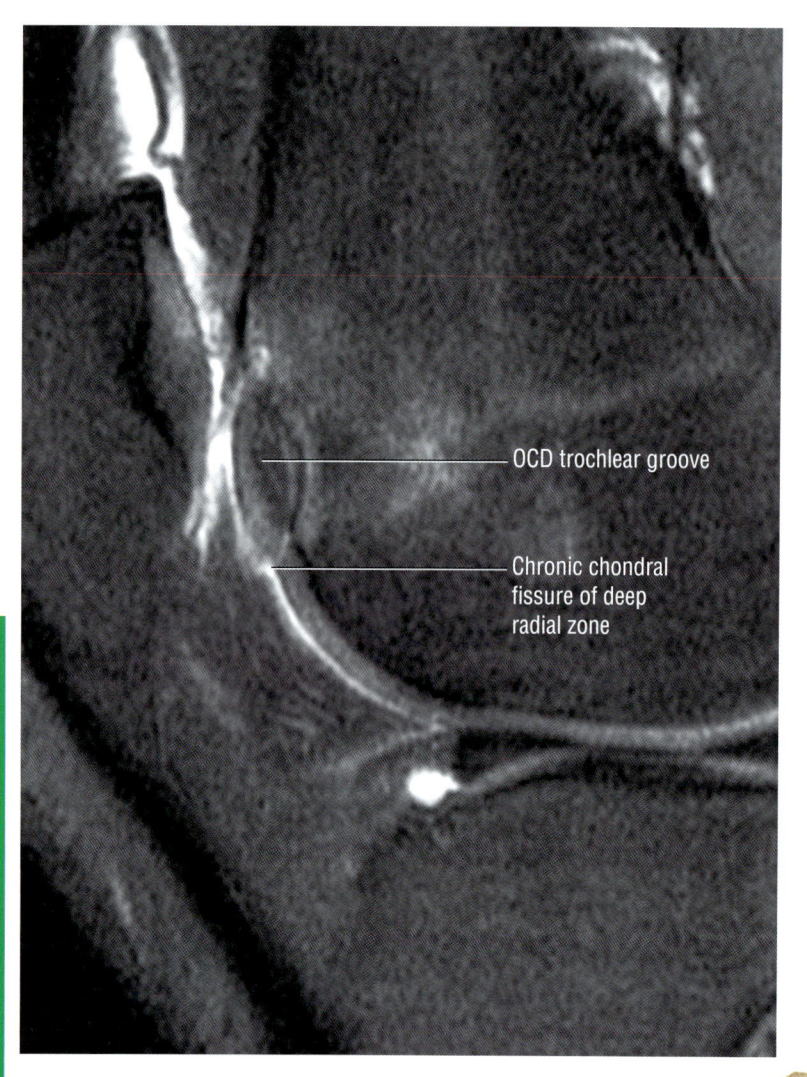

FIGURE 8.103 Clinically stable osteochondritis dissecans of the lateral femoral condyle with chronic fissure of deep radial zone articular cartilage at the inferior aspect of the fragment. There is no hyperintense marrow reaction, and the trochlear groove surface is congruent. Sagittal FS PD FSE image.

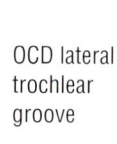

FIGURE 8.104 A lateral view color illustration of osteochondritis dissecans (OCD) of the anterior aspect of the lateral femoral condyle.

General Pathologic Conditions Affecting the Knee

- Delamination
- Trochlear groove osteochondritis dissecans
- Chondral delamination
- Subchondral cystic change and edema in trochlear groove osteochondritis dissecans

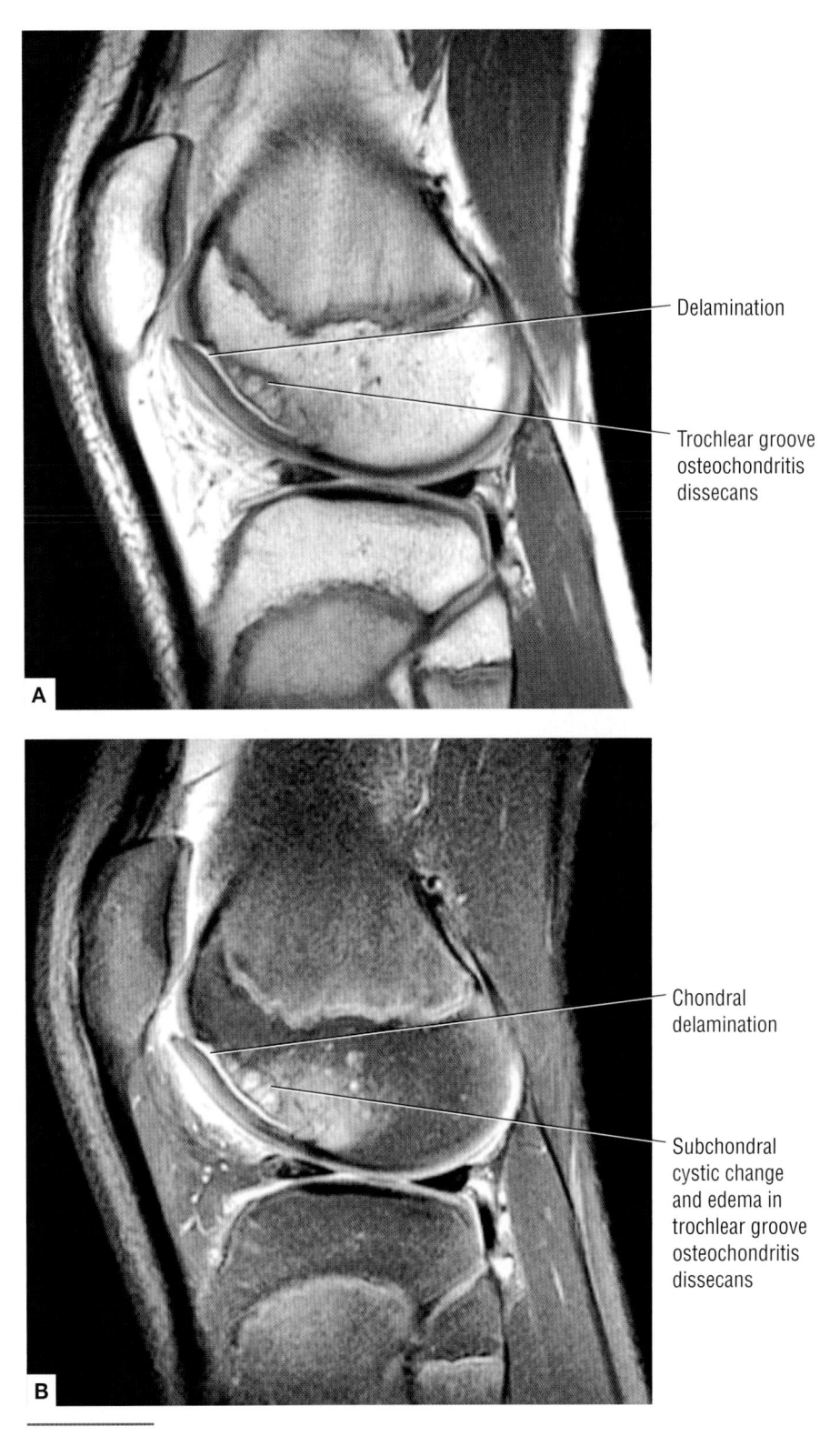

FIGURE 8.105 Anterolateral femoral condyle osteochondritis dissecans with delamination of trochlear groove articular cartilage on sagittal PD FSE (**A**) and FS PD FSE (**B**) images.

Osteochondritis Dissecans

FIGURE 8.106 In situ osteochondral fragment in osteochondritis dissecans (OCD) with an intact overlying chondral surface.

FIGURE 8.107 The development of an osteocartilaginous flap in osteochondritis dissecans (OCD).

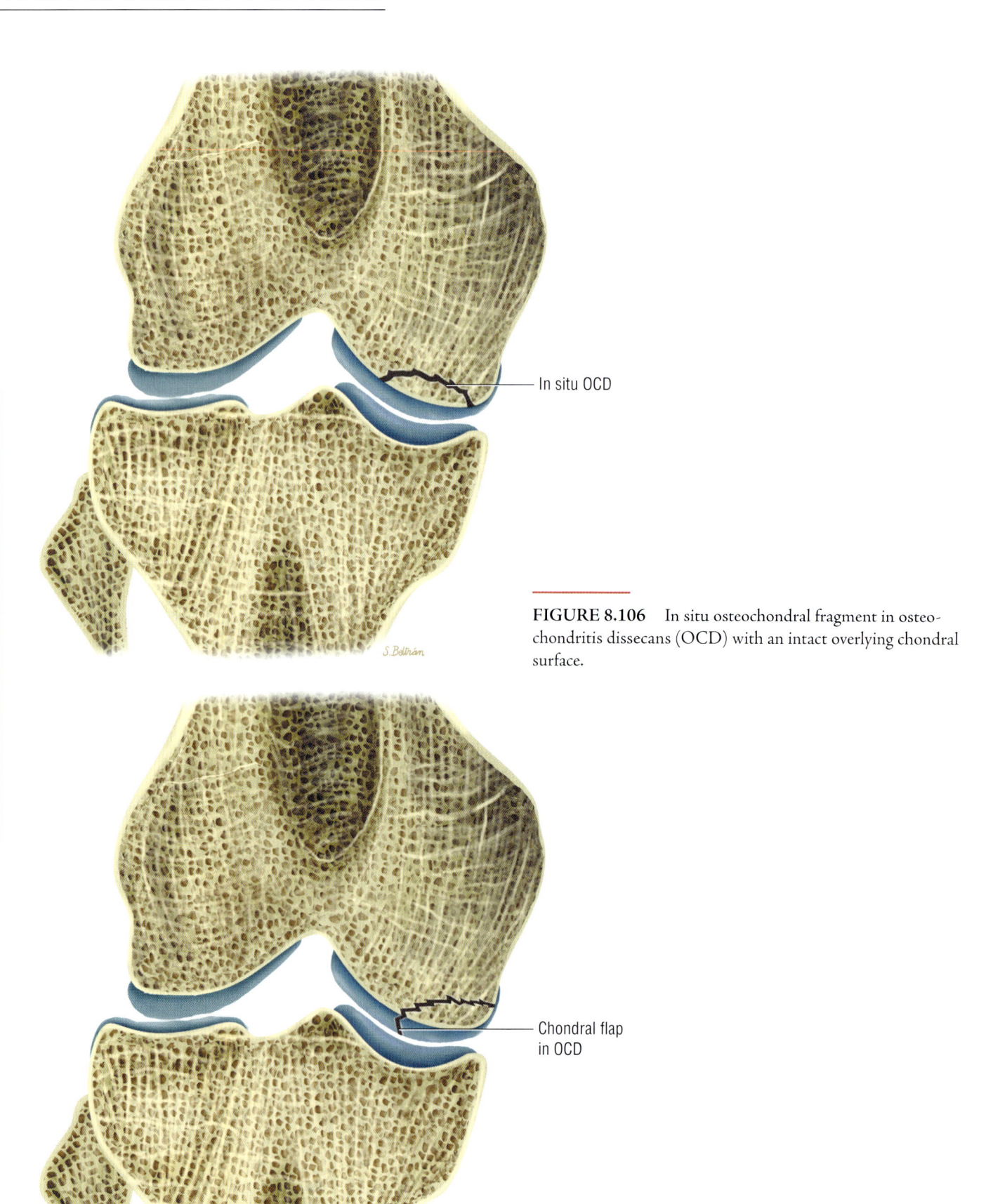

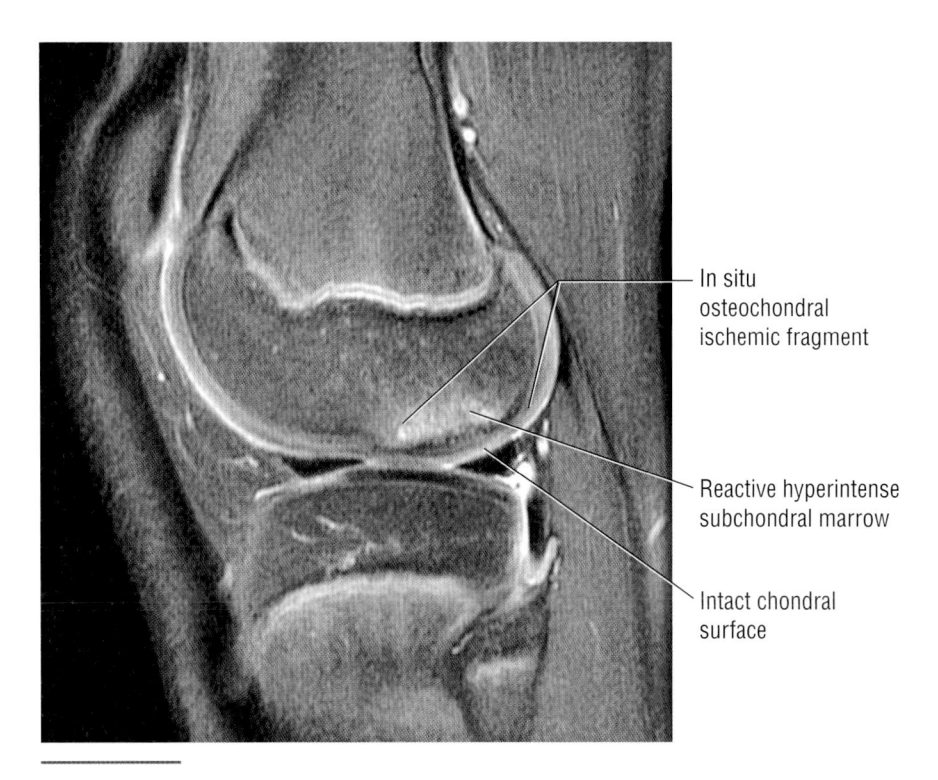

General Pathologic Conditions Affecting the Knee

FIGURE 8.108 Intact articular cartilage with reactive edema at subchondral interface with an in situ osteochondral segment on a sagittal FS PD FSE image.

- In situ osteochondral ischemic fragment
- Reactive hyperintense subchondral marrow
- Intact chondral surface

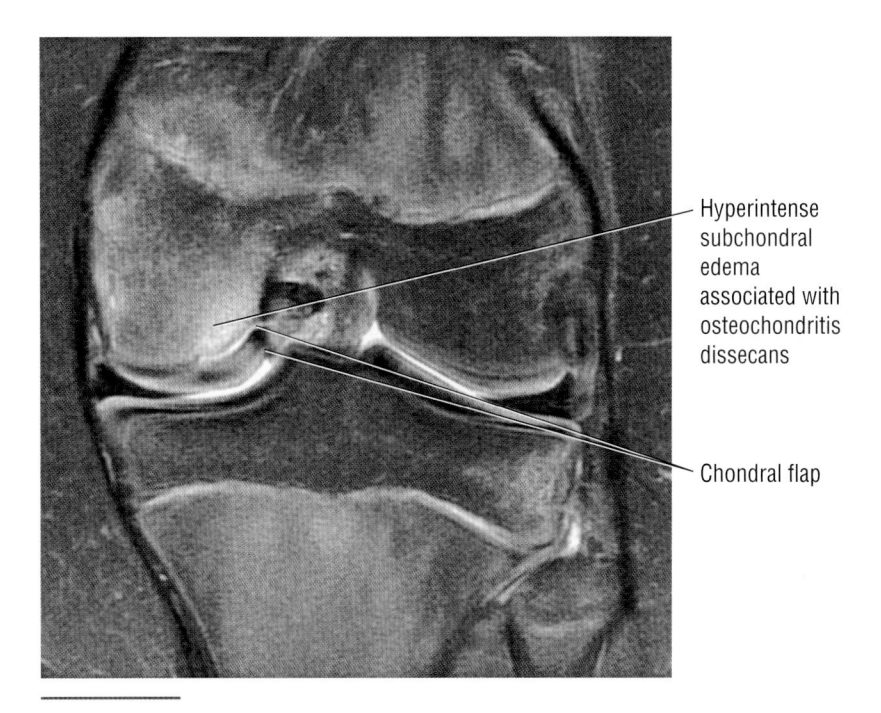

FIGURE 8.109 Coronal FS PD FSE showing fluid undermining the articular cartilage and producing an osteocartilaginous flap in osteochondritis dissecans of the medial femoral condyle.

- Hyperintense subchondral edema associated with osteochondritis dissecans
- Chondral flap

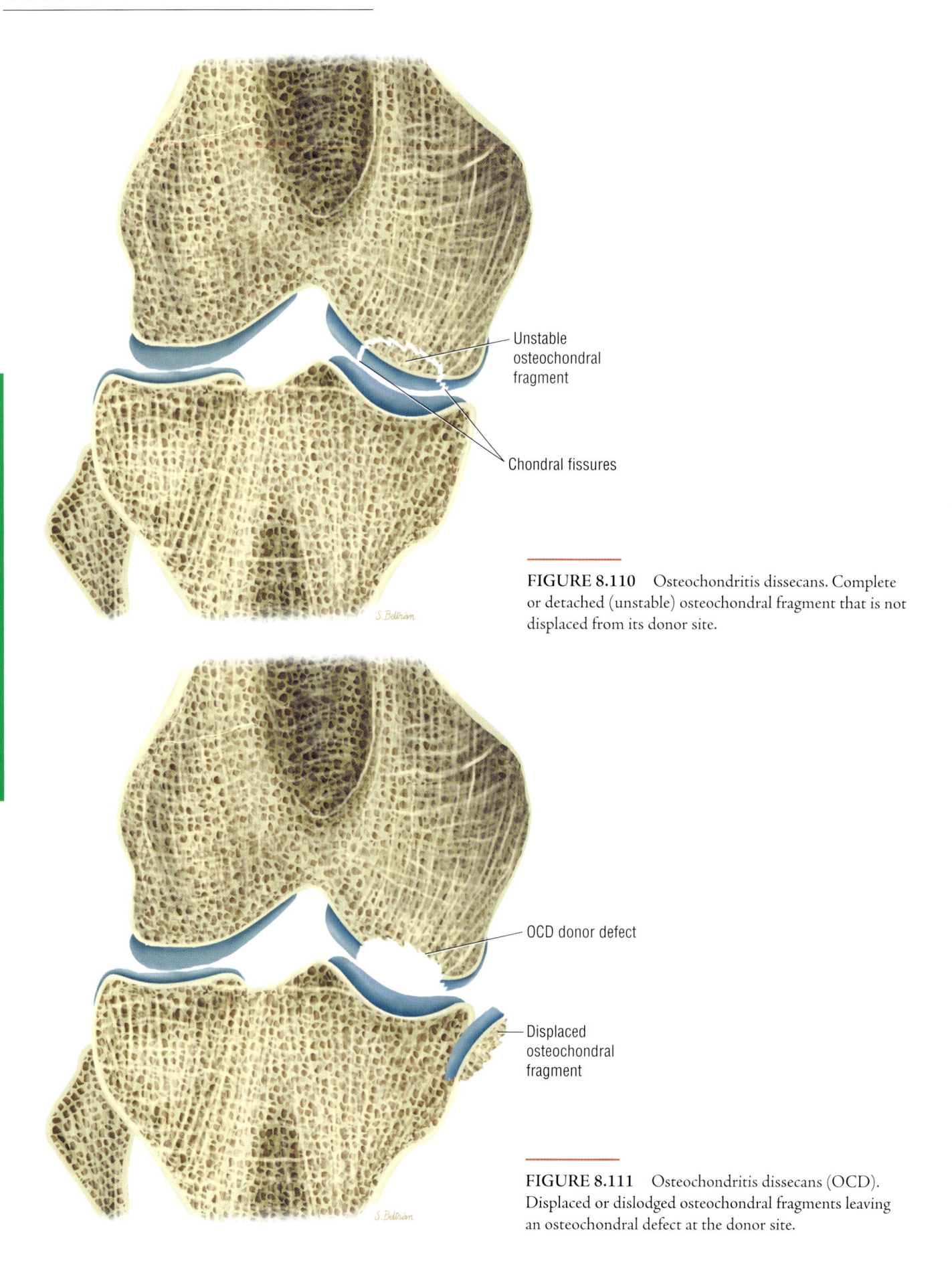

Osteochondritis Dissecans

FIGURE 8.110 Osteochondritis dissecans. Complete or detached (unstable) osteochondral fragment that is not displaced from its donor site.

FIGURE 8.111 Osteochondritis dissecans (OCD). Displaced or dislodged osteochondral fragments leaving an osteochondral defect at the donor site.

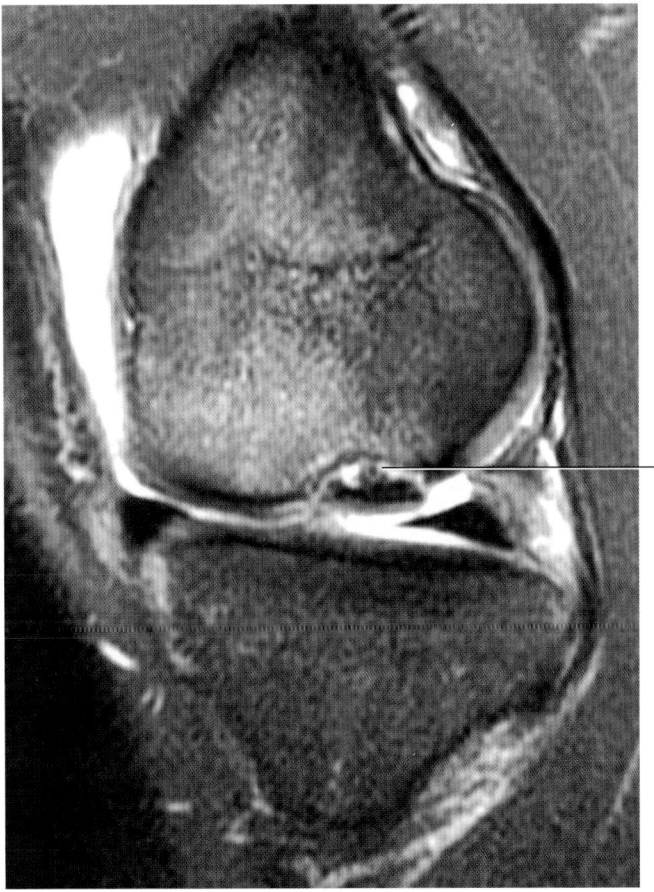

General Pathologic Conditions Affecting the Knee

FIGURE 8.112 Sagittal FS PD FSE image of detached and unstable osteochondral fragment circumferentially surrounded by fluid.

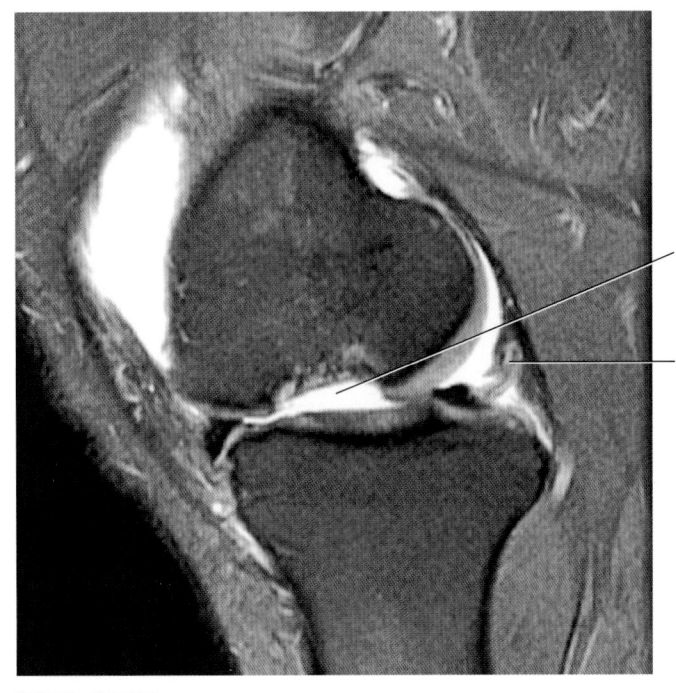

FIGURE 8.113 Fluid-filled donor site on sagittal FS PD FSE image.

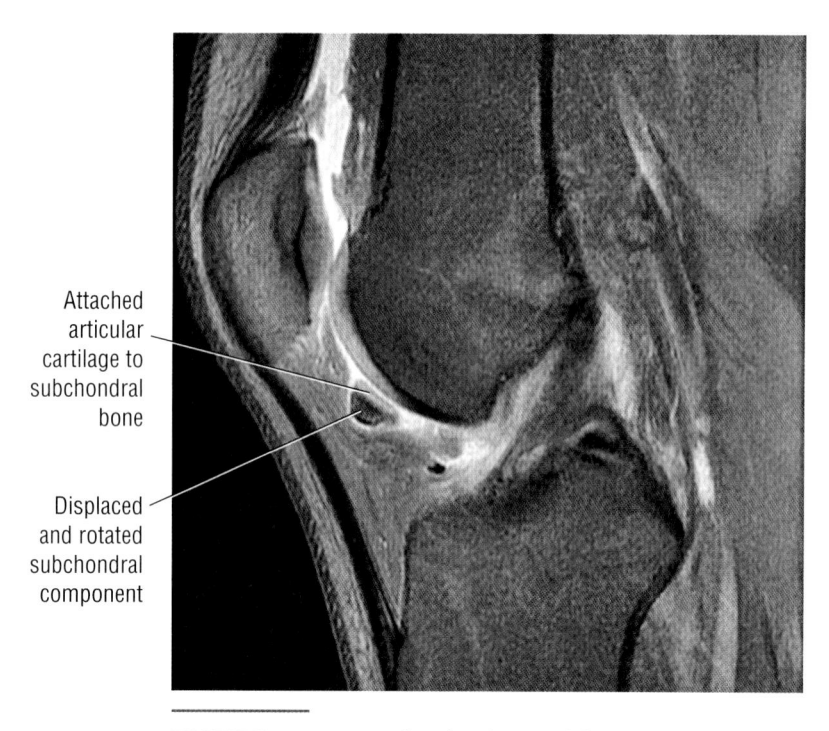

FIGURE 8.114 Displaced and rotated free fragment in osteochondritis dissecans. The articular cartilage and subchondral bone components are identified on a sagittal FS PD FSE image.

- Attached articular cartilage to subchondral bone
- Displaced and rotated subchondral component

- Chronic OCD with marrow fat signal intensity
- Incorporation of involved osteochondral segment
- Congruous articular cartilage surface

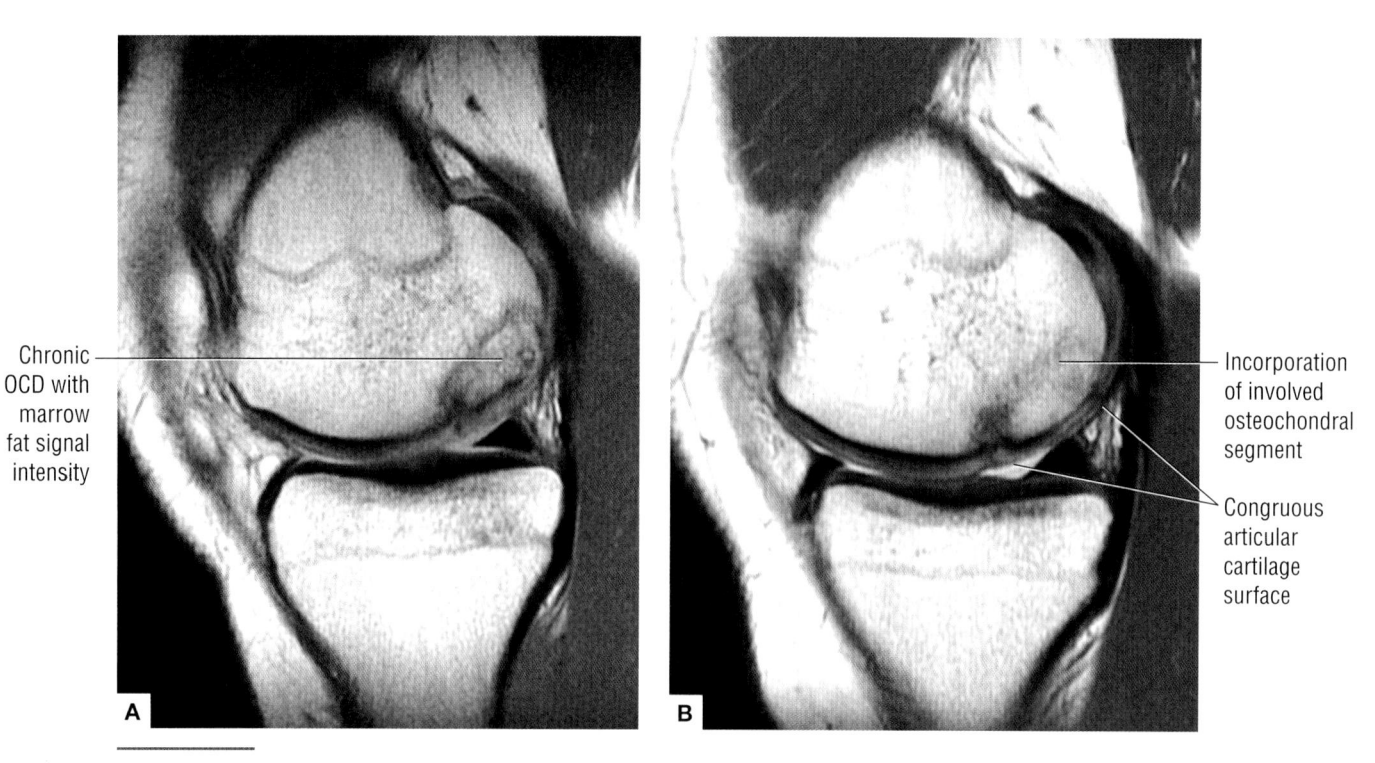

FIGURE 8.115 Healing phase of osteochondritis dissecans (OCD) with marrow fat signal intensity in the osteochondral fragment. Progressive incorporation is seen over a 3-year interval. (**A**) Sagittal PD FSE image. (**B**) Sagittal PD FSE image taken 3 years later.

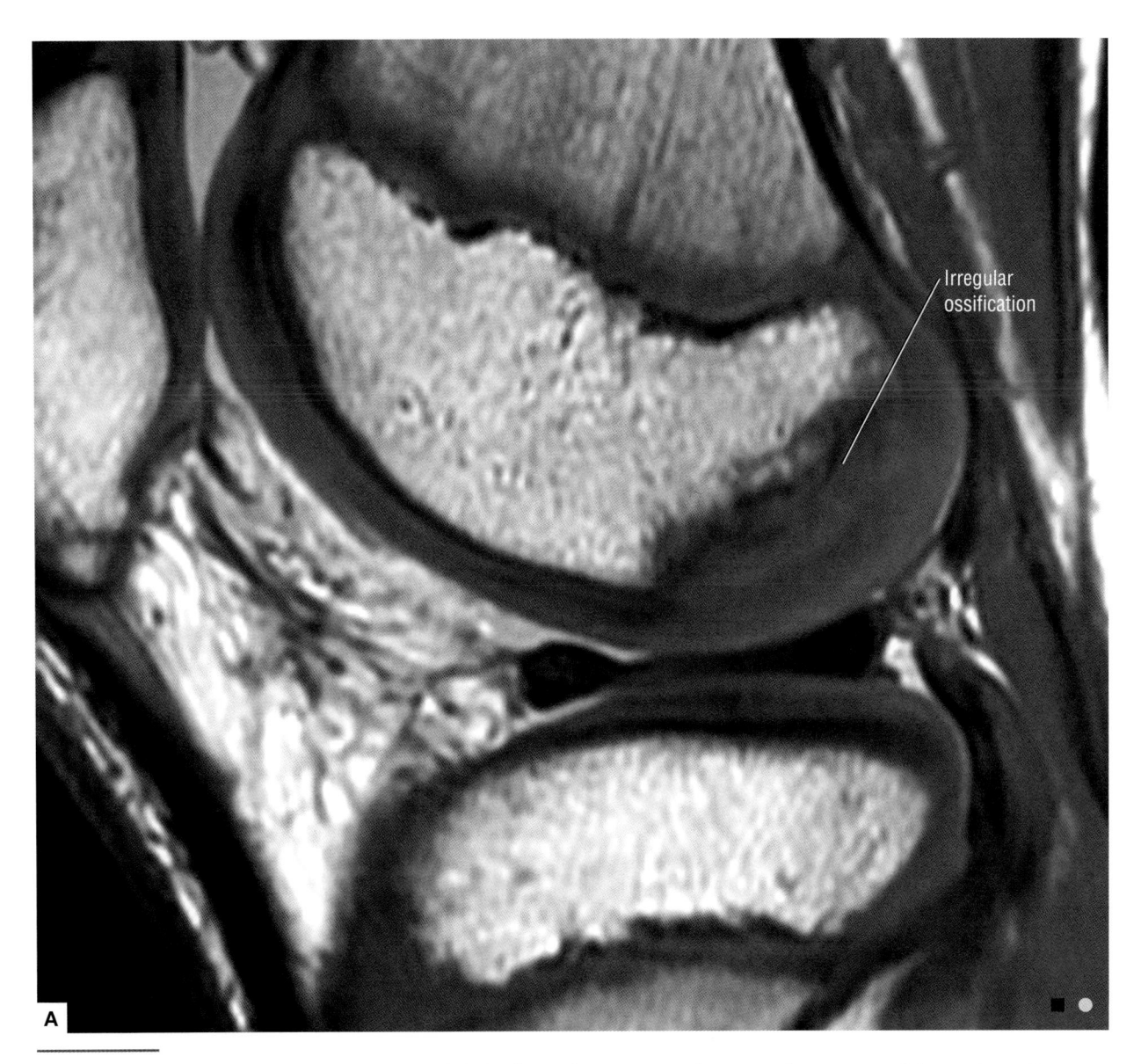

FIGURE 8.116 Endochondral ossification of the body epiphysis may produce irregular margins of the epiphysis. In comparison, osteochondritis dissecans (OCD) is usually (75% of cases) in the lateral aspect of the medial femoral condyle with a peak incidence at age 12 to 13 years compared to a range of 3 to 13 years in this normal developmental ossification. Early epiphyseal ossification may be associated with femoral abnormal heterogeneity. Because of the cystic changes of the subchondral bone, these cases should be followed with a subsequent study to document proper skeletal maturation. Normal variation of ossification occurs at an early age of OCD of 12 to 13 years. Sagittal PD- (**A**) and FS PD- (**B**) weighted images. (*Continued*)

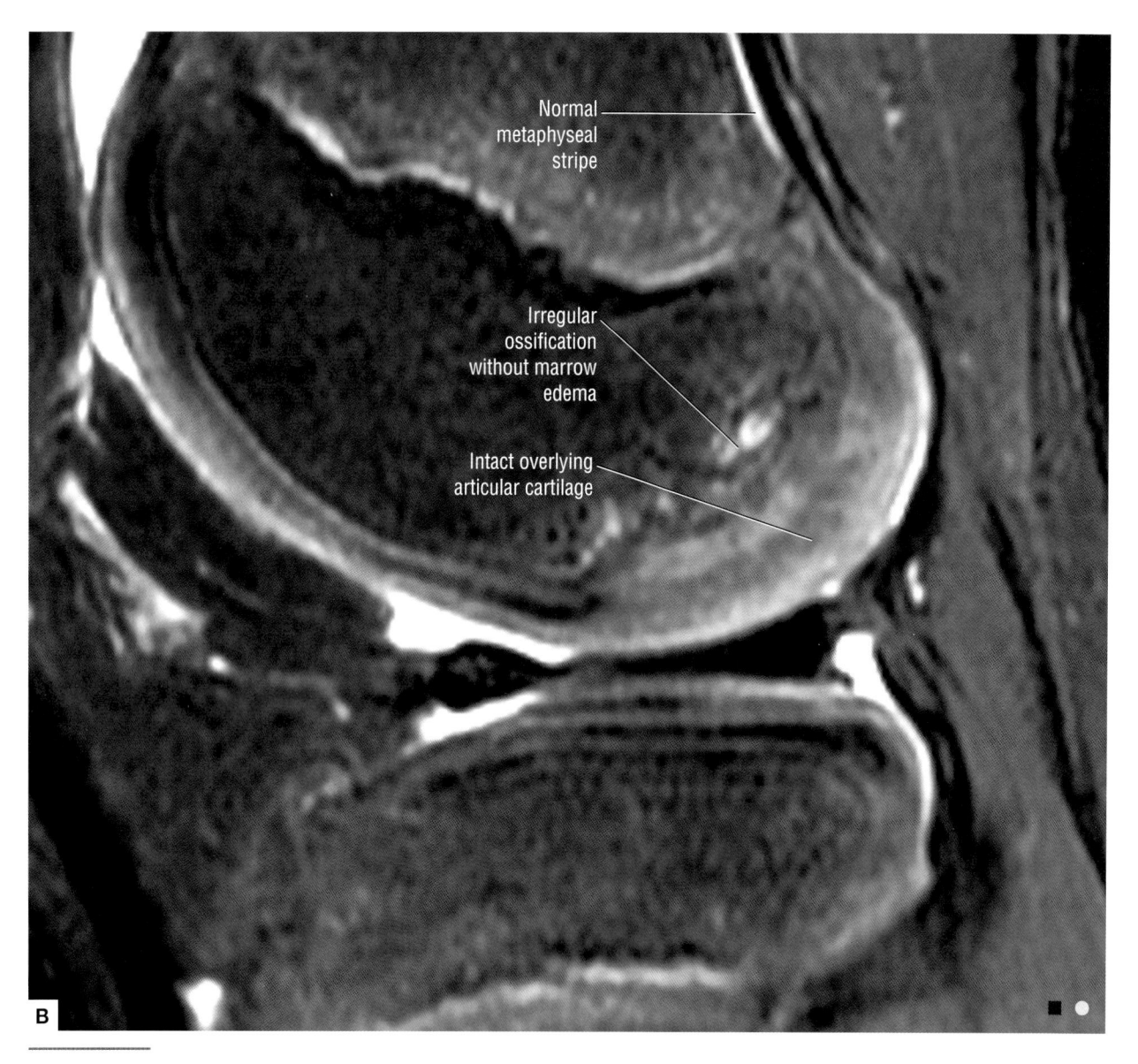

FIGURE 8.116 (*Continued*) Irregular ossification of lateral femoral condyle epiphysis. Frequently bilateral but may be asymmetric. Lateral femoral condyle location is more common than medial femoral condyle. Simulates OCD.

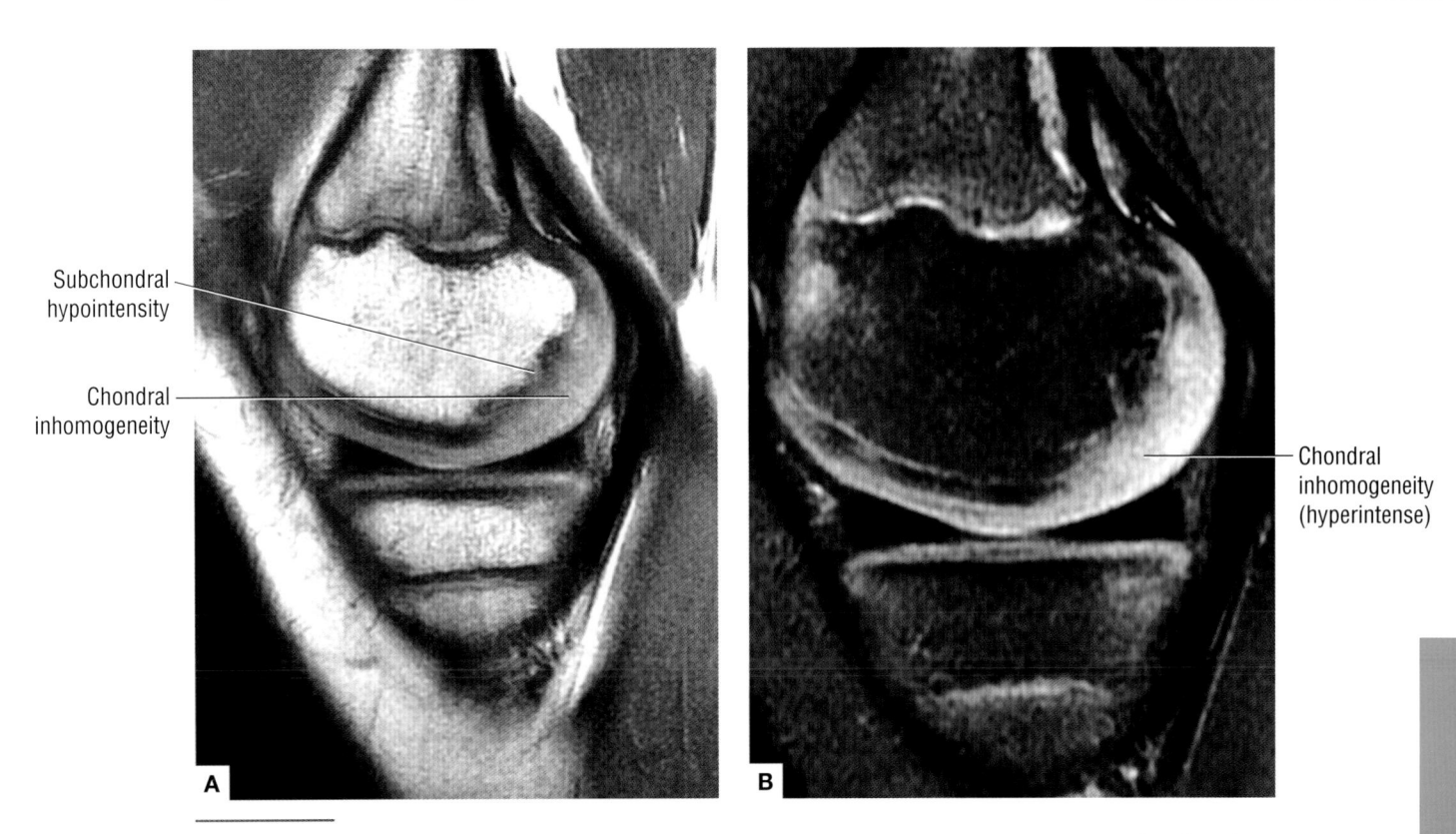

General Pathologic Conditions Affecting the Knee

FIGURE 8.117 (**A**) Hypointense subchondral sclerotic irregularity of the medial femoral condyle (epiphysis) on a sagittal PD FSE image. (**B**) Corresponding FS PD FSE image with overlying chondral inhomogeneity in normal epiphyseal development.

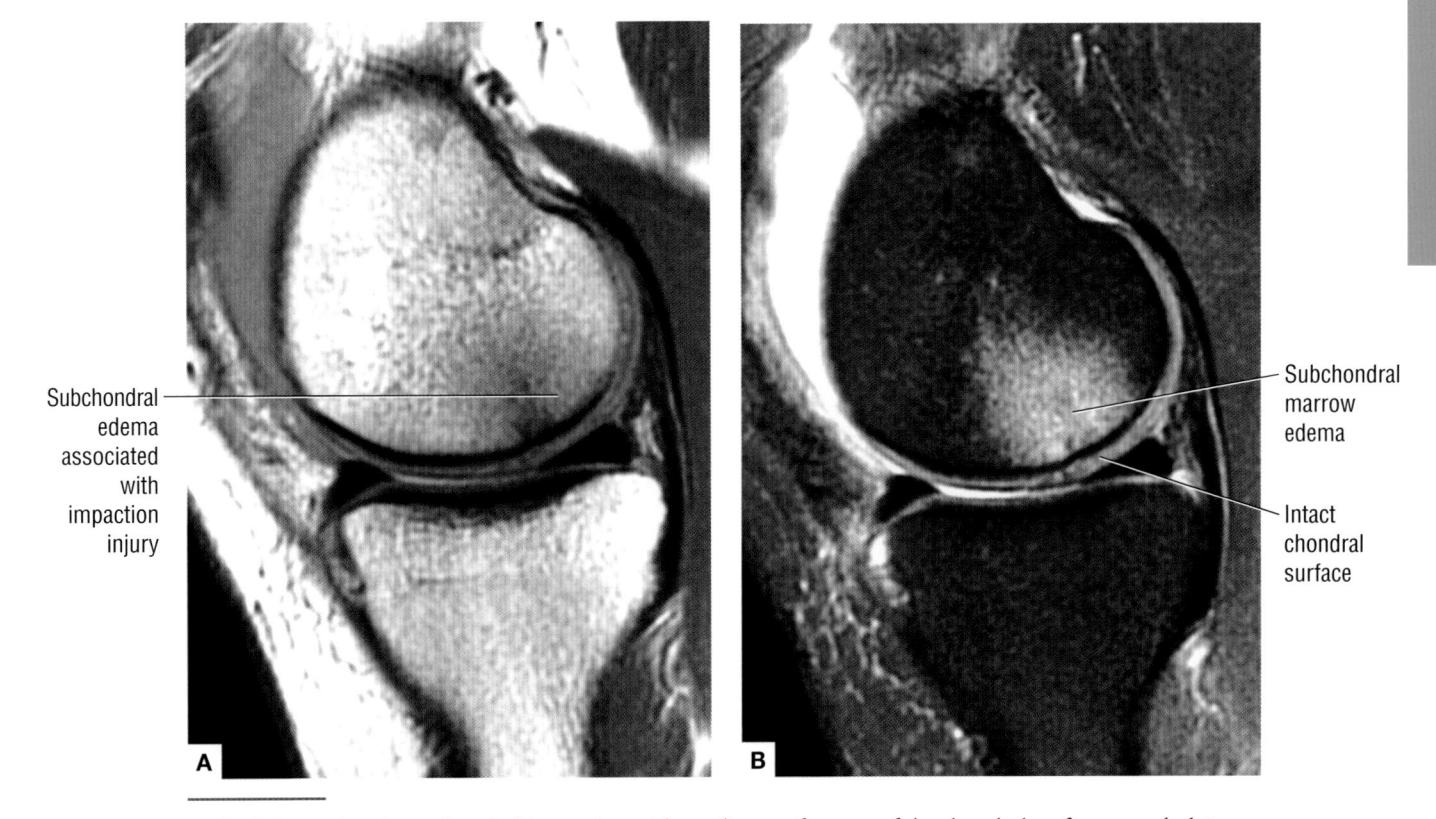

FIGURE 8.118 Osteochondral impaction without discrete fracture of the chondral surface or underlying subchondral bone on (**A**) sagittal PD FSE and (**B**) sagittal FS PD FSE images.

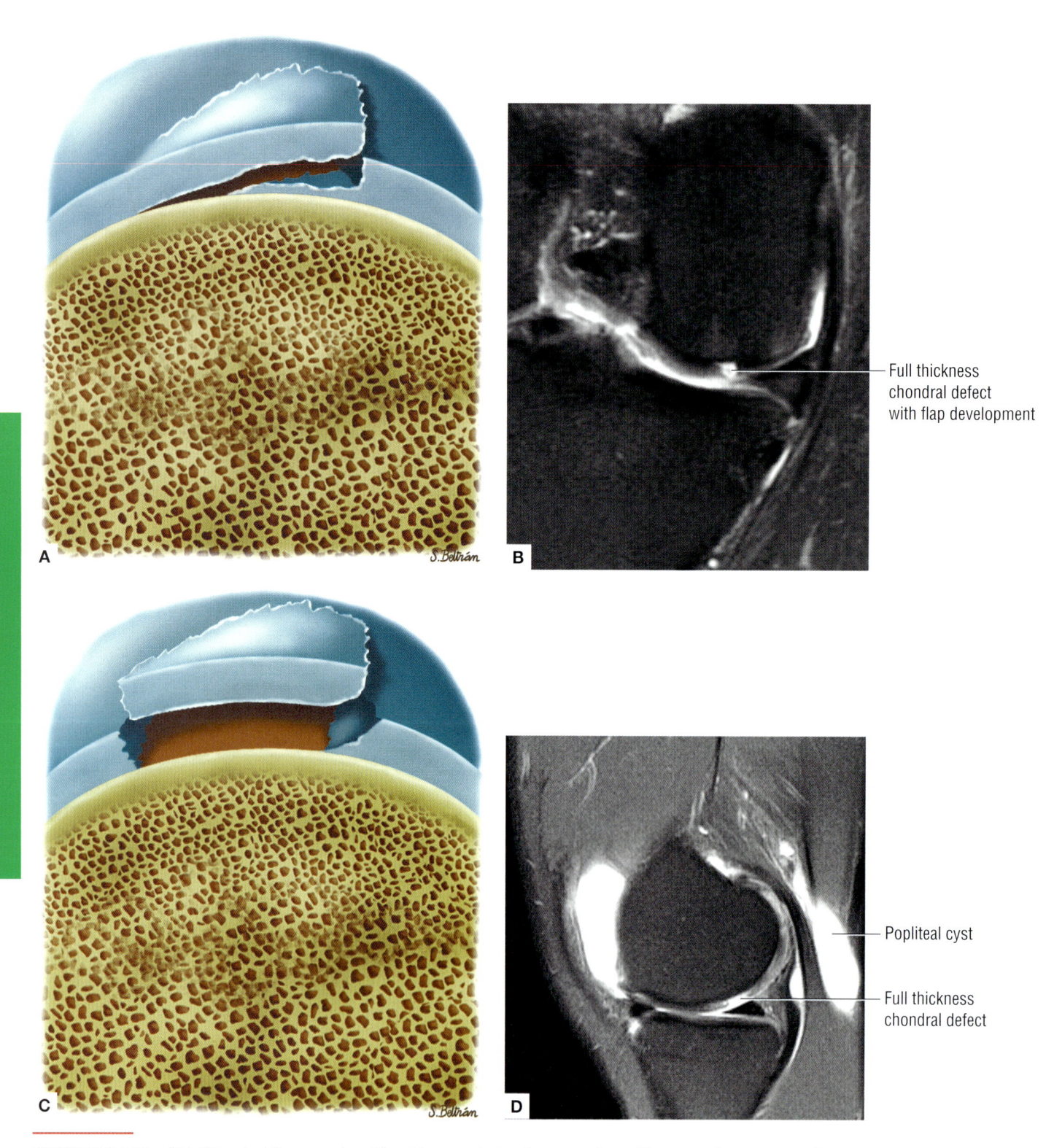

FIGURE 8.119 (**A**) Chondral flaps, produced by either a twisting force or a direct blow, are often associated with ligament tears. (**B**) Corresponding medial femoral condyle full thickness chondral flap on a coronal FS PD FSE image. (**C**) Chondral fractures or separations such as chondral flaps are associated with athletic injuries. The fragment either remains in situ or becomes displaced and is seen as an intraarticular loose body. (**D**) Full thickness medial femoral condylar defect on a sagittal FS PD FSE image.

- Surgical options for chondral injuries include débridement, abrasion with microfracture, osteochondral plugs (OATS), osteochondral allografts, and chondrocyte implantation.
- *Surface débridement*
    - Has good to excellent results at 5 years in 66% of cases
    - Indications for chondral resurfacing techniques: focal defects of femur and patella, no malalignment, intact meniscus, posttraumatic defects, and no evidence of bipolar lesions
- *Microfracture* is a marrow-stimulating technique that results in formation of a combination of fibrocartilage and hyaline cartilage.
    - Also known as *Steadman technique*
    - Cost-effective, and 97% of patients show improvement at follow-up
- *Mosaicplasty*
    - Cartilage transfer procedure used to resurface grade 4 defect with cartilage plug
    - Multiple small plugs, approximately 4mm in size, used to distribute force across a broad area
- *Osteochondral autograft transfer system (OATS)*
    - Type of mosaicplasty
    - Use of larger plugs, 6 to 10mm, to cover larger surface areas with greater stability
    - Favorable results reported in 80% to 94% of OATS procedures
    - *Osteochondral allografts (allograft OATS)* also used for large defects, tumors, and osteochondritis dissecans, but are subject to greater likelihood of infection-related complications than autograft implantation
- *Autologous chondrocyte implantation (ACI or Genzyme procedure)*
    - Cells obtained from cloned chondrocytes and used to repair large defects (>15mm) of femur, patella, and trochlea
    - Used for unipolar lesion in normally aligned knee with intact meniscus and no inflammatory disease
    - Expensive and may be complicated by detachment of patch
    - Biopsies in knees treated with ACI (versus OATS) show that more of the reparative tissue is fibrocartilage, which is not as desirable as hyaline cartilage repair.

- Newer techniques with binding the chondrocytes in a glue without using a perichondral flap.
- Collagen matrix scaffold for chondrocyte implantation to produce a more uniform distribution of cells in the chondral defect
- Hyaluronate-based polymer has been used to provide a biodegradable 3D biologic scaffold colonized with chondrocytes.

■ Current recommendations
- Débridement alone for lesions of non-weight-bearing surfaces
- Débridement or microfracture for lesions smaller than 5mm
- Microfracture or OATS for defects 5 to 15mm
- OATS, Genzyme, or allografts for lesions 15 to 20mm
- Genzyme or allografts for defects larger than 20mm
- Articular cartilage stem cell paste graft as an alternative to microfracture

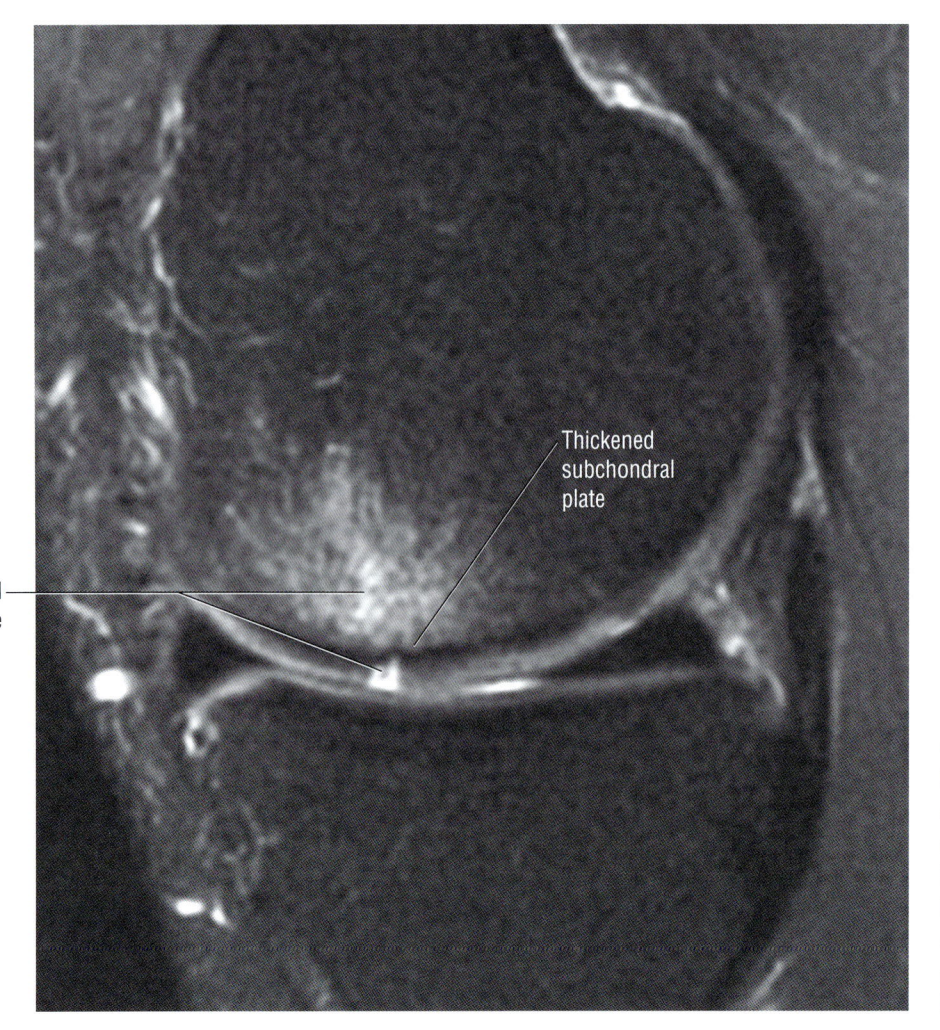

FIGURE 8.120 Osteochondral fracture with large area of reactive subchondral bone in response to increased loading from a discrete smaller full thickness chondral fracture. Sagittal FS PD FSE image.

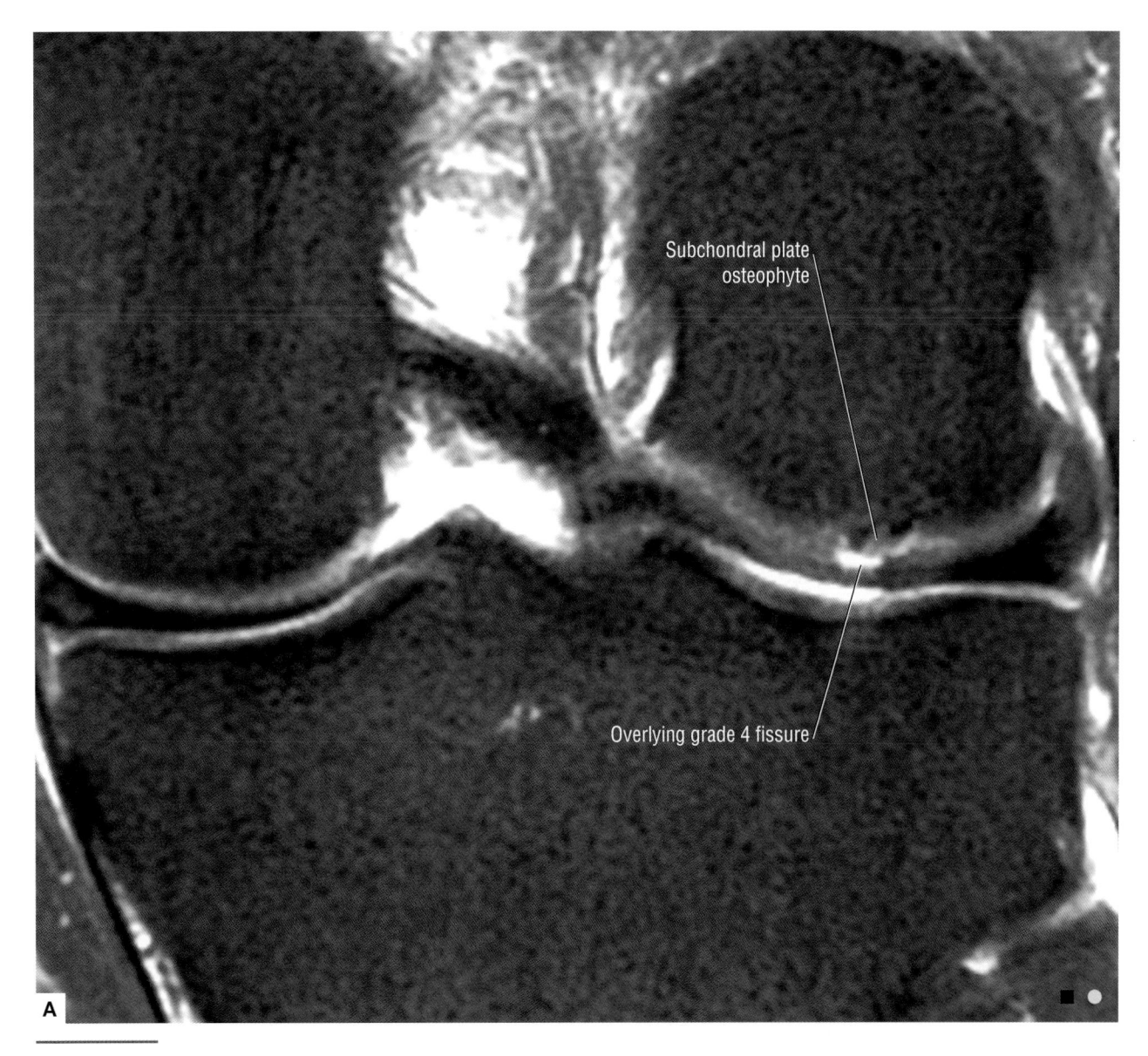

General Pathologic Conditions Affecting the Knee

FIGURE 8.121 Subchondral plate osteophyte is indicator of overlying chondral pathology. The sharp interface of a shear fracture is seen in a traumatic episode. A free chondral fragment may display a thin layer of adherent subchondral plate. (**A**) Coronal FS PD FSE image. (*Continued*)

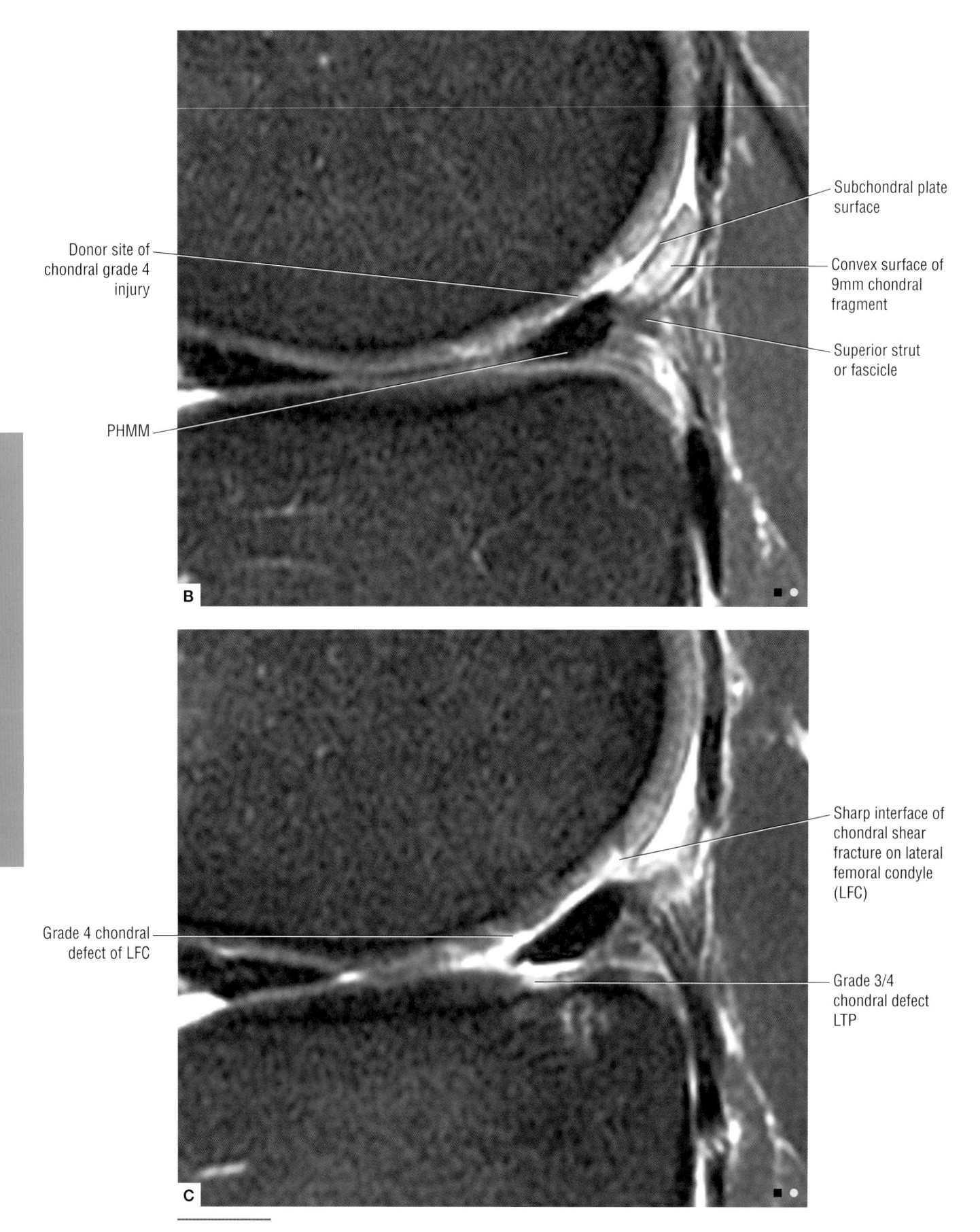

FIGURE 8.121 *(Continued)* **(B, C)** Sagittal FS PD FSE images.

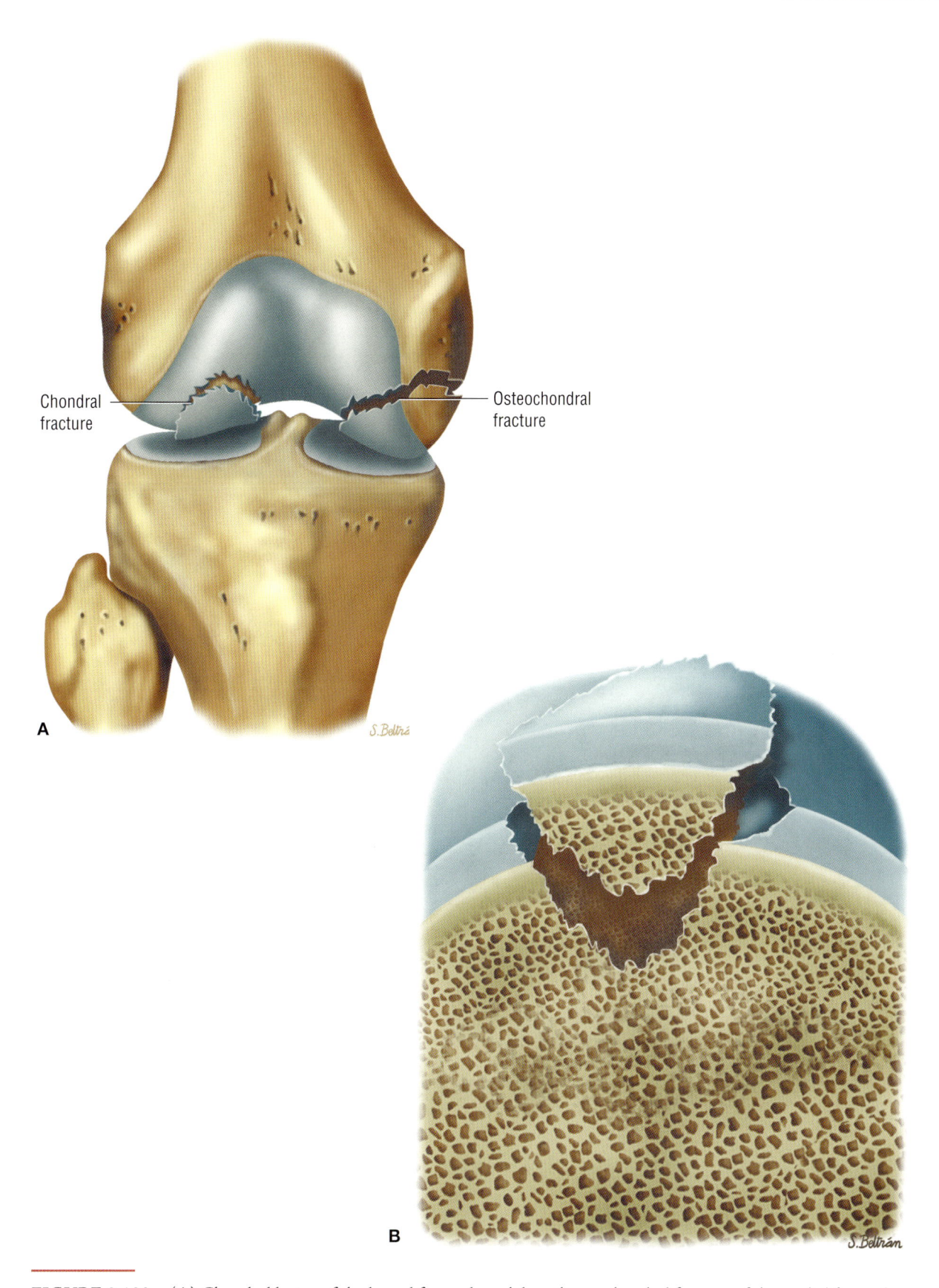

General Pathologic Conditions Affecting the Knee

FIGURE 8.122 (**A**) Chondral lesion of the lateral femoral condyle and osteochondral fracture of the medial femoral condyle. Osteochondral fractures often occur in an adolescent population, where there is no well-defined articular cartilage tidemark and stresses are transmitted directly to the subchondral bone. In the skeletally mature patient, the tidemark functions as a weak transitional zone and allows the transference of forces, resulting in a chondral fracture. (**B**) Osteochondral fracture with involvement of both chondral and subchondral bone with fracture extension across the subchondral plane presenting as osteochondritis dissecans.

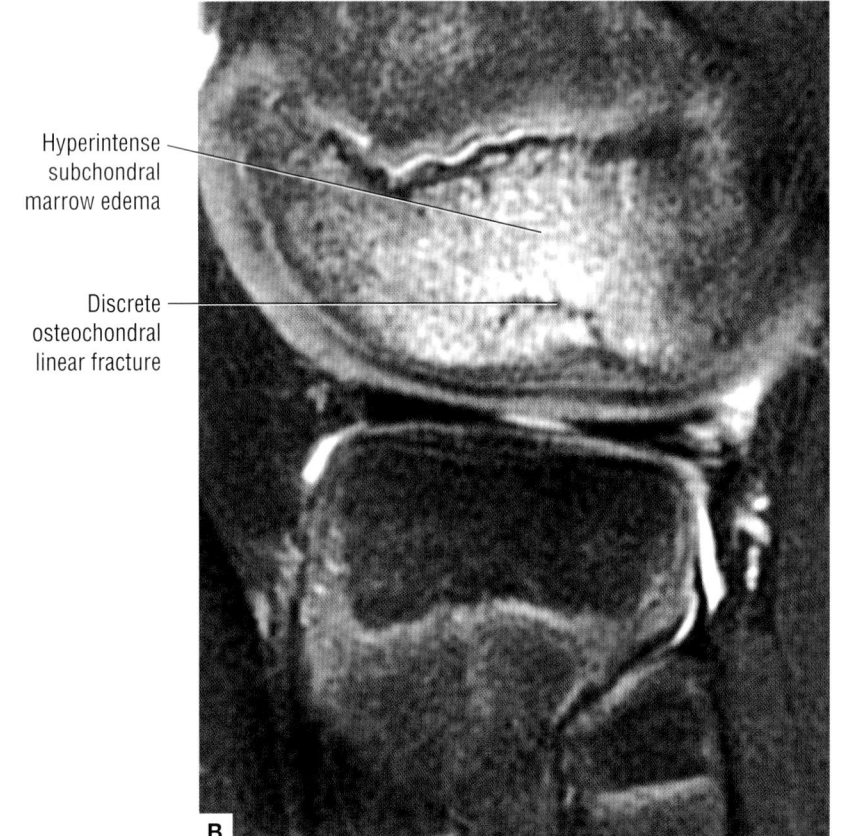

FIGURE 8.123 Lateral femoral condyle osteochondral fracture in a skeletally immature knee on (**A**) coronal PD FSE and (**B**) sagittal FS PD FSE images.

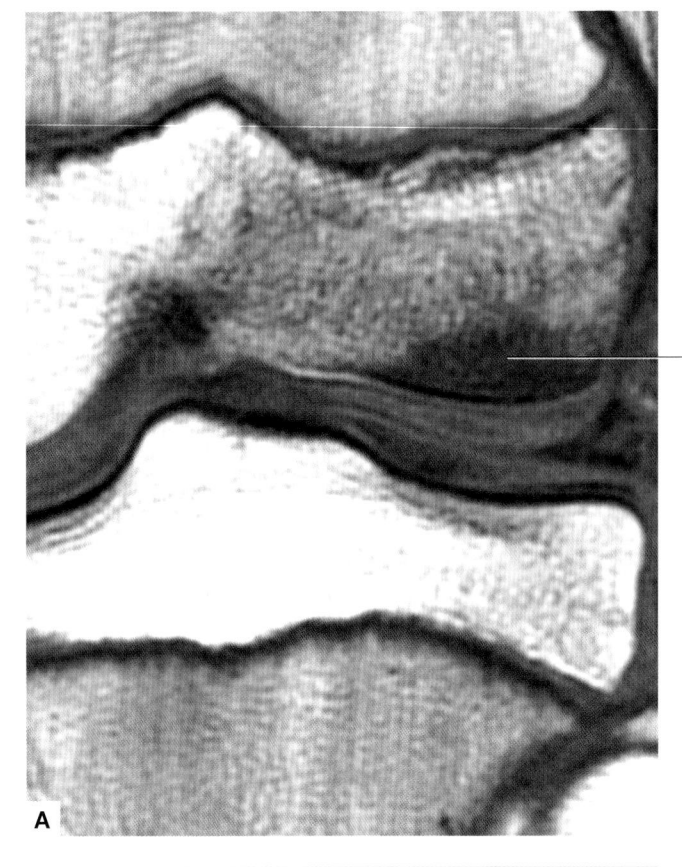

Delamination of Articular Cartilage

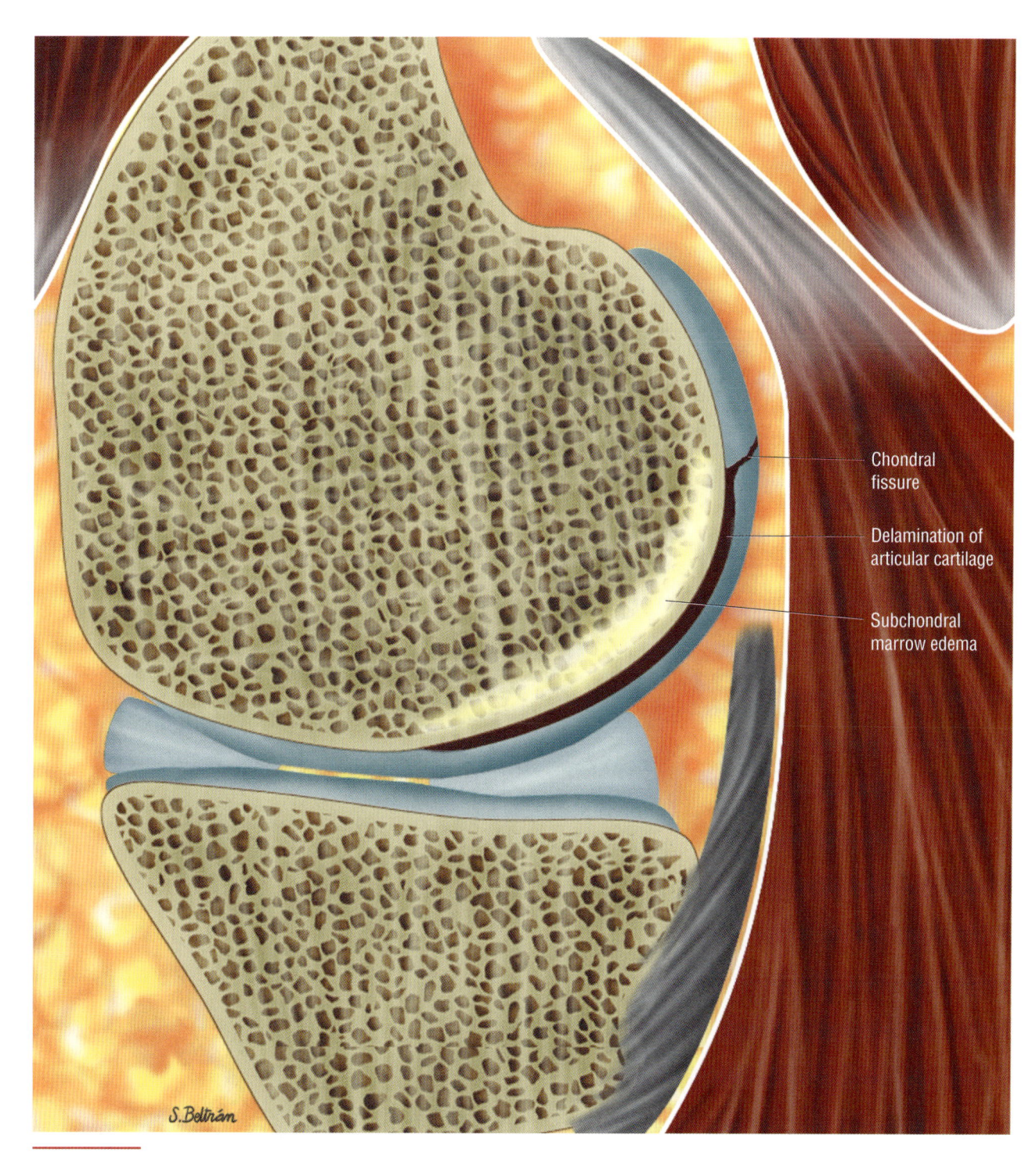

FIGURE 8.124 Delamination of articular cartilage with a fluid interface between the long-segment chondral flap of delamination and the deeper subchondral plate.

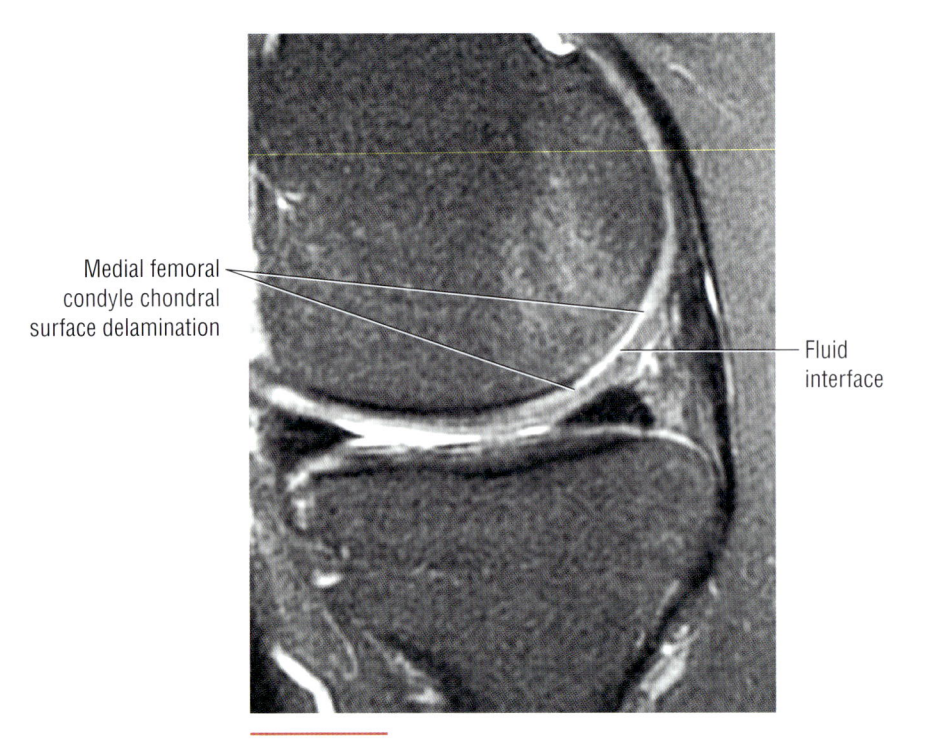

FIGURE 8.125 Sagittal FS PD FSE image showing chondral delamination of the medial femoral condyle.

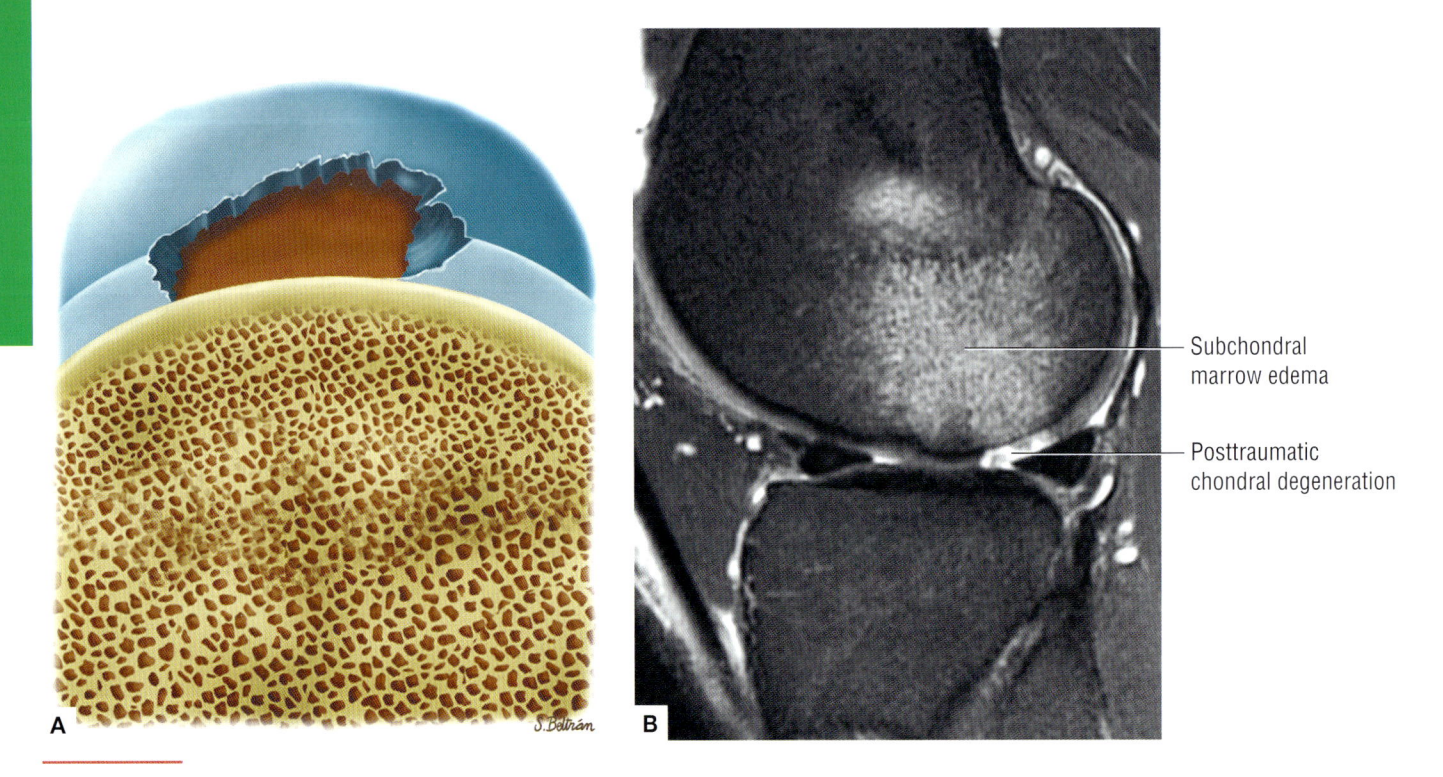

FIGURE 8.126 (A) In chondromalacia or degenerative chondrosis, the margins of the chondral lesion are less sharply defined or shallow than those seen in chondral flaps and fractures. (B) Posttraumatic chondrosis of the lateral femoral condyle with irregular chondral margins and reactive subchondral edema on a sagittal FS PD FSE image.

General Pathologic Conditions Affecting the Knee

Articular Cartilage Composition and Structure

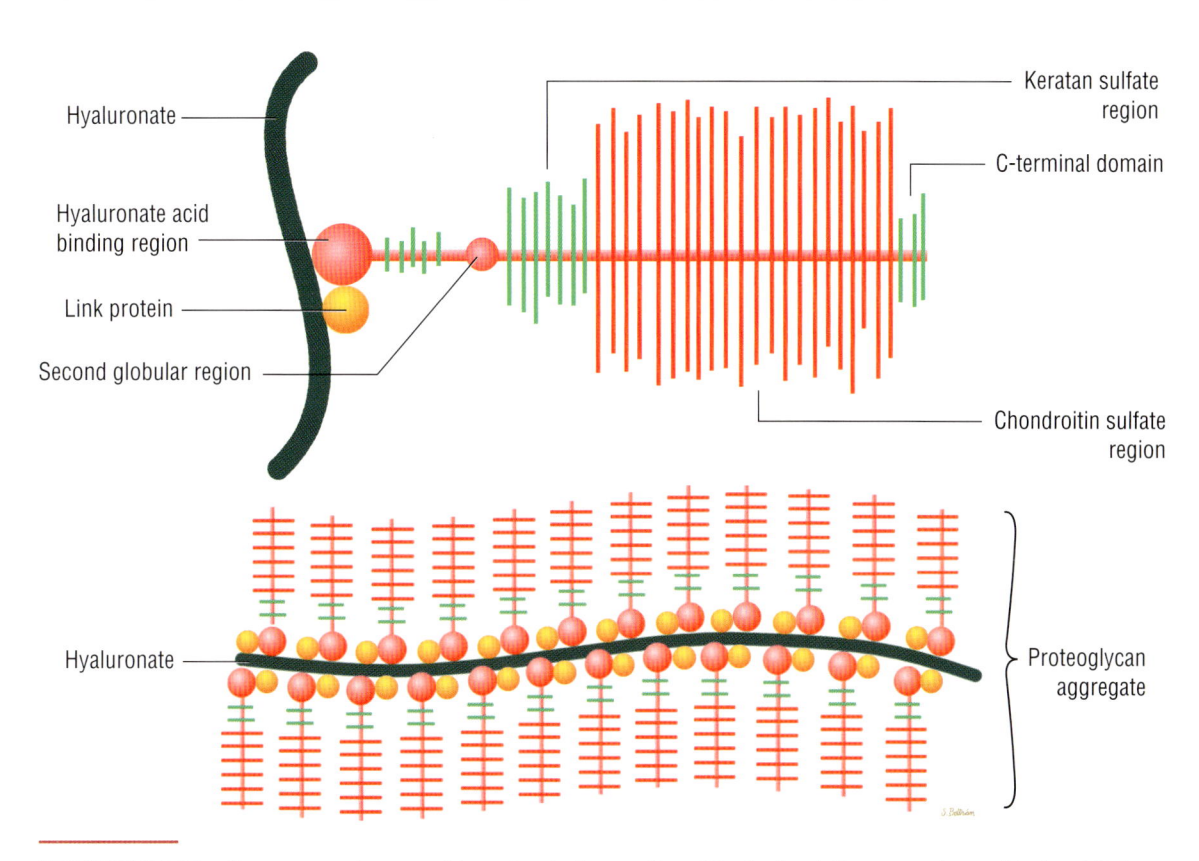

FIGURE 8.127 Structure and composition of articular cartilage. The hydrophilic proteoglycans bind and link to both small- and large-diameter collagen fibers. The glycosaminoglycans of the proteoglycan aggregate include both chondroitin and keratin sulfate.

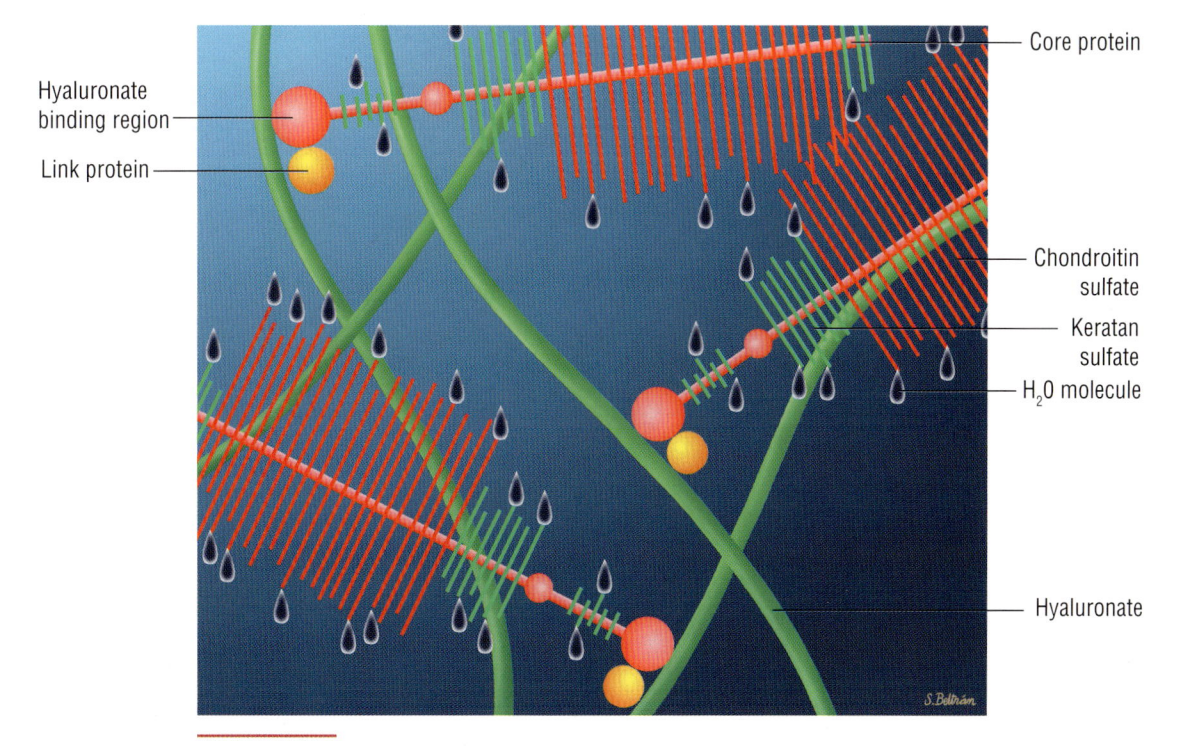

FIGURE 8.128 Aggrecan monomers with hydrophilic chondroitin sulfate and keratin sulfate chains are attached to a core protein backbone. The link proteins bind aggrecan monomers to hyaluronic acid.

Zonal Anatomy of Articular Cartilage

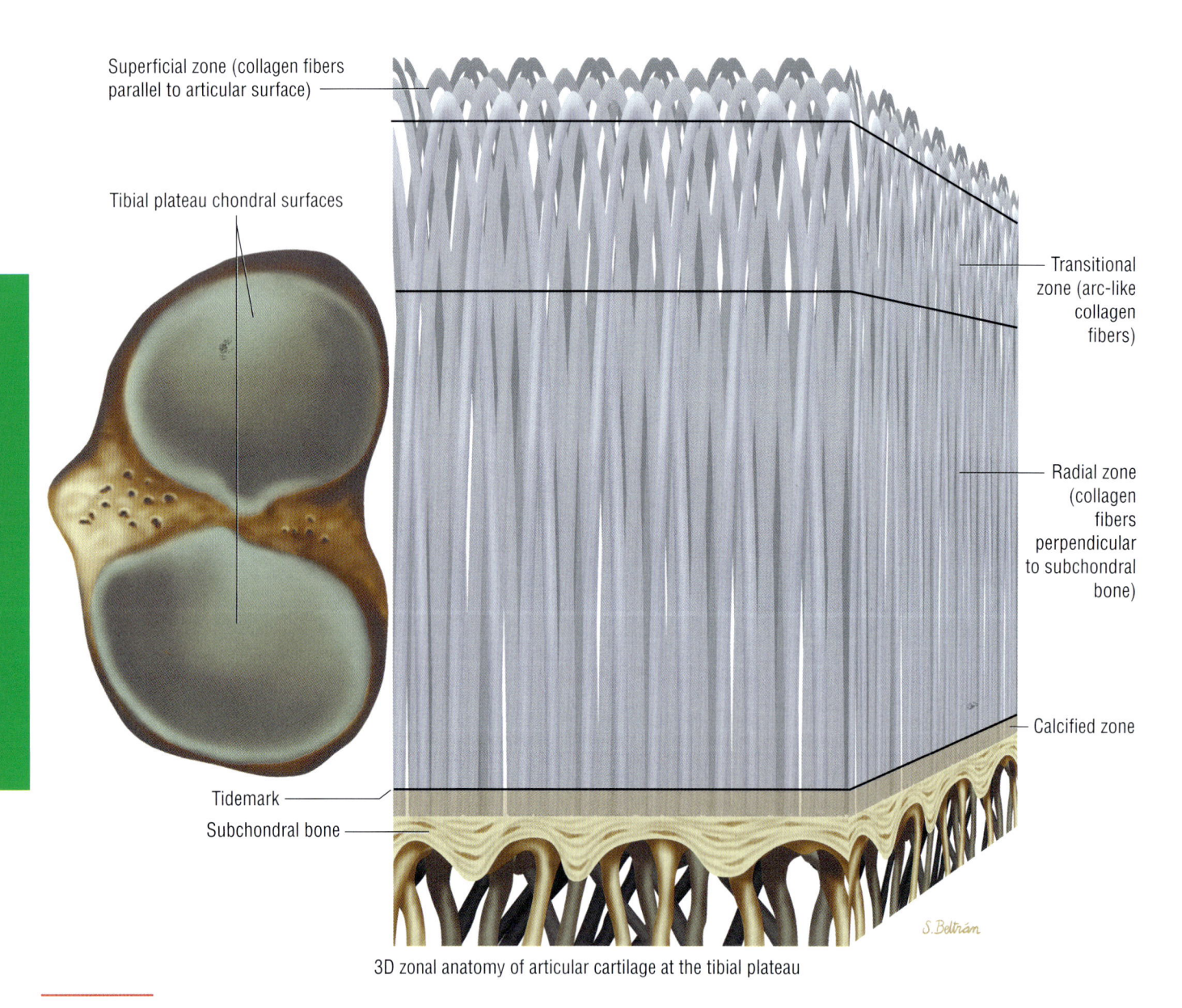

FIGURE 8.129 Zonal anatomy of the articular cartilage demonstrating the superficial, transitional, radial, and calcified zones. Tibial plateau chondral surfaces are shown as representative chondral surfaces.

General Pathologic Conditions Affecting the Knee

Cartilage Matrix and dGEMRIC

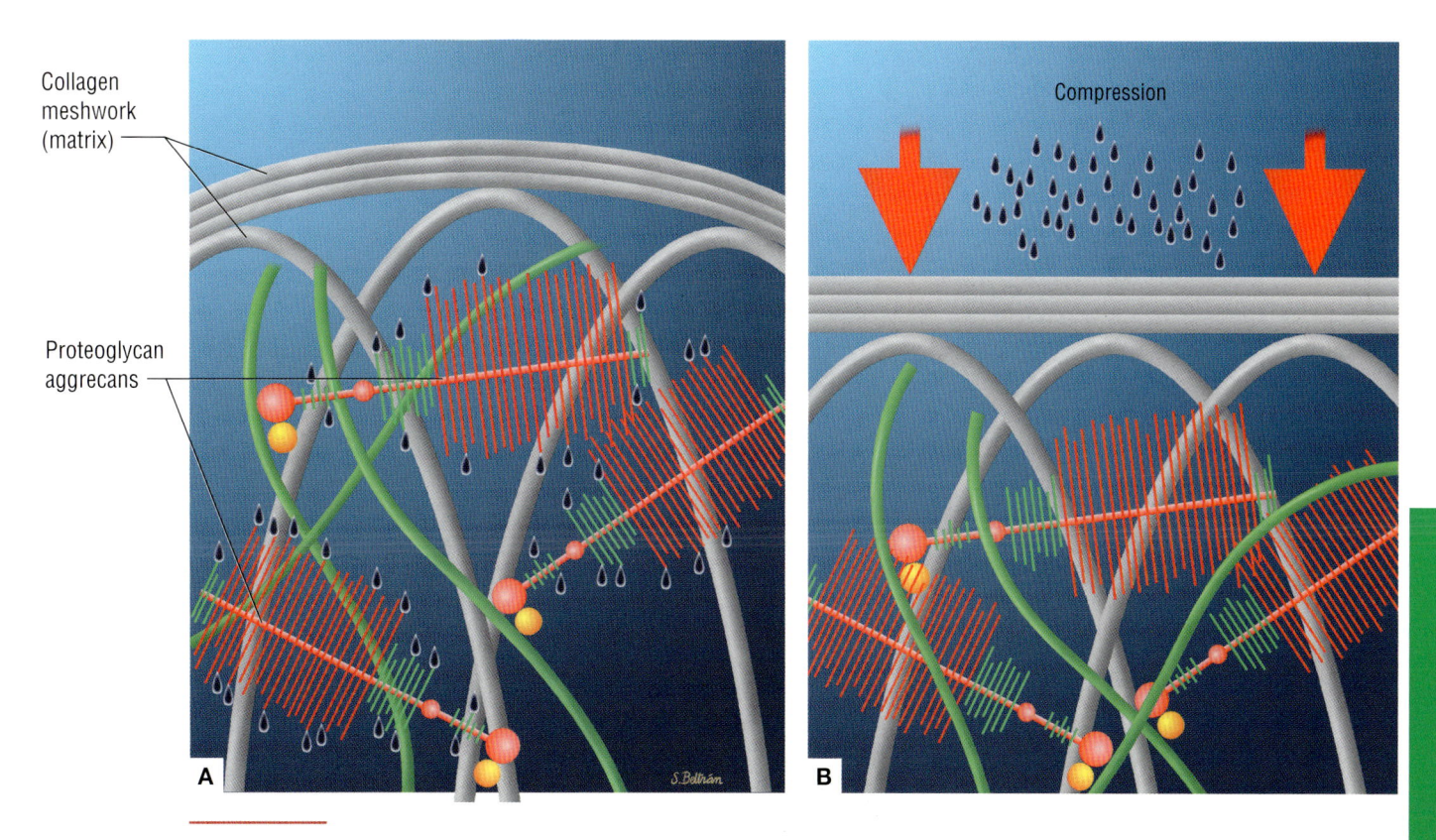

FIGURE 8.130 (**A**) Matrix volume is maintained by negatively charged glycosaminoglycan chains, which repel each other and attract water. Osmotic swelling is limited by the tensile strength of the collagen network. (**B**) The effect of matric compression pushes glycosaminoglycan side chains together, releasing water and decreasing pressure and the repulsive force generated by the increased negative charge density relative to the externally applied compressive force.

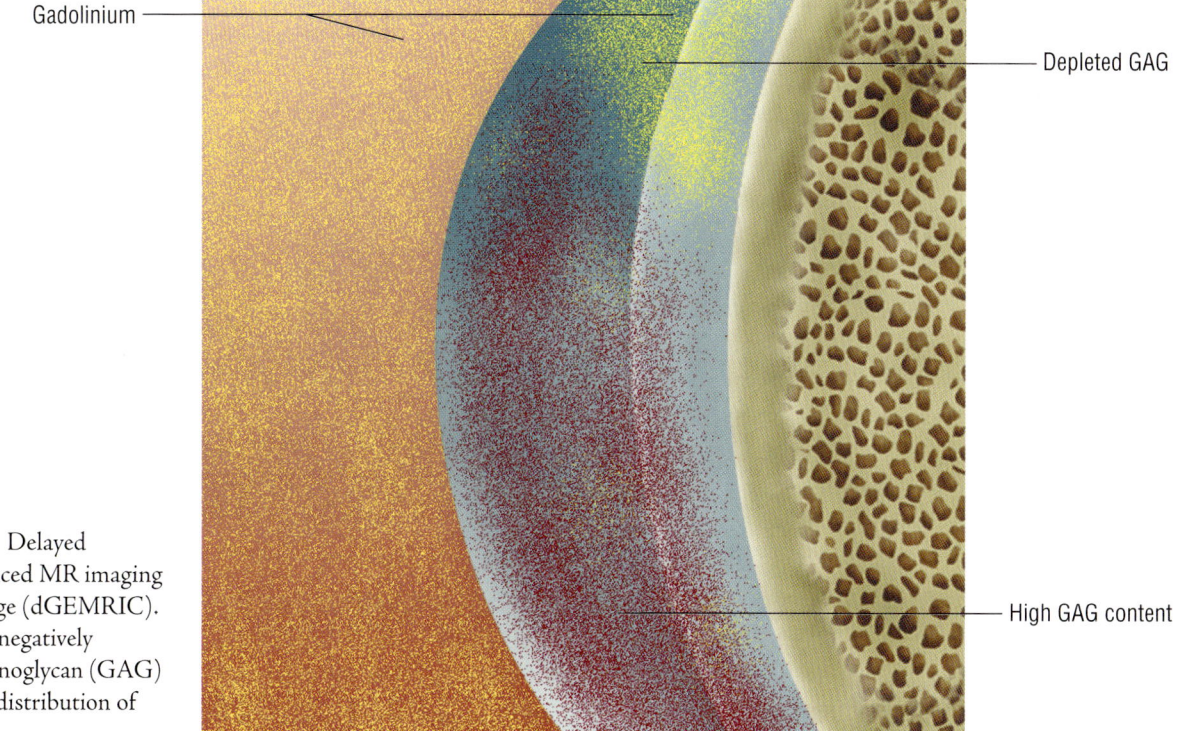

FIGURE 8.131 Delayed gadolinium-enhanced MR imaging of articular cartilage (dGEMRIC). Areas of depleted negatively charged glycosaminoglycan (GAG) show the greatest distribution of gadolinium.

Zonal Anatomy of Articular Cartilage

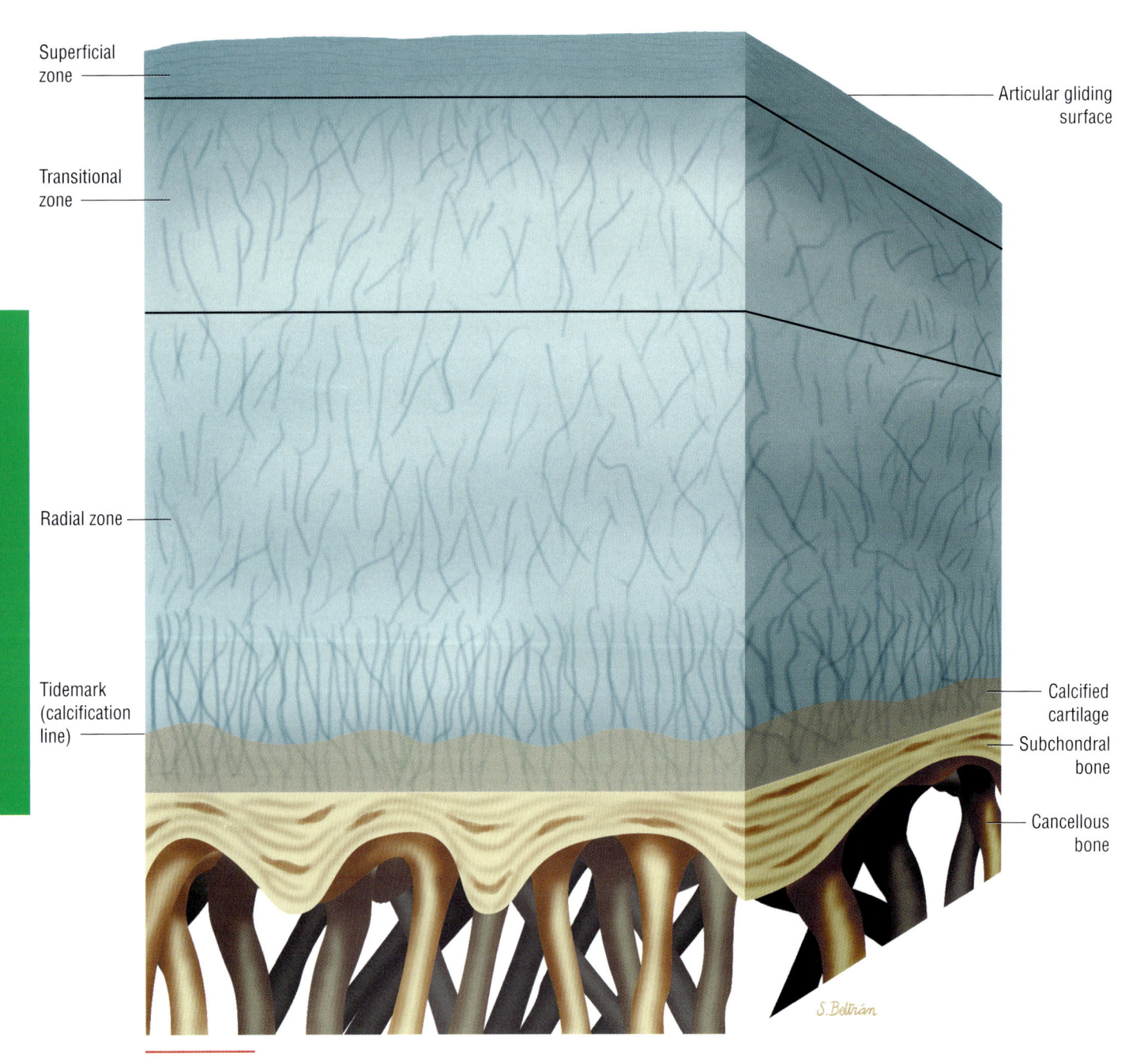

FIGURE 8.132 The collagen fibers of the radial zone are oriented perpendicular to the subchondral plate and anchor articular cartilage to bone. Collagen fibers form arcades in the transitional zone and are directed parallel to the surface in the superficial zone.

General Pathologic Conditions Affecting the Knee

FIGURE 8.133 Reference between conventional fluid-sensitive sequence FSE image (**A**), T2-map (**B**), and T1 rho map (**C**) of the articular cartilage. T2 and T1 rho are acquired using the same 3D fast spin-echo acquisition approach with T2 prep and T1 rho prep, respectively. Both T2 and T1 rho quantification are promising methods for probing early stage biochemical change in cartilage. (**A**) Anatomy reference with FR (fast recovery) FSE image through the lateral compartment.

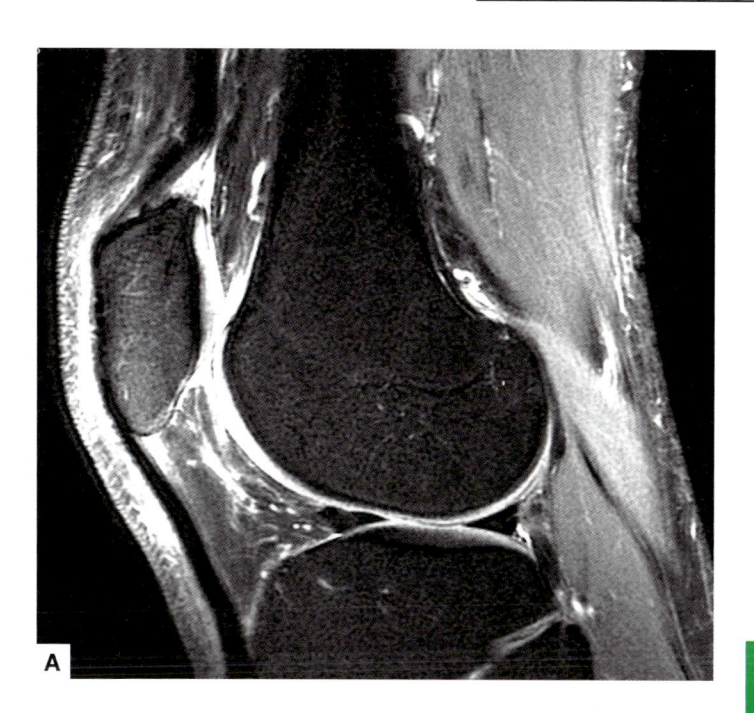

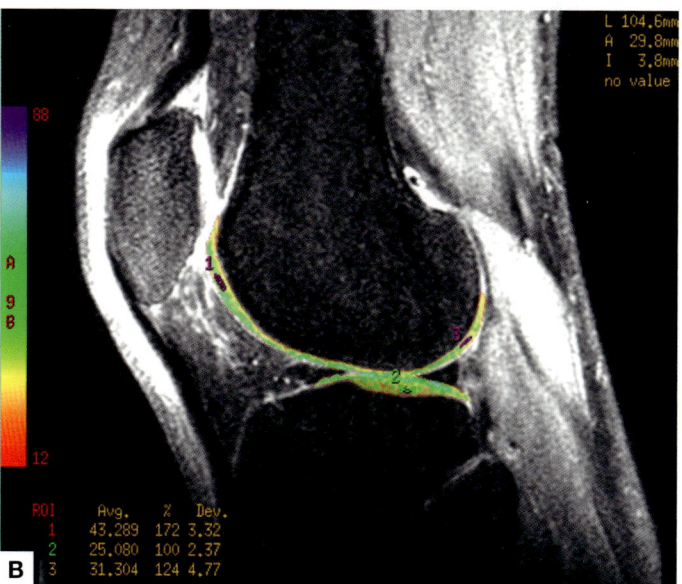

FIGURE 8.133 (**B**) T2 map of lateral compartment cartilage. T2 is primarily used for quantification of changes associated with collagen.

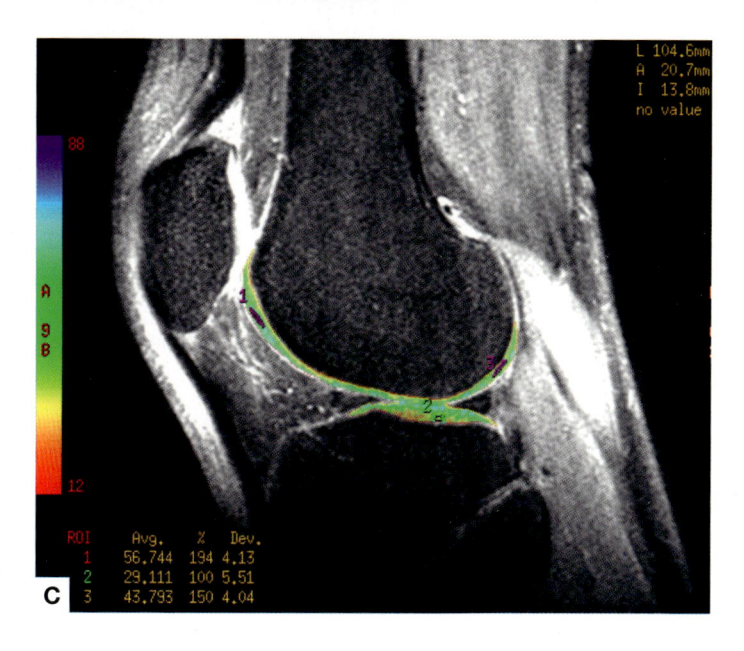

FIGURE 8.133 (**C**) T1 rho map of lateral compartment cartilage. T1 rho describes spin-lattice relaxation in the rotating frame, and its change may reflect the changes of the extracellular matrix including proteoglycan loss.

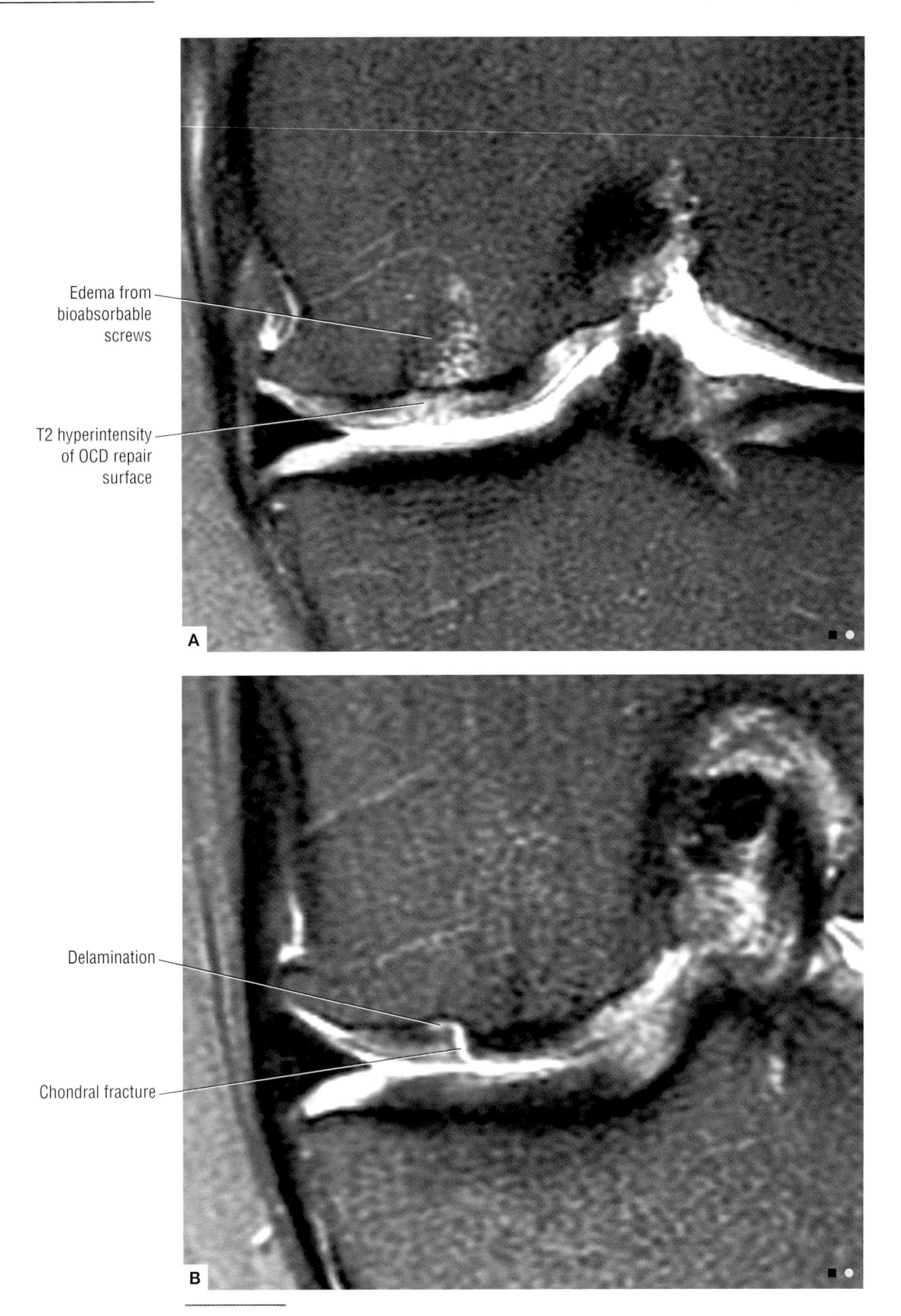

FIGURE 8.134 Failure of a treated (arthroscopic fixation) osteochondritis dissecans with bioabsorbable screws. The chondral fracture and basilar delamination are identified by the direct influx of hyperintense joint fluid. (**A, B**) Coronal FS PD FSE images.

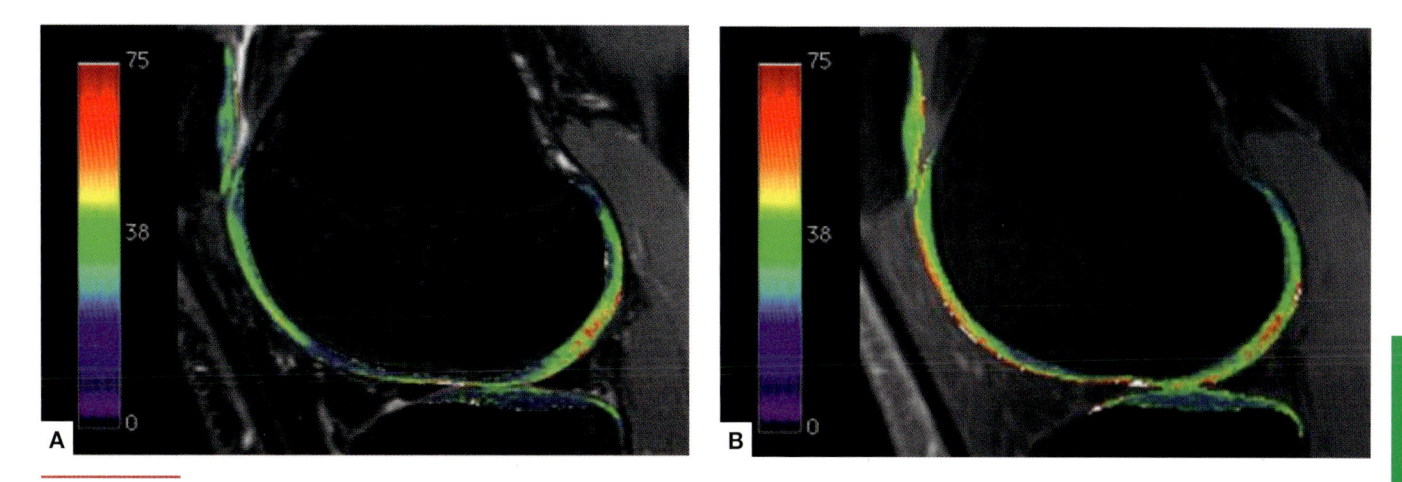

General Pathologic Conditions Affecting the Knee

FIGURE 8.135 T2 and T1 rho maps: T2 maps show collagen organization and hydration. T1 rho maps are correlated with glycosaminoglycan content. While T1 rho is an important marker for changes in articular cartilage, it may not be specific to just GAG or collagen orientation. (**A**) T2 map. (**B**) T1 rho. (Courtesy of Garry E. Gold, MD, Stanford Department of Radiology.)

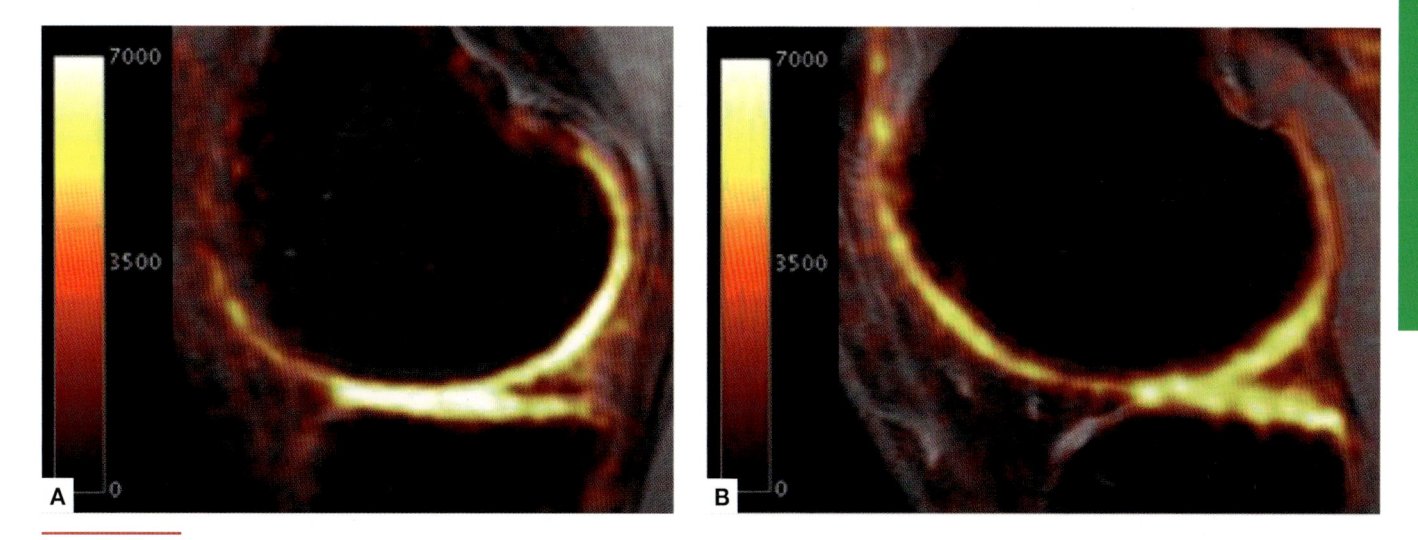

FIGURE 8.136 Sodium images: Sodium is a marker for cartilage glycosaminoglycan. These were acquired at 3T and overlaid on a proton MR image. Sodium resolution was $1 \times 1 \times 4$ mm. (**A**) Sodium medial color scale. (**B**) Sodium lateral color scale. (Courtesy of Garry E. Gold, MD, Stanford Department of Radiology.)

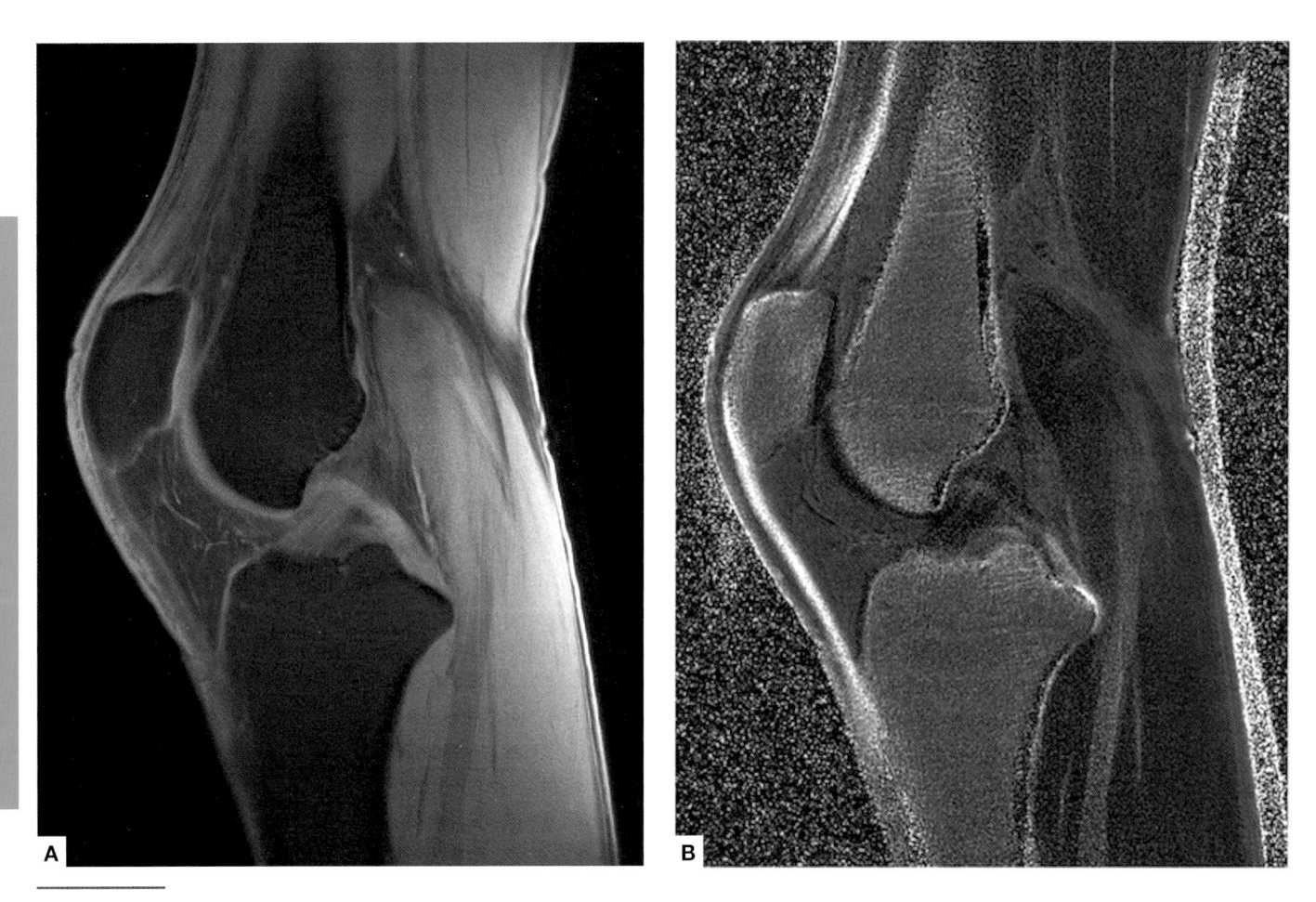

FIGURE 8.137 Ultrashort (UTE) images: water image acquired with a TE of 100msec. R2* map shows the short T2 tissues and suppresses signal from longer tissues such as joint fluid. **(A)** UTE water image. **(B)** UTE knee R2* map. UTE pulse sequences allow the detection of signal from the knee structures with short T2s, such as cortical bone. (Courtesy of Garry E. Gold, MD, Stanford Department of Radiology.)

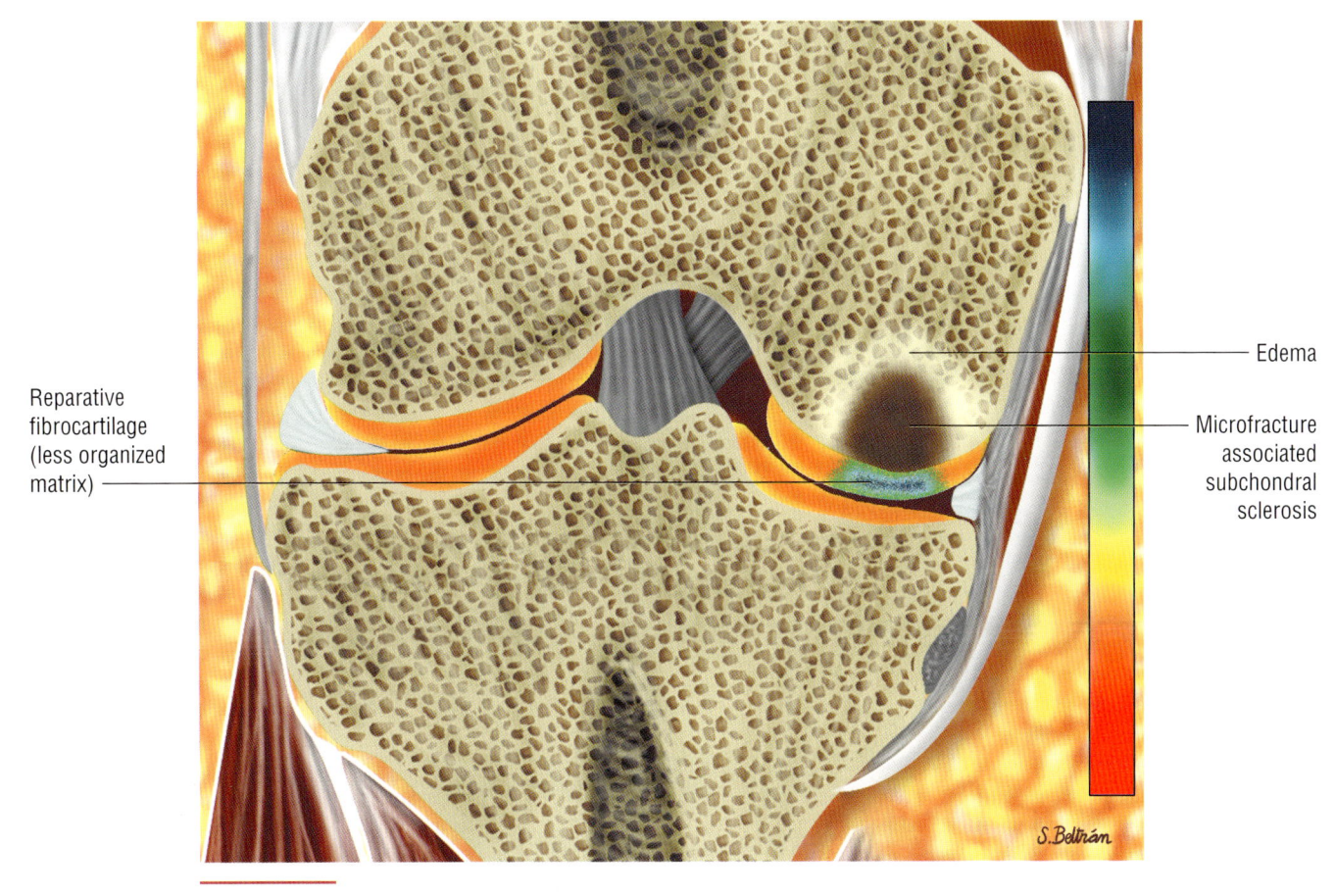

General Pathologic Conditions Affecting the Knee

FIGURE 8.138 Reparative fibrocartilage with prolongation of T2 relaxation times several months following a microfracture procedure illustrated in a coronal section.

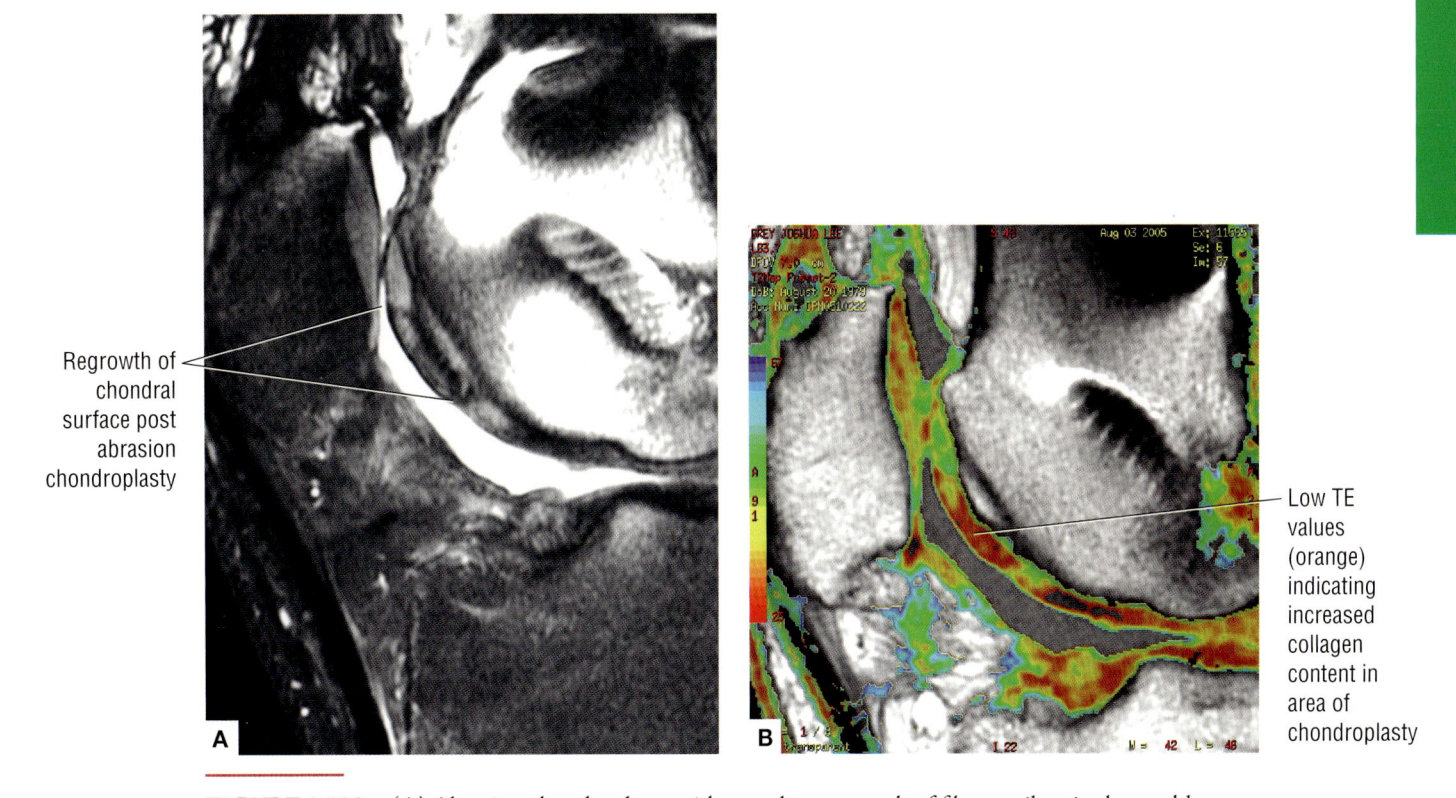

FIGURE 8.139 (**A**) Abrasion chondroplasty with complete regrowth of fibrocartilage in the trochlear groove on sagittal FS PD FSE image. (**B**) T2 mapping showing normal collagen-rich tissue associated with shorter T2 values (orange) in treated area.

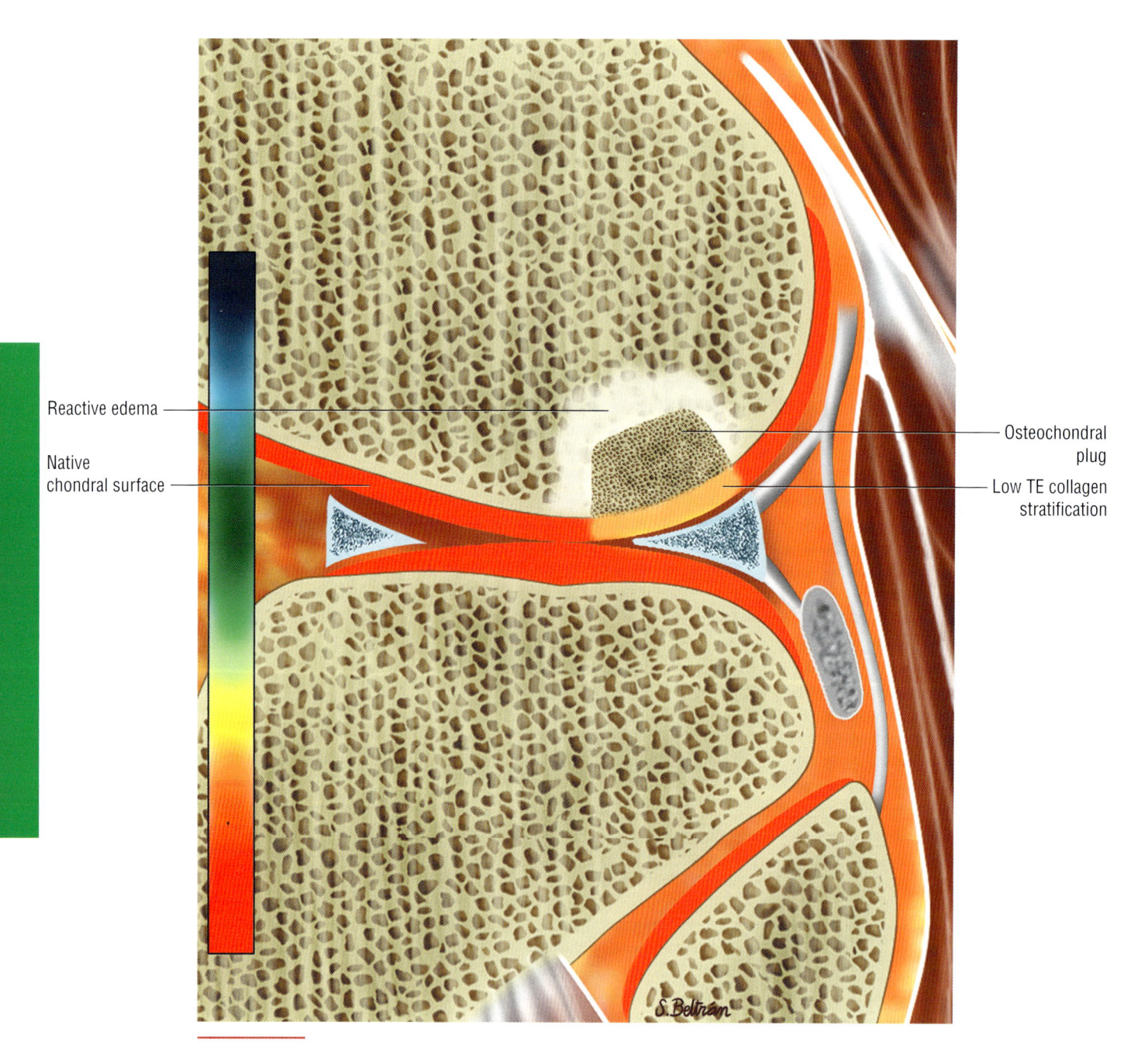

FIGURE 8.140 Osteochondral autograft transfer system (OATS) of the lateral femoral condyle with low TE value stratification of the chondral surface illustrated in sagittal section. The subchondral osseous component of the osteochondral plug is not proud and effectively restores the curvature of the overlying chondral surface.

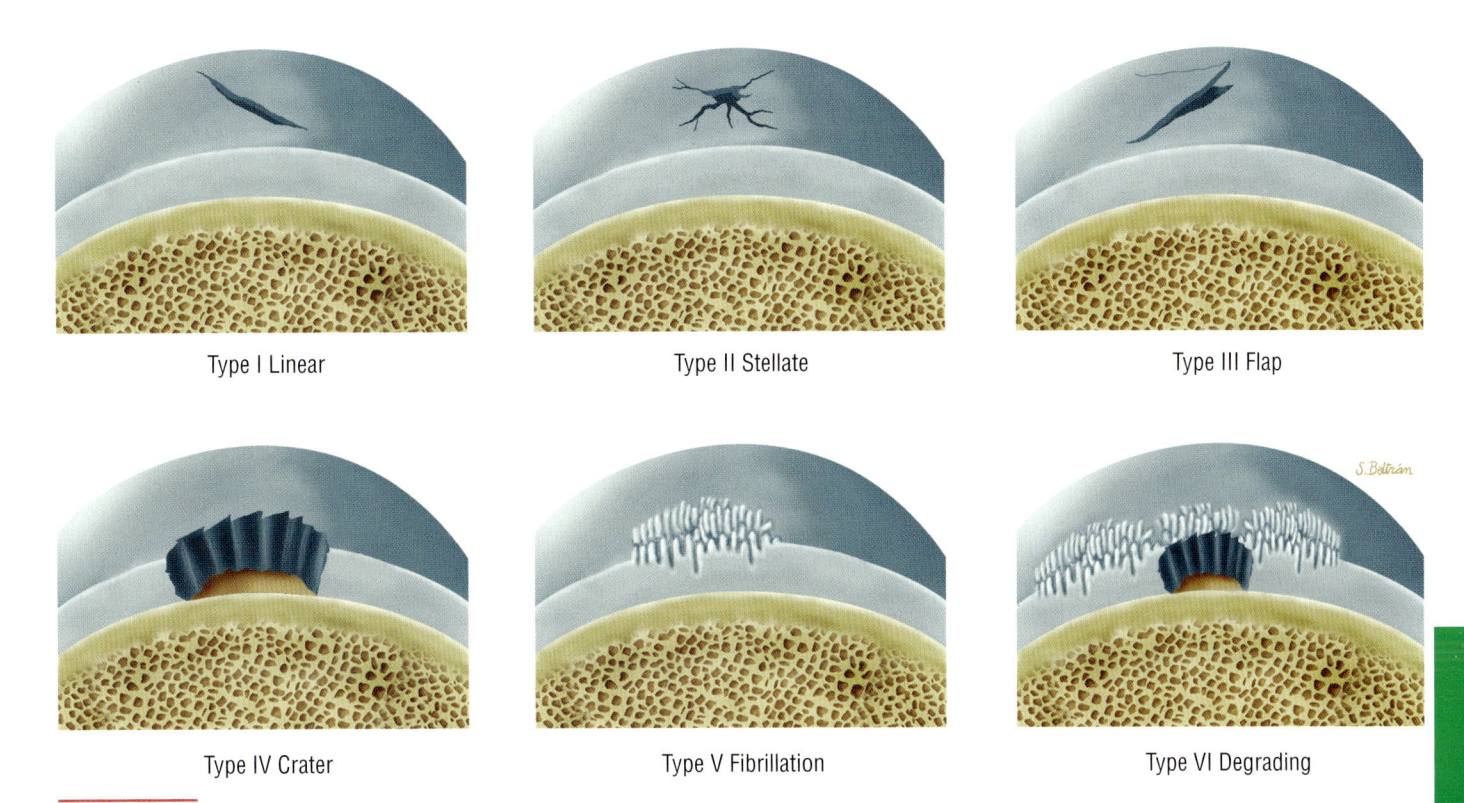

General Pathologic Conditions Affecting the Knee

| Type I Linear | Type II Stellate | Type III Flap |
| Type IV Crater | Type V Fibrillation | Type VI Degrading |

FIGURE 8.141 Classification of articular cartilage injury as developed by Baurer and Jackson.

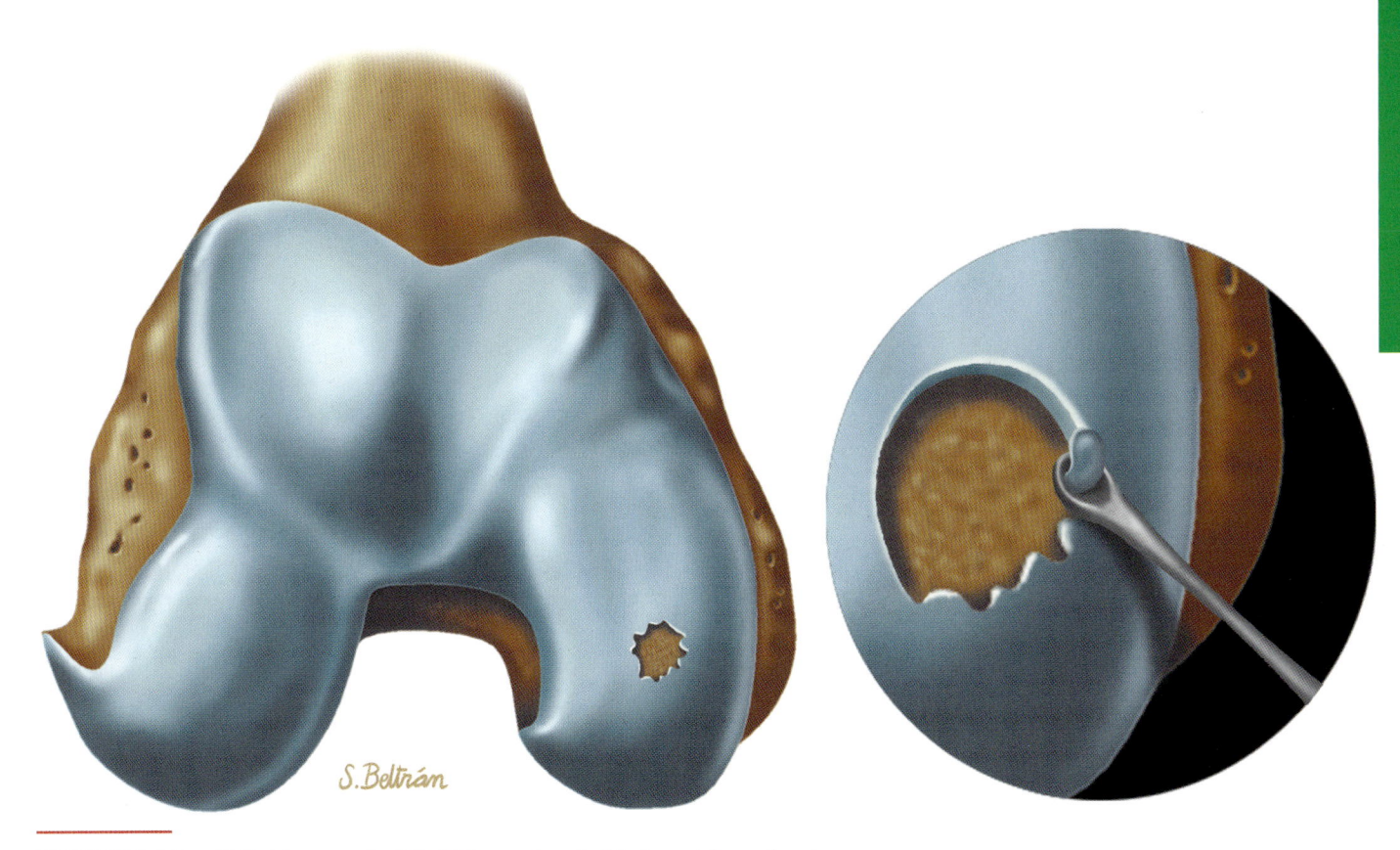

FIGURE 8.142 Débridement of a full thickness chondral lesion without abrasion.

Treatment of Chondral Lesions

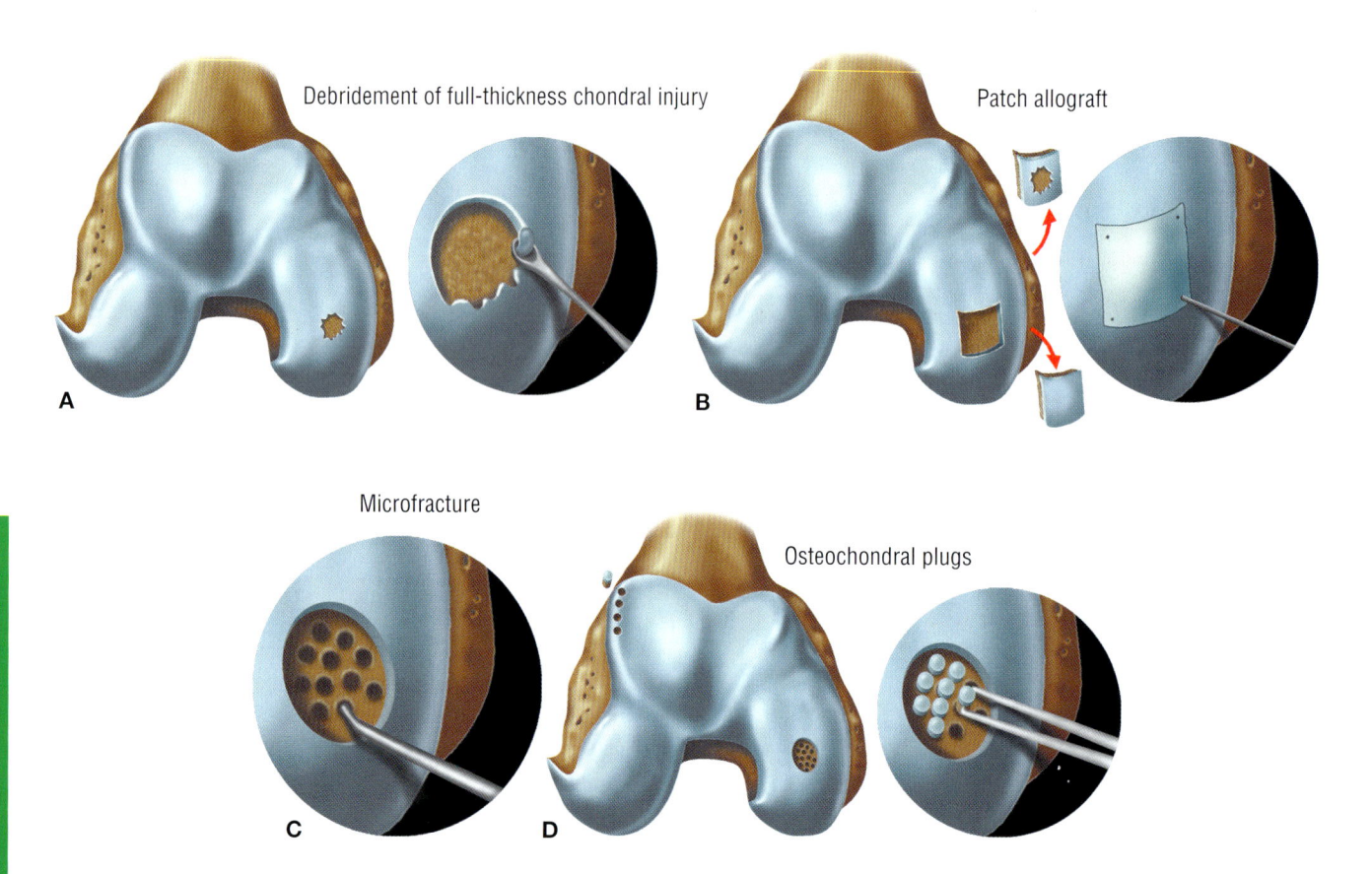

FIGURE 8.143 Cartilage resurfacing procedures. (**A**) Abrasion chondroplasty with débridement of a full thickness chondral defect. (**B**) Patch or shell allograft using a matched osteochondral graft. (**C**) Microfracture using surgical awls to penetrate the subchondral bone up to 4mm. (**D**) Osteochondral plugs harvested and transferred as a mosaicplasty. (Based on Miller MD, Howard RF, Plancher KD. *Surgical Atlas of Sports Medicine*. Philadelphia, PA: Saunders, Elsevier; 2003.)

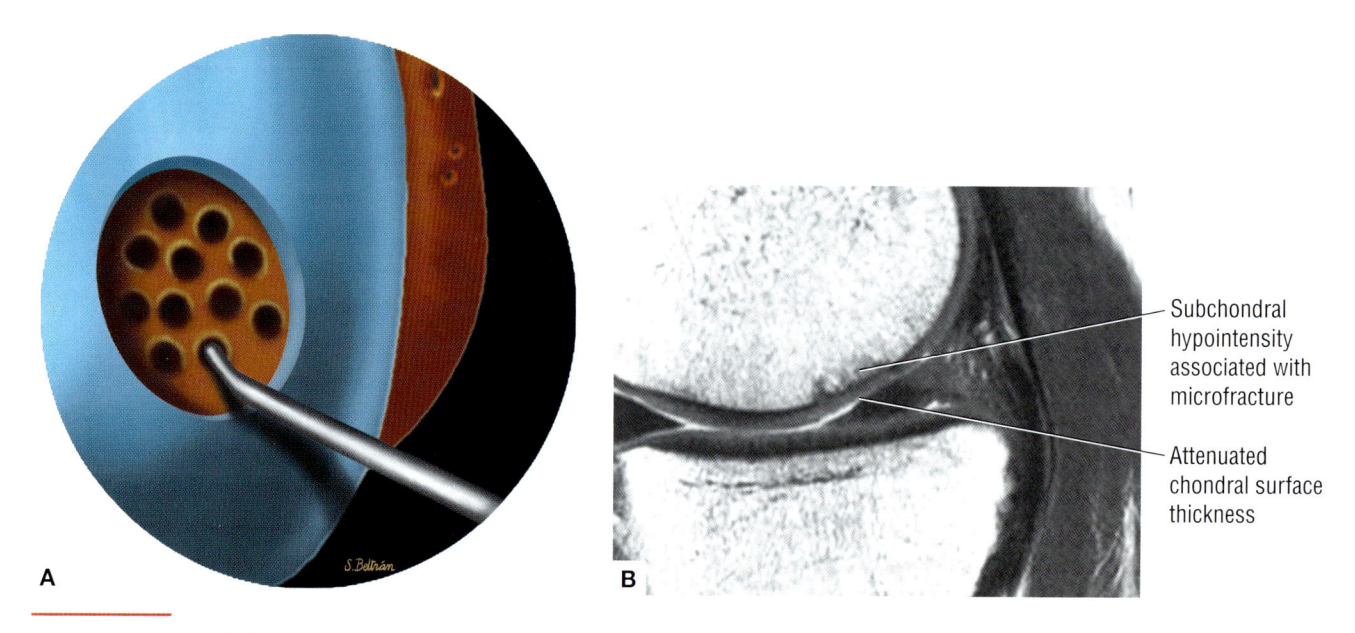

FIGURE 8.144 (**A**) Microfracture technique with the creation of subchondral holes using a specialized awl to penetrate the subchondral plate. This technique is performed after débridement of the lesion, including the calcified cartilage layer. The awl is inserted to a depth of approximately 4mm to facilitate the formation of a superclot. (**B**) Microfracture with partial regrowth of a new hybrid surface of hyaline and fibrocartilage on a sagittal PD FSE image.

General Pathologic Conditions Affecting the Knee

Donor site of osteochondral transfer

Recipient site of plug

Biocart implant

Congruous fit of donor osteochondral transfer

Biocart repair implant

Chondral degeneration (overload) between osteochondral transfer plug and Biocart scaffold

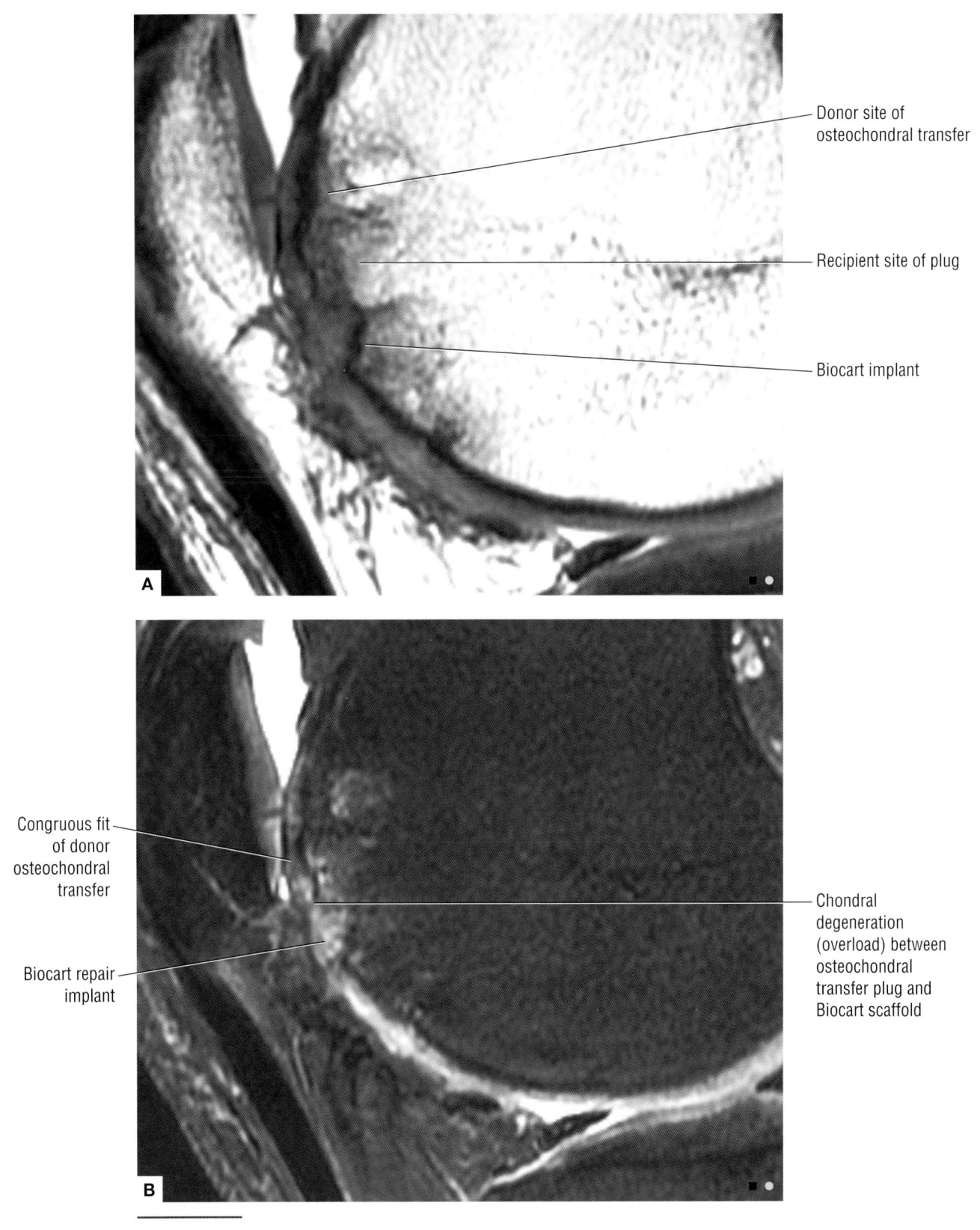

FIGURE 8.145 Donor (most superior on lateral femoral condyle) and recipient region (inferior to donor region) of osteochondral transplant plug. There is excellent congruency of the subchondral plate and chondral surface without a proud or irregular transition. Inferior to OATS is a third site representing a Biocart matrix-assisted autologous chondrocyte implant. The articular cartilage repair implant is composed of autologous cells embedded within a fibrin and hyaluronic scaffold. The chondral surface is more irregular in the Biocart implant comparing the precise press fit of the osteochondral transfer to the region of the Biocart. Sagittal PD (**A**) and FS PD (**B**) images. *(Continued)*

Donor site

Recipient site location of plug

Region of Biocart matrix implant

Proper fit (congruency of recipient site of osteochondral transfer plug)

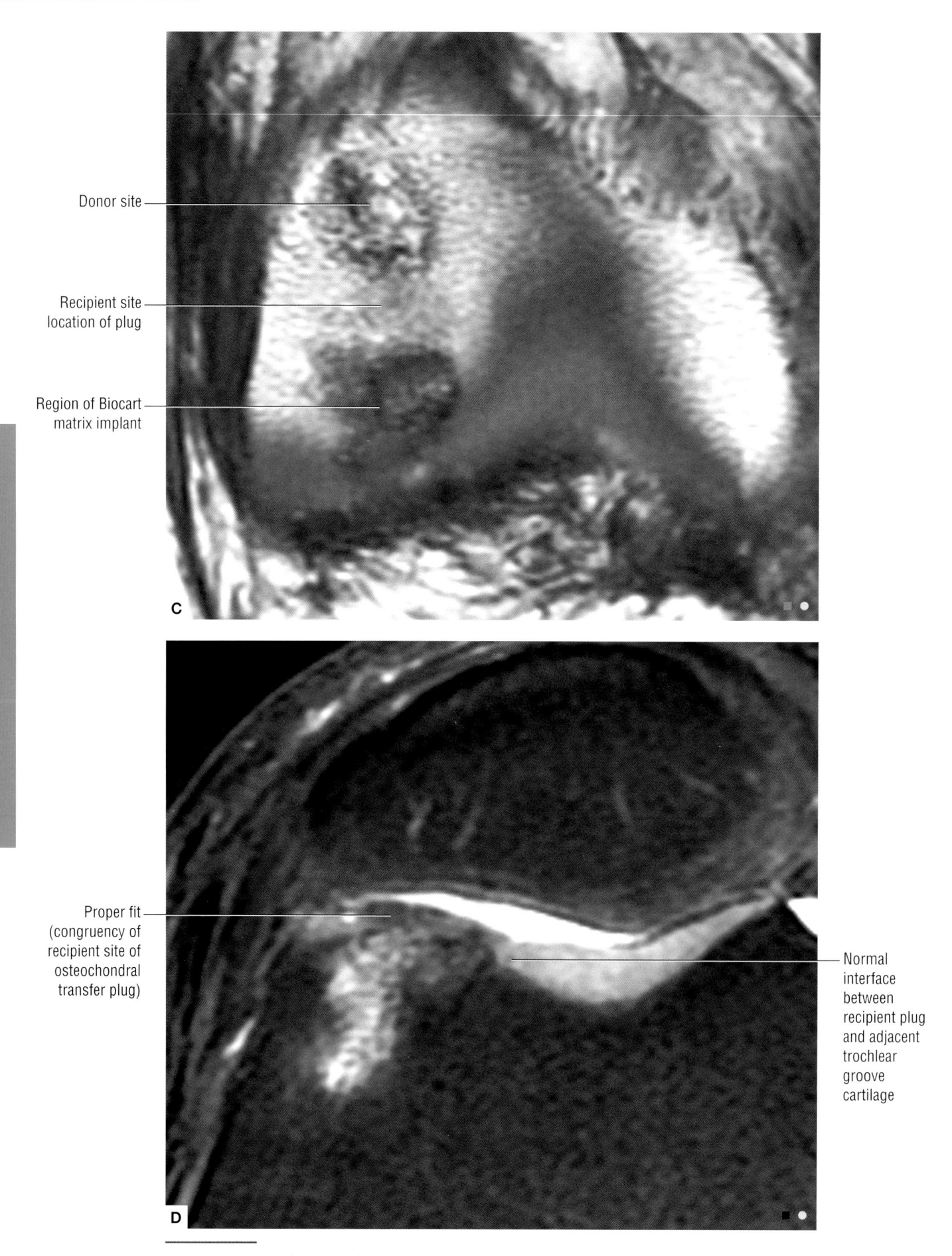

Normal interface between recipient plug and adjacent trochlear groove cartilage

FIGURE 8.145 (*Continued*) Axial PD (**C**) and FS PD (**D**) images.

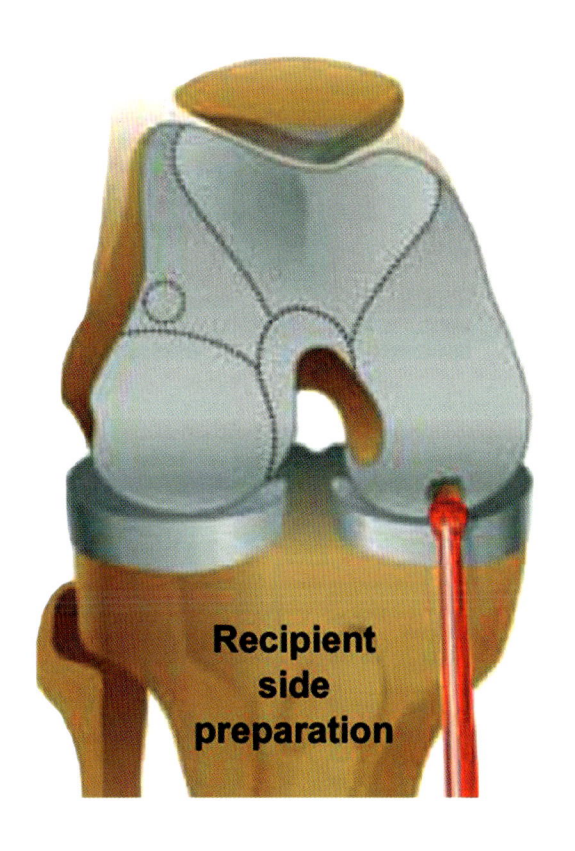

FIGURE 8.146 Preparation of the recipient side of the osteochondral transplant. The defect should be left surrounded by well-defined walls of stable normal hyaline cartilage to receive the plugs and stop progression of the lesion. (Reprinted from Fu FH. *Master Techniques in Orthopaedic Surgery: Sports Medicine*. Philadelphia, PA: Lippincott Williams & Wilkins; 2010, with permission.)

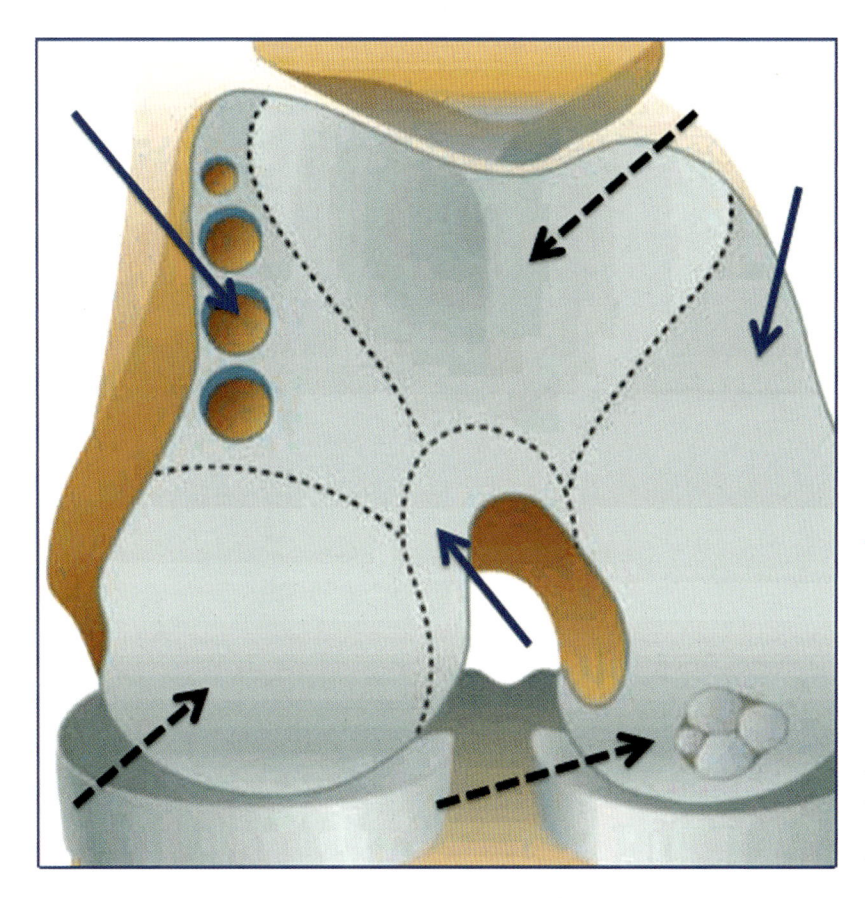

FIGURE 8.147 Donor regions are marked with *blue arrows*. Recipient regions are marked with *dashed arrows*. Donor regions may be chosen depending on their shape and congruency with the recipient side. (Reprinted from Fu FH. *Master Techniques in Orthopaedic Surgery: Sports Medicine*. Philadelphia, PA: Lippincott Williams & Wilkins; 2010, with permission.)

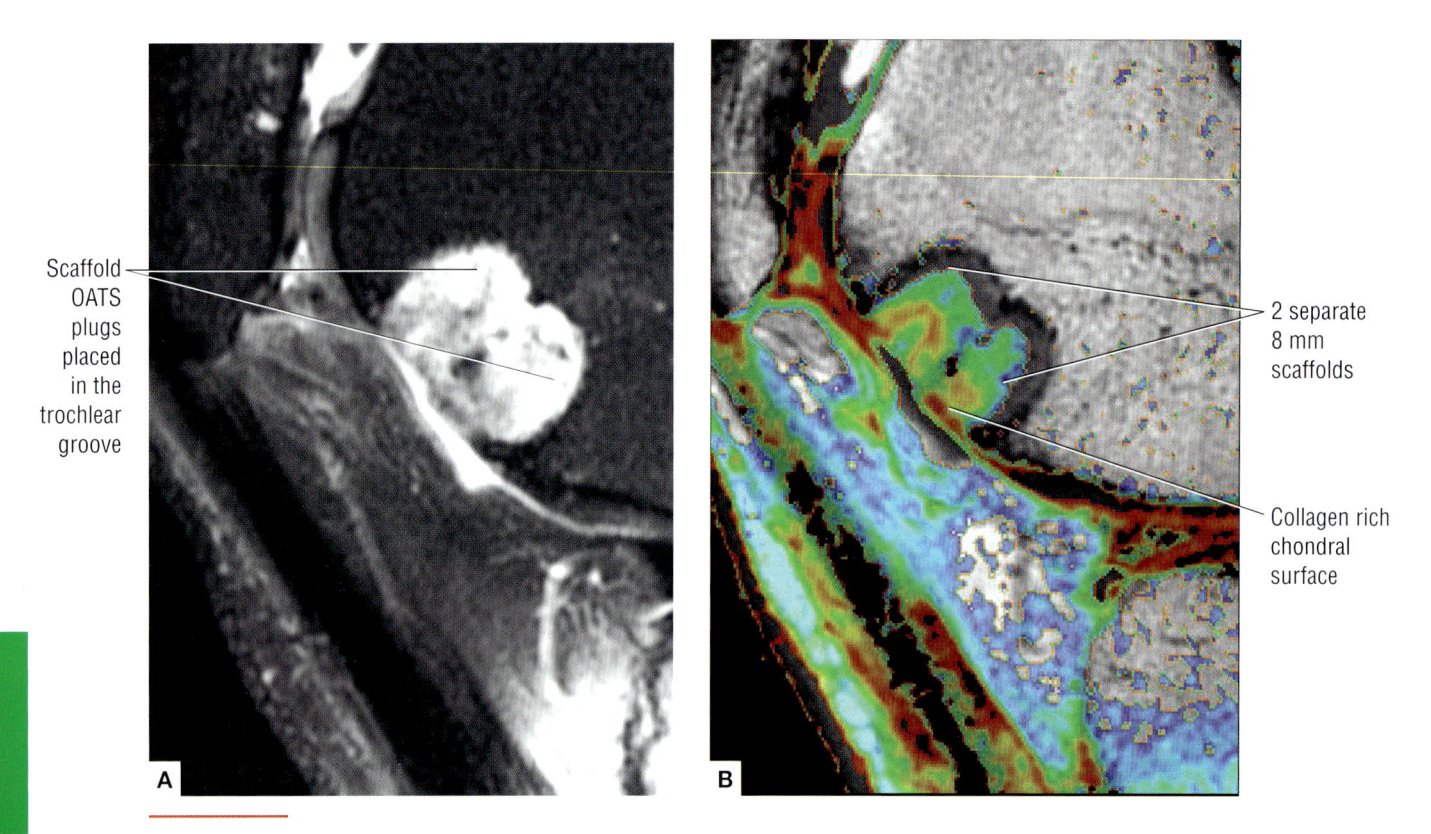

FIGURE 8.148 (**A**) Sagittal FS PD FSE image of two OATS scaffold grafts placed in the trochlear groove. The bioabsorbable polymer scaffolds are hyperintense on FS PD FSE images. (**B**) Sagittal T2 map documents chondral surface regrowth with lower TE values (orange) in the more inferior scaffold OATS graft.

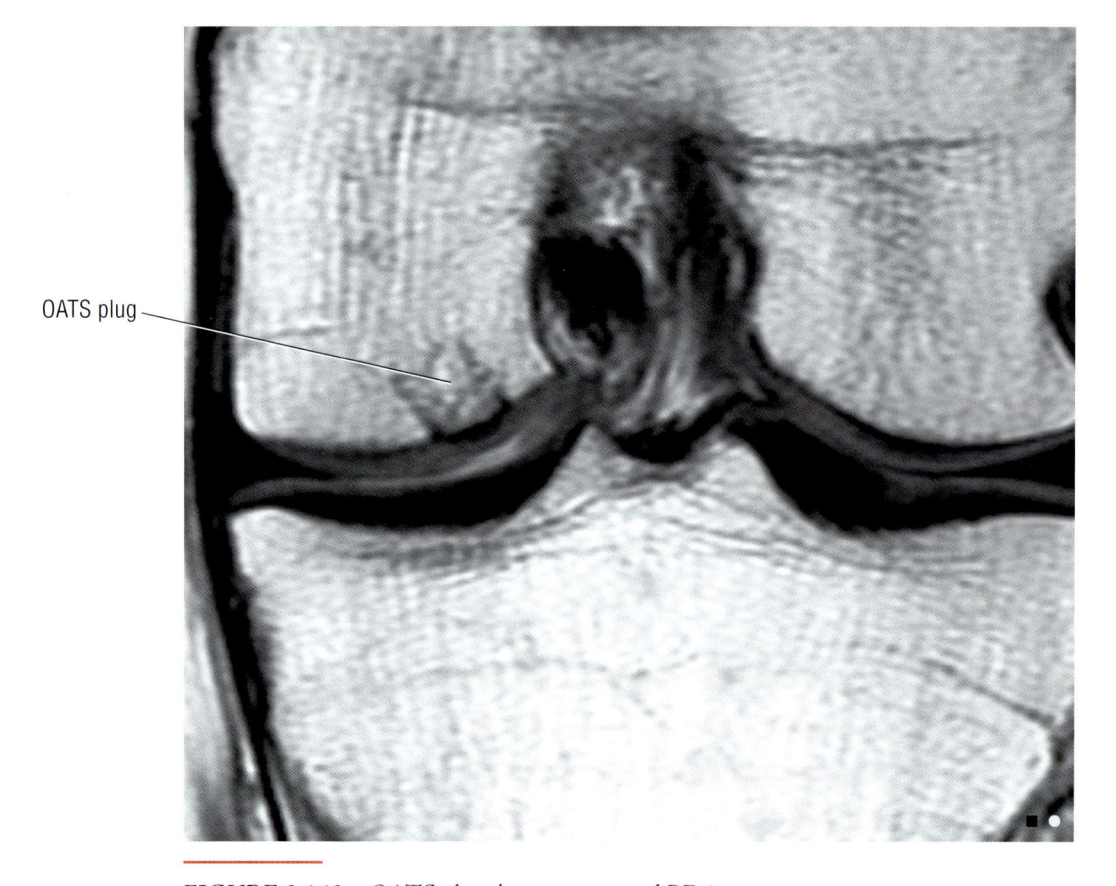

FIGURE 8.149 OATS plug shown on coronal PD image.

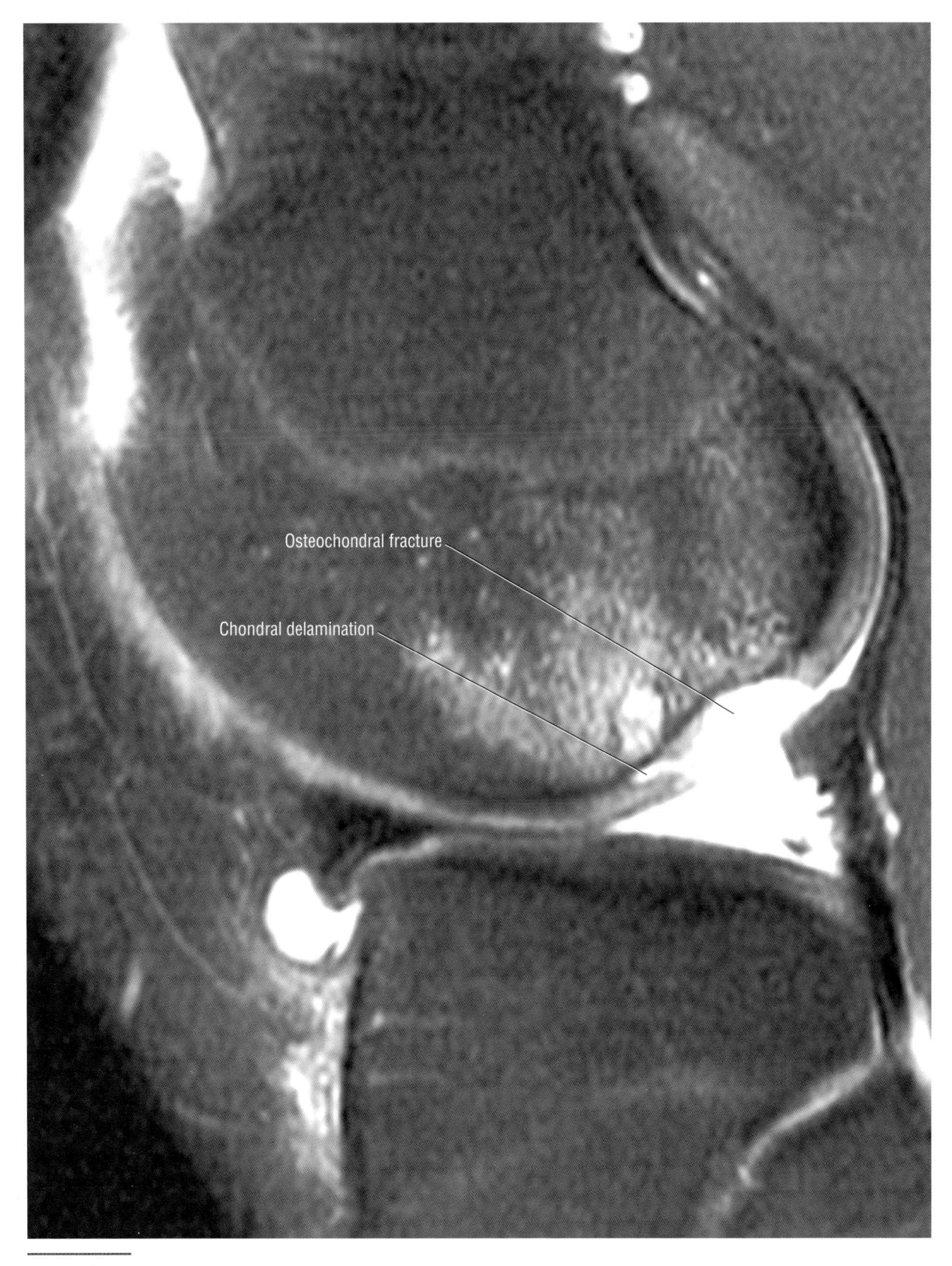

FIGURE 8.150 Large osteochondral defect with unstable flap of articular cartilage at its inferior margin. Sagittal FS PD FSE image.

Articular Cartilage Stem Cell Paste Graft

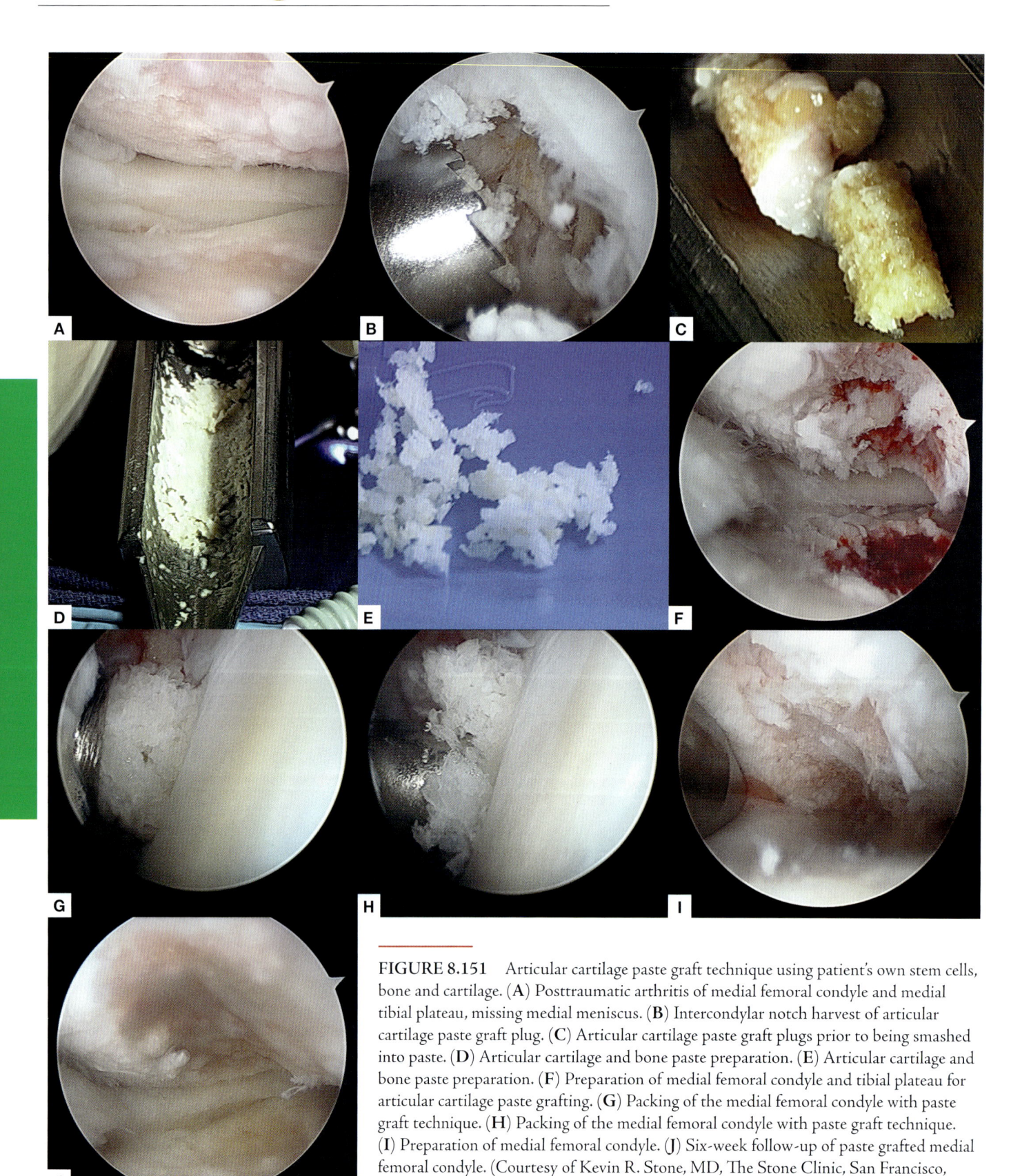

FIGURE 8.151 Articular cartilage paste graft technique using patient's own stem cells, bone and cartilage. (**A**) Posttraumatic arthritis of medial femoral condyle and medial tibial plateau, missing medial meniscus. (**B**) Intercondylar notch harvest of articular cartilage paste graft plug. (**C**) Articular cartilage paste graft plugs prior to being smashed into paste. (**D**) Articular cartilage and bone paste preparation. (**E**) Articular cartilage and bone paste preparation. (**F**) Preparation of medial femoral condyle and tibial plateau for articular cartilage paste grafting. (**G**) Packing of the medial femoral condyle with paste graft technique. (**H**) Packing of the medial femoral condyle with paste graft technique. (**I**) Preparation of medial femoral condyle. (**J**) Six-week follow-up of paste grafted medial femoral condyle. (Courtesy of Kevin R. Stone, MD, The Stone Clinic, San Francisco, California.)

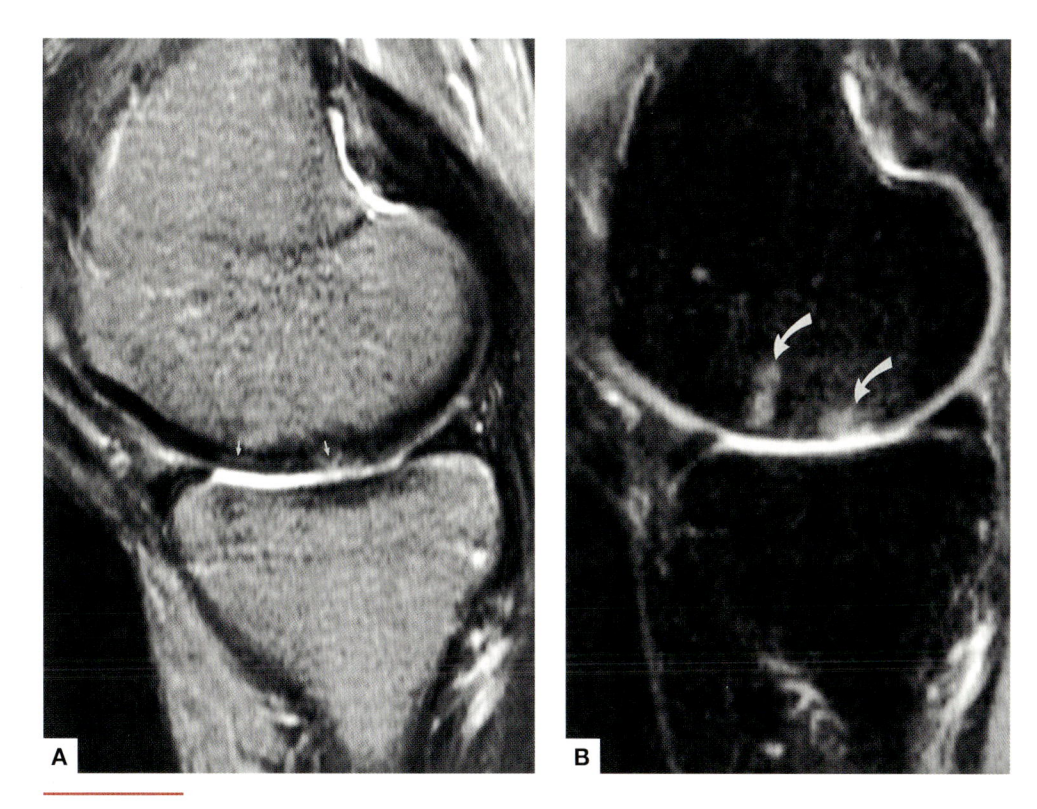

General Pathologic Conditions Affecting the Knee

FIGURE 8.152 Application of the microfracture technique is documented on (**A**) an FSE version of an echo-planar imaging (EPI) image and (**B**) a sagittal STIR image. The microfracture technique is used to create a neofibrocartilaginous surface to replace the damaged hyaline articular cartilage. The EPI image exaggerates the thickness of the subchondral plate as a result of a chemical-shift artifact and allows identification of vascular areas (*straight arrows*) as distinguished from the reactive subchondral marrow edema (*curved arrows*) seen on the STIR image.

Reactive subchondral edema
OATS autograft
Chondral/fibrocartilage regrowth

Collagen associated TE values (orange color) in OATS autograft

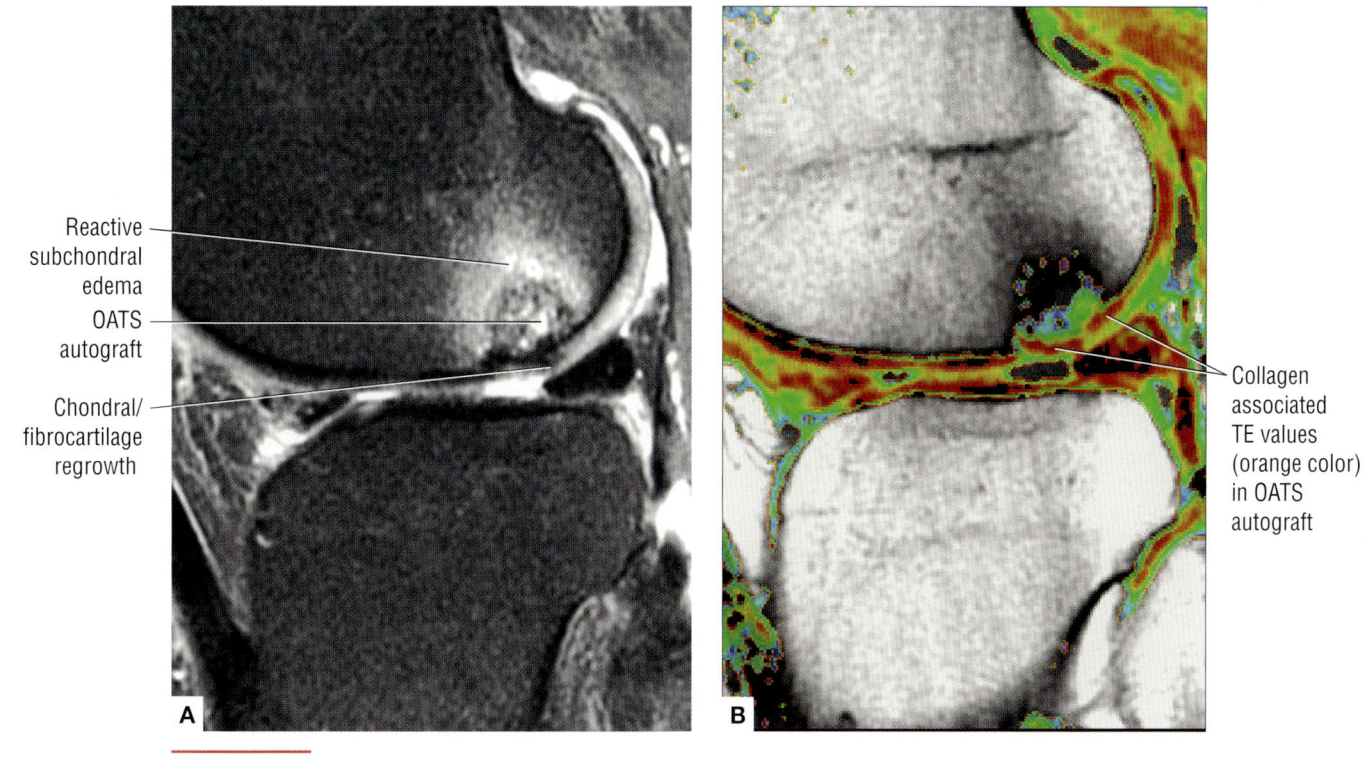

FIGURE 8.153 (**A**) Sagittal FS PD FSE image of osteochondral autograft transfer system (OATS) of the lateral femoral condyle. (**B**) Corresponding T2 map with collagen development associated with low TE values (orange).

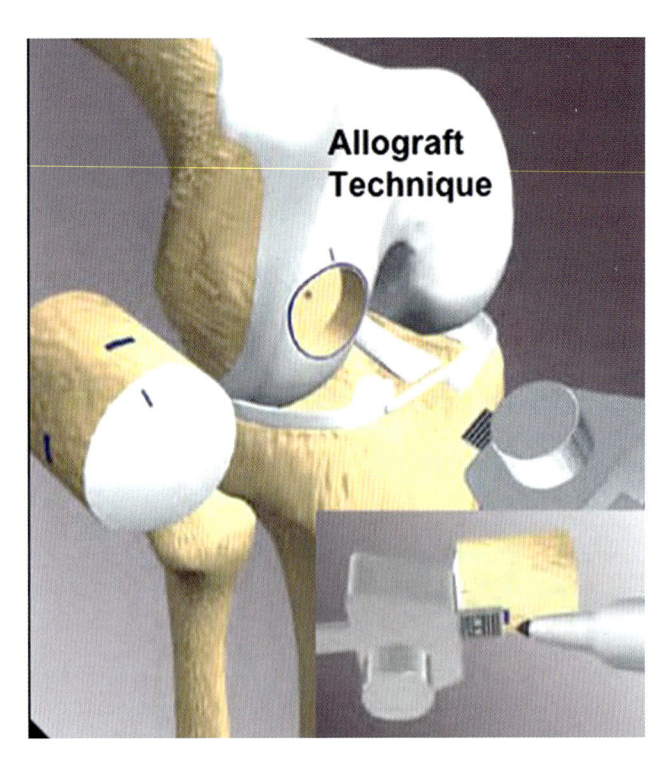

FIGURE 8.154 Osteochondral allograft dowel technique. This technique is similar to the autograft technique where the surgeon is able to insert single or multiple osteochondral allograft plugs into the defect, matching the curvature of the lesion. Note the importance of marking the allograft in order to match the original curvature of the recipient site as accurately as possible. (Reprinted from Fu FH. *Master Techniques in Orthopaedic Surgery: Sports Medicine*. Philadelphia, PA: Lippincott Williams & Wilkins; 2010, with permission.)

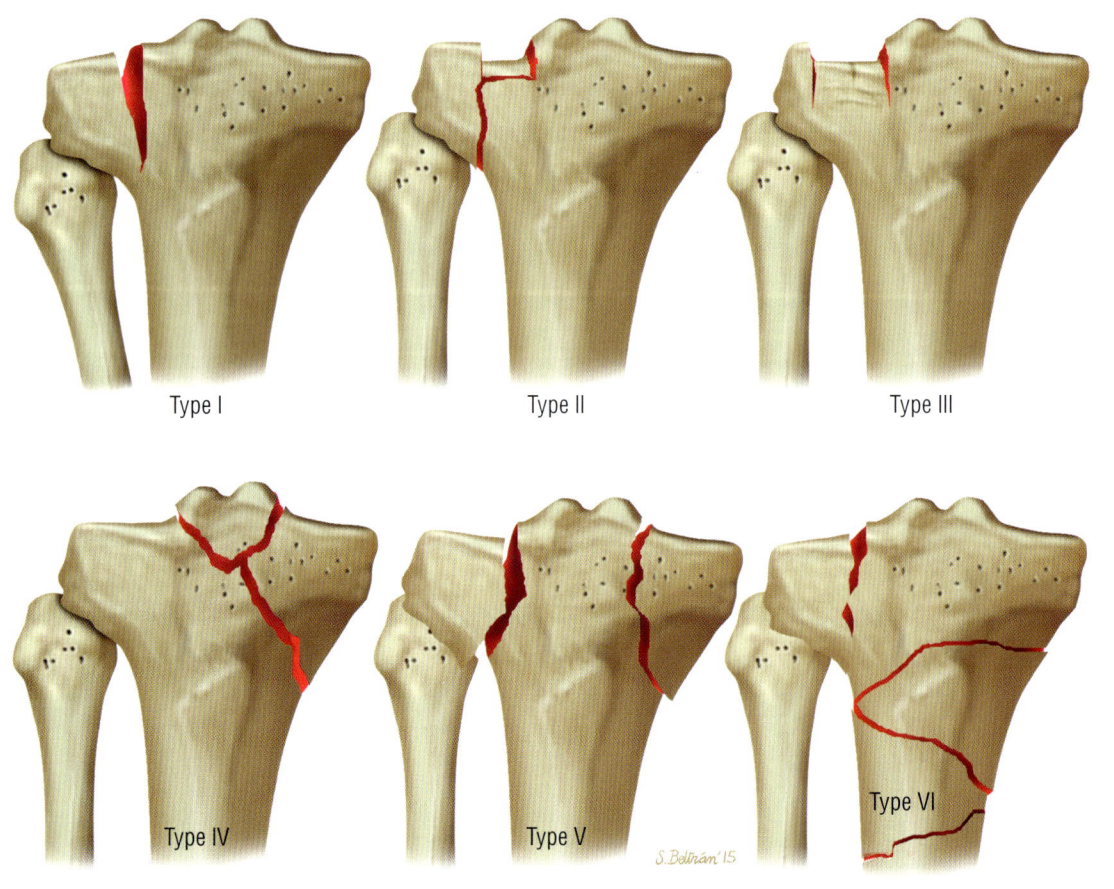

FIGURE 8.155 Schatzker (similar to Hohl system) classification of tibial plateau fractures. Schatzker system types of tibial plateau fractures are based on the involvement of the medial and/or lateral tibial plateaus. Type I: lateral tibial plateau split; type II: lateral tibial plateau split depression; type III: lateral plateau central depression; type IV: medial plateau; type V: bicondylar split; and type VI: plateau and proximal diaphysis. Plateau depression, split fragments, and soft tissue injury including meniscal disruption and entrapment are demonstrated on MR imaging. MR offers the advantage over CT in the characterization of secondary nondisplaced fracture extensions as well as soft tissue constraint injuries.

Fractures

Key Concepts

- Fracture morphology and associated edema may be underestimated on PD FSE or conventional T2-weighted images.

- Red marrow heterogeneity should not extend to epiphysis.

- In reflex sympathetic dystrophy, FS PD FSE or STIR images are needed to appreciate marrow hyperintensity.

Osseous Fractures and Bone Contusions

- Knee fractures can involve femoral condyle, the tibial plateau, or patella.[469]

- Tibial plateau fractures most frequent, predominantly with lateral plateau involvement[28]

- Mechanism of injury

    - Most common cause is impaction of anterior portion of lateral femoral condyle in valgus injury.

    - Axial loading, or pure compressive force, produces impaction or compression fracture of plateau.

    - Pure valgus force results in split condylar fracture.

    - Valgus compressive force responsible for frequent occurrence of lateral tibial condylar plateau fractures with tears of medial meniscus, ACL, and medial collateral ligament (MCL)

- Radiographic evaluation

    - Fractures of knee can be identified on MR in patients with negative findings on conventional radiographs.

    - MR imaging is equivalent or superior to two-dimensional computed tomography (CT) reconstruction for displaying fracture morphology.[45]

    - Subsequent plain-film radiography often shows areas of sclerosis or periosteal reaction at fracture site initially identified on MR.

MR Appearance of Osseous Fractures and Bone Contusions

- Most common MR pattern is sharp, well-defined, linear segments of decreased signal intensity in distal femur or proximal tibia.

- In acute fracture, associated fluid or hemorrhage demonstrates increased signal intensity on conventional T2, FS PD-weighted FSE, and STIR images.

- GRE T2 contrast images may also demonstrate hyperintensity in acute fractures.

- Fractures with diffuse areas of associated low signal intensity on T2-weighted images demonstrate increased signal intensity with long TR and TE settings.
    - Reflects prolonged T2 values in edematous or hemorrhagic marrow

- STIR images more sensitive than GRE T2*-weighted images and conventional T2-weighted images in identifying subacute fractures with associated marrow edema

- T2*-weighted contrast may be useful in displaying acute fracture morphology when extensive marrow hemorrhage obscures detail on T1-weighted or STIR images.

- Chronic fractures remain low in signal intensity with variable TR and TE parameters.

- In animal models, posttraumatic growth plate abnormalities, including changes in cartilage, transphyseal vascularity, and bone bridge formation, can be detected with MR imaging.[218,370]

- Metaphyseal–diaphyseal junction in physis should not be mistaken for a transverse linear fracture.[221]

- Discontinuity of physis may occur with trauma or epiphysiodesis.[359]

- In the adult, physeal line or scar does not demonstrate increased signal intensity on T2-weighted images.

- In a child, chemical-shift artifact may display bright signal intensity parallel with physis.

- The acute fracture line is usually hypointense compared to adjacent T2 hypointense marrow in acute fractures.

- The actual site of fracture or linear fracture line is hyperintense in subacute fractures. Subchondral bone may persist with T2 hyperintensity.

Stress Fractures

- Common in proximal tibia
- MR imaging can differentiate from neoplastic processes.
- Linear segment of stress fracture usually accompanied by marrow edema
- Lack of soft tissue mass, cortical destruction, and characteristic marrow extension effectively exclude tumor from differential diagnosis.
- Rarely, stress fracture is obscured on MR by reactive edema.
    - High-resolution and thin-section CT required to identify it
- Pathologic fractures complicating nonossifying fibromas may occur in adolescents and are more common in distal femoral diaphysis.

Contusions (Bone Bruise)

- Diffuse or localized pattern of low signal intensity on T1-weighted images without defined fracture line
- At sites of microtrauma or impaction of trabecular bone[326]
- Recognition of occult subchondral fractures is important because osteochondral sequelae with significant cartilage damage may develop.[501]
- In an acute or subacute setting, increased signal intensity is seen on T2, FS PD-weighted FSE, or STIR images, before the appearance of sclerosis on plain-film radiographs.[480]
- Normal metaphyseal–diaphyseal low-signal-intensity red marrow inhomogeneity should not be mistaken for a contusion.
    - Frequently seen in female patients
    - Should not cross the physeal scar into subchondral bone
    - Reconversion of yellow to red marrow associated with increased demand for hematopoiesis
    - May also be seen in sickle cell– or thalassemia-related hemolytic anemias and marrow proliferative or replacement disorders
    - On T1-weighted images, marrow replacement disorders usually demonstrate hypointensity equal to or lower than muscle.
    - STIR images or heavily T2-weighted images (>3000msec for conventional T2 and >5000msec for FS PD-weighted FSE images) may demonstrate varying degrees of increased signal intensity.

- Morphology of bone contusions characterized into three types based on T1- or intermediate-weighted images[295]
    - Type I: diffuse decrease in signal intensity in metaphyseal and epiphyseal areas
    - Type II: interruption of low-signal-intensity cortical line
    - Type III: localized decrease in signal intensity in subchondral bone
- Type I and II lesions are difficult to detect on radiography and arthroscopy and are frequently associated with ACL and collateral ligament injuries.
- Pathologic fracture may be complicated by internal hemorrhage that obscures underlying lesion.

Tibial Plateau Fractures

- Hohl classification
    - Minimally displaced (i.e., <4mm of depression or displacement) or displaced[190]
    - Displaced fractures further subdivided into local compression, split compression, total condylar depression, split rim, and bicondylar fractures
- MR allows articular cartilage characterization
- Supracondylar, condylar, or intercondylar
- Nondisplaced, impacted, displaced, or comminuted
- Description of subchondral plate depression should include area or region of maximum depression.
- Secondary fracture lines transmitted from the point of impact should be identified.
- Identify entrapped meniscal tissue or torn attachments.

Patellar Fractures

- Must be differentiated from bipartite patellar morphology
- Vertical, transverse, or comminuted[418]

General Pathologic Conditions Affecting the Knee

Lateral Plateau Fracture

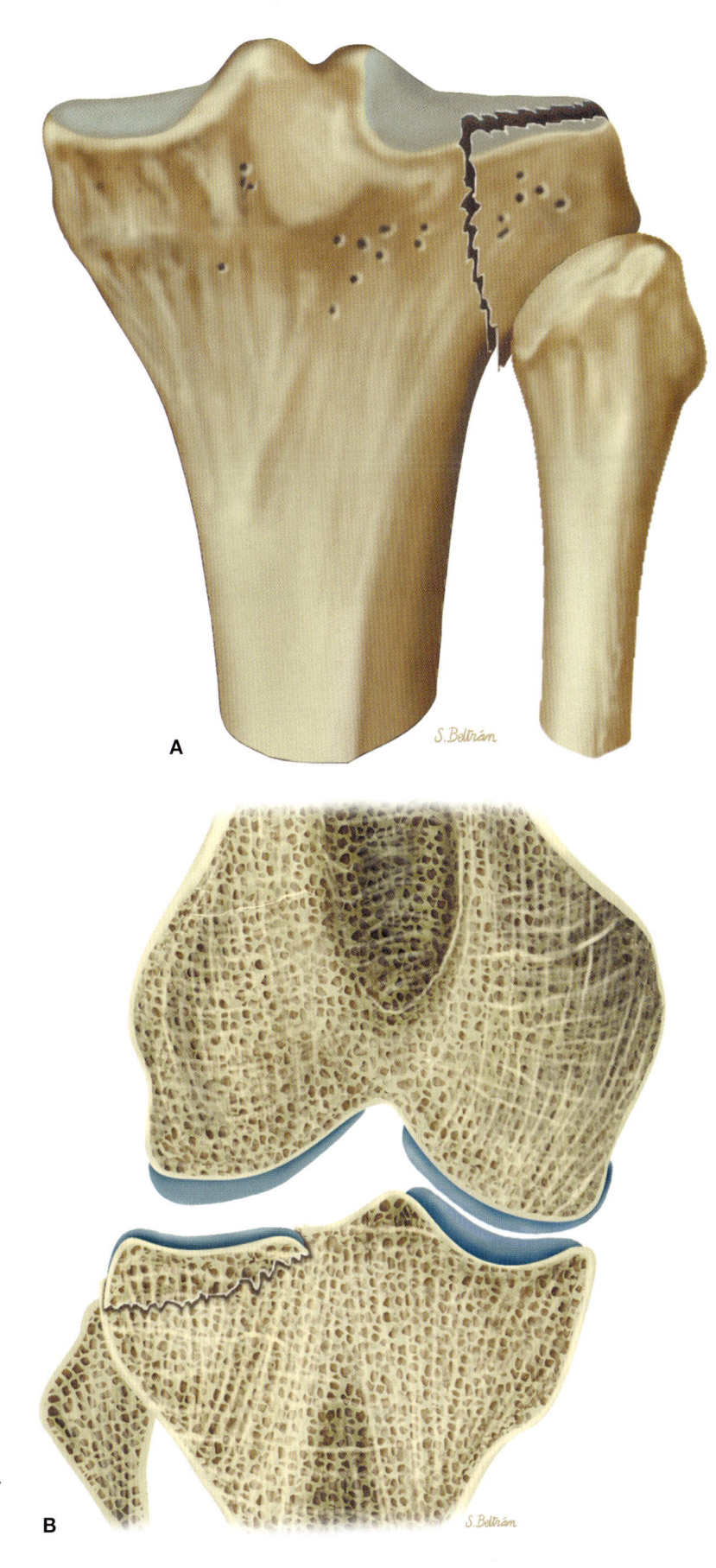

FIGURE 8.156 (A) Nondisplaced split fracture of the lateral tibial plateau (Hohl type I fracture). (B) Local central depression with medial-to-lateral fracture extension shown on a coronal color section. This corresponds to a type II tibial plateau fracture in the Hohl classification scheme.

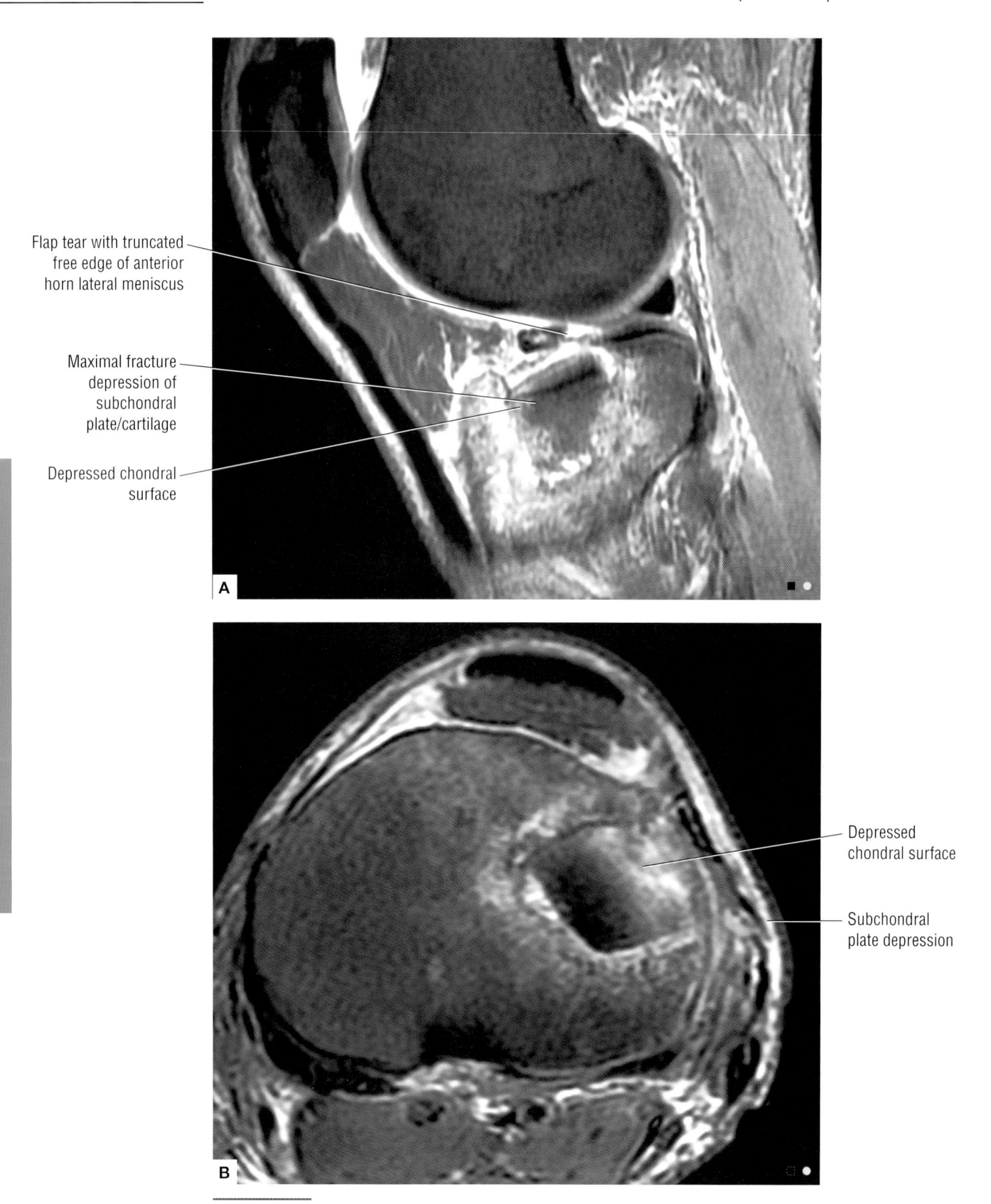

FIGURE 8.157 Lateral plateau split-depression fracture with associated tear of the anterior horn of the lateral meniscus. Precise area of plateau depression is determined by comparing sagittal/coronal with axial images. Sagittal (**A**) and axial (**B**) FS PD FSE images.

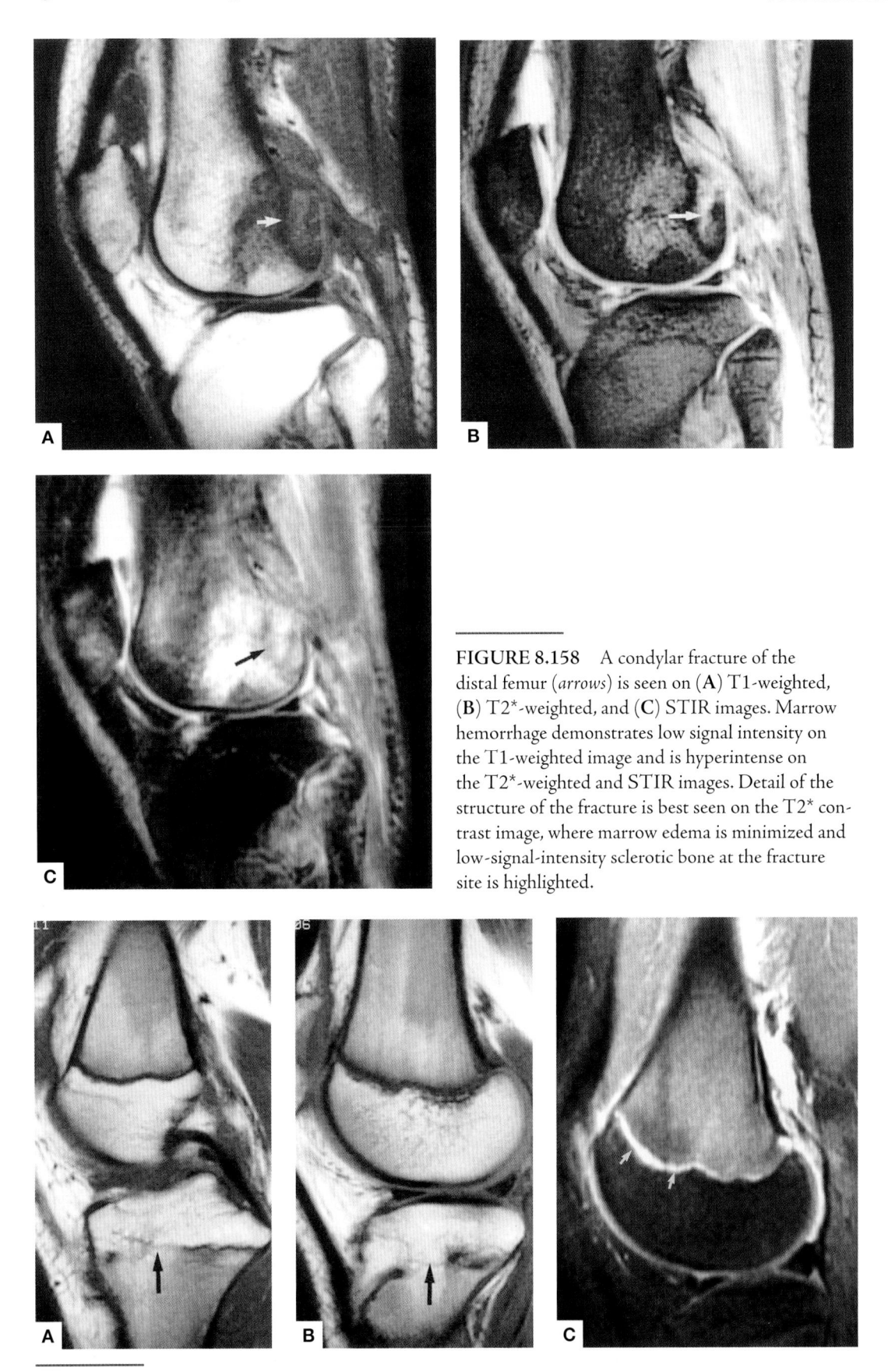

FIGURE 8.158 A condylar fracture of the distal femur (*arrows*) is seen on (**A**) T1-weighted, (**B**) T2*-weighted, and (**C**) STIR images. Marrow hemorrhage demonstrates low signal intensity on the T1-weighted image and is hyperintense on the T2*-weighted and STIR images. Detail of the structure of the fracture is best seen on the T2* contrast image, where marrow edema is minimized and low-signal-intensity sclerotic bone at the fracture site is highlighted.

FIGURE 8.159 Epiphysiodesis is used to treat leg-length inequality. Interruption (*arrows*) of the normal low-signal-intensity physeal plates in the (**A**) medial and (**B**) lateral aspects of the proximal tibia is seen on T1-weighted sagittal images. (**C**) In another patient, physeal trauma is shown as a hyperintense line following the contour of the anterior lateral femoral condyle and physis (*arrows*). There is no epiphyseal involvement on this FS T2-weighted FSE sagittal image.

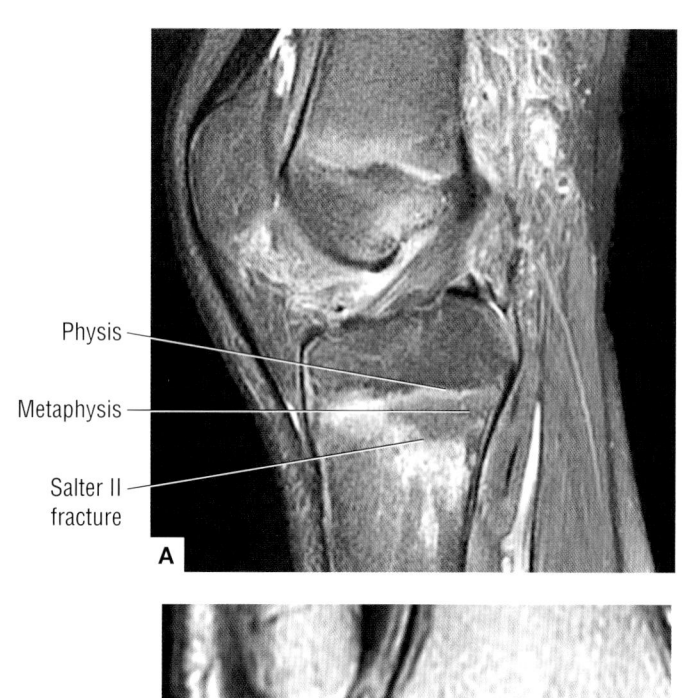

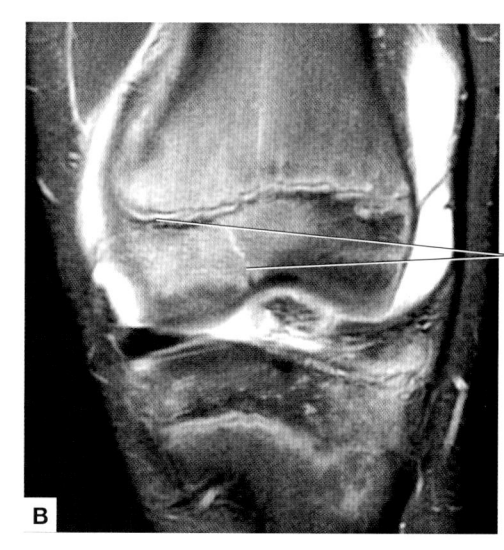

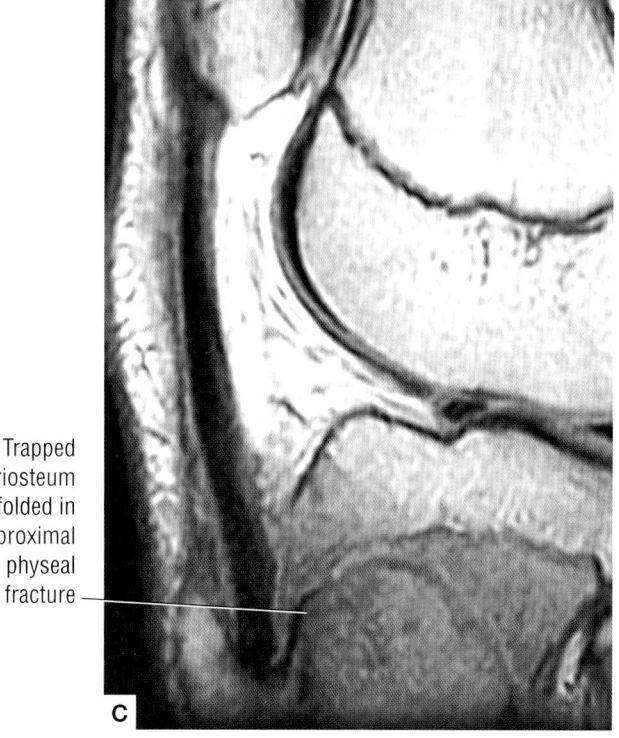

FIGURE 8.160 (**A**) Salter-Harris type II fracture through the growth plate of the proximal tibia and metaphysis on a sagittal FS PD FSE image. (**B**) Salter-Harris type III fracture through the physis with perpendicular extension through the epiphysis of the distal femur on a coronal FS PD FSE image. (**C**) Trapped periosteum flipped into the anterior proximal tibial physis on a sagittal PD FSE image.

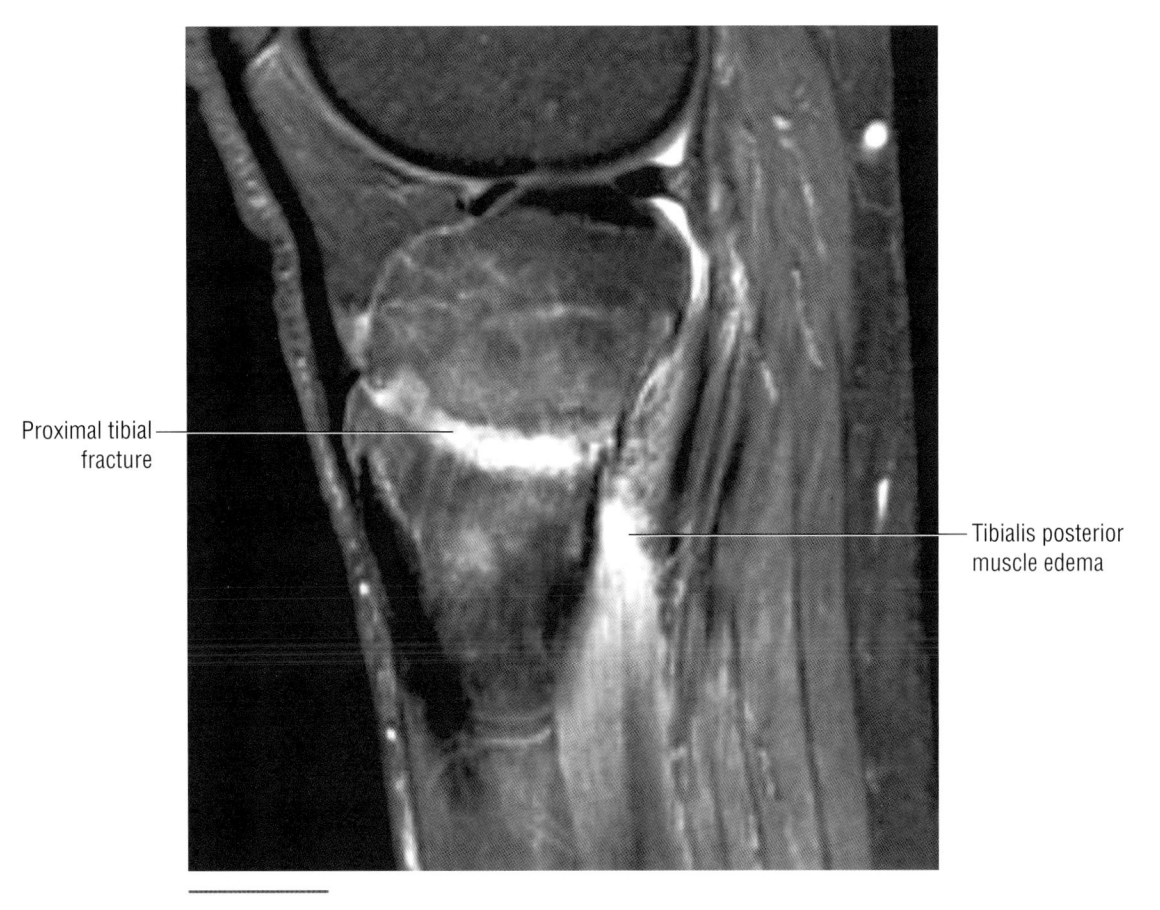

General Pathologic Conditions Affecting the Knee

FIGURE 8.161 Fracture of the proximal third of the tibia associated with tibialis posterior muscle edema. Compartment syndrome and malalignment are potential complications of nonarticular proximal tibial fractures. Sagittal FS PD FSE image.

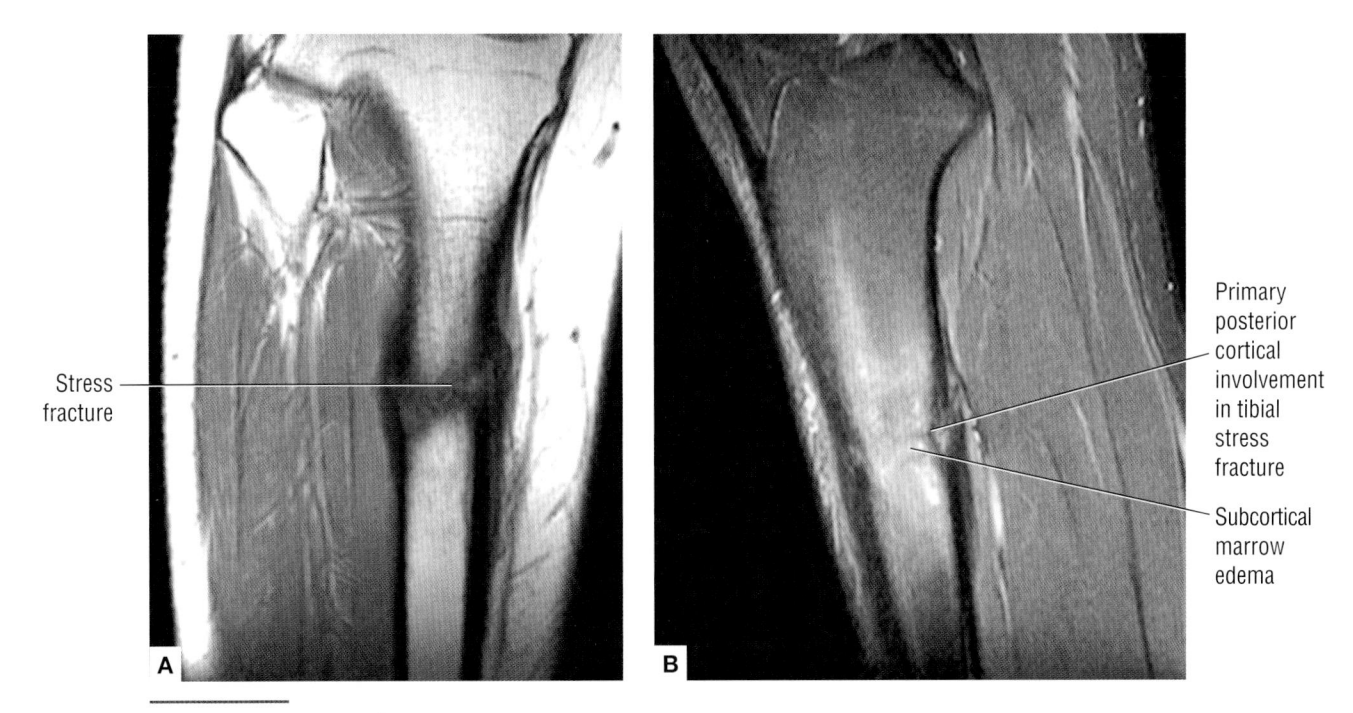

FIGURE 8.162 Stress fracture of the posterior cortex of the tibial diaphysis in a 20-year-old is seen on (**A**) coronal PD FSE and (**B**) sagittal FS PD FSE images. The posterior coronal image shows medial-to-lateral fracture extension. The sagittal image, however, accurately demonstrates intact (stable) bone stock anterior to the involved posterior cortex.

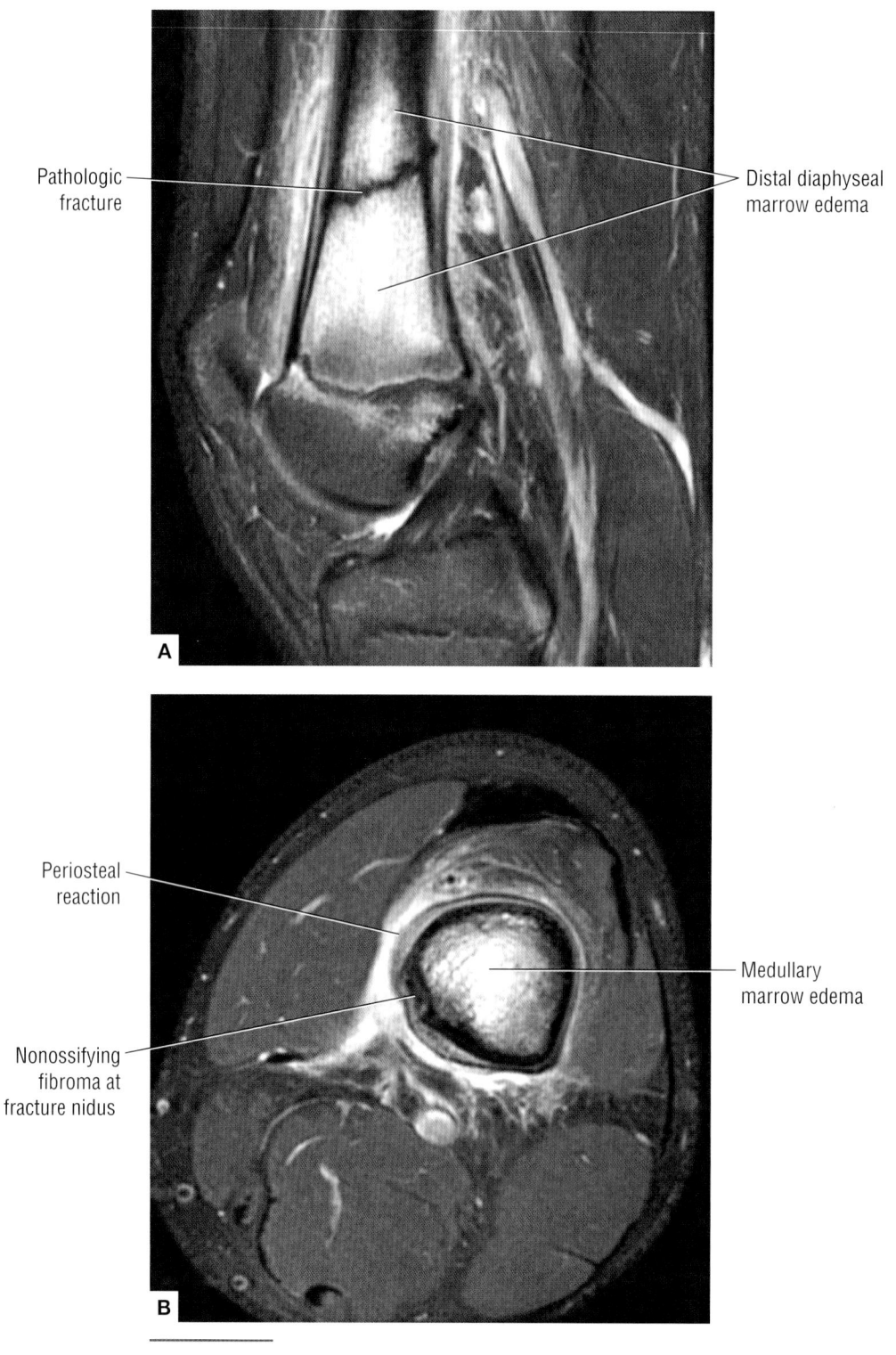

FIGURE 8.163 Pathologic fracture of the distal femoral diaphysis as a complication of a posterior nonossifying fibroma on (**A**) sagittal FS PD FSE and (**B**) axial FS PD FSE images.

General Pathologic Conditions Affecting the Knee 1011

— Subchondral stress fracture

Marrow edema prominent adjacent to fracture —

— Linear morphology of subchondral fracture

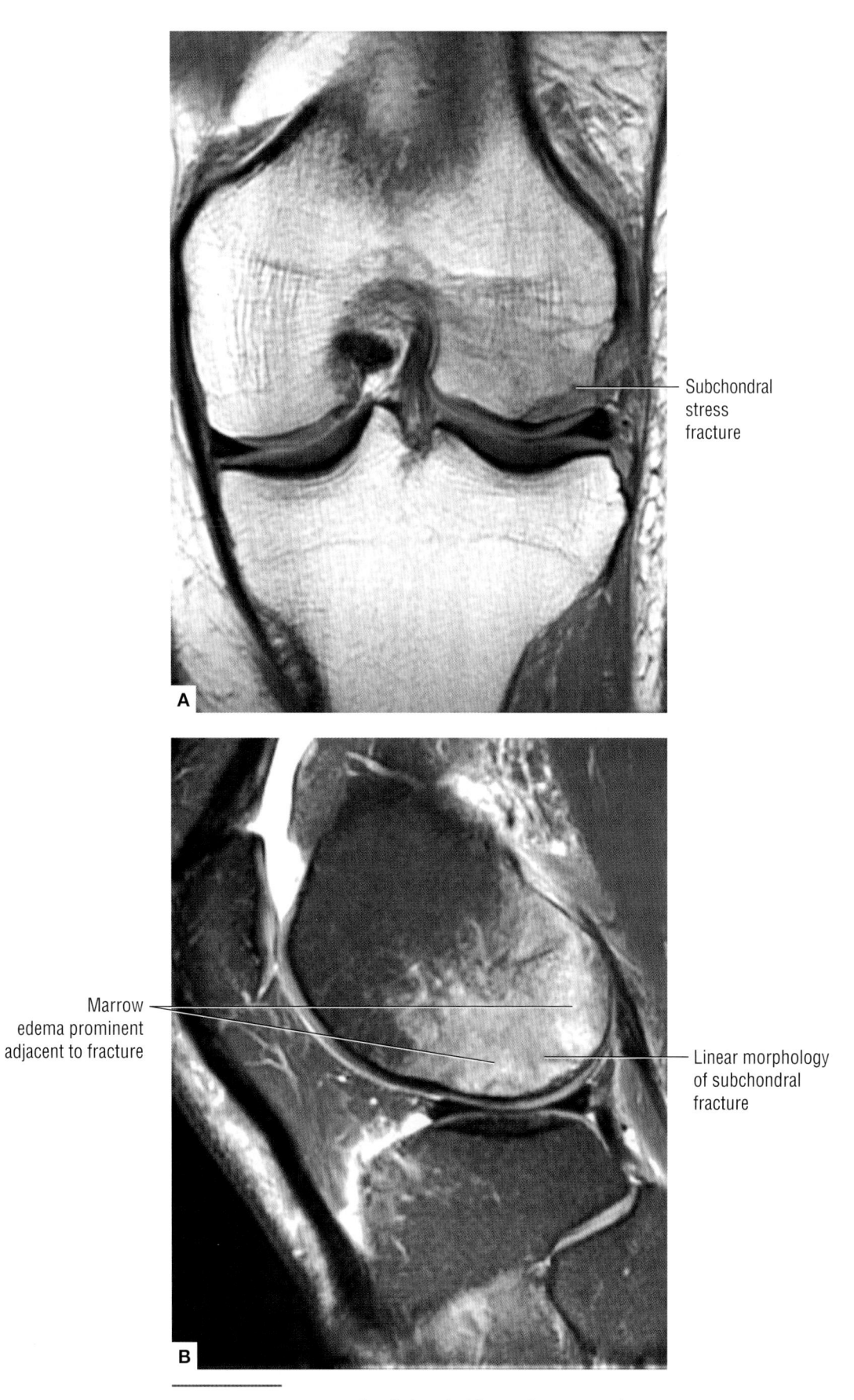

FIGURE 8.164 Occult subchondral linear fracture involving the lateral aspect of the lateral femoral condyle on (**A**) coronal T1-weighted and (**B**) sagittal FS PD FSE images. Reactive marrow edema is hyperintense on the FS PD FSE image (**B**).

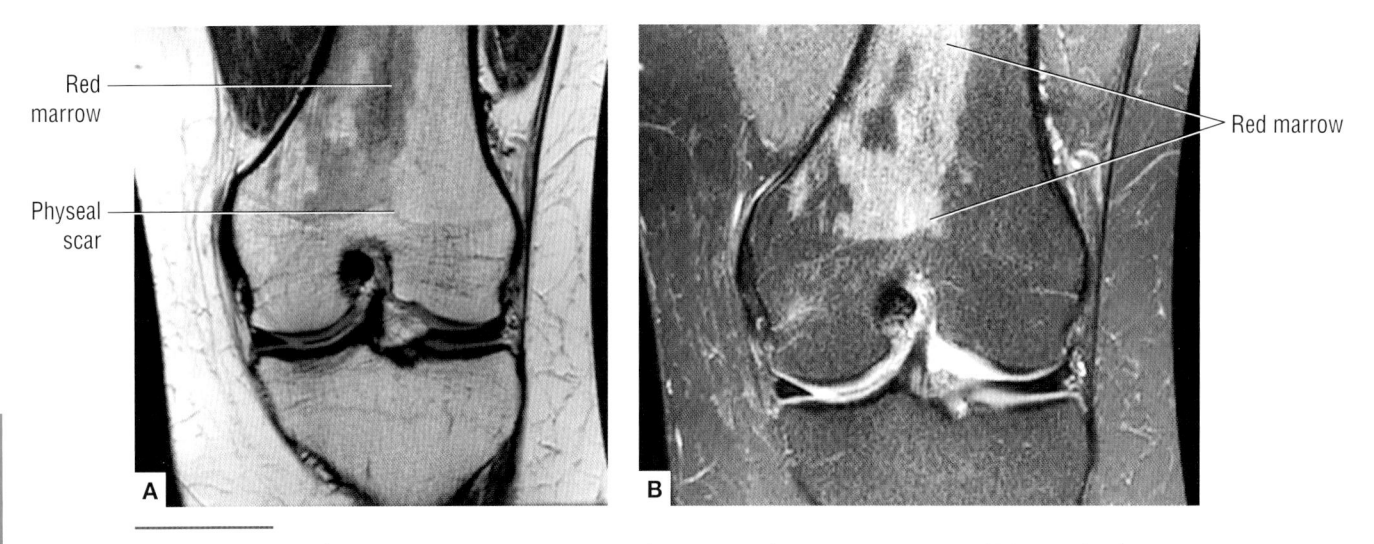

FIGURE 8.165 (**A**) Normal red marrow intermediate in signal intensity on a coronal T1-weighted image. (**B**) Relatively hyperintense signal intensity on a coronal FS PD FSE image.

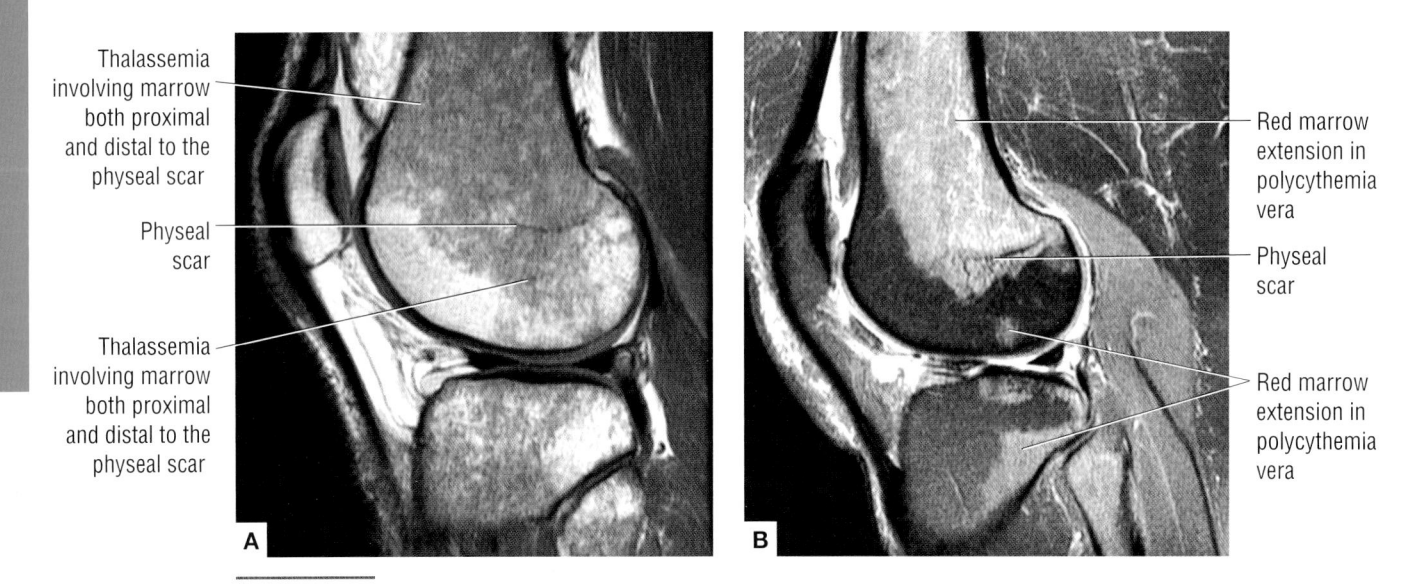

FIGURE 8.166 (**A**) Thalassemia with hypointense marrow extending distal to the femoral physeal scar and proximal to the tibial physeal scar. Thalassemia is caused by an inherited abnormality in globin production and is characterized by ineffective erythropoiesis, hemolysis, and anemia. (**B**) Abnormal extension of red marrow distal to the femoral physeal scar and proximal to the physeal scar of the tibia and fibula in polycythemia vera. Hyperplasia of the cellular elements of marrow, primarily erythrocytes, is characteristic and may result in complete replacement of marrow fat elements.

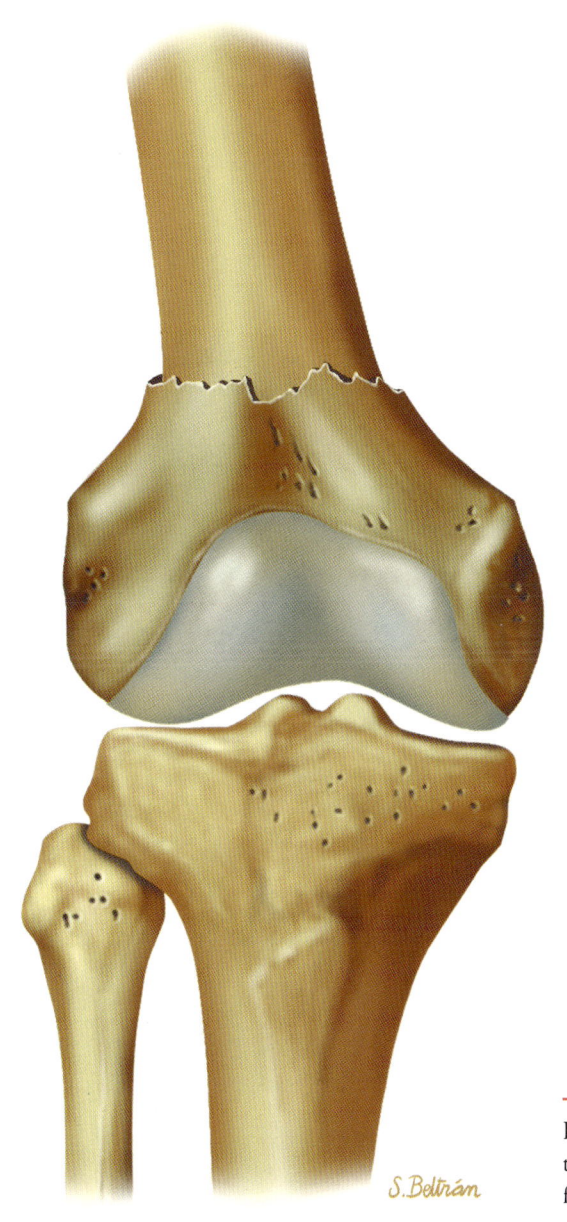

General Pathologic Conditions Affecting the Knee

FIGURE 8.167 Impacted supracondylar fracture of the distal femur. Fractures of the distal femur are classified as supracondylar, condylar, or intercondylar.

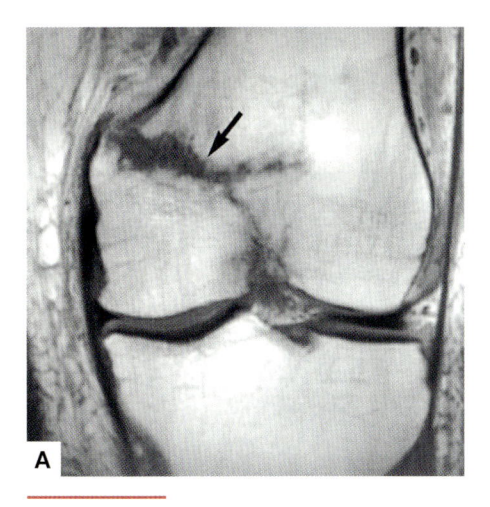

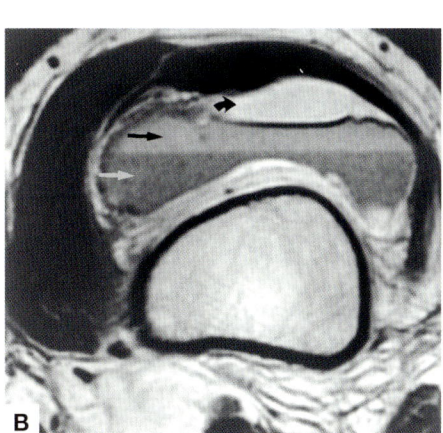

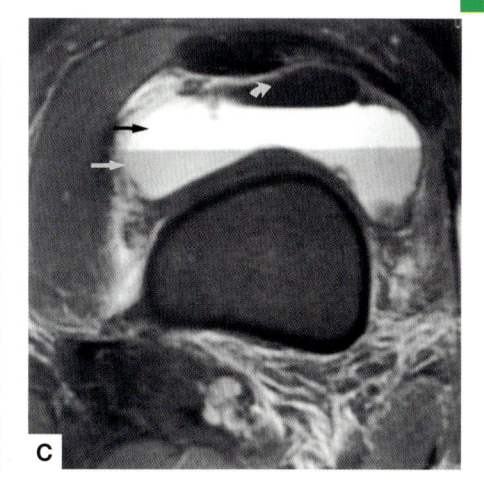

FIGURE 8.168 (A) T1-weighted coronal image of a medial femoral condylar fracture (*arrow*). Lipohemarthrosis with fat–serum–cellular layering is identified in a hemorrhagic effusion on a (B) T1-weighted axial image and (C) FS T2-weighted FSE axial image. *Straight white arrow*, cellular layer; *straight black arrow*, serum layer; *curved arrow*, fat layer. Hemarthrosis is commonly seen in ACL tears and osteochondral fractures. The supernatant layer of hemorrhage is bright on long-TR/TE sequences, whereas the cellular layer is dark on short- and long-TR/TE protocols. The fat layer is hypointense on the FS T2-weighted FSE sequence (C).

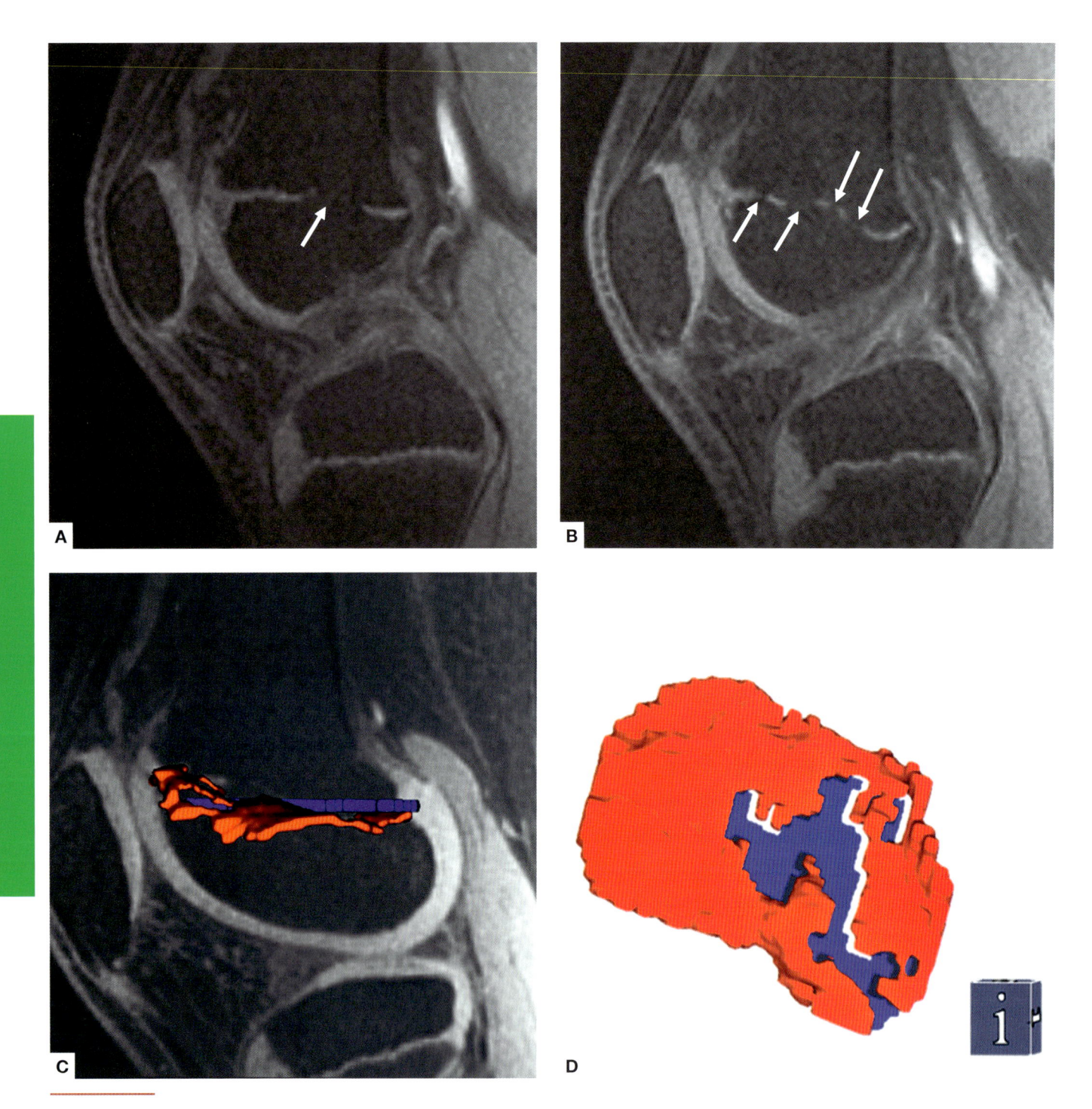

FIGURE 8.169 (**A, B**) Coronal 3D T1-weighted gradient echo MR images of the knee with fat suppression in an 8-year-old boy with a history of femoral fracture 1 year prior, instrumented with pins, which were subsequently removed. Clinical concern was growth arrest. There are several foci of osseous bar formation at the distal femoral physis (*arrows*). (**C**) Coronal 3D T1-weighted gradient echo MR image with fat suppression, and superimposed 3D physeal model. Red indicates the normal unfused physis, and blue represents the bar. (**D**) A 3D model of the physis has been "extracted" from the planar images. The area of the unfused physis and bar can be calculated from the 3D model. Physis area: 2153.4mm^2, bar area: 332.2mm^2, percent bar: 15.4%. (Courtesy of Hollis G. Potter, MD, Hospital for Special Surgery, New York, NY.)

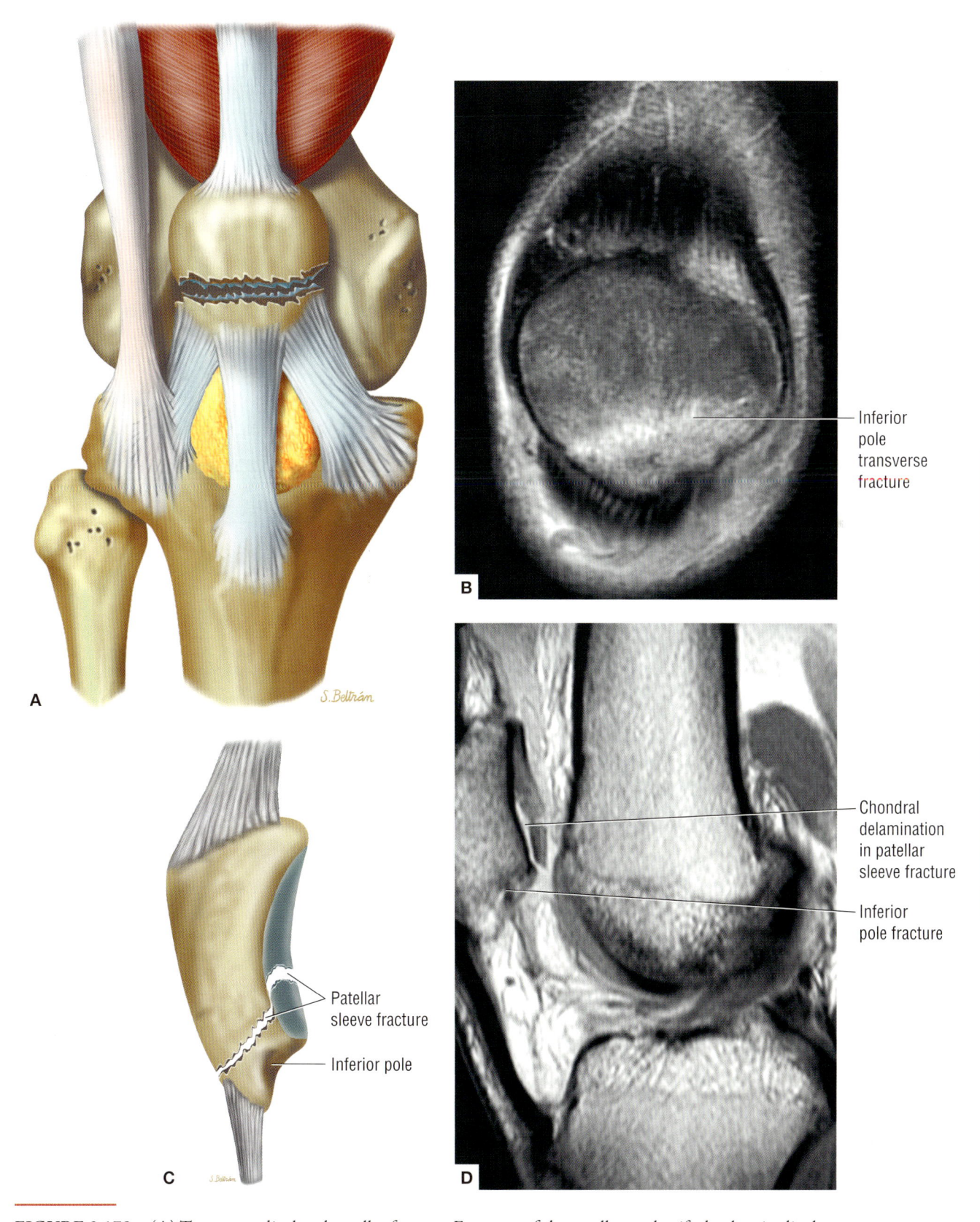

FIGURE 8.170 (**A**) Transverse displaced patellar fracture. Fractures of the patella are classified as longitudinal (vertical), transverse (nondisplaced or displaced), comminuted (nondisplaced or displaced), and superior margin avulsion type. (**B**) Inferior pole transverse fracture of the patella on a coronal FS PD FSE. Patellar sleeve fracture on a (**C**) color graphic sagittal view and (**D**) sagittal PD FSE image. A separate type of patellar fracture, classified as a patellar sleeve fracture, involves the inferior pole with fracture extension and delamination of the articular cartilage. The patellar sleeve fracture is an osteochondral fracture in children and adolescents that may involve any aspect of the patella. Inferior pole involvement is usually associated with indirect trauma such as forceful contraction of the quadriceps with the knee in flexion.

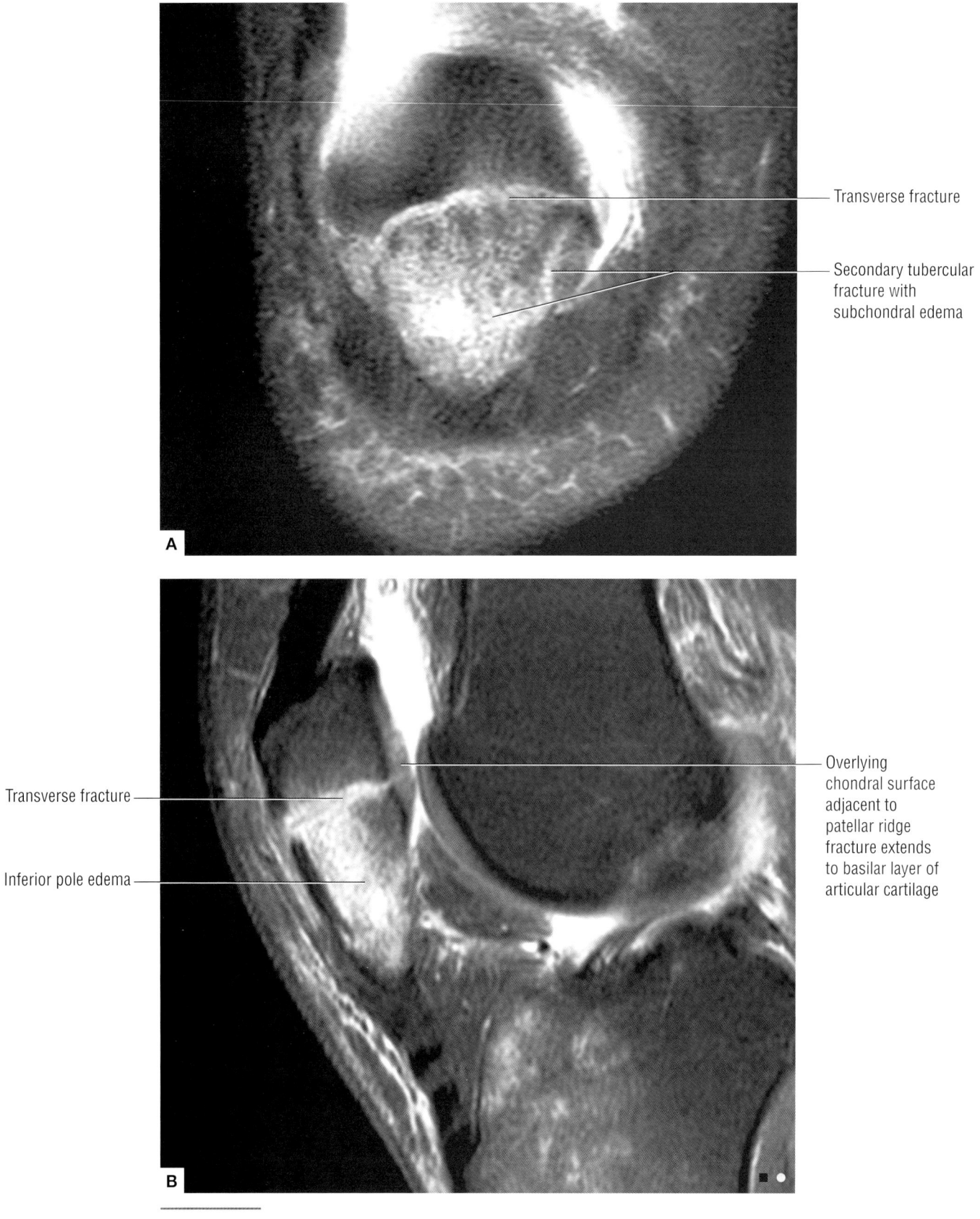

FIGURE 8.171 Central nondisplaced transverse patellar fracture. Transverse fractures usually occur in the central or distal third of the patella. Patellar fractures occur as a result of direct and indirect trauma. Coronal (**A**) and sagittal (**B**) FS PD FSE images.

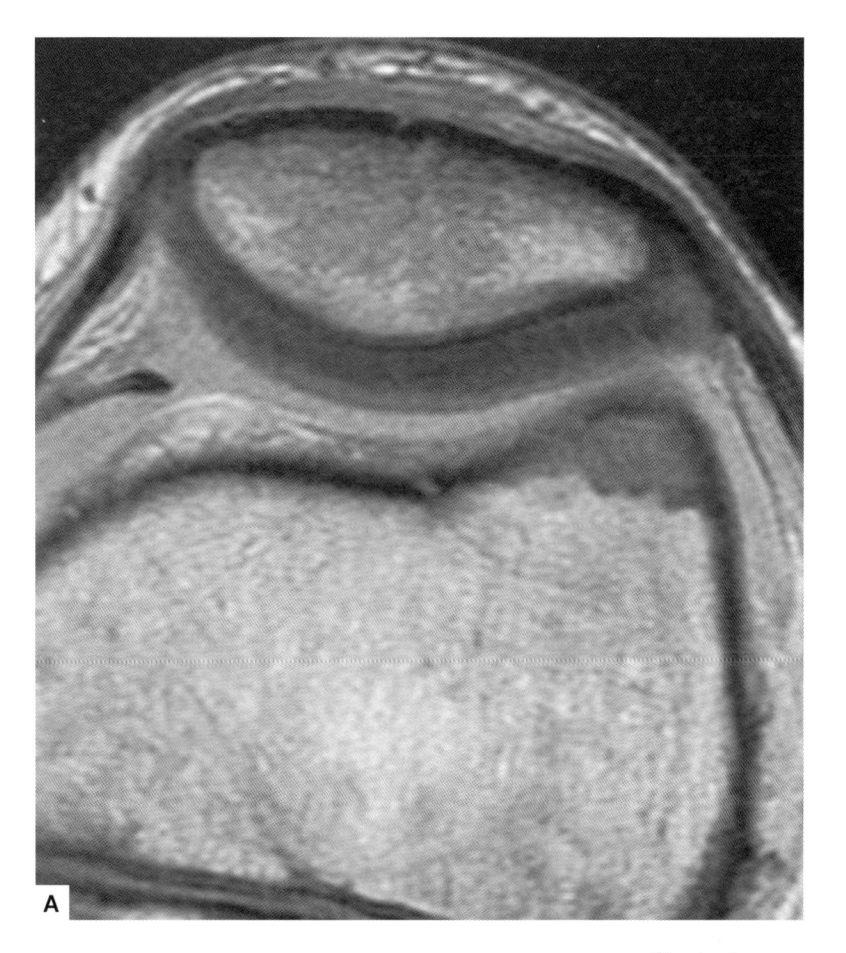

General Pathologic Conditions Affecting the Knee

Short axis vertical fracture

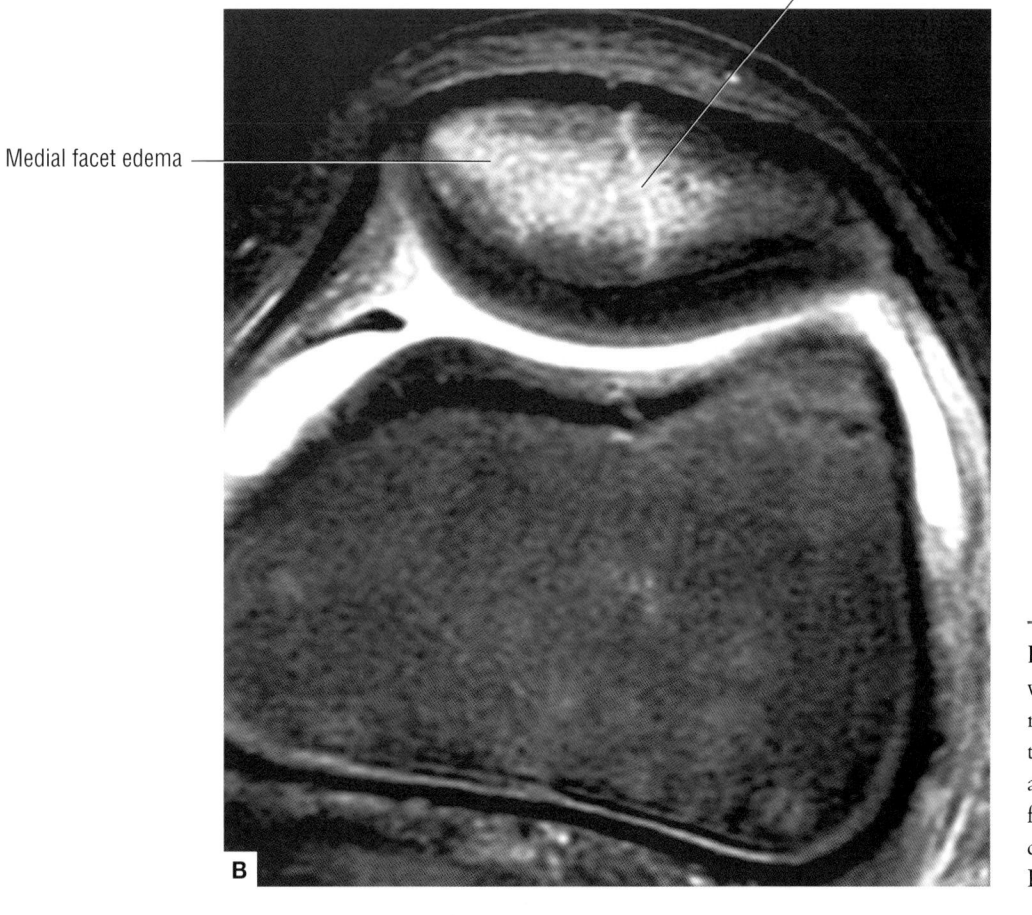

Medial facet edema

FIGURE 8.172 Nondisplaced vertical fracture of the patella as a result of a direct blow to the anterior knee. Patellar fractures may also occur from indirect tension forces generated by the quadriceps contraction. Axial PD (**A**) and FS PD (**B**) images.

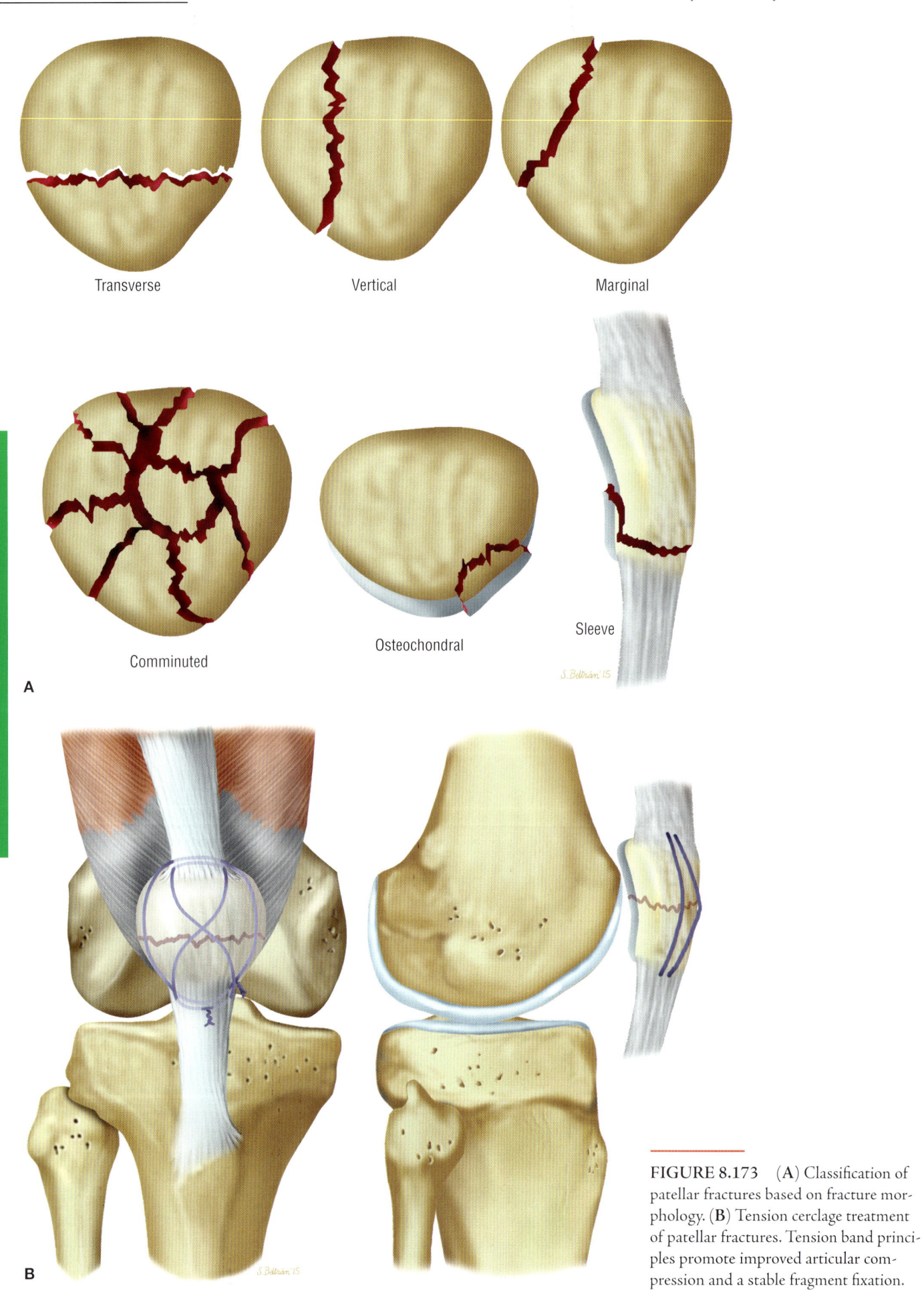

Transverse   Vertical   Marginal

Comminuted   Osteochondral   Sleeve

A

B

FIGURE 8.173 (**A**) Classification of patellar fractures based on fracture morphology. (**B**) Tension cerclage treatment of patellar fractures. Tension band principles promote improved articular compression and a stable fragment fixation.

Lipohemarthrosis

- May be identified in fractures involving patella, femur, or tibia
- T1 and FS PD FSE images useful in identifying fluid–fluid layers

Compartment Syndrome

- Known complication of trauma
- Identified on MR images by presence of edema that is limited to specified muscle group or groups[29]
- Edema may be replaced with fatty atrophy after chronic denervation.

Complex Regional Pain Syndrome

- Also known as Sudeck's atrophy or reflex sympathetic dystrophy
- May also occur as a complication of fracture
- Chronic pain disorder of the sympathetic nervous system
- Usually a result of trauma or a complication of surgery, infection, casting, or splinting
- Two types
    - Type I: replaces the name "reflex sympathetic dystrophy"
    - Type II: replaces the term "causalgia," occurs after a nerve injury (although findings are not necessarily limited to distribution of injured nerve)
- Diffuse juxtaarticular low signal intensity on T2-weighted images represents aggressive osteoporosis that develops with or without the presence of an associated fracture.[259]
- Increased signal intensity secondary to hyperemic bone marrow edema on STIR and FS PD FSE images[392]
- STIR imaging sequences are more sensitive and may define increased signal intensity in hyperemic bone in patients with negative findings on T2- or T2*-weighted images.

Infection

Key Concepts

- Secondary signs of joint sepsis include intermediate-signal-intensity synovial thickening and irregular fat-pad sign with or without fat-pad edema.
- Marrow edema may not be visualized until osseous extension and/or soft tissue tracts develop.
- Hyperintensity of subchondral bone on T2* GRE in the absence of trauma is associated with osteomyelitis in the setting of joint sepsis.

Infection

- Capsular distention and joint effusions can be seen but are nonspecific findings.[392]
- Septic joint may be further characterized by intraarticular debris and synovitis from hematogenous seeding.
- Inhomogeneity of joint fluid and irregular fat-pad sign with enhancing thickened synovium seen in early stages of joint sepsis
- Subchondral changes progress from hyperemia adjacent to inflamed synovium to osteomyelitis.
- Postsurgical knee infections, direct contamination from steroid injections, and penetrating trauma are all causes of adult osteomyelitis.

Osteomyelitis in Children

- Mottled pattern of yellow marrow stores in epiphyseal center of femur or tibia
- Appearance should not be confused with coarsened trabecular pattern seen in Paget's disease.[396]
- Metaphysis, an active site of bone formation in children, may show signal abnormalities (low signal on T1, bright signal on T2 or STIR images) restricted to this region.[407]
- Infectious tract with fluid may simulate pathologic or stress fractures or infarction.
    - When associated with extensive surrounding edema, may be confused with tumor

Multifocal Osteomyelitis

- Seeding of distal femur and proximal humerus identified on MR as a central nidus of high-intensity marrow and calcified sequestra of low signal intensity
- Marrow infiltration and soft tissue extension of osteomyelitis on STIR and FS T2-weighted FSE images[127]
- Cellulitis best identified on either STIR or FS T2-weighted FSE images

Chronic Infection

- Low-signal-intensity *rim sign* (in cases resulting from trauma)[127]
- Rim of fibrous tissue or reactive bone

Subacute Osteomyelitis

- Brodie's abscess
    - Focus of involvement of osteomyelitis is hyperintense on STIR and FS PD-weighted FSE images.
    - Sclerotic margin displays low signal intensity on all pulse sequences.
- Sequestrum or necrotic bone adjacent to or associated with osteomyelitis can be visualized as low-signal-intensity fragment on MR images.
    - Areas of edema or fluid may be associated with sequestrum.

Differential Diagnosis

- Differential diagnosis for Brodie's abscess usually includes osteoid osteoma and stress fracture.
- Selective muscle denervation or myositis may mimic infection.
- Muscular dystrophy, in contrast, may produce fatty infiltration of multiple muscle groups with limited muscle sparing.
- Joint swelling and deformity also seen in dysplasia epiphysealis hemimelica (commonly known as Trevor's disease)
    - Irregular ossification and asymmetrical metaphyseal widening may be mistaken for joint destruction.

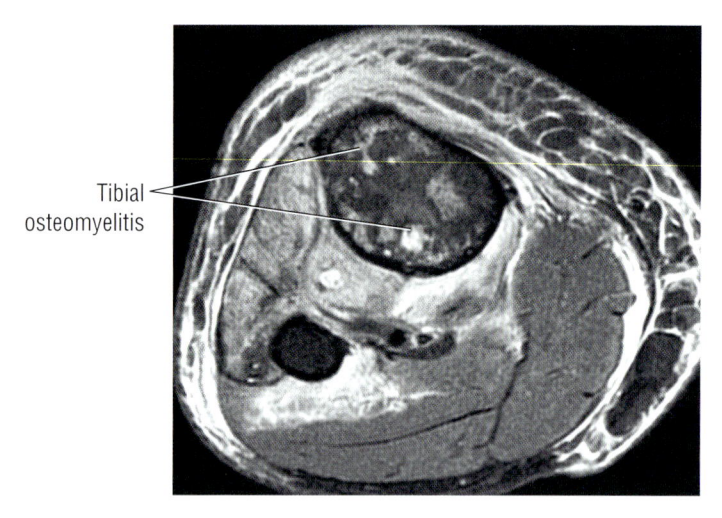

FIGURE 8.174 Anterolateral soft tissue infection associated with tibial osteomyelitis in a diabetic. Compartment syndrome and diabetic myonecrosis may produce similar MR findings. Involved muscle groups include the tibialis anterior, the extensor digitorum longus, the tibialis posterior, the popliteus, and the soleus.

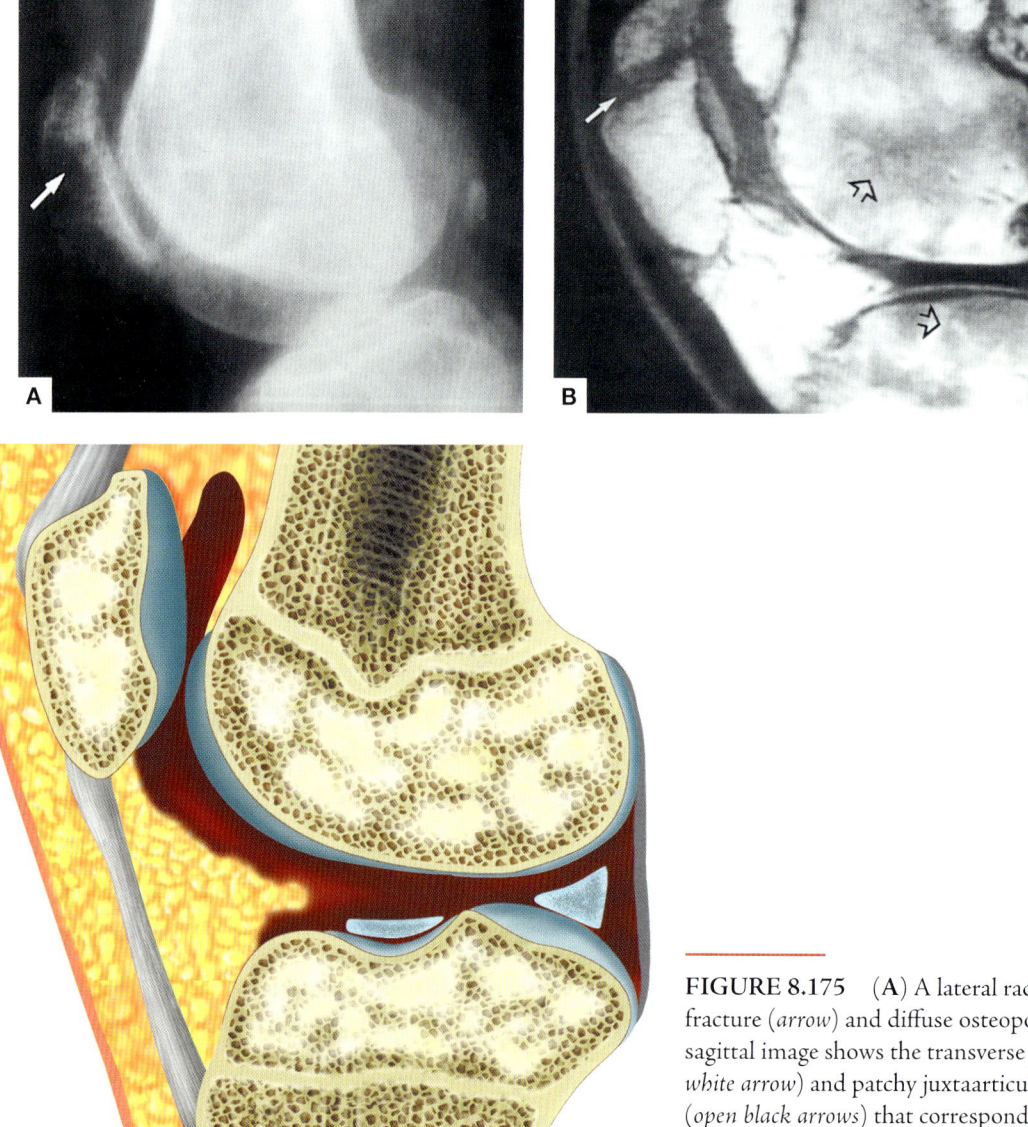

FIGURE 8.175 (**A**) A lateral radiograph shows a patellar fracture (*arrow*) and diffuse osteoporosis. (**B**) A T1-weighted sagittal image shows the transverse patellar fracture (*solid white arrow*) and patchy juxtaarticular low signal intensity (*open black arrows*) that correspond with aggressive osteoporosis in complex regional pain syndrome (CRPS). (**C**) CRPS with subchondral and subarticular osteoporosis involving the patellar distal femur and proximal tibia. This pattern of signal change is not characteristic of infection.

General Pathologic Conditions Affecting the Knee

Osteomyelitis

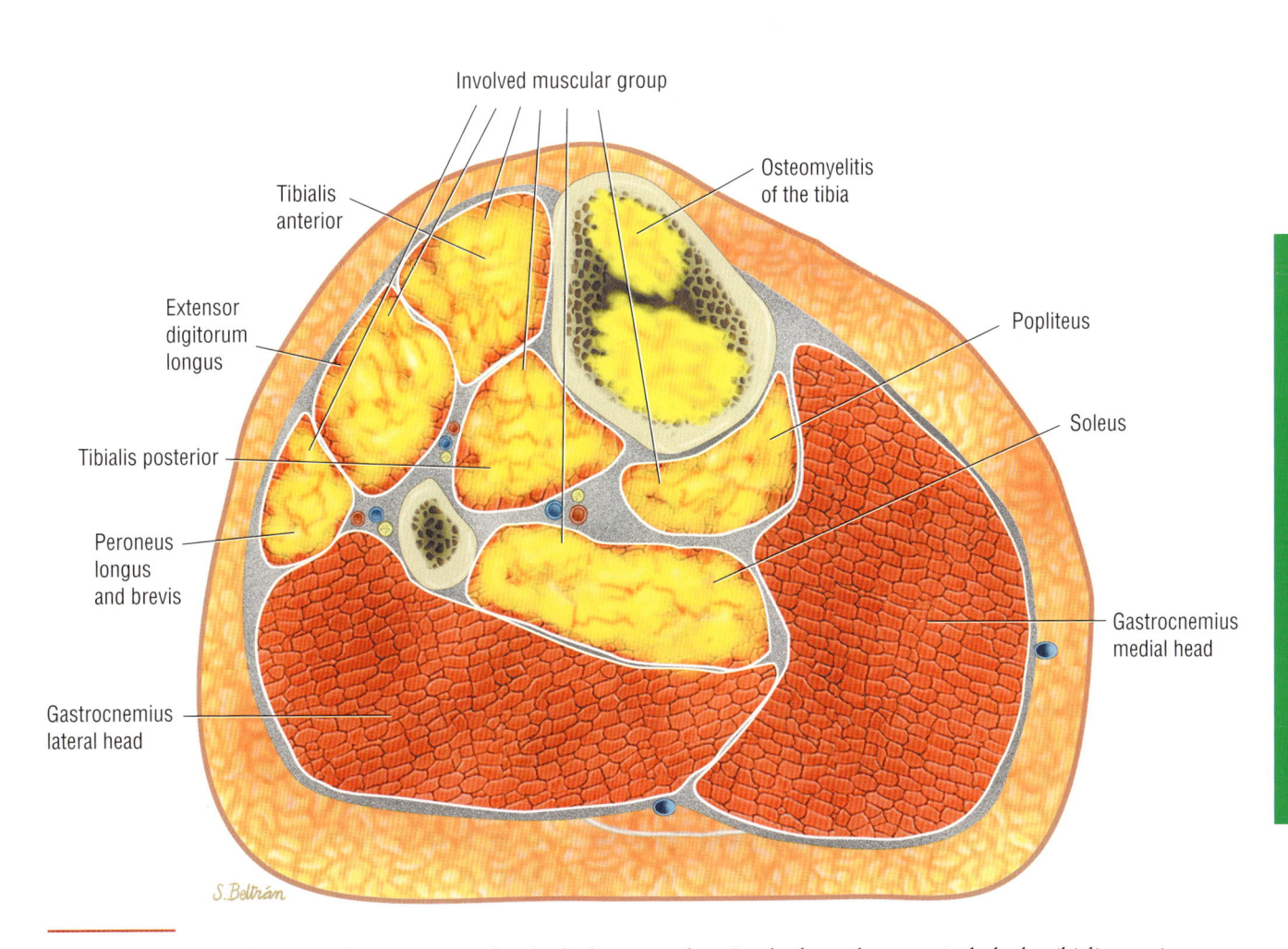

FIGURE 8.176 Soft tissue infection associated with tibial osteomyelitis. Involved muscle groups include the tibialis anterior, extensor digitorum longus, tibialis posterior, popliteus, and soleus.

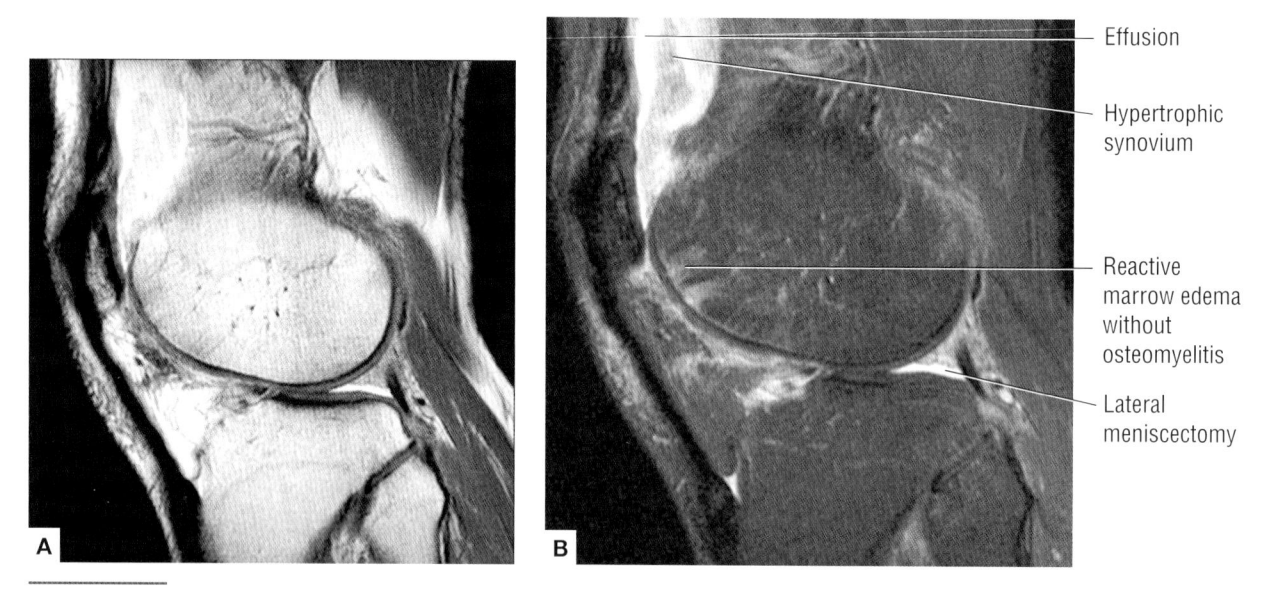

FIGURE 8.177 Post–lateral meniscectomy staphylococcal infection with hypertrophic synovial effusion and synovitis on (**A**) sagittal PD FSE and (**B**) sagittal FS PD FSE images.

Labels (B): Effusion; Hypertrophic synovium; Reactive marrow edema without osteomyelitis; Lateral meniscectomy

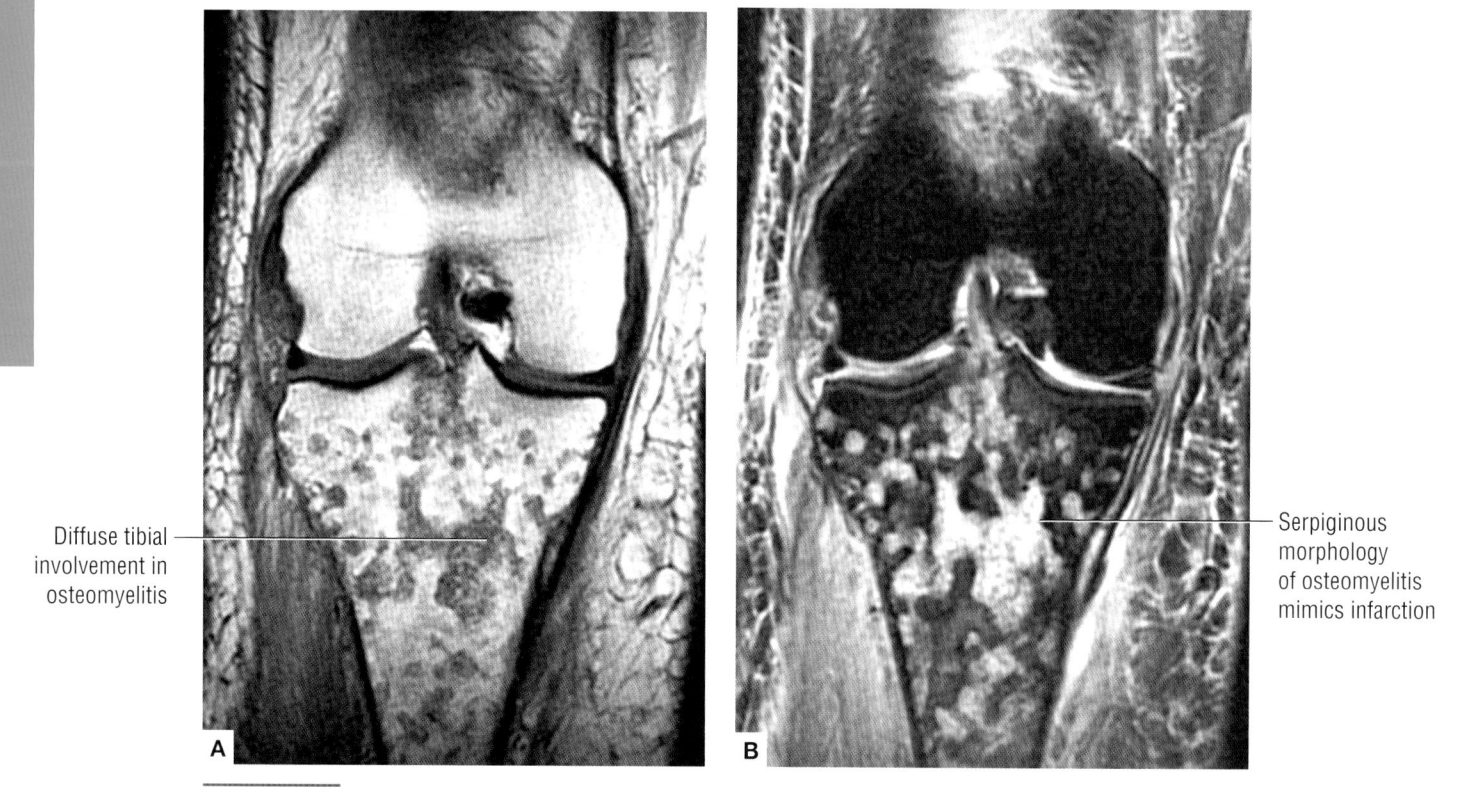

FIGURE 8.178 Staphylococcal osteomyelitis in a diabetic patient as seen on (**A**) coronal T1-weighted FSE and (**B**) coronal FS PD FSE images. The serpiginous involvement of the tibia simulates tibial infarction.

Labels: Diffuse tibial involvement in osteomyelitis; Serpiginous morphology of osteomyelitis mimics infarction

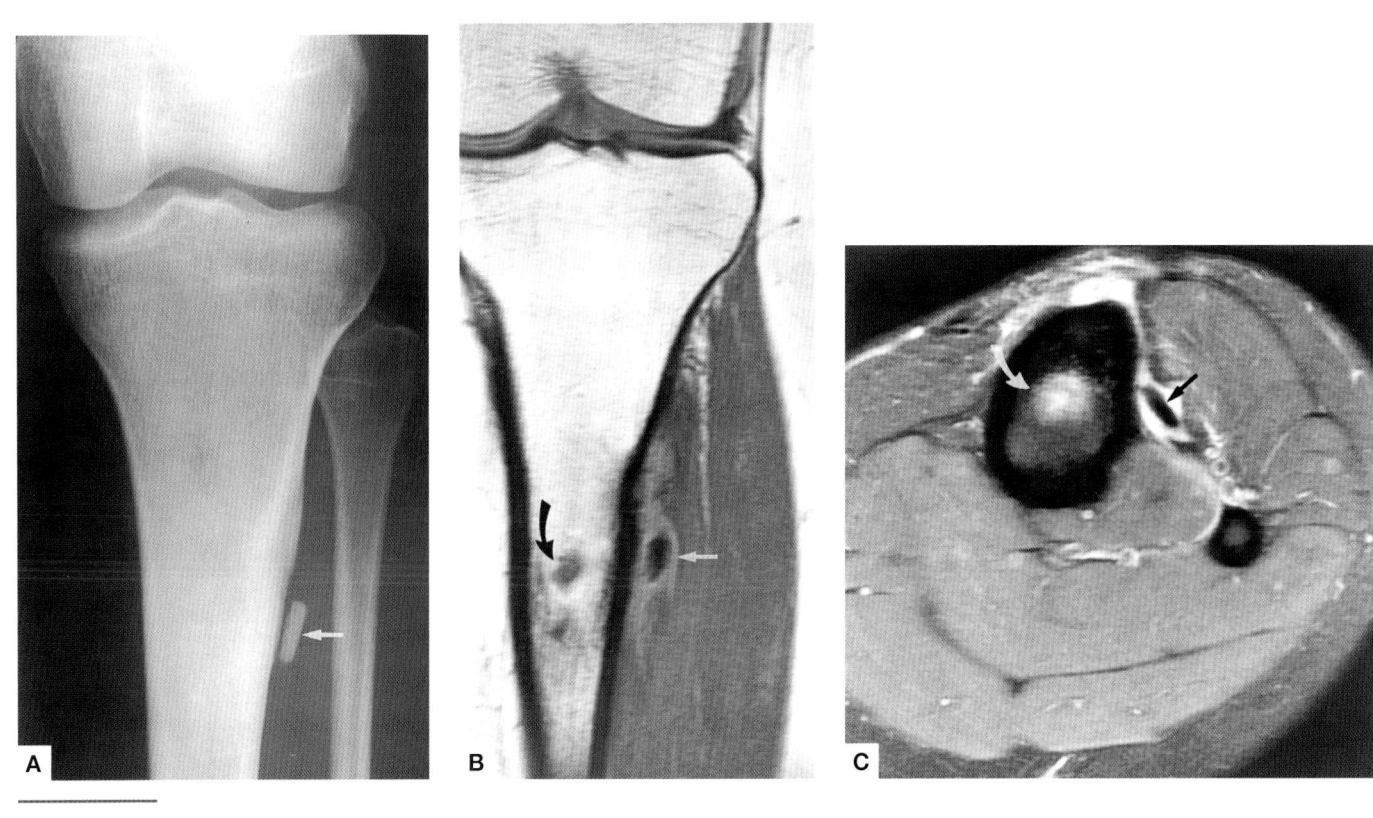

General Pathologic Conditions Affecting the Knee

FIGURE 8.179 Chronic active osteomyelitis with a sequestrum (*straight arrow*) adjacent to the lateral tibial cortex. An anteroposterior radiograph (**A**) demonstrates irregularity of the lateral tibial cortex, the presence of the sequestrum, and medullary bone sclerosis. The active infection within the medullary cavity (*curved arrow*) is seen as hypointense foci on a T1-weighted coronal image (**B**) and as a hyperintense area on the FS T2-weighted FSE axial image (**C**). Note the chronically infected fluid associated with the sequestrum, which tracks anterolateral to the tibia. The sequestrum (*straight arrow*) is hypointense on both the T1 (**B**) and the FS T2-weighted FSE (**C**) images.

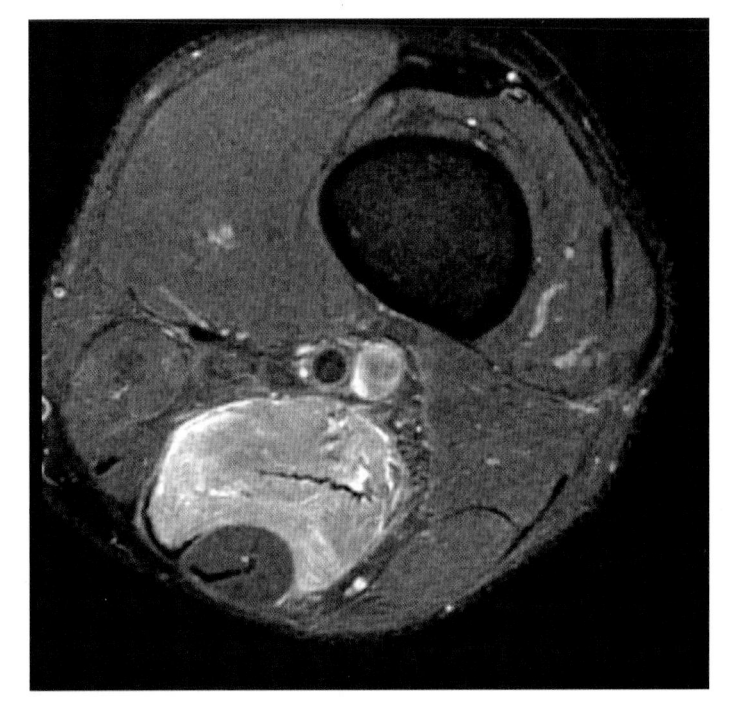

FIGURE 8.180 Semimembranosus hyperintensity in acute denervation is seen on this axial FS PD FSE image. The semimembranosus receives a sciatic motor nerve distribution.

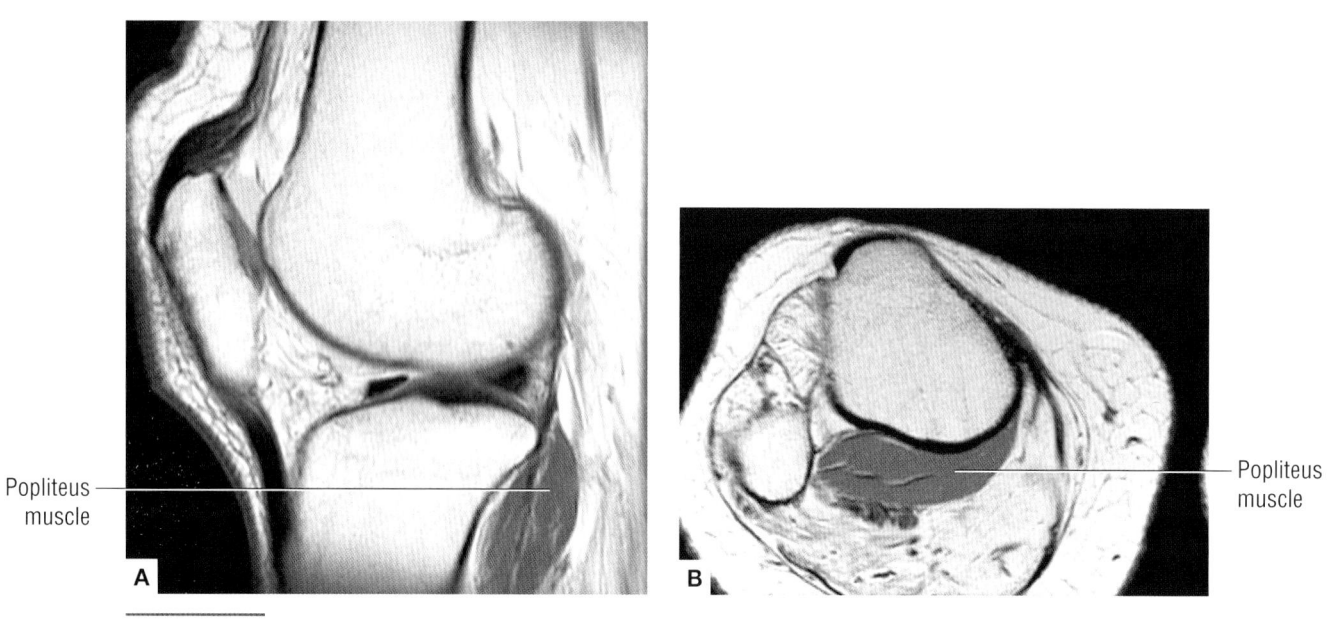

FIGURE 8.181 Muscular dystrophy with preservation of the popliteus muscle on sagittal (**A**) and axial (**B**) PD FSE images. Severe fatty infiltration of all other muscle compartments is demonstrated.

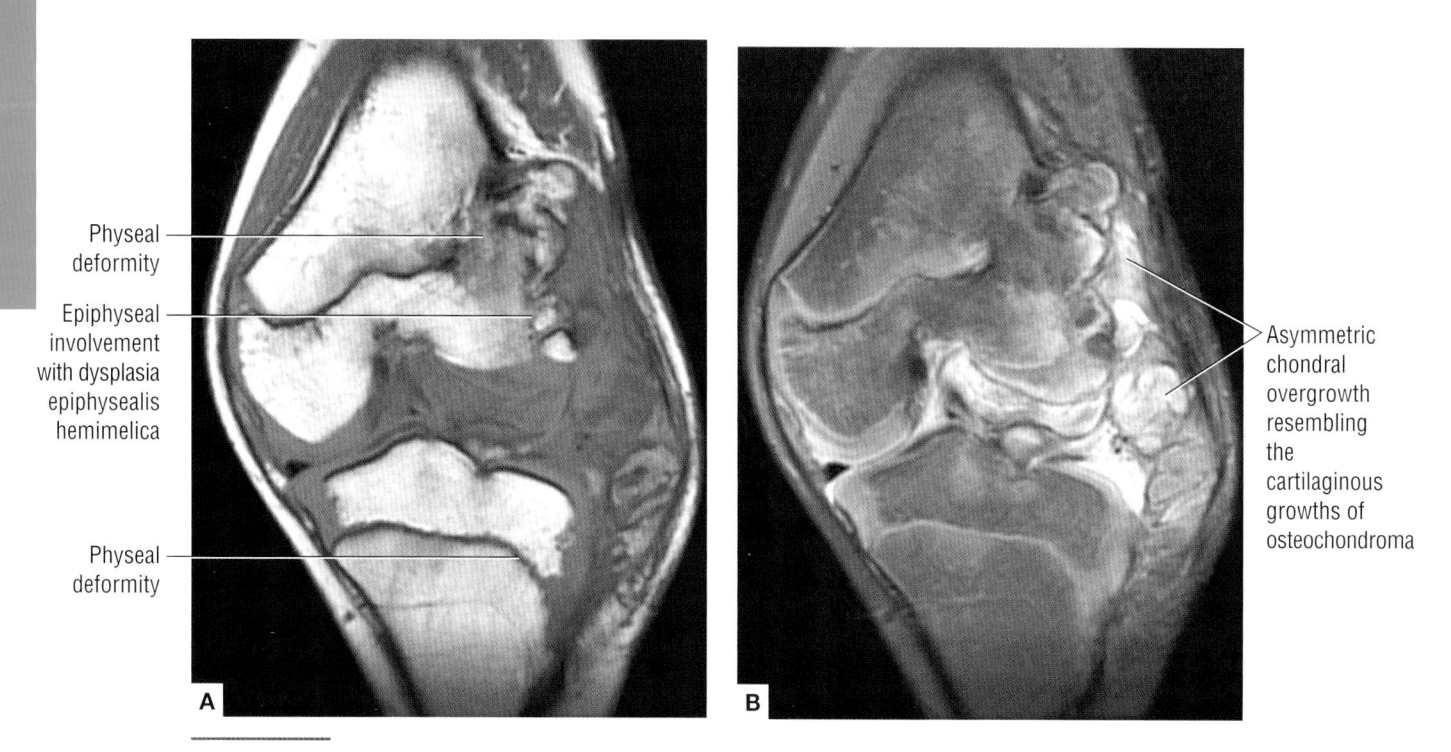

FIGURE 8.182 T1 (**A**) and FS PD FSE (**B**) coronal images of Trevor's disease simulating asymmetric joint destruction.

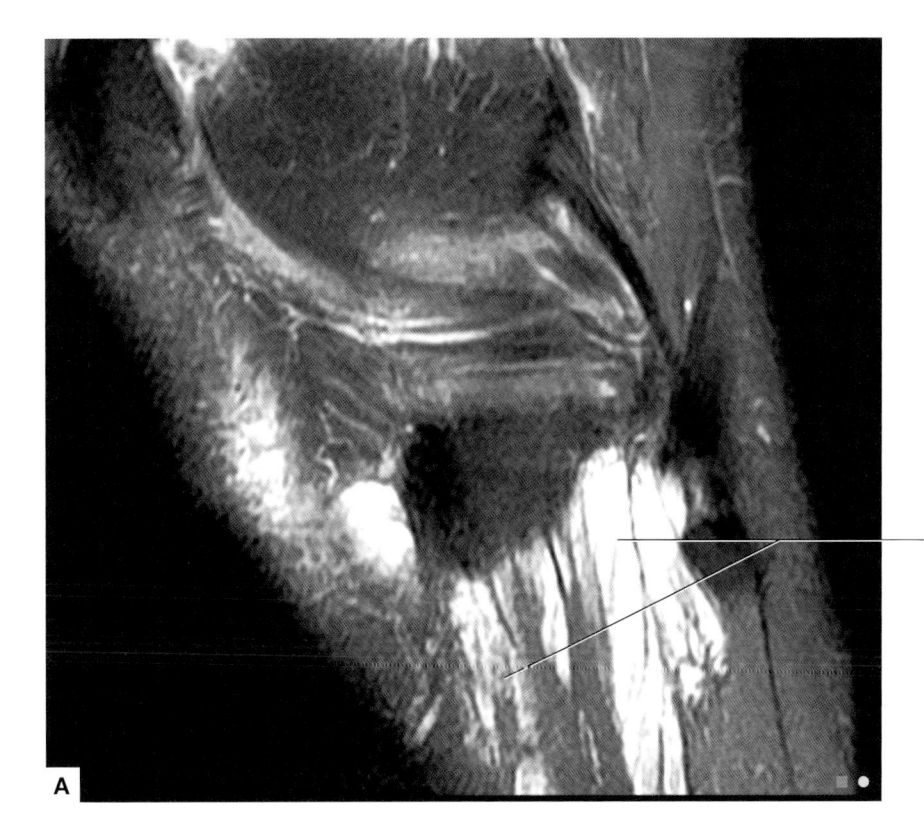

General Pathologic Conditions Affecting the Knee

Vascular malformation with hyperintense tubular structures

Vascular malformation anterolateral compartment

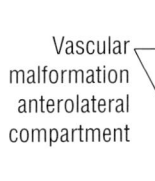

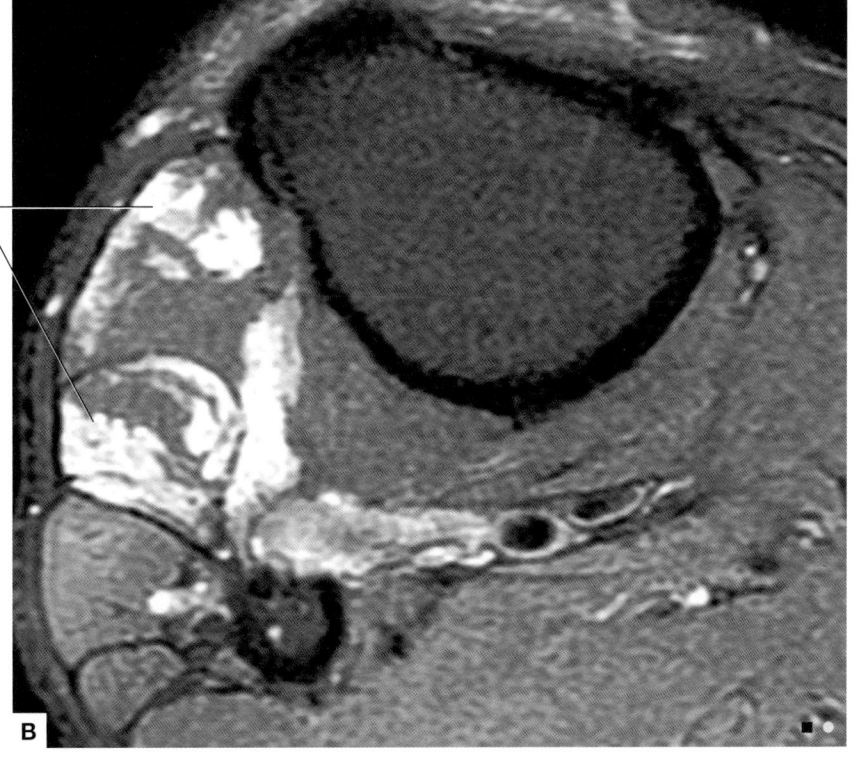

FIGURE 8.183 Skeletal muscle is a common location for hemangioma of deep soft tissue. Although rare, hemangiomas may be associated with other pathologies including Kasabach-Merritt syndrome (consumptive coagulopathy), tumor-induced osteomalacia, Gorham disease (osteolysis), and Maffucci syndrome with multiple enchondromatosis. Vascular malformation of the anterolateral compartment. As these lesions are present from birth and do not involute spontaneously vascular malformations is a more accurate term than hemangiomas when affecting the musculoskeletal system. Vascular malformations of muscle may cause pain and swelling. Sagittal (**A**) and axial (**B**) FS PD FSE images.

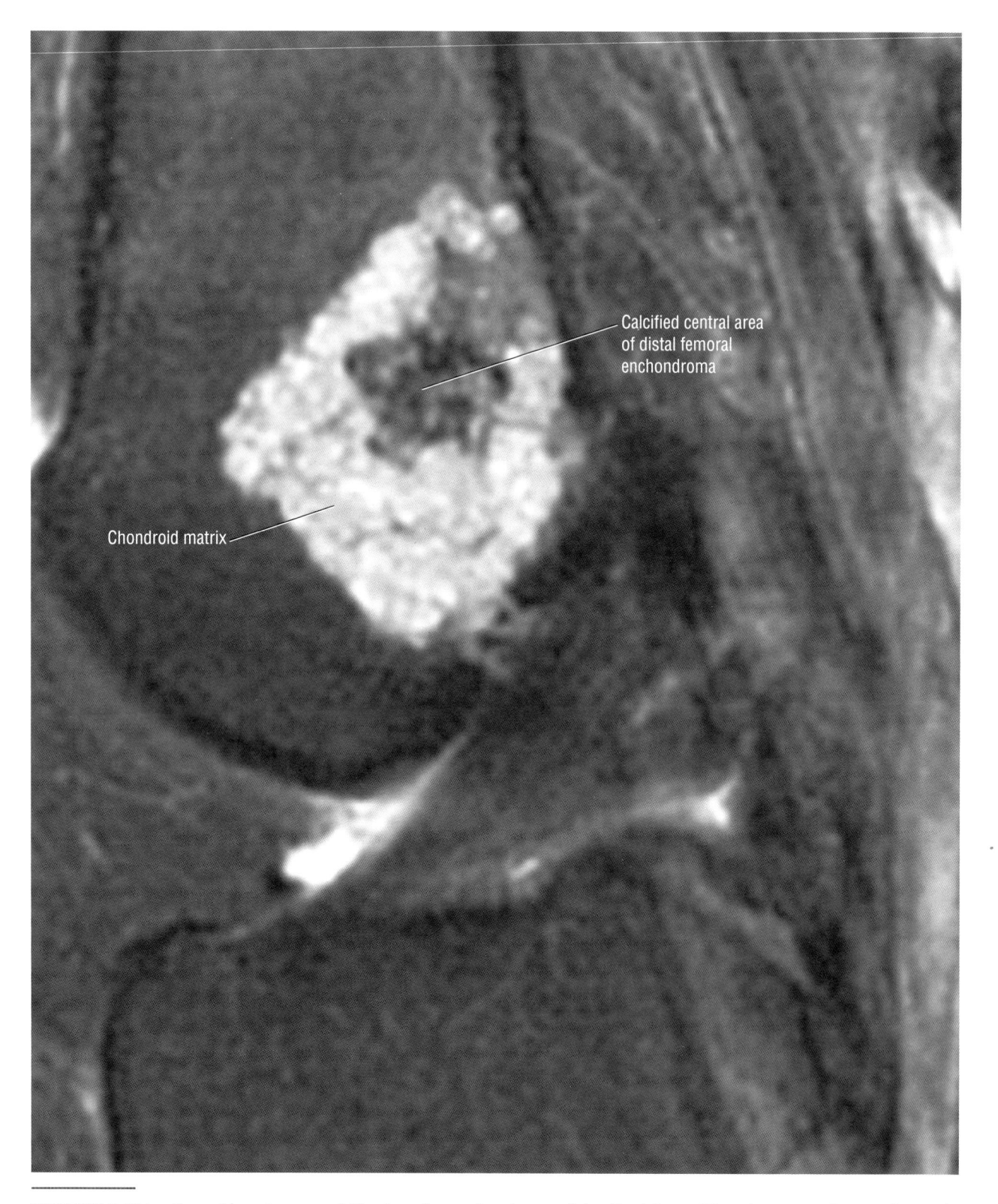

FIGURE 8.184 Central hypointense calcification of an enchondroma of the distal femur. These lesions are frequently ovoid and have well-defined margins. An enchondroma is a benign medullary cartilaginous neoplasm. Chondroid matrix is high signal on T2-weighted images. Sagittal PD FSE image.

References

1. Aarvold A et al. MRI performed on dedicated knee coils is inaccurate for the measurement of tibial tubercle trochlear groove distance. *Skeletal Radiol* 2014;43(3):345–349.
2. Abe S, Kurosaka M, Iguchi T, et al. Light and electron microscopic study of remodeling and maturation process in autogenous graft for anterior cruciate ligament reconstruction. *Arthroscopy* 1993;9(4):394–405.
3. Adam G, Bohndorf K, Drobnitzky M, Guenther RW. MR imaging of the knee: three-dimensional volume imaging combined with fast processing. *J Comput Assist Tomogr* 1989;13(6):984–988.
4. Adam G, Dammer M, Bohndorf K, et al. Rheumatoid arthritis of the knee: value of gadopentetate dimeglumine-enhanced MR imaging. *AJR Am J Roentgenol* 1991;156(1):125–129.
5. Ahmad SS et al. The hundred most-cited publications in orthopaedic knee research. *J Bone Joint Surg Am* 2014;96(22):e190.
6. Aichroth PM, Al-Duri Z. Dislocation and subluxation of the patella: an overview. In: Aichroth PM, Cannon WD, eds. *Knee Surgery: Current Practice*. London, United Kingdom: Martin Dunitz; 1992:354.
7. Aichroth PM, Patelin D. Congenital discoid lateral meniscus in children: an overview and current clinical perspectives. In: Aichroth M, Cannon WD, eds. *Knee Surgery: Current Practice*. London, United Kingdom: Martin Dunitz; 1992:521.
8. Alcala-Galiano A et al. Imaging of posterior cruciate ligament (PCL) reconstruction: normal postsurgical appearance and complications. *Skeletal Radiol* 2014;43(12):1659–1668.
9. Alizai H et al. Cartilage lesion score: comparison of a quantitative assessment score with established semiquantitative MR scoring systems. *Radiology* 2014;271(2):479–487.
10. Allenspach R, Stampanoni M, Bischof A. Magnetic domains in thin epitaxial Co/Au(111) films. *Phys Rev Lett* 1990;65(26):3344–3347.
11. Anderson JE. *Grant's Atlas of Anatomy*. 8th ed. Baltimore, MD: Williams & Wilkins; 1983.
12. Andrews JR, Edwards JC, Satterwhite YE. Isolated posterior cruciate ligament injuries. History, mechanism of injury, physical findings, and ancillary tests. *Clin Sports Med* 1994;13(3):519–530.
13. Apple JS, Martinez S, Hardaker WT, et al. Synovial plicae of the knee. *Skeletal Radiol* 1982;7(4):251–254.
14. Applegate GR, Flannigan BD, Tolin BS, Fox JM, Del Pizzo W. MR diagnosis of recurrent tears in the knee: value of intraarticular contrast material. *AJR Am J Roentgenol* 1993;161(4):821–825.
15. Arnoczky SP, Cooper TG, Stadelmaier DM, Hannafin JA. Magnetic resonance signals in healing menisci: an experimental study in dogs. *Arthroscopy* 1994;10(5):552–557.
16. Arnoczky SP, Warren RF. Microvasculature of the human meniscus. *Am J Sports Med* 1982;10(2):90–95.
17. Arnoczky SP, Warren RF. The microvasculature of the meniscus and its response to injury. An experimental study in the dog. *Am J Sports Med* 1983;11(3):131–141.
18. Arnoczky SP, Warren RF, Ashlock MA. Replacement of the anterior cruciate ligament using a patellar tendon allograft. An experimental study. *J Bone Joint Surg Am* 1986;68(3):376–385.
19. Au KS, Chan KC. Variations in (Ca2+ + Mg2+)-ATPase, its inhibitor protein and calmodulin of density (age) separated rabbit erythrocytes. *Biochim Biophys Acta* 1983;761(3):291–295.
20. Auge WK, Kaeding CC. Bilateral discoid medial menisci with extensive intrasubstance cleavage tears: MRI and arthroscopic correlation. *Arthroscopy* 1994;10(3):313–318.
21. Barber FA. Snow skiing combined anterior cruciate ligament/medial collateral ligament disruptions. *Arthroscopy* 1994;10(1):85–89.
22. Barnes CL, McCarthy RE, VanderSchilden JL, McConnell JR, Nusbickel FR. Discoid lateral meniscus in a young child: case report and review of the literature. *J Pediatr Orthop* 1988;8(6):707–709.
23. Bateni C, Bindra J, Haus B. MRI of sports injuries in children and adolescents: what's different from adults. *Curr Radiol Rep* 2014;2(5):1–12.
24. Bay BK et al. Repair of large cortical defects with block coralline hydroxyapatite. *Bone* 1993;14(3):225–230.
25. Beltran J, Noto AM, Mosure JC, Bools JC, Zuelzer W, Christoforidis AJ. Meniscal tears: MR demonstration of experimentally produced injuries. *Radiology* 1986;158(3):691–693.
26. Bencardino JT et al. MR imaging of complications of anterior cruciate ligament graft reconstruction. *Radiographics* 2009;29(7):2115–2126.
27. Bermejo A et al. MR imaging in the evaluation of cystic-appearing soft-tissue masses of the extremities. *Radiographics* 2013;33(3):833–855.
28. Berquist TH. Imaging of Orthopaedic Trauma and Surgery. Philadelphia, PA: WB Saunders; 1986.
29. Berquist TH. *Magnetic Resonance Imaging of the Musculoskeletal System*. New York, NY: Raven Press; 1987.
30. Bessette GC, Hunter RE. The anterior cruciate ligament. *Orthopedics* 1990;13(5):551–562.

31. Bikkina RS, Tujo CA, Schraner AB, Major NM. The "floating" meniscus: MRI in knee trauma and implications for surgery. *AJR Am J Roentgenol* 2005;184(1):200–204.
32. Bittersohl B et al. Spectrum of T2* values in knee joint cartilage at 3 T: a cross-sectional analysis in asymptomatic young adult volunteers. *Skeletal Radiol* 2014;43(4):443–452.
33. Bjorkengren AG, Geborek P, Rydholm U, Holtås S, Petterson H. MR imaging of the knee in acute rheumatoid arthritis: synovial uptake of gadolinium-DOTA. *AJR Am J Roentgenol* 1990;155(2):329–332.
34. Blackman AJ et al. Correlation between magnetic resonance imaging and clinical outcomes after cartilage repair surgery in the knee: a systematic review and meta-analysis. *Am J Sports Med* 2013;41(6):1426–34.
35. Blais RE, LaPrade RF, Chaljub G, Adesokan A. The arthroscopic appearance of lipoma arborescens of the knee. *Arthroscopy* 1995;11(5):623–627.
36. Bloecker K et al. Correlation of semiquantitative vs quantitative MRI meniscus measures in osteoarthritic knees: results from the Osteoarthritis Initiative. *Skeletal Radiol* 2014;43(2):227–232.
37. Boden BP, Moyer RA, Betz RR, Sapega AA. Arthroscopically-assisted anterior cruciate ligament reconstruction: a follow-up study. *Contemp Orthop* 1990;20(2):187–194.
38. Boks SS et al. Follow-up of posttraumatic ligamentous and meniscal knee lesions detected at MR imaging: systematic review. *Radiology* 2006;238(3):863–871.
39. Bonilla-Yoon I et al. The Morel-Lavallée lesion: pathophysiology, clinical presentation, imaging features, and treatment options. *Emerg Radiol* 2014;21(1):35–43.
40. Bonnin M, Amendola A, Bellemans J, et al, eds. *The Knee Joint: Surgical Techniques and Strategies*. Paris, France: Springer; 2012.
41. Boutin RD, Januario JA, Newberg AH, et al. MR imaging features of osteochondritis dissecans of the femoral sulcus. *AJR Am J Roentgenol* 2003;180(3):641–645.
42. Boynton MD, Fadale PD. The basic science of anterior cruciate ligament surgery. *Orthop Rev* 1993;22(6):673–679.
43. Bradley DM, Bergman AG, Dillingham MF. MR imaging of cyclops lesions. *AJR Am J Roentgenol* 2000;174(3):719–726.
44. Brandser EA, Riley MA, Berbaum KS, et al. MR imaging of anterior cruciate ligament injury: independent value of primary and secondary signs. *AJR Am J Roentgenol* 1996;167(1):121–126.
45. Broderick LS, Turner DA, Renfrew DL, et al. Severity of articular cartilage abnormality in patients with osteoarthritis: evaluation with fast spin-echo MR vs arthroscopy. *AJR Am J Roentgenol* 1994;162(1):99–103.
46. Bron EE et al. Image registration improves human knee cartilage T1 mapping with delayed gadolinium-enhanced MRI of cartilage (dGEMRIC). *Eur Radiol* 2013;23(1):246–252.
47. Brossmann J, Muhle C, Schröder C, et al. Patellar tracking patterns during active and passive knee extension: evaluation with motion-triggered cine MR imaging. *Radiology* 1993;187(1):205–212.
48. Brown SM, Muroff LR, Bradley WG. Ultrafast kinematic MR imaging of the knee: increased sensitivity with a quadriceps loading device. *J Magn Reson Imaging* 1993;Suppl(S29).
49. Buckwalter JA, Martin J. Degenerative joint disease. *Clin Symp* 1995;47(2):1–32.
50. Buckwalter KA et al. MR imaging of meniscal tears: narrow versus conventional window width photography. *Radiology* 1993;187(3):827–830.
51. Burk DL, Dalinka MK, Kanal E, et al. Meniscal and ganglion cysts of the knee: MR evaluation. *AJR Am J Roentgenol* 1988;150(2):331–336.
52. Burk DL, Kanal E, Brunberg JA, et al. 1.5-T surface-coil MRI of the knee. *AJR Am J Roentgenol* 1986;147(2):293–300.
53. Burk DL et al. Recent advances in magnetic resonance imaging of the knee. *Radiol Clin North Am* 1990;28(2):379–393.
54. Burstein D, Gray M. New MRI techniques for imaging cartilage. *J Bone Joint Surg Am* 2003;85-A(Suppl 2):70–77.
55. Buss DD, Min R, Skyhar M, et al. Nonoperative treatment of acute anterior cruciate ligament injuries in a selected group of patients. *Am J Sports Med* 1995;23(2):160–165.
56. Calvo RD, Steadman JR, Sterling JC, et al. Managing plica syndrome of the knee. *Phys Sports Med* 1990;18(7):64.
57. Camacho MA. The double posterior cruciate ligament sign. *Radiology* 2004;233(2):503–504.
58. Campbell SE, Sanders TG, Morrison WB. MR imaging of meniscal cysts: incidence, location, and clinical significance. *AJR Am J Roentgenol* 2001;177(2):409–413.
59. Campos JC, Chung CB, Lektrakul N, et al. Pathogenesis of the Segond fracture: anatomic and MR imaging evidence of an iliotibial tract or anterior oblique band avulsion. *Radiology* 2001;219(2):381–386.
60. Canale T. *Campbell's Operative Orthopaedics*. 10th ed. Vol. 3. Philadelphia, PA: Mosby; 2003.
61. Cannon WD, Morgan CD. Meniscal repair. *J Bone Joint Surg* 1994;76(2):294–311.
62. Cannon WD, Vittori JM. Basic arthroscopy. In: Aichroth PM, Cannon WD, eds. *Knee Surgery: Current Practice*. London, United Kingdom: Martin Dunitz; 1992:54.
63. Cannon WD, Vittori JM. The incidence of healing in arthroscopic meniscal repairs in anterior cruciate ligament-reconstructed knees versus stable knees. *Am J Sports Med* 1992;20(2):176–181.
64. Cannon WD, Vittori JM. Meniscal repair. In: Aichroth PM, Cannon WD, eds. *Knee Surgery: Current Practice*. London, United Kingdom: Martin Dunitz; 1992:71.
65. Carrillon Y, Abidi H, Dejour D, et al. Patellar instability: assessment on MR images by measuring the lateral trochlear inclination-initial experience. *Radiology* 2000;216(2):582–585.
66. Cerabona F, Sherman MF, Bonamo JR, Sklar J. Patterns of meniscal injury with acute anterior cruciate ligament tears. *Am J Sports Med* 1988;16(6):603–609.
67. Chang EY et al. Morphologic characterization of meniscal root ligaments in the human knee with magnetic resonance microscopy at 11.7 and 3 T. *Skeletal Radiol* 2014;43(10):1395–1402.
68. Chen W et al. Accuracy of 3-T MRI using susceptibility-weighted imaging to detect meniscal tears of the knee. *Knee Surg Sports Traumatol Arthrosc* 2015;23(1):198–204.

References

69. Cherney S. Disorders of the knee. In: Dee R, ed. *Principles of Orthopaedic Practice*. New York, NY: McGraw-Hill; 1989:1283.
70. Cherney S. The knee. In: Dee R, ed. *Principles of Orthopaedic Practice*. New York, NY: McGraw-Hill; 1989:1054.
71. Choi JY et al. Posterior medial meniscus root ligament lesions: MRI classification and associated findings. *AJR Am J Roentgenol* 2014;203(6):1286–1292.
72. Choi YS, Potter HG, Chun TJ. MR imaging of cartilage repair in the knee and ankle. *Radiographics* 2008;28(4):1043–1059.
73. Ciccotti MG, Lombardo SJ, Nonweiler B, Pink M. Non-operative treatment of ruptures of the anterior cruciate ligament in middle-aged patients. Results after long-term follow-up. *J Bone Joint Surg Am* 1994;76(9):1315–1321.
74. Claes S et al. Anatomy of the anterolateral ligament of the knee. *J Anat* 2013;223(4):321–328.
75. Clancy WG, Shelbourne KD, Zoellner GB, Keene JS, Reider B, Rosenberg TD. Treatment of knee joint instability secondary to rupture of the posterior cruciate ligament. Report of a new procedure. *J Bone Joint Surg Am* 1983;65(3):310–322.
76. Coll JP et al. Best cases from the AFIP: lipoma arborescens of the knees in a patient with rheumatoid arthritis. *Radiographics* 2011;31(2):333–337.
77. Conway WF, Hayes CW, Loughran T, et al. Cross-sectional imaging of the patellofemoral joint and surrounding structures. *Radiographics* 1991;11(2):195–217.
78. Costa CR, Morrison WB, Carrino JA. Medial meniscus extrusion on knee MRI: is extent associated with severity of degeneration or type of tear? *AJR Am J Roentgenol* 2004;183(1):17–23.
79. Cothran RL, Major NM, Helms CA, Higgins LD. MR imaging of meniscal contusion in the knee. *AJR Am J Roentgenol* 2001;177(5):1189–1192.
80. Council on Scientific Affairs (American Medical Association), Advisory Panel on Standard Nomenclature of Athletic Injuries; American Medical Association. *Standard Nomenclature of Athletic Injuries*. Chicago, IL: American Medical Association; 1998.
81. Coupens SD, Yates CK, Sheldon C, Ward C. Magnetic resonance imaging evaluation of the patellar tendon after use of its central one-third for anterior cruciate ligament reconstruction. *Am J Sports Med* 1992;20(3):332–335.
82. Covey CD, Sapega AA. Injuries of the posterior cruciate ligament. *J Bone Joint Surg Am* 1993;75(9):1376–1386.
83. Covey DC, Sapega AA. Anatomy and function of the posterior cruciate ligament. *Clin Sports Med* 1994;13(3):509–518.
84. Crema MD et al. Articular cartilage in the knee: current MR imaging techniques and applications in clinical practice and research. *Radiographics* 2011;31(1):37–61.
85. Crues JV et al. Meniscal tears of the knee: accuracy of MR imaging. *Radiology* 1987;164(2):445–448.
86. Crues JV, Ryu R, Morgan FW. Meniscal pathology. The expanding role of magnetic resonance imaging. *Clin Orthop Relat Res* 1990;(252):80–87.
87. Crues JV, Shellock FG. *Magnetic Resonance Imaging of the Knee*. New York, NY: Raven Press; 1987.
88. Crues JV, Stoller DW. The menisci. In: Mink JH, Reicher MA, Crues JV, eds. *MRI of the Knee*. New York, NY: Raven Press; 1993:91.
89. Dandy DJ. Chondral and osteochondral lesions of the femoral condyles. In: Aichroth PM, Cannon WD, eds. *Knee Surgery: Current Practice*. London, United Kingdom: Martin Dunitz; 1992:443.
90. Dehaven KEASP. Meniscal repair. *J Bone Joint Surg* 1994;76(1):140–152.
91. DeLee JC, Drez D, Miller MD. *Orthopaedic Sports Medicine: Principles and Practice*. 2nd ed. New York, NY: WB Saunders; 2003.
92. Delfaut EM et al. Fat suppression in MR imaging: techniques and pitfalls. *Radiographics* 1999;19(2):373–382.
93. De Maeseneer M et al. Distal insertions of the semimembranosus tendon: MR imaging with anatomic correlation. *Skeletal Radiol* 2014;43(6):781–791.
94. De Maeseneer M, Shahabpour M, Van Roy F, et al. MR imaging of the medial collateral ligament bursa: findings in patients and anatomic data derived from cadavers. *AJR Am J Roentgenol* 2001;177(4):911–917.
95. De Maeseneer M, Van Roy F, Lenchik L, et al. Three layers of the medial capsular and supporting structures of the knee: MR imaging-anatomic correlation. *Radiographics* 2000;20(Spec No):83–89.
96. De Maeseneer M, Van Roy P, Shahabpour M, et al. Normal anatomy and pathology of the posterior capsular area of the knee: findings in cadaveric specimens and in patients. *AJR Am J Roentgenol* 2004;182(4):955–962.
97. d'Entremont AG et al. Using the dGEMRIC technique to evaluate cartilage health in the presence of surgical hardware at 3T: comparison of inversion recovery and saturation recovery approaches. *Skeletal Radiol* 2014;43(3):331–344.
98. Desai MA et al. Clinical utility of dual-energy CT for evaluation of tophaceous gout. *Radiographics* 2011;31(5):1365–1375.
99. De Smet AA, Fisher DR, Graf BK, Lange RH. Osteochondritis dissecans of the knee: value of MR imaging in determining lesion stability and the presence of articular cartilage defects. *AJR Am J Roentgenol* 1990;155(3):549–553.
100. De Smet AA et al. Diagnosis of meniscal tears of the knee with MR imaging: effect of observer variation and sample size on sensitivity and specificity. *AJR Am J Roentgenol* 1993;160(3):555–559.
101. De Smet AA, Norris MA, Yandow DR, et al. MR diagnosis of meniscal tears of the knee: importance of high signal in the meniscus that extends to the surface. *AJR Am J Roentgenol* 1993;161(1):101–107.
102. De Smet AA et al. MR diagnosis of meniscal tears: analysis of causes of errors. *AJR Am J Roentgenol* 1994;163(6):1419–1423.
103. Deutsch A, Veltri DM, Altchek DW, et al. Symptomatic intraarticular ganglia of the cruciate ligaments of the knee. *Arthroscopy* 1994;10(2):219–223.
104. Deutsch AD, Shellock FG, Mink JH. Imaging of the patellofemoral joint: emphasis on advanced techniques. In: Fox JM, Pizzo WD, eds. *The Patellofemoral Joint*. New York, NY: McGraw-Hill; 1993.
105. Deutsch AL, Mink JH. The postoperative knee. In: Mink JH, Reicher MA, Crues JV, eds. *MRI of the Knee*. New York, NY: Raven Press; 1993:237.

106. Deutsch AL, Mink JH, Fox JM, et al. Peripheral meniscal tears: MR findings after conservative treatment or arthroscopic repair. *Radiology* 1990;176(2):485–488.
107. Deutsch AL, Shellock FG. The extensor mechanism and patellofemoral joint. In: Mink JH, Reicher MA, Crues JV, eds. *MRI of the Knee*. New York, NY: Raven Press; 1993:189.
108. Dickason JM, Del Pizzo W, Blazina ME, et al. A series of ten discoid medial menisci. *Clin Orthop Relat Res* 1982;168:75–79.
109. Diederichs G, Issever AS, Scheffler S. MR imaging of patellar instability: injury patterns and assessment of risk factors. *Radiographics* 2010;30(4):961–981.
110. Dietrich TJ et al. End-stage extension of the knee and its influence on tibial tuberosity-trochlear groove distance (TTTG) in asymptomatic volunteers. *Knee Surg Sports Traumatol Arthrosc* 2014;22(1):214–218.
111. Dillon EH et al. Follow-up of grade 2 meniscal abnormalities in the stable knee. *Radiology* 1991;181(3):849–852.
112. Dillon EH et al. The clinical significance of stage 2 meniscal abnormalities on magnetic resonance knee images. *Magn Reson Imaging* 1990;8(4):411–415.
113. Disler DG, McCauley TR, Kelman CG, et al. Detection of knee hyaline cartilage defects using fat-suppressed three-dimensional spoiled gradient-echo MR imaging: comparison with standard MR imaging and correlation with arthroscopy. *AJR Am J Roentgenol* 1995;165(2):377–382.
114. Disler DG, Peters TL, Muscoreil SJ, et al. Fat-suppressed spoiled GRASS imaging of knee hyaline cartilage: technique optimization and comparison with conventional MR imaging. *AJR Am J Roentgenol* 1994;163(4):887–892.
115. Dodds AL et al. The anterolateral ligament: anatomy, length changes and association with the Segond fracture. *Bone Joint J* 2014;96-B(3):325–331.
116. Dodds JA, Arnoczky SP. Anatomy of the anterior cruciate ligament: a blueprint for repair and reconstruction. *Arthroscopy* 1994;10(2):132–139.
117. Dorsay TA, Helms CA. Bucket-handle meniscal tears of the knee: sensitivity and specificity of MRI signs. *Skeletal Radiol* 2003;32(5):266–272.
118. Dowdy PA, Vellet A, Fowler P, et al. Magnetic resonance imaging of the partially torn anterior cruciate ligament: an in vitro animal model with correlative histopathology. *Clin J Sport Med* 1994;4(3):187–191.
119. Drape JL, Thelen P, Gay-Depassier P, Silbermann O, Benacerraf R. Intraarticular diffusion of Gd-DOTA after intravenous injection in the knee: MR imaging evaluation. *Radiology* 1993;188(1):227–234.
120. Duncan JB, Hunter R, Purnell M, Freeman J. Meniscal injuries associated with acute anterior cruciate ligament tears in alpine skiers. *Am J Sports Med* 1995;23(2):170–172.
121. Dupuis CS et al. Injuries and conditions of the extensor mechanism of the pediatric knee. *Radiographics* 2009;29(3):877–886.
122. Edmonson AS, Crenshaw AH. *Campbell's Operative Orthopaedics*. Vol. 2. St. Louis, MO: C. V. Mosby Company; 1980.
123. Ekman EF et al. Magnetic resonance imaging of iliotibial band syndrome. *Am J Sports Med* 1994;22(6):851–854.
124. Elias DA, White LM, Fithian DC. Acute lateral patellar dislocation at MR imaging: injury patterns of medial patellar soft-tissue restraints and osteochondral injuries of the inferomedial patella. *Radiology* 2002;225(3):736–743.
125. England E et al. Cysts of the anterior horn lateral meniscus and the ACL: is there a relationship? *Skeletal Radiol* 2015;44(3):369–373.
126. Eppley RA. Medial patellar subluxation. In: Fox JM, Pizzo WD, eds. *The Patellofemoral Joint*. New York, NY: McGraw-Hill; 1993:149.
127. Erdman WA, Tamburro F, Jayson HT, et al. Osteomyelitis: characteristics and pitfalls of diagnosis with MR imaging. *Radiology* 1991;180(2):533–539.
128. Escobedo EM, Mills WJ, Hunter JC. The "reverse Segond" fracture: association with a tear of the posterior cruciate ligament and medial meniscus. *AJR Am J Roentgenol* 2002;178(4):979–983.
129. Fanelli GC. Posterior cruciate ligament injuries in trauma patients. *Arthroscopy* 1993;9(3):291–294.
130. Fanelli GC, Giannotti BF, Edson CJ. The posterior cruciate ligament arthroscopic evaluation and treatment. *Arthroscopy* 1994;10(6):673–688.
131. Feagin JA, Curl WW. Isolated tear of the anterior cruciate ligament: 5-year follow-up study. *Am J Sports Med* 1976;4(3):95–9100.
132. Feller JF, Rishi M, Hughes EC. Lipoma arborescens of the knee: MR demonstration. *AJR Am J Roentgenol* 1994;163(1):162–164.
133. Ferrer-Roca O, Vilalta C. Lesions of the meniscus. Part II: horizontal cleavages and lateral cysts. *Clin Orthop Relat Res* 1980;(146):301–307.
134. Fetto JF, Marshall JL. Medial collateral ligament injuries of the knee: a rationale for treatment. *Clin Orthop Relat Res* 1978;132:206–218.
135. Fetto JF, Marshall JL. The natural history and diagnosis of anterior cruciate ligament insufficiency. *Clin Orthop Relat Res* 1980;147:29–38.
136. Fezoulidis I, Neuhold A, Wicke L, et al. [MRT of the status following augmentation plasty of the anterior cruciate ligament using carbon fibers]. *Radiologe* 1989;29(11):550–553.
137. Ficat RF, Hungerford DS. *Disorders of the Patellofemoral Joint*. Baltimore, MD: Williams & Wilkins; 1977.
138. Fischer SP, Fox JM, Del Pizzo W, et al. Accuracy of diagnoses from magnetic resonance imaging of the knee. A multi-center analysis of one thousand and fourteen patients. *J Bone Joint Surg Am* 1991;73(1):2–10.
139. Fitzgerald SW, Remer EM, Friedman H, et al. MR evaluation of the anterior cruciate ligament: value of supplementing sagittal images with coronal and axial images. *AJR Am J Roentgenol* 1993;160(6):1233–1237.
140. Fitzgibbons RE, Shelbourne KD. "Aggressive" nontreatment of lateral meniscal tears seen during anterior cruciate ligament reconstruction. *Am J Sports Med* 1995;23(2):156–159.
141. Flors L et al. MR imaging of soft-tissue vascular malformations: diagnosis, classification, and therapy follow-up. *Radiographics* 2011;31(5):1321–1340.
142. Forbes JR, Helms CA, Janzen DL. Acute pes anserine bursitis: MR imaging. *Radiology* 1995;194(2):525–527.
143. Fowler PJ. Bone injuries associated with anterior cruciate ligament disruption. *Arthroscopy* 1994;10(4):453–460.
144. Fox JM. Techniques and preliminary results in arthroscopic anterior cruciate prosthesis. In:

53rd Annual Meeting of the American Academy of Orthopaedic Surgeons. New Orleans, LA, 1986.
145. Fox MG et al. MR imaging of fibroma of the tendon sheath. *AJR Am J Roentgenol* 2003;180(5): 1449–1453.
146. Frija G et al. Grossly normal knee menisci: correlations with pathology and magnetic resonance imaging. *Diagn Interv Radiol* 1989;1:29–34.
147. Fu FH. *Master Techniques in Orthopaedic Surgery Sports Medicine*. Philadelphia, PA: Lippincott Williams & Wilkins; 2000.
148. Fu FH, Harner CD, Johnson DL, Miller MD, Woo SL. Biomechanics of knee ligaments. Basic concepts and clinical application. *Instr Course Lect* 1993;75:1716–1727.
149. Fujikawa K. Discoid meniscus in children. In: Aichroth PM, Cannon WD, eds. *Knee Surgery: Current Practice*. London, United Kingdom: Martin Dunitz; 1992:530.
150. Fulkerson JP, Hungerford DS. *Disorders of the Patellofemoral Joint*. 2nd ed. Baltimore, MD: Williams & Wilkins; 1990.
151. Fulkerson JP et al. Attachment of epiphyseal cartilage cells and 17/28 rat osteosarcoma osteoblasts using mussel adhesive protein. *J Orthop Res* 1990;8(6):793–798.
152. Fullerson JP. Patellar malalignment. In: Aichroth PM, Cannon WD, eds. *Knee Surgery: Current Practice*. London, United Kingdom: Martin Dunitz; 1992:389.
153. Gagliardi JA, Chung EM, Chandnani VP, et al. Detection and staging of chondromalacia patellae: relative efficacies of conventional MR imaging, MR arthrography, and CT arthrography. *AJR Am J Roentgenol* 1994;163(3):629–636.
154. Gallimore GW, Harms SE. Knee injuries: high-resolution MR imaging. *Radiology* 1986; 160(2):457–461.
155. Garcia-Valtuille R, Abascal F, Cerezal L, et al. Anatomy and MR imaging appearances of synovial plicae of the knee. *Radiographics* 2002;22(4): 775–784.
156. Garner HW, Ortiguera CJ, Nakhleh RE. Pigmented villonodular synovitis. *Radiographics* 2008; 28(5):1519–1523.
157. Garrett JC, Steensen RN, Stevensen RN. Meniscal transplantation in the human knee: a preliminary report. *Arthroscopy* 1991;7(1):57–62.
158. Garver P et al. Epiphyseal sclerosis in renal osteodystrophy simulating osteonecrosis. *AJR Am J Roentgenol* 1981;136(6):1239–1241.
159. Geissler WB, Whipple TL. Intraarticular abnormalities in association with posterior cruciate ligament injuries. *Am J Sports Med* 1993;21(6): 846–849.
160. George M, Wall EJ. Locked knee caused by meniscal subluxation: magnetic resonance imaging and arthroscopic verification. *Arthroscopy* 2003;19(8): 885–888.
161. Gill KG, Nemeth BA, Davis KW. Magnetic resonance imaging of the pediatric knee. *Magn Reson Imaging Clin N Am* 2014;22(4):743–763.
162. Girgis FG, Marshall JL, Monajem A. The cruciate ligaments of the knee joint. Anatomical, functional and experimental analysis. *Clin Orthop Relat Res* 1975;106:216–231.
163. Glashow JL et al. Double-blind assessment of the value of magnetic resonance imaging in the diagnosis of anterior cruciate and meniscal lesions. *J Bone Joint Surg Am* 1989;71(1):113–119.
164. Glazebrook KN et al. Case-control study to estimate the performance of dual-energy computed tomography for anterior cruciate ligament tears in patients with history of knee trauma. *Skeletal Radiol* 2014;43(3):297–305.
165. Gold GE, McCauley TR, Gray ML, Disler DG. What's new in cartilage? *Radiographics* 2003; 23(5):1227–1242.
166. Gondim Teixeira PA et al. Linear signal hyperintensity adjacent to the subchondral bone plate at the knee on T2-weighted fat-saturated sequences: imaging aspects and association with structural lesions. *Skeletal Radiol* 2014;43(11):1589–1598.
167. Gottsegen CJ et al. Avulsion fractures of the knee: imaging findings and clinical significance. *Radiographics* 2008;28(6):1755–1770.
168. Grelsamer RP, Cartier P. Comprehensive approach to patellar pathology. *Contemp Orthop* 1990;20(5):493–501.
169. Grimberg A et al. Deep lateral notch sign and double notch sign in complete tears of the anterior cruciate ligament: MR imaging evaluation. *Skeletal Radiol* 2015;44(3):385–391.
170. Grimm NL et al. Osteochondritis dissecans of the knee: pathoanatomy, epidemiology, and diagnosis. *Clin Sports Med* 2014;33(2):181–188.
171. Grood ES. Placement of knee ligament grafts. In: Aichroth PM, Cannon WD, eds. *Knee Surgery: Current Practice*. London, United Kingdom: Martin Dunitz; 1992:116.
172. Grover JS, Bassett LW, Gross ML, Seeger LL, Finerman GA. Posterior cruciate ligament: MR imaging. *Radiology* 1990;174(2):527–530.
173. Guerra J, Newell JD, Resnick D, Danzig LA. Pictorial essay: gastrocnemio-semimembranosus bursal region of the knee. *Am J Roentgenol* 1981;136(3):593–596.
174. Gutierrez LB et al. MR imaging near metallic implants using MAVRIC SL: initial clinical experience at 3T. *Acad Radiol* 2015;22(3):370–379.
175. Gylys-Morin VM, Graham TB, Blebea JS, et al. Knee in early juvenile rheumatoid arthritis: MR imaging findings. *Radiology* 2001;220(3): 696–706.
176. Gylys-Morin VM, Hajek PC, Sartoris DJ, Resnick D. Articular cartilage defects: detectability in cadaver knees with MR. *AJR Am J Roentgenol* 1987;148(6):1153–1157.
177. Hallen LG, Lindahl O. The "screw-home" movement in the knee-joint. *Acta Orthop Scand* 1966;37(1):97–106.
178. Hamada M et al. Usefulness of magnetic resonance imaging for detecting intrasubstance tear and/or degeneration of lateral discoid meniscus. *Arthroscopy* 1994;10(6):645–653.
179. Harner CD, Xerogeanes JW, Livesay GA, et al. The human posterior cruciate ligament complex: an interdisciplinary study. Ligament morphology and biomechanical evaluation. *Am J Sports Med* 1995;23(6):736–745.
180. Hartzman S et al. MR imaging of the knee. Part II. Chronic disorders. *Radiology* 1987;162(2): 553–557.
181. Hauger O et al. Characterization of the "red zone" of knee meniscus: MR imaging and histologic correlation. *Radiology* 2000;217(1):193–200.
182. Hayes CW, Sawyer RW, Conway WF. Patellar cartilage lesions: in vitro detection and staging with MR imaging and pathologic correlation. *Radiology* 1990;176(2):479–483.

183. Helito CP et al. MRI evaluation of the anterolateral ligament of the knee: assessment in routine 1.5-T scans. *Skeletal Radiol* 2014;43(10):1421–1427.
184. Henderson IJ et al. Prospective clinical study of autologous chondrocyte implantation and correlation with MRI at three and 12 months. *J Bone Joint Surg Br* 2003;85(7):1060–1066.
185. Henning CE, Yearout KM, Vequist SW, Stallbaumer RJ, Decker KA. Use of the fascia sheath coverage and exogenous fibrin clot in the treatment of complex meniscal tears. *Am J Sports Med* 1991;19(6):626–631.
186. Herman LJ, Beltran J. Pitfalls in MR imaging of the knee. *Radiology* 1988;167(3):775–781.
187. Herzog RJ, Silliman JF, Hutton K, et al. Measurements of the intercondylar notch by plain film radiography and magnetic resonance imaging. *Am J Sports Med* 1994;22(2):204–210.
188. Ho YY et al. Postoperative evaluation of the knee after autologous chondrocyte implantation: what radiologists need to know. *Radiographics* 2007;27(1):207–220.
189. Hodler J, Haghighi P, Trudell D, Resnick D. The cruciate ligaments of the knee: correlation between MR appearance and gross and histologic findings in cadaveric specimens. *AJR Am J Roentgenol* 1992;159(2):357–360.
190. Hohl M. Managing the challenge of tibial plateau fractures. *J Musculoskeletal Med* 1991;8:70–86.
191. Hohl M, Hong YN, Schopfer P. Acid- and enzyme-mediated solubilization of cell-wall beta-1.3,beta-1.4-d-glucan in maize coleoptiles: implications for auxin-mediated growth. *Plant Physiol* 1991;95(4):1012–1018.
192. Horton LK, Jacobson JA, Lin J, Hayes CW. MR imaging of anterior cruciate ligament reconstruction graft. *AJR Am J Roentgenol* 2000;175(4):1091–1097.
193. Howe MA, Buckwalter KA, Braunstein EM, Wojtys EM. Case report 483: discoid lateral meniscus (DLM), medially displaced, with complex tear. *Skeletal Radiol* 1988;17(4):293–294.
194. Howell SM, Barad SJ. Knee extension and its relationship to the slope of the intercondylar roof. Implications for positioning the tibial tunnel in anterior cruciate ligament reconstructions. *Am J Sports Med* 1995;23(3):288–294.
195. Howell SM, Berns GS, Farley TE. Unimpinged and impinged anterior cruciate ligament grafts: MR signal intensity measurements. *Radiology* 1991;179(3):639–643.
196. Howell SM, Knox KE, Farley TE, Taylor MA. Revascularization of a human anterior cruciate ligament graft during the first two years of implantation. *Am J Sports Med* 1995;23(1):42–49.
197. Howell SM, Taylor MA. Failure of reconstruction of the anterior cruciate ligament due to impingement by the intercondylar roof. *J Bone Joint Surg Am* 1993;75(7):1044–1055.
198. Huang BK et al. Injury of the gluteal aponeurotic fascia and proximal iliotibial band: anatomy, pathologic conditions, and MR imaging. *Radiographics* 2013;33(5):1437–1452.
199. Huang G-S, Lee CH, Chan WP, et al. Acute anterior cruciate ligament stump entrapment in anterior cruciate ligament tears: MR imaging appearance. *Radiology* 2002;225(2):537–540.
200. Huang G-S, Lee CH, Chan WP, et al. Localized nodular synovitis of the knee: MR imaging appearance and clinical correlates in 21 patients. *AJR Am J Roentgenol* 2003;181(2):539–543.
201. Huang G-S, Yu JS, Munshi M, et al. Avulsion fracture of the head of the fibula (the "arcuate" sign): MR imaging findings predictive of injuries to the posterolateral ligaments and posterior cruciate ligament. *AJR Am J Roentgenol* 2003;180(2):381–387.
202. Hughston JC, Andrews JR, Cross MJ, Moschi A. Classification of knee ligament instabilities. Part I. The medial compartment and cruciate ligaments. *J Bone Joint Surg Am* 1976;58(2):159–172.
203. Hughston JC et al. Classification of knee ligament instabilities. Part II. The lateral compartment. *J Bone Joint Surg Am* 1976;58(2):173–179.
204. Hughston JC, Bowden JA, Andrews JR, Norwood LA. Acute tears of the posterior cruciate ligament. Results of operative treatment. *J Bone Joint Surg Am* 1980;62(3):438–450.
205. Hughston JC, Deese M. Medial subluxation of the patella as a complication of lateral retinacular release. *Am J Sports Med* 1988;16(4):383–388.
206. Indelicato PA. Nonoperative management of complete tears of the medial collateral ligament. *Orthop Rev* 1989;18(9):947–952.
207. Indelicato PA, Bittar ES. A perspective of lesions associated with ACL insufficiency of the knee. A review of 100 cases. *Clin Orthop Relat Res* 1985;198:77–80.
208. Insall J. "Chondromalacia patellae": patellar malalignment syndrome. *Orthop Clin North Am* 1979;10(1):117–127.
209. Insall JN, Scott WN. *Surgery of the Knee*. 3rd ed. Vol. 1. Philadelphia, PA: Churchill Livingstone; 2001.
210. Insall JN, Scott WN. *Surgery of the Knee*. Philadelphia, PA: Churchill Livingstone; 2001:913–1004.
211. Insall JN, Scott WN. *Surgery of the Knee*. Philadelphia, PA: Churchill Livingstone; 2001:1355–1397.
212. Jackson DW, Gasser SI. Tibial tunnel placement in ACL reconstruction. *Arthroscopy* 1994;10(2):124–131.
213. Jackson DW et al. Magnetic resonance imaging of the knee. *Am J Sports Med* 1988;16(1):29–38.
214. Jadhav SP et al. Comprehensive review of the anatomy, function, and imaging of the popliteus and associated pathologic conditions. *Radiographics* 2014;34(2):496–513.
215. Jaimes C et al. MR imaging of normal epiphyseal development and common epiphyseal disorders. *Radiographics* 2014;34(2):449–471.
216. Jans LBO et al. Evolution of femoral condylar ossification at MR imaging: frequency and patient age distribution. *Radiology* 2011;258(3):880–888.
217. Janzen DL et al. Cystic lesions around the knee joint: MR imaging findings. *AJR Am J Roentgenol* 1994;163(1):155–161.
218. Jaramillo D, Shapiro F, Hoffer FA, et al. Posttraumatic growth-plate abnormalities: MR imaging of bony-bridge formation in rabbits. *Radiology* 1990;175(3):767–773.
219. Javadpour SM, Finegan PJ, Glacken P. Anatomy of the posterior cruciate ligament and its length patterns during knee flexion. *Clin J Sport Med* 1994;4(2):125–132.
220. Jee W-H, McCauley TR, Kim JM, et al. Meniscal tear configurations: categorization with MR imaging. *AJR Am J Roentgenol* 2003;180(1):93–97.
221. Jelinek JS, Kransdorf MJ, Shmookler BM, et al. Giant cell tumor of the tendon sheath: MR findings in nine cases. *AJR Am J Roentgenol* 1994;162(4):919–922.

222. Johnson DL, Swenson TM, Livesay GA, Aizawa H, Fu FH, Harner CD. Insertion-site anatomy of the human menisci: gross, arthroscopic, and topographical anatomy as a basis for meniscal transplantation. *Arthroscopy* 1995;11(4):386–394.
223. Johnson DL, Warner JJ. Diagnosis for anterior cruciate ligament surgery. *Clin Sports Med* 1993;12(4):671–684.
224. Johnson DP, Eastwood DM, Witherow PJ. Symptomatic synovial plicae of the knee. *J Bone Joint Surg Am* 1993;75(10):1485–1496.
225. Johnson RL. Anatomy and biomechanics of the knee. In: Chapman MW, ed. *Operative Orthopaedics*. Philadelphia, PA: JB Lippincott; 1993:2039.
226. Johnston YE, Duray PH, Steere AC, et al. Lyme arthritis. Spirochetes found in synovial microangiopathic lesions. *Am J Pathol* 1985;118(1):26–34.
227. Jones CD, Keene GC, Christie AD. The popliteus as a retractor of the lateral meniscus of the knee. *Arthroscopy* 1995;11(3):270–274.
228. Jouben LM, Steele RJ, Bono JV. Orthopaedic manifestations of Lyme disease. *Orthop Rev* 1994;23(5):395–400.
229. Juhng S-K, Lee JK, Choi SS, et al. MR evaluation of the "arcuate" sign of posterolateral knee instability. *AJR Am J Roentgenol* 2002;178(3):583–588.
230. Justice WW, Quinn SF. Error patterns in the MR imaging evaluation of menisci of the knee. *Radiology* 1995;196(3):617–621.
231. Kaneko K, De Mouy EH, Robinson AE. Distribution of joint effusion in patients with traumatic knee joint disorders: MRI assessment. *Clin Imaging* 1993;17(3):176–178.
232. Kang CN, Lee SB, Kim SW. Symptomatic ganglion cyst within the substance of the anterior cruciate ligament. *Arthroscopy* 1995;11(5):612–615.
233. Kaplan EB. Dorsal dislocation of the metacarpophalangeal joint of the index finger. *J Bone Joint Surg Am* 1957;39(5):1081–1086.
234. Kaplan EB. The embryology of the menisci of the knee joint. *Bull Hosp Joint Dis* 1955;16(2):111–124.
235. Kaplan PA, Gehl RH, Dussault RG, et al. Bone contusions of the posterior lip of the medial tibial plateau (contrecoup injury) and associated internal derangements of the knee at MR imaging. *Radiology* 1999;211(3):747–753.
236. Kaplan PA et al. MR of the knee: the significance of high signal in the meniscus that does not clearly extend to the surface. *AJR Am J Roentgenol* 1991;156(2):333–336.
237. Karzel RP. Arthroscopic diagnosis and treatment of cruciate and collateral ligament injuries. In: Scott W, ed. *Arthroscopy of the Knee*. Philadelphia, PA: WB Saunders; 1990:131.
238. Karzel RP, Friedman MJ. Anterior cruciate ligament reconstruction using central one-third of the patellar tendon. In: Aichroth PM, Cannon WD, eds. *Knee Surgery: Current Practice*. London, United Kingdom: Martin Dunitz; 1992:138.
239. Kaushik S, Erickson JK, Palmer WE, et al. Effect of chondrocalcinosis on the MR imaging of knee menisci. *AJR Am J Roentgenol* 2001;177(4):905–909.
240. Kennedy JC, Fowler PJ. Medial and anterior instability of the knee. An anatomical and clinical study using stress machines. *J Bone Joint Surg Am* 1971;53(7):1257–1270.
241. Kennedy JC, Grainger RW. The posterior cruciate ligament. *J Trauma* 1967;7(3):367–377.
242. Kennedy JC, Hawkins RJ, Willis RB, Danylchuck KD. Tension studies of human knee ligaments. Yield point, ultimate failure, and disruption of the cruciate and tibial collateral ligaments. *J Bone Joint Surg Am* 1976;58(3):350–355.
243. Kennedy JC, Weinberg HW, Wilson AS. The anatomy and function of the anterior cruciate ligament. As determined by clinical and morphological studies. *J Bone Joint Surg Am* 1974;56(2):223–235.
244. Kent RH, Pope CF, Lynch JK, Jokl P. Magnetic resonance imaging of the surgically repaired meniscus: six-month follow-up. *Magn Reson Imaging* 1991;9(3):335–341.
245. Kezdi-Rogus PC, Lomasney LM. Radiologic case study. Plain film manifestations of ACL injury. *Orthopedics* 1994;17(10):967–973.
246. Khan N et al. Increasing lateral tibial slope: is there an association with articular cartilage changes in the knee? *Skeletal Radiol* 2014;43(4):437–441.
247. Kijowski R et al. Evaluation of the articular cartilage of the knee joint: value of adding a T2 mapping sequence to a routine MR imaging protocol. *Radiology* 2013;267(2):503–513.
248. Kijowski R et al. MRI characteristics of healed and unhealed peripheral vertical meniscal tears. *AJR Am J Roentgenol* 2014;202(3):585–592.
249. Kim HK et al. Age and sex dependency of cartilage T2 relaxation time mapping in MRI of children and adolescents. *AJR Am J Roentgenol* 2014;202(3):626–632.
250. Kim JM, Ma CB. Quantitative MRI of the ACL-injured and reconstructed knee. *Clin Sports Med* 2013;32(1):21–36.
251. Kim Y-J et al. Assessment of early osteoarthritis in hip dysplasia with delayed gadolinium-enhanced magnetic resonance imaging of cartilage. *J Bone Joint Surg Am* 2003;85-A(10):1987–1992.
252. Kindynis P, Haller J, Kang HS, et al. Osteophytosis of the knee: anatomic, radiologic, and pathologic investigation. *Radiology* 1990;174(3 Pt 1):841–846.
253. Kirsch MD, Fitzgerald SW, Friedman H, Rogers LF. Transient lateral patellar dislocation: diagnosis with MR imaging. *AJR Am J Roentgenol* 1993;161(1):109–113.
254. Kohn D, Moreno B. Meniscus insertion anatomy as a basis for meniscus replacement: a morphological cadaveric study. *Arthroscopy* 1995;11(1):96–103.
255. Konig H, Sieper J, Wolf KJ. Rheumatoid arthritis: evaluation of hypervascular and fibrous pannus with dynamic MR imaging enhanced with Gd-DTPA. *Radiology* 1990;176(2):473–477.
256. Kornick J et al. Meniscal abnormalities in the asymptomatic population at MR imaging. *Radiology* 1990;177(2):463–465.
257. Kottal RA, Vogler JB 3rd, Matamoros A, et al. Pigmented villonodular synovitis: a report of MR imaging in two cases. *Radiology* 1987;163(2):551–553.
258. Krause WR, Pope MH, Johnson RJ, Wilder DG. Mechanical changes in the knee after meniscectomy. *J Bone Joint Surg Am* 1976;58(5):599–604.
259. Kressel HY. *Magnetic Resonance Annual*. New York, NY: Raven Press; 1986.
260. Kujala UM, Osterman K, Kormano M, et al. Patellofemoral relationships in recurrent patellar dislocation. *J Bone Joint Surg Br* 1989;71(5):788–792.
261. Kulkarni MV, Drolshagen LF, Kaye JJ, et al. MR imaging of hemophiliac arthropathy. *J Comput Assist Tomogr* 1986;10(3):445–449.

262. Kummel BM. The treatment of patellofemoral problems. *Prim Care* 1980;7(2):217–229.
263. Kursunoglu-Brahme S, Resnick D, Magnetic resonance imaging of the knee. *Orthop Clin North Am* 1990;21(3):561–572.
264. Kursunoglu-Brahme S et al. Jogging causes acute changes in the knee joint: an MR study in normal volunteers. *AJR Am J Roentgenol* 1990;154(6):1233–1235.
265. Ladak A et al. MRI findings in patients with tibial nerve compression near the knee. *Skeletal Radiol* 2013;42(4):553–559.
266. Lance E, Deutsch AL, Mink JH. Prior lateral patellar dislocation: MR imaging findings. *Radiology* 1993;189(3):905–907.
267. Lance V et al. MR imaging characteristics and clinical symptoms related to displaced meniscal flap tears. *Skeletal Radiol* 2015;44(3):375–384.
268. Lancourt JE, Cristini JA. Patella alta and patella infera. Their etiological role in patellar dislocation, chondromalacia, and apophysitis of the tibial tubercle. *J Bone Joint Surg Am* 1975;57(8):1112–1115.
269. LaPrade RF, Burnett QM 2nd. Femoral intercondylar notch stenosis and correlation to anterior cruciate ligament injuries. A prospective study. *Am J Sports Med* 1994;22(2):198–202.
270. Larson RL. Subluxation-dislocation of the patella. In: Kennedy JC, ed. *The Injured Adolescent Knee*. Baltimore, MD: Williams & Wilkins; 1979:161.
271. Laurin CA, Dussault R, Levesque HP. The tangential x-ray investigation of the patellofemoral joint: x-ray technique, diagnostic criteria and their interpretation. *Clin Orthop Relat Res* 1979;144:16–26.
272. Lawson JP, Rahn DW. Lyme disease and radiologic findings in Lyme arthritis. *AJR Am J Roentgenol* 1992;158(5):1065–1069.
273. Le Blanche AF et al. Histomorphometric evaluation of (198)Au endovascular brachytherapy in a renal artery restenosis model in rabbits. *AJR Am J Roentgenol* 2002;179(3):611–618.
274. Lecas LK, Helms CA, Kosarek FJ, Garret WE. Inferiorly displaced flap tears of the medial meniscus: MR appearance and clinical significance. *AJR Am J Roentgenol* 2000;174(1):161–164.
275. Lee JK, Yao L, Phelps CT, et al. Anterior cruciate ligament tears: MR imaging compared with arthroscopy and clinical tests. *Radiology* 1988;166(3):861–864.
276. Lee K, Siegel MJ, Lau DM, Hildebolt CF, Matava MJ. Anterior cruciate ligament tears: MR imaging-based diagnosis in a pediatric population. *Radiology* 1999;213(3):697–704.
277. Lee SH, Petersilge CA, Trudell DJ, et al. Extrasynovial spaces of the cruciate ligaments: anatomy, MR imaging, and diagnostic implications. *AJR Am J Roentgenol* 1996;166(6):1433–1437.
278. Lektrakul N, Skaf A, Yeh L, et al. Pericruciate meniscal cysts arising from tears of the posterior horn of the medial meniscus: MR imaging features that simulate posterior cruciate ganglion cysts. *AJR Am J Roentgenol* 1999;172(6):1575–1579.
279. Levinsohn EM, Baker BE. Prearthrotomy diagnostic evaluation of the knee: review of 100 cases diagnosed by arthrography and arthroscopy. *AJR Am J Roentgenol* 1980;134(1):107–111.
280. Li DK, Adams ME, McConkey JP. Magnetic resonance imaging of the ligaments and menisci of the knee. *Radiol Clin North Am* 1986;24(2):209–227.
281. Lim PS, Schweitzer ME, Bhatia M, et al. Repeat tear of postoperative meniscus: potential MR imaging signs. *Radiology* 1999;210(1):183–188.
282. Linden B. The incidence of osteochondritis dissecans in the condyles of the femur. *Acta Orthop Scand* 1976;47(6):664–667.
283. Linden B, Nilsson. Strontium-85 uptake in knee joints with osteochondritis dissecans. *Acta Orthop Scand* 1976;47(6):668–671.
284. Lindgren PG, Willen R. Gastrocnemio-semimembranosus bursa and its relation to the knee joint. I. Anatomy and histology. *Acta Radiol Diagn (Stockh)* 1977;18(5):497–512.
285. Link TM, Steinbach LS, Ghosh S, et al. Osteoarthritis: MR imaging findings in different stages of disease and correlation with clinical findings. *Radiology* 2003;226(2):373–381.
286. Lintner DM, Kamaric E, Moseley JB, Noble PC. Partial tears of the anterior cruciate ligament. Are they clinically detectable? *Am J Sports Med* 1995;23(1):111–118.
287. Liu SH, Osti L, Mirzayan R. Ganglion cysts of the anterior cruciate ligament: a case report and review of the literature. *Arthroscopy* 1994;10(1):110–112.
288. Llauger J, Palmer J, Rosón N, et al. Nonseptic monoarthritis: imaging features with clinical and histopathologic correlation. *Radiographics* 2000;20(Spec No):263–278.
289. Logue JN, Fox JM. Residential health study of families living near the Drake Chemical Superfund site in Lock Haven, Pennsylvania. *Arch Environ Health* 1986;41(4):222–228.
290. Lombardo SJ, Bradley JP. Arthroscopic diagnosis and treatment of patellofemoral disorders. In: Scott W, ed. *Arthroscopy of the Knee*. Philadelphia, PA: WB Saunders; 1990:155.
291. Loos WC, Fox JM, Blazina ME, et al. Acute posterior cruciate ligament injuries. *Am J Sports Med* 1981;9(2):86–92.
292. Loosli A, Oshimo T. Conservatively treated anterior cruciate ligament injuries: activities, symptoms, and roentgenographic changes. *Clin J Sport Med* 1994;4(4):228–232.
293. Lotke PA, Ecker ML. Osteonecrosis-like syndrome of the medial tibial plateau. *Clin Orthop Relat Res* 1983;176:148–153.
294. Lyle NJ, Sampson MA, Barrett DS. MRI of intermittent meniscal dislocation in the knee. *Br J Radiol* 2009;82(977):374–379.
295. Lynch TC, Crues JV 3rd, Morgan FW, et al. Bone abnormalities of the knee: prevalence and significance at MR imaging. *Radiology* 1989;171(3):761–766.
296. MacIntosh DL, Darby JA. Lateral substitution reconstruction. In Proceedings of the Canadian Orthopaedic Association. *J Bone Joint Surg Br* 1976;58:142.
297. MacKay JW, Godley KC, Toms AP. MRI signal-based quantification of subchondral bone at the tibial plateau: a population study. *Skeletal Radiol* 2014;43(11):1567–1575.
298. MacLeod TD et al. Magnetic resonance analysis of loaded meniscus deformation: a novel technique comparing participants with and without radiographic knee osteoarthritis. *Skeletal Radiol* 2015;44(1):125–135.
299. Magee T. Accuracy of 3-Tesla MR and MR arthrography in diagnosis of meniscal retear

300. Magee T et al. MR arthrography of postoperative knee: for which patients is it useful? *Radiology* 2003;229(1):159–163.
301. Magee T, Shapiro M, Williams D. Usefulness of simultaneous acquisition of spatial harmonics technique for MRI of the knee. *AJR Am J Roentgenol* 2004;182(6):1411–1415.
302. Mandelbaum BR, Finerman GA, Reicher MA, et al. Magnetic resonance imaging as a tool for evaluation of traumatic knee injuries. Anatomical and pathoanatomical correlations. *Am J Sports Med* 1986;14(5):361–370.
303. Mansour R et al. The iliotibial band in acute knee trauma: patterns of injury on MR imaging. *Skeletal Radiol* 2014;43(10):1369–1375.
304. Markhardt BK, Gross JM, and Monu J. Schatzker classification of tibial plateau fractures: use of CT and MR imaging improves assessment. *Radiographics* 2009;29(2):585–597.
305. Marks KE, Bentley G. Patella alta and chondromalacia. *J Bone Joint Surg Br* 1978;60(1):71–73.
306. Matcuk GR Jr et al. Superolateral hoffa fat pad edema and patellofemoral maltracking: predictive modeling. *AJR Am J Roentgenol* 2014;203(2):W207–W212.
307. Mattrey RF et al. Perfluorochemicals as gastrointestinal contrast agents for MR imaging: preliminary studies in rats and humans. *AJR Am J Roentgenol* 1987;148(6):1259–1263.
308. Maywood RM, Murphy BJ, Uribe JW, Hechtman KS. Evaluation of arthroscopic anterior cruciate ligament reconstruction using magnetic resonance imaging. *Am J Sports Med* 1993;21(4):523–527.
309. McCauley TR. MR imaging evaluation of the postoperative knee. *Radiology* 2005;234(1):53–61.
310. McCauley TR, Elfar A, Moore A, et al. MR arthrography of anterior cruciate ligament reconstruction grafts. *AJR Am J Roentgenol* 2003;181(5):1217–1223.
311. McCauley TR, Kornaat PR,. Jee WH. Central osteophytes in the knee: prevalence and association with cartilage defects on MR imaging. *AJR Am J Roentgenol* 2001;176(2):359–364.
312. McCauley TR, Moses M, Kier R, et al. MR diagnosis of tears of anterior cruciate ligament of the knee: importance of ancillary findings. *AJR Am J Roentgenol* 1994;162(1):115–119.
313. McDaniel WJ, Dameron TB. Untreated ruptures of the anterior cruciate ligament. A follow-up study. *J Bone Joint Surg Am* 1980;62(5):696–705.
314. McLoughlin RF, Raber EL, Vellet AD, Wiley JP, Bray RC. Patellar tendinitis: MR imaging features, with suggested pathogenesis and proposed classification. *Radiology* 1995;197(3):843–848.
315. McMonagle JS et al. Tram-track appearance of the posterior cruciate ligament (PCL): correlations with mucoid degeneration, ligamentous stability, and differentiation from PCL tears. *AJR Am J Roentgenol* 2013;201(2):394–399.
316. Merchant AC. Radiologic evaluation of the patellofemoral joint. In: Aichroth PM, Cannon WD, eds. *Knee Surgery: Current Practice*. London, United Kingdom: Martin Dunitz; 1992:380.
317. Mesgarzadeh M et al. MR imaging of the knee: expanded classification and pitfalls to interpretation of meniscal tears. *Radiographics* 1993;13(3):489–500.
318. Mesgarzadeh M, Sapega AA, Bonakdarpour A, et al. Osteochondritis dissecans: analysis of mechanical stability with radiography, scintigraphy, and MR imaging. *Radiology* 1987;165(3):775–780.
319. Miller MD, Harner CD. Posterior cruciate ligament injuries. Current concepts in diagnosis and treatment. *Physician Sports Med* 1993;21:38.
320. Miller MD, Howard RF, Plancher KD. *Surgical Atlas of Sports Medicine*. Philadelphia, PA: Saunders; 2003.
321. Miller MD, Howard RF, Plancher KD. *Surgical Atlas of Sports Medicine*. Philadelphia, PA: Saunders; 2003:123–128.
322. Miller MD, Johnson DL, Harner CD, Fu FH. Posterior cruciate ligament injuries. *Orthop Rev* 1993;22(11):1201–1210.
323. Mink JH. Pitfalls in interpretation. In: Mink JH, Reicher MA, Crues JV, eds. *MRI of the Knee*. New York, NY: Raven Press; 1993:433.
324. Mink JH, Deutsch A. The knee. In: Mink JH, Deutsch A, eds. *MRI of the Musculoskeletal System: A Teaching File*. New York, NY: Raven Press; 1990:251.
325. Mink JH, Deutsch AL. Magnetic resonance imaging of the knee. *Clin Orthop Relat Res* 1989;244:29–47.
326. Mink JH, Deutsch AL. Occult cartilage and bone injuries of the knee: detection, classification, and assessment with MR imaging. *Radiology* 1989;170(3 Pt 1):823–829.
327. Mink JH, Levy T, Crues JV. Tears of the anterior cruciate ligament and menisci of the knee: MR imaging evaluation. *Radiology* 1988;167(3):769–774.
328. Mirowitz SA. Fast scanning and fat-suppression MR imaging of musculoskeletal disorders. *AJR Am J Roentgenol* 1993;161(6):1147–1157.
329. Moeser P, Bechtold RE, Clark T, et al. MR imaging of anterior cruciate ligament repair. *J Comput Assist Tomogr* 1989;13(1):105–109.
330. Mohankumar R et al. Meniscal ossicle: posttraumatic origin and association with posterior meniscal root tears. *AJR Am J Roentgenol* 2014;203(5):1040–1046.
331. Mohankumar R, White LM, Naraghi A. Pitfalls and pearls in MRI of the knee. *AJR Am J Roentgenol* 2014;203(3):516–530.
332. Møller BN, Krebs B, Jurik AG. Patellofemoral incongruence in chondromalacia and instability of the patella. *Acta Orthop Scand* 1986;57(3):232–234.
333. Morgan CD, Kalman VR, Grawl DM. Definitive landmarks for reproducible tibial tunnel placement in anterior cruciate ligament reconstruction. *Arthroscopy* 1995;11(3):275–288.
334. Mori Y, Kubo M, Okumo H, Kuroki Y. A scanning electron microscopic study of the degenerative cartilage in patellar chondropathy. *Arthroscopy* 1993;9(3):247–264.
335. Mosher TJ, Dardzinski BJ, Smith MB. Human articular cartilage: influence of aging and early symptomatic degeneration on the spatial variation of T2—preliminary findings at 3 T. *Radiology* 2000;214(1):259–266.
336. Mosher TJ, Smith H, Dardzinski BJ, et al. MR imaging and T2 mapping of femoral cartilage: in vivo determination of the magic angle effect. *AJR Am J Roentgenol* 2001;177(3):665–669.
337. Motamedi D et al. Thermal ablation of osteoid osteoma: overview and step-by-step guide. *Radiographics* 2009;29(7):2127–2141.

338. Muhle C, Ahn JM, Yeh L, et al. Iliotibial band friction syndrome: MR imaging findings in 16 patients and MR arthrographic study of six cadaveric knees. *Radiology* 1999;212(1):103–110.
339. Mulcahy H, Chew FS. Current concepts in knee replacement: complications. *AJR Am J Roentgenol* 2014;202(1):W76–W86.
340. Mulcahy H, Chew FS. Current concepts in knee replacement: features and imaging assessment. *AJR Am J Roentgenol* 2013;201(6):W828–W842.
341. Munshi M, Pretterklieber ML, Kwak S, et al. MR imaging, MR arthrography, and specimen correlation of the posterolateral corner of the knee: an anatomic study. *AJR Am J Roentgenol* 2003;180(4):1095–1101.
342. Murphey MD et al. From the radiologic pathology archives imaging of osteonecrosis: radiologic-pathologic correlation. *Radiographics* 2014;34(4):1003–1028.
343. Murphey MD et al. Pigmented villonodular synovitis: radiologic-pathologic correlation. *Radiographics* 2008;28(5):1493–1518.
344. Murphey MD et al. Imaging of synovial chondromatosis with radiologic-pathologic correlation. *Radiographics* 2007;27(5):1465–1488.
345. Murphy BJ, Hechtman KS, Uribe JW, et al. Iliotibial band friction syndrome: MR imaging findings. *Radiology* 1992;185(2):569–571.
346. Murphy BJ, Smith RL, Uribe JW, et al. Bone signal abnormalities in the posterolateral tibia and lateral femoral condyle in complete tears of the anterior cruciate ligament: a specific sign? *Radiology* 1992;182(1):221–224.
347. Muscolo DL, Makino A, Costa-Paz M, Ayerza MA. Localized pigmented villonodular synovitis of the posterior compartment of the knee: diagnosis with magnetic resonance imaging. *Arthroscopy* 1995;11(4):482–485.
348. Negendank WG et al. Magnetic resonance imaging of meniscal degeneration in asymptomatic knees. *J Orthop Res* 1990;8(3):311–320.
349. Newman AP, Daniels AU, Burks RT. Principles and decision making in meniscal surgery. *Arthroscopy* 1993;9(1):33–51.
350. Ng AW et al. MRI diagnosis of ACL bundle tears: value of oblique axial imaging. *Skeletal Radiol* 2013;42(2):209–217.
351. Nguyen JC et al. MR imaging–based diagnosis and classification of meniscal tears. *Radiographics* 2014;34(4):981–999.
352. Niitsu M, Anno I, Fukubayashi T, et al. Tears of cruciate ligaments and menisci: evaluation with cine MR imaging. *Radiology* 1991;178(3):859–864.
353. Nogalski MP, Bach BR. A review of early anterior cruciate ligament surgical repair or reconstruction. Results and caveats. *Orthop Rev* 1993;22(11):1213–1223.
354. Nottage WM, Matsuura PA. Management of complete traumatic anterior cruciate ligament tears in the skeletally immature patient: current concepts and review of the literature. *Arthroscopy* 1994;10(5):569–573.
355. Noyes FR, Barber-Westin SD. Surgical reconstruction of severe chronic posterolateral complex injuries of the knee using allograft tissues. *Am J Sports Med* 1995;23(1):2–12.
356. Noyes FR, Mooar LA, Moorman CT 3rd, McGinniss GH. Partial tears of the anterior cruciate ligament. Progression to complete ligament deficiency. *J Bone Joint Surg Br* 1989;71(5):825–833.
357. Nusman CM et al. Distribution pattern of MRI abnormalities within the knee and wrist of juvenile idiopathic arthritis patients: signature of disease activity. *AJR Am J Roentgenol* 2014;202(5):W439–W446.
358. Oberlander MA, Shalvoy RM, Hughston JC. The accuracy of the clinical knee examination documented by arthroscopy. A prospective study. *Am J Sports Med* 1993;21(6):773–778.
359. Ogilvie-Harris DJ, Giddens J. Hoffa's disease: arthroscopic resection of the infrapatellar fat pad. *Arthroscopy* 1994;10(2):184–187.
360. O'Meara PM. The basic science of meniscus repair. *Orthop Rev* 1993;22(6):681–686.
361. Østergaard M, Gideon P, Wieslander S, et al. Pannus-induced destruction of joint cartilage and subchondral bone. visualization and staging by MRI. *Magn Reson Materials Phys Biol Med* 1994;2(2):91–100.
362. Outerbridge RE. The etiology of chondromalacia patellae. *J Bone Joint Surg Br* 1961;43-B:752–757.
363. Panni AS. Overuse injuries of the extensor mechanism in athletes. *Clin Sports Med* 2002;21(3):483–498.
364. Park HJ et al. Medial meniscal root tears and meniscal extrusion transverse length ratios on MRI. *Br J Radiol* 2012;85(1019):e1032–e1037.
365. Park HJ et al. Comparison between arthroscopic findings and 1.5-T and 3-T MRI of oblique coronal and sagittal planes of the knee for evaluation of selective bundle injury of the anterior cruciate ligament. *AJR Am J Roentgenol* 2014;203(2):W199–W206.
366. Park HJ et al. A practical MRI grading system for osteoarthritis of the knee: association with Kellgren-Lawrence radiographic scores. *Eur J Radiol* 2013;82(1):112–117.
367. Parker AW, Drez D, Cooper JL. Anterior cruciate ligament injuries in patients with open physes. *Am J Sports Med* 1994;22(1):44–47.
368. Pearlstone JR, Smillie LB. The binding sites of rabbit skeletal troponin-I on troponin-T. *Can J Biochem* 1980;58(8):649–654.
369. Peltola EK, Lindahl J, Koskinen SK. The reverse Segond fracture: not associated with knee dislocation and rarely with posterior cruciate ligament tear. *Emerg Radiol* 2014;21(3):245–249.
370. Peterfy CG, Majumdar S, Lang P, et al. MR imaging of the arthritic knee: improved discrimination of cartilage, synovium, and effusion with pulsed saturation transfer and fat-suppressed T1-weighted sequences. *Radiology* 1994;191(2):413–419.
371. Peterfy CG, van Dijke CF, Janzen DL, et al. Quantification of articular cartilage in the knee with pulsed saturation transfer subtraction and fat-suppressed MR imaging: optimization and validation. *Radiology* 1994;192(2):485–491.
372. Peterson JJ, Kransdorf MJ, Bancroft LW, Murphey MD. Imaging characteristics of cystic adventitial disease of the peripheral arteries: presentation as soft-tissue masses. *AJR Am J Roentgenol* 2003;180(3):621–625.
373. Petri M et al. Influence of rupture patterns of the medial patellofemoral ligament (MPFL) on the outcome after operative treatment of traumatic patellar dislocation. *Knee Surg Sports Traumatol Arthrosc* 2013;21(3):683–689.
374. Poletti SC, Gates HS 3rd, Martinez SM, Richardson WJ. The use of magnetic resonance imaging in the diagnosis of pigmented villonodular synovitis. *Orthopedics* 1990;13(2):185–190.

375. Polly DW et al. The accuracy of selective magnetic resonance imaging compared with the findings of arthroscopy of the knee. *J Bone Joint Surg Am* 1988;70(2):192–198.
376. Polster JM et al. Rheumatoid arthritis: evaluation with contrast-enhanced CT with digital bone masking. *Radiology* 2009;252(1):225–231.
377. Quinn SF, Brown TR, Szumowski J. Menisci of the knee: radial MR imaging correlated with arthroscopy in 259 patients. *Radiology* 1992;185(2):577–580.
378. Rahmouni A, Chosidow O, Mathieu D, et al. MR imaging in acute infectious cellulitis. *Radiology* 1994;192:493–496.
379. Rajgopal A. *Knee Surgery*. New Delhi, India: Jaypee Brothers Medical; 2014.
380. Rak KM, Gillogly SD, Schaefer RA, Yakes WF, Liljedahl RR. Anterior cruciate ligament reconstruction: evaluation with MR imaging. *Radiology* 1991;178(2):553–556.
381. Raunest J, Hotzinger H, Burrig KF. Magnetic resonance imaging (MRI) and arthroscopy in the detection of meniscal degenerations: correlation of arthroscopy and MRI with histology findings. *Arthroscopy* 1994;10(6):634–640.
382. Recht MP, Kramer J. MR imaging of the postoperative knee: a pictorial essay. *Radiographics* 2002;22(4):765–774.
383. Recht MP, Kramer J, Marcelis S, et al. Abnormalities of articular cartilage in the knee: analysis of available MR techniques. *Radiology* 1993;187(2):473–478.
384. Recht MP, Piraino DW, Cohen MA, et al. Localized anterior arthrofibrosis (cyclops lesion) after reconstruction of the anterior cruciate ligament: MR imaging findings. *AJR Am J Roentgenol* 1995;165(2):383–385.
385. Recht MP, Resnick D. MR imaging of articular cartilage: current status and future directions. *AJR Am J Roentgenol* 1994;163(2):283–290.
386. Recondo JA, Salvador E, Villanúa JA, et al. Lateral stabilizing structures of the knee: functional anatomy and injuries assessed with MR imaging. *Radiographics* 2000;20(Spec No):91.
387. Reicher MA. The spectrum of knee joint disorders. In: Mink H, Reicher MA, Crues JV, eds. *MRI of the Knee*. New York, NY: Raven Press; 1993:333.
388. Reicher MA, Bassett LW, Gold RH. High-resolution magnetic resonance imaging of the knee joint: pathologic correlations. *AJR Am J Roentgenol* 1985;145(5):903–909.
389. Reicher MA, Hartzman S, Bassett LW, et al. MR imaging of the knee. Part I. Traumatic disorders. *Radiology* 1987;162(2):547–551.
390. Reinig JW, McDevitt ER, Ove PN. Progression of meniscal degenerative changes in college football players: evaluation with MR imaging. *Radiology* 1991;181(1):255–257.
391. Resnick D, Niwayama G. *Diagnosis of Bone and Joint Disorders*. 2nd ed. Philadelphia, PA: W.B. Saunders; 1988.
392. Resnick D, Niwayama G. *Diagnosis of Bone and Joint Disorders*. 2nd ed. Vol. 3. Philadelphia, PA: WB Saunders; 1988.
393. Resnick D, Niwayama G. *Internal Derangement of Joints. Diagnosis of Bone and Joint Disorders*. 2nd ed., Vol. 5. Philadelphia, PA: WB Saunders; 1988.
394. Ricklin P, Rüttimann A, Buono SD. *Meniscus Lesions: Diagnosis, Differential Diagnosis, and Therapy*. 2nd ed. New York, NY: Thieme; 1983.
395. Riddle RD et al. Sonic hedgehog mediates the polarizing activity of the ZPA. *Cell* 1993;75(7):1401–1416.
396. Roberts MC, Kressel HY, Fallon MD, et al. Paget disease: MR imaging findings. *Radiology* 1989;173(2):341–345.
397. Robertson PL, Schweitzer ME, Bartolozzi AR, Ugoni A. Anterior cruciate ligament tears: evaluation of multiple signs with MR imaging. *Radiology* 1994;193(3):829–834.
398. Rockwood CA, Green DP, Bucholz RW, et al. *Rockwood and Green's Fractures in Adults*. 4th ed. Philadelphia, PA: Lippincott Williams & Wilkins; 1996.
399. Rodrigo JL, Gershwin ME. Management of the arthritic joint. In: Chapman MW, ed. *Operative Orthopaedics*. Philadelphia, PA: JB Lippincott; 1993.
400. Roemer FW et al. Can structural joint damage measured with MR imaging be used to predict knee replacement in the following year? *Radiology* 2015;274(3):810–820.
401. Rose PM, Demlow TA, Szumowski J, Quinn SF. Chondromalacia patellae: fat-suppressed MR imaging. *Radiology* 1994;193(2):437–440.
402. Rosenberg TD. Arthroscopic diagnosis and treatment of meniscal disorders. In: Scott W, ed. *Arthroscopy of the Knee*. Philadelphia, PA: WB Saunders; 1990:67.
403. Rosenberg TD, Paulos LE. Arthroscopic surgery of the knee. In: Chapman MW, ed. *Operative Orthopaedics*. Philadelphia, PA: J.B. Lippincott; 1993:2403.
404. Rosenberg TD, et al. Arthroscopic surgery of the knee. In: Chapman MW, ed. *Operative Orthopaedics*. Philadelphia, PA: JB Lippincott; 1988:1585.
405. Rosenberg TD, Paulos LE, Parker RD, et al. The forty-five-degree posteroanterior flexion weight-bearing radiograph of the knee. *J Bone Joint Surg Am* 1988;70(10):1479–1483.
406. Roth C et al. Quadriceps fat pad signal intensity and enlargement on MRI: prevalence and associated findings. *AJR Am J Roentgenol* 2004;182(6):1383–1387.
407. Rubenstein JD, Kim JK, Morova-Protzner I, et al. Effects of collagen orientation on MR imaging characteristics of bovine articular cartilage. *Radiology* 1993;188(1):219–226.
408. Rubin DA, Harner CD, Costello JM. Treatable chondral injuries in the knee: frequency of associated focal subchondral edema. *AJR Am J Roentgenol* 2000;174(4):1099–1106.
409. Rubin DA, Kneeland JB, Listerud J, Underberg-Davis SJ, Dalinka MK. MR diagnosis of meniscal tears of the knee: value of fast spin-echo vs conventional spin-echo pulse sequences. *AJR Am J Roentgenol* 1994;162(5):1131–1135.
410. Runyan BR et al. Cyclops lesions that occur in the absence of prior anterior ligament reconstruction. *Radiographics* 2007;27(6):e26.
411. Ruwe PA et al. Can MR imaging effectively replace diagnostic arthroscopy? *Radiology* 1992;183(2):335–339.
412. Ryu RK, Ting AJ. Arthroscopic treatment of meniscal cysts. *Arthroscopy* 1993;9(5):591–595.
413. Samim M et al. MRI of anterior knee pain. *Skeletal Radiol* 2014;43(7):875–893.
414. Sanders TG, Linares RC, Lawhorn KW, Tirman PF, Houser C. Oblique meniscomeniscal ligament: another potential pitfall for a meniscal tear—anatomic description and appearance at MR imaging in three cases. *Radiology* 1999;213(1):213–216.

415. Sanders TG, Medynski MA, Feller JF, Lawhorn KW. Bone contusion patterns of the knee at MR imaging: footprint of the mechanism of injury. *Radiographics* 2000;20(Spec No):135–151.
416. Santyr GE, Mulkern RV. Magnetization transfer in MR imaging. Relaxometry and Biophysics Committee. *J Magn Reson Imaging* 1995;5(1):121–124.
417. Sapega AA, Covey DC. The biomechanics of femoral and tibial posterior cruciate ligament graft placement. *Clin Sports Med* 1994;13(3):553–559.
418. Savage L, Garth WP. Intra-articular synovial cyst of the knee originating from a chondral fracture of the medial femoral condyle. A case report. *J Bone Joint Surg Am* 1994;76(9):1394–1396.
419. Schonholtz GJ, Koenig TM, Prince A. Bilateral discoid medial menisci: a case report and literature review. *Arthroscopy* 1993;9(3):315–317.
420. Schutzer SF, Ramsby GR, Fulkerson JP. Computed tomographic classification of patellofemoral pain patients. *Orthop Clin North Am* 1986;17(2):235–248.
421. Schweitzer ME, Tran D, Deely DM, Hume EL. Medial collateral ligament injuries: evaluation of multiple signs, prevalence and location of associated bone bruises, and assessment with MR imaging. *Radiology* 1995;194(3):825–829.
422. Scott WR. Innovation in medical care organizations: a synthetic review. *Med Care Rev* 1990;47(2):165–192.
423. Seebacher JR, Inglis AE, Marshall JL, Warren RF. The structure of the posterolateral aspect of the knee. *J Bone Joint Surg Am* 1982;64(4):536–541.
424. Shapiro GS, Fanton GS. Intraarticular hemangioma of the knee. *Arthroscopy* 1993;9(4):464–466.
425. Shaw JA, Murray DG. The longitudinal axis of the knee and the role of the cruciate ligaments in controlling transverse rotation. *J Bone Joint Surg Am* 1974;56(8):1603–1609.
426. Sheehan SE et al. A biomechanical approach to interpreting magnetic resonance imaging of knee injuries. *Magn Reson Imaging Clin N Am* 2014;22(4):621–648.
427. Shellock FG. Kinematic MRI evaluation of the joints. In: Stoller DW, ed. *Magnetic Resonance Imaging in Orthopaedics and Rheumatology*. Philadelphia, PA: JB Lippincott; 1993.
428. Shellock FG, Crues JV. Temperature, heart rate, and blood pressure changes associated with clinical MR imaging at 1.5 T. *Radiology* 1987;163(1):259–262.
429. Shellock FG, Deutsch AL, Mink JH. Identification of medial subluxation of the patella in a dancer using kinematic MRI of the patellofemoral joint: a case report. *Kinesiol Med Dance* 1991;13:1.
430. Shellock FG, Kim S, Mink JH. "Functional" patella alta determined by axial plane imaging of the patellofemoral joint: association with abnormal patellar alignment and tracking [abstract]. *J Magn Reson Imaging* 1992;2(S1):93.
431. Shellock FG, Mink JH, Deutsch A, Fox JM, Ferkel RD. Evaluation of patients with persistent symptoms after lateral retinacular release by kinematic magnetic resonance imaging of the patellofemoral joint. *Arthroscopy* 1990;6(3):226–234.
432. Shellock FG, Mink JH, Deutsch A, Pressman BD. Kinematic magnetic resonance imaging of the joints: techniques and clinical applications. *Magn Reson Q* 1991;7(2):104–135.
433. Shellock FG, Mink JH, Deutsch AL. Kinematic magnetic resonance imaging for evaluation of patellar tracking. *Physician Sports Med* 1989;17:99.
434. Shellock FG, Mink JH, Deutsch AL, Fox JM. Patellar tracking abnormalities: clinical experience with kinematic MR imaging in 130 patients. *Radiology* 1989;172(3):799–804.
435. Shellock FG, Mink JH, Deutsch AL, et al. Effect of a patellar realignment brace on patellofemoral relationships: evaluation with kinematic MR imaging. *J Magn Reson Imaging* 1994;4(4):590–594.
436. Shellock FG, Mink JH, Deutsch AL, et al. Evaluation of patellar alignment and tracking: comparison between kinematic MR imaging and "true" dynamic Hyperscan MR imaging [abstract]. *J Magn Reson Imaging* 1992;2(S1):148–149.
437. Shellock FG, Mink JH, Fox JM. Patellofemoral joint: kinematic MR imaging to assess tracking abnormalities. *Radiology* 1988;168(2):551–553.
438. Shellock FG, Morisoli S, Kanal E. MR procedures and biomedical implants, materials, and devices: 1993 update. *Radiology* 1993;189(2):587–599.
439. Sherman PM, Sanders TG, Morrison WB, et al. MR imaging of the posterior cruciate ligament graft: initial experience in 15 patients with clinical correlation. *Radiology* 2001;221(1):191–198.
440. Sheybani EF et al. Imaging of juvenile idiopathic arthritis: a multimodality approach. *Radiographics* 2013;33(5):1253–1273.
441. Silverman JM, Mink JH, Deutsch AL. Discoid menisci of the knee: MR imaging appearance. *Radiology* 1989;173(2):351–354.
442. Simpfendorfer C, Polster J. MRI of the knee: what do we miss? *Curr Radiol Rep* 2014;2(4):1–14.
443. Singson RD, Feldman F, Staron R, Kiernan H. MR imaging of displaced bucket-handle tear of the medial meniscus. *AJR Am J Roentgenol* 1991;156:121–124.
444. Slaughter AJ et al. Clinical orthopedic examination findings in the lower extremity: correlation with imaging studies and diagnostic efficacy. *Radiographics* 2014;34(2):e41–e55.
445. Smillie LS. *Diseases of the Knee Joint*. 2nd ed. London, United Kingdom: Churchill Livingstone; 1980.
446. Smith DK, Gilula LA, Amadio PC. Dorsal lunate tilt (DISI configuration): sign of scaphoid fracture displacement. *Radiology* 1990;176(2):497–499.
447. Smith DS et al. Anesthetic management of acutely ill patients during magnetic resonance imaging. *Anesthesiology* 1986;65(6):710–711.
448. Smith KL, Daniels JL, Arnoczky SP, et al. Effect of joint position and ligament tension on the MR signal intensity of the cruciate ligaments of the knee. *J Magn Reson Imaging* 1994;4(6):819–822.
449. Sofka CM et al. Magnetic resonance imaging of total knee arthroplasty. *Clin Orthop Relat Res* 2003;(406):129–135.
450. Sonin AH, Fitzgerald SW, Friedman H, et al. Posterior cruciate ligament injury: MR imaging diagnosis and patterns of injury. *Radiology* 1994;190(2):455–458.
451. Sonin AH, Fitzgerald SW, Hoff FL, et al. MR imaging of the posterior cruciate ligament: normal, abnormal, and associated injury patterns. *Radiographics* 1995;15(3):551–561.
452. Sonin AH, Pensy RA, Mulligan ME, Hatem S. Grading articular cartilage of the knee using fast spin-echo proton density-weighted MR imaging without fat suppression. *AJR Am J Roentgenol* 2002;179(5):1159–1166.

References

453. Sonnery-Cottet B et al. Arthroscopic identification of the anterolateral ligament of the knee. *Arthrosc Tech* 2014;3(3):e389–392.
454. Souryal TO, Freeman TR. Intercondylar notch size and anterior cruciate ligament injuries in athletes. A prospective study. *Am J Sports Med* 1993;21(4):535–539.
455. Speer KP, Warren RF, Wickiewicz TL, et al. Observations on the injury mechanism of anterior cruciate ligament tears in skiers. *Am J Sports Med* 1995;23(1):77–81.
456. Spiers AS, Meagher T, Ostlere SJ, Wilson DJ, Dodd CA. Can MRI of the knee affect arthroscopic practice? A prospective study of 58 patients. *J Bone Joint Surg Br* 1993;75(1):49–52.
457. Spinner RJ, Atkinson JL, Scheithauer BW, et al. Peroneal intraneural ganglia: the importance of the articular branch. Clinical series. *J Neurosurg* 2003;99(2):319–329.
458. Spritzer CE, Vogler JB, Martinez S, et al. MR imaging of the knee: preliminary results with a 3DFT GRASS pulse sequence. *AJR Am J Roentgenol* 1988;150(3):597–603.
459. Stanford W, Phelan J, Kathol MH, et al. Patellofemoral joint motion: evaluation by ultrafast computed tomography. *Skeletal Radiol* 1988;17(7):487–492.
460. Stanitski CL, Harvell JC, Fu F. Observations on acute knee hemarthrosis in children and adolescents. *J Pediatr Orthop* 1993;13(4):506–510.
461. Stark DD, Crues JV. Remote diagnosis raises efficiency of radiology. *Diagn Imaging* 1993;15(11):91–98.
462. Steinbach L. MRI of the knee. *Magnetic Resonance Imaging Clinics of North America* 2014;22(4):xii.
463. Stoller DW. MRI in juvenile rheumatoid (chronic) arthritis. In: *Meeting of the Association of University Radiologists*. Charleston, SC, 1987.
464. Stoller DW. Three-dimensional rendering and classification of meniscal tears disarticulated from 3-D FT images. In: *9th Annual Meeting of the Society of Magnetic Resonance in Medicine*. New York, NY, 1990.
465. Stoller DW, Genant HK. Magnetic resonance imaging of the knee and hip. *Arthritis Rheum* 1990;33(3):441–449.
466. Stoller DW, Genant HK. MRI of pigmented villonodular synovitis. In: *Abstract in American Roentgen Ray Society*. San Francisco, CA; 1988.
467. Stoller DW, Helms CA, Genant HK. Gradient echo MR imaging of the knee. In: *Annual Meeting of the Radiologic Society of North America*. Chicago, IL; 1987.
468. Stoller DW, Martin C, Crues JV 3rd, Kaplan L, Mink JH. Meniscal tears: pathologic correlation with MR imaging. *Radiology* 1987;163(3):731–735.
469. Stoller DW, Mink JH. MRI detection of knee fractures. Abstract presented in Miami, FL, 1987.
470. Stoller DW, Tirman PFJ, Bredella MA, eds. *Diagnostic Imaging: Orthopaedics*. Salt Lake City, UT: Amirsys; 2004.
471. Stone K, Walgenbach A. Meniscal allografting: the three-tunnel technique. *Arthroscopy*. 2003;19: 426–430.
472. Strobel M. Anatomy, proprioception and biomechanics. In: Strobel M, Stedtfeld H, eds. *Diagnostic Evaluation of the Knee*. Berlin/Heidelberg: Springer-Verlag; 1990:2.
473. Strobel M, Stedtfeld H. *Diagnostic Evaluation of the Knee*. Berlin, Germany: Springer Verlag; 1990.
474. Studler U et al. Anterior cruciate ligament reconstruction by using bioabsorbable femoral cross pins: MR imaging findings at follow-up and comparison with clinical findings. *Radiology* 2010; 255(1):108–116.
475. Sueyoshi Y, Shimozaki E, Matsumoto T, Tomita K. Two cases of dorsal defect of the patella with arthroscopically visible cartilage surface perforations. *Arthroscopy* 1993;9(2):164–169.
476. Sulkowski U et al. Clinical aspects and therapy of achalasia exemplified by a case of dolicho-esophagus. *Med Klin* 1990;85(10):624–628.
477. Sutter R et al. Is dedicated extremity 1.5-T MRI equivalent to standard large-bore 1.5-T MRI for foot and knee examinations? *AJR Am J Roentgenol* 2014;203(6):1293–1302.
478. Taneja AK et al. MRI features of the anterolateral ligament of the knee. *Skeletal Radiol* 2015;44(3): 403–410.
479. Tarhan NC, Chung CB, Mohana-Borges AV, Hughes T, Resnick D. Meniscal tears: role of axial MRI alone and in combination with other imaging planes. *AJR Am J Roentgenol* 2004;183(1):9–15.
480. Tervonen O, Dietz MJ, Carmichael SW, Ehman RL. MR imaging of knee hyaline cartilage: evaluation of two- and three-dimensional sequences. *J Magn Reson Imaging* 1993;3(4):663–668.
481. Tiderius CJ et al. Delayed gadolinium-enhanced MRI of cartilage (dGEMRIC) in early knee osteoarthritis. *Magn Reson Med* 2003;49(3):488–492.
482. Tobler TH. Makroskopische und histologische befund am kniegeluk meniscus in verschiedenen lebensaitern [In German]. *Schweiz Med Wochenschr* 1926;56:1359.
483. Torstensen ET, Bray RC, Wiley JP. Patellar tendinitis: a review of current concepts and treatment. *Clin J Sport Med* 1994;4(2):77–82.
484. Tsavalas N, Karantanas AH. Suprapatellar fat-pad mass effect: MRI findings and correlation with anterior knee pain. *AJR Am J Roentgenol* 2013;200(3):W291–W296.
485. Tschirch FTC, Schmid MR, Pfirrmann CW, et al. Prevalence and size of meniscal cysts, ganglionic cysts, synovial cysts of the popliteal space, fluid-filled bursae, and other fluid collections in asymptomatic knees on MR imaging. *AJR Am J Roentgenol* 2003;180(5):1431–1436.
486. Tung GA, Davis LM, Wiggins ME, Fadale PD. Tears of the anterior cruciate ligament: primary and secondary signs at MR imaging. *Radiology* 1993;188(3):661–667.
487. Turek SL. *Orthopaedics: Principles and Their Application*. 4th ed. Philadelphia, PA: JB Lippincott; 1984.
488. Turner DA, Prodromos CC, Petasnick JP, Clark JW. Acute injury of the ligaments of the knee: magnetic resonance evaluation. *Radiology* 1985; 154(3):717–722.
489. Turner DA et al. Truncation artifact: a potential pitfall in MR imaging of the menisci of the knee. *Radiology* 1991;179(3):629–633.
490. Tyrrell RL et al. Fast three-dimensional MR imaging of the knee: comparison with arthroscopy. *Radiology* 1988;166(3):865–872.
491. Umans H et al. Posterior horn medial meniscal root tear: the prequel. *Skeletal Radiol* 2014;43(6): 775–780.
492. Umans H, Wimpfheimer O, Haramati N, et al. Diagnosis of partial tears of the anterior cruciate ligament of the knee: value of MR imaging. *AJR Am J Roentgenol* 1995;165(4):893–897.

493. Vahey TN, Bennett HT, Arrington LE, Shelbourne KD, Ng J. MR imaging of the knee: pseudotear of the lateral meniscus caused by the meniscofemoral ligament. *AJR Am J Roentgenol* 1990;154(6):1237–1239.
494. Vahey TN, Broome DR, Kayes KJ, Shelbourne KD. Acute and chronic tears of the anterior cruciate ligament: differential features at MR imaging. *Radiology* 1991;181(1):251–253.
495. Vahey TN, Hunt JE, Shelbourne KD. Anterior translocation of the tibia at MR imaging: a secondary sign of anterior cruciate ligament tear. *Radiology* 1993;187(3):817–819.
496. Vande Berg BC, Malghem J, Poilvache P, Maldague B, Lecouvet FE. Meniscal tears with fragments displaced in notch and recesses of knee: MR imaging with arthroscopic comparison. *Radiology* 2005;234(3):842–850.
497. van Tiel J et al. Delayed gadolinium-enhanced MRI of the meniscus (dGEMRIM) in patients with knee osteoarthritis: relation with meniscal degeneration on conventional MRI, reproducibility, and correlation with dGEMRIC. *Eur Radiol* 2014;24(9):2261–2270.
498. Varich LJ, Laor T, Jaramillo D. Normal maturation of the distal femoral epiphyseal cartilage: age-related changes at MR imaging. *Radiology* 2000;214(3):705–709.
499. Vaughan WH, Williams JL. Familial achalasia with pulmonary complications in children. *Radiology* 1973;107(2):407–409.
500. Vellet AD, Marks P, Fowler P, Munro T. Accuracy of nonorthogonal magnetic resonance imaging in acute disruption of the anterior cruciate ligament. *Arthroscopy* 1989;5(4):287–293.
501. Vellet AD, Marks PH, Fowler PJ, Munro TG. Occult posttraumatic osteochondral lesions of the knee: prevalence, classification, and short-term sequelae evaluated with MR imaging. *Radiology* 1991;178(1):271–276.
502. Veltri DM, Deng XH, Torzilli PA, Warren RF, Maynard MJ. The role of the cruciate and posterolateral ligaments in stability of the knee. A biomechanical study. *Am J Sports Med* 1995;23(4):436–443.
503. Veltri DM, Warren RF. Operative treatment of posterolateral instability of the knee. *Clin Sports Med* 1994;13(3):615–627.
504. Veltri DM, Warren RF. Posterolateral instability of the knee. *J Bone Joint Surg Am* 1994;76(3):460–472.
505. Vergis A, Gillquist J. Graft failure in intra-articular anterior cruciate ligament reconstructions: a review of the literature. *Arthroscopy* 1995;11(3):312–321.
506. Viana SL, Machado BB, Mendlovitz PS. MRI of subchondral fractures: a review. *Skeletal Radiol* 2014;43(11):1515–1527.
507. Vincent JP et al. The anterolateral ligament of the human knee: an anatomic and histologic study. *Knee Surg Sports Traumatol Arthrosc* 2012;20(1):147–52.
508. Voto SJ et al. Ankle arthroscopy: neurovascular and arthroscopic anatomy of standard and trans-achilles tendon portal placement. *Arthroscopy* 1989;5(1):41–46.
509. Warren RF. Primary repair of the anterior cruciate ligament. *Clin Orthop Relat Res* 1983;172:65–70.
510. Watanabe AT, Carter BC, Teitelbaum GP, Seeger LL, Bradley WG Jr. Normal variations in MR imaging of the knee: appearance and frequency. *AJR Am J Roentgenol* 1989;153(2):341–344.
511. Watanabe BM, Howell SM. Arthroscopic findings associated with roof impingement of an anterior cruciate ligament graft. *Am J Sports Med* 1995;23(5):616–625.
512. Watanabe Y, Moriya H, Takahashi K, et al. Functional anatomy of the posterolateral structures of the knee. *Arthroscopy* 1993;9(1):57–62.
513. Watt I, Tasker T. Pitfalls in double contrast knee arthrography. *Br J Radiol* 1980;53(632):754–759.
514. Weber WN, Neumann CH, Barakos JA, et al. Lateral tibial rim (Segond) fractures: MR imaging characteristics. *Radiology* 1991;180(3):731–734.
515. Weiner B, Rosenberg N. Discoid medial meniscus: association with bone changes in the tibia. A case report. *J Bone Joint Surg Am* 1974;56(1):171–173.
516. Weiss KL, Morehouse HT, Levy IM. Sagittal MR images of the knee: a low-signal band parallel to the posterior cruciate ligament caused by a displaced bucket-handle tear. *AJR Am J Roentgenol* 1991;156:117–119.
517. Weissman B, Sledge CB. *Orthopedic Radiology*. Philadelphia, PA: Saunders; 1986.
518. Westrich GH, Hannafin JA, Potter HG. Isolated rupture and repair of the popliteus tendon. *Arthroscopy* 1995;11(5):628–632.
519. White EA et al. Coronal plane fracture of the femoral condyles: anatomy, injury patterns, and approach to management of the Hoffa fragment. *Skeletal Radiol* 2015;44(1):37–43.
520. White LM, Schweitzer ME, Weishaupt D, et al. Diagnosis of recurrent meniscal tears: prospective evaluation of conventional MR imaging, indirect MR arthrography, and direct MR arthrography. *Radiology* 2002;222(2):421–429.
521. White LM et al. Cartilage T2 assessment: differentiation of normal hyaline cartilage and reparative tissue after arthroscopic cartilage repair in equine subjects. *Radiology* 2006;241(2):407–414.
522. Wiberg G. Roentgenographs and anatomic studies on the femoropatellar joint: with special reference to chondromalacia patellae. *Acta Orthopaedica* 1941;12(1–4):319–410.
523. Williams JL, Cliff MM, Bonakdarpour A. Spontaneous osteonecrosis of the knee. *Radiology* 1973;107(1):15–19.
524. Williams PL. *Gray's Anatomy*. 37th ed. Edinburgh, United Kingdom: Churchill Livingstone; 1989.
525. Wilson R. Arthroscopic anatomy. In: Scott W, ed. *Arthroscopy of the Knee*. Philadelphia, PA: WB Saunders; 1990.
526. Wodicka R et al. MRI evaluation of the anterolateral ligament of the knee in the setting of ACL rupture. *Orthopaedic Journal of Sports Medicine*, 2014;2(2 Suppl).
527. Wolff SD, Chesnick S, Frank JA, et al. Magnetization transfer contrast: MR imaging of the knee. *Radiology* 1991;179(3):623–628.
528. Woo SL, Hollis JM, Adams DJ, Lyon RM, Takai S. Tensile properties of the human femur-anterior cruciate ligament-tibia complex. The effects of specimen age and orientation. *Am J Sports Med* 1991;19(3):217–225.
529. Wright DH, De Smet AA, Norris M. Bucket-handle tears of the medial and lateral menisci of the knee: value of MR imaging in detecting displaced fragments. *AJR Am J Roentgenol* 1995;165(3):621–625.

530. Yao L, Gai N, Boutin RD. Axial scan orientation and the tibial tubercle-trochlear groove distance: error analysis and correction. *AJR Am J Roentgenol* 2014;202(6):1291–1296.
531. Ye X et al. Electrochemical behaviour of gold, silver, platinum and palladium on the glassy carbon electrode modified by chitosan and its application. *Talanta* 1998;47(5):1099–1106.
532. Yocum LA, Kerlan RK, Jobe FW, et al. Isolated lateral meniscectomy. A study of twenty-six patients with isolated tears. *J Bone Joint Surg Am* 1979;61(3):338–342.
533. Yoon MA et al. High prevalence of abnormal MR findings of the distal semimembranosus tendon: contributing factors based on demographic, radiographic, and MR features. *AJR Am J Roentgenol* 2014;202(5):1087–1093.
534. Yu JS, Popp JE, Kaeding CC, Lucas J. Correlation of MR imaging and pathologic findings in athletes undergoing surgery for chronic patellar tendinitis. *AJR Am J Roentgenol* 1995;165(1):115–118.
535. Yu JS, Salonen DC, Hodler J, et al. Posterolateral aspect of the knee: improved MR imaging with a coronal oblique technique. *Radiology* 1996;198(1):199–204.
536. Yulish BS, Lieberman JM, Strandjord SE, et al. Hemophilic arthropathy: assessment with MR imaging. *Radiology* 1987;164(3):759–762.
537. Yulish BS, Yulish BS, Montanez J, Goodfellow DB, et al. Chondromalacia patellae: assessment with MR imaging. *Radiology* 1987;164(3):763–766.
538. Zanetti M, Pfirrmann CW, Schmid MR, Romero J, Seifert B, Hodler J. Patients with suspected meniscal tears: prevalence of abnormalities seen on MRI of 100 symptomatic and 100 contralateral asymptomatic knees. *AJR Am J Roentgenol* 2003;181(3):635–641.
539. Zarins B, Rowe CR. Combined anterior cruciate-ligament reconstruction using semitendinosus tendon and iliotibial tract. *J Bone Joint Surg Am* 1986;68(2):160–177.

Index

Page numbers with italicized *f* indicates figures or images.

A

Abrasion. *See also* Microfracture
  with microfracture, 971
    for chondral lesions, 973
  of perimeniscal synovium, meniscal repair and, 329
Abrasion chondroplasty
  with débridement, 992*f*
  with fibrocartilage regrowth in trochlear groove, 989*f*
Accessory head of gastrocnemius muscle, 919*f*
Acetabulum, superior rim of, rectus femoris and, 68*f*
Achilles tendon, 75, 490, 517, 572*f*
Achondroplasia, patella baja and, 801
ACI (autologous chondrocyte implantation), 973
ACL. *See* Anterior cruciate ligament
Acufex ACL tip guide positioning, 254*f*
Acute meniscal flap tears, 258
Adductor magnus tendon (AMT), 584*f*, 596*f*
  attachments of, 767
  MPFL course and, 756*f*
  MPFL reattachment with, 750
  Pellegrini-Stieda disease and, 612
  thigh muscle innervation and, 63*f*
Adductor tubercle, 142*f*, 767, 768*f*
Adiabatic spectral inversion recovery technique (ASPIR), 12, 22
Adolescents
  chondromalacia patellae and, 706
  Osgood-Schlatter disease and, 817
  osteochondral fractures in, 971, 977, 978*f*
  osteochondritis dissecans and, 951
  patellar sleeve fracture in, 1015
  Sinding-Larsen-Johansson syndrome and, 818
  stress fractures with nonossifying fibromas in, 1003
Adults
  arthritis in, MR imaging of, 845
  knee degeneration, popliteal cysts and, 116
  meniscal vascularity in, 154, 162
  osteochondral fractures in, 971
  osteochondritis dissecans in, 956*f*
  osteomyelitis in, 1020
  physeal line or scar signal intensity in, 1002
  primary and secondary ACL tear findings in, 440
  tibial spine avulsions in, 472
Adventitious bursa, ITB syndrome and cystic fluid collection in, 794*f*–795*f*
Adventitious mucoid cysts, 917*f*
Age of patient. *See also* Adolescents; Adults; Children
  ACL treatment methods and, 487
  articular cartilage desiccation and, 897
  articular cartilage T2 values and, 849
  chondromalacia and
    with basal degeneration, 711, 731
    with superficial degeneration, 712, 732*f*
  chronic degenerative quadriceps tendon and, 837
  cystic adventitial disease and, 917*f*
  MCL failure loads and, 602
  meniscal repairs and, 330–331
  osteochondritis dissecans and, 949
  patellar tendon tears and, 800
  quadriceps tendon tears and, 833
  spontaneous osteonecrosis and, 933
Aggrecan, 845, 847, 848*f*, 897, 981*f*, 983*f*
AHLM. *See* Anterior horn lateral meniscus
AHMM. *See* Anterior horn medial meniscus
Alar fold. *See also* Lateral alar fold
  suprapatellar pouch and, 90*f*
ALB. *See* Anterolateral band or bundle
Alcoholism, 933, 946
All-inside meniscus repair, 211*f*, 338, 340*f*
Allograft OATS, 973
Allograft tissue, ACL reconstruction using, 490
Allograft transplants
  ACL, with stem cells, 539*f*
  bridge technique, 343*f*
  for cartilage resurfacing, 992*f*
  of meniscus, 326, 331
  for mid-substance and femoral avulsions, 556
  osteochondral, 971, 973
  for osteonecrosis, 936
  preparation, 342*f*–343*f*
  for segmental meniscus reconstruction, 348*f*
Alpine hunter's cap patellar deformity, 701
American Medical Association Ligament Injury Classification System, 444
AMT. *See* Adductor magnus tendon
Anemias. *See also* Sickle cell anemia
  hemolytic, thalassemia and, 1003
Angioblastic hyperplasia, quadriceps tendon tears and, 834
Angiogenesis, patellar tendinosis and, 798
Animal models, MR imaging of posttraumatic growth plate abnormalities in, 1002
Ankylosing spondylosis, in children, 866
Ankylosis, rheumatoid arthritis and, 870, 876*f*
Annefacts, 302–303. *See also* Artifacts
Anterior aponeurotic expansion, 644*f*
Anterior arm, biceps femoris tendon, 644*f*, 646*f*
Anterior arm, long head of biceps femoris, 655, 668*f*
Anterior compartment, osseous injuries, PCL and, 540
Anterior cruciate ligament (ACL), 163*f*. *See also* Anteromedial bundle; Posterolateral bundle
  acute stump entrapment, 444, 446*f*–447*f*
  with AM and PL bundle disruption, 402*f*

Anterior cruciate ligament (*continued*)
  anatomy
    anterior, knee in partial flexion and, 93*f*
    axial intercondylar, 410*f*
    in cross-section, 35
    double-bundle, 408*f*, 413*f*
    fiber-bundle striations of, 45
    functional, 77*f*, 397–398, 403*f*–405*f*
    origin, 37*f*
    posterior, knee in partial flexion and, 93*f*
  anterior horn medial meniscus vs., 306
  anterior horn of lateral meniscus and, 157
  anterior meniscofemoral ligament variant vs., 927*f*
  axial image, 38*f*–39*f*
    checklist, 113, 140*f*
  biomechanics, 412
  coronal image, 54, 60*f*, 89*f*
    anteromedial bundle of, 54
    checklist, 99, 119*f*
    distal insertion, 59*f*
    lateral meniscus root tears and, 246
    posterolateral bundle of, 54
    proximal origin, 60*f*–61*f*
  cysts, 455, 456*f*–460*f*, 464*f*
  deficient, MR referral for meniscal tear and, 288
  degenerative joint disease and, 174
  disruption, amorphous meniscal signal and, 307
  double-bundle distal insertions, 164*f*
  double-bundle footprint, 509*f*
  footprint measurement, 510*f*
  grafts, isometry and, 489
  graphic depiction, 413*f*
  Hoffa's fat pad and, 856*f*
  infrapatellar plica vs., 922
  injuries
    acute, appearance in, 441–442
    acute, lateral meniscus tear repair and, 329
    bone contusion Types I and II and, 1004
    bucket-handle meniscal tears and, 213, 427*f*
    classification of, 424
    clinical assessment, 424, 425*f*–428*f*, 429
    collateral venous flow after, 693*f*
    complex meniscal flap tears and, 258
    diagnosis, 429
    lateral meniscus and MCL injuries and, 423
    MCL injuries and, 599
    mechanisms, 416, 417*f*–423*f*, 424
    MR accuracy in detection of, 486
    multiligament, 685*f*–687*f*, 691*f*
    posterolateral corner injuries and, 691*f*
    proximal osseous avulsion, 435*f*
    secondary tibial restraints and, 583
    tibial eminence fractures and
      displaced, 432*f*, 434*f*
      nondisplaced, 431*f*
      partially displaced, 433*f*
    tibial spine avulsions and, 472–473
  key concepts, 397
  lateral meniscus and, 164*f*
  lateral meniscus bucket-handle tears and, 215, 231*f*
  longitudinal meniscal tears and, 203
  medial meniscus tears and, 210*f*
  meniscal transplantation and, 331
  meniscectomy and, 154
  MR imaging
    key concepts, 436
    normal characteristics of, 437–438
    techniques for, 436–437
  oblique intermeniscal ligaments and, 321*f*
  osseous injuries and, key concepts, 470
  pathology, 119*f*
  pivot-shift test, 428*f*
  popliteal fossa view, 87*f*
  popliteus complex and, 645*f*
  popliteus hiatus area and, 680*f*
  posterolateral corner injuries and, key concepts, 465
  reconstruction
    bone–patellar tendon–bone, 490, 494*f*, 515*f*
    complications
      scarring, 526*f*–527*f*
      tunnel and pretibial cysts, 538*f*
    double-bundle, 504*f*, 506*f*, 510–511, 511*f*–514*f*
    epiphyseal tunnels and, 498*f*
    failure
      cyclops lesion and, 524*f*–525*f*
      dislodged interference screw, 515*f*, 535*f*
      femoral bone plug and, 503*f*, 532*f*
      fractured interference screw, 537*f*
      pin extrusion, 536*f*
      transtibial technique and, 497*f*
    ganglion cysts and, 529*f*
    goals and techniques, 490–491, 494*f*–496*f*
    gracilis muscle and, 73
    graft impingement and, 492, 501, 516
      roof, 520–521, 530*f*
      side wall, 522
    graft revascularization, 493
    graft revision, 519*f*
    graft tunnel motion, 518*f*
    hamstring muscles and, 71
    key concepts, 489
    meniscal implants and, 326
    meniscal repairs and, 328, 338
    modified, 498*f*
    MR evaluation of
      graft impingement, 501, 515*f*
      image recommendations, 499–501
      key concepts, 499
      postoperative, 516–517
    over-the-top position for, 502*f*
    retears of, 485*f*, 528*f*, 531*f*, 533*f*
    stem cells and, 539*f*
    synovial thickening and, 523*f*, 536*f*
    tibial footprint preparation, 511*f*
    unimpinged, 528*f*
    vertical orientation of, 497*f*
    without impingement, 503*f*
  repair, 488
  sagittal image, 42, 50*f*–51*f*, 92*f*
    anteromedial bundle of, 44–45
    checklist, 106, 129*f*
    medial to lateral direction, 44
    origin to insertion of, 44
    PCL on same section as, 45
    PCL signal intensity vs., 45
    posterolateral bundle of, 44–45
    through medial compartment, 83*f*
  sMCL and, 590*f*
  sprains
    diagnosing, 425*f*
    with intact ligament morphology, 463*f*
    parallel fiber orientation and, 463*f*
    sagittal image, 106
  surgery, patella baja and, 801
  tears
    acute, 443*f*
    AM and PL bundles and, 507*f*
    AM bundle rupture and, 448
    anterior flap lateral meniscus fragment and, 234*f*
    arcuate ligament and, 643*f*
    chronic, 439, 452*f*, 453
    complex bucket-handle, 232*f*
    coronal image, 99
    grade 3
      displaced lateral meniscus root tear and, 278*f*
      displaced meniscal flap tear into notch and, 279*f*
      fluid between LFC and proximal fibers of, 426*f*

Index

MCL grade 3 tear and, 625f–626f
medial meniscus bucket-handle tear and, 226f
meniscocapsular separations and, 372f–373f
O'Donoghue's triad and, 417f
retracted fibers of, 421f
twisting injury, 414f
hemarthrosis and, 1013
inferior popliteomeniscal fascicle and, 667f
interstitial, 422f, 441, 454f
key concepts, 439–440
knee dislocation and, 572f
knee laxity and, 419f
lateral meniscus root tears and, 246
LCL tears and, 669f
MCL sprain and, 600f
mechanism of injury, 1001
middle third, 423f
evaluation of, 420f
multiligament injuries and, 575f–577f
near meniscocapsular junction, 368f
osseous injuries with, 470–473, 473f–485f
partial, 424, 444, 448
PCL injuries and, 547, 556
peripheral meniscal vertical tear and, 208f
pitfalls interpreting findings on, 455
popliteal cysts and, 916
posterolateral corner injuries and, 465–466, 468f–469f, 679f–680f
posteromedial medial tibial osseous contusions or fractures and, 367
proximal attachment of, 418f
with proximal fiber discontinuity, 428f
sagittal image, 106
signs of, 440
subacute, 452f, 453
surgery for PCL tears and, 556
tibial footprint, 508f
tibial insertion sites for, 401f
transverse ligament and, 304
treatment of injuries to, 487–488
vascular supply, 399f–400f
Anterior division of obturator nerve, thigh muscle innervation and, 63f
Anterior drawer sign, 424, 442, 443f, 453, 486
Anterior flipped meniscus, pitfalls interpreting findings on, 311
Anterior horn. See also Anterior horn lateral meniscus; Anterior horn medial meniscus
meniscal transplantation and, 331
of meniscus, 154
innervation, 163
Anterior horn–body junction, of meniscus, radial tears and, 240f–241f
Anterior horn lateral meniscus (AHLM)
ACL and PCL insertion sites in, 401f
anatomy, 33
functional, 77f
anteriorly displaced bucket fragment, 235f
attachments, 157
axial image, 39f–40f
bicompartmental bucket-handle tears and, 230f
central rhomboid attachment of, meniscal tear vs., 306, 316f
coronal image, 55, 59f, 100
articular cartilage and, 101
discoid menisci and, 290w
flap tears, 1006f
intrameniscal cysts and, 385f
pitfalls interpreting findings on, 306
pseudohypertrophy of, 311
sagittal image, 44, 48f, 165f
central attachment, 49f
intrameniscal signal intensity tear, 148f
transverse ligament and, 77f, 156, 304–305, 305f
trochlear groove cartilage and, 105
Anterior horn medial meniscus (AHMM)
ACL and PCL insertion sites in, 401f
ACL differentiation from, 306
anatomy, 156
popliteus tendon and, 186f
axial image, 77f
bucket-handle tears and, 214, 220f
bicompartmental, 230f
displaced, 222f, 224f–225f
displaced fragment, 229f
coronal image, 55, 58f–59f, 100
articular cartilage and, 101
discoid menisci and, 290
joint capsule and, 581
sagittal image, 52f
checklist, 103, 125f
superior flap displacement, 274f
transverse ligament and, 77f, 156, 300f
trochlear groove cartilage and, 105
Anterior inferior iliac spine, rectus femoris and, 68f
Anterior intermediate iliotibial fibers, 81
Anterior megahorn discoid meniscus, 291
Anterior meniscofemoral ligament, 310, 926f–927f. See also Ligament of Humphrey
Anterior patellar surface, 699
Anterior popliteofibular ligament, 657
Anterior superior iliac spine, 72, 72f, 81
Anterior superior pes anserinus, 72f
Anterior tibial artery, 85f, 169f
Anterior tibial intercondylar area, ACL and, 398
Anterior tibial recurrent artery, 169f, 644f, 646f
Anterior tibial spine, mid-coronal sections of, 55
Anterior tibial subluxation, 423, 442
Anterior tibiofibular ligament, 653f
Anteroinferior popliteomeniscal fascicle, 108, 157, 657
Anterolateral band or bundle (ALB), 44, 540, 541f, 546f, 562f
Anterolateral femoral condyle, ITB friction syndrome and, 787
Anterolateral femoral diaphysis, vastus intermedius and, 67f
Anterolateral joint capsule, 643f
Anterolateral rotary instability test, 424
Anteromedial bundle (AMB)
ACL in extension and, 403f
ACL partial or incomplete tears and, 448
ACL reconstruction and, 510f, 514f
ACL tears and, 507f
of anterior cruciate ligament, 99
coronal image, 54
disruption
anterior drawer sign and, 424
grade 3 ACL with, 402f
in extension, 398, 407f
fat signal between PL bundle and, 413f
femoral footprint, 409f
in flexion, 402, 407f
fractured, ACL roof impingement and, 520–521
hypointense, PLB tear and, 449f–450f
knee flexion and, 509f
medial meniscus and, 164f
MR imaging, 438
nonisometric in flexion-extension motion, 404f
PL bundle injury and, 451f
PL bundle tear and, 406f
posterolateral bundle tear and, 404f
reconstruction, postoperative patellar tendon and, 522
sagittal image, 44, 106
tears in PLB vs., 448
tibial footprint, 403f, 405f, 408f, 510f
preparation for ACL reconstruction, 511f–513f
Anteromedial tibial crest, 42

Anteroposterior motion, medial
  meniscectomy and, 154
Apex, meniscal. *See also* Free edge,
    of meniscus
  blunting
    bucket-handle tears of lateral
      meniscus and, 234f
    complex tears and, 286f
    coronal images, 302
    partial meniscectomy and,
      334
    radial tears and, 239
  degeneration, signal intensity
    and, 176
  fraying and signal intensity in,
    307, 316f
  horizontal cleavage tears and,
    183–184, 199f, 202f
  intercondylar notch and, 154
Apley grinding test, 173
Apophysis
  Osgood-Schlatter disease and,
    817, 819f
  Sinding-Larsen-Johansson
    syndrome and, 823f
ARC (Autocalibrating
    Reconstruction for
    Cartesian imaging), 21
Arciform fascia, 827f, 829
Arcuate complex. *See also*
    Posterolateral complex
  PCL injuries and, 542
Arcuate ligament
  anatomy, 637, 643f, 677f
  arcuate sign and, 470
  avulsion fracture and, 483f
  axial image, 40f
    popliteus tendon and, 115
    posterior fibula head fracture
      and, 145f
  injuries, 674f, 676f
  lateral collateral ligament and,
    636, 649f
  lateral limb, 665f
  medial limb, 661f, 677f
    tears, 669f
  popliteal fossa view, 87f
  popliteus tendon and, 665f
  posterior coronal image, 85f
  posterolateral complex and, 637
  posterolateral corner and, 465,
    672f
  posterolateral corner injuries and,
    467f–468f
  sagittal image, 42, 47f–48f, 108,
    126f
    medial limb of, 46
    posterior capsule and, 49f
  sprains, 664f
  superficial dissection from
    posterior perspective, 85f
  tears, 660f
    lateral compartment
      contusions and, 473f
Arcuate popliteal ligament, 54, 87f,
    647f
Arcuate sign, 470, 473, 540, 553
Array Spatial Sensitivity Encoding
    Technique (ASSET), 20
Arteritis, bone infarcts and, 946

Arthritis. *See also* Juvenile chronic
    arthritis; Lyme arthritis;
    Osteoarthritis; Rheumatoid
    arthritis
  degenerative
    early, 896f
    end-stage, 900f
  inflammatory
    chondromalacia patellae and,
      706
    Hoffa's fat pad and, 857
    meniscal tears and, 173
    popliteal cysts and, 916
  meniscus and, 154
  MR imaging, 845
  patellofemoral, 711, 733f
  pes anserinus bursitis and, 612
  posttraumatic, 482
  septic, 857
  symmetric, rheumatoid arthritis
    and, 869
Arthrofibrosis
  ACL reconstruction and, 499,
    526f–527f
  scarring of Hoffa's fat pad and,
    111
Arthrography
  of discoid meniscus, 293
  of joint effusions, 912
  magnetic resonance
    of articular cartilage, 851
    of chondromalacia, 713
      grading classification of,
        716–717
    with contrast, of articular
      cartilage, 723f
    free fluid in plane of meniscal
      repair and, 338
    joint effusions and, 911
    meniscal resections and, 336
    of meniscal tears vs., 181
    of post–primary meniscal
      repairs, 333
Arthroplasty
  total joint, 870
  unicompartmental, for
    osteonecrosis, 936
Arthroscopic rasping, 180
Arthroscopic resection, as partial
    meniscectomy,
    349f
Arthroscopy
  of ACL graft-side wall
    impingement, 522
  of ACL injuries, 429–430, 486,
    508f
  of bone contusion Types I and
    II, 1004
  for closed meniscal tears, 301
  of discoid meniscus, 292
  of dorsal defect of patella, 743
  instrumentation, 194f
  of lipoma arborescens, 908
  of medial patellar facet softening,
    723f
  for meniscal cysts, 380
  meniscal healing and signal
    intensity with,
    337–338
  for meniscal root repair, 330

meniscal stability testing with,
    330
  meniscal tear detection accuracy
    using, 288
  meniscal tears stable to probing
    with, 330
  MR grade 3 signal intensity
    extension to stable rim
    and, 204
  of osteochondritis dissecans
    stages, 948
  partial ACL tears and, 448
  of patellar dislocations, 750
  of PCL, 551
  of PCL injuries, 548
  Shahriaree's chondromalacia
    grading system with, 712
  variations in MR accuracy vs.,
    289
Arthrosis
  after meniscectomy, 335, 359f,
    361f
  degenerative
    chondral fissures and, 896f
    meniscal transplantation and,
      331
  patellofemoral joint, 709f, 711,
    721f
Arthrotomy, of PCL, 551
Articular branch
  of common peroneal nerve,
    904f–906f
    interneural ganglia and, 907
    superior tibiofibular joint
      ganglia and, 913
  of descending geniculate artery,
    169f
Articular cartilage
  anatomy
    composition and structure,
      981f
    extracellular matrix, 845
    posterior surface of patella
      and, 94f
    zonal, 982f, 984f
  in children, 853
  chondral fractures of, 971
  chondrocalcinosis of, 390f, 392f
  chondromalacia patellae and,
    706, 711–713, 716, 717f
  coronal plane checklist, 101, 122f
  cruciate ligament injuries and,
    423
  degeneration
    ACL deficiencies and, 487
    arthritis and, 896f
    patellar malalignment and, 698
    PCL deficiencies and, 547, 568
  evaluation, 847
  excessive lateral pressure
    syndrome and, 704
  healed osteochondritis dissecans
    and, 948
  hemophilia and, 891
  hydration, osteoarthritis and, 897
  imaging, 849–853, 985f, 987f
    motion correction pulse
      sequences and, 150
    MR arthrography with
      contrast, 723f

Index

injuries
　Baurer and Jackson
　　classification, 991f
　vacuum phenomenon and, 312
juvenile chronic arthritis and,
　866, 867f
loss, meniscectomy and, 335
Lyme arthritis and, 892
medial meniscus flap tear and,
　283f
meniscal tears and, 100
osteoarthritis and, 898, 900f
osteochondral defect with
　unstable flap, 997f
osteochondritis dissecans and,
　744, 947, 949
osteonecrosis and, 936
patellar
　evaluation of, 714–715
　medial plica and erosion or
　　abrasion of, 923
pathology, 122f, 849
posttraumatic chondral
　hyperintensity and, 109
repair
　meniscal implants and, 326
　MPFL reconstruction and,
　　777f–778f
sagittal plane checklist, 104, 127f
stem cell paste graft, 974, 998f
tears, patellar tendinosis and, 798
tibial, meniscocapsular
　separations and, 366
Articular gliding surface, 984f
Articularis genu muscle, vastus
　intermedius and, 67
Articular surface. *See also specific
　associated surfaces*
of meniscus, 175
of patella, 699
Artifacts
calcium pyrophosphate dihydrate
　deposition disease and,
　388
chemical-shift, 43, 150, 944,
　999f, 1002
concave peripheral meniscal edge
　as, 309
dielectric, 3.0T imaging and,
　19–20
ghost, blurring by FSE sequences
　and, 176
peripheral signal, 302–303
pulsation, popliteal artery and,
　314, 314f
streaking, PROPELLER and, 15
susceptibility, 17, 914
vacuum phenomenon, 312, 324f
Ascending transverse branch,
　femoral nerve
rectus femoris and, 68f
vastus intermedius and, 67f
vastus lateralis and, 65f
vastus medialis and, 66f
Ascites, dielectric effect and, 20
ASPIR (Adiabatic Spectral
　Selective Inversion
　Recovery), 12, 22
ASSET (Array Spatial Sensitivity
　Encoding Technique), 20

Asymptomatic persons
discoid meniscus and, 291
lateral meniscus tears in, ACL
　reconstruction and, 330
meniscal tears in, MR studies
　and, 288
Athletic participation. *See also
　Sports injuries*
ACL treatment methods and,
　487–488
pes anserinus bursitis and, 612
tibiofibular joint dislocation and,
　907
Atypical popliteal cysts, 913
Augmentation
for Achilles tendon repairs, 75
carbon fiber, of ACL, 517
for interstitial LCL injuries, 671
intraarticular, primary ACL
　repair and, 488
for mid-substance and femoral
　avulsions, 556
for PCL reconstruction, 571
for posterolateral injuries, 466
Autocalibrating Reconstruction for
　Cartesian imaging (ARC),
　21
Autogenous bone pegs, 949
Autogenous tissue, ACL
　reconstruction using, 490
Autografts
for ACL reconstruction, 490–
　491, 493, 495f–496f, 517
for medial patellofemoral
　ligament reconstruction,
　771f–772f
Autologous chondrocyte
　implantation (ACI), 973
Avascular inner edge, of meniscus,
　flap tears of, 259
Avascular zone, of meniscus
tear healing in, 328
tear repair and, 329
Avulsion fractures, anterior superior
　iliac spine and, 72
Avulsions
ACL injuries as, 472
ACL-related ligament injury and,
　483f
epicondylar attachment of MCL,
　616f–617f
of LCL and biceps femoris, 636,
　673f
MCL injuries and, 611, 624f
multiligament injuries and,
　576f–577f
PCL injuries and, 553, 556, 560f
PCL injuries as, 547–548
proximal osseous ACL, 435f
repair of, 487–488
displaced, 560
Segond fractures and, 471–472
tibial eminence, ACL injuries
　and, 430, 442
Awls, surgical, microfracture with,
　992f
Axial loading, fractures and, 1001
Axial plane images
of ACL acute injuries, 441
of ACL injuries, 436, 438, 486

ACL tear diagnosis and, 440
checklist for meniscal
　degeneration or tears,
　112–116, 137f–145f
of discoid meniscus, 294
of medial plicae, 921
MR accuracy in meniscal tear
　detection on, 288
of oblique popliteal ligament, 603
of patellar dislocations, 749
of PCL, normal, 551
of retinacula, 751
of transverse ligament, 304, 305f

B

Baker's cysts, 913. *See also* Popliteal
　cysts
Band-like morphology, of ACL,
　410f
Basal degeneration
chondromalacia with, 711, 720f,
　731f
superficial extension of, 732f
Baseball, Segond fractures and, 472
Basketball
ACL injuries and, 424
indirect head of rectus femoris
　injuries risk and, 68
medial meniscal tears and, 329
posterior horn remnant, chondral
　delamination and, 363f
Segond fractures and, 472
twisting injury, 414f
Baurer and Jackson classification, of
　articular cartilage injuries,
　991f
Biceps femoris muscle
anatomy, 639f
　functional, 69, 69f
axial image, 36f–38f
coronal image, 60f–62f
edema between ITB and, 791f
injuries, lateral stabilization and,
　663
long head, 63f, 81f, 108
posterolateral corner injuries and,
　675f–676f
sagittal image, 47f–48f
short head, 81f, 108, 644f
strain, PCL tear and, 569f
tendinous attachments to fibular
　head, 638
Biceps femoris tendon
acute ACL tears and, 443f
anatomy, 34, 639f, 641f, 643f,
　647f, 650f
attachments of, 636
augmentation of interstitial LCL
　injuries with, 671, 671f
axial image, 36f–41f
coronal image, 60f–62f
posterior, 85f
fibular collateral ligament and,
　637
graft reinforcement of LCL with,
　692f
injuries
avulsions, LCL avulsion, PCL
　tear and, 673f

Biceps femoris tendon (*continued*)
  fracture avulsion, 689*f*–690*f*
  multiligament, 685*f*–687*f*
  osseous avulsion, 688*f*
  strain, PCL tear and, 569*f*
 intercondylar notch and, 455*f*
 ITB and, 81*f*
 ITB friction syndrome and, 796*f*
 lateral collateral ligament and, 636, 640*f*, 653, 653*f*
  insertion, sagittal image, 46
 long head, 644*f*, 646*f*, 655, 668*f*
 popliteal fossa view, 87*f*
 posterolateral corner and, 465
 sagittal image, 42, 108, 126*f*
 semitendinosus muscle origin and, 71*f*
 short head, 63*f*, 108, 646*f*, 656
Bicondylar split (Type V), 1000*f*
Bifurcate ridge, AM and PL bundle femoral insertion sites and, 409*f*
Bilaminar morphology
 of articular cartilage, 851
 of patellar articular cartilage, 714, 722*f*
Bioabsorbable polymer scaffolds, 996*f*
Bioabsorbable screws, 986*f*
Biocart matrix-assisted autologous chondrocyte repair, chondral degeneration after, 993*f*–994*f*
Biomechanics
 ACL reconstruction and, 489
  hamstring autograft for, 498*f*
 of cruciate ligaments, 412
 of medial collateral ligament, 602
  scarring, 635
 of patellofemoral joint, 782*f*–783*f*
 of posterior cruciate ligament, 546*f*
Bipartite patella
 accessory ossification of, 822*f*
 characteristics and treatment, 744
 chondromalacia underlying synchondrosis and, 740*f*
 classification by location of, 741
 dorsal defect of patella and, 743
 fracture differentiation from, 1004
 lateral facet, 739*f*
 Sinding-Larsen-Johansson syndrome and, 818
Biters, arthroscopic, 194*f*
Blistering
 chondromalacia and, 711–712, 716, 718*f*–719*f*
  basal degeneration of deep layer and, 731*f*
 chondrocalcinosis and, 730*f*
 medial facet of patellar articular surface, 722*f*
Blood supply. *See* Vascular supply
Blumensaat angle, ACL tears and, 439–440

Blumensaat line, 418*f*, 426*f*
 ACL graft impingement and, 501
 ACL tears and, 440
Blunting. *See* Apex, meniscal; Free edge, of meniscus
Blurring
 cartilage–fluid interface imaging and, 851
 CUBE and, 11
 echo spacing and, 5, 6*f*, 147
 echo time and, 13, 149, 176
 echo train length and, 9, 146, 150
 MAVRIC SL PD and, 17
 parallel imaging and, 20
 receiver bandwidth and, 150
Body
 of lateral meniscus, 55
 of medial meniscus, 55
 of meniscus, 154
  innervation, 163
  inside-out technique for repair of, 328
  low-signal-intensity, 165*f*
  tear repair and, 329
Body coils, peripheral signal artifacts and, 302
Bone, rheumatoid arthritis and, 869
Bone bridge block, 343*f*
Bone contusions, 1001. *See also* Contusions
Bone infarcts. *See also* Osteonecrosis
 characteristics, 944
 fibroblastic reactive tissue and, 945
 imaging, 946*f*
 metaphyseal, serpiginous border of, 944*f*
 osteomyelitis in children and, 1020
 osteomyelitis mimicking, 1024*f*
 rheumatoid arthritis and, 870
 subchondral, 945*f*
Bone–patellar tendon–bone grafts, 490, 494*f*, 515*f*, 517, 539*f*, 572*f*
Bone plugs. *See also* Osteochondral plugs
 ACL reconstruction using, 491, 515*f*
 chondral resurfacing with, 971, 973
 dislodged, 520–521, 532*f*, 535*f*
Bone remodeling, osteoarthritis and, 898
Bone susceptibility effect, 813*f*
Borrelia burgdorferi, 892
Bowtie appearance
 of discoid meniscus, 293
 of medial meniscus, 43
 of meniscus, 103, 153, 165*f*
  bucket-handle tears and, 214
 of synovium-lined meniscal fascicles, 46
Brace, dynamic patellar, dislocations and, 750
Brodie's abscess, 743, 1021
Bucket-handle tears
 bicompartmental, 230*f*
 broken, 213
 complex, 43, 232*f*

 displaced, 292, 329
 flap tear mimicking, 283*f*
 fragment, Segond fracture and, 478*f*
 of lateral meniscus, 231*f*, 233*f*–235*f*
 of medial meniscus
  ACL graft failure and, 503*f*
  ACL injuries and, 427*f*
  displaced, 213, 217*f*–225*f*
  grade 3 ACL tear and, 226*f*
  partial meniscectomy of, 228*f*
  with truncated posterior horn, 229*f*
 of meniscus, 114, 191*f*
  arthroscopic images, 193*f*
  characteristics, 213–216
  flap tears vs., 259
  inside-out repair of, 338
  longitudinal tears and, 204
  oblique meniscofemoral ligaments mistaken for, 311, 323*f*
  posterior horn mistaken for, 311
Buckling, meniscal, simulated vs. true, 312
Bungee effect, 518*f*
Bursa of Voshell, 630*f*
Bursitis
 axial image, 116
 deep infrapatellar, 116, 828*f*, 829, 831*f*
 medial collateral ligament, 612, 630*f*
 pes anserinus, 612, 633*f*–634*f*, 935
 prepatellar bursa, 829
 traumatic, meniscal cysts and, 379

C

Caisson's decompression sickness, 933
Calcification
 of bone infarcts, 944
 cartilaginous, calcium oxalate and, 389
 endochondroma of distal femur and, 1028*f*
 Hoffa's disease and, 862*f*
 patellar tendinosis and, 807*f*
Calcified zone of articular cartilage, 714, 849, 851, 982*f*, 984*f*
Calcium pyrophosphate dihydrate deposition disease (CPDD), 388–389
Cancellous bone, articular cartilage and, 846*f*, 984*f*
Cancellous grooves, for osteochondritis dissecans, 949
Capacious hiatus, 684*f*
Capillary hyperplasia, diffuse pigmented villonodular synovitis and, 878
Capsular arm, 646*f*
Capsular attachment, peripheral vertical tear of medial meniscus mistaken for, 313

Index

Capsule
  anterior perspective, 92f
  overlying meniscus, pes anserinus tendon and, 78f
  posterior removed, 85f–86f, 88f
  sagittal image, 82f
  sagittal plane dissection, 42
  vastus medialis and, 66f
Capsulorrhaphy, 747
Carbon fiber, for ACL allografts, 490, 517
CartiGram (T2 mapping), 10, 11f
Cartilage. See also specific types of cartilage
  rheumatoid arthritis and, 869
Cartilage intermediate layer protein (CILP), 897
Cartilage oligomeric matrix protein (COMP), 897
Cast immobilization
  complex regional pain syndrome and, 1019
  patellar dislocations and, 750
Catching, synovial plicae and, 921
Causalgia, 1019
Celery stalk appearance, of ganglion cysts, 455, 461f
Cell growth factors, meniscal tear healing and, 328
Cell nutrition, meniscal, 162
Cellulitis, multifocal osteomyelitis and, 1021
Central notch, ACL course in, 410f
Cerebral palsy, patella alta and, 801
Changing slope sign of flap tears, 269f
  central notch displacement in, 270f
Channel counts, MR imaging and, 4
Chemical-shift artifacts or techniques
  bone infarcts and, 944
  in children, 1002
  cortical bone and, 43
  echo-planar imaging and, 999f
  hyaline articular cartilage and, 850
  receiver bandwidth and, 150
  3.0T imaging and, 18
Children. See also Adolescents; Juvenile chronic arthritis
  ACL reconstruction in, 517
  ACL tears in, primary and secondary findings, 440
  articular cartilage in, 853
  chemical-shift artifact signal intensity in, 1002
  cruciate ligament injuries in, 423
  discoid meniscus and, 291
    complete and, 296f
  meniscal vascularity in, 154, 162
  MR imaging of arthritis in, 845
  MR imaging of osteochondritis dissecans in, 949
  osteochondral fractures in, 971, 978f

  osteochondritis dissecans and, 951, 958f
  early epiphyseal ossification and, 967f–968f
  treatment, 949
  osteomyelitis in, 1020
  other rheumatic diseases of, 866
  patellar sleeve fracture in, 1015
  popliteal cysts in, 914
  subchondral epiphyseal hypointensity in, 948
  unfused physis after femoral fracture repair in, 1014f
Chondral bone. See also Chondral fractures
  Grade 4 loss, displaced meniscal flap tear and, 275f
  loss, osteoarthritis and, 899f
Chondral defects, raw and segmented MRI of, 26f
Chondral degeneration
  after medial meniscectomy, 174f
  osteoarthritis and, 899f
Chondral delamination. See also Delamination
  after partial meniscectomy, 363f
  in articular cartilage, 997f
  of lateral femoral condyle, 163f
  in patellar sleeve fracture, 1015f
Chondral erosion
  crabmeat, 137f, 717, 728f, 731f
  partial lateral meniscectomy and, 360f
  of subchondral bone, 101
  suprapatellar bursa and, 105
Chondral flaps
  articular cartilage delamination and, 979f
  ligament tears and, 970f
  MR evaluation of, 972
  osteochondritis dissecans and, 962f–963f
Chondral fractures, 971, 974f, 977f, 986f, 1006f. See also Chondral bone; Chondral lesions; Osteochondral lesions
Chondral inhomogeneity, normal epiphyseal development and, 969f
Chondral lesions
  articular cartilage and, 122f
  débridement without abrasion of, 991f
  key concepts, 971
  meniscal tears and, 173
  MR accuracy in detection of, 288
  MR evaluation of, 972
  subchondral plate osteophyte and, 975f–976f
  surgical evaluation of, 972–974
  treatment of, 992f
Chondral resurfacing techniques, 971
Chondral surfaces, imaging, 851
Chondrocalcinosis, 303f, 388–389, 389f–392f, 730f
Chondrocytes
  in articular cartilage, 847
  matrix disruption and, 849

  decreased, meniscal degeneration and, 187f
  implantation of, 971, 973–974
  regenerative, meniscus healing and, 180
Chondroitin, 845
Chondroitin sulfate region, of articular cartilage, 981f
Chondromalacia
  altered organization of collagen and, 715f
  axial vs. sagittal images of, 32
  cartilage damage and, 697
  chondral flaps vs., 972, 980f
  discoid meniscus and, 293
  fractures vs., 972, 980f
  key concepts, 706
  lateral patellar facet, 697
  loose bodies in joint effusion and, 116
  medial patellar facet, medial plica and, 921, 925f, 929f
  patellar, 706
    alternative classification, 710f
    cartilage changes in, 716, 717f–719f
    chondrocalcinosis and, 730f
    chronic degenerative, 736f
    crabmeat erosion and, 731f
    grade 1, 719f
    grade 2, 718f, 720f, 724f–725f
    grade 4, 717f, 721f, 733f–734f
    medial patellar facet and, 728f
    MR appearance of, 711–712
    MR imaging protocols, 712–713
    Outerbridge classification, 709f
    with superficial degeneration, 725f, 732f
    synchondrosis and, 740f
  patellofemoral, irregular infrapatellar fat-pad sign and, 858
  patellofemoral mechanics and, 783f
  reactive bone marrow edema and, 109
  stages of, 855f
  treatment of, 743
Chondromatosis, 382f, 871f, 898, 902f, 908
Chondroplasty, 743, 989f
Chondrosis, 572
  degenerative, chondral flaps or fractures vs., 980f
CILP (cartilage intermediate layer protein), 897
Cine-MR imaging, patellar tracking using, 746
Circular cross-section, of PCL, 410f
Circumferential (C) zone
  of meniscal fibrocartilage and, 159
  of meniscus, 166f
  radial meniscal tear extending to, 286f
Circumferential collagen fibers
  meniscal hoop tension and, 159
  in middle layer of meniscus, 161, 168f

Circumflex fibular artery, 644f, 646f
Cleavage tears
  horizontal
    of meniscus, 114, 197f–198f
      meniscal cysts and, 377–378
      mucoid ACL and, 462f
    of PHMM, 198f–201f
  intrasubstance, discoid meniscus and, 294
  intrasubstance degenerative, arthroscopy of, 289
Clergyman's knee, 829
Clicking
  discoid meniscus and, 291
  knee extension, ganglion cysts and, 455
  meniscal pathology and, 173
  synovial plicae and, 921
Clinical knee examination, MR imaging accuracy vs., 288
Clip injury, 415–416
Closed chondromalacia, 709f, 716
Coagulopathy, consumptive, 1027
Coapted flap tears, of meniscus, 257, 261f, 263f, 269f
Collagen
  ACL healing capacity and, 429
  in articular cartilage, 846f, 982f, 984f
  chondromalacia patellae and, 716, 729f
  in cruciate ligaments, 411
  degeneration, patellar tendinosis and, 798
  direction of, in meniscus, 161
  meniscal hoop tension and, 159
  in patellar articular cartilage, 714–715, 715f
  in patellar facet articular cartilage, 721f
  patellar tendinosis and, 807f–808f
  T2 map for changes with, 985f
Collagen bundle zones, of meniscus, 159–160, 167f
Collagen matrix scaffold, 974
Collagen meshwork (matrix), 983f
Collagen network, osteoarthritis and, 897
Collagen type I, in meniscus, 161
Collagen type II
  in articular cartilage, 847
  in articular cartilage extracellular matrix, 845
  in meniscus, 161
  proteoglycan complexes and, 848f
Collagen type IX, 847
Collagen type XI, 847
Collagen vascular disease, 866, 946
Collateral ligaments. See also Lateral collateral ligament; Medial collateral ligament
  axial image, 115
  coronal image, 54
  coronal plane checklist, 98
  injuries, bone contusion Types I and II and, 1004
  PCL injuries and, 547

Combined ganglia, tibiofibular joint and, 907
Comminuted fractures
  patellar, 1004, 1015, 1018f
  tibial plateau, 1004
Common peroneal nerve
  anatomy, 641f, 647f, 649f, 904f
  interneural ganglia and, 905f–906f, 907
Compartment syndrome, 1009, 1019, 1022f
Complete discoid meniscus, 290, 294, 296f–297f
Complete discoid tear, of meniscus, 191f
Complex meniscal tears, 191f. See also Meniscal degeneration and tears
  arthroscopic images, 193f
  flap
    ACL injuries and, 258
    descriptions of, 255
    MR accuracy in detection of, 159, 288
  with radial, flap, and longitudinal components, 282f
  radial, peripheral extension to circumferential zone, 286f
  with radial and flap components, 196f, 281f
  with truncated free edge flap and longitudinal components, 284f
Complex regional pain syndrome (CRPS), 1019, 1022f
Compressive forces
  on articular cartilage, menisci and, 172
  circumferential fibers or bundles of meniscus and, 159, 161
  fractures and, 1001
  longitudinal meniscal tears and, 204
  meniscal cysts and, 377
Computed tomography (CT), two-dimensional, fracture morphology and, 1001
Concave articular surface, of lateral patellar facet, 697
Concave superior surface
  of discoid-like meniscus, 298f–299f
  discoid meniscus and, 290
  incomplete discoid meniscus and, 295f
  of meniscus, 153
Condylar fractures
  of distal femur, 1013f
  split, 1001
Condylar tibial plateau fractures, 1004
Condylopatellar limiting grooves, 94f
Condylopatellar sulcus, lateral notch sign and, 471
Congenital deformities
  discoid meniscus and, 291
  secondary osteoarthritis and, 897

Congruence angle, 745–746
Connective tissue, red zone of meniscal fibrocartilage vs., 162
Consumptive coagulopathy, 1027
Contact hyperextension injuries, 416
Contact stress
  meniscectomy and, 174, 335, 359f
  patellar malalignment and, 698
Contrast
  interarticular, postoperative meniscus and, 333
  intraarticular, osteochondritis dissecans and, 947
  PROPELLER and, 15
Contrast agents. See also Gadolinium contrast; Intravenous contrast
  articular cartilage imaging and, 845
  gadolinium–diethylene triamine pentaacetic acid, 460f, 723f, 858, 870
  MR imaging and, 3
Contrast-enhanced imaging, 853
Contrecoup injuries
  contusions
    of ACL, posteroinferior corner tear of PHMM and, 374f
    after ACL rupture, 472
    of medial tibial plateau, 212f, 368f, 482f
  fractures, of medial tibial plateau, peripheral meniscal vertical tear and, 208f
  impaction, posteromedial crush injury and, 473
  meniscocapsular separations and, 481f
  posteromedial tibial plateau osseous injuries as, 470
Contusions. See also Bone contusions
  ACL injuries and, 439
  ACL tears and, 440, 445f
    acute, 443f
    chronic, 452f
    lateral compartment and, 470–471
  characteristics, 1003–1004
  coronal plane checklist, 102
  lateral femoral condyle, 477f, 612
  lipohemarthrosis and, 912
  MCL sprains and, 604
  medial patellofemoral ligament, 757f
    tears and, 759f–760f
  patellar dislocations and, 749
  PCL injuries and, 540
    hyperextension, 550f
    tears, 553, 557f, 559f, 563f–564f
  posterolateral tibial plateau, 418f
  posteromedial tibial plateau, 439
  signal intensity variations, 471
  subacute ACL tears and, 453
  trabecular bone, signal intensity of, 324f
  valgus injury and, 599

Convex articular surface
  medial patellar facet, 697
  patellar, 699
Core decompression, for osteonecrosis, 936
Core protein, in articular cartilage, 981f
Coronal plane images
  of ACL injuries, 436, 438, 486
  of ACL tears, 439–441
  of deep capsular layer, 367
  of joint effusions, 911
  of lateral plica, 930
  of medial collateral ligament, 603
  of meniscal degeneration or tears
    checklist, 98–102, 117f–124f
    grade 2 vs. grade 3 signal intensity and, 302
    MR accuracy in detection of, 288
  of meniscofemoral ligaments, 310
  of PCL, normal, 551
  of PCL injuries, 552
  pseudo–bucket-handle tears and, 311
Coronary ligaments, 108, 154, 156, 658
Coronary recess
  meniscal flap tears and, 100, 257–258
  displaced, 271f, 275f–277f
Cortical bone
  coronal plane checklist, 102
  femoral and tibial attachments of MCL and, 55
  T1-weighted medial sagittal images and, 43
  tibial and femoral, sagittal image, 43
  UTE pulse sequences and, 988f
  visualization of, 487
COX-2 (cyclooxygenase 2), 798
CPDD (calcium pyrophosphate dihydrate deposition disease), 388–389
Crabmeat patellar cartilage, 137f, 717, 728f, 731f
Crater articular cartilage injuries (Type IV), 991f
Creep, cruciate ligaments and, 412
Crepitus, retropatellar, 744
CRPS (complex regional pain syndrome), 1019, 1022f
Cruciate fascicles, 411, 440, 442
Cruciate ligaments. See also Anterior cruciate ligament; Posterior cruciate ligament
  arthroscopic reconstruction, osteonecrosis and, 936
  associated intraarticular pathology, 423
  axial plane checklist, 114, 140f
  biomechanics, 412
  injuries
    mechanisms of
      ACL, 416, 417f–422f, 423
      key concepts, 415
      posterolateral corner injuries and, 671
    meniscal tears and, 423
  microanatomy, 411
  sprains, 106
  vascular supply, 399f–400f
Crural fascia, 589f
Crystals, CPDD, 389, 391f
C-shape
  of fibrocartilaginous meniscus, 153
  of lateral meniscus
    axial image, 114
    sagittal image, 46
  of medial meniscus, 34, 166f
    axial image, 114
  of medial vs. lateral meniscus, 156
C-terminal domain, of articular cartilage, 981f
CTL spine coil, peripheral signal artifacts and, 302
CUBE, 11–13, 12f, 21
Cutting, meniscal injury due to, 172
Cycling, iliotibial band friction syndrome and, 787
Cyclooxygenase 2 (COX-2), 798
Cyclops lesion
  ACL reconstruction and, 499, 524f–525f
  ACL roof impingement and, 520
  acute ACL stump entrapment and, 444
Cyclops nodule, Hoffa's fat pad and, 134f
Cystic adventitial disease, of popliteal artery, 914, 917f
Cystic fluid collection, ITB friction syndrome and, 787, 795f
Cysts. See also Ganglia; Meniscal cysts; Microcystic areas; Popliteal cysts; Subchondral cysts
  ACL, 456f
  adventitious mucoid, 917f
  atypical
    axial image of joint fluid, 144f
    key concepts, 913
  chondromalacia and, 711, 713, 721f
  discoid meniscus and, 291
  extraneural, osteoarthritis and, 901f
  fluid-filled, hemophilia and, 891
  Hoffa's fat pad and, potential maltracking and, 783f
  intercondylar notch, 455, 459f–460f
    chronic ACL tears and, 439
  interosseous, in children, imaging of, 853
  intrameniscal, 377, 385f, 387f
  intraneural tibiofibular, 914
  intraosseous, hemophilia and, 891
  parameniscal, 377, 379, 384f–385f, 387f
  patellar, chondromalacia and, 711, 713
  quadriceps tendon, 837f
  subarticular, juvenile chronic arthritis and, 866
  synovial, 377, 379
  tibial tunnel and pretunnel, 538f
  tibiofibular, 379
Cytokines, articular cartilage degradation and, 849

D
Dacron, knitted, for ACL allografts, 490
Dashboard injuries, 415, 547, 557f, 560f
Débridement
  arthroscopic, 455, 936
  for chondral lesions, 973–974
  of chondral lesion without abrasion, 991f
  meniscal, biter and shaver for, 194f
  for osteochondritis dissecans, 949
  of torn MPFL, 750
Deep artery of thigh, 65f–68f, 73f
Deep capsular layer, 367, 376f, 590f
Deep capsular ligament, 156, 583
Deep fascia, medial aspect of knee and, 581
Deep femoral artery, 69f–71f
Deep infrapatellar bursa
  anatomy, 828f
  bursitis, 116, 828f, 829, 831f
  Osgood-Schlatter disease and, 819f
  sagittal image, 50f–51f, 92f
Deep lateral retinaculum layer, 751
Deep layer fibers of quadriceps tendon, 56
  partial tear, 840f
Deep layer of articular cartilage, 851. See also Deep zone of articular cartilage
Deep medial collateral ligament (dMCL), 581. See also Medial capsular ligament
  anatomy, 79f, 597f
    functional, 583, 589f–590f
  axial image, 115
  biomechanics of, 602
  coronal image, 117f
  intercondylar notch and, 455f
  joint capsule and, 581
  layer 2 and, 596f
  MCL tears and, 613f
  posteromedial corner and, 591f
  sagittal image, 107
  sMCL and, 622f
  tears, 615f
Deep peroneal nerve, 64f, 904f, 907
Deep transverse retinaculum, 642f, 751, 784f
Deep venous thrombosis, 664, 917
Deep zone of articular cartilage, 714, 720f, 722f, 847. See also Deep layer of articular cartilage
Deer ticks, Lyme arthritis and, 892
DEFT (driven equilibrium Fourier transform) imaging, 851
Degeneration, chronic, meniscal tears and, 172

Degenerative arthrosis, meniscal transplantation and, 331
Degenerative meniscal tears, 191f
 flap, 258
Degrading articular cartilage injuries (Type VI), 991f
Delamination. *See also* Chondral delamination
 of articular cartilage, 979f
 basilar, of deep radial zone cartilage, 720f
 with deep radial zone hyperintensity and subchondral edema, 737f
 of medial femoral condyle surface, 980f
 medial patellar facet chondral surface, 763f
 MR evaluation of, 972
 osteochondritis dissecans and, 961f, 986f
 subchondral edema and, 720f
Delayed gadolinium-enhanced MR imaging of cartilage (dGEMRIC), 713, 983f
Demineralization, juxtaarticular, rheumatoid arthritis and, 869
Descending geniculate (genicular) artery, 63f, 169f
Descending transverse branch, femoral artery, 65f–68f
dGEMRIC (delayed gadolinium-enhanced MR imaging of cartilage), 713, 983f
Diabetes mellitus, 800, 909, 1022f, 1024f
Diaphyseal bone infarcts, 944
Dicalcium phosphate dihydrate, cartilaginous calcifications and, 389
Dielectric artifacts, 3.0T imaging and, 19–20
Diffuse pigmented villonodular synovitis, 877–878, 885f–886f, 888f
Diffusion-weighted imaging, 853
Direct arm
 biceps femoris muscle, 638, 644f, 646f
 long head of biceps femoris muscle, 655, 668f, 672f
 short head of biceps femoris muscle, 656, 668f
Direct blow. *See also* Trauma
 chondral flaps and, 970f
 dislocations and, 757
 to flexed knee, 416, 555f
 osteochondral fractures and, 971
 patellar fractures and, 1016, 1017f
Discoid meniscus
 characteristics, 290–292
 complete vs. incomplete, 294
 differential diagnosis of, 292
 illustrations and examples of, 295f–300f
 imaging findings in evaluation of, 293
 key concepts, 290

 lateral
  osteochondritis dissecans of, 948
  parameniscal cysts and, 379, 384f
 meniscal tears and, 173
 treatment of, 292
Dislocations. *See also* Knee, dislocations
 patella, vastus medialis and, 66
 patellofemoral joint, 292
 PCL rupture and, 547–549
 tibiofibular joint, 292, 781f, 907
Displaced bucket-handle tears of medial meniscus, 213, 217f–223f
Displaced tibial plateau fractures, 1004
Displacement, meniscus and, 154
Dissecting popliteal cysts, 914
Dissections, meniscal cysts and, 377–378, 384f
Distal aponeurosis, 655
Distal femur articular cartilage, knee extension and, 33
Distal metaphysis, medial collateral ligament and, 55
Distal quadriceps tendinosis, 109
Distal quadriceps tendon, 109
Divergent tunnel technique, for ACL graft revision, 519f
Dixon technique, 23
dMCL. *See* Deep medial collateral ligament
Donor site
 for osteochondral transplants, 993f–994f
 preparation, 995f
Dorsal defect of patella, 742f, 743
Dorsiflexion injuries, 555f
Double ACL sign, 258
Double-bundle technique, 504f, 506f, 511, 511f–514f, 572f
Double-decker pattern, meniscal flap tears and, 255, 268f, 273f
Double delta sign
 bicompartmental bucket-handle tears and, 230f
 flap tear mimicking bucket-handle tear and, 283f
 lateral meniscal bucket-handle tear and, 231f
 lateral meniscus version, 235f
 meniscal bucket-handle tears and, 214, 217f–220f, 223f–226f
 sagittal MR images of bucket-handle tear and, 213
Double PCL sign, 213–214, 219f–220f
Double vertical longitudinal bucket-handle tears, 213
Driven equilibrium Fourier transform (DEFT) imaging, 851
DTPA. *See* Gadolinium–diethylene triamine pentaacetic acid

Dysplasia epiphysealis hemimelica, 1021, 1026f
Dysplastic meniscus. *See* Discoid meniscus

E
Ecchymosis, 614
Echo-planar imaging (EPI), 999f
Echo time (TE)
 cartilage–fluid interface imaging and, 851
 chronic fractures and, 1002
 imaging protocols, 149
 intrameniscal signal intensity and, 176
 magic-angle phenomenon and, 313
 meniscal degeneration and tears and, 176
 MR imaging and, 5, 6f
Echo train length (ETL), 5, 150
Edema. *See also* Hyperintense edema; Subchondral edema
 ACL graft failure and, 534f
 ACL injuries and
  acute, 441
  chronic tears, 453
  MR imaging of, 437
 bioabsorbable screws and, 986f
 compartment syndrome and, 1019
 Hoffa's disease and, 862f
 Hoffa's fat pad and, 134f, 697
 hyperintense
  subchondral fracture and, 938f, 940f
  subchondral stress fracture and, 1011f
 ITB friction syndrome and, 115, 790f
 ITB syndrome and, 788, 792f, 794f–795f
 joint sepsis and, 1020
 MCL sprains and, 600f, 603, 605f, 608f
 MCL tear and, 619f
 in medial femoral condyle subchondral ischemia, 364f
 medial retinaculum tears and, 751
 osteochondritis dissecans and, 949, 963f
 patellar dislocations and, 748
 patellar tendinosis and, 797f, 805f
 patellar tendon tears and, 800, 802f–803f
 PCL injuries and, MR imaging of, 552
 posterior fibular styloid, 145f
 posterolateral corner injuries and, 466, 467f
 posttraumatic diffuse meniscal, 307, 317f
 posttraumatic meniscal, 307, 317f
 quadriceps tendon tears and, 841f
 stress-related, coronal plane checklist, 102

Index

styloid, popliteofibular ligament avulsion and, 681f
subcortical, 1009f
superficial to intact MCL, 764f–765f
T2-weighted images of, 1001
Effusions. See Joint fluid or effusions
Ehlers-Danlos syndrome, 917f
Elastic components of cruciate ligaments, 411
Elastin, in meniscal fibrocartilage, 161
Electrocautery, of ACL tibial footprint, 508f
11 o'clock position, for ACL reconstruction, 489, 496f
Elmslie-Trillat procedure, 830
Elongation
 of ACL grafts, 521
 of cruciate ligaments, 412
ELPS. See Excessive lateral pressure syndrome
Empty lateral wall, 484f
Empty notch sign, 452f, 453
Enchondromatosis, Maffucci syndrome with, 1027
Endo-Button, 498f
Endochondroma, femoral, calcification and, 1028f
Endoplasmic retinaculum, in fibrochondrocytes, 159
Endothelial cells, patellar tendinosis and, 805f
End-stage chondromalacia, 711
EPI (echo-planar imaging), 999f
Epicondylopatellar band, 751, 784f
Epiligament, of cruciate ligaments, 411
Epiphyseal bone infarcts, 944–945
Epiphyseal plate, osteochondritis dissecans and, 958f
Epiphyseal tunnels, ACL reconstruction using, 498f
Epiphysiodesis, 1002, 1007f
Epiphysis
 juvenile chronic arthritis and, 866
 maturation of
  chondral inhomogeneity and, 969f
  osteochondritis dissecans and, 967f–968f
  subchondral hypointensity and, 933
  red marrow heterogeneity and, 1001
Epitenon, of cruciate ligaments, 411
ETL (echo train length), 5, 150
Excessive lateral pressure syndrome (ELPS), 697, 704–706, 751–752, 783f, 786f
Extensor digitorum longus muscle
 anatomy, 639f, 641f
 coronal image, 59f–60f
 extraneural ganglia and, 906f
 infection in diabetic and, 1022f
 ITB and, 81f
 leg muscle innervation and, 64f
 osteomyelitis and infection in, 1023f
 sagittal image, 47f

Extensor mechanism
 coronal image, 54
 patellofemoral joint and, 697
Extensor muscle injuries, magnetic resonance evaluation of, 834
External iliac artery, 65f–68f
External rotation. See Knee rotation
Extraarticular ACL reconstruction, 490, 517
Extracapsular ligament, 157
Extracellular matrix
 of articular cartilage, 845, 847
 of meniscus, 159
Extraneural ganglia, 904f–906f, 907
Extraneural tibiofibular cysts, 914

F
Fabella, 588f, 640f, 660f, 666f, 677f
Fabellofibular ligament. See also Short lateral ligament
 anatomy, 638, 649f, 677f
  proximal course of, 660f
 arcuate sign and, 470
 attachment of, 666f, 672f
 lateral collateral ligament and, 636
 lateral limb of arcuate ligament and, 665f
 posterolateral complex and, 637
 posterolateral corner and, 465
 sagittal image, 42, 108
Fabellopopliteal ligament, 638, 660f
False-positive MR findings
 ACL pathology and, 429
 in meniscal degeneration and tears, 288
Familial calcium pyrophosphate dihydrate deposition disease, 388
Fascia, long head of biceps femoris tendon and, 655
Fascia lata, 636, 703
Fascicle tears, 308, 318f
Fascioplasty, 747
Fast low-angle–shot techniques, hyaline articular cartilage and, 850
Fast recovery fast spin-echo (FRFSE) sequence
 for chondral lesions, accuracy of, 288
 fat saturation images, sagittal image, 9f
 MR imaging and, 5
Fast spin-echo (FSE) sequence, 302
 meniscal degeneration and tears and, 176
 MR imaging and, 5
 PROPELLER vs., 16f
Fat
 pigmented villonodular synovitis and, 877
 sagittal image, knee joint, 82f
 saturation
  adiabatic spectral inversion recovery technique in CUBE and, 12
 CUBE and, 12f

suppression
 MAVRIC SL Fluid and, 17
 spectral selective fat saturation, 21
 uniform, MR imaging and, 3
 water excitation in 3D MERGE and, 14
Fatigue fractures of collagen meshwork, 897
Fat pad. See Hoffa's infrapatellar fat pad
Fat-pad impingement syndrome, 173
Fatty villonodular proliferation, lipoma arborescens and, 908
Femoral artery, 169f
 biceps femoris and, 69f
 gracilis muscle and, 73f
 rectus femoris and, 68f
 sartorius muscle and, 72f
 semitendinosus muscle and, 71f
 vastus intermedius and, 67f
 vastus lateralis and, 65f
 vastus medialis and, 66f
Femoral articular cartilage, osteoarthritis and, 43
Femoral cartilage, segmentation example, 26f
Femoral condyles, 94f. See also Lateral femoral condyle; Medial femoral condyle
 anterior cruciate ligament and, 99
 capsule covering, lateral collateral ligament and, 80f
 cartilage surface, 101, 104
 chondromalacia patellae and, 706
 complete discoid meniscus and, 294
 fractures, 1001
 hemophilia and surface of, 891
 medial plica and erosion or abrasion of, 923
 meniscectomy and changes in, 335
 meniscus and, 153, 155
 meniscus body and, 103
 sagittal image, 109
 spontaneous osteonecrosis and, 937f
 trochlear groove cartilage and, 105
Femoral epicondylar attachment
 hemorrhage, MCL avulsion, 611, 616f
 MCL avulsion fracture and, 617f
 medial collateral ligament and, 55
Femoral nerve
 rectus femoris and, 68f
 sartorius muscle and, 72f
 thigh muscle innervation and, 63f
 vastus intermedius and, 67f
 vastus lateralis and, 65f
 vastus medialis and, 66f
Femoral osteotomy, for knee subluxation or dislocations, 747

Femoral trochlear groove
  anatomy, 699, 701, 701f
  dysplastic
    lateral patellar subluxation and, 704
    lateral patellar tilt and, 705
    patellar height relative to, 702–703, 702f
    patellar malalignment and abnormal tracking and, 698
    patellofemoral joint contact areas and, 707f
Femoral tunnels
  ACL graft impingement and, 501
  ACL reconstruction and
    bone–patellar tendon–bone, 515f
    graft revision, 519f
    over-the-top position in, 397
    placement, 489, 491, 494f
    preparation, 512f
    side wall impingement, 522
  footprint measurement, 511f
  medial patellofemoral ligament reconstruction and, 771f–772f
Femorotibial gliding, fibrocartilaginous menisci and, 153
Femur
  ACL and posterior translation of, 402
  ACL attachment to, 405f
    avulsion repair and, 487
    disruption to, 414f
  anatomy
    functional, patellar surface, 77f
    knee in partial flexion and, 93f
  axial image, 36f–37f
  compensatory varus alignment with internal rotation of, 472
  condylar fracture of distal, 1007f
  cortical bone, tibial cortical bone vs., 43
  cruciate ligamentous tissue and, 411
  dMCL and motion of, 583
  endochondroma of, calcification and, 1028f
  flexion, gastrocnemius muscle and, 75
  footprint, 510f
  fractures
    lipohemarthrosis and, 1019
    pathologic, nonossifying fibroma and, 1010f
  hyaline articular cartilage signal intensity of, 43
  knee capsule and ligaments and, 92f
  lateral supracondylar line of, 76f
  multifocal osteomyelitis and, 1021
  patellofemoral joint flexion and, 703
  popliteofibular ligament and, 638
  posterior cruciate ligament and, 542
  rotation, during flexion and extension, 172
  sagittal image, 50f–51f, 92f
  tibia relative to, ACL tears and, 468f–469f
Fibrillation
  in articular cartilage, 849
  chondromalacia and, 711–712, 728f
  false interpretation as meniscal tears of, 289
  pitfalls interpreting findings on, 307, 316f
Fibrillation articular cartilage injuries (Type V), 991f
Fibrin clots, 328–329
Fibrinoid necrosis, 807f
Fibroblasts
  ACL graft revascularization and, 493
  patellar tendinosis and, 805f
Fibrocartilage
  discoid meniscus and, 291
  repair of, 973
  reparative, 989f
  zone of, 411
Fibrocartilaginous menisci, 153
Fibrocartilaginous nodule, ACL roof impingement and, 520
Fibrochondrocytes, meniscus and, 159
Fibromas, nonossifying, 1003, 1010f
Fibrosis
  acute ACL stump entrapment and, 444
  hemophilia and, 891
  Hoffa's disease and, 857, 862f
  hypointense signal on T1/PD images and, 737
  postoperative, Hoffa's fat pad and, 860f
Fibrovascular repair tissue, signal intensity in healing menisci and, 338
Fibula
  anatomy
    anterior view, knee in partial flexion and, 93f
    biceps femoris muscle insertion at head of, 69f
    knee capsule and ligaments and, 92f
    knee in partial flexion and, 93f
    superior aspect of, 672f
  arcuate ligament and, 661f
  contusion, ACL reinjury and, 485f
  coronal image, 60f–62f
  popliteofibular ligament and, 638
  posterolateral corner and, 466
  sagittal image, 47f
Fibular collateral ligament
  anatomy, 637, 639f
    functional, 77f
    insertion for, 41f
  axial image, 37f–40f, 115
  coronal image, 54f, 61f
  high-signal-intensity fat and MR images of, 35
  intercondylar notch and, 455f
  lateral meniscus and, 157
  popliteus complex and, 645f
  posterior coronal image, 85f
  sagittal image, 42, 108
Fibular head
  anatomy, 41f, 86f
  avulsion fractures, 470, 473, 483f, 556, 689f–690f
  discoid meniscus and, 293
  fracture, popliteofibular ligament and, 683f
  LCL and biceps femoris attachment to, 636
  posterior fracture of, 145f
  posterolateral corner injuries and, 674f, 676f
Fibular styloid
  arcuate ligament and, 42
  avulsion fractures, 470
  PCL injury and, 568f
  fabellofibular ligament and, 42
  fracture, PCL injury and, 563f–564f
  fractured elliptical fragment of, 473
Ficat and Hungerford classification, of patellar facet configurations, 701
Field of view (FOV), 17, 302–303
Fish-mouth tears, meniscal, 183, 198f
Fissuring
  chondromalacia and, 711, 724f, 726f–727f, 729f
  degenerative arthrosis and, 896f
  osteochondritis dissecans and, 950f, 960f
  superficial, chondral lesions and, 972
Flap articular cartilage injuries (Type III), 991f
Flap tears
  of body/posterior horn medial meniscus
    displaced into coronary recess, 275f
    meniscal cyst development and, 287f
    vertical superior folding and, 280f
  complex, PCL tear and, 565f
  of inferior meniscal surface, blunted surface and, 265f
  of medial meniscus
    displaced, PCL injuries and, 566f
    meniscal cysts and, 380f
    radial tear and, 281f
    vertical, inferior displacement of, 268f
  of meniscal free edge
    changing slope sign of, 269f
    with longitudinal component, 284f
  of meniscus, 114, 186, 289f
    characteristics, 255, 257–259
    coapted, 261f
    displaced
      into coronary recess, 271f, 277f

discoid meniscus and, 292
into notch, 279f
oblique meniscomeniscal ligaments mistaken for, 311
displaced bucket-handle tears and, 225f
graphic depiction, 191f, 256f
horizontal, meniscal cysts and, 378
horizontal and vertical, 190f
horizontal tear and cyst and, 202f
horizontal tears and, 184–185
longitudinal tears and, 204
mimicking bucket-handle tear, 283f
with radial and longitudinal components, 282f
as radial tear in longitudinal direction, 196f
repair of, 331
of posterior horn medial meniscus, 155f, 260f
coapted, 263f
displaced, 264f
displaced into popliteal hiatus, 285f
meniscotibial displaced, 271f–272f
Flexion. *See* Knee flexion; Thigh flexion
Floating meniscus, meniscocapsular separations and, 368, 375f
Fluid. *See also* Edema; Joint fluid or effusions
ACL injuries and, 426f–427f, 430
ACL tears and, 419f
chronic, 439, 484f
hypotense distal ligament and, 485f
LCL tears and, 669f
meniscocapsular separations and, 481f
subacute, 453
acute fractures and imaging of, 1002
fractures and extension of, 971
inhomogeneity of, joint sepsis and, 1020
MCL sprains and, 605f
of meniscal cysts, 379
osteochondritis dissecans and, 947, 965f
posterolateral corner injuries and, 466, 467f
synovial masses and, imaging of, 857
Fluid-filled cysts, hemophilia and, 891
Fluid-sense pulse sequences, 150, 338, 438
Focal fat pad edema, 111
Foot, flexion of, 75–76
Football
ACL injuries and, 415, 424
iliotibial band friction syndrome and, 787
indirect head of rectus femoris injuries risk and, 68
medial meniscal tears and, 329
osteochondral fractures and, 971
PCL injuries and, 547
FOV (field of view), 17, 302–303
Fractures. *See also* Contusions; Osteonecrosis; Stress fractures
ACL graft bundles, 520–521
ACL graft failure and, 534f
ACL injuries and, 430, 439
tibial eminence, 431f
acute line hypotensity in, 1002
chondral, 971
MR evaluation of, 972
chondromalacia patellae and, 706
complex regional pain syndrome and, 1019
coronal plane checklist, 102, 123f
impacted supracondylar, of femur, 1013f
insufficiency, 934–935, 940f
sagittal plane checklist, 133f
subchondral, 938f
intraarticular patellar, 748
key concepts, 1001
lateral tibial plateau, 679f–680f, 1005f
lipohemarthrosis and, 912
mechanism of injury, 1001
MR appearance of, 1002
nondisplaced compression, 612
nonossifying fibroma and, 1010f
osteochondral
cartilage damage and, 697
characteristics, 971
MR evaluation of, 972
patellar, 1004
patellar dislocations and, 774f
patellar medial margin, 748
radiographic evaluation of, 1001
sagittal image, subchondral plate and, 109
Salter-Harris type II, 1008f
Salter-Harris type III, 1008f
sites, 1001
subacute, hyperintensity in, 1002
subchondral
ACL tears and, 482f
ischemia-related, 941f
linear, 1011f
spontaneous osteonecrosis and, 933–935, 937f, 943f
tibial plateau, 1004, 1005f
Fragmentation
chondromalacia and, 712, 715f, 717, 730f
with basal degeneration, 711
osteochondritis dissecans and, 739f, 949, 962f
nondisplaced, 964f
Fragments, chondral, 898, 901f–902f. *See also* Loose bodies
Fragments, fracture
posterolateral corner injuries and, 475f–476f
of Segond fractures, 472
Fragments, osteochondral, osteoarthritis and, 898
Fragments, postoperative meniscal, 334, 337
Fraying
false interpretation as meniscal tears of, 289
pitfalls interpreting findings on, 307, 316f
Free edge, of meniscus
blunted
flap tears and, 256f, 257
with longitudinal component, 284f
partial meniscectomy and, 350f, 353f–354f
radial tear extending to circumferential zone and, 286f
fibrillation or fraying mistaken for tear in, 316f
flap tears of, 255, 262f–263f, 289f
changing slope sign of, 269f
foreshortened inferior surface and, 266f
radial tears and, 103, 195f, 236f, 240f–243f, 245f
transverse zone of meniscal fibrocartilage and, 160
FRFSE sequence. *See* Fast recovery fast spin-echo sequence
FS 3D spoiled gradient recalled (SPGR) technique
of articular cartilage, 855f
articular cartilage and, 850
FSE sequences. *See* Fast spin-echo sequence
FS PD FSE
of ACL acute injuries, 441
of ACL injuries, 437, 486
of ACL partial tears, 448
of articular cartilage, 845
avulsion injuries, ACL tears and, 442
of bone contusions, 471, 1003
of cartilage–fluid interface, 851
of chondral lesions, 971–972
of chondromalacia, 706, 712, 716, 855f
of complex regional pain syndrome, 1019
defining meniscal outline using, 307
of diffuse pigmented villonodular synovitis, 886f
of discoid meniscus, 294
fluid tracking after meniscectomy using, 334
of ganglion cysts, 455
of hyaline articular cartilage, 849–850
imaging after meniscectomy, 335
of ITB syndrome, 787
of joint effusions, 911
of lateral tibial plateau chondral erosion, 854f
of lipoma arborescens, 908
of MCL tears, 611
of medial collateral ligament, 603
meniscal vs. capsular signal intensity using, 313

FS PD FSE (continued)
  of normal red marrow, T1-weighted images vs., 1012f
  of osseous fractures and bone contusions, 1002
  of osteochondral lesions, 972
  of osteochondritis dissecans, 947, 953f–954f
  of patellar articular cartilage, 721f
  of patellar tendinosis, 799, 809f
  of PCL, 551
  of PCL partial tears, 552
  of postoperative meniscus, 334
  of reflex sympathetic dystrophy, 1001
  of rheumatoid arthritis, 869
Fulcrum effect, patella and, 699
Fulkerson osteotomy, 738f, 830

G
Gadolinium contrast. See also Delayed gadolinium-enhanced MR imaging of cartilage
  ACL graft-side wall impingement and, 522
  articular cartilage imaging and, 851
  delayed enhanced MR imaging of cartilage with, 713
  hemorrhage differential diagnosis with, 834
  intravenous
    bone infarcts and, 944
    osteochondritis dissecans and, 947
    pannus tissue and, 870
  joint effusions and, 912
  meniscal cysts and, 380
  postoperative meniscus and, 147, 337, 362f
Gadolinium–diethylene triamine pentaacetic acid (DTPA)
  intercondylar notch cysts and, 460f
  MR arthrography of articular cartilage with, 723f
  pannus tissue and, 858
  rheumatoid arthritis and, 870
GAG. See Glycosaminoglycans
Ganglia (ganglion cysts). See also Anterior cruciate ligament, cysts; Intercondylar notch cysts
  ACL reconstruction and, 529f
  ACL tears and, 455
  anterior cruciate ligament and, 457f
  extraneural, tibiofibular joint and, 904f–906f, 907
  horizontal meniscal tears and, 377
  intercondylar notch, 459f–460f
  intraneural, articular branch of common peroneal nerve and, 905f–906f
  key concepts, 917
  tibiofibular joint arthrosis and, 907

Ganglion cyst stalk, 917
Gangrene, popliteal artery aneurysm and, 918
Gas, intraarticular, vacuum phenomenon and, 324f
Gastrocnemius lateral head muscle
  anatomy, 641f
  sagittal image, 47f
Gastrocnemius lateral head tendon, 650f
  sagittal image, 47f
Gastrocnemius medial head muscle
  axial image, 37f, 39f
Gastrocnemius medial head tendon
  axial image, 37f, 39f
  posteromedial corner and, 591f–592f
  sagittal image, 52f
  sMCL and, 596f
Gastrocnemius muscle
  accessory head, 919f
  anatomy, 34, 79f
  anatomy, functional, 75, 75f
  ITB and, 81f
  knee joint sagittal image, 82f
  lateral head
    axial image, 37f, 39f–41f
    coronal image, 60f–62f
    leg muscle innervation and, 64f
    posterolateral corner and, 465
    injuries, 676f
    sagittal image, 46
    tendon, fabellofibular ligament and, 666f
  medial head
    axial image, 38f, 41f, 79f
    collateral venous flow after injury in, 693f
    coronal image, 60f–62f
    leg muscle innervation and, 64f
    popliteal cysts and, 913
    popliteal fossa view, 87f
    posterior coronal image, 85f
    sagittal image, 52f–53f, 79f
    origin, sagittal image, 107
    popliteal fossa view, 87f
Gastrocnemius tendon
  lateral head, axial image, 39f–41f
  medial head
    axial image, 38f
    popliteal cysts and, 915f–916f
    posteromedial capsule and, 367
Gaucher's disease
  bone infarcts and, 946
  spontaneous osteonecrosis and, 933
GE Healthcare acronyms, 27
Geniculate (genicular) artery, 169f
Genu valgum, miserable malalignment syndrome and, 780f
Genzyme procedure, 973–974
Gerdy's tubercle, 102
  avulsion fractures, 556
  iliotibial tract to, 81f
  coronal plane checklist, 124f
  ITB syndrome and, 792f, 796f
Ghost artifacts, blurring by FSE sequences and, 176

Ghost ligament, axial image, collateral ligaments rupture and, 115
Ghost meniscus
  displaced root tears and, 246, 250f–252f
  sagittal image, 103
Giant cells, multinucleated
  diffuse pigmented villonodular synovitis and, 878
  pigmented villonodular synovitis and, 877, 881f
Giving way of knee, meniscal pathology and, 173
Glide test, of patella, 773f
Gliding zone of articular cartilage, 714, 847, 984f
  high-signal intensity of, 851
Glue
  chondrocyte binding with, 974
  meniscal tear healing and, 328
Glycosaminoglycans (GAG)
  in articular cartilage, 713, 845, 848f, 981f
  cartilage matrix compression and, 983f
  in cruciate ligaments, 411
  mapping distribution of, 853
  T1 rho maps correlated with, 987f
Godfrey test, 559f
Golgi complexes, in fibrochondrocytes, 159
Goose foot. See Pes anserinus
Gorham disease, 1027
Gout
  bone infarcts and, 946
  tophaceous, 878, 889f–890f
  pseudo, 388
Gracilis muscle
  anatomy, 34, 79f
  functional, 73, 73f
  axial image, 36f, 40f
  coronal image, 61f
  superficial medial collateral ligament and, 590f
  thigh muscle innervation and, 63f
Gracilis tendon
  anatomy, 79f
  autograft of
    for ACL reconstruction, 490–491, 495f
    postoperative imaging, 517
    for medial patellofemoral ligament reconstruction, 771f–772f
  axial image, 36f–39f, 41f, 79f
  coronal image, 62f
  intercondylar notch and, 455f
  knee subluxation or dislocation and, 747
  MCL tears and, 621f, 623f–624f
  medial collateral ligament and, 587f, 593f
  pes anserinus and, 632f
  pes anserinus bursitis and, 612, 633f–634f
  pes anserinus tendons and, 78f
  posterior coronal image, 85f

Index

posterior oblique ligament and, 629f
posteromedial corner and, 591f–592f
ruptured, 598f
sagittal image, 42, 53f, 79f, 131f
sMCL and, 590f, 596f, 622f
Gradient echo (GRE) sequences
 of ACL graft failure, 521
 of ACL injuries, 437
 of ACL partial tears, 448
 of articular cartilage, 851
 chondral imaging and, 845
 of chondromalacia, 713
 cortical and trabecular bone and, 487
 CPDD and false-positive tears on, 389
 of hyaline articular cartilage, 850
 MR imaging and, 6
 of osseous fractures and bone contusions, 1002
 of osteochondritis dissecans, 953f–954f
 of patellar tendinosis, 809f
 of PCL partial tears, 552
 of pigmented villonodular synovitis, 888f
 postoperative meniscal MR imaging and, 334
 of subacute and chronic hemorrhage, 914
Grafting techniques
 ACL reconstruction, 489–491, 494f–498f
  bone–patellar tendon–bone, 490, 494f, 515f
  dislodged bone plug, 503f, 532f
  double-bundle, 504f, 506f, 511, 511f–514f
  graft tunnel and fixation, 505f
  impingement of, 492, 501, 516–517
   retears and, 485f, 528f, 531f, 533f–534f
  roof, 520–521, 530f
  side wall, 522
  MR evaluation of, 499–501
  over-the-top position for, 397, 502f, 517
  revision, 519f
  stem cells and, 539f
  synovial thickening and, 523f, 536f
  tunnel motion, 518f
 medial patellofemoral ligament reconstruction, 771f–772f
 of meniscus, 326, 331, 342f–343f, 348f
  stem cells and, 347f
 patellar tendon reconstruction, 801
 PCL reconstruction, 556, 572f
 posterolateral corner repair, 692f
 postoperative imaging, 516–517
 revascularization of, 493, 516, 556

Granulation tissue
 chondral and osteochondral lesions and, 972
 chronic PCL tears and, 130f
 hypointense signal on T1/PD images and, 737
 osteochondritis dissecans and, 947
 patellar tendon repair and, 813f
 rheumatoid arthritis and, 870
Greater saphenous vein, 595f
 axial image, 36f, 38f–41f
 coronal image, 60f–62f
 leg muscle innervation and, 64f
 posterior oblique ligament and, 629f
 thigh muscle innervation and, 63f
Greater trochanter, vastus lateralis and, 65f
GRE sequences. See Gradient echo sequences
Ground substance, chondromalacia and, 712
Gymnastics, ACL injuries and, 423

H
Half-moon patella, 701
Hamstring muscles
 biceps femoris of, 69, 69f
 knee stabilization and, 107
 sagittal image, knee joint, 82f
 semimembranosus, 70, 70f
 semitendinosus, 71, 71f
 spasms, pseudo-locking and, 173
Hamstring tendons. See Gracilis tendon; Semitendinosus tendon
Headaches, Lyme arthritis and, 892
Healed osteochondritis dissecans, 948
Healing response technique, for ACL injuries, 488
Hemangiomas, 379, 908, 1027f
Hemarthrosis
 ACL injuries and, 430
 acute ACL tears and, 424, 442
 hemorrhagic effusion and, imaging, 1013f
 lateral femoral condyle fracture and, 912f
 MCL injuries and, 611
 PCL injuries and, 547
 peripheral meniscal tears and, 329
Hematoma
 meniscal tear healing and, 328
 subacute, quadriceps tendon tears and, 834
Hematopoiesis, reconversion of yellow to red marrow in, 1003
Hemipatella, 701
Hemoglobinopathies, spontaneous osteonecrosis and, 933
Hemophilia
 Hoffa's fat pad and, 857
 irregular infrapatellar fat-pad sign and, 858
 key concepts, 891
 MR findings, 891, 893f
 pathology, 891

Hemorrhage
 acute ACL tears and, 442
 acute fractures and imaging of, 1002
 bone contusions and, 1004
 condylar fracture of distal femur and, 1007f
 hemophilia and, 891, 893f
 with hemosiderin deposition, pigmented villonodular synovitis and, 881f
 Hoffa's disease and, 862f
 hypointense signal on T1/PD images and, 737
 interosseous, in children, imaging of, 853
 MCL injuries and, 611, 616f
 MCL sprains and, 603
 MCL tears and, 624f
 medial retinaculum tears and, 751
 MR imaging of ACL injuries and, 437
 MR imaging of PCL injuries and, 552
 pain in meniscal tears and, 172
 patellar tendon repair and, 813f
 patellar tendon tears and, 800, 802f, 812f
 PCL injuries and, 553
 pes anserinus bursitis and, 612
 posterolateral corner injuries and, 468f, 676f
 prepatellar bursa and, 827f
 quadriceps tendon tears and, 834
 subacute ACL tears and, 453
Hemorrhagic effusions
 hemarthrosis and
  lateral femoral condyle fracture and, 912f
  medial condylar fracture and, 1013f
 irregular infrapatellar fat-pad sign and, 858, 911–913
 popliteal cysts and, 913
 suprapatellar plica and, 922, 928f
Hemorrhagic popliteal cysts, 913
Hemosiderin
 hemophilia and, 891, 893f
 imaging, in pannus tissue, 886f
 pigmented villonodular synovitis and, 877–878, 880f, 883f–886f
 paramagnetic effect of, 887f–888f
 suprapatellar plica and, 928f
 synovial proliferation with, 881f
Hepatosplenomegaly, juvenile chronic arthritis and, 865
Heterotopic bone, T1 PD images for, 138f
High-resolution imaging
 at 3.0T, advantages of, 18
 using MR techniques, 3
High-signal-intensity fat
 lateral and fibular collateral ligaments and, 35
 posterior horn medial meniscus and posterior capsule and, 44

Hip, functional anatomy of, 65f–68f, 71f–72f
Histiocytes, diffuse pigmented villonodular synovitis and, 877
Histofibroblastic hyperplasia, pigmented villonodular synovitis and, 877
Hoffa's disease, 857, 859f, 862f
Hoffa's infrapatellar fat pad. *See also* Infrapatellar fat pad; Irregular Hoffa's infrapatellar fat-pad sign
 ACL reconstruction and cyclops lesion, 525f
  dislodged graft debris, 535f
  scarring, 526f–527f
 ACL roof impingement and, 520
 ACL tears and nodular soft mass near, 445f
 acute ACL stump entrapment and, 444, 446f
 acute ACL tears and, 442
 anatomy, 34, 647f
 anterior mid-coronal sections of, 55–56
 axial image, 38f–40f, 112
 contour edge of, 856f
 contour irregularities, ACL injuries and, 430
 coronal image, 57f–58f
 deep infrapatellar bursitis and, 828f, 829
 edema
  excessive lateral pressure syndrome and, 752, 786f
  Lyme arthritis and, 892
  Osgood-Schlatter disease and, 817
  patellar tendinosis and, 797f, 805f
  potential maltracking and, 783f
  Sinding-Larsen-Johansson syndrome and, 821f, 823f
 excessive lateral pressure syndrome and, 697
 free edge
  evaluation of, 857
  irregular contour of, 858, 859f
  pigmented villonodular synovitis and, 887f
  restoration after ACL subacute tear, 452f
  synovitis of, 419f
  transverse ligament and, 300f
 ganglion cysts and, 917
 hemophilia and, 891
 infrapatellar plica and, 922
 irregularity, joint effusion and, 911
 ITB and, 81f
 joint effusion and, 135f
 low-signal-intensity tissue bordering, 35
 Lyme arthritis and, 892
 medial plica and, 923
 meniscal cysts and, 384f–385f
 pigmented villonodular synovitis and, 877–878, 879f
 postoperative fibrosis of, 860f
 sagittal image, 45, 48f–51f, 111
 sagittal plane checklist, 104, 134f
 scar tissue fibrosis and, 522
 transverse ligament and, 304
 vascular supply to ACL and PCL and, 400
Hohl classification, for tibial plateau fractures, 1000f, 1004, 1005f
Hoop stresses
 circumferential fibers of meniscus and, 161
 meniscal transplantation and, 331
Hoop tension
 meniscal, circumferential collagen fibers and, 159
 radial tears and, 161
 segmental meniscectomy and, 174
Horizontal meniscal tears
 about, 182–183
 characteristic findings, 184–186
 cleavage, 114, 197f–198f
  instability of one leaf in, 331
  meniscal cysts and, 377–378
  mucoid ACL and, 462f
 fish-mouth, 183, 198f
 flap tears and, 202f, 255, 257
 graphic depiction, 191f
 meniscal cysts and, 199f–202f, 381f, 383f
 primary meniscal repair and, 330
Horizontal sutures, 341f
Housemaid's knee, 829
Humerus, multifocal osteomyelitis and, 1021
Humphrey ligament. *See* Ligament of Humphrey
Hyaline articular cartilage
 in children, imaging of, 853
 femoral and tibial, 43
 imaging signal intensity of, 849
 osteoarthritis and, 939f
 repair of, 973, 999f
 rheumatoid arthritis and, 870
Hyaluronan, 847, 848f
Hyaluronate, 981f
Hyaluronate acid binding region, of articular cartilage, 981f
Hyaluronate-based polymer, 974
Hyaluronic acid, ganglion cysts and, 917
Hydrogen nuclei, dephasing of, low signal intensity of meniscal tissue and, 175
Hydroxyapatite, cartilaginous calcifications and, 389
Hyperemia
 joint sepsis and, 1020
 osteonecrosis and, 935
 reactive, after meniscectomy, 335
Hyperextension
 ACL injuries and, 416
 contusions and, 553
 injury mechanics, 414f, 415
 PCL injuries and, 547, 549f–550f
 posterolateral bundle of ACL and, 397
 posterolateral corner injuries and, 466
 sMCL and, 582
Hyperflexion
 anterolateral bundle sprain, PCL and, 562f
 PCL injuries and, 549f
Hyperintense edema
 after partial meniscectomy, 355f–357f
 coronal plane checklist, 123f–124f
 postoperative meniscus, signal intensity and, 333
 recurrent meniscal tears and, 355, 358f
Hyperplasia of marrow elements, thalassemia and, 1012f
Hyperpronation, miserable malalignment syndrome and, 780f
Hypertrophy, synovial, meniscal tears and, 180
Hypointense sclerosis, coronal plane checklist, 123f

I

IDEAL, 12f, 13–14
Idiopathic osteonecrosis of the knee, 933
Iliotibial band (ITB). *See also* Iliotibial band friction syndrome; Iliotibial band syndrome
 ACL graft failure and, 537f
 ACL reconstruction using, 490, 517
 acute tibial Segond fracture and, 668f
 anatomy, 639f, 642f–644f, 647f, 654, 784f, 787, 789f
 attachment of, 81f
 avulsion injuries, Segond fractures and, 472
 axial image, 37f–40f
  checklist, 145f
 coronal image, 58f–60f, 89f
  checklist, 102, 124f
  lateral patellar retinaculum and, 56
 extraarticular ACL reconstruction using, 490
 Hoffa's infrapatellar fat pad and, 35
 injuries, 675f
 intercondylar notch and, 455f
 lateral collateral ligament and, 636
 patellar subluxation or dislocations and, 745
 popliteal fossa view, 87f
 posterolateral corner and, 465
 sagittal image, 108
  insertion, 47f
 Segond fractures and, 478f–479f
 tears, MR imaging of, 664

Iliotibial band friction syndrome (ITBFS), 102, 115, 145f, 787, 790f–791f
Iliotibial band syndrome
 clinical presentation and assessment, 788
 edema and thickening in, 792f
 edema in, 794f–795f
 graphic depiction, 793f–794f
 key concepts, 787
 lateral femoral pin extrusion and, 536f
 treatment, 788
Iliotibial tract (ITT). See Iliotibial band
Immobilization, for MR imaging, 4
Immunoglobulin (Ig) G, Lyme arthritis and, 892
Immunoglobulin (Ig) M, Lyme arthritis and, 892
Impacted tibial plateau fractures, 1004
Impaction forces
 fractures and, 1001
 subchondral edema and, 969f
 tibial spine avulsions and, 473
Incomplete discoid meniscus, 290, 294, 295f
 tears, 191f
Indirect knee injuries
 dislocations, 747, 757
 osteochondral fractures, 971
 patellar fractures and, 1016–1017
Infants. See also Children
 articular cartilage in, 853
Infection
 chondromalacia patellae and, 706
 chronic, 1021
 complex regional pain syndrome and, 1019
 coronal plane checklist, 102
 joint effusions and, 911
 key concepts, 1020
 secondary osteoarthritis and, 897
 soft tissue, 1022f
 staphylococcal, 1024f
Inferior fascicle
 gross anatomic specimen, 320f
 imaging, 308, 318f
 of lateral meniscus, 157
Inferior genicular artery, 400
Inferior lateral genicular artery, 644f, 646f
Inferior meniscal surface (leaf)
 anatomy, 153
 blunting, partial meniscectomy and, 333
 degenerative flap tears of, 258
 flap tear of
  blunted surface and, 265f
  radial tear and, 281f
  central notch displacement and, 270f
  and deficiency, 262f–263f
  surface, 265f
  truncated and foreshortened, 266f
 horizontal cleavage tear and, 197f

preferential resection in partial meniscectomy, 349f
 tears extending to, resection priority for, 333
 transverse zone of meniscal fibrocartilage and, 160, 166f
Inferior patellar pole
 axial image, 38f
 bipartite, 741
 edema of, patellar tendinosis and, 797f, 809f
 osseous fragment, 813f
 osteitis, rheumatoid arthritis and, 873f
 patellar tendon tears and, 800, 811f
 Sinding-Larsen-Johansson syndrome and, 818, 821f, 823f
 transverse fracture of, 1015
Inferior popliteomeniscal fascicle
 anatomy, 638
 imaging, 651f
 normal deficiency, 319f
 popliteus tendon and, 46
 posterolateral corner injuries and, 664f
 tears, ACL tear and, 667f
Inferior popliteomeniscal ligament, 666f
Inferior posterior patellar surface, 699
Inferior pubis ramus, gracilis muscle origin and, 73f
Inferocentral osteochondritis dissecans, 951f
Inflammation
 hemophilia and, 891
 Hoffa's disease and, 857
 joint effusions and, 911
 Osgood-Schlatter disease and, 817
 osteoarthritis and, 897
 patellar tendinosis and, 798
 rheumatoid arthritis and, 868f, 870, 873f–874f
 synovial, 857
  pigmented villonodular synovitis and, 881f
Inflammatory bowel disease, arthritis associated with, in children, 866
Infrapatellar bursa, Hoffa's fat pad and, 856f
Infrapatellar bursitis, 829
Infrapatellar fat pad. See also Hoffa's infrapatellar fat pad
 sagittal image, 82f
 suprapatellar pouch and, 90f
Infrapatellar fat-pad sign. See also Irregular Hoffa's infrapatellar fat-pad sign
 Hoffa's disease vs., 857
Infrapatellar plica. See also Ligamentum mucosum
 anatomy, 921
 anterior meniscofemoral ligament mistaken for, 310, 927f
 anterior perspective, 920f

characteristics, 922
 sagittal image, 50f–51f
 checklist, 111, 136f
Inguinal ligament, sartorius muscle and, 72f
Insall and Salvati's ratio of patellar height to femoral trochlear groove, 702f
Insall's classification, for patellofemoral disorders, 697, 727
Inside-out meniscus repair, 328, 338, 339f
Instability. See also Stability
 acceptance of, ACL treatment and, 487
 ACL, MR imaging of, 486
 ACL roof impingement and, 520
 anterolateral rotary test of, 424
 of chondral or osteochondral lesions, 972
 chondromalacia patellae and, 706
 irregular infrapatellar fat-pad sign and, 858
 partial ACL tears and, 486
 patellar, Alpine hunter's cap deformity and, 701
 patellar tendinosis and, 798
 patellofemoral, meniscal tears and, 173
 patellofemoral, patellar tilt and, 755f
 patellofemoral joint, 698
  femoral trochlear groove and, 701
 posterolateral
  surgical reconstruction and, 671
  types of, 662
 posteromedial, PCL injuries and, 547
 primary ACL repair and, 488
 sports activity goals, ACL repair and, 488
Insufficiency fractures, 133f
 of medial femoral condyle, 940f
 sagittal plane checklist, 133f
 spontaneous osteonecrosis and, 934–935
 subchondral, 938f
Intercondylar eminence, 94f
Intercondylar fossa side walls, ACL graft impingement and, 501
Intercondylar fractures
 of distal femur, 1013f
 of tibial plateau, 1004
Intercondylar notch
 ACL graft impingement and, 492, 496f
 ACL reconstruction and, 491
 acute ACL stump entrapment and, 444
 anatomy, 94f, 455f
 anterior and posterior horns of medial meniscus and, 43
 anterior cruciate ligament and, 44, 408f
 anterior horn lateral meniscus and, 306
 axial image, 113–114

Intercondylar notch (continued)
  bucket-handle tears and, 213, 215
  chronic ACL tears and, 453
  complete discoid meniscus and, 291
  discoid-like meniscus and, 299f
  discoid meniscus and, 293–294
  flap tear mimicking bucket-handle tear and, 283f
  infrapatellar plica and, 922
  joint effusion and, 110
  juvenile chronic arthritis and, 866
  meniscal bucket-handle tears and, 214, 217f
  meniscal flap tears and, 100
  meniscus and, 154
  osteochondritis dissecans and, 952f, 955f
  posterior, loose bodies in, 116
  posterior horn root attachment of menisci and, 44
  Wrisberg variant of discoid meniscus and, 292, 297f
Intercondylar notch cysts, 455, 459f–460f. *See also* Ganglia
  chronic ACL tears and, 439
Intercondylar roof, ACL graft impingement and, 501, 516–517, 520, 530f
Intermediate layer of quadriceps tendon, partial tear, 840f
Intermediate oblique aponeurotic layer, 825f–827f, 829
Intermediate-signal-intensity bursa, posterior horn medial meniscus and, 156
Intermeniscal ligaments, 321f
Internal rotation. *See* Knee rotation
International Cartilage Repair Society (ICRS) articular cartilage classification, 104
Interosseous membrane, superficial dissection from posterior perspective, 85f
Interstitial tears
  of anterior cruciate ligament, 422f, 441
  patellar tendinosis and, 798
  patellar tendon, 804f
  of posterior cruciate ligament, 540, 548, 559f, 562f, 571f
  imaging, 552
Intertrochanteric line, vastus medialis and, origin, distal half, 66f
Intraarticular ACL reconstruction, 490, 517
Intraarticular augmentation. *See* Augmentation
Intraarticular gas, vacuum phenomenon and, 324f
Intraarticular polyester ligament augmentation device, 488
Intraligamentous bursa, 603
Intraligamentous thickening, MCL sprains and, 606f–608f
Intrameniscal cysts, 377, 385f
  lateral meniscus horizontal tear and, 387f

Intrameniscal signal conversion, 334, 383f
Intraneural ganglia
  articular branch of common peroneal nerve and, 905f–906f
  tibiofibular joint and, 907
Intraneural tibiofibular cysts, 914
Intraosseous cysts, hemophilia and, 891
Intravenous (IV) contrast
  atypical popliteal cysts and, 110
  joint effusions and, 911
  peripheral meniscal vascularity and, 162
  postoperative meniscus and, 337
  rheumatoid arthritis and, 869
Inversion recovery sequences
  MAVRIC SL Fluid and, 17
  MR imaging and, 6
Iridocyclitis, 865
Iron, paramagnetic effect of, pigmented villonodular synovitis and, 878, 887f
Irregular Hoffa's infrapatellar fat-pad sign
  early juvenile chronic arthritis and, 866
  hemophilia and, 891, 893f
  joint sepsis and, 1020
  Lyme arthritis and, 895f
  osteoarthritis and, 897, 900f
  rheumatoid arthritis and, 870
  synovitis with, 859f
  synovium evaluation and, 858
Ischial avulsion fractures, hamstrings and, 70f
Ischial tuberosity
  biceps femoris muscle origin and, 69f
  semimembranosus muscle origin and, 70f
  semitendinosus muscle origin and, 71f
Isometry
  for ACL reconstruction, 489–491, 496f
  medial collateral ligament and, 582
  in PCL, 542
Isotropic arrangement, of collagen, 851
Isotropic resolution, using MR techniques, 3
ITB. *See* Iliotibial band
ITBFS (iliotibial band friction syndrome), 102, 115, 145f, 787, 790f–791f
ITT. *See* Iliotibial band
Ixodes ticks, 892

J

Jagerhut patella, 753f
Joint articular cartilage, 169f
Joint capsule
  ACL cysts and, 456f, 459f
  anatomy, 79f, 597f, 642f, 647f
  degenerative arthrosis and, 896f

diffuse pigmented villonodular synovitis and, 885f
ganglion cysts and, 917
ITB and, 81f
lateral meniscus and, 157
Lyme arthritis and, 894f
MCL injuries and, 611
medial aspect of knee and, 581
osteoarthritis and, 901f
pannus tissue, rheumatoid arthritis and, 874f
perimeniscal capillary plexus and, 162
peripheral, for surgical access, 325f
peripheral meniscus and, 153
pigmented villonodular synovitis and, 878, 882f, 886f
popliteal fossa view, 87f
popliteus hiatus area and, 680f
posterior horn medial meniscus and, 156
posteromedial corner and, 591f
rheumatoid arthritis and, 868f, 876f
suprapatellar pouch and, 90f
Joint dissection, axial MR imaging, 32
Joint fluid or effusions. *See also* Edema
  ACL roof impingement and, 520
  after total meniscectomy, 335
  axial plane checklist, 116, 144f
  chronic ACL tears and, 453
  diffuse pigmented villonodular synovitis and, 885f
  grade 3 signal intensity and, 301
  hyaline articular cartilage imaging and, 850
  key concepts, 911
  Lyme arthritis and, 895f
  MCL injuries and, 611
  meniscal pathology and, 173
    signal intensity of, 176
  meniscal tears and, recurrent, 355
  meniscocapsular separations and, 366
  MR appearance of, 911–912
  Osgood-Schlatter disease and, 817, 819f
  patellar bursae and, 825
  patellar dislocations and, 749
  PCL injuries and, 556
  popliteal cysts and, 913
  popliteus tendon sheath signaling and, 308
  rheumatoid arthritis and, 870, 871f, 873f–874f
  sagittal image
    absence of, collapsed patellar bursa and, 45
    checklist, 110, 135f
  staphylococcal infection and, 1024f
  transverse ligament and, 304
Joint function, meniscal transplantation and, 331
Joint line tenderness, discoid meniscus and, 291

Index

Joint locking. *See also* Locking
  lateral meniscus bucket-handle tears and, 215
  longitudinal meniscal tears and, 204
Joint replacement, MR assessment of articular cartilage and, 898
Joint sepsis, secondary signs of, 1020
Joint stabilization. *See also* Stability
  hamstring muscles and, 107
  menisci and, 172
Joint swelling, Brodie's abscess and, 1021
Jumper's knee, 798–799, 810f
Jumping sports, eccentric contraction of extensor mechanism and, 820
Juvenile chronic arthritis
  key concepts, 865
  MR studies of, 866
  patella baja and, 801
  popliteal cysts and, 914
  suprapatellar synovial hypertrophy and, 867f
  synovial enhancement in, 863f
  types of, 865
Juxtaarticular demineralization, rheumatoid arthritis and, 869

K

Kaplan fibers, 81, 654
Kasabach-Merritt syndrome, 1027
Keratan sulfate region, of articular cartilage, 845, 981f
Kick. *See* Direct blow
Kissing impaction fractures, 471
Kissing lesions, patellofemoral chondromalacia, 734f
Knee. *See also* Articular cartilage; Knee extension; Knee flexion; Knee rotation; *under* joint
  anatomy
    functional, 68
    lateral aspect, layer 1, 636, 641f
    lateral aspect, layer 2, 636, 642f
    lateral aspect, layer 3, 636, 643f, 649f
    medial aspect, layer 1, 581, 595f
    medial aspect, layer 2, 581, 596f
    medial aspect, layer 3, 581, 597f
    medial osseous landmarks, 599f
    normal, 32–62
      axial image, 32–35, 36f–41f
      coronal image, 54–56, 57f–62f
      sagittal image, 42–46, 47f–53f
  dislocations
    ACL injuries and, 548
    classification of, 573f
    multiligament injuries and, 572f, 688f, 691f
  general pathology affecting, 850
  introduction, 845
  laxity
    ACL tears and, 419f
    LCL tears and, 670f
    MR imaging of ACL injuries and, 437
    PCL adhesions, attachments, or subacute tears and, 424
    testing instruments, 429
  leg muscle innervation and, 64f
  muscles related to, 63–94
  thigh muscle innervation and, 63f
  total replacement, for osteonecrosis, 936
Knee extension
  ACL and, 397
  ACL cross-sectional area and, 398
  ACL roof impingement and, 520–521
  acute ACL stump entrapment and, 444
  anterolateral bundle of PCL and, 546f
  discoid meniscus and, 291
  iliotibial band and, 793f
  load transmission in, 172
  medial collateral ligament and, 585f
  MR imaging of ACL injuries and, 437
  pain, ganglion cysts and, 455
  patellar contact zones with, 782f
  patellofemoral joint and, 703
  posterolateral bundle of ACL and, 398
  posteromedial bundle of PCL and, 546f
  superolateral movement of patella in, 32
Knee flexion
  ACL and, 397
  ACL cross-sectional area and, 398
  ACL footprint and, 508f
    double-bundle, 509f
  ACL graft impingement and, 492
  ACL reconstruction and, 496f, 512f
    tibial tunnel placement, 516
  acute, quadriceps tendon tears and, 833
  anterolateral and posteromedial bands of PCL and, 540
  anteromedial bundle of ACL and, 398
  chronic PCL tears and, 553
  direct blow with, 416, 555f
  femoral attachment of ACL and, 402
  ITB syndrome and, 793f–794f
  lateral femoral contusions and, 471
  load transmission in, 172
  medial collateral ligament and, 585f, 599
  medial patellofemoral ligament and, 768f
  MR imaging of ACL injuries and, 437
  partial, posterior cruciate ligament and, 44
  patellar contact zones with, 782f
  patellar malalignment and abnormal tracking and, 698
  patellofemoral joint and, 703
  patellofemoral joint contact areas and angle of, 707f
  patellofemoral mechanics, 782f–783f
  PCL injuries and, 555f
  PCL rupture, meniscofemoral ligaments and, 542
  Pisani's sign and, 379
  plical impingement on medial femoral condyle and, 923
  popliteus muscle and, 74
  posterolateral corner and, 466
  sMCL and, 582
  suprapatellar plica and, 921
  tibiofibular joint dislocation and, 781f
  weight-bearing surface for, 104
Knee joint. *See under* joint
Knee rotation. *See also* Leg rotation
  AHLM foreshortening and, 306
  lateral femoral condyle elongation on MR imaging and, 436
  LCL and posterolateral structures and, 659
  meniscal tear findings and, 301
  meniscofemoral ligament mimicking meniscal pathology and, 310
  pseudo–bucket-handle tears and, 311
  twisting injury from, 414f
Krackow-Bunnell weave technique, 839, 840f
Krackow locking stitches, 812f
K-space sampling, 851
KT-1000 arthrometer, 429, 532f
KT-2000 arthrometer, 429, 532f

L

Lachman's test, 419f, 424, 442, 443f, 486
Laser-assisted arthroscopic surgery, osteonecrosis and, 936
Lateral alar fold, 930f
  lateral plica vs., 930, 931f
Lateral aponeurosis, 655
Lateral aponeurosis expansion, 644f, 646f
Lateral bifurcate ridge, AM and PL bundle femoral insertion sites and, 409f, 508f
Lateral capsular ligaments, lateral collateral ligament and, 636
Lateral capsule, 649f

Lateral circumflex branch, femoral
nerve, vastus lateralis and,
65f
Lateral circumflex femoral artery
rectus femoris and, 68f
vastus intermedius and, 67f
vastus medialis and, 66f
Lateral collateral ligament (LCL)
ACL tears and, 669f
ACL tears and coronal image
of, 442
acute ACL tears and, 443f
anatomy, 642f–644f, 646f, 648f,
653
anterior oblique band of, Segond
fractures and, 472
attachment of, 672f
axial image, 37f
checklist, 115, 143f
biceps femoris muscle strain and,
569f
biceps femoris tendon and, 668f
sagittal image, 46
biomechanics, 658–659
coronal image, 54
checklist, 98, 118f
dissection from lateral aspect, 80f
edema between ITB and, 791f
high-signal-intensity fat and MR
images of, 35
iliotibial band and, 784f
injuries, 673f–676f
distal course interruption, 691f
fracture avulsion of fibular
head attachment,
689f–690f
location and mechanism of,
662
MR imaging, 663
multiligament, 685f–688f,
691f
treatment of, 671, 671f
ITB and, 81f
ITB syndrome and, 793f–794f
joint capsule and, 86f
key concepts, 636
knee capsule and ligaments and,
92f
knee in partial flexion and, 93f
lateral femoral condyle and, 640f
lateral meniscal cysts and, 378
lateral meniscus and, 126f, 157
MR appearance of, 663
osseous avulsion, 670f, 688f
pathology, 118f
popliteal fossa view, 87f
popliteofibular ligament and,
652f
popliteus tendon and, 650f
posterior view, 88f
posterolateral corner and, 465,
672f
injuries, 468f, 676f
repair, 692f
sagittal plane dissection, 42
Segond fracture and, 479f
structural layers, 636–637
superficial dissection from
anterior, 91f
suprapatellar pouch and, 90f
tears
knee dislocation and, 572f
from lateral fibular head, 639f
multiligament injuries and,
575f–577f
partial, with laxity, 670f
Lateral combined knee dislocations,
573f
Lateral compartment
anatomy, 647f
contusions, 473f
ACL tears and, 439, 486
O'Donoghue's triad and, 417f
PCL injuries and, 563f–564f
osseous injuries, 470–471, 480f
PCL injuries and, 547
sagittal image, 83f
Lateral compartment cartilage, 101
sagittal image checklist, 104
Lateral condyle, plicae and, 920f
Lateral facet, on posterior patella,
94f
Lateral femoral condylar groove,
648f
Lateral femoral condylar notch,
separation from sulcus
terminalis, 471
Lateral femoral condyle (LFC)
ACL origin on, 35
ACL proximal attachment to,
397–398
ACL tears and, 129f, 418f–419f,
440
articular cartilage loss, PHLM
remnant and, 360f
axial image, 37f–39f, 112
bone infarcts of, 945f
chondral degeneration of, 899f
chondral delamination of, 163f
chondral fracture on, 977f
chondral shear fracture on, 976f
chondrocalcinosis and, 303f
chondromalacia and, 733f
contusions
ACL tears and, 480f, 684f
acute ACL tears and, 443f
MCL injuries and, 612
medial patellofemoral ligament
tear and, 757f, 759f–760f
patellar dislocations and, 749,
774f
MPFL disruption and, 761f
coronal image, 58f–62f
lateral collateral ligament and,
98
discoid meniscus and, 293
edema between ITB and, 791f
elongation, on MR imaging of
ACL injury, 436
erosion
ganglion cysts and, 455
hemophilia and, 893f
pannus tissue and, 875f
excessive lateral pressure and,
783f
fractures
ACL injuries and, 430
hemorrhagic effusion and,
912f
loose body and, 775f
patellar dislocations and, 748,
774f
subchondral linear, 1011f
gastrocnemius muscle origin
and, 75f
graphic depiction, 640f
hypoplastic femoral sulcus and,
745
intercondylar notch and, 113
ITB friction syndrome and, 793f,
796f
joint capsule and, 86f
lateral collateral ligament and,
653
lateral compartment contusions
and, 470
lateral head of gastrocnemius
muscle and, 46
osseous contusions of, 474f
osteochondral autograft transfer
system (OATS) of,
990f
osteochondritis dissecans of, 948,
958f
chronic chondral fissure, 960f
discoid meniscus and, 292
early epiphyseal ossification
and, 967f–968f
inferocentral, 959f
patellar dislocation and, 758f
pigmented villonodular synovitis
and, 886f
popliteus muscle origin and, 74f
popliteus tendon and, 74
posterior view, 88f
posttraumatic chondrosis of,
980f
sagittal image, 47f–49f
shear injury during dislocation,
762f–763f
spontaneous osteonecrosis and,
933
subchondral edema, medial
retinaculum tear and,
776f
weight-bearing surface of
osteochondritis dissecans and,
958f
osteonecrosis and, 935
Lateral femoral condyle articular
cartilage, 48f
Lateral femoral condyle cartilage
coronal image, 59f–60f
sagittal image, 47f, 49f
Lateral gastrocnemius muscle, 644f,
646f–647f
Lateral gastrocnemius tendon,
647f–648f
anatomy, 655–656
posterolateral corner injuries and,
664f
sagittal image, 108
Lateral geniculate artery, 162
Lateral gutter, plicae and, 920f
Lateral head gastrocnemius muscle,
sagittal image, 48f–49f
Lateral inferior genicular artery,
169f
Lateral intercondylar ridge, ACL
footprint and, 409f, 508f

Index

Lateral intermuscular septum
  biceps femoris muscle origin and, 69f
  vastus lateralis obliquus fibers and, 65f
Lateral joint capsule, lateral collateral ligament and, 636
Lateral knee compartment, anterior mid-coronal sections of, 55–56
Lateral margin bipartite patella, 741
Lateral meniscocapsular ligaments, sagittal image, 108
Lateral meniscus. *See also* Anterior horn lateral meniscus; Posterior horn lateral meniscus
  ACL injuries and, 424
  anatomy, 33, 157–158, 642f, 647f
    normal, 34
  anterior cruciate ligament and, 164f
  anterior view, knee in partial flexion and, 93f
  arthrosis after meniscectomy of, 335, 361f
  axial plane checklist, 114, 141f
  body
    coronal image, 60f
    sagittal image, 47f
  central rhomboid attachment of, transverse ligament and, 304
  complete discoid, 296f
  coronal image, 54, 89f
  coronary ligament to, 108
  discoid, medial discoid meniscus vs., 290
  discoid-like, 298f–299f
  discoid meniscus and, 293
  double delta sign of bucket-handle tear, 235f
  floating meniscus and, 368, 375f
  incomplete discoid, 295f
  injuries, ACL and MCL injuries and, 423
  knee in partial flexion and, 93f
  lateral collateral ligament and, 80f, 636
  meniscal flounce in, simulated vs. true, 312
  meniscofemoral ligaments and, 309, 322f
  meniscotibial attachment of, 476f
  morphology, 180
  normal superior deficiency of PMF in, 158f, 319f
  osteoarthritis and, 901f
  parameniscal cysts and, 378
  partial meniscectomy of, subchondral sclerosis and, 360f
  plicae and, 920f
  popliteal fossa view, 87f
  popliteus complex and, 645f
  popliteus hiatus area and, 680f
  popliteus muscle and, 74
  popliteus tendon and, 166f
  posterior root attachment, coronal image, 60f–61f
  posterior view, 88f, 93f
  posterolateral corner and, 466
  reconstruction of, allograft for, 348f
  removal, degenerative joint changes and, 172
  root attachment, ACL insertion vs., 410
  sagittal image, 46
    checklist, 103, 126f
  suprapatellar pouch and, 90f
  tears
    all-inside repair of, 211f, 340f
    allograft transplant for, 343f
    asymptomatic, ACL reconstruction and, 330
    bicompartmental bucket-handle, 230f
    bucket-handle, 215–216, 231f–234f
      displaced complex, 477f
      pseudohypertrophy of anterior horn and, 311
    flap, 255
      displaced, in popliteus tendon sheath, 258, 282f
      displaced, reactive plateau edema and, 258
    horizontal cleavage, cyst and, 201f
    horizontal fish-mouth, 198f
    longitudinal, 206f, 211f
    osteoarthritis and, 899f–900f
    peripheral, obliquity of popliteus tendon sheath vs., 308, 320f
    radial, 240f–241f
      meniscal cyst and, 386f
    repair characteristics, 329
    root, 246, 254f
      arthroscopic repair of, 330
      displaced, with ACL tear, 278f
    suturing, 341f
    transverse or oblique, 172
  vascularity of, at popliteal hiatus, 162
  vascularized synovial fringe of, 163
  Wrisberg-ligament type discoid, 291
Lateral middle facet, 697
Lateral notch sign, 471
Lateral oblique intermeniscal ligament, 321f
Lateral patellar facet
  about, 700
  axial image, 37f
    checklist, 112, 137f
  bipartite dysplasia of, 739f
  cartilage repair for, 777f–778f
  chondromalacia underlying synchondrosis of, 740f
  concave articular surface, 697
  coronal image, 57f
  excessive lateral pressure syndrome and, 752f, 785f
  Fulkerson osteotomy and, 738f
  knee extension and, 33
  lateral patellar subluxation and, 704
  lateral patellar tilt and, 704–705
  lateral retinacular release and, 786f
  medial aspect of
    chondromalacia and chondrocalcinosis and, 730f
    fissuring, 727f
    osteochondritis dissecans of, 739f
  sagittal image, 49f, 128f
  superficial chondral erosion, 732f
Lateral patellar fascicle, lateral retinaculum and, 751
Lateral patellar ligament, static patellofemoral joint stabilizing by, 703
Lateral patellar plica, 930, 930f–931f. *See also* Lateral plicae
Lateral patellar retinaculum, 641f, 647f
Lateral patellar subluxation, 744
Lateral patellofemoral angle, 745
Lateral patellofemoral ligament, 703, 752f
Lateral patellofemoral recesses, loose bodies in, 116
Lateral patellotibial ligament, 752f
Lateral plicae, 930, 930f
  anterior perspective, 920f
  vertical or vertical oblique, 932f
Lateral retinaculum
  anatomy, 639f, 642f, 784f
  attachments, 35
  axial image, 37f–38f
    checklist, 112, 139f
  coronal image, 57f
    ITB blends with, 56
  disease, patella baja and, 801
  focal fat pad edema and, 111
  iliotibial tract and, 81f
  insufficient, medial patellar subluxation and, 705
  ITB and, 81f
  lateral patellar subluxation and, 704
  lateral plica and, 930
  longitudinal, knee capsule and ligaments and, 92f
  osseous avulsion of, 785f
  patellar stability and, 779f
  release
    knee subluxation or dislocations and, 747
    thickening and scarring and, 786f
  static patellofemoral joint stabilizing by, 703
  tight, ELPS and, 751–752
  transverse, knee capsule and ligaments and, 92f
  vastus lateralis muscle and, 751
Lateral superior geniculate (genicular) artery, 36f, 49f, 169f
Lateral supracondylar line of femur
  biceps femoris muscle origin and, 69f
  plantaris muscle origin and, 76f

Lateral synovial recess, ITB syndrome and, 788
Lateral tibial articular facet
  anatomy, 700–701, 701f
  knee extension and, 32
Lateral tibial condyle, 88f
Lateral tibial cortex, chronic active osteomyelitis and, 1025f
Lateral tibial plateau
  axial image, 40f
  central depression fracture (Type III), 1000f
  chondral degeneration and, 101
  chondral erosion, 854f
    partial meniscectomy and, 360f
  chondrocalcinosis and, 303f
  contusions, ACL tears and, 445f, 477f, 528f
  cupping, discoid meniscus and, 293
  displaced, acute ACL tear and, 443f
  fractures, 1001, 1005f
    ACL injuries and, 430, 482f
    posterolateral corner injuries and, 679f–680f
    pigmented villonodular synovitis and, 886f
  posterior, fracture in, 322f
  posterolateral corner injuries and, 676f
  sagittal image
    cartilage, 47f
    popliteofibular ligament and, 46
  split depression fracture (Type II), 1000f, 1005f–1006f
  split fracture (Type I), 1000f, 1005f
  spontaneous osteonecrosis and, 933
  trabecular contusion, 682f
Lateral tibial plateau articular cartilage, 94f
  coronal image, 59f–62f
  sagittal image, 48f–49f, 104
Lateral trochlear groove, 37f
Lateral trochlear groove cartilage
  axial image, 38f
  coronal image, 58f
  ELPS and, 752
  sagittal image, 48f
Lateral tuberosity, knee subluxation or dislocations and, 747
Lax bundles, ACL graft, 520
Lax meniscus, simulated vs. true, 312
Layer 1
  of lateral aspect of knee, 636, 641f
  of medial aspect of knee, 581, 595f. see also deep fascia
Layer 2
  of lateral aspect of knee, 636, 642f
  of medial aspect of knee, 581, 596f
Layer 3
  of lateral aspect of knee, 636, 643f, 649f
  of medial aspect of knee, 581, 597f
LCL. See Lateral collateral ligament
Leg extension
  vastus intermedius and, 67f
  vastus lateralis and, 65f
  vastus medialis and, 66f
Leg muscle innervation, 64f
Leg rotation. See also Knee rotation
  ACL injuries and, 416
  gracilis muscle and, 73
  miserable malalignment syndrome and, 780f
  PCL injuries and, 547
  popliteus muscle and, 74
Lesser saphenous vein, leg muscle innervation and, 64f
LFC. See Lateral femoral condyle
Ligament augmentation device, intraarticular polyester, 488
Ligamentization, ACL graft revascularization and, 493, 517, 524f
Ligament of Humphrey
  anatomy, normal, 33–34
  coronal image, 54
  displaced medial meniscal bucket-handle tear and, 227f
  interstitial PCL tear and, 571f
  normal, PCL injuries mistaken for, 548
  PHLM attachment to medial femoral condyle and, 321f, 323f
  pitfalls interpreting findings on, 309–311
  popliteal fossa view, 87f
  popliteus complex and, 645f
  posterior cruciate ligament and, 157, 542, 543f–545f
  sagittal image, 50f–51f
    PCL and, 44, 106, 322f
Ligament of Wrisberg. See also Wrisberg variant of discoid meniscus
  anatomy, normal, 33–34
  attached to displaced PHLM, 476f
  coronal image, 54
  intact, 297f
  PCL interstitial tear and, 562f
  peripheral tear of PHLM vs., 301
  PHLM attachment to medial femoral condyle and, 321f, 323f
  pitfalls interpreting findings on, 309–311
  popliteal fossa view, 87f
  popliteus complex and, 645f
  posterior cruciate ligament and, 157, 542, 543f–545f
  posterior view, 93f
  sagittal image, PCL and, 44, 106
Ligament stretching, of posterior cruciate ligament, 548
Ligamentum mucosum. See also Infrapatellar plica
  acute ACL injuries on arthrography and, 430
  anterior meniscofemoral ligament vs., 926f
  location of, 920f
  MR imaging, 438, 921
  vascular supply to ACL and PCL and, 400
Ligamentum patellae
  cruciate ligaments and, 77f
  lateral collateral ligament and, 80f
  pes anserinus tendons and, 78f
  sagittal image, 82f
  superficial dissection from anterior, 91f
Linea aspera
  biceps femoris muscle origin and, 69f
  lateral aspect, vastus lateralis and, 65f
  vastus intermedius and, 67f
Linear articular cartilage injuries (Type I), 991f
Link protein, 847, 981f
Lipohemarthrosis
  bone contusion or fracture and, 912
  characteristics, 1019
  in hemorrhagic effusion, imaging of, 1013f
Lipoma, meniscal cysts and, 379
Lipoma arborescens, 908, 909f–910f
Load-bearing function
  ACL and, 424
  ACL elongation and, 412
  ACL injuries and, 416
  in ACL with extension, 402
  condylar meniscus contact area and, 359f
  hoop tension in segmental meniscectomy and, 174
  lateral femoral condyle contusion and, 763f
  lateral meniscus tear repair and, 329
  MCL–bone complex and, 635
  medial meniscus flap tear and, 283f
  meniscus and, 154, 159
  osteonecrosis treatment and, 936
  PCL and, 546f
  posterior horn remnant, chondral delamination and, 363f
Localized nodular pigmented villonodular synovitis, 878, 879f–880f
Localized nodular synovitis, 877
Localized pigmented villonodular synovitis, 111, 877, 883f–884f
Locking. See also Joint locking
  discoid meniscus and, 291
  in fixed flexion, meniscal tears and, 173
  synovial plicae and, 921
Loculations, meniscal cysts and, 377, 379

Index

Longitudinal loading, circumferential fibers or bundles of meniscus and, 159
Longitudinal meniscal tears. *See also* Flap tears
  ACL tears and, 373f
  characteristics, 203–204
  classification of, 182, 186
  with flap and radial components, 282f
  graphic depiction, 191f
  horizontal tears and, 184
  inside-out repair of, 338
  of medial meniscus, 208f
  surface types, 205f–207f
  with truncated free edge flap component, 284f
  vertical, 195f
  repair of, 329, 339f–341f
Longitudinal patellar fractures, 1015
Longitudinal splitting, radial collagen fibers in transverse zone of meniscus and, 160
Loose bodies
  axial image, 144f
  coronal image
    appearance and location, 102
    joint spaces in articular cartilage and, 101
  intercondylar notch signal mistaken for, 312
  in joint fluid/effusion, 110, 116
  medial and lateral articular cartilage, 104
  meniscal tears and, 173
  osteoarthritis and, 898, 900f–901f
  osteochondritis dissecans and, 948
  patellar dislocations and, 775f
  popliteal cysts and, 903f, 913
  pseudo, pitfalls interpreting findings on, 312
  synovial chondromatosis and, 902f–903f
  transient lateral subluxation of patella and, 112
Lupus erythematosus, systemic
  bone infarcts and, 946
  in children, 866
  spontaneous osteonecrosis and, 933
Lyme arthritis, 858, 892, 894f–895f
Lymphadenopathy, juvenile chronic arthritis and, 865

M

MacIntosh lateral substitution over-the-top ACL repair, 517
Maffucci syndrome, 1027
Magic-angle phenomenon, 313, 551, 715
Magnetic resonance (MR) imaging. *See also specific muscles or sites*
  of ACL injuries, 429
    accuracy of, 486
    key concepts, 436
    normal characteristics of, 437–438
    tears, partial vs. complete and, 448
    techniques for, 436–437
  of ACL reconstruction
    postoperative, 516–517
    patellar tendon, 522
    roof impingement and, 520–521
    side wall impingement and, 522
  acquisition time for, 7
  advanced applications for, 10–18, 11f–14f, 16f–17f
  after ACL reconstruction, 514f
  after meniscal transplantation, 332
  after meniscectomy, 334–336
  of aneurysmal sacs, 918
  of articular surfaces, 849
  artifacts, 302–303
  of atypical cysts, 914
  basic pulse sequences in, 5–6, 6f
  of bone infarcts, 944
  of calcium pyrophosphate dihydrate deposition disease, 388
  of chondromalacia, 712–713
  cine imaging, patellar tracking using, 746
  clinical diagnosis factors using, 3
  of discoid meniscus, 290, 292, 294
  of dorsal defect of patella, 743
  equipment and surface coil variations, 289
  of extensor muscle injuries, 834
  fat suppression and, 21–23
  fat surrounding transverse ligament and, 304
  of fractures, 1001
  fraying vs. tearing meniscus and, 307
  of hemophilia, 891
  image enhancement filters, 23–24
  of juvenile chronic arthritis, 866
  kinematic
    patellar tracking using, 746
    of patellofemoral joint, 703–705
  of knee anatomy, normal, 31–62
  knee rotation and, 306
  of lateral collateral ligament, 663
  of lipoma arborescens, 908
  of Lyme arthritis, 892
  of medial collateral ligament, 603–604, 604f–610f
    associated findings, 611–612
  of medial plicae, 923
  of meniscal cysts, 378
  meniscal tear detection accuracy using, 288–289
  of meniscofemoral ligaments, 310
  of meniscus
    degeneration and tears, 175–181
    flap, signal direction and, 258
    grade 2 vs. grade 3 signal intensity and, 301–302
    grading system, 176–180
    signal intensity and, 175–176
    postoperative, 333
    protocols for, 146–147, 148f
    middle perforating collagen fibers vs. adjacent meniscal tissue on, 160
  of Osgood-Schlatter disease, 817
  of osseous fractures and bone contusions, 1002
  of osteoarthritis, 898
  of osteochondritis dissecans, 949
  of osteonecrosis, 935–936
  parallel imaging for, 20–21
  of patellar dislocations, 748–749
  of patellar tendinosis, 799–800
  of patellar tendon tears, 801
  of patellofemoral joint, kinematic, 703–705
  of PCL, normal, 551
  of PCL injuries, 556
    protocols, 551–552
    tears, 540
  of pigmented villonodular synovitis, 878
  of plicae, 921
    medial, 923
  of popliteal cysts, 864f, 914
  positioning for, 4
  of post–primary meniscal repair, 333
  of quadriceps tendon and tears, 839
  of quadriceps tendon tears, 834
  of rheumatoid arthritis, 869–870
  scan parameters, 7–9, 9f
  segmentation in, 25, 26f
  sequence and parameter acronyms, 27
  signal intensity in healing menisci and, 337–338
  of Sinding-Larsen-Johansson syndrome, 818
  SNR in, 8
  spatial resolution for, 7
  speckled signal, central rhomboid attachment of AHLM and, 306, 316f
  of stress fractures, 1003
  3-T imaging considerations, 18–20
  of thrombosis, 918
  of tibial plateau fractures, 1004
  trade-offs for, 8–9, 9f
  uniformity corrections, 23–24
  variations in arthroscopy accuracy vs., 289
Magnetic susceptibility, 3.0T imaging and, 19
Magnetization transfer contrast, articular cartilage imaging and, 851
Malaise, Lyme arthritis and, 892
Malalignment
  nonarticular tibial fractures and, 1009
  patella realignment procedures, 830
  patellar tendinosis and, 798

Malalignment syndrome, variable cartilage damage and, 697
Maquet's procedure, 747, 779f, 830
Marginal patellar fractures, 1018f
Marrow. *See also* Subchondral edema
   coronal plane checklist, 123f
   in corticated ossicle, MR imaging of, 389
   edema
      juvenile chronic arthritis and, 866
      osteonecrosis and, 935
   ischemic subchondral, 364f
   metaphyseal–diaphyseal low-signal-intensity red marrow inhomogeneity, 1003
   multifocal osteomyelitis and, 1021
   red, in polycythemia vera, 1012f
   sagittal plane checklist, 109, 133f
   Segond fracture fragments and, 472
   T1-weighted medial sagittal images and, 43
Marrow fat, 146
Marrow proliferative disorders, 1003
Marrow replacement disorders, imaging, 1003
MARS high-resolution sequence, 17
Matrix proteins, noncollagenous, 845
Matrix resolution, imaging protocols, 150
MAVRIC SL, 17–18, 18f
   parallel imaging and, 21
MAVRIC SL Fluid, 17
MAVRIC SL PD, 17
MCL. *See* Medial collateral ligament
McMurray test
   discoid meniscus and, 291
   meniscal tears and, 173
Mechanical loading. *See also* Load-bearing function
   meniscus and, 154
Medial capsular ligament, 366. *See also* Deep medial collateral ligament
   anatomy, 654
   joint capsule and, 581
Medial capsule
   disruption, anterior drawer sign and, 424
   tears, MCL rupture and, 599
Medial circumflex artery, gracilis muscle and, 73
Medial collateral ligament (MCL)
   anatomy, 34, 584f–590f
      functional, 77f, 581–583
      oblique fibers, 79f
   attachments of, 767
   avulsion, meniscotibial ligament avulsion and, 376f
   axial image, 37f, 39f–40f
   checklist, 115, 142f
   biomechanics of, 602
   bursitis, 612, 630f
   coronal image, 55, 60f, 89f
      checklist, 98, 117f
   cut, proximal fibers of, 79f
   displaced flap tear and, 277f
   epicondylar attachment, avulsion fracture, 616f–617f
   in flexion, 585f
   healing and treatment, 635
   incarcerated into medial compartment, 620f
   infolding in distal avulsion of, 624f
   injuries
      ACL and lateral meniscus injuries and, 423
      classification of, 601–602
      location and mechanism of, 599, 599f–600f
      in O'Donoghue's triad, 417f
      O'Donoghue's triad and, 416
      treatment of ACL injuries and, 635
   insertion for, 41f
   key concepts, 581
   knee capsule and ligaments and, 92f
   laxity, 581
   longitudinal medial meniscal tear and, 227f
   longitudinal meniscal tears and, 203
   magnetic resonance appearance of, 603–604
   magnetic resonance imaging, associated findings, 611–612
   medial meniscal attachment to, 156
   medial patellofemoral ligament and, 756f
      medial retinacular tear and, 773f
   meniscocapsular separations and, 368
   meniscofemoral ligament tear and, 371f
   ossification, Pellegrini-Stieda disease and, 627f
   pathology, 117f
   PCL injuries and, 556
   pes anserinus and, 632f
   pes anserinus tendons and, 78f
   pes tendons and, 593f–598f
   popliteal fossa view, 87f
   posterior oblique ligament and, 586f
   posterior view, 88f, 93f
   posteromedial corner, 591f–592f
      injuries, 602
   sagittal image, 42–43, 53f, 107, 131f
   secondary stability by ACL of, 412, 412f
   sprains, 600f, 606f–608f
      classification of, 601
      grade 3, 610f
      tears of MPFL and medial retinaculum vs., 764f–765f
   superficial dissection from anterior, 91f
   suprapatellar pouch and, 90f
   tears
      assessment, 588
      chronic, 611–612
      classification of, 601
      complete, 604
      coronal image, 98
      in deep capsular layer, 376f
      grade 2, 604
      grade 3, 476f, 604, 604f, 610f
         ACL grade 3 tear and, 625f–626f
         with femoral ligamentous stump, 615f
         ligament discontinuity and, 613f–614f
      knee dislocation and, 572f
      laxity and, 581, 620f–621f
      with ligament folding, 624f
      with ligament laxity, 623f
      ligamentous, 606f
      mechanism of injury, 1001
      meniscocapsular separations and, 367, 369f
      MR referral and, 288
      multiligament injuries and, 575f–577f
      partial, 603–604
      retracted distal, 618f–619f
      valgus hyperextension stress and, 751
   vascular supply, 169f
Medial collateral ligament (MCL) bursa, pitfalls interpreting findings on, 313
Medial combined knee dislocations, 573f
Medial compartment
   cartilage, 101
      sagittal plane checklist, 104
   contusions, 473
   dislodged ACL graft debris and, 535f
   LCL and posterolateral structures and, 659
   PCL deficiencies and, 547
   transplantation preparation, 343f
Medial condyle, 587f
   plicae and, 920f
   synovial capsule of, 601
Medial epicondyle of femur
   anatomy, 79f
   marked on skin, 768f
   medial collateral ligament and, 142f
   MPFL course and, 756f
   MPFL reattachment to, 750
Medial facet. *See* Medial patellar facet
Medial femoral condyle
   articular cartilage stem cell paste graft preparation for, 998f
   avascular necrosis, PCL reconstruction and, 556
   axial image, 38f–39f, 112
   bone infarcts of, 945f–946f
   chondral degeneration and, 101
   chondral delamination, 980f

Index

chondral flap, 970f
chondrosis of, 572
coronal image, 58f–62f
    triangular attachment of PCL and, 55
defect, full thickness, 970f
edema
    subchondral fracture and, 938f
    in subchondral ischemia of, 364f
erosion, pannus tissue and, 875f
flap tear and, 256f
    edema extension to, 275f
fractures
    insufficiency, 940f
    subchondral edema and, 938f, 941f
gastrocnemius muscle origin and, 75f
Gillquist view of posteromedial knee and, 252f
intercondylar notch and, 113
knee extension and, 32
MCL injuries and, 599
MCL origin and, 115
medial patellofemoral ligament and, 748
medial plica impingement of, 923, 924f
meniscal bucket-handle tears and, 217f, 223f
meniscal root tear and, 249f
obstructed arthroscopic visualization of PHMM and, 289
osteochondral fracture on, 977f
osteochondritis dissecans of, 947–948, 950f
    inferocentral, 959f
osteonecrosis, 939f
posterior cruciate ligament origin and, 35, 540, 541f
posterior oblique ligament and, 629f
posterior view, 88f
sagittal image, 52f–53f
    posterior cruciate ligament and, 44
    vastus medialis muscle and, 43
sagittal plane checklist, 127f
tibial plateau contact area with, 359f
tibial spine avulsions and, 472
tophaceous gout and, 890f
unstable osteochondritis dissecans, 953f–954f
weight-bearing surface of osteochondritis dissecans and, 951f–952f
    osteonecrosis and, 935
    spontaneous osteonecrosis and, 933
Medial femoral condyle cartilage
coronal image, 58f–60f
sagittal image, 52f
Medial gastrocnemius, 584f
Medial genicular vein, 85f
Medial geniculate (genicular) artery, 85f, 162. See also Middle geniculate artery

Medial head gastrocnemius muscle
gastrocnemius muscle origin and, 75f
plantaris tendon and, 76
sagittal image, 50f–51f
strains of, 75
Medial inferior genicular artery, 53f, 169f
Medial intercondylar tubercle, ACL attachment and, 398
Medial linea aspera, vastus medialis and, 66f
Medial margin fracture of patella, 748
Medial meniscus. See also Anterior horn medial meniscus; Posterior horn medial meniscus
anatomy, 156, 169f, 584f
    normal, 34
    popliteus tendon and, 186f
anterior view, knee in partial flexion and, 93f
axial plane checklist, 114, 141f
body of, 53f, 60f
coronal image, 89f
discoid, lateral discoid meniscus vs., 290
discoid meniscus and, 293
floating meniscus and, 368
graft for, 342f
injuries, in O'Donoghue's triad, 416
lateral meniscus mobility vs., 158
medial collateral ligament and, 55, 587f, 589f–590f
meniscal cysts and, 378, 380f
meniscectomy, anteroposterior motion and, 154
meniscocapsular separations and, 366–368
meniscotibial dMCL rupture and, 583
morphology, 180
partial meniscectomy
    and load transference in, 359f
    subchondral edema after, 336f
partial volume averaging fat and structures in concavity of, 309
plicae and, 920f
popliteal fossa view, 87f
popliteus complex and, 645f
posterior cruciate ligament and, 164f
posterior root attachment
    coronal image, 60f–61f
    sagittal image, 125f
posterior view, 88f, 93f
posteromedial corner and, 591f
resection, degenerative joint changes and, 172
reverse Segond fractures and, 574f
root attachment of, PCL and, 545f
sagittal image, 43–44
    checklist, 103, 125f
small bursa between deep layer of MCL and, 55

tears
ACL tears and, 210f, 484f–485f
bucket-handle, 213–215, 217f–230f
    ACL injuries and, 427f
complex, 286f
degenerative, 588f
flap, 260f
    ACL with AM and PL bundle disruption and, 402f
    blunted body and, 267f
    blunted inferior surface and, 268f
    central notch displacement in, 270f
    cyst development and, 287f
    displaced into coronary recess, 276f
    medial tibial plateau edema and, 283f
    PCL injuries and, 566f
    radial tear and, 281f
    superior rotation in, 273f–274f
    vertical superior folding of, 280f
football and basketball injuries and, 329
horizontal, 200f
longitudinal, 206f, 208f–210f, 227f
MCL rupture and, 599
mechanism of injury, 1001
O'Donoghue's triad and, 417f
PCL injuries and, 553
peripheral, posteromedial crush injury and, 473
peripheral vertical, 209f
peripheral vertical, capsular attachment mistaken for, 313
posteroinferior corner, ACL disruption and, 307
posteromedial tibial plateau osseous injuries and, 470
radial with peripheral extension, 244f
root, 246
    arthroscopic repair of, 330
    displaced, 247f, 250f–253f
    Gillquist view of, 252f
    nondisplaced, 248f–249f
    with residual meniscotibial ligament, 250f
tibial attachment sites, 164f
transplantation, three-tunnel technique for, 344f–345f
vascularized synovial fringe of, 163
Medial oblique intermeniscal ligament, 321f
Medial odd facet, 697
Medial patella, rectus femoris origin and, 68f
Medial patellar facet, 700, 715f
axial image, 37f
    checklist, 112, 137f
basal degeneration in inferior central ridge near, 732f
blister, 722f

Medial patellar facet (continued)
  chondral softening, 722f–723f
  chondromalacia, medial plica and, 921, 925f, 929f
  contusions, 757f
    patellar dislocations and, 749, 759f–760f
  convex articular surface, 697
  crabmeat erosion of, 728f
  fractures, patellar dislocations and, 766f, 774f
  graphic depiction, 590f
  knee extension and, 33
  lateral aspect, fissuring of, 727f
  medial patellofemoral ligament reconstruction and, 771f–772f
  medial plica impingement of, 923
  osteochondritis dissecans of, 744
  patellar dislocation and, 758f
  posterior, 94f
  sagittal image, 128f
Medial patellar fascicle, medial retinaculum and, 751
Medial patellar margin, medial patellofemoral ligament and, 748
Medial patellar plica, 590f, 923. See also Medial plica
Medial patellar retinaculum, 591f, 595f–596f
  injuries, patellar subluxation or dislocations and, 745
Medial patellar subluxation, 744
Medial patellofemoral ligament (MPFL)
  contusions, 757f
  disruption, patellar dislocations and, 747–748, 750
  graphic depiction, 756f
  knee flexion and, 768f
  medial patellotibial ligament and, 756f
  reconstruction, 771f–772f, 777f–778f
  tears
    deep layer of, detachment or, 757f
    MCL sprain vs., 764f–765f
    patellar dislocation and, 759f–761f, 767f
    vastus medialis obliquus tears and, 769f–770f
Medial patellofemoral recesses, loose bodies in, 116
Medial patellotibial ligament, 756f
Medial plica
  anatomy, 921
  anterior perspective, 920f
  axial image, 37f, 112, 137f
  characteristics, 923
  medial patellar facet chondromalacia and, 925f
  sagittal plane checklist, 111, 136f
  shelf-like, 921, 925f, 929f
  Type C, 924f
Medial retinaculum
  anatomy, 79f
  attachments, 35
    vastus medialis and, 56
  axial image, 37f, 40f
  checklist, 112, 139f
  bilaminar morphology of, 748, 779f
  coronal image, 57f, 59f, 117f
  deep layer, 590f
  disruption, patellar dislocation and, 748–749
  Hoffa's infrapatellar fat pad and, 35
  joint capsule and, 581
  longitudinal, knee capsule and ligaments and, 92f
  medial patellofemoral ligament fibers and, 756f, 770f
  medial patellofemoral ligament tear and, 757f
  patellar dislocations and, 750, 758f
  patellar stability and, 779f
  sMCL and, 622f
  static patellofemoral joint stabilizing by, 703
  tears, 614f
    axial image, 112
    chondral degeneration after, 776f
    MCL sprain vs., 764f–765f
    medial patellofemoral ligament and, 773f
    partial, 779f
    patellar dislocations and, 766f, 774f–775f
    patellar tendon tears and, 811f
    vastus medialis obliquus tears and, 769f–770f
    tight, medial patellar subluxation and, 705
  tophaceous gout and, 890f
  transverse, knee capsule and ligaments and, 92f
  vastus medialis muscle and, 751
  vastus medialis obliquus and, 755f
Medial superior genicular artery, 36f, 169f
Medial supracondylar line, vastus medialis and, 66f
Medial tibial articular facet, 32, 700–701, 701f
Medial tibial condyle, 55, 88f
Medial tibial plateau
  complex tear and subchondral edema of, 282f
  contusions, 229f
    contrecoup, longitudinal meniscal tear and, 212f
    PCL tear and, 563f–564f
    posterolateral corner injury and, 683f
  flap tear and, 256f
  edema of, 271f
  subchondral edema of, 264f, 283f
  fractures
    contrecoup, peripheral meniscal vertical tear and, 208f
    PCL tear and, 574f
    Type IV, 1000f
  Gillquist view of posteromedial knee and, 252f
  meniscal root tear and, 249f
  meniscus remnant and erosion of, 360f
  osteonecrosis, 939f
    spontaneous, 933
  sagittal image, 107
Medial tibial plateau articular cartilage, 94f
  coronal image, 58f–62f
  sagittal image, 52f, 104
Medial trochlear groove cartilage, axial image, 38f
Median patellar ridge, axial image, 37f
Median patellar ridge cartilage
  axial image, 112
  sagittal image, 50f–51f
Mediopatellar plica, 921. See also Medial plica
Men
  cystic adventitial disease and, 917f
  osteochondritis dissecans and, 947
Meniscal cavitations
  complete discoid meniscus and, 296f
  discoid meniscus and, 294
Meniscal contusion, use of term, 307, 317f
Meniscal cysts, 377–380
  chondromatosis mimicking, 382f
  deep radial tears and, 330
  discoid meniscus and, 292, 294
  flap tears of body/PHMM and, 287f
  horizontal cleavage tears or flap tears and, 183
  horizontal tears and, 185, 185f, 199f–202f, 381f, 383f, 387f
  meniscal remnant or postrepair meniscus and, 334
  mucoid ACL and, 462f
  partial meniscectomy and, 356f–357f
  popliteal cysts and, 916f
  radial tears and, 386f
Meniscal degeneration and tears. See also Meniscectomy; Recurrent meniscal tears
  ACL injuries and, 416, 423, 486
  ACL reconstructions and, 487
  ACL treatment methods and, 487
  acute trauma vs. degenerative, 180
  axial image confirmation of, 114
  calcium pyrophosphate dihydrate deposition disease and, 388–389
  chronic PCL injuries and, 572
  circumferential, axial image, 32
  classification of, 182f–194f
    circumferential or surface patterns, 186

Index

cross-sectional patterns, 182–183
horizontal, 184–185, 185f
key concepts, 182
longitudinal, 182
clinical signs, 173
closed tears
attenuated grade 3 signal intensity in, 175, 192f, 301
confined fibrocartilage separation in, 191f
complex, coronal images and, 43
differential diagnosis, 173
discoid meniscus and, 291
flap tears, 155f
axial image, 181f
classification of, 182
coronal image, 100
sagittal image, 103
focal or globular degeneration, 187f
grade 1 signal intensity, 175, 177
grade 2 signal intensity, 175, 177–179
intrasubstance degeneration, 188f
MR accuracy in detection of, 288
mucinous degeneration and, 190f
grade 3 signal intensity, 175, 179–181
gradient echo (GRE) for, 175
horizontal tears, 184–186
meniscocapsular separations, 366–368, 368f–376f
MR accuracy in detection of, 288–289
MR findings, 175–181
classification of, 182
pathogenesis and clinical presentation, 172–174
PCL injuries and, 547
pitfalls interpreting findings on, 301–314, 314f–320f
popliteal cysts and, 916
popliteus hiatus area and, 157, 158f
radial tears
classification of, 182
coronal image, 100
free edge, 103, 195f, 236f, 240f–243f
hoop tension and, 161
repair
MR appearance after, 337–338
popliteal artery location and, 35
retear indicators, after meniscectomy, 336
sagittal plane images and, 42
secondary, ACL deficiencies and, 487
short tau inversion recovery for, 175
spontaneous osteonecrosis and, 935

T1 for, 175
T2 for, 175
tear patterns, 195f–287f
axial images and identification of, 183
bucket-handle, 213–216
medial meniscus, 217f–230f
complex, 196f
flap, 196f, 247, 255, 256f, 257–259, 259f–287f
horizontal, 197f–202f
longitudinal, 203–204, 205f–212f
radial, 195f, 236f, 237–238, 240f–245f
radial root, 246–247, 247f–254f
vertical longitudinal, 195f
tear rim widths and repair of, 329
treatment options, 327–332
vacuum phenomenon and, 312
Meniscal fibrocartilage
ACL and PCL insertion sites in, 401f
complete discoid meniscus and, 294, 296f
confined separation in closed tear and, 191f
discoid meniscus and, 291
flap tears of, 255, 262f
grade 2 intrasubstance degeneration, 188f
idealized structure, 168f
intrasubstance degeneration and tear in, 190f
load transmission by, 172
osteoarthritis and, 898
red zone of, connective tissue vs., 162
root attachments, 55
Meniscal flounce
lateral, sagittal image, 324f
meniscal tear findings and, 301
simulated vs. true, 312
Meniscal folding, redundant, 324f
simulated vs. true, 312
Meniscal ossicles, 389, 393f
Meniscal rasping, meniscal repair and, 329
Meniscal remnants
graphic depiction, 352f
imaging of, 351f, 353f–354f
intrameniscal signal conversion and, 334, 351f
medial tibial plateau erosion and, 360f
PHMM, retear of, 358f
recurrent meniscal tears and, 355
Meniscal replacement, 326
for meniscal tears, 328
Meniscal roots
coronal image, 100
Gillquist view of posteromedial knee and, 252f
innervation, 163
Meniscal transplantation, 331–332
graft preparation for, 342f–343f
for tears, 328

three-tunnel technique for, 332f, 344f–345f
stem cells and, 347f
Meniscectomy
arthroscopic medial, osteonecrosis and, 936
complete, sequelae, 174
degenerative arthrosis and, 331
for discoid meniscus, 294
lateral, popliteus tendon vs. retained posterior horn remnant after, 309
with medial meniscal fibrocartilage loss, 174f
for meniscal tears, 328
MR appearance after, 334–336
partial
defects, partial meniscal implants and, 326
for discoid meniscus, 292
displaced bucket-handle medial meniscus tear, 228f
for flap tears, 259
graphic depiction, 349f–350f
ischemic change in medial femoral condyle and, 364f
for lateral meniscus bucket-handle tears, 216
for longitudinal tears, 204
medial meniscus load-bearing and, 359f
normal posterior horn remnant after, 357f
primary meniscal repair vs., 183
remnant imaging after, 351f, 353f–354f
signal intensity and, 351f
Smith's groups, 335
subchondral erosion and, 360f
tear identification in meniscal remnants after, 333
tear morphology and extension to free edge, 330
recurrent meniscal tears after, 355f–356f
staphylococcal infection after, 1024f
total
degenerative joint changes and, 172
Wrisberg variant of discoid meniscus and, 292
Meniscocapsular injury
ACL disruption and, 307
sagittal image, 131f
tear repair characteristics, 329
Meniscocapsular junction
circumferential zone and, 159
edema between ITB and, 791f
peripheral meniscus imaging at, 289, 325f
peripheral vertical longitudinal tear near, 368f
popliteus tendon and, 157
sagittal FS PD FSE vs. gradient echo image of, 189f
Meniscocapsular ligaments, sagittal image, 107

Meniscocapsular separations, 366–368
   ACL tears and, 372f–373f
   complete, 374f
   posteromedial tibial plateau osseous injuries and, 470, 480f–481f
   tibial spine avulsions and, 473
Meniscocapsular tears, peripheral, MCL bursa mistaken for, 313
Meniscocruciate ligament, transverse ligament and, 305
Meniscofemoral ligaments. See also Ligament of Humphrey; Ligament of Wrisberg
   coronal image, 54
   of deep MCL, 156
   displaced flap tear fragment in coronary recess and, 276f
   disruption, MCL sprain and, 369f
   graphic depiction, 321f
   joint capsule and, 86f
   lateral joint line and, 369f
   lateral meniscus, normal, and, 322f
   location of, 370f
   longitudinal meniscal tears and, 204
   meniscal flap tears and, 114
   meniscal root tear and, 254f
   meniscocapsular separations and, 366, 368
   MR appearance of, 603
   MR imaging, 551
   of PCL, 542, 543f–545f
   PCL injuries and, 557f
   Pellegrini-Stieda ossification in, 629f
   pitfalls interpreting findings on, 309–311
   posterior horn attachments to PCL and, 157
   sagittal image, 106–107
   as static medial stabilizers, 589f
   tears, 609f, 614f
      MCL tear and, 371f, 619f
      O'Donoghue's triad and, 417f
      tibial meniscal attachment and, 154
Meniscofemoral recess
   flap tear extension into, 267f
   meniscal flap tears and, 100
Meniscotibial attachments, meniscal transplantation and, 331
Meniscotibial ligaments
   avulsion, MCL avulsion and, 376f
   bursitis, 630f
   discoid morphology and, 290
   lateral joint line and, 369f
   meniscal flap tears and, 114
   meniscal root tears and, 250f, 252f–253f
   meniscocapsular separations and, 366
   MR appearance of, 603
   sagittal image, 107
   sprain, meniscal tears and, 173
   as static medial stabilizers, 589f
   tears
      MCL sprain and, 600f
      meniscofemoral ligament and, 376f
      tibial meniscal attachment and, 154
Meniscotibial recess. See Coronary recess
Meniscus (menisci). See also Lateral meniscus; Medial meniscus; Peripheral meniscus; Postoperative meniscus; under Meniscal
   ACL injuries and anterior tibial translation by, 486
   anatomy, 153–155, 165f
      of circumferential surface and attachments, 33–35
      sagittal vs. axial images of, 32
   attachments of, 77f
   avascular inner edge, flap tears of, 259
   axial plane checklist, 114, 141f
   capsule overlying, 78f
   central tapering, discoid meniscus and, 293
   chondrocalcinosis of, 390f, 392f
   coronal plane checklist, 100, 121f
   discoid, 290–300
   dissection from lateral aspect, 80f
   dMCL and, 583
   evaluation protocols, 146–148, 148f
      application and techniques for, 149–150
   hypoplastic, juvenile chronic arthritis and, 866
   injuries
      avulsions
         of posteroinferior corner, 375f
         from tibial plateau, 367
      patellar dislocations and, 749
   joint capsule and, 86f
   magnetic resonance imaging of, 153–155
   microstructure, 159–160
   morphology, 180
   neuroanatomy, 163
   osteonecrosis and, 936
   pathology, 121f
      miscellaneous, 365
   perimeniscal capillary plexus radial vessels to, 171f
   posterior medial retraction and, 84f
   radial diameter, discoid meniscus and, 294
   reconstruction, segmental, 348f
   sagittal image, 82f, 147
   structural layers, 161
   synovium-lined fascicles of, 46
   tibial plateau fractures and entrapped, 1004
   vascular supply, 162–163, 163f, 169f, 171f
      arthroscopic rasping and, 180

Metabolic disorders, secondary osteoarthritis and, 897
Metal, MR imaging and distortion around, 3
Metaphyseal bone infarcts, 944, 944f
Metaphyseal–diaphyseal junction, transverse linear fractures vs., 1002
Metaphyseal–diaphyseal low-signal-intensity red marrow inhomogeneity, 1003
Metaphysis
   asymmetrical widening, Brodie's abscess and, 1021
   fractures, 1008f
   osteomyelitis in children and, 1020
Microcystic areas. See also Cysts
   hypointense signal on T1/PD images and, 737
Microfracture. See also Abrasion
   application of, 999f
   for chondral lesions, 974
   fibrocartilage and hyaline cartilage formation with, 973
   partial tears of proximal ACL and, 488
   subchondral sclerosis and, 989f
   using surgical awls, 992f
Microtears, patellar tendinosis and, 798, 806f, 809f
Middle geniculate artery, 398, 399f–400f. See also Medial genicular artery
Middle layer, of meniscus, 161
Middle perforating collagen fibers
   horizontal mucinous degeneration and, 167f
   horizontal oriented intrasubstance degeneration along, 160, 160f
   in meniscal fibrocartilage, 168f
   in meniscus central plane, 166f
   MR imaging, 178
Mid-third capsular ligament, anatomy, 654
Midtrochlear groove, axial image, 37f
Midtrochlear groove cartilage
   axial image, 38f
   sagittal image, 51f
Mineralized cartilage, zone of, 411
Miserable malalignment syndrome, 780f
Mitochondria, in fibrochondrocytes, 159
Mobility
   disrupted posterosuperior fascicle and, 158
   of lateral meniscus, 157
   of medial meniscal attachment to MCL and, 156
Mononuclear cells, pigmented villonodular synovitis and, 877
Morel-Lavallée lesion, axial image, 116

Morning stiffness, rheumatoid arthritis and, 869
Mosaicplasty, 973
  with osteochondral plugs, 992f
Motorcycle injury, posterolateral corner and, 683f
Mottled appearance of yellow marrow, osteomyelitis and, 1020
MPFL. See Medial patellofemoral ligament
MR. See Magnetic resonance imaging
Mucinous meniscal degeneration
  grade 2 intrasubstance, 188f
  grade 2 signal intensity, 190f
  horizontal, 167f
Mucoid degeneration
  of ACL, 129f
    without secondary injury signs, 462f
    ACL cysts and, 455, 458f, 461f
    ACL sprain vs., 463
    chronic ACL tears and, 439
    patellar tendinosis and, 804f–808f
Mucopolysaccharides
  ganglion cysts and, 917
  sulfated, chondromalacia and, 712
Multichannel coils, dielectric effect and, 20
Multiligament injuries, 575f–577f, 685f–687f
  knee dislocations and, 572f, 688f, 691f
Multi-NEX imaging, CUBE and, 12
Multipartite patella, 741f, 744
Muscle denervation
  mimicking Brodie's abscess, 1021
  semimembranosus, 1025f
Muscular dystrophy
  Brodie's abscess vs., 1021
  popliteus muscle and, 1026f
Musculoskeletal (MSK) imaging
  magnetic resonance
    advanced applications for, 10–18, 11f–14f, 16f–17f
    basic pulse sequences in, 5–6, 6f
    clinical diagnosis factors using, 3
    fat suppression and, 21–23
    image enhancement filters, 23–24
    parallel imaging for, 20–21
    positioning for, 4
    scan parameters for, 7–9, 9f
    segmentation in, 25, 26f
    sequence and parameter acronyms, 27
    3-T imaging considerations, 18–20
    uniformity corrections, 23–24
  parallel imaging and, 21
  practical guide to
    high-resolution for, 3
    instrumentation, surface coils in, 3

Musculotendinous junctions
  sports and distal injuries to, 68
  strains and, 69
Myofibroblasts, cruciate ligaments and, 411
Myonecrosis, diabetic, soft tissue infection and, 1022f
Myositis, mimicking Brodie's abscess, 1021
Myositis ossificans, 834
Myotendinous unit strains, 636

N

Narrow neck, of popliteal cysts, 913. See also Popliteal cyst stalk
Necrosis. See also Osteonecrosis
  hypointense signal on T1/PD images and, 737
Neoplasms
  bony lesions, dorsal defect of patella and, 743
  coronal plane checklist, 102
  differential diagnosis of, 834
  osteomyelitis in children vs., 1020
  soft tissue, popliteal cysts vs., 917
Neovascularization, quadriceps tendon tears and, 834
Neurovascular injuries
  evaluation, knee dislocation and, 548
  tibial tunnel preparation for PCL reconstruction and, 556
9:30 position, for ACL reconstruction, 491, 496f
Noble's test, 788
Nodular pigmented villonodular synovitis, 877
Noncoapted flap tears, of meniscus, 257
Noncollagenous matrix proteins, 845
Noncontact dislocations, 757
Noncontact injuries
  ACL, 416, 417f, 424
  knee, 747
Nondisplaced flap tears. See Coapted flap tears, of meniscus
Nondisplaced tibial plateau fractures, 1004
Nonisometric structure
  of ACL, 397
    two-bundle, 402
  of AM and PL bundles, 404f
  of PCL, 542
Nonoperative treatment
  of ACL injuries, 487
  of avulsion fractures, 560f
  of MCL sprains, 635
  of meniscal tears, 328
  of patellar dislocations, 750
  of PCL injuries, 556
Nonorthogonal plane, MR imaging of ACL injuries using, 486
No phase wrap (NPW) imaging, CUBE and, 12
Notchplasty, 491–492, 530f

O

OATS. See Osteochondral autograft transfer system
Ober's test, 788
Oblique meniscofemoral ligaments, mistaken for displaced flap tears, 311, 323f
Oblique popliteal ligament (OPL)
  anatomy, 588f, 594f, 637, 643f
  attachment of, 601
  coronal image, 54
  joint capsule and, 86f, 581
  MR imaging, 603
  popliteal fossa view, 87f
  sagittal image, 42
  superficial dissection from posterior aspect, 85f
Oblique tears, of meniscus, 186, 255, 257. See also Flap tears
  repair of, 330
  transverse ligament simulating, 304
Obturator artery, 73f
Obturator nerve, 73f
  anterior division of, 63f
Occupation of patient, ACL treatment methods and, 487
OCD. See Osteochondritis dissecans
Odd facet, patellar, 700
O'Donoghue's triad, 415–416, 417f, 423
Off-isocenter image quality, MR imaging and, 3
Older patients. See also Age of patient
  ACL treatment in, 487
Oligoarthritis, 869, 892
1 o'clock position, for ACL reconstruction, 489
Open chondromalacia, 715f, 731f
Open meniscal repair, 327
OPL. See Oblique popliteal ligament
Orthogonal plane, MR imaging of ACL injuries using, 486
Orthotics, ITB syndrome and, 788
OSF (oversampling factor), PROPELLER and, 15
Osgood-Schlatter disease, 109, 132f, 799, 817, 819f–820f
O-shape, of lateral meniscus, 166f
Osmotic swelling, cartilage matrix and, 983f
Osseous bar formation, after femoral fracture in boy, unfused physis and, 1014f
Osseous structures
  anterior cruciate ligament and, 470
  coronal plane checklist, 102, 123f
  injuries
    ACL tears and, 470–473, 473f–485f
    PCL tears and, 553
Ossification disorders
  bipartite patella, 739f–741f, 743–744
  Brodie's abscess and, 1021
  heterotopic, of patellar tendon, 138f

Ossification disorders (continued)
    patella, accessory ossification, 740f, 744
    Pellegrini-Stieda disease, 611–612, 627f–629f
Osteitis inferior pole, rheumatoid arthritis and, 873f
Osteoarthritis. See also Arthritis
    ACL deficiencies and, 487
    after meniscectomy, 335
    cartilage damage and, 697
    degenerative, 900f–901f
    early chondral degeneration due to, 845
    femoral articular cartilage and, 43
    inflammatory, irregular infrapatellar fat-pad sign and, 858
    key concepts, 897
    lipoma arborescens and, 909
    MR findings, 898
    osteonecrosis vs., 935
    PCL and PLC injuries and, 659
    PCL injuries and, 556
    popliteal cysts and, 916
    pyrophosphate arthropathy and, 388
    three-dimensional articular pulse sequences of, 713
Osteoarthrosis, 900f
Osteochondral allograft dowel technique, 1000f
Osteochondral allografts, 971
Osteochondral autograft transfer system (OATS), 971, 973
    coronal PD image, 996f
    donor site and recipient site for, 993f–994f
    of lateral femoral condyle, 990f, 999f
    scaffold plug placement in trochlear groove, 996f
Osteochondral defects, transient lateral subluxation of patella and, 112
Osteochondral fractures, 971, 974f
    in articular cartilage, 997f
    hemarthrosis and, 1013
    in skeletal immature patient, 978f
Osteochondral injury
    meniscal root tear and, 250f
    patellar dislocations and, 749
    posterolateral corner injuries and, 678f
Osteochondral lesions
    fractures, 971
        of LFC, ACL injuries and, 430
    key concepts, 971
    loose bodies in joint effusion and, axial image, 116
    MR evaluation of, 972
    surgical evaluation of, 972–974
Osteochondral patellar fractures, 1018f
Osteochondral plugs, 971. See also Bone plugs; Osteochondral autograft transfer system
    donor site and recipient site for, 993f–994f
    mosaicplasty with, 992f
    subchondral osseous component of, 990f
Osteochondritis
    meniscal tears and, 173
    patellofemoral, 721f
Osteochondritis dissecans (OCD)
    cartilage damage and, 697
    characteristics, 947
    chondral flaps and, 962f–963f
    chronic chondral fissure, 960f
    dorsal defect of patella and, 743
    early epiphyseal ossification and, 967f–968f
    extended pattern, 951f
    fragmentation, 962f
        displaced, 956f, 964f, 966f
    healing of, signal intensity and, 933, 966f
    inferocentral, 951f, 959f
    of lateral femoral condyle, discoid meniscus and, 292
    with lateral patellar fragmentation, 739f
    MR imaging, 949
    osteochondral fracture presenting as, 977f
    osteonecrosis vs., 935
    patellar, 744
    pathology, 947–948
    reactive edema and, 963f
    repair failure, bioabsorbable screws and, 986f
    in situ, reactive edema and, 963f
    subchondral cysts and, 957f
    treatment, 949
    unstable, 953f–955f
        fluid surrounding, 965f
        nondisplaced and displaced, 964f
Osteochondroma, Trevor's disease resembling, 1026f
Osteochondromatosis, 903f
Osteochondrosis
    Osgood-Schlatter disease and, 817, 819f
    Sinding-Larsen-Johansson syndrome and, 818
Osteolysis, 1027
Osteoma, osteoid, Brodie's abscess vs., 1021
Osteomalacia, tumor-induced, 1027
Osteomyelitis
    chronic active, with sequestrum, 1025f
    joint sepsis and, 1020
    multifocal, 1021
    staphylococcal, 1024f
    subacute, 1021
    tibial, soft tissue infection and, 1023f
Osteonecrosis. See also Bone infarcts
    clinical history of, 934
    convex upper border of, 942f
    coronal plane checklist, 102
    differential diagnosis of, 935
    juvenile chronic arthritis and, 866
    key concepts, 933
    of medial femoral condyle, 939f
    MR patterns of, 935–936
    pathogenesis theories, 934
    radiographic classification of, 935
    risk
        insufficiency fractures and, 940f
        subchondral fractures and, 941f
    spontaneous, 933–934
    stress fractures vs., 941f
    subacute osteomyelitis in, 1021
    treatment of, 936
Osteopenia
    rheumatoid arthritis and, 870
    subchondral, rheumatoid arthritis and, 868f
Osteophytes
    articular cartilage matrix disruption and, 849
    degenerative arthrosis and, 896f
    osteoarthritis and, 898
Osteophytic spurring, 379
    osteoarthritis and, 898, 899f
Osteophytosis, rheumatoid arthritis and, 870
Osteoporosis
    diffuse, patellar fracture and, 1022f
    excessive lateral pressure and, 783f
    rheumatoid arthritis and, 869
    subchondral, rheumatoid arthritis and, 868f
Osteotomy
    femoral, 747
    Fulkerson, 738f, 830
    tibial, 326, 936
Outerbridge classification
    of chondromalacia, 709f, 711, 727
    of joint cartilage breakdown, 104
Outerbridge's ridge, knee extension and, 33
Outside-in meniscus repair, 338
Oversampling factor (OSF), PROPELLER and, 15
Over-the-top position for ACL reconstruction, 502f, 517
    femoral tunnel in, 397
Overuse syndromes, 697

P

Paget's disease, osteomyelitis in children and, 1020
Pain
    ACL repair and, primary, 488
    ACL roof impingement and, 520
    chondromalacia patellae and, 706
    deep venous thrombosis and, 917
    diffuse pigmented villonodular synovitis and, 885f
    discoid meniscus and, 291
    ganglion cysts and, 455
    Hoffa's disease and, 857
    ITB syndrome and, 788
    lateral patellar release for, 830
    longitudinal meniscal tears and, 204
    Lyme arthritis and, 892
    meniscal cysts and, 379

Index

meniscal ossicle and, 393
meniscal tears and, 172
horizontal, 185
lateral, bucket-handle tears, 215
synovial ingrowth and, 180
meniscocapsular separations and, 366
miserable malalignment syndrome and, 780*f*
osteochondritis dissecans of, 744
osteonecrosis and, 934
patellofemoral
after ACL reconstruction, 491
meniscal tears and, 173
Sinding-Larsen-Johansson syndrome and, 818
synovial plicae and, 921
Wrisberg variant of discoid meniscus and, 292
Pancreatitis, bone infarcts and, 946
Pannus tissue
hemophilia and, 891
hemosiderin imaging in, 886*f*
Hoffa's fat pad and, 135*f*
rheumatoid arthritis and, 868*f*, 869–870, 873*f*–874*f*
tendinomuscular marginal erosions and, 875*f*
Pants-over-vest technique
for lax intact lax medial patellofemoral ligament, 750
for patellar tendon repair, 813*f*
Parallel imaging, 20–21
Paramagnetic effect of iron, pigmented villonodular synovitis and, 878, 887*f*–888*f*
Parameniscal cysts
about, 377
differential diagnosis of, 379
discoid meniscus and, 384*f*
intrameniscal and, 385*f*
lateral meniscus, 387*f*
Paratenon, of cruciate ligaments, 411
Parrot beak tear, graphic depiction, 191*f*
Partial meniscal implants, 326
Partial volume averaging, pitfalls interpreting findings on, 309
Partial volume effect, MR imaging of ACL injuries and, 436, 438
Patch allograft, for cartilage resurfacing, 992*f*
Patella. *See also* Lateral patellar facet; Medial patella; Medial patellar facet; *under* Patellar
accessory ossification of, 740*f*, 744
anatomy, 79*f*, 699–701
knee in partial flexion and, 93*f*
median ridge, 37*f*
reflected downwards, 90*f*
articular cartilage of
MR imaging of, 35
PCL injuries and, 547

axial image, 37*f*
central movement of, 782*f*
dislocations
complete, 753*f*
contusions and, 758*f*
imaging evaluation, 746
lateral femoral condyle contusion and, 762*f*–763*f*
medial patellofemoral ligament avulsion and, 761*f*
medial patellofemoral ligament tear and, 759*f*–760*f*
MR findings, 748–749
multiple injuries with, 766*f*
radiographic measurements, 745–746
transient, 774*f*–775*f*
traumatic, 747–750
treatment, 747
types, 744
displaced, patellar tendon rupture and, 811*f*–812*f*
dorsal defect of, 742*f*, 743
dysplastic
lateral patellar subluxation and, 704
lateral patellar tilt and, 705
fractures, 1001, 1004, 1015*f*–1017*f*
after ACL reconstruction, 491
classification of, 1018*f*
lipohemarthrosis and, 1019
osteoporosis and, 1022*f*
tension cerclage treatment of, 1018*f*
transverse displaced, 1015*f*
glide test, 773*f*
height relative to femoral trochlear groove, 702–703, 702*f*
high-riding, patellar tendon tears and, 800
Jagerhut defect of, 753*f*
juvenile chronic arthritis and, 866
knee capsule and ligaments and, 92*f*
knee in partial flexion and, 93*f*
lateral collateral ligament and, 636
lateral release of, 830
lateral retinaculum and iliotibial band, 783*f*–784*f*
lateral tilting of, 704–705
marked on skin, 768*f*
medial patellofemoral ligament reconstruction and, 777*f*–778*f*
miserable malalignment syndrome and, 780*f*
pes anserinus tendons and, 78*f*
posterior surface of, articular cartilage and, 94*f*
rectus femoris and, 68*f*
redislocation, 750
resurfacing, for chondromalacia, 743
sagittal image, 48*f*–51*f*, 82*f*, 92*f*
subluxation, 744–747
congruence angle and, 745–746

ELPS and, 786
imaging evaluation, 746
lateral, 704
lateral-to-medial, 705
medial, 705
osteochondritis dissecans and, 744
patellar dislocations and, 749
radiographic measurements, 745–746
transient lateral, axial image, 112
treatment of, 747
trochlear dysplasia and, 754*f*
superficial dissection from anterior, 91*f*
superolateral movement in knee extension, 32
trochlear groove cartilage and, 105
vastus intermedius and, 67*f*
vastus medialis and, 66*f*
dislocation and, 66
Wiberg type-2, 753*f*
Patella adentro, 705
Patella alta
characteristics, 702–703, 702*f*, 801
chondromalacia patellae and, 706
lateral patellar subluxation and, 704
lateral-to-medial subluxation of, 705
patellar subluxation or dislocations and, 745
patellar tendinosis and, 815*f*
patellar tendon rupture and, 814*f*
patellar tendon tears and, 802*f*
sagittal image, 109
Patella baja
characteristics, 703, 801
polio and, 816*f*
postoperative patellar tendon and, 522
quadriceps tendon rupture and, 841*f*
sagittal image, 109
Patellar anastomosis, 169*f*
Patellar bone, 825*f*
Patellar bursae. *See also* Prepatellar bursae; Superficial infrapatellar bursa
absence of, 45
Patellar cysts, chondromalacia and, 711, 713
Patellar facet articular cartilage, 94*f*
Patellar facets
axial plane checklist, 137*f*
chondromalacia and, 706
Patellar ridge. *See also* Secondary ridge, patellar; Transverse ridges, patellar
patellar alignment and tracking and, 703
Patellar sleeve fracture, 818, 1015*f*, 1018*f*
Patellar tendinitis, acute, 810*f*

Patellar tendinosis
   axial image, 138f
   graphic depiction, 797f
   GRE vs. FS PD FSE imaging, 809f
   key concepts, 798
   MR findings, 799–800
   with mucoid degeneration, 804f–808f
   Osgood-Schlatter disease and, 817, 820f
   patellar tendinopathy vs., 808
   prepatellar edema and, 803f
   quadriceps tendinosis and, 838f
   sagittal image, 109
   Sinding-Larsen-Johansson syndrome and, 822f

Patellar tendon
   ACL reconstruction using, 490, 493
   anatomy, 79f, 591f, 641f–642f, 647f
   axial image, 38f–40f
      checklist, 112, 138f
      near insertion, 41f
   buckling, chronic ACL tears and, 453
   coronal image, 57f
   cystic fluid collection in, 795f
   edges, 768f
   gouty tophi and, 878
   Hoffa's infrapatellar fat pad and, 35
   ITB and, 81f
   knee capsule and ligaments and, 92f
   knee in partial flexion and, 93f
   Lyme arthritis and, 892
   midsagittal sections, 45
   Osgood-Schlatter disease and, 817, 819f
   partial detachment, patellar dislocation and, 748
   patellectomy and, 738f
   postoperative MR imaging, 522
   rupture, 812f–813f
      Krackow locking stitches for, 812f
      patella alta and, 814f
      retinacular tears and, 811f
   sagittal image, 42, 49f–51f
      checklist, 109, 132f
   scar tissue fibrosis and, 522
   soft tissue–like mass of, 878
   static patellofemoral joint stabilizing by, 703
   tears, 802f–804f, 810f–811f
      key concepts, 800
      MR findings, 801
      retears of, 813f–814f
      retinacular tears and, 751
      treatment of, 801
   tophaceous gout and, 890f
   vastus intermedius and, 67f
   vastus lateralis and, 65f

Patellar tendon–to-patella ratio, patella alta and, 801

Patellar tilt
   assessment, 755f
   ELPS and, 751–752
   issues due to, 746
   movement and, 782f
   patellar dislocations and, 749
   quadriceps tendon insufficiency and, 839

Patellectomy, 738f, 743, 747, 830

Patellofemoral compartment
   axial image, 112
   sagittal image, 42

Patellofemoral disease, 32

Patellofemoral disorders
   Insall's classification, 697
   vastus medialis and, 66

Patellofemoral index, 745–746

Patellofemoral joint
   anatomy, 699
   biomechanics, 782f–783f
   chondromalacia of, 706
      alternative classification, 711f
      Outerbridge classification, 709f, 711
   chondrosis of, 571f
   dislocation, discoid meniscus and, 292
   dorsiflexion injuries, 555f
   extension, 703
   extensor mechanism and, 697
   key concepts, 697
   kinematic MR imaging of, 703–705
   knee flexion angle and contact areas of, 707f
   LCL and posterolateral structures and, 658–659
   malalignment and abnormal tracking, 698
   medial and lateral patellar retinacular attachments and, 35
   pain and instability, meniscal tears and, 173
   pathokinematics, 704–705
   subluxation
      chondromalacia patellae and, 706
      discoid meniscus and, 292
   surgical procedures, 830

Patellofemoral ligaments, lateral collateral ligament and, 636

Patellotibial band, 751, 784f

Patellotibial ligament, 642f

Patient criteria. See also Adolescents; Adults; Age of patient; Children
   for meniscal transplantation, 331

Patient motion
   MR imaging and, 3, 150
   PROPELLER and, 15

Pauciarticular juvenile chronic arthritis, 865

Pebble-shaped patella, 701

Pediatric population. See Children

Pellegrini-Stieda disease
   characteristics, 611–612
   femoral attachment of MCL ossification and, 627f
   MCL ossification and, 629f
   sMCL ossification and, 628f

Perforating branches of deep femoral artery
   biceps femoris and, 69f
   semimembranosus muscle and, 70f
   semitendinosus muscle and, 71f

Perforating collagen fibers. See Middle perforating collagen fibers

Pericarditis, juvenile chronic arthritis and, 865

Perimeniscal capillary plexus
   geniculate artery and, 169f
   meniscocapsular separations and, 366
   of meniscus, 162, 170f
   radial vessels to meniscus from, 171f

Perimeniscal capsular plexus, meniscal repair and, 329

Periosteal reaction at fracture site, radiography of, 1001

Periosteum, trapped in tibial physeal fracture, 1008f

Peripheral embolization, popliteal artery aneurysm and, 918

Peripheral meniscocapsular tears, MCL bursa mistaken for, 313

Peripheral meniscus
   anatomy, 153
      continuous bowtie appearance, 165f
   attachments, pain from tearing of, 172
   circumferential zone, free edge anterior to tear site, 245f
   flap tears of, 155f
   innervation, 163
   longitudinal flap tears and, 255
   longitudinal tears and, 203
   at meniscocapsular junction, imaging of, 289
   perimeniscal capillary plexus of, 170f
   tears
      conditions for, 329
      contrecoup forces and, 367
      MCL injuries and, 611

Peripheral signal artifacts, 302–303

Peritenon edema, patellar tendinosis and, 797f, 799

Peroneal artery
   gastrocnemius muscle and, 75f
   leg muscle innervation and, 64f
   perimeniscal capillary plexus and, 169f

Peroneal branch of sciatic nerve, biceps femoris muscle and, 69

Peroneal nerve
   axial image, 36f–41f
   long head of biceps and, 644f
   MR imaging of, 35
   sagittal image, 48f
   short head of biceps tendon and, 646f
   thigh muscle innervation and, 63f

Peroneal vein, leg muscle innervation and, 64f

Index

Peroneus longus muscle
    anatomy, 639f, 641f, 644f
    coronal image, 62f
    ITB and, 81f
    leg muscle innervation and, 64f
Pes anserinus
    anatomy, 632f
    coronal image, 58f
    extraarticular ACL reconstruction using, 490
    medial collateral ligament and, 582
    perimeniscal capillary plexus and, 169f
    posterior inferior, semitendinosus muscle insertion at, 71
Pes anserinus bursitis, 612, 633f–634f
    osteonecrosis vs., 935
Pes anserinus tendons
    abduction stability and, 591
    ganglion cysts and, 917
    MCL tears and, 611
    medial aspect
        deep MCL exposure, 79f
        with superficial dissection, 78f
    sagittal image, 42, 131f
Pes tendons
    marked on skin, 768f
    medial patellofemoral ligament and, 756f
    sMCL and, 622f
Phased-array coils, peripheral signal artifacts and, 302
Phased Array Uniformity Enhancement (PURE), 23
Philips acronyms, 27
PHMM. *See* Posterior horn medial meniscus
Physeal scar, thalassemia involving marrow and, 1012f
Physeal spine fractures, 173
Physical examination, of ACL injuries, 429
Physiologic imaging techniques, 853
Physis
    discontinuity, trauma or epiphysiodesis and, 1002
    fractures, 1008f
    trauma, 1007f
    Trevor's disease and deformity of, 1026f
    unfused, after femoral fracture repair in boy, 1014f
Pigmented villonodular synovitis (PVNS)
    heterogenous mass in, 881f
    histologic photomicrograph of, 879f
    Hoffa's fat pad and, 857, 879f
    irregular infrapatellar fat-pad sign and, 858
    key concepts, 877
    lipoma arborescens vs., 908
    lobular mass in, 882f
    localized, 883f–884f
    localized or nodular, 880f, 882f
    MR findings, 878
    tophaceous gout vs., 889f–890f

Pisani's sign, 379
Pivoting
    during deceleration, ACL injuries and, 416
    in knee extension, osteochondral fractures and, 971
Pivot shift injury, 415
Pivot-shift test, 424, 428f
    ACL reconstruction and, 491, 497f
    reverse, 548
Plantarflexion
    gastrocnemius muscle and, 75
    plantaris muscle and, 76
    posterior cruciate ligament injuries, 555f
Plantaris muscle
    anatomy, functional, 76, 76f
    axial image, 37f–40f
    peroneal nerve and, 35
    popliteal fossa view, 87f
    posterolateral corner injuries and, 676f
    sagittal image, 47f–49f
    strain and edema, 682f
Plantaris tendon
    anatomy, functional, 76
    axial image, 37f
Plicae
    disorders, variable cartilage damage and, 697
    key concepts, 921
    lateral patellar, 930, 930f–932f
    sagittal plane checklist, 111, 136f
    types of, 920f
Plica syndrome, 173, 921
Point tenderness, ITB syndrome and, 788
Polio
    patella alta and, 815f
    patella baja and, 801, 816f
Polyarthritis, rheumatoid arthritis and, 869
Polyarticular arthritis, Lyme arthritis and, 892
Polyarticular juvenile chronic arthritis, 865
Polycythemia vera, red marrow in, thalassemia and, 1012f
Polymer, hyaluronate-based, 974
Polymorphic rounded cells, diffuse pigmented villonodular synovitis and, 878
Polypropylene, braided, as ACL allograft material, 490
Polytetrafluoroethylene, as ACL allograft material, 490
Pop, audible, at time of ACL tears, 424
Popliteal artery
    anatomy, 647f
    aneurysm, 918f
        popliteal or atypical cysts vs., 914, 917f
        thrombosed, 917f
    anterior, cruciate ligaments' vascular supply and, 399f
    axial image, 36f–40f
    coronal image, 61f–62f
    of low-signal-intensity, 54

    fibular collateral ligament and, 637
    gastrocnemius muscle and, 75f
    intercondylar sagittal view, 45
    meniscal repair and, 35
    patent, 572f
    perimeniscal capillary plexus and, 169f
    pitfalls interpreting findings on, 314, 314f
    plantaris muscle and, 76f
    popliteus muscle and, 74f
    sagittal image, 50f
        knee joint, 82f
    thigh muscle innervation and, 63f
    thrombosed, 917f
    thrombosed aneurysm, 918f
Popliteal artery entrapment syndrome, 914, 919f
Popliteal cysts
    axial image, 144f
    imaging methods and, 864f
    juvenile chronic arthritis and, 866
    key concepts, 913
    location of, 915f
    loose bodies in, 116
    medial, 903f
    meniscal cysts and, 916f
    rheumatoid arthritis and, 870
    treatment of, 917
    types, 110
Popliteal cyst stalk, 913, 915f
Popliteal fossa
    cysts and, 914
    popliteus tendon and, 87f
Popliteal hiatus
    lateral meniscus vascularity at, 162
    meniscal fascicles and, 126f, 308, 318f, 321f
    meniscal flap tear displaced into, 285f
    meniscal tears and, 157, 158f
    of posterolateral corner, 680f
Popliteal oblique ligament, 602
Popliteal tendinitis, meniscal tears and, 173
Popliteal vein
    anatomy, 647f
    axial image, 36f–37f
    coronal image, 60f–62f
    of low-signal-intensity, 54
    intercondylar sagittal view, 45
    meniscal repair and, 35
    patent, 572f
    sagittal image, 49f
        knee joint, 82f
    thigh muscle innervation and, 63f
Popliteofibular ligament (PFL)
    anatomy, 638, 652f, 657
    arcuate sign and, 470
    attachment of, 672f
    avulsion fracture and, 483f
    avulsions, 674f
        styloid edema and, 681f
    fibular head fracture and, 683f
    fibular styloid fracture and, 563f–564f
    injuries, 664
        sprains, 669f

Popliteofibular ligament (*continued*)
   lateral collateral ligament and, 636, 649*f*
   popliteus complex and, 657
   popliteus hiatus area and, 680*f*–681*f*
   popliteus tendon and, 115, 651*f*
   posterior fibula head fracture and, 145*f*
   posterolateral complex and, 637
   posterolateral corner and, 465, 672*f*
   posterolateral structure injuries and, 660*f*
   sagittal image, 46, 47*f*, 126*f*
   tears, 691*f*
Popliteomeniscal fascicles (PMF)
   disruption, ACL tear and, 684*f*
   lateral compartment contusions and, 473*f*
   lateral meniscus stability and, 659
   normal superior deficiency of, 158*f*, 318*f*
   posterolateral corner and, 465
   sulcus fracture and, 475*f*–476*f*
Popliteomeniscal ligaments, 318*f*
Popliteus capsular hiatus, arcuate ligament and, 42
Popliteus complex
   anatomy, 645*f*, 657
   sagittal image, 108
Popliteus muscle
   ACL cysts and, 459*f*
   anatomy, 644*f*
      functional, 74, 74*f*
      normal, 34
   arcuate ligament and, 661*f*
   axial image, 41*f*
   coronal image, 60*f*–62*f*
   course of, MR imaging of, 308
   fascia, 601
   infection and
      in diabetic, 1022*f*
      osteomyelitis, 1023*f*
   lateral head of gastrocnemius muscle and, 46
   leg muscle innervation and, 64*f*
   MR imaging, 664
   muscular dystrophy and, 1026*f*
   popliteal fossa view, 87*f*
   popliteus complex and, 657
   popliteus hiatus area and, 680*f*
   posterolateral corner and, 465, 672*f*
      injuries, 466, 467*f*
   posteromedial corner and, 592*f*
   sagittal image, 48*f*–52*f*
   strains, 636
      displaced tibial eminence fracture and, 432*f*
      PCL injury and, 568*f*
   tears, 660*f*
      posterolateral corner injuries and, 468*f*
Popliteus recess, posterolateral attachment of lateral meniscus and, 157

Popliteus tendon. *See also* Popliteus tendon sheath
   acute ACL tears and, 443*f*
   anatomy, 647*f*
      functional, 77*f*
      gross, lateral meniscus and, 166*f*
   arcuate ligament and, 665*f*, 677*f*
   attachments of, 648*f*
      function of, 158
      lateral collateral ligament, 650*f*
   axial image, 39*f*–40*f*, 144*f*
      LCL origin along lateral femoral condyle and, 115
   coronal image, 54, 60*f*–61*f*
   course of, MR imaging of, 308, 666*f*
   division of medial meniscus and, 186*f*
   fabellofibular ligament and, 666*f*, 677*f*
   free edge radial tear of lateral meniscus and, 236*f*
   inferior and superior popliteal fascicles and, 308, 320*f*
   inferior popliteomeniscal fascicle and, 46
   injuries, 675*f*–676*f*, 678*f*
      multiligament, 685*f*–687*f*
   intercondylar notch and, 455*f*
   ITB friction syndrome and, 793*f*–794*f*
   joint capsule and, 86*f*
   lateral collateral ligament and, 636, 640*f*, 649*f*
   lateral meniscus and, 157, 158*f*
   lateral meniscus oblique tear and, 320*f*
   longitudinal meniscal tears and, 207*f*
   MR imaging, 664
   multiligament injuries and, 576*f*–577*f*
   osseous avulsion, 691*f*
   pitfalls interpreting findings on, 308–309, 317*f*–318*f*
   popliteal fossa view, 87*f*
   popliteofibular ligament and, 46, 651*f*–652*f*
   popliteus complex and, 645*f*
   popliteus hiatus area and, 680*f*
   popliteus muscle and, 74
   posterolateral complex and, 637
   posterolateral corner and, 465
   posterolateral corner injuries and, 466, 664*f*
   posterolateral structure injuries and, 660*f*
   sagittal image, 46, 47*f*–48*f*, 82*f*
      checklist, 108, 126*f*
   sMCL and, 596*f*
   strain, PCL injury and, 568*f*
   superficial dissection from posterior perspective, 85*f*
   vertical longitudinal meniscal tears and, 204
Popliteus tendon sheath
   displaced lateral meniscus flap tear and, 258, 282*f*
   loose bodies in, 116

   signal intensity interpretation, 308, 317*f*
   variable thickness of, 308
Popping knee syndrome, Wrisberg variant of discoid meniscus and, 290
Positive PCL angle, 440
Positive PCL sign, 440
Positive posterior femoral line sign, 440
Posterior capsule
   arcuate ligament and, 49*f*
   contact hyperextension injuries and, 416
   coronal image, 54
   rupture, displaced tibial eminence fracture and, 432*f*
   sagittal image, 50*f*–51*f*
   tears, MCL rupture and, 599
Posterior cruciate ligament (PCL). *See also* Anterolateral band or bundle
   ACL cysts and, 456*f*, 461*f*
   ACL reconstruction and, 496*f*, 517
   anatomy, 541*f*
      axial intercondylar, 410*f*
      in cross-section, 35
      functional, 77*f*, 540, 542, 543*f*–545*f*
      tibial insertion, 40*f*, 401*f*
      triangular attachment, 55
   anterior and posterior horns of medial meniscus and, 33
   avulsion fractures and, 560*f*
   axial image, 38*f*–39*f*
      checklist, 113–114, 140*f*
   biomechanics, 546*f*
   bucket-handle fragment and, 227*f*
   chronic ACL tears and, 453
   contact hyperextension injuries and, 416
   coronal image, 54, 60*f*–61*f*
      checklist, 99, 120*f*
      distal insertion, 62*f*
      proximal origin, 60*f*
   footprint, 540
   Hoffa's fat pad and, 856*f*
   hypointense, ACL sprain and, 425*f*
   iliotibial band and, 654
   injuries
      adhesions, laxity and, 424
      arcuate sign and, 473
      arthroscopic evaluation, 548
      associated findings, 556, 568
      chondromalacia patellae and, 706
      clinical diagnosis, 548
      flexion, 555*f*
      hyperextension, 550*f*
      LCL and posterolateral structures and, 659
      location and mechanism of, 547–548, 549*f*, 662
      MR imaging, 551–553
      treatment, 556
      types of, 552, 557*f*

intercondylar notch cysts and, 460f
key concepts, 540
knee in partial flexion and, 44, 93f
laxity and subacute tears, adhesions or attachments in, 424
ligament of Wrisberg diameter and, 309
ligaments of Wrisberg and Humphrey and, 33–34
medial collateral ligament and, 587f
medial meniscus and, 164f
  bucket-handle tears, 217f
popliteal fossa view, 87f
popliteus complex and, 645f
popliteus hiatus area and, 680f
positive angle of, ACL tears and, 440
positive sign of, ACL tears and, 440
posterior horn medial meniscus and, 156
posterior view, 88f
posteromedial corner and, 591f–592f
reconstruction, revascularization after, 556
sagittal image, 42, 50f–51f
  ACL on same section as, 45
  ACL signal intensity vs., 45
  checklist, 106, 130f
  medial to lateral direction, 44
  through medial compartment, 83f
sprains
  posterolateral corner injuries and, 664f
  sagittal image, 106, 554f
tears
  biceps femoris muscle–tendon strain and, 569f
  bucket-handle, 221f–222f, 224f
    complex, 232f
    displaced, 220f
    medial meniscus and, 217f
  chronic, 570f
    imaging, 553
  complete, imaging, 552
  grade 3, 546f, 558f, 560f
    complex flap tear and, 565f
  incidence of, 547
  interstitial, 540, 548, 559f, 562f, 571f
    imaging, 552
  knee dislocation and, 572f
  laxity and, 424
  LCL and biceps femoris tendon avulsions and, 673f
  mid-substance, 561f
  multiligament injuries and, 575f–577f
  partial, 540, 554f, 567f
    imaging, 552
  posterolateral corner injuries and, 465–466

reconstruction, 571f–572f
reverse Segond fractures and, 574f
sagittal image, 106, 322f
valgus stress test and, 635
vascular supply, 399f–400f
Posterior drawer exam, 548, 559f, 567
Posterior femoral condyle
  axial image, 37f
  coronal image, 54
    checklist, chondral abnormalities and, 101
  cortex, posteromedial capsule and, 367
  medial collateral ligament and, 55
  sagittal plane checklist, 104, 127f
Posterior fibular ligament, posterior view, 93f
Posterior fibular styloid edema, 145f
Posterior horn. See also Posterior horn lateral meniscus; Posterior horn medial meniscus
  after primary repair, intrasubstance signal intensity and, 362f
  meniscal transplantation and, 331
  meniscotibial attachment of, root tears and, 246
  of meniscus, 154
    innervation, 163
    inside-out repair of, 328, 339f
  remnant
    flap tear, chondral delamination and, 363f
    imaging methods, 361f
    normal appearance of, 357f
Posterior horn–body junction, of meniscus, radial tears and, 240f, 244f
Posterior horn lateral meniscus (PHLM)
  ACL and PCL insertion sites in, 401f
  attachments, 157, 321f
  bicompartmental bucket-handle tears and, 230f
  coronal image, 55, 60f–62f
  discoid menisci and, 290
  displaced
    anterior flap lateral meniscus fragment and, 234f
    toward AHLM, 324f
  fabellofibular ligament and, 666f
  foreshortened, 235f
  ligament of Wrisberg vs., 301
  meniscofemoral ligaments and, 54, 542, 543f, 545f
  oblique intermeniscal ligaments and, 321f
  popliteus tendon sheath signaling and, 308, 317f
  posterolateral corner injuries and, 679f–680f
  remnant, articular cartilage loss and, 360f

root attachment, 89f
  ACL insertion vs., 410
  avulsed, 476f
  sagittal image, 50f, 103, 108
sagittal image, 48f–49f, 165f
tears
  disrupted posterosuperior fascicle and, 158
  O'Donoghue's triad and, 416
  vertical, popliteus tendon sheath and, 309
uncovered, ACL tears and, 439
vascularity of, complex tear repairs and, 328
Posterior horn medial meniscus (PHMM)
  ACL and PCL insertion sites in, 401f
  anatomy, 33, 156, 584f
    popliteus tendon and, 186f
  axial image, 39f–40f, 77f
  blunted, inferiorly displaced flap tear and, 268f
  coronal image, 55, 60f–62f
  checklist, 99
  deficient, lateral meniscus with, 114
  discoid menisci and, 290
  foreshortened inferior surface of, 267f
  grade 1 signal intensity, 187f
  grade 3 signal intensity in, 181
  meniscal ossicle and, 393f
  meniscocapsular separations and, 374f
  obstructed arthroscopic visualization of, 289
  popliteal cysts and, 916
  posteromedial capsule interface with, 367
  posteromedial corner injuries and, 602
  root attachment, 89f
  sagittal image, 44, 52f
    checklist, 103, 125f
    medial limb of arcuate ligament and, 46
  tears
    bucket-handle, 214, 218f, 221f, 223f, 225f
      bicompartmental, 230f
      complex, 232f
      at capsular attachment of, 366
    flap, 155f, 181f, 255, 259f–260f
      coapted, 263f
      displaced, 264f
      displaced into popliteal hiatus, 285f
      meniscal cyst and, 287f
      superior surface extension in, 274f
      truncated and foreshortened inferior surface, 266f
      vertical graft orientation for, 262f
    horizontal cleavage, 198f
      cyst formation and, 199f–201f
      inferior surface, 172

Posterior horn medial meniscus (*continued*)
   longitudinal, 212*f*
      ACL tears and, 373*f*
   osseous injuries and, 482
   peripheral, tibial spine avulsions and, 473
   popliteal cysts and, 913
   root
      displaced, 251*f*–253*f*
      ghost meniscus, 250*f*–251*f*, 253*f*
      nondisplaced, 248*f*–249*f*
   truncated, bucket-handle tears with, 229*f*
Posterior iliotibial fibers, 81
Posterior intercondyloid fossa, tibial, posterior cruciate ligament and, 540
Posterior lateral femoral condyle cartilage
   axial image, 37*f*–38*f*
   coronal image, 60*f*–62*f*
   sagittal image, 48*f*
Posterior medial femoral condyle cartilage
   axial image, 37*f*–38*f*
   coronal image, 60*f*–62*f*
   sagittal image, 52*f*
Posterior medial tibia, semitendinosus muscle insertion at, 71*f*
Posterior medial tibial condyle, semimembranosus muscle insertion and, 70*f*
Posterior meniscofemoral ligament, 310.
   See also Ligament of Wrisberg
Posterior oblique band or bundle, 540
Posterior oblique ligament (POL)
   anatomy, 79*f*, 584*f*, 586*f*–587*f*, 590*f*
   axial image, 115
   injuries, 602
   joint capsule and, 581
   medial collateral ligament and, 635
   posterior medial retraction and, 84*f*
   sagittal image, 131*f*
Posterior patellar articular cartilage, sagittal image, 45
Posterior patellar surface, 699
Posterior pes anserinus, gracilis muscle insertion and, 73*f*
Posterior popliteofibular ligament, 657
Posterior root lateral meniscus, 158
Posterior root medial meniscus, axial image, 39*f*
Posterior sag sign, 548, 552, 559*f*
Posterior spring sign, lateral meniscus bucket-handle tears and, 216
Posterior tibial artery
   axial image, 41*f*
   gastrocnemius muscle and, 75*f*
   leg muscle innervation and, 64*f*

   perimeniscal capillary plexus and, 169*f*
   sagittal image, 49*f*
Posterior tibial intercondylar fossa, posterior horn medial meniscus and, 156
Posterior tibial veins
   axial image, 41*f*
   leg muscle innervation and, 64*f*
Posterior tibiofibular ligament, popliteal fossa view, 87*f*
Posteroinferior corner
   avulsion, 375*f*
   tear, of PHMM, ACL contrecoup contusion and, 374*f*
Posteroinferior popliteomeniscal fascicles, 657
   popliteus muscle and, 74
   sagittal image, 108
Posterolateral bundle (PLB)
   ACL in extension and, 403*f*
   ACL reconstruction and, 510*f*
   ACL tears and, 507*f*
   of anterior cruciate ligament, 99
   avulsed and lax, 451*f*
   coronal image, 54
   disruption, grade 3 ACL with, 402*f*
   in extension, 398, 407*f*
   fat signal between AM bundle and, 413*f*
   femoral footprint, 409*f*
   in flexion, 407*f*
   fractured, ACL roof impingement and, 520–521
   knee flexion and, 509*f*
   medial meniscus and, 164*f*
   MR imaging, 438
   nonisometric in flexion-extension motion, 404*f*
   as resistance to hyperextension, 397
   sagittal image, 44, 106
   tears, 404*f*, 406*f*, 449*f*–450*f*
   tears in AMB vs., 448
   tibial footprint, 403*f*, 405*f*, 408*f*, 510*f*
   preparation for ACL reconstruction, 511*f*–513*f*
Posterolateral capsule, injuries, chronic ACL tears and, 453
Posterolateral complex.
   See also Arcuate complex
   ACL injuries and, 424
   anatomical components, 637
   PCL injuries and, 542
Posterolateral corner (PLC)
   attachments, 672*f*
   axial plane checklist, 115, 145*f*
   components, 465
   coronal plane checklist, 124*f*
   injuries, 465–466, 475*f*–476*f*, 553, 673*f*–691*f*
   collateral venous flow after, 693*f*
   multiligament, 685*f*–688*f*, 691*f*

   sprain, 467*f*
   treatment of, 671, 692*f*
   key concepts, 636
   PCL injuries and, 568, 568*f*
   popliteal hiatus region, 680*f*
   primary repair, 692*f*
   sagittal plane checklist, 108, 126*f*
Posterolateral instability
   surgical reconstruction and, 671
   types of, 662
Posterolateral joint capsule, 643*f*
Posterolateral ligaments, arcuate sign and, 473
Posterolateral tibial plateau contusions, 418*f*, 477*f*
   ACL reinjury and, 485*f*
   acute ACL tears and, 443*f*, 474*f*
   lateral compartment contusions and, 470
   nondisplaced fracture, ACL disruption and, 477*f*
Posteromedial band or bundle
   mid-substance PCL tear and, 561*f*
   PCL anatomy and, 540, 541*f*, 546*f*
Posteromedial calcaneus, plantaris muscle insertion and, 76*f*
Posteromedial capsule (PMC), 581
   anatomy, 601–602
   axial image, 115
   injuries, 602
   PHMM interface with, 367
   sagittal image, 107
   valgus stress and, 582
Posteromedial compartment, valgus stress test and, 635
Posteromedial corner
   anatomy, 591*f*–592*f*, 601–602
   injuries, 602
   sagittal plane checklist, 107, 126*f*, 131*f*
Posteromedial crush injury, contrecoup impaction and, 473
Posteromedial tibial plateau contusions or fractures
   ACL rupture and, 470
   ACL tears and, 439, 480*f*–481*f*
   tibial spine avulsions and, 472
Posterosuperior calcaneus, gastrocnemius muscle insertion and, 75*f*
Posterosuperior popliteomeniscal fascicle, 657
   of lateral meniscus, 157
   popliteus hiatus area and, 680*f*
Posterosuperior popliteomeniscal fascicles
   popliteus muscle and, 74
   sagittal image, 108
Postmeniscal transplants, vertical meniscal tears vs., 325*f*
Postoperative meniscus, 333–364
   after flap tear resection, 259
   gadolinium and, 147
   key concepts, 333

Index

Posttraumatic chondral hyperintensity, sagittal image, 109
Posttraumatic chondrosis, 980f
Posttraumatic meniscal edema, use of term, 307, 317f
Prefemoral fat body, sagittal image, 50f–51f
Prepatellar bursae
  anatomy, 824f–826f
  fluid, 827f
  gouty tophi and, 889f
  Hoffa's fat pad and, 856f
  key concepts, 825
  sagittal image, 92f
  subaponeurotic, 825f–826f
  subcutaneous, 825f–826f
  subfascial, 825f–826f
Prepatellar bursitis, 697, 829
  axial image, 116
Pretibial cysts, 538f
Primary ACL repair
  for mid-substance tears, 488
  MR evaluation of, 499
Primary chondromatosis, 898
Primary meniscal repair, 361f
  complete meniscectomy vs., 174
  gadolinium after, 147
  horizontal tears and, 330
  intrasubstance signal intensity and, 361f–362f
  MR image after, 337
  for peripheral vertical tears, 183
  postoperative signal intensity, 338
  tear morphology and location and, 183
Primary osteoarthritis, 897
Primary posterolateral corner repair, 692f
Profunda femoris artery
  semitendinosus muscle and, 71f
  vastus intermedius and, 67f
  vastus medialis and, 66f
PROPELLER, 15–16, 16f
  parallel imaging and, 21
Proprioception, meniscus and, 155
Prostaglandins (prostaglandin E2), 798
Proteins, noncollagenous in meniscal fibrocartilage, 161
Proteoglycan complex, collagen fibers and, 848
Proteoglycans
  in articular cartilage, 713, 847, 981f, 983f
    matrix disruption and, 849
  chondromalacia patellae and, 716
  in cruciate ligaments, 411
  load-bearing function and, 159
  osteoarthritis and, 897
  in patellar articular cartilage, 714
  patellar tendinosis and, 807f
  water-binding, hyaline articular cartilage and, 849
Proton density (PD)
  ACL injury diagnosis and, 486
  of hyaline articular cartilage, 849
  imaging contrast and, 3
  PCL imaging and, 551

Proton density (PD), fast-spin echo (FSE) sequences, of articular cartilage, 845
Proximal medial tibia
  gracilis muscle insertion and, 73f
  sartorius muscle insertion and, 72f
Proximal meniscal surface, 153
  anatomy, 153
Proximal posterior tibia, popliteus muscle insertion and, 74f
Proximal realignment, of patella, 830
Proximal tibiofibular joint, posterior view, 88f
Pseudo–bucket-handle tears, pitfalls interpreting findings on, 311
Pseudogout, 388
Pseudohypertrophy of anterior horn, pitfalls interpreting findings on, 311
Pseudo-locking, meniscal tears and, 173
Pseudo loose bodies, pitfalls interpreting findings on, 312
Pseudomass
  MR imaging of ACL injuries and, 436
  nodular, ACL tear and, 445f
Pseudo-subluxation, of patellofemoral joint in extension, 703
Pseudo-tears
  of meniscus, truncation artifacts and, 303
  of transverse ligament, AHLM vs., 306
  vertical, of PHLM mimicking meniscal insertion of meniscofemoral ligament, 310
Psoriasis, lipoma arborescens and, 909
Psoriatic arthritis, in children, 866
Pubis, body of, gracilis muscle origin and, 73f
Pulsation artifacts, popliteal artery and, 314, 314f
PURE (Phased Array Uniformity Enhancement), 23–24
Pure anterior knee dislocations, 573f
Pure posterior knee dislocations, 573f
Pyrophosphate arthropathy, 388

Q

Quadriceps active test, 548
Quadriceps angle (Q angle)
  chondromalacia patellae and, 706
  patellar subluxation or dislocations and, 745
Quadriceps femoris tendon
  anatomy, 79f
  ITB and, 81f
  thigh muscle innervation and, 63f
  vastus medialis and, 66f
Quadriceps mechanism, 699, 811

Quadriceps muscles. *See also specific muscles*
  contraction, ACL injuries and, 424
  dynamic patellofemoral joint stabilizing by, 703
  hypertrophy, discoid meniscus and, 291
  imbalance, medial patellar subluxation and, 705
  quadriceps tendon tears and, 833–834
  tears, treatment of, 839
  weakness, after ACL reconstruction, 491
  windless effect of, 782f
Quadriceps rehabilitation, patellar dislocations and, 750
Quadriceps retinaculum, lateral collateral ligament and, 636
Quadriceps tendon
  atrophy, patella alta and, 801
  axial image, 36f
  checklist, 112, 138f
  coil repositioning for more proximal pathology, 56
  coronal image, 57f
  cyst, 837f
  deep surface of, vastus intermedius and, 67f
  gouty tophi and, 878
  intermediate layer of, 56
  Lyme arthritis and, 892
  midsagittal sections, 45
  MR imaging, 839
  patella and, 699
  patellar stability and, 779f
  patellar tendon tear extension into, 814f
  patellectomy and, 738f
  rupture
    patella baja and, 816f
    superior patellar pole and, 838f
  sagittal image, 42, 48f–51f
    checklist, 109, 132f
    for correct orientation, 56
    knee joint, 82f
  tears
    coronal oblique images of, 56
    MR imaging, 839
    partial, 840f
    patellar tendon tears vs., 800
    propagation from medial to lateral, 56
    retinacular tears and, 751
    tendinosis and, 832f, 833–834, 835f, 837f–838f, 841f
    treatment of, 839
  trilaminar model of, 840
  vastus medialis and, 66f

R

R2* map, ultrashort images with, 988f
Radial (radial tie) fibers
  circumferential collagen fibers and, 159
  from circumferential peripheral zone, 167f
  in meniscal fibrocartilage, 168f
  meniscal structure and, 161

Radial collagen fibers, 160
Radial meniscal tears, 114, 186.
  See also Flap tears
  characteristics, 237–238,
      240f–245f
  classification of, 182
  coronal image, 100
  displaced bucket-handle tears
      and, 225f
  fibrillation or fraying mistaken
      for, 316f
  with flap and longitudinal
      components, 282f
  flap tear and, 281f
  flap tears vs., 259
  free edge, 103, 195f, 236f
      common locations for,
      240f–243f
  graphic depiction, 191f
  hoop tension and, 161
  meniscal cysts and, 386f
  repair of, 330
  root-type, 246–247
Radial vessels, from perimeniscal
    capillary plexus to meniscus,
    171f
Radial zone of articular cartilage,
    714–715, 722f, 982f, 984f
  characteristics, 846f, 847
  hyperintensity, chondromalacia
      and, 729f
  imaging, 851
Radiofrequency (RF) coils, options
    for, 4
Radiography
  of ACL injuries, 430
  of bone contusion Types I and
      II, 1004
  of discoid meniscus, 292, 298f
  of meniscal calcifications, 388
  of osseous fractures and bone
      contusions, 1001
  of osteonecrosis stages, 935
  of patellar malalignment and
      abnormal tracking, 698
  of patellofemoral congruence,
      745–746
  of popliteal cysts, 864f
  of tibial tunnels, 511f
Range of motion
  patellar dislocations and, 750
  Sinding-Larsen-Johansson
      syndrome and, 818
Rash, circular erythematous, Lyme
    arthritis and, 892
Receive-only coils, MR imaging
    and, 4
Receiver bandwidth (RBW)
    imaging protocols, 150
Recipient site
  for osteochondral transplants,
      993f–994f
  preparation, 995f
Recreational athletes. See also
    Athletic participation;
    Sports injuries
  ACL treatment and, 487–488
Rectangular tunnel technique,
    for ACL reconstruction,
    515f

Rectus femoris muscle
  anatomy, functional, 68
  coronal image, 56
  injuries, 67
  knee capsule and ligaments and,
      92f
  longitudinal fibers, 825f–826f,
      829
  quadriceps tendon tears and,
      833–834
  tears, 836f
  thigh muscle innervation and, 63f
  vastus medialis and, 66f
Rectus femoris tendon, coronal
    image, 56
Recurrent meniscal tears
  after meniscectomy, 336,
      355f–356f
  direct signs of, 355
Red marrow heterogeneity,
    epiphysis and, 1001
Red-red vascular zone, of meniscus,
    162, 163f
  meniscal repairs and, 338
  tear healing in, 328
Red-white vascular zone, of
    meniscus, 162, 171f
Reflected head, of rectus femoris,
    68f
Reflex sympathetic dystrophy, 522,
    697, 1019
  imaging, 1001
Regenerated meniscal tissue, after
    meniscectomy, 335
Renal transplantation
  bone infarcts and, 946
  spontaneous osteonecrosis and,
      933
Repetition time (TR)
  cartilage–fluid interface imaging
      and, 851
  chronic fractures and, 851
  imaging protocols, 149
Retears
  of ACL, 485f, 528f, 531f,
      533f–534f
  meniscal
      after primary repair, 337
      indicators, after meniscectomy,
          336
      of posterior horn remnant,
          361f
      of posterior horn remnant
          medial meniscus, 358f
Retinaculum. See also Lateral
    retinaculum; Medial
    retinaculum
  axial plane checklist, 139f
Reverse pivot-shift test, 548
Reverse Segond fractures
  PCL tear and, 560f, 574f
  posterior cruciate ligament, 540,
      553
Rheumatoid arthritis
  characteristics, 869
  chondromatosis mimicking, 871f
  chronic, 876f
  irregular infrapatellar fat-pad
      sign and, 858
  key concepts, 869

  lipoma arborescens and, 909
  lipoma arborescens vs., 908
  MR findings, 870
  pannus tissue in, 868f, 872f
  patellar tendon tears and, 800
  popliteal cysts and, 914
Rheumatoid factor, 869
Rheumatoid nodules, 869
Rim sign, 1021
Running
  ACL cysts and, 464f
  iliotibial band friction syndrome
      and, 787–788
  ITB syndrome and, 793f–794f
  pain, ganglion cysts and, 455
Ruptured popliteal cysts, 914

S

Sacrotuberous ligament, biceps
    femoris muscle origin and,
    69f
Saddle-bag appearance, coronal
    images of joint effusions
    and, 911
Sagittal plane images
  of ACL injuries, 436–438, 486
      acute, 441
  of ACL tears, 439–440
      chronic, 453
  of AHLM and intercondylar
      notch, 306
  of chondromalacia, 713
  of deep capsular layer, 366–367
  of discoid meniscus, 293
  of inferior and superior popliteus
      fascicles, 308
  of ligament of Humphrey, 310
  of meniscal degeneration or tears
      checklist, 103–111, 125f–136f
      MR detection accuracy, 288
  of oblique popliteal ligament,
      603
  of PCL, normal, 551
  of PCL injuries, 552
  peripheral signal artifacts and,
      302
  of plicae, 921
  of pseudo–bucket-handle tears,
      311
  of round transverse ligament, 305
  of transverse ligament, 304
Sakakibara arthroscopic classification
    for medial plica, 923
Salter-Harris type II fracture, 1008f
Salter-Harris type III fracture,
    1008f
Saphenous branch of descending
    geniculate artery, 169f
Saphenous nerve
  leg muscle innervation and, 64f
  thigh muscle innervation and, 63f
Saphenous vein, axial image, 37f
Sartorius fascia, 581, 622f
Sartorius muscle
  anatomy, 34, 79f, 587f
      functional, 72, 72f
  axial image, 36f–40f
  coronal image, 60f–62f
  posterior coronal image, 85f

posterior oblique ligament and, 629f
sagittal image, 53f
superficial dissection from anterior, 91f
thigh muscle innervation and, 63f
Sartorius tendon
  anatomy, 79f
  axial image, 38f, 41f, 79f
  intercondylar notch and, 455f
  knee subluxation or dislocation and, 747
  MCL tears and, 621f, 623f–624f
  medial collateral ligament and, 593f
  pes anserinus and, 632f
  pes anserinus bursitis and, 612, 633f–634f
  pes anserinus tendons and, 78f
  posterior oblique ligament and, 629f
  posteromedial corner and, 591f–592f
  sagittal image, 42, 53f, 79f
  sMCL and, 590f, 596f
Saucerization, for discoid meniscus, 292
Saupe's accessory ossification of patella types, 744
Scarring
  fibrous, pigmented villonodular synovitis and, 877
  of Hoffa's fat pad, 111, 134f, 526f–527f
  of lateral retinaculum, 786f
  of medial collateral ligament, 635
  physeal, thalassemia involving marrow and, 1012f
  postoperative meniscus, signal intensity and, 333, 338
Schatzker classification, of tibial plateau fractures, 1000f
Sciatic nerve
  biceps femoris muscle and, 69, 69f
  common peroneal nerve and, 904f, 906f
  ganglia and, 907
  semimembranosus muscle and, 70f, 1025f
  semitendinosus muscle and, 71f
  thigh muscle innervation and, 63f
SCIC (Surface Coil Intensity Correction), 23–24
Sclerosis
  articular cartilage matrix disruption and, 849
  in children, subchondral signal intensity and, 853
  hypointense signal on T1/PD images and, 737
  peripheral, bone infarct and, 946f
  radiographic, 335, 1001
  rheumatoid arthritis and, 876f
  subchondral
    after meniscectomy, 361f
    after partial meniscectomy, 359f–360f
    coronal plane checklist, 123f

degenerative arthrosis and, 896f
dorsal defect of patella and, 742f
juvenile chronic arthritis and, 867f
osteoarthritis and, 898
osteoarthrosis and, 900f
osteochondritis dissecans and, 949, 958f
osteonecrosis and, 935
patellar, 706
rheumatoid arthritis and, 870
trochlear groove, 734f
Screw-home mechanism
  function of, 158
  osseous contribution to, 33
  regulation of, 402
Screws
  interference
    ACL reconstruction using, 491
    dislodged, 515f, 535f
    fractured, 537f
  internal fixation, for osteochondritis dissecans, 949
Secondary bursa, ITB syndrome and cystic fluid collection in, 794f–795f
Secondary chondromatosis, 898
Secondary fracture lines, tibial plateau fractures and, 1004
Secondary osteoarthritis, 897
Secondary ridge, patellar, 700
  lateral patellar subluxation and, 704
Secondary vertical collagen fibers, transverse zone of meniscal fibrocartilage and, 160
Segmentation, of MR images, 25, 26f
Segond avulsions, 656
  short head of biceps femoris and, 656
Segond fractures
  ACL injuries and, 430
  acute, lateral tibia, 668f
  avulsion forces and, 470
  characteristics, 471–472
  iliotibial tract and, 478f–479f
  reverse, posterior cruciate ligament, 540, 553
  short head of biceps femoris and, 108
Semilunar cartilages, anatomy, 153
Semimembranosus muscle
  anatomy, functional, 70
  axial image, 36f–37f, 39f
  coronal image, 60f–62f
  denervation, 1025f
  with expansion to capsule, 40f
  as hamstring muscle, 69
  origin of, 107
  popliteal fossa view, 87f
  posterior medial retraction and, 84f
  sagittal image, 49f–52f
  thigh muscle innervation and, 63f
Semimembranosus muscle–tendon junction tears, 598f

Semimembranosus tendon
  anatomy, 34, 584f
  axial image, 36f–38f
  coronal image, 60f–62f
  expansion, 598f
  medial collateral ligament and, 587f, 593f–594f
  oblique popliteal ligament and, 588f
  popliteal cysts and, 913, 915f–916f
  posterior coronal image, 85f
  posteromedial capsule and, 601
  posteromedial corner and, 591f–592f, 601
  reverse Segond fractures and, 553
  ruptured and retracted, 626f
  sagittal image, 52f, 131f
  superficial dissection from posterior aspect, 85f
  superficial medial collateral ligament and, 590f, 622f
Semitendinosus muscle
  anatomy, 79f
  functional, 71
  axial image, 39f–40f
  as hamstring muscle, 69
  superficial dissection from anterior, 91f
  thigh muscle innervation and, 63f
Semitendinosus tendon
  ACL reconstruction using, 490–491, 495f
  postoperative imaging, 517
  anatomy, 34, 79f
  axial image, 38f, 41f, 79f
  coronal image, 61f–62f
  intercondylar notch and, 455f
  knee subluxation or dislocation and, 747
  MCL tears and, 621f, 623f–624f
  medial collateral ligament and, 593f
  patellar tendon reconstruction with, 801
  pes anserinus and, 632f
  pes anserinus bursitis and, 612, 633f–634f
  pes anserinus tendons and, 78f
  popliteal cysts and, 913
  posterior coronal image, 85f
  posteromedial corner and, 591f–592f
  ruptured, 598f
  ruptured and retracted, 626f
  sagittal image, 42, 52f–53f, 79f, 131f
  sMCL and, 590f, 596f, 622f
SENSE, 20
Septations
  ACL cysts and, 456f–457f
  ganglion cysts and, 917
  intercondylar notch cysts and, 459f
  meniscal cysts and, 377, 379, 384f
  pes anserinus bursitis and, 612
  popliteal cysts and, 913

Septic arthritis, 857
Septum completum, of suprapatellar plicae, 922
Septum extinctum, of suprapatellar plicae, 922
Septum perforatum, of suprapatellar plicae, 922
Septum residual, of suprapatellar plicae, 922
Sequestrum
　chronic active osteomyelitis with, 1025f
　subacute osteomyelitis in, 1021
Sesamoid bone, patella and, 699
Shahriaree's chondromalacia arthroscopic grading system, 712
Sharpshooter, with zone-specific cannula attachments, 341f
Shavers, arthroscopic, 194f
Shaving, arthroscopic, 743
Shear (shearing) forces
　abnormal, meniscal damage and, 172
　chondral fractures and, 975f–976f
　chronic, flap tears after trauma and, 255
　osteochondral fractures and, 971
　patellar dislocation and lateral femoral condyle contusion, 762f–763f
　patellar malalignment and, 698
　tibial spine avulsions and, 473
Shear stress
　horizontal cleavage tears and, 197f
　superficial layer of meniscus and, 161
Shell allograft, for cartilage resurfacing, 992f
Shock absorption, meniscus and, 154
Short biceps lateral aponeurosis, 656
Short lateral ligament. See also Fabellofibular ligament
　anatomy, 638
　posterolateral corner and, 465
Short tau inversion recovery (STIR)
　of bone contusions, 471
　of meniscus, 175
　of Segond fractures, 472
Shuttle suture, for ACL graft placement, 512f
Sickle cell anemia
　bone infarcts and, 946
　reconversion of yellow to red marrow in, 1003
Side chains proteoglycan, 848f
Siemens acronyms, 27
Signal-to-noise ratio (SNR), 8, 20
Sinding-Larsen-Johansson syndrome, 801, 818, 821f–823f
Single-bundle technique, for PCL reconstruction, 572
Single vertical longitudinal tears, 213

Skiing
　ACL injuries and, 416, 424
　acute ACL injuries, axial images of, 441
　osteochondral fractures and, 971
　Segond fractures and, 472
Sleeve fracture, patellar, 818, 1015f, 1018f
Sloppy ACL sign, 548
sMCL. See Superficial medial collateral ligament
Snapping knee syndrome
　discoid meniscus and, 291–292
　Wrisberg variant of discoid meniscus and, 290
SNR (signal-to-noise ratio), 8, 20
Soccer
　indirect head of rectus femoris injuries risk and, 68
　lateral meniscal tears and, 329
　tibiofibular joint dislocation and, 781f
Sodium magnetic resonance (MR) imaging
　of articular cartilage, 853
　cartilage glycosaminoglycan and, 987f
Softening of articular cartilage
　arthroscopy of, 723f
　chondromalacia and, 706, 709f–710f, 711–712, 716, 719f, 722f
　patellar cysts and, 713
Soft tissue
　infection, 1022f
　multifocal osteomyelitis and, 1021
Soft tissue mass
　nodular, ACL tear and, 455f
　patellar tendon and, 878
　popliteal cysts and, 917
　suprapatellar, suprapatellar plicae and, 922
Soleus muscle
　anatomy, 641f, 644f
　imaging, 651f
　infection in diabetic and, 1022f
　ITB and, 81f
　leg muscle innervation and, 64f
　osteomyelitis and infection in, 1023f
　plantaris tendon and, 76
　strain, 690f
　superficial dissection from posterior perspective, 85f
SONK (spontaneous osteonecrosis of knee), 942f–943f
SPAIR (Spectral Selective Adiabatic Inversion Recovery), 22
Specific absorption rate (SAR), 3.0T imaging and, 19
Speckled MR signal, central rhomboid attachment of AHLM and, 306, 316f
Spectral Presaturation with Inversion Recovery (SPIR), 22
Spectral Selective Adiabatic Inversion Recovery (SPAIR), 22
Spectral selective fat saturation, 21

SPGR (spoiled gradient echo) sequence, 6, 855f
Spin-echo imaging, of articular cartilage, 851
SPIR (Spectral Presaturation with Inversion Recovery), 22
Splinting, complex regional pain syndrome and, 1019
Spoiled gradient echo (SPGR) sequence, 6, 855f
Spondyloarthropathies, seronegative, in children, 866
Spongialization realignment procedures, for chondromalacia, 743
Spontaneous osteonecrosis, 933–935, 937f
Spontaneous osteonecrosis of knee (SONK), 942f–943f
Sports injuries. See also Athletic participation; specific sports
　ACL injuries and, 415, 423
　avulsion fractures at anterior superior iliac spine, 72
　gastrocnemius muscle, 75
　indirect head of rectus femoris and, 68
　ischial tuberosity and, 70
　Morel-Lavallée lesion, 116
　pain, ganglion cysts and, 455
　PCL rupture and, 547, 549f
　peripheral meniscal tears and, 329
　quadriceps tendon tears and, 833
　Segond fractures and, 472
　tibial spine avulsions and, 473
Sprains
　anterior cruciate ligament
　　diagnosing, 425f
　　with intact ligament morphology, 463f
　　with ligamentous splaying, 454f
　anterolateral bundle, PCL and, 562f
　cruciate ligaments, 106
　medial collateral ligament, 369f, 606f–608f, 610f
　　acute, 603
　　healing, 635
　posterior cruciate ligament, 550f
　posterolateral corner, 467f
　valgus injury and, 599
Squatting
　joint pain and meniscal pathology with, 173
　meniscal injury due to, 172
SSFP (steady-state free precession) imaging, 851
Stability. See also Instability
　biceps femoris muscle injuries and, 663
　medial patellofemoral ligament and, 767
　meniscal, arthroscopic testing of, 330
　of patella, 779f
　secondary, ACL and, 412

Index

Stacked leaflet pattern, meniscal flap tears and, 255
Staphylococcal infection, 1024f
Star artifacts, 302–303
Steadman technique, 973
Steady-state free precession (SSFP) imaging, 851
Stellate articular cartilage injuries (Type II), 991f
Stem cells
　ACL allograft with, 539f
　articular cartilage paste graft with, 998f
　three-tunnel meniscal transplantation and, 347f
Steroids
　bone infarcts and, 944, 946
　injection contamination, infection and, 1020
　for ITB syndrome, 788
　quadriceps tendon weakening and, 837
　spontaneous osteonecrosis and, 933–934
Stiffness
　of cruciate ligaments, 412
　MCL–bone complex and, 635
　morning, rheumatoid arthritis and, 869
　primary ACL repair and, 488
Still's disease, 865
Stippled pattern, of osteochondritis dissecans in children, 949
STIR (short TI inversion recovery) sequences, 21–22
　of articular cartilage and subchondral bone, 851
　of bone contusions, 1003
　of chondromalacia, 713
　of complex regional pain syndrome, 1019
　discoid meniscus and, 294
　imaging after meniscectomy, 335
　of lipoma arborescens, 908
　of osseous fractures and bone contusions, 1002
　of osteochondritis dissecans, 949
　of patellar tendinosis, 799
　of reactive subchondral marrow edema, 999f
　of reflex sympathetic dystrophy, 1001
Straight head, of rectus femoris, 68f
Streaking artifacts, PROPELLER and, 15
Strengthening, patellar dislocations and, 750
Stress fractures
　Brodie's abscess vs., 1021
　characteristics, 1003
　coronal plane checklist, 123f
　osteomyelitis in children and, 1020
　osteonecrosis vs., 935, 941f
　patellar, Sinding-Larsen-Johansson syndrome and, 818
　sagittal plane checklist, 133f
　subchondral, 1011f
　of tibial diaphysis, 1009f

Stress-related edema, coronal plane checklist, 102
Stress relaxation, cruciate ligaments and, 412
Stress testing, medial collateral ligament injuries and, 601
Subarticular cysts, juvenile chronic arthritis and, 866
Subchondral bone
　articular cartilage and, 846f, 982f
　calcified zone of, 849
　chondral erosion of, 101
　chondral lesions and, 972
　chondromalacia patellae and, 706, 711, 717
　　low-signal-intensity, 713
　　with superficial degeneration, 712
　coronal plane checklist, 102
　fracture, ACL tear and displaced meniscal flap tear, 279f
　imaging, 851
　joint sepsis and, 1020
　osteochondritis dissecans and, 947
　sagittal image, 109
　　checklist, 104, 133f
　T2 hyperintensity of, 1002
　Wiberg patella types and, 700
Subchondral cysts
　articular cartilage matrix disruption and, 849
　diffuse pigmented villonodular synovitis and, 886f
　hemophilia and, 891
　juvenile chronic arthritis and, 866
　osteoarthritis and, 898
　osteochondritis dissecans and, 957f–958f
　patellofemoral osteochondritis and, 721f
　rheumatoid arthritis and, 869
Subchondral edema
　after partial medial meniscectomy, 336f
　articular cartilage delamination and, 979f
　central lateral femoral condyle, 477f
　chondromalacia and, 717, 717f
　　chronic degenerative, 736f
　　hypointense signal compared to, 726f
　delamination injury and, 737f
　dislodged ACL graft debris and, 535f
　lateral femoral condyle, patellar dislocation and, 766f
　marrow, rheumatoid arthritis and, 870
　MCL tear and ACL tear, 625f
　medial facet and, 758f
　medial femoral condyle, flap tear and, 270f
　medial meniscus flap tear and, 283f
　medial tibial plateau, flap tear and, 264f
　meniscectomy and, 335

　Osgood-Schlatter disease and, 819f
　osteoarthritis and, 899f–900f
　osteochondral fracture and, 477f
　osteochondritis dissecans and, 950f
　PCL injuries and, 553
　　fibular styloid fracture and, 564f
　sagittal image, 109, 128f, 133f
　tibial, meniscal root tear and, 252f
　of trochlear groove, 734f
Subchondral ischemia, in medial femoral condyle, edema and, 364f
Subchondral plate
　bone infarcts and weakening of, 945
　sagittal image, 128f
　split-depression fracture and, 1006f
Subchondral sclerosis. See Sclerosis, subchondral
Subfascicular units, of cruciate ligaments, 411
Subgastrocnemius bursa, posteromedial capsule and, 367
Subpopliteal recess, 647f
Sudeck's atrophy, 1019
Sulcus
　anatomic patellar alignment and, 745
　condylopatellar, lateral notch sign and, 471
　terminalis
　　depression of, 477f
　　fractures, 475f–476f
　　lateral femoral condylar notch separation from, 471
　of trochlear groove, 701, 701f
Sulcus angle, 745
Superficial degeneration, chondromalacia with, 712, 725f
Superficial fissures, chondral lesions as, 972
Superficial infrapatellar bursa, 824f, 827f
　bursitis, 829
　　axial image, 116
　　key concepts, 825
Superficial lateral retinaculum layer, 751
Superficial layer
　of meniscus, 161
　of quadriceps tendon, 56
Superficial medial collateral ligament (sMCL)
　anatomy, 596f–597f
　　functional, 582–583, 586f, 588f–590f
　axial image, 115, 142f
　biomechanics of, 602
　bursitis, 630f–631f
　displaced flap tear fragment in coronary recess and, 276f
　dMCL and, 583
　intercondylar notch and, 455f

1085

Superficial medial collateral ligament (*continued*)
  medial aspect of knee and, 581
  ossification, Pellegrini-Stieda disease and, 628f
  popliteus complex and, 645f
  posterior oblique ligament and, 629f
  posteromedial corner and, 591f
  sagittal image, 107
  sprains, 603
Superficial oblique retinaculum, 642f, 751, 784f
Superficial peroneal nerve
  leg muscle innervation and, 64f
  normal course of, 904f
Superficial transverse fascial layer, 825f–826f
Superficial zone of articular cartilage, 714, 982f, 984f
  characteristics, 846f, 847
  chondromalacia and, 720f
  chondromalacia and extension into, 732f
Superior (s) leaflets
  horizontal cleavage tear and, 197f
  transverse zone of meniscal fibrocartilage and, 160, 166f
Superior fascicle
  gross anatomic specimen, 320f
  imaging, 308, 319f
  of lateral meniscus, 157, 318f
Superior lateral supracondylar line, vastus intermedius and, 67f
Superior medial genicular artery, 169f
Superior meniscal surface
  anatomy, 153
  flap tears of, 277f
    changing slope sign and, 269f
    double-decker pattern, 273f
Superior patellar pole, 838f
Superior popliteomeniscal fascicle, 638
  arcuate ligament and, 677f
  coronal image, 319f
  imaging, 651f
  medial limb of arcuate ligament and, 661f
  sagittal image, 46
  posterolateral corner injuries and, 467f, 676f
  sagittal image, 319f
Superior popliteomeniscal ligament, 666f
Superior posterior patellar surface, 699
Superior tibiofibular joint
  axial image, 41f
  coronal image, 62f
  sagittal image, 47f
Superior-to-inferior (S-I) direction, peripheral signal artifacts and, 302–303
Superolateral bipartite patella, 741, 741f
Superolateral facet, semimembranosus muscle origin and, 70f
Superolateral suprapatellar plica, 922
Superomedial suprapatellar plica, 922
Supracondylar fractures
  of distal femur, 1013f
  of tibial plateau, 1004
Suprapatellar bursa (fat body, pouch)
  axial image, 36f–37f
  capsule extending into, 78f
  chondral erosion of, 105
  diffuse pigmented villonodular synovitis and, 885f
  fluid, sagittal image, 48f
  graphic depiction, 590f
  Hoffa's fat pad and, 856f
  joint effusion and, 110
  joint interior and, 90f
  juvenile chronic arthritis and, 866, 867f
  knee joint, 82f
  lipoma arborescens and, 910f
  loose bodies in, 116
  medial and lateral reflections of, 35
  pigmented villonodular synovitis and, 887f
  rheumatoid arthritis and, 873f
  sagittal image, 42, 47f, 49f–51f
Suprapatellar cord, 922
Suprapatellar membrane, 922
Suprapatellar plicae
  anatomy, 921
  anterior perspective, 920f
  characteristics, 922
  sagittal plane checklist, 111, 136f
  Type I, 922
  Type II, 922
  Type III, 922
  Type IV, 922
Suprapatellar recess, joint effusions and, 911
Suprapatellar septum, 921
Supratrochlear tubercle, knee extension and, 33
Surface Coil Intensity Correction (SCIC), 23–24
Surface concavity
  of discoid-like meniscus, 298f–299f
  of discoid meniscus, 290
  incomplete discoid meniscus and, 295f
  of meniscus, 153
Surface débridement. *See* Débridement
Surface layer, of meniscus, 161
Surgery, for ACL and PCL injuries, 556
Surgical access, to peripheral joint capsule, 325f
Surgical awls, microfracture with, 992f
Susceptibility artifacts
  MAVRIC SL and, 17
  subacute and chronic hemorrhage and, 914
Suturing
  for ACL graft placement, 512f
  for avulsion LCL injuries, 671
  Krackow-Bunnell weave technique for, 839, 840f
  for meniscal transplantation, 342f–343f
  in red-red meniscal vascular zone, 328
  Sharpshooter for, 341f
  for torn MPFL, 750
  vertical mattress, 338
Synchondrosis, chondromalacia of lateral facet cartilage and, 740f
Synovectomy, 870
Synovial bleeding, meniscal tear healing and, 328
Synovial chondromatosis
  lipoma arborescens vs., 908
  osseous bodies and, 903f
  osteoarthritis and, 898, 902f
Synovial cysts, 377, 379
Synovial fluid. *See also* Joint fluid or effusions
  cell nutrition of meniscus and, 162
  diffusion, ACL grafting and, 516
  joint effusion, grade 3 signal intensity and, 301
  macerated meniscus, signal intensity and, 307
  meniscal degeneration and tears and, 175–176
  meniscus and, 154
  tophaceous gout and, 890f
Synovial hypertrophy, 857
Synovial impingement, meniscus and, 155
Synovial lesions or tumors, meniscal tears and, 173
Synovial membrane
  ACL graft revascularization and, 493
  hyperplasia, diffuse pigmented villonodular synovitis and, 878
Synovial plicae, 921
Synovial sarcoma
  meniscal cysts and, 379
  quadriceps tendon tears vs., 834
Synovitis
  ACL injuries and, 430
  ACL tears and, 485f
    hypotense distal ligament and, 484f
  acute ACL tears and, 442
  chondromalacia patellae and, 706
  chronic ACL tears and, 439, 452f, 453
  diffuse pigmented villonodular synovitis and, 885f
  early juvenile chronic arthritis and, 866
  Hoffa's fat pad and, 134f–135f, 419f, 856f, 857
  inflammatory, lipoma arborescens vs., 908
  ITB friction syndrome and, 115

Index

joint, chondral lesions and, 104
joint effusions and, 911
joint sepsis and, 1020
localized pigmented villonodular, 111, 877
osteoarthritis and, 900f
prepatellar, 144f
sagittal image, 110–111
staphylococcal infection and, 1024f
subacute ACL tears and, 453
transient, in children, 866
Synovium
 of ACL, 397
 axial image, 37f, 112
 contrast-enhanced image of, 861f
 hemophilia and, 891
 hypertrophy of, 871f
  Lyme arthritis and, 892
  rheumatoid arthritis and, 870
 inflammatory, rheumatoid arthritis and, 871f
 intermediate-signal, chronic PCL tears and, 130f
 intermediate-signal hypertrophy of, 861f
 irregular infrapatellar fat-pad sign and, 858
 juvenile chronic arthritis and enhancement of, 863f, 866
 lipoma arborescens and, 908, 909f
 peripheral, meniscal repair and, 329
 posterior cruciate ligament and, 540
 postoperative Hoffa's fat pad fibrosis and, 860f
 rheumatoid arthritis and, 869
 thickened
  ACL reconstruction and, 523f, 536f
  chondral erosions and, 875f
  Lyme arthritis and, 894f
  rheumatoid arthritis and, 873f–874f
Synthetic scaffold implants, of meniscus, 326
Synthetic tissue, ACL reconstruction using, 490
Systemic-onset juvenile chronic arthritis, 865

T
T1 rho map
 of articular cartilage, 985f
 of collagen organization and hydration, 987f
T1-weighted images
 of ACL injuries, 437, 486
 of bone contusion types, 1004
 of ganglion cysts, 917
 of hyaline articular cartilage, 849
 of lipoma arborescens, 908
 of normal red marrow, 1012f
 of osseous fractures and bone contusions, 1002
 of pannus tissue, 858
 of PCL, 551

T2*-weighted images. See also Gradient echo sequences
 bone susceptibility effect, 813f
 contrast, 3, 6
 3D MERGE and, 14
T2 mapping, 10, 11f
 of articular cartilage, 845, 853, 985f
 chondromalacia and, 712–713
 of collagen development, 999f
 of collagen organization and hydration, 987f
 of lateral compartment cartilage, 985f
T2-weighted images
 of ACL acute injuries, 441
 of ACL injuries, 437, 486
 of bone contusions, 1003
 of chondromalacia patellae, grade 2, 729f
 of complex regional pain syndrome, 1019
 fracture morphology and, 1001
 of ganglion cysts, 917
 of hyaline articular cartilage, 850
 of osseous fractures and bone contusions, 1002
 of osteochondritis dissecans, 949
 of patellar tendinosis, 799
 of popliteus tendon sheath, 308
TE. See Echo time
Tendinitis
 after ACL reconstruction, 491, 522
 patellar, 810f
 popliteal, meniscal tears and, 173
Tendinomuscular rheumatoid arthritis, 870
Tendinosis, 697. See also Patellar tendinosis
 distal quadriceps, 109
 quadriceps tendon tears and, 832f, 835f, 837f–838f, 841f
Tennis leg, medial head gastrocnemius strains in, 75
Tension cerclage treatment, of patellar fractures, 1018f
Tensor fasciae latae muscle, 81, 789f
Thalassemia, 1003, 1012f
Thigh, medial aspect adductors of, 73
Thigh flexion
 gracilis muscle and, 73
 semitendinosus muscle and, 72
 vastus lateralis and, 65f
 vastus medialis and, 66f
Thigh muscle innervation, 63f
3D fast spin-echo (FSE) sequence, 5. See also CUBE; MAVRIC SL
3D MERGE, 14–15, 14f
Three-dimensional (3D) high-resolution imaging, 851. See also FS PD FSE
Three-dimensional (3D) MR imaging
 of articular cartilage, 850
 of articular pulse sequences, 713
 of discoid meniscus, 298f
 meniscal tear detection accuracy using, 288

Three-point Dixon technique, 23
Three-tunnel technique
 for meniscal transplantation, 332, 332f, 344f–345f
 stem cells and, 347f
Thrombosis
 deep venous, 664, 917
 popliteal artery, 917f
  aneurysm, 918f
Tibia
 ACL and anterior translation of, 402
 ACL and PCL insertion sites in, 401f
 ACL attachment to, 398, 405f
  avulsion repair and, 487
 anterior displacement, ACL tears and, 439
 anterior drawer sign, ACL tears and, 453
 anterior translation
  LCL and posterolateral structures and, 658
  measuring, 532f
 anterolateral, ACL insertion at, 113
 axial image, 41f
 condylar surface, fibrocartilaginous menisci and, 153
 coronal image, 58f–62f
 cruciate ligamentous tissue and, 411
 displacement
  ACL injuries and, 416
  tibial spine avulsions and, 472
 dMCL and motion of, 583
 femur relative to
  ACL tears and, 468f–469f
  cortical bone and, 43
 fractures
  acute Segond, 668f
  lipohemarthrosis and, 1019
  patellar tendon tears and, 810f
  proximal, tibialis posterior muscle edema and, 1009f
 hemophilia and surface of, 891
 hyaline articular cartilage signal intensity of, 43
 intercondylar area of, axial image, 40f
 intercondylar fossa of, anterior horn medial meniscus and, 156
 knee capsule and ligaments and, 92f
 knee in partial flexion and, 93f
 lateral collateral ligament and, 80f
 medial collateral ligament and, 582, 587f
 osteomyelitis in diabetic, 1022f
  staphylococcal, 1024f
 patellofemoral joint flexion and, 703
 periosteum trapped in physeal fracture of, 1008f
 peripheral blood supply to meniscus and, 169f
 posterior cruciate ligament and, insertion site, 401f, 540–541f

1087

Tibia (continued)
  posterior drop-back of, PCL and, 548
  posterior extrusion, rheumatoid arthritis and, 871f
  posterior translation
    LCL and posterolateral structures and, 658
    PCL injuries and, 568
  sagittal image, 47f–53f, 92f
  screw-home mechanism and, 33
  Segond fracture, ACL tear and, 478f
  stress fractures, 1003, 1009f
  subluxation
    bone contusions and, 471
    supine ACL tear imaging and, 453
Tibial branch of sciatic nerve, hamstring muscles and, 69
Tibial cartilage, segmentation example, 26f
Tibial collateral ligament. See also Medial collateral ligament
  bursitis, 631f
  coronal image, 55
  posterior oblique ligament and, 629f
Tibial condyles, 94f. See also Lateral tibial condyle; Medial tibial condyle
  erosion of, meniscal cysts and, 379
  superficial dissection from anterior, 91f
Tibial eminence
  avulsions, ACL injuries and, 430, 442
  fractures, ACL injuries and
    displaced, 432f, 434f
    nondisplaced, 431f
    partially displaced, 433f
Tibialis anterior muscle
  anatomy, 641f
  axial image, 41f
  coronal image, 60f
  extraneural ganglia and, 906f
  infection in diabetic and, 1022f
  ITB and, 81f
  leg muscle innervation and, 64f
  osteomyelitis and infection in, 1023f
  sagittal image, 47f–48f
Tibialis posterior muscle
  edema, tibial fracture and, 1009f
  infection in diabetic and, 1022f
  leg muscle innervation and, 64f
  osteomyelitis and infection in, 1023f
Tibial marginal spurring, meniscectomy and, 335
Tibial nerve
  anatomy, 647f
  axial image, 36f–41f
  at femoral condyles, 35
  gastrocnemius muscle and, 75f
  leg muscle innervation and, 64f
  plantaris muscle and, 76f
  popliteus muscle and, 74f

  sagittal image, 49f
  thigh muscle innervation and, 63f
Tibial osteotomy
  meniscal implants and, 326
  for osteonecrosis, 936
Tibial plateau. See also Lateral tibial plateau; Medial tibial plateau
  anatomy, 34
  anterior and posterior horns of lateral meniscus and, 33
  articular cartilage stem cell paste graft preparation for, 998f
  avulsions, PCL tears and, 556
  cartilage surface, 101
  chondral surfaces, 982f
  complete discoid meniscus and, 294
  discoid menisci and, 290
  displaced flap tears and reactive edema of, 258
  fractures, 1001
    Hohl classification, 1004
    Schatzker classification, 1000f
  large radial or root tears and, 247
  medial femoral condyle contact area with, 359f
  meniscus body and, 103
  semimembranosus and semitendinosus tendons and, 34
  3D articular cartilage zonal anatomy at, 982f
Tibial plateau articular facets, knee extension and, 32
Tibial spine avulsions, 472–473
Tibial spine fractures, meniscal tears and, 173
Tibial tubercle
  anatomy, 94f
  axial image, 41f
  elevation, for chondromalacia, 743
  Elmslie-Trillat procedure and, 830
  Fulkerson osteotomy of, 738f
  Osgood-Schlatter disease and, 817, 819f
  pes anserinus tendons and, 78f
  superficial dissection from anterior, 91f
  transfers, 830
Tibial tubercle–trochlear groove (TT-TG) distance, 754f
Tibial tuberosity
  deep infrapatellar bursitis and, 829
  elevation (Maquet's procedure), 747, 779f
  by patellar tendon, vastus medialis and, 66f
  vastus intermedius and, 67f
Tibial tunnels
  ACL graft impingement and, 501, 516
  ACL graft motion and, 518f
  ganglion cysts and, 529f
  for PCL reconstruction, neurovascular injury and, 556

  placement, ACL reconstruction and, 489, 491, 494f, 496f, 515f
  preparation, 511f–513f
  pretunnel cysts and, 538f
Tibiofibular cysts, 379
Tibiofibular joint
  anatomy, 642f
  congenital subluxation of, discoid meniscus and, 292
  cysts and, 914
  dislocations, 781f
    degenerative arthrosis and, 907
  extraneural ganglia and, 904f–906f
  osteoarthritis and, 898
  sagittal image, 126f
  subluxation or dislocation, discoid meniscus and, 292
Tidemark, articular cartilage, 846f, 847, 982f, 984f
  in adolescents, 977
Tophaceous gout, 878, 889f–890f
Tophaceous pseudogout, 388
Total joint arthroplasty, 870
Total meniscal implants, 326
TR. See Repetition time
TR (transmit/receive) coils, 4
Trabecular bone
  contusions
    multiligament injuries and, 575f
    signal intensity of, 324f
  coronal plane checklist, 102, 123f
  fractures
    ACL tear and, 482
    edema and, 534f
    inferior popliteomeniscal fascicle and, 667f
    nondisplaced, 470
  visualization of, 487
Track and field injuries, indirect head of rectus femoris injuries' risk and, 68
Transitional zone of articular cartilage, 714, 722f, 982f, 984f
  characteristics, 846f, 847
  hyperintensity, chondromalacia and, 729f
  imaging, 851
Transmit/receive (TR) coils, 4
Transplantation. See Meniscal transplantation
Transverse (T) zone
  of meniscal fibrocartilage and, 160
  of meniscus, 166f
Transverse intermeniscal ligament, longitudinal meniscal tears and, 204
Transverse ligament
  ACL and, 398
  AHLM near, 306, 318f
  AHLM vs. pseudo-tears of, 306, 315f
  anatomy, 33–34, 77f, 591f, 647f
  anterior horn of medial meniscus and, 156
  axial and sagittal images, 300f

lateral meniscus, ACL and, 305f
meniscal bucket-handle tears and, 217f, 220f, 225f
oblique intermeniscal ligaments and, 321f
pitfalls interpreting findings on, 304–305
plicae and, 920f
Transverse linear fractures, metaphyseal–diaphyseal junction vs., 1002
Transverse patellar fractures, 1004, 1015f–1016f, 1018f
Transverse patellofemoral ligament, 642f
Transverse ridges, patellar, 700
lateral patellar subluxation and, 704
Transverse superficial fascia, gouty tophi and, 889f
Transverse synovial arcuate fold, 930f
Trauma. *See also* Direct blow; Indirect knee injuries
acute, meniscal tears and, 172
bipartite or multipartite patella and, 741
bone infarcts and, 946
bucket-handle tears and, 213
chondral fractures and, 975f–976f
chondromalacia and basal degeneration after, 711
chondromalacia patellae and, 706
chondrosis of lateral femoral condyle and, 980f
chronic, Pellegrini-Stieda disease and, 611–612
chronic repetitive, quadriceps tendon tears and, 833
complex meniscal tears and, 183
complex regional pain syndrome and, 1019
diffuse increased intrameniscal signal intensity after, 307, 317f
direct blow to flexed knee, 416, 555f
Hoffa's disease and, 857
joint effusions and, 911
longitudinal meniscal tears and, 203
meniscal cysts and, 377
osteochondral fractures and, 971
osteochondritis dissecans and, 947, 958f
osteonecrosis and, 934
patellar dislocations and, 747–750
patellar tendon tears and, 800, 813f
PCL injuries and, 547, 549f, 555f, 566f
penetrating, infection and, 1020
physis discontinuity and, 1002
posterolateral corner injuries and, 466, 683f, 688f
rim sign and, 1021

secondary osteoarthritis and, 897
Sinding-Larsen-Johansson syndrome and, 818, 823f
synovial lining and, 857
trochlear groove chondral signal hyperintensity and, 735f
Traumatic vascular channels, for meniscal tear healing, 328
Trevor's disease, 1021, 1026f
Triangular appearance
of ACL reconstruction, 495f
of Hoffa's fat pad, 111
of meniscal horns
coronal plane checklist, 100
sagittal image, 43, 46, 103
of PCL attachment, coronal image, 55
Trifurcation, of iliotibial band, 789f
Trilaminar appearance, of articular cartilage, 851
Trilaminar model of prepatellar bursae, 825f–826f
Tripartite patella, 744
Triple vertical longitudinal bucket-handle tears, 213
Trochlear groove
ACL graft impingement and, 492
chondromalacia
chronic degenerative, 736f
infrapatellar plica and, 111, 922
osteoarthritis and, 43
depth of, 745
dysplasia and, 754f
knee extension and, 33
patellar dislocations and, 749
subchondral sclerosis of, 734f
tibial tubercle distance and, 754f
traumatized, chondral signal hyperintensity in, 735f
Trochlear groove cartilage
axial plane checklist, 112, 137f
MPFL reconstruction and, 777f–778f
osteochondritis dissecans and, 960f–961f
sagittal image, 50f
checklist, 105, 128f
femoral condyle cartilage and, 104
Truncation artifacts, 303
TT-TG (tibial tubercle–trochlear groove) distance, 754f
Tumors. *See also* Neoplasms
osteomyelitis in children vs., 1020
Turf injuries, 416
Twisting
chondral flaps due to, 970f
medial patellar facet chondral surface and, 763f
meniscal injury due to, 172
2:30 position, for ACL reconstruction, 491, 496f
Two-bundle nonisometric structure, of ACL, 402, 408f
Two-point Dixon technique, 23

U

Ulcers
chondromalacia and, 712, 717, 718f
with basal degeneration, 711
popliteal artery aneurysm and, 918
Ultrashort (UTE) images, water images with, 988f
Undersurface tear, meniscal, arthroscopic images, 193f
Unicondylar arthroplasty, 898
Unlocking of knee. *See also* Joint locking; Locking mechanics, 158
U-shape
of infrapatellar plica, 111
of intercondylar notch, 113
Uveitis, chronic, 865

V

Vacuum phenomenon, 312, 324f
Valgus angulation
chondromalacia patellae and, 706
MCL tear and ACL tear and, 626f
PCL and, 542
Valgus impaction
fractures and, 1001
MCL tear and ACL tear, 625f
Valgus load, pivot shift injury and, 415
Valgus movement, MCL and, 582
Valgus stress
ACL injuries and, 416
hyperextension, retinacular tears and, 751
medial collateral ligament and, 582–583, 599, 601
Valgus stress test, 635
Varus angulation, PCL and, 542
Varus load, medial compartment contusions and, 473
Varus motion, LCL and posterolateral structures and, 658
Vascular malformations, 1027f
Vascular supply
cruciate ligaments, 399f–400f
middle geniculate artery and, 398
healing response technique and, 488
medial collateral ligament, 169f
menisci, 162–163, 163f, 169f, 171f
arthroscopic rasping and, 180
Vascular zone, of meniscus, 162, 163f, 171f
tear healing in, 328
tear repair and, 329
Vastus intermedius muscle
anatomy, functional, 67
injuries of, 67
knee capsule and ligaments and, 92f
quadriceps tendon tears and, 833–834
rectus femoris tear and, 836f

Vastus intermedius muscle (*continued*)
   thigh muscle innervation and, 63*f*
   vastus medialis and, 66*f*
Vastus intermedius tendon, quadriceps tears and, 833
Vastus lateralis muscle
   anatomy, 639*f*, 641*f*–642*f*, 644*f*
      functional, 65*f*
   axial image, 36*f*
   coronal image, 58*f*–60*f*
      intermediate layer, 56
   injuries of, 67
   ITB and, 81*f*, 790*f*
   ITB friction syndrome and, 790*f*
   knee capsule and ligaments and, 92*f*
   lateral retinaculum and, 751
   quadriceps tendinosis and, 832*f*
   quadriceps tendon tears and, 833–834
   retinacula and, 139*f*
   sagittal image, 47*f*–48*f*
   thigh muscle innervation and, 63*f*
   vastus medialis and, 66*f*
Vastus lateralis obliquus (VLO) fibers, vastus lateralis and, 65*f*
Vastus lateralis tendon, 36*f*, 65*f*, 112, 745, 786*f*
Vastus medialis extensor aponeurosis tendon, 591
Vastus medialis muscle
   anatomy, 79*f*, 589*f*, 595*f*
      functional, 66*f*
   axial image, 36*f*
   coronal image, 56, 57*f*–60*f*
      intermediate layer, 56
   hypoplasia, 701
   injuries of, 67
   knee capsule and ligaments and, 92*f*
   medial retinaculum and, 751
   pes anserinus tendons and, 78*f*
   posterior oblique ligament and, 629*f*
   quadriceps tendinosis and, 832*f*
   quadriceps tendon and, 66*f*
   quadriceps tendon tears and, 833–834
   retinacula and, 139*f*
   sagittal image, 43, 52*f*–53*f*
   superficial dissection from anterior, 91*f*
   tears, 838*f*
   thigh muscle innervation and, 63*f*
Vastus medialis obliquus (VMO)
   injuries, 769*f*–770*f*
      patellar dislocation and, 66
   lateral retinacular release and, 786*f*
   medial patellofemoral ligament and, 756*f*, 767, 768*f*
   medial retinaculum and, 755*f*
   miserable malalignment syndrome and, 780*f*
   patella stabilized by, 748
   strain, medial retinaculum and MPFL tear, 760*f*
Vastus medialis tendon, 36*f*, 57*f*, 112, 838*f*
Venous malformations, popliteal or atypical cysts vs., 914
Venous occlusion, popliteal artery aneurysm and, 918
Vertical mattress sutures, 338, 341*f*
Vertical meniscal tears, 182–183, 191*f*
   with contrecoup medial tibial plateau fracture, 208*f*
   flap tears and, 255
   longitudinal, 195*f*, 207*f*
      repair of, 329, 339*f*–341*f*
   of PHLM mimicking meniscal insertion of meniscofemoral ligament, 310
   postmeniscal transplant vs., 325*f*
Vertical patellar fractures, 1004, 1015, 1017*f*–1018*f*
Villous lipomatous proliferation of synovium, 909*f*–910*f*
Viscoelastic behavior, of cruciate ligaments, 412
VLO. *See* Vastus lateralis obliquus
VMO. *See* Vastus medialis obliquus

W

Water molecules
   in articular cartilage, 981*f*
   cartilage matrix compression and, 983*f*
   joint effusion, grade 3 signal intensity and, 301
   trapped, meniscal degeneration and tears and, 175–176
   ultrashort images of, 988*f*
Weight bearing. *See* Load-bearing function
Weight lifting, iliotibial band friction syndrome and, 787
White-white vascular zone, of meniscus, 162, 171*f*
   tear healing in, 328
Wiberg patella types, 700, 708*f*, 753*f*
Windless effect, 782*f*
Windshield wiper effect, 518*f*
Women
   insufficiency fractures and, 940*f*
   metaphyseal–diaphyseal low-signal-intensity red marrow inhomogeneity, 1003
   spontaneous osteonecrosis and, 933
Wrestling, lateral meniscal tears and, 329
Wrisberg ligament. *See* Ligament of Wrisberg
Wrisberg variant of discoid meniscus, 290–292, 297*f*

X

Xanthoma cells, pigmented villonodular synovitis and, 877, 881*f*
Xenograft tissue, ACL reconstruction using, 490

Y

Yield load, cruciate ligaments and, 412

Z

Zidorn classification of suprapatellar plicae, 922
Zone of fibrocartilage, 411
Zone of mineralized cartilage, 411

STOLLER'S
Orthopaedics and Sports Medicine Series
Series Editor: David W. Stoller, MD, FACR

Stoller's Orthopaedics and Sports Medicine
The Shoulder

Stoller's Orthopaedics and Sports Medicine
The Knee

Stoller's Orthopaedics and Sports Medicine
The Hip

Stoller's Orthopaedics and Sports Medicine
The Wrist and Hand

Stoller's Orthopaedics and Sports Medicine
The Elbow

Stoller's Orthopaedics and Sports Medicine
The Foot and Ankle

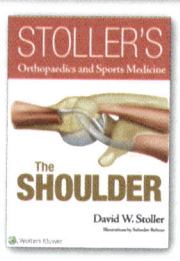

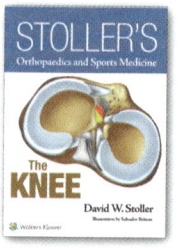

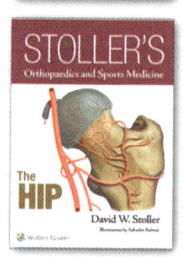